Carroll C. Lupton, M.D.
12-6-39

ESSENTIALS
OF
PATHOLOGY

ESSENTIALS OF PATHOLOGY

BY

LAWRENCE W. SMITH, M.D.

PROFESSOR OF PATHOLOGY, TEMPLE UNIVERSITY SCHOOL OF MEDICINE;
FORMERLY ASSISTANT PROFESSOR OF PATHOLOGY, HARVARD
MEDICAL COLLEGE; AND, ASSOCIATE PROFESSOR
OF PATHOLOGY, CORNELL UNIVERSITY
MEDICAL SCHOOL.

AND

EDWIN S. GAULT, M.D.

ASSOCIATE PROFESSOR OF PATHOLOGY, TEMPLE UNIVERSITY
SCHOOL OF MEDICINE

WITH A FOREWORD BY

JAMES EWING, M.D.

MEMORIAL HOSPITAL, NEW YORK CITY

D. APPLETON-CENTURY COMPANY
INCORPORATED

NEW YORK   LONDON

TO

WILLIAM N. PARKINSON, M.D.

THROUGH WHOSE ENTHUSIASTIC COÖPERATION

THIS VOLUME HAS BEEN MADE POSSIBLE,

THESE PAGES ARE GRATEFULLY

DEDICATED.

PREFACE

The past quarter of a century has seen almost unbelievable advances in the field of medicine. From a relatively simple "art" medicine has been expanded to a highly specialized and complex "science." As a result, medical education has had to adapt itself to these changes. Formerly, it had been actually possible to impart to the student the major part of our detailed medical information within the four year period of his medical school career. To-day, with the extraordinary expansion of our knowledge, it has become more and more obvious that instruction in medicine must be restricted to absolute *essentials*.

It has seemed to us that a thorough grounding in the fundamental *principles* of pathology is of greater value to the student than any attempt at encyclopedic presentation of the subject. He will have ample opportunity to apply this basic knowledge to each clinical case as it presents during his hospital and dispensary years, and thus learn the almost infinite variation in pattern of the more elaborate superstructure of disease.

With this thought in mind, this textbook has been prepared. In it, we have departed from the time-honored method of presentation of the subject in several particulars:

1. First, we believe that, in the limited time at the disposal of the student to-day, a textbook should be *practical*. We have, therefore, emphasized those things which we believe to be fundamental and essential. No attempt has been made to cover the entire field, and of necessity, there have been many omissions of less important conditions.

2. In controversial subjects, we have attempted to follow a middle course, wherever possible, in presenting those views which are generally accepted, rather than to stress too much, theories in which the pendulum has not yet come to rest.

3. The Pathology of parasitic infestations is given rather more than the usual amount of attention. As time and space recede with modern transportation, the diseases of Asia, Africa, South America and Europe assume an ever greater importance, and tropical medicine becomes a problem for every practitioner of medicine, so a consideration of its pathology is a matter of practical necessity.

4. Tumors are likewise emphasized to a rather greater extent than is customary. Cancer, in scarcely more than two decades, has risen from seventh to second place as a cause of death, which seems adequate explanation for the position of importance it assumes in this volume. The physician should be as familiar with the natural history of the various neoplastic diseases as he is with the several infectious diseases. Their manifestations are as variable and pleomorphic as the cells of which they are composed, and their etiology is perhaps more complex a problem than that of any other group of diseases.

5. In the general arrangement of the material in the book, the more familiar and orthodox division of the discussion into (1) general pathology, (2) tumors, and (3) systemic pathology, is followed. It has been our experience that this division of material into a consideration of first, basic fundamental processes (general pathology), to be followed by their application in the lesions of the various organ systems (special pathology), has proved less confusing to the beginning student than the presentation of the subject from the more theoretically ideal standpoint of etiology.

6. The various subjects in the chapters, as far as possible, follow a uniform arrangement. In general, there is a concise discussion of the subject at the beginning, which is followed by carefully selected illustrative case histories, complete with their associated gross and microscopic pathology. In this way we attempt to correlate, as far as possible, the clinical findings on the basis of pathology.

The case-history method of teaching is probably the oldest method known, but for some obscure reason, curiously, it has never been applied to the teaching of pathology, except in the later years of the student's work, in the form of clinicopathologic conferences. It seems to us that this correlation should be begun with the student's first concept of pathology, and we have attempted to utilize the case-history method as a means of vitalizing the study of pathology. Appendicitis, pneumonia, tuberculosis, nephritis, and cancer thus become problems affecting an actual patient, not merely abstract morbid pictures.

It will be remembered that up to the time the student begins the study of pathology he has been building a secure foundation through a study of the *normal*—a knowledge of *form,* through embryology, histology and gross anatomy, a knowledge of *function,* through physiology and chemistry. With his introduction to pathology he begins his study of disease —*abnormal* form and function—upon which is based his subsequent interpretation of clinical signs and symptoms. Thus, pathology bridges the broad abyss of the preclinical and the clinical aspects of medicine.

By definition, pathology represents the scientific study of the alterations of cell function and form which go to make up disease. Similarly, clinical medicine may be defined as the art and science of interpreting the signs and symptoms of disturbed function or relationships of those same fundamental processes, and of atempting by some type of therapy to readjust those abnormal states. It is only through the clinician's thorough and sound knowledge of pathology that even a modicum of success follows.

From these comments it becomes apparent that pathology and medicine are merely two different methods of approach to the same problem. It is with this concept in mind, we believe, that the teaching of pathology should be undertaken to-day in an attempt to correlate the underlying pathologic processes on the one hand, and the visible evidence of disease on the other. To this end, the case-history method of presentation has been adopted.

7. To assist the student in visualizing the underlying alterations in form and function, the pictorial method has been employed, more extensively, perhaps, than is generally found. It has likewise seemed of some definite value to introduce a number of roentgenograms and gross pathological pictures in an attempt to correlate the appearance of the lesions with the miscroscopic histology, for the obvious reason that the x-ray picture is again a method of demonstrating pathological alteration in form and functional capacity of an organ.

8. Even the format has been changed in order to maintain the integral relationship of the individual case reports and the illustrative material. This has resulted in the development of what almost might be termed a concise "atlas of histopathology," together with case histories, which the student can have readily available throughout his medical school career to refresh his memory, as clinical problems in medicine and surgery confront him.

9. In addition to the usual index, for the convenience of the student, an index of the cases and associated illustrations has been incorporated. Also, for the convenience of the student, blank pages for notes have been inserted either for use in the lecture room or in the laboratory as he studies his own histopathological material.

10. Finally, after much consideration, it has been decided that no useful purpose is served by the addition of any extensive bibliography. References are made, from time to time, to recent reviews regarding controversial subjects, but otherwise, it is believed that the student would do better to consult more encyclopedic reference books. From a questionnaire compiled over the past ten years, it has been found that less than two per cent of students make use of such appended bibliographies. They rarely have sufficient time to read more than the required factual material. Should they wish to delve deeper into any given subject, it requires more extensive research than the already outdated literature suggested in the ordinary textbook.

We wish to take this opportunity to acknowledge our indebtedness and gratitude to the many individuals, who have aided us in one way or another in the assembling of the material and the preparation of this book. It is impossible to mention them all by name, but to the members of the department of pathology, Drs. Frank W. Konzelmann, Ernest A. Aegerter, Hershel C. Lennon and David B. Fishback go our especial thanks. To Dr. W. Edward Chamberlain for his generous contribution of the numerous x-ray films; to Dr. W. Wayne Babcock, Dr. Temple S. Fay, Drs. Chevalier and C. L. Jackson, and all the other members of the clinical staff of Temple University Hospital for the use of the material in the great majority of the clinical cases; to Dr. Jefferson W. Clark, Dr. R. Philip Custer and Dr. Helena Riggs, as well as to the several heads of the clinical services for the use of autopsy material and clinical abstracts from the Philadelphia General Hospital likewise goes our sincere appreciation.

To Dr. Walter J. Crocker, head of the hematology laboratory at the Philadelphia General Hospital belongs the credit for unselfishly placing at our disposal the colored plates illustrating the several blood dyscrasias. To Dr. Eleanor H. Valentine, hematologist at the Methodist Hospital, goes our unbounded admiration and gratitude for the preparation of these colored illustrations of the various blood diseases and the plate of the blood and tissue cells in inflammation. To Etta Piotti, medical illustrator extraordinary, goes the credit for the other colored histologic plates. To Mr. William J. Taylor goes our thanks for his invaluable help in the preparation of many of the gross photographs. The photomicrographs, with few exceptions, were taken by the authors from the actual case material.

Much of the material presented here has been collected personally from many sources over a period of many years. The tropical material came largely from the Philippines and our gratitude goes back to the coöperative spirit of the members of the staff of the Philippine General Hospital and the Medical School of the University of the Philippines, who aided in its accumulation. To Dr. James Ewing, especially, and to the staff of the New York Hospital and that of the Willard Parker Hospital in New York, we are likewise indebted beyond measure for the opportunities afforded by our long and close asociation, in acquiring a very considerable amount of valuable material which is presented here.

In the preparation of the manuscript, our particular thanks are due to Mr. Edwin S. Gault, Sr. for his invaluable assistance, and to Miss Anna M. St. Germain for her untiring, and uncomplaining secretarial efforts in its compilation. And finally, to our publishers, D. Appleton-Century Company, goes our appreciation for their painstaking efforts in the production of the finished volume.

LAWRENCE W. SMITH
EDWIN S. GAULT

FOREWORD

Various devices have been employed to take the teaching of pathology out of the realm of abstract philosophy and make it an effective force in the professional equipment of the medical student. None of these devices has proven so efficient as the study of case reports interpreted in the light of gross pathological data and analyzed by the methods of histopathology. When the student listens to a theoretical classification of the nephritides he burdens his memory with a series of abstractions of which, without repeated iteration and reiteration, he remembers nothing, whereas when he begins with the dramatic story of a case of Bright's disease, detailing the patient's struggles against hypertension, edema, and terminal uremia, and connects the renal changes with these incidents, the whole case becomes an impressive, consecutive, and highly significant picture of which he finds it difficult to forget anything.

In the present treatise, Dr. Smith and his collaborators have succeeded, to an admirable degree, in covering the broad field of pathology from the standpoint of the student's needs and the laws of psychology. They balance the clinical picture with as much theoretical data as it will carry and make it possible for the student to undertake histopathological interpretation with interest and intelligence. The very numerous illustrations are uniformly of a high order and in their context readily understood. While this laboratory textbook will show its highest value when the sections presented actually represent cases observed, the method employed will not lose its efficiency in any laboratory course. One may therefore predict a wide popularity for such a treatise and an improvement in the general results of the teaching of pathology to medical students where it may be introduced.

JAMES EWING

CONTENTS

ESSENTIALS OF PATHOLOGY

CHAPTER I
RETROGRADE PROCESSES
FATTY METAMORPHOSIS

The metabolism of fat is one of the most important general physiological functions of the body. Its pathological manifestations correspondingly represent some of the most fundamental disturbances of these normal body functions. These range all the way from endocrine and nutritional abnormalities through such apparently unrelated conditions as gall-bladder disease, diabetes, cirrhosis of the liver and the like, up to widespread degenerative changes of the entire vascular system commonly known as hardening of the arteries or arteriosclerosis. These are spoken of generically as fatty metamorphosis.

To intelligently approach the problems of pathological fat in disease, it is necessary to review briefly the essentials of its behavior in health. Much of our knowledge regarding normal fat metabolism is still in a transitional state, but certain facts are firmly established. Fats (lipins) occur in two major forms in the body—one as neutral or visible fat, in the fat depots of the body (the subcutaneous tissue, mesentery, omentum, etc.), the other as invisible, tissue or cellular fat (the lipoids—including the cholesterins, the phosphatides, the cerebrosides and the lipochromes).

The depot fat or adipose tissue represents *saturated* esters of glycerin with fatty acids (principally stearic, palmitic and oleic) and is derived largely from ingested fat. To a limited extent, fat may be formed also from carbohydrates in the course of their breakdown, and theoretically, at least, indirectly, from the amino acid decomposition products of proteins. The ingested fat is broken down in the intestine by lipolytic ferments, converted into soluble soaps, carried by the blood stream to the tissues and there resynthesized by the cells. The function of the liver seems to be in the nature of a middleman, temporarily storing and preparing the fat until it can be distributed, either to the tissue cells if needed for their metabolism, or to the depot cells (adipose tissue) if supplied in excess, for more permanent storage, and subsequent withdrawal for body requirements.

The tissue fats or lipoids, unlike the depot fats contain *unsaturated* fatty acids in combination with the cytoplasm of the tissue cells and serve a multitude of functions in the growth and activity of the cell. Most important among the lipoids is cholesterol, which is a universal cell constituent. This substance is certainly necessary for the maintenance of life, and yet our knowledge of its source, its behavior and its significance is still rudimentary or at best, fragmentary. Here perhaps lies the key to longevity, for senility, with its blood vessel degenerative changes is linked inseparably with disturbances of cholesterol metabolism, and yet this relationship thus far is still largely hypothetical.

Pathologically, fatty metamorphosis is divided into two major forms: (1) fatty *infiltration,* which (except in the liver) is characterized by the deposition of abnormal amounts of neutral (depot) fat, *between* the normal tissue cells; and (2) fatty *degeneration,* in which the lipoid substance of the cells (invisible fat) is converted into visible neutral fat and fatty acids, as part of the general picture of cell injury. This latter process is spoken of as fat *phanerosis,* and is one of the most significant general pathologic degenerative processes, always being indicative of impaired functional capacity of the cell, although not necessarily irreversible. In the case of the liver, as might be expected, *all* fatty changes, both infiltrative and degenerative, are seen microscopically as being *intra*cellular.

Fatty Infiltration

Fatty infiltration in general is the result of the ingestion of excessive amounts of fat and insufficient exercise to burn up this excess. In addition, at times it may be due to an inadequate endocrine control

PLATE I

FATTY INFILTRATION

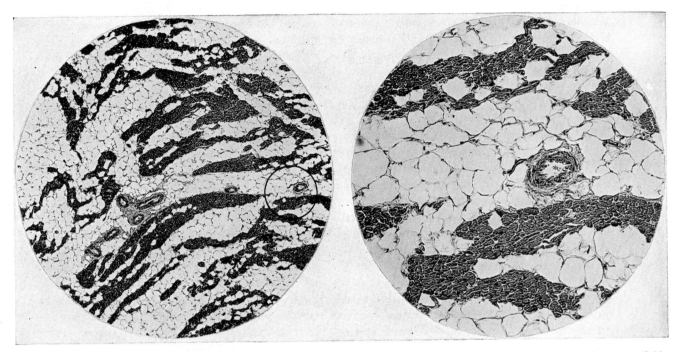

Fig. 1.—Heart: Fatty Infiltration.—Case 1.—Low power photomicrograph of section through heart muscle, between the bundles of which deposition of fat has occurred. App. 30 x.

Fig. 2.—Heart: Fatty Infiltration.—Case 1.—High power field of Fig. 1. Infiltration has occurred within the interstitial tissue. Muscle fibers are atrophied. App. 100 x.

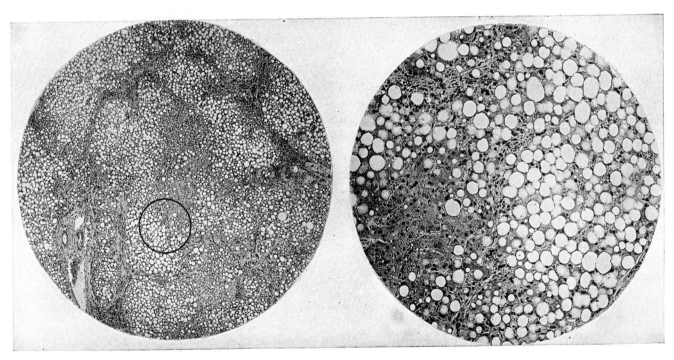

Fig. 3.—Liver: Fatty Infiltration.—Case 2.—Infiltration of liver cells with large fat globules of varying size. Process is seen to be more extensive at periphery of lobules. App. 30 x.

Fig. 4.—Liver: Fatty Infiltration.—Case 2.—High power view from Fig. 3. Infiltration of liver cells by large single fat globules is seen with the nuclei pushed to the side. App. 100 x.

of fat metabolism. Thus we find with pituitary disorders (Fig. 621) very characteristic forms of obesity. The same may be said to a less extent of certain disorders of the thyroid and adrenals. Following the climacteric, with the diminution in ovarian function, obesity is also prone to follow. Aside from these specific glandular disorders, obesity is almost entirely the result of unintelligence, laziness and lack of will power on the part of the individual in respect to diet and exercise.

Fatty Degeneration

In fatty degeneration, on the other hand, we are dealing with a strictly pathologic process, the result in the last analysis, of tissue or *cellular anoxemia*. This may be due to direct interference with the circulation mechanically from obstruction to the blood flow. It may be the result of severe anemia, the blood cells failing to sufficiently oxygenate the tissues through loss of the oxygen carrying substance, hemoglobin. This is especially seen in the heart muscle (Fig. 5). And finally, it may be the result of circulating toxins whether bacterial or chemical in origin. In fatty degeneration the total amount of fat may not be actually increased in an organ by chemical analysis, but the fat has been converted into visible form so that it appears histologically greatly increased in amount as we examine it under the microscope. From a practical consideration, in fatty degeneration the fat tends to occur in finely divided form giving the cytoplasm of the cell a foamy appearance in the usual hematoxylin and eosin stained slide. This is due, of course, to the fact that the actual fat being alcohol-soluble has been dissolved out of the tissue in preparing the slide so that only the vacuoles where the fat was present can be seen. In the liver particularly, but also to a less extent in other tissue cells, the larger vacuoles which we see are more likely to represent infiltration of the cell, although such a differentiation is largely artificial and one of degree rather than of difference, and furthermore of relatively little practical importance.

Histologic Demonstration of Fats

For the actual demonstration of the various lipins, formalin-fixed or fresh tissue cut by frozen section and stained by fat-soluble dyes such as Sudan III or Scharlach R (Fig. 13 and 14) is the most generally satisfactory method. Polychrome stains, of which Nile Blue sulphate is the one most commonly employed, are used to differentiate the various lipoid fractions through differences in the staining reactions; neutral fat staining blue and the various lipoids ranging from old rose to lavender. Finally, fixation of the fat by osmic acid (Fig. 8 and 518), so that paraffin preparations may be made in the usual manner is still one of the best ways of demonstrating certain of the lipins, although requiring a much longer time and presenting one serious objection, the question of expense.

Illustrative Cases

CASE 1. (Ref. #S-48)
Diagnosis.—Heart—fatty infiltration.
Patient was an obese, middle-aged white married woman, 48 years of age, who was admitted to the hospital complaining of severe right-sided upper abdominal pain, which radiated posteriorly to the right scapular region. This had been accompanied by marked nausea and several attacks of vomiting.
Present Illness.—Patient's illness began with a severe type of colic-like pain in the right side of the abdomen radiating toward the umbilicus and to the right scapular region. The pain was excruciating and knife-like in character and was accompanied by nausea and vomiting. She called a physician, who gave her an opiate to quiet the pain and referred her to the hospital with the presumptive diagnosis of gallbladder disease complicated by the presence of gall stones.

Past History.—The history in general had been irrelevant. She had had all the usual childhood diseases except diphtheria. She had been well all her life, never having required medical care except for minor digestive upsets and occasional upper respiratory infections.
In reviewing her systems the history brought out the following facts of interest: Gastro-intestinal System: Patient had always had an unusually hearty appetite and had eaten far in excess of her caloric requirements. She had had her menopause three years ago and since that time she had shown an almost steady progressive increase in weight. At one time she attempted to reduce by the use of thyroid tablets but developed such definite symptoms of thyrotoxicosis that she was forced to give this up. Her weight three years ago was 135; her weight on admission was 190. For the past several years, she had had occasional attacks of what she called "indigestion," char-

PLATE II

RETROGRADE PROCESSES

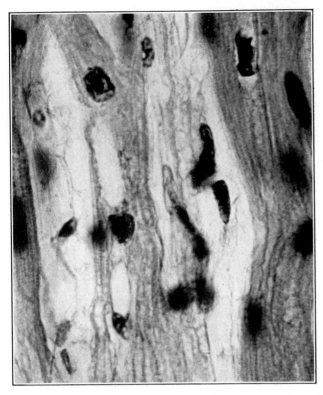

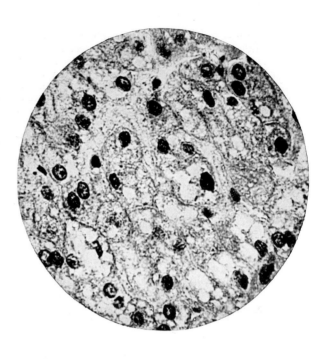

FIG. 5.—HEART: FATTY DEGENERATION.—CASE 217.—Section of heart muscle, with numerous, varying-sized, irregular globules of fat within the pale, swollen muscle cylinders. The striations are lost and the nuclei are pyknotic. App. 800 x.

FIG. 6.—LIVER: FATTY DEGENERATION.—CASE 3.—Section from a case of eclampsia with the finely vacuolated appearance of the cells due to the presence of multiple small fat globules. App. 600 x.

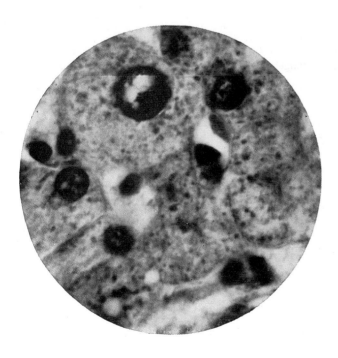

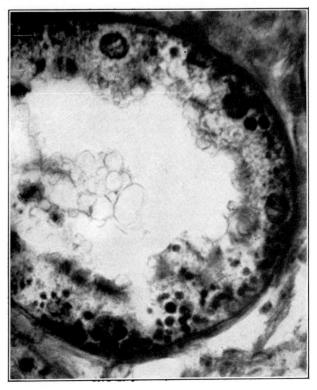

FIG. 7.—LIVER: CLOUDY SWELLING (PARENCHYMATOUS, GRANULAR DEGENERATION).—CASE 174 (LOBAR PNEUMONIA).—The cells which are swollen and stain palely contain numerous albuminous granules in their cytoplasm. App. 800 x.

FIG. 8.—KIDNEY: FATTY DEGENERATION.—CASE 5.—Osmic acid preparation. The cell outlines of the convoluted tubule shown are indistinct. The cytoplasm is filled wih albuminous granules and numerous varying-sized fat globules which appear black. App. 800 x.

acterized by flatulence, belching, the feeling of distention and discomfort in her upper abdomen and occasional attacks of nausea, but never accompanied by vomiting. She had the impression that fatty foods, especially fried foods, tended to aggravate this condition. Cardiorespiratory System.—She had never had any upper respiratory diseases of importance, and she had never been heart conscious except during the period she was taking thyroid when she had marked palpitation, which was the chief reason she gave up this therapy. Genito-urinary System. —Her menstrual history had been entirely normal. Her menses began at the age of fourteen and were regular up to her menopause. She was married and had had three normal children, who are now fully grown.

Physical Examination.—Patient was an obese, middle-aged woman lying in bed, with a tense, anxious expression. She appeared moderately jaundiced especially as observed in the sclerae. Her head was normal in shape. Pupils were regular and equal. Her eyes, ears, nose and throat were negative. Chest was symmetrical, with large, heavy, pendulous breasts. Lungs were clear throughout. Heart was apparently normal. Due to the obesity, it was difficult by percussion to establish the exact measurements. There were no murmurs and the sounds were distant. Abdomen was extremely obese and lax. There was definite tenderness and spasm in the right upper quadrant. Due to the obesity none of the abdominal organs could be palpated. Gynecologic examination was negative.

Laboratory Examination.—Red blood cells 3,500,000; hemoglobin 70%; white blood cells 14,000 with 82% polynuclears. Stool examination showed a definitely diminished bile content, although the stools were not entirely clay colored. Bile was present in the urine. The urine otherwise was negative. Van den Bergh: Direct was positive; indirect was delayed.

On the basis of the physical examination and laboratory findings a diagnosis of chronic cholecystitis with cholelithiasis and partial obstruction of the common duct was made and operation advised.

Operative History.—Patient was operated upon and a large gall stone measuring 1.5 cm. in diameter found in the ampulla where it acted as a ball valve. There was moderate thickening of the gallbladder and evidence of secondary infection with pus in the lumen.

Subsequent History.—Patient developed a secondary peritonitis and after a stormy week died of this infection.

Autopsy Findings.—At autopsy, the obvious cause of death was found to be a generalized peritonitis, the result of the gallbladder infection which had disseminated throughout the abdominal cavity. The outstanding feature of the entire case was the extreme obesity of the patient. This was especially marked in the fat depots of the mesentery, omentum and subcutaneous tissues, but in addition was notable in the pericardium and in the retroperitoneal tissues. The heart was moderately enlarged and showed acute dilatation, heart failure being the immediate cause of death, but really only a contributory factor in respect to the infection. The heart weighed 450 grams. There were no valvular lesions. The myocardium, on section, showed gross streaking with fat which infiltrated from the pericardial surface almost throughout the wall. The other lesions were those of secondary toxic changes, the result of the infection.

Microscopic Description of the Heart.—Sections through the heart muscle show the presence of a very diffuse deposition of fat between the heart fibers. This apparently arises from the epicardial fat and has grown in along the course of the blood vessels and connective tissue septa where it has been deposited in large amounts. As a result, the muscle bundles tend to show atrophy and secondary degenerative changes in part due to an inadequate blood supply insulated as they are by this heavy fat deposit. (See Fig. 1 and 2.)

CASE 2. (Ref. #S-222, 122 and 42)

Diagnosis.—Liver—fatty infiltration.

Patient was a colored woman 49 years of age, who was admitted to the hospital with a history of chronic cardiac disease. On the day before admission she developed slight difficulty with speech and suddenly noted numbness in the left arm, hand and leg. This was followed by an acute attack of pain in the chest associated with marked dyspnea.

Physical Examination.—On admission showed an extremely dyspneic, cyanotic, middle-aged woman, with marked edema of the lower extremities. There was a partial right facial paralysis with deviation of the tongue. The heart was enlarged 14 cms. to the left of the midsternal line with the apex in the 6th interspace. Gallop rhythm. Blood pressure 210/150. Left arm was nearly flaccid. Both legs showed nearly complete flaccid paralysis. Chest: Lungs—râles were present at both bases.

Laboratory Findings.—Wassermann negative. Chemistry within normal limits.

Course.—She developed a marked accumulation of fluid and 1200 c.c. were withdrawn from the two sides of the chest. She remained in the hospital for about six months, slowly progressing downhill, with her cardiac condition becoming more marked, and ultimately died of cardiac failure.

Autopsy Findings.—Showed a generalized accumulation of fluid in the body cavities: about 300 c.c. in the pericardium, 1000 c.c. in each side of the chest, 6000 c.c. in the peritoneum. Heart: Weighed 520 gm. Marked hypertrophy and right-sided dilatation. Marked coronary sclerosis with a terminal early infarction. There was evidence of an old infarct with marked thinning in the left ventricular wall at the apex. There was also evidence of an old chronic mitral valvulitis with a terminal acute bacterial endocarditis. Lungs: Showed several small hemorrhagic infarcts in the lower lobes. Spleen: Showed a picture of chronic passive congestion with an anemic infarct. Liver: Showed a suggestive beginning cirrhosis with a rather marked fatty infiltration and some suggestion of chronic passive congestion. The kidneys showed moderate toxic nephrosis. In addition, there was noted a large peptic ulcer in the midportion of the stomach on the lesser curvature.

Microscopic Description of Liver.—Sections taken from the liver are studied in two ways. One section of the liver is fixed in formalin and frozen section preparations made, which are stained with Scharlach R to demonstrate the appearance of the fat in the liver cells. The usual liver lobulation can be made out with the central vein, the radiating cords of liver cells and the portal areas serving as topographical landmarks. The fat is observed as droplets of varying size stained a brilliant orange-red. These are found within the cytoplasm of the liver cells. In many places these droplets have pushed the nucleus to one side of the cell producing an almost "signet ring" appearance. The nucleus, however, retains its normal features other than a tendency here and there to be slightly compressed. The characteristic large nucleolus may be observed and the chromatin granules are normal in size and arrangement. The distribution of this fatty substance is found to be chiefly in the peripheral and midzonal portions of the lobule rather than around the central vein and may be explained in part on the basis of an anoxemia of the liver cells due to circulatory stasis. In Figures 3 and 4, may be seen liver tissue from the same case prepared in the usual manner and stained by hematoxylin and eosin. This has been run through alcohols to dehydrate the tissues for sectioning and, as a result, the fat being soluble appears as vacuoles instead of droplets. The general appearance of the liver by this method is, therefore, somewhat lacy. It will be noted that the vacuoles are for the most part large and occupy the major portion of the cytoplasm of the cell. There is considerable variation in their size. However, the tendency is for the smaller droplets to fuse and form the larger masses. By this method of preparation the preservation of the liver cells is better observed than in the frozen section slide.

CASE 3. (Ref. #S-127)

Diagnosis.—Liver—fatty degeneration.

Patient is a young white woman 27 years of age who was admitted to the hospital with the following history: She had been under observation in the prenatal clinic and was in her eighth month of pregnancy. Her physician was called at 5 A.M. and told that the patient had fallen out of bed, hitting her head against the bedpost. She was found semicomatose and in the interval had had two convulsions. She was rushed to the hospital and a spinal tap was done. She had one convulsion on the way to the hospital and another shortly after the spinal tap. Blood pressure 178/118. Spinal puncture was repeated and this time a blood-tinged fluid was obtained. She became deeply cyanotic with rapid, shallow respirations. There was considerable frothy, bloody fluid regurgitated from her mouth. She became more and more toxic and comatose, with several convulsive seizures and died about twelve hours after admission to the hospital.

The entire onset was sudden, because she had been examined in the clinic only a week before at which time her blood pressure and urine findings were within normal limits, and she presented no evidence of toxemia.

Autopsy Findings.—An obese young woman, white, weighing around two hundred pounds. On opening the abdomen, the liver was seen to be about 5 cm. below the costal margin and its capsule appeared tense. On section, the liver was found to show marked fatty degeneration and was yellow in color. Scattered throughout the entire liver were seen many small, irregular sized and shaped red hemorrhagic patches (Fig. 473, 474 and 482) measuring from 0.5 to 1 cm. in diameter. The pericardial cavity contained about 120 c.c. of bloody fluid which came from a varicosity of one of the pericardial vessels. The heart itself was pale; otherwise negative. The spleen, pancreas and adrenals were normal. Kidneys were normal in size. On section they were very pale in the cortex and deeply congested in the pyramids. The uterus contained a 2400 gm. dead male fetus. The head was opened in the usual way and a fracture found at the base of the petrous portion of the right temporal bone extending into the right transverse sinus. This was the source of a rather diffuse hemorrhage over the convex surface of both hemispheres, more marked on the left and at the base of the brain.

Microscopic Description of Liver.—The section from the liver may be seen in Figure 6 where the characteristic fine vacuolization of the cells may be observed. The most marked fatty changes are noted around the central portion of the lobule in contradistinction to the preceding case. The liver cells acquire a foamy appearance of their cytoplasm as a result, rather than the coarsely vacuolated lacy effect of simple fatty infiltration. This process is fairly diffuse throughout the liver substance although more marked in the central areas. In addition, it will be noted that there are numerous areas of necrosis and hemorrhage scattered throughout the liver lobule. These tend to be distributed near the periphery of the lobule in relation to the portal circulation rather than around the central vein. Many of them, however, are of sufficient size to encroach upon the central portion of the lobule. There is a marked necrosis of the liver cells in these areas, which is evidenced by the cytoplasm of the cells taking a strong eosinophilic stain in contradistinction to the purplish color of the normal cells. In many places these cells have actually become disintegrated and the fragments of cytoplasm stain even more intensely with the eosin. There is a secondary leukocytic infiltration in an attempt to remove the necrotic cellular debris. The other feature of the picture is the hemorrhage where rupture of vessels or sinuses has occurred with diffusion of red cells into the stromal tissue spaces and even into the necrotic liver cells. This combination of acute focal necrosis and hemorrhage is essentially pathognomonic for the condition known as eclampsia.

CHAPTER II

RETROGRADE PROCESSES (*Continued*)

GLYCOGENIC, HYDROPIC AND MUCOID DEGENERATION

PART I

DISTURBANCES OF CARBOHYDRATE METABOLISM

The only visually demonstrable form of carbohydrate occurs as glycogen, a water-soluble isomer of glucose. This is distributed normally throughout most of the body tissues. It is stored particularly in the striated muscles of the body to the extent of about forty-four per cent where it is instantly available for oxidation when called upon through muscular activity. It is secondarily stored in the liver where about thirty-eight per cent of the total glycogen is normally found. Here it is synthesized by the liver cells from the circulating blood sugar and stored in the form of glycogen.

Glycogen may be stained by Best's carmine method and appears as red granules in the cytoplasm of the cells (Fig. 15). It likewise may be stained by iodine and appears a brownish-red by this method. Being water-soluble, tissues require fixation in absolute alcohol to prevent the loss of the glycogen in the preparation of permanent sections. Normally, after a meal high in carbohydrates, the cytoplasm of the liver cells may be found almost completely filled with minute, rather uniformly sized glycogen granules and may be similarly demonstrated in striated musculature.

Under pathological conditions the demonstration of glycogen is helpful in establishing a diagnosis in two diseases; namely, diabetes and secondarily, von Gierke's disease. In severe diabetes the normal stored glycogen largely disappears from the cytoplasm of the liver and muscle cells. Due to the lowered threshold of glucose excretion, glycogen is apt to be seen in the epithelium of the renal tubules, especially in Henle's loop cells (Fig. 9) where absorption takes place from the highly concentrated sugar in the urine. Likewise, in diabetes, for some poorly understood reason, the nuclei of the liver cells are likely to undergo degenerative changes with swelling of the nucleus and the accumulation of glycogen within the nucleus itself. Thus, the presence of spherical, irregularly sized carmine staining droplets of glycogen within the nuclei of the liver cells is diagnostic of the condition "diabetes" to all intents and purposes.

In von Gierke's disease we are dealing with a condition in which there is an abnormal mechanism relating to carbohydrate metabolism. Apparently the liver and other body tissues are capable of manufacturing glycogen but are incapable of resynthesizing it for utilization as glucose. The result is that the liver and other organs increase steadily in size as a result of the accumulation of glycogen within the substance of the cells. This curious disease is usually seen in infancy or early childhood and is, as far as the reported cases are concerned, invariably fatal.

ILLUSTRATIVE CASE

CASE 4. (Ref. #S-209)

Diagnosis.—Liver and kidney—Diabetes; glycogenic infiltration.

Patient was a ten-year-old white male child, who was admitted to the hospital in coma.

Present Illness.—The patient was known to have had diabetes for approximately one and one-half years and had been under the care of a physician intermittently.

The mother, who was herself a mild diabetic, had been attempting to maintain his carbohydrate balance as far as possible on a dietary basis in the same way that she had been able to control her own disease. At times, however, this had proved inadequate, and she had been obliged to resort to the use of insulin. This had not been accurately gauged on the basis of blood sugar determinations, but rather in a haphazard fashion upon the basis

PLATE III
RETROGRADE PROCESSES (Continued)

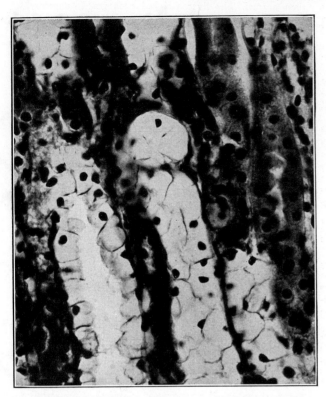

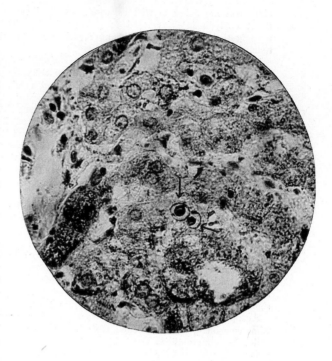

FIG. 9.—KIDNEY: GLYCOGENIC INFILTRATION.—CASE 4, DIABETES.—Tubular epithelium of Henle's loop, distended with glycogen which appears unstained. (Glycogen, being water-soluble, is lost by routine technical methods.) App. 400 x.

FIG. 10.—LIVER: GLYCOGENIC INFILTRATION.—CASE 4, DIABETES.—(Best's carmine stain.) Characteristic, pathognomonic, intra-nuclear infiltration by glycogen and normal intracytoplasmic glycogen storage. (See also colored Plate IV—Fig. 15 and 16.) App. 600 x.

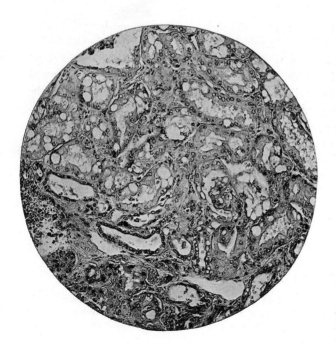

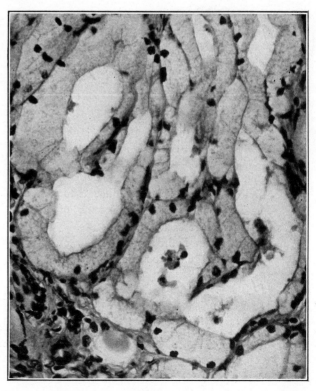

FIG. 11.—KIDNEY: HYDROPIC DEGENERATION.—CASE 5, TOXIC NEPHROSIS.—Convoluted tubular epithelial cells with hydropic vacuolization of their cytoplasm. Nuclei tend to be displaced basally. App. 100 x.

FIG. 12.—KIDNEY: HYDROPIC DEGENERATION.—An almost imperceptible "skeining" of the cytoplasm of the cell is observed as a result of edema in the early stages in contradistinction to fatty, glycogenic and advanced hydropic degeneration. App. 400 x.

of the presence of an appreciable amount of urinary sugar, and symptoms which led the mother to believe the child was not doing as well as usual, notably increased thirst (polydipsia), increased frequency of micturition, a suggestion of beginning air hunger and marked lassitude.

For the past five days she had been increasing the dose of insulin by twenty units a day until during the twenty-four hours preceding admission, the child had received 100 units.

Physical Examination.—The patient was a somewhat emaciated, pale, white male child, who appeared his given age. He was in profound coma with convulsive twitchings of his extremities. Owing to the critical state of the patient no complete physical examination was done at the time of admission other than a very cursory examination of his heart and lungs, which showed no significant abnormalities.

Laboratory Findings.—Blood was taken for a blood sugar analysis and showed only 40 mgm. of carbohydrate per 100 c.c. of blood.

Subsequent Course.—A presumptive diagnosis of insulin shock was made and therapy instituted to combat the depleted carbohydrate balance by the intravenous administration of glucose and fluids. In spite of this treatment, the patient developed a succession of convulsions shortly after admission and died two hours later.

Autopsy Findings.—The body was that of a somewhat emaciated, well developed ten-year-old white male child. No abnormalities were found at the time of autopsy other than very striking congestion of all the viscera. .The pancreas itself weighed 35 grams, seemed somewhat soft in consistency and rather more yellow than normal. The liver weighed 1300 gm. It appeared edematous and congested and on section the cut surface bulged slightly over the capsule.

Microscopic Examination of Liver.—Microscopic section of the liver presents a typical picture of diabetes in the tissue fixed in absolute alcohol and sectioned with the view of preventing the dissolving out of any glycogen present. Careful search, particularly around the central portions of each lobule, showed many large, swollen nuclei with the chromatin gathered around the nuclear membrane tending to intensify it. In places, actual rupture of the nucleus appears to have taken place. Scattered throughout these swollen liver nuclei are found many granules which stain intensely red. These vary considerably in size, some of them nearly filling the entire nucleus, others appearing in multiple form and being much smaller in size. Presumably due to the use of insulin over a period of one and one-half years and the administration of glucose shortly before the patient's death, a moderate amount of glycogen can be demonstrated in the cytoplasm of the liver cells much as in normal liver tissue. (Fig. 10 and 16.)

In preparations from the liver and kidney made in the usual manner by formalin fixation and the ordinary hematoxylin and eosin stain, the glycogen has been dissolved and only the empty vacuolated spaces where it was present may be demonstrated. In the kidney this is very prominent, showing a marked selectivity for the Henle's loops (Fig. 9). In the liver it is difficult to differentiate the fine vacuolization of the cytoplasm of the cell from the appearance sometimes seen in fatty degeneration except that unlike the fatty vacuoles there is not the sharp, spherical arrangement so typical of the former.

PART II

HYDROPIC DEGENERATION

By the term "hydropic degeneration" is meant the pathological accumulation of fluid *within* a cell. This is in contradistinction to the term "edema" by which is meant accumulation *between* cells, especially in the connective tissue supporting stroma, even separating the collagen fibrils. It represents a retrograde degenerative process which is frequently seen accompanying other rather profound fatty and albuminous degenerative cytoplasmic changes of cells. Indeed, at times it may be difficult to always differentiate true hydrops from some of these other changes where vacuolization occurs. Typically, a cell showing true hydrops contains one or more poorly defined, irregularly outlined vacuoles which, as a result of their size, may cause nuclear distortion although this latter feature is very likely to be missing. If the cell is fortunately cut in the proper plane after fixation, a minute fibrin clot may be observed within the vacuole. This identifies the nature of the fluid as having the blood serum as an origin. Such hydropic degeneration is seen most often in association with various types of inflammation accompanied by edema. In general, this hydropic degeneration is of relatively little significance except as in relation to the other degenerative changes. In itself, it is usually a reversible reaction and does not indicate necessarily cell injury to the degree where necrobiosis of the cell is likely to occur.

ILLUSTRATIVE CASE

CASE 5. (Ref. #S-80)
Diagnosis.—Kidney—acute toxic nephrosis with granular, fatty and hydropic degeneration of the epithelium.

Patient was a 65-year-old white female, who was admitted to the hospital following a fall down a flight of stairs, where she was found unconscious.

PLATE IV

INFILTRATIONS AND DEGENERATIONS

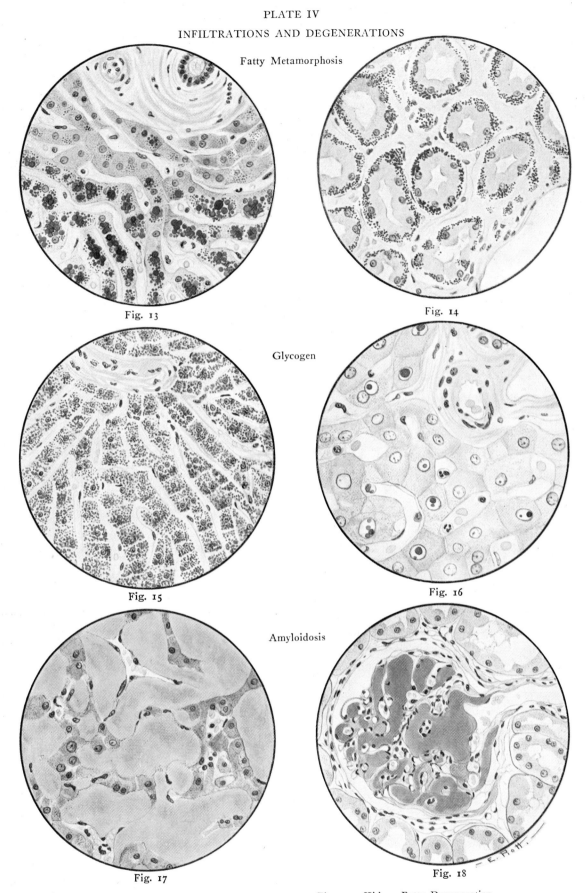

Fatty Metamorphosis

Fig. 13   Fig. 14

Glycogen

Fig. 15   Fig. 16

Amyloidosis

Fig. 17   Fig. 18

Fig. 13.—Liver-Fatty Infiltration   Fig. 14.—Kidney-Fatty Degeneration
Fig. 15.—Liver-Glycogen Storage (Infiltration)   Fig. 16.—Liver-Diabetes, Nuclear Glycogen
Fig. 17.—Liver-Amyloid Infiltration   Fig. 18.—Kidney-Glomerulus-Amyloid

PLATE V

RETROGRADE PROCESSES—MUCOID DEGENERATION

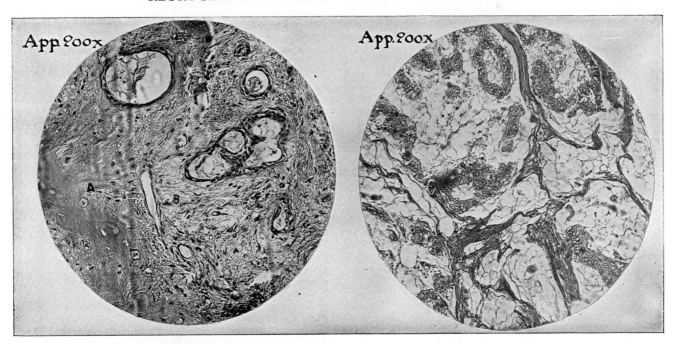

FIG. 19.—PAROTID GLAND TUMOR: MUCOID DEGENERATION.—CASE 9.—Basophilic epithelial mucinous material is seen in acinar structures, pseudochondromucinous changes of stroma at "A," and typical myxomatous degeneration at "B."

FIG. 20.—COLON: ADENOCARCINOMA.—MUCINOUS DEGENERATION.—CASE 6.—Intra- and extracellular masses of basophilic-staining, epithelial mucin, the product of tumor cell degeneration.

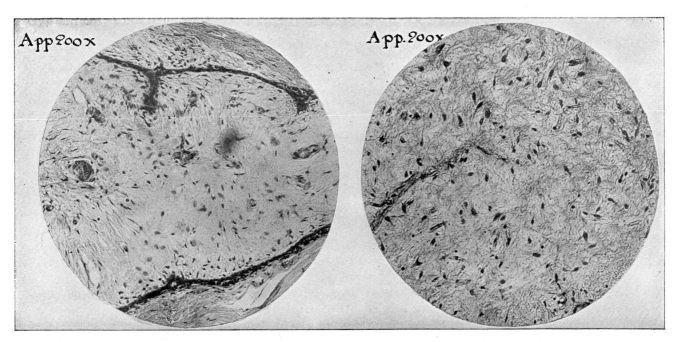

FIG. 21.—BREAST: ADENOFIBROMA.—MYXOMATOUS DEGENERATION.—CASE 8.—Wide separation of the nuclei of the stroma, with swelling of the intercellular collagen which presents the characteristic basophilic reaction of mucin may be readily observed.

FIG. 22.—RETROPERITONEAL FIBROMYXOMA.—CASE 7.—Cells tend to be stellate and resemble primitive umbilical cord myxoblasts. Intercellular matrix composed of swollen fibrillae showing marked myxomatous degeneration.

Present Illness.—Began about six months ago with increasing dyspnea on exertion. There had been an increase in the size of the patient's abdomen during this period and she had complained of intermittent attacks of girdle-like pains around her waist. There was in her history a suggestion of possible chronic alcoholism with a good many attacks of acute gastritis associated with nausea and vomiting. In the past few months these had been accompanied not infrequently by the raising of blood. She had not been able to be sure whether this was true hematemesis or whether it was hemoptysis, as she had had a persistent cough during most of this same period. At the time of her fall she was attempting to go down stairs to the kitchen, apparently lost consciousness and fell, as she had no recollection of the intervening period until she awoke in the hospital.

Past History.—She remembered nothing significant in her family history. Her father and mother both died when she was a small child and she knew practically nothing of them. She did not remember whether or not she had the usual childhood diseases. She had had an appendectomy ten years ago. Other than that, she had had fairly good health with the usual quota of mild upper respiratory infections.

Physical Examination.—The patient was an obese, middle-aged white female extremely dyspneic and acutely ill. Numerous ecchymoses were noted from her chest to her feet, the result of her fall. Head and scalp were negative. There was a profuse, purulent discharge from her nose. Eyes: There was a purulent bilateral conjunctivitis. Pupils were regular and equal. Mouth showed marked oral sepsis. There was intense congestion of the pharynx. Chest: There was tenderness over the lower right costal cage with dullness and flatness in the upper portion of the right side anteriorly. Here tactile fremitus was increased. There was definite bronchial breathing and there were numerous coarse râles. The heart was moderately enlarged apparently, although percussion was not satisfactory. Sounds were of poor quality. The rhythm was completely irregular. There were no murmurs. Blood pressure 105/0. Abdomen was obese but otherwise apparently negative. Extremities were negative.

Laboratory Findings.—Red blood cells 2,800,000; hemoglobin 60%. White blood cells 22,000 with 85% polynuclears. Urinalysis: moderate trace of albumin; many pus cells seen in the sediment, otherwise negative. Sputum examination: There was a rusty-colored, mucoid sputum obtained which, on culture, yielded a pneumo-coccus. Urea nitrogen 40 mgm. on admission which rose to 92 mgm.

Subsequent Course.—Temperature on admission 102°; pulse 80; respirations 30. During the course of the next few days, the patient's condition varied somewhat from time to time, but her general progress was definitely down hill. Temperature became septic ranging from 99° to 105°. Pulse rose to 130 or 140 and respirations climbed to 45 and 50. She was delirious a good deal of the time, showing any mental alertness only at intervals. Such history as was obtained was largely from a sister with whom she lived. She died five days after admission with a diagnosis of lobar pneumonia following her injury, complicated by a cirrhosis of the liver and renal failure.

Autopsy Findings.—The body was that of an obese, middle-aged white woman showing external ecchymoses as noted in the history. There was marked myocardial degeneration with right cardiac dilatation. There was diffuse, confluent, right upper lobe pneumonia apparently more of bronchopneumonic than lobar type. The kidneys showed severe toxic nephrosis. The liver showed a moderate portal cirrhosis. There were esophageal varices present. There was a chronic cholecystitis with cholelithiasis. The cause of death was felt to be primarily the post-traumatic pneumonia, but this was obviously influenced extensively by the portal cirrhosis picture.

Microscopic Description of Kidney.—Sections through the kidney in this case are of particular interest in studying the degenerative changes which affect the tubules. The picture is one of very marked degeneration with hydropic, albuminous and fatty degenerative changes all present. In Fig. 11 and 12, it is of particular interest to observe the distribution of these various degenerative lesions. The convoluted tubular epithelium is particularly found to be the site of diffuse, granular, albuminous change whereas lower down along the course of the tubule more striking fatty and hydropic lesions are observed. The fatty degeneration is characterized by very fine vacuolization of the cytoplasm of the renal tubular epithelium. More pertinent to the discussion in hand is the presence of coarse vacuolization in certain of these cells. These coarse vacuoles are very large for the most part, are found in the cytoplasm of epithelial cells and definitely impinge upon the nuclei causing at times considerable distortion. Very little actual necrosis of the renal epithelium is noted, however, in spite of the very extensive degenerative picture present.

PART III

Mucoid (Mucinous and Myxomatous) Degeneration

In many inflammatory conditions affecting mucous epithelium as well as in many tumors both of connective tissue and epithelial origin we find degenerative changes of the cells associated with the excessive production of mucin. This is spoken of inexactly as mucoid degeneration. For convenience the two types occurring in epithelial and connective tissue are separately designated by the terms "mucinous" and "myxomatous" respectively, having but one factor in common, the presence of true mucin as distinguished from para- or pseudomucin, which is found only in certain tumors of the ovary.

Mucin may be described as a slimy, gelatinous material which is normally secreted by the goblet cells of the gastro-intestinal tract, by the primitive myxomatous cells of the umbilical cord and by the cells lining the joint and bursal cavities. There are probably many variations in the exact chemical composition of this material, but it has certain outstanding reactions by which it may be identified. It is readily precipitated by acetic acid and by alcohol and may be redissolved by the addition of alkali. It likewise has a characteristic staining affinity for basic dyes and may be well demonstrated by a special mucicarmine stain where it appears as red strands or amorphous masses.

Pathologically, increased mucin production is found in many inflammatory conditions, particularly those affecting the mucous membranes which contain goblet cells. In the milder forms of such inflammatory response the condition is spoken of as catarrhal inflammation and represents merely an increased secretory activity on the part of the cell. In certain tumors of epithelial origin, particularly those of the stomach and large intestine, less frequently those found in the breast, there is a true mucoid degeneration of the cells in which the cytoplasm of the cell becomes enormously distended with mucoid material reaching a point ultimately where the nucleus is destroyed by compression and anoxemia. This is followed by actual rupture of the cell membrane and the deposition of this excessive mucoid material in the interstitial stroma where it largely replaces all of the normal structures. Such tumors are inaccurately spoken of as colloid carcinomas because of the gelatinoid appearance of this mucoid material, which grossly resembles the colloid secretion of the thyroid gland.

In connective tissue, we may also see myxomatous degeneration of the collagen under certain inflammatory conditions. More often, however, such degenerative changes of the connective tissue cells are best seen in tumors arising from the group of connective-tissue-derived cells. Rarely, a true myxoblastic tumor arising from embryonal stellate myxoblasts may occur. More often, however, the picture is one of a retrograde degenerative picture of more completely differentiated connective tissue cells. Almost any fibrous tissue tumor may at times present this picture of myxomatous change. Not infrequently in epithelial tumors such as adenofibromata of the breast, leiomyomata of the uterus or indeed in any carcinoma, similar myxomatous degeneration of the connective tissue supporting stroma may result, particularly when the blood supply is interfered with. Thus, myxomatous degeneration may be compared in the last analysis to a retrograde process comparable to fatty degeneration, and resulting largely from an inadequate supply of oxygen to maintain cytologic metabolism.

ILLUSTRATIVE CASES

CASE 6. (Ref. #S-223)

Diagnosis.—Mucous carcinoma of the colon.

Patient was a 47-year-old white male, who was admitted to the hospital because of persistent constipation, and the presence of a mass which tended to protrude from the anal orifice with defecation. This was accompanied by considerable pain.

Present Illness.—The history dated back for about six months when the patient first noted a moderate tendency for constipation from which he had never suffered in the past. This had increased steadily in severity during this period and at times he had been unable to evacuate his colon in spite of a marked desire on his part. He had noticed that his stool tended to occur in almost ribbon fashion and to be blood-streaked frequently, although he had never had any actual hemorrhage from the rectum. There had been a bulging mass which had at times protruded from his anal orifice and which he had considered to be hemorrhoids and for that reason had paid no undue attention to these symptoms. During this six-months period, however, the patient had noted loss of weight of approximately 25 pounds. He had felt this was due to diminished food intake because of a loss of appetite and a fear of pain with defecation.

Past History.—Patient's past history was essentially irrelevant in respect to his present illness. His mother died of carcinoma of the breast at the age of 54. His father died of pneumonia at the age of 72. As far as he recalled, he had the usual childhood diseases, but had never had any severe gastro-intestinal disturbances. He had never been hospitalized for any illness and had had no operations.

A review of his systems was negative.

Physical Examination.—The patient was a well developed, middle-aged white male with a somewhat anxious facies. He showed evidence of some recent loss of weight with his skin somewhat dry and wrinkled. His head was negative. Eyes, ears, nose and throat were entirely negative. Chest was symmetrical. The lungs were clear. The heart was not enlarged. There were no murmurs. Abdomen was markedly distended and tympanitic throughout. There was no visible peristalsis. The muscle tone was poor. There were no areas of localized tenderness or muscle spasm. There was no definite rigidity. Proctoscopic examination revealed a large cauliflower-like mass just within the anal orifice approximately 2 or 3 cm. above the sphincter. This showed superficial ulceration but appeared freely movable and there was no gross fixation of the bowel wall in the pelvis. Operation was advised for the removal of the tumor.

Operative History.—The patient was operated on by perineal approach and a proctosigmoidectomy was performed removing the entire tumor mass as well as approximately 15 cm. of the bowel.

Subsequent Course.—Post-operative history was complicated by the development of a urethral vesical fistula which, however, was satisfactorily repaired. No recurrence of the tumor mass had occurred at the end of a three-year period and the patient had regained his normal weight and appeared in his usual good health.

Pathological Report.—*Gross Description:* Specimen consisted of a section of large bowel approximately 18 cm. in length. This was opened longitudinally and a large, polypoid tumor mass measuring 12 cm. in diameter was noted about 3 cm. above the anal ring. This was pedunculated in appearance with a broad base. Superficially it had an ulcerated, cauliflower appearance, and on section was gelatinous in consistency. There was no gross evidence of invasion of the wall of the rectum.

Microscopic Description.—(Fig. 20) Histologically, the picture is typical of the so-called mucous or colloid type of adenocarcinoma of gastro-intestinal origin. The tumor cells are found as nests embedded in great masses of mucoid material, which is almost homogeneous in appearance save for delicate, thread-like septa representing both interstitial stroma and cell membrane rests. The nuclei are extremely distorted for the most part, and the cell outlines are made out with great difficulty. Here and there some persistence of the true grandular arrangement of the cells is found, indicative of its origin. There is a certain amount of myxomatous degeneration of the connective tissue stroma. Occasional atypical nuclear figures are observed. There is definite microscopic invasion of the deeper structures at the point of origin of the tumor. It is evidently of a slow-growing type and of a relatively low-grade malignancy.

Case 7. (Ref. #S-239)

Diagnosis.—Retroperitoneal fibromyxoma.

Patient was a 47-year-old white female, who was admitted to the hospital because of abdominal pain and discomfort, accompanied by metrorrhagia.

Present Illness.—Began approximately six months before her admission. She complained of vague, indefinite abdominal pain and discomfort. She had always been constipated and at the outset tended to feel that this constipation was the cause of her symptoms. However, the liberal use of relatively radical cathartics failed to show any improvement in her picture and she developed considerable frequency of urination and a marked metrorrhagia. This was accompanied by fatigability and a feeling of weakness. She felt that her abdomen was increasing in size and as the symptoms were increasing in severity she finally went to a physician, who sent her to the hospital for study.

Past History.—Her past history was irrelevant. As a child she had the usual contagious diseases.

A review of her systems showed nothing of particular significance other than the history of chronic constipation. Her menstrual history had always been normal up to the past six months. Menses began at the age of 13 and had been regular. She had had three normal pregnancies. During the past six months, however, her periods had been irregular and there had been more or less constant flowing. She had attributed this to her probable menopause. Cardiovascular history was negative. Genito-urinary history was entirely negative except for her recent frequency.

Physical Examination.—Patient was a well developed and nourished middle-aged white woman. The head was normal. Eyes, ears, nose and throat were negative except

for the fact that the tonsils were moderately hypertrophied. The chest was negative. The lungs were clear throughout. The heart was slightly enlarged. There was a diastolic murmur heard over the mitral area, which was transmitted to the axilla. Abdomen: Showed very marked enlargement. There was no rigidity, muscle spasm or tenderness. Due to the distention, deep palpation was difficult, but there appeared to be a large mass about the size of a football, arising more or less in the midline but tending to be somewhat more prominent on the left. Rectal and gynecologic examinations were negative.

Laboratory Findings.—Red blood cells 4,600,000; hemoglobin 11 grams. White blood cells 8,100 with 50% polynuclears, 38% lymphocytes, 9% monocytes, 3% eosinophiles. Urinalysis negative.

Operative History.—Exploratory laparotomy with the intention of removal of the tumor, if possible, was advised. At operation, a large retroperitoneal tumor was found embedded in the root of the mesentery and apparently arising in the midline. This was fairly well defined from the surrounding tissues and was removed without much difficulty.

Pathological Report.—*Gross Description.*—The tumor is a large, flabby mass of gelatinoid, edematous appearing tissue measuring about 35 cm. in diameter and weighing 5700 gm. On section it is pinkish in color, glistening in appearance and resembles colloid in its translucency. It is partially surrounded by a thin connective tissue membrane. On section, the cut surface seems to be in a "gel" state, so fluid that it almost seems to pour out on the table top, but still held together by a delicate stroma and a membranous-like capsule. There is no evidence of necrosis or hemorrhage.

Microscopic Description.—(Fig. 22) The entire tumor is made up of a mass of loosely woven, fine, delicate connective tissue fibrils. Interspersed in this mass of fibrils are scattered, bipolar, spindle-shaped nuclei. Here and there, certain of these nuclei have a definite stellate appearance as if representing much more primitive myxoblasts. The entire structure is uniform in multiple sections taken from various parts of the tumor. It resembles closely a true tumor of myxoblastic origin, but in view of the age of the patient and the location of the tumor, it is felt that this should better be classified as a tumor of connective tissue origin with very extensive myxomatous degeneration, realizing that many pathologists would classify the lesion as either a myxoma or a myxofibroma. At all events it represents the most characteristic histologic picture of a tumor of myxoblastic origin which is ordinarily encountered and the argument as to its exact terminology would appear to be one of academic importance only.

Case 8. (Ref. #S-108)

Diagnosis.—Adenofibroma.

Patient was a young unmarried girl of twenty-two years, who went to her physician because of a small nodule in her left breast.

Present Illness.—Patient noted, while bathing, a definite small mass in her left breast. Because of the intensive campaign being waged against cancer, she became worried and went to her physician for examination. In all other respects her history was essentially negative. At the time of examination, the patient's menses had been present fourteen days earlier.

Past History.—Patient had a normal developmental history. She had suffered the usual childhood diseases. She had never had any symptoms relating to her cardio-respiratory system other than occasional colds. Her gastro-intestinal history was negative except for an attack of acute appendicitis for which she was operated upon three years ago. Her menstrual history had begun at the age of twelve and had always been regular at twenty-eight day intervals, lasting four or five days. It had not been associated with any dysmenorrhea.

Physical Examination.—The patient was a well developed, well nourished young woman. Her head was normal. Her eyes, ears, nose and throat were negative. Chest was symmetrical. Breasts were relatively small and firm. The abdomen was negative except for an old scar 4 cm. in length in the right lower quadrant. Examination of the breasts revealed a small, firm mass in the lateral lower quadrant of her left breast. This was approximately 3 cm. in diameter. It was not adherent to the skin and showed no attachment to the nipple. It was freely movable. It appeared sharply demarcated from the surrounding breast tissue. A tentative, pre-operative diagnosis of adenofibroma was made and excision advised.

Operative History.—The nodule was excised under local anesthesia and frozen section diagnosis made at the time of operation. A benign fibroadenoma was the diagnosis and the wound was closed without drainage.

Subsequent Course.—The patient, one year later, showed nothing but a small linear scar in the fold of the breast. No recurrence or other tumor masses were noted.

Pathological Report.—*Gross Description.*—Specimen consisted of an almost spherical, well encapsulated, firm, whitish nodule 3.5 cm. in diameter. This could readily be shelled out of a rather dense connective tissue capsule. On section, it had a trabeculated appearance and was almost pure white in color save for minute grayish streaks or dots apparently representing the glandular structures.

Microscopic Description.—(Fig. 21) Sections microscopically through the tumor present a somewhat variable picture in different areas. In one part of the slide there is a rather definite glandular hyperplasia with small acini lined by cuboidal epithelial cells, which in places are two or three cells deep. These are normal in appearance and show no evidence of neoplastic degeneration, and there is no invasion of the underlying stroma. This suggests a premenstrual hyperplasia in association with ovarian hormonal activity. Surrounding these acini is a loose connective tissue stroma, which shows very marked myxomatous change, the collagen occurring as blue staining threads arranged in a loose meshwork. In other portions of the slide, we find the tumor more of the typical so-called intracanalicular picture. Here there are distorted tubules, which show encroachment upon their lumen by dense connective tissue proliferation. These areas of connective tissue are almost hyalinized and stain intensely with eosin instead of hematoxylin, as in the previously described areas. The epithelium in these acini and ducts appears similar, but compressed, leaving little or no lumen demonstrable.

CASE 9. (Ref. #S-220)
Diagnosis.—Parotid gland—"mixed" tumor.
Patient was a white male, aged thirty, who was ad-

mitted to the hospital because of swelling at the angle of the jaw on the left side of some three or four months' duration.

Present Illness.—Patient first noticed this swelling between three and four months before admission. It had been steadily but slowly increasing in size. It had been more inconvenient than actually painful, although palpation revealed a moderate amount of tenderness. It had interfered somewhat with his speech and with the motion of his jaw so that it had bothered him considerably while eating. His history in other respects was essentially negative.

Past History.—Patient had never had any previous illness requiring hospitalization. He suffered the usual childhood diseases. A review of his systems was essentially negative. He had had no significant upper respiratory infections. His gastro-intestinal picture was entirely negative. His cardiovascular history was likewise irrelevant. His genito-urinary history was entirely negative. He denied venereal infection.

Physical Examination.—Patient was a well developed, well nourished young white male. Head was normal in contour. His eyes were negative. The pupils were regular and reacted normally. The ears themselves were negative, but on the left side in the angle of the jaw involving the parotid region and thus causing some distortion of the lobe of the ear and the contour of the face in this region was found a firm, discrete, rather circumscribed tumor mass approximately 4 cm. in its greatest diameter. It seemed fairly movable and did not appear to be definitely attached to the bone at any point. On palpation it was moderately tender. There was no fluctuation noted. Examination of the nose and throat was essentially negative, although it was difficult for the patient to open his mouth sufficiently for satisfactory examination of the pharynx. The rest of the physical examination was essentially negative. Lungs were clear throughout. The heart was not enlarged and showed no murmurs. The abdomen was normal in contour. The extremities were negative.

Laboratory Findings.—Red blood cells 4,800,000; hemoglobin 85%. White blood cells 8,600 with 64% polynuclears. Urinalysis negative.

The patient was advised to have this tumor mass removed on the basis of a tentative diagnosis of a so-called "mixed" tumor of the parotid gland.

Operative History.—The tumor was removed as completely as possible surgically. It was found to be rather intimately related to both the 5th and 7th nerves in its deeper portions. The greater part of the tumor appeared fairly well encapsulated, although it was somewhat adherent to the surrounding subcutaneous tissues. At the base this adherence was more marked and it was uncertain whether the entire capsular portion of the deeper pole was entirely removed surgically as the under surface of the operative specimen was ragged.

Subsequent Course.—The patient remained free from symptoms for a period of about one and one-half years. At that time he again noted a recurrent swelling in the operative field and returned to the hospital for further treatment. The recurrent tumor was similarly surgically removed with a resulting partial facial paralysis, as it was felt better to attempt its radical excision rather than to save the nerve. Further history on this patient will be followed with great interest, but at the present time he appears free from any recurrence.

Pathological Report.—*Gross Description.*—Specimen consisted of a rounded, irregularly nodular mass of firm, grayish yellow tissue with a fairly well defined fibrous capsule. On cross section, several small foci of hemorrhage and necrosis were noted and numerous small cystic areas were seen. The tumor measured approximately 4 cm. in its greatest diameter.

Microscopic Description.—(Fig. 19) The outstanding histopathological findings in this tumor are those associated with the so-called "mixed" character of the cells. One's impression is that these tumors must be of both epithelial and mesothelial origin, as one find nests of epithelial cells which in places definitely form acini. In other places they occur in sheets and no definite glandular arrangement is identified. In places the epithelial cells tend to show a squamous metaplasia. More striking per-haps than this epithelial feature of the tumor is the stromal factor. Characteristically this tumor shows a curious pseudocartilaginous matrix with connective tissue cells in varying stages of development. Most of the collagen and much of the cartilaginous matrix show marked myxomatous degeneration. It is because of the extent of this stromal reaction, which appears to be an integral part of the tumor rather than merely an accompanying stromal desmoplasia, that the term "mixed" tumor has arisen. In this particular case mucoid degeneration of both epithelial cells and the connective tissue cells may readily be observed. The tumor histologically shows a very low grade appearance of malignancy, but both from experience and from the subsequent history in this case we anticipate a progressive recurrence until frank malignant degeneration occurs.

CHAPTER III

RETROGRADE PROCESSES (*Continued*)

CLOUDY SWELLING (PARENCHYMATOUS AND GRANULAR DEGENERATION); HYALINE DEGENERATION AND AMYLOID INFILTRATION

PART I

DISTURBANCES OF PROTEIN METABOLISM

Just as cells normally may be demonstrated to contain fat or carbohydrate, so do they contain certain protein substances which, under pathological conditions, may show demonstrable morphologic changes by which we may estimate the type of disturbance associated with protein metabolism. Normally most parenchymatous organs show in their cytoplasm small granules scarcely visible as a rule to the naked eye. Not only in the epithelial cells, but also in the striated musculature, both in the heart and peripheral muscles, may these albuminous granules be demonstrated. That they are of an albu-

minous nature is usually accepted on the basis that they may be dissolved by acetic acid, but are not altered by any of the fat solvents. One of the most satisfactory places to study these changes in the protein granules of the cells is to be found in the kidney where they are perhaps most readily observed, especially in the convoluted tubules of the renal unit. There are numerous terms applied to these degenerative changes which range through more or less progressive stages. First among these terms must be mentioned cloudy swelling (Fig. 7), or granular (parenchymatous) degeneration.

Cloudy Swelling

This is a term applied to certain granular changes occurring in the cytoplasm of the cells, chiefly of parenchymatous organs and especially in relation to many infectious diseases such as typhoid, pneumonia, diphtheria and so forth. It is a toxic degeneration of the albuminous material which is characterized by what is believed by many to be a swelling of the mitochrondria and the secretory granules of the cells; by others a hydropic degeneration of the colloid proteins of the cytoplasm of the cell. Grossly, such tissues appear somewhat swollen and have a parboiled, opaque appearance. Its differentiation from simple postmortem changes of a similar nature

is extremely difficult. It represents one of the mildest and earliest demonstrable degenerative changes of cells and is usually a reversible reaction if the etiologic toxic factor is removed; otherwise, it may go on to more extensive changes and even to cell death. The term cloudy swelling is one the importance of which has been much overemphasized. In the marked cases it is perfectly readily recognized microscopically but in the milder stages it is a term which is frequently misused and should perhaps be deleted from the histologic vocabulary, reserving it only as a gross term as Virchow originally applied it, if only to avoid confusion for the beginning student.

Illustrative Cases

In the preceding chapter a case of toxic nephrosis (Case 5) was described in which fatty and hydropic changes were present. It was commented that in

addition to these degenerative features very marked granular degeneration of the convoluted tubular epithelium was also present. This corresponds to

PLATE VI
RETROGRADE PROCESSES—HYALINE DEGENERATION

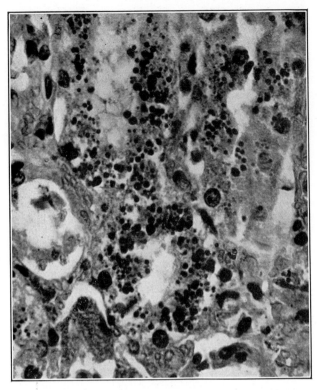

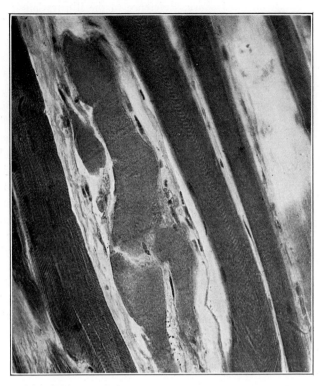

Fig. 23.—Kidney: Hyaline ("Colloid") Degeneration.—Cf. Cases 3 and 5.—(Phloxin-methylene-blue stain) Marked hyaline degeneration of renal convoluted tubular epithelium evidenced by multiple, varying-sized, highly refractile, globular, basophilic-staining bodies, many extruded into the tubule lumen. App. 400 x.

Fig. 24.—Striated Muscle: "Zenker's" Degeneration.—Case 12.—A swollen and distorted muscle fiber showing loss of striation and nuclear detail, and with a vitreous, homogeneous, intensely eosinophilic-staining cytoplasm indicative of advanced hyaline degeneration. App. 200 x.

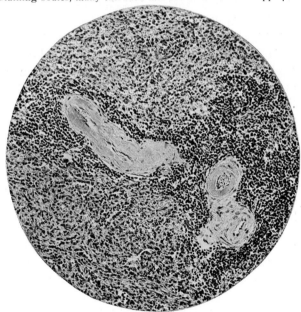

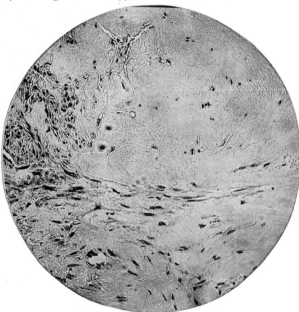

Fig. 25.—Spleen: Hyaline Degeneration of Blood Vessels.—Case 11.—Vessel walls present an homogeneous, translucent, swollen appearance due to hyaline degeneration of the intima and media of the vessel wall. App. 100 x. (See also colored Plate CXIV, Fig. 382.)

Fig. 26.—Uterus: Leiomyoma.—Hyaline Degeneration.—Case 10.—The intercellular collagen of the tumor, through an inadequate blood supply, presents a pale, eosin-staining, homogeneous, structureless, highly refractile appearance. (Hyaline degeneration.) App. 100 x.

the terminology of cloudy swelling which has been outlined above. Reference to the illustrations (Fig. 11, 12 and 23) will show the presence of a marked increase in size of the normal cell granules so that the entire cell appears somewhat swollen, encroaching upon the lumen of the tubule and causing actual distention of the cell membrane. This is typical of a rather marked example of this condition. It may also be observed in Case 3 Fig. 6 which was presented in Chapter I. Identical diffuse granular degeneration of the renal convoluted tubular epithelium may be observed in that case, but in addition more extensive degenerative features are also to be noted. In certain of the tubules will be found very much larger, coarser granules which vary considerably in size. They apparently tend to fuse to form larger granules. With the usual hematoxylin and eosin preparation these stain intensely with the eosin. In sections stained by eosin-methylene blue, it will be found that they have an intense affinity for the alkaline methylene blue in contradistinction to the usual albumin granules which continue to take the eosin stain (Fig. 23). For this reason these larger granules have frequently been spoken of as. *colloid degeneration* because of their translucent appearance and staining reactions comparable to those seen in the thyroid secretion. Just what the chemical composition of these particular protein granules is has not been demonstrated but they are generally classed as one of a group of hyaline substances. In the kidney these hyaline droplets attain such a size from swelling and fusion that rupture of the cell membrane not infrequently results and these masses of amorphous hyaline material are discharged into the lumen of the tubule where they fuse to form hyaline casts. This may be considered as a progressive degenerative lesion following in severity the changes described under cloudy swelling or granular degeneration. They are seen particularly in severe toxic conditions such as diphtheria or as in this case, eclampsia, and are likely to be associated with irreversible cell injury going on to actual cell death.

PART II

HYALINE DEGENERATION

By the term hyaline degeneration is meant a number of conditions which have one feature in common, a gross translucency with a somewhat glassy appearance. There are probably a wide variety of actual chemical disturbances involved in the various forms of hyaline degeneration. The condition is found both in epithelial cells and in tissues of connective tissue origin. It is notably observed in degenerative lesions of blood vessel walls. We have already observed what might be considered as a form of hyaline degeneration in a consideration of the more marked toxic albuminous degeneration of the renal epithelium as described in the preceding case. At this time it will suffice merely to indicate some of the more common forms of hyaline degeneration as we see them and reserve more detailed discussion of these lesions to a later time when they will be taken up in relation to the various organ systems. In the blood vessels we have perhaps one of the most familiar examples of hyaline degeneration. This is especially prominent in the spleen, in the brain and in many cases of degenerative diseases of the kidney. In tumors we are very apt to find it involving the collagenous stroma. It is very commonly observed in the myomatous tumors of the uterus. In inflammatory lesions associated with various infections, particularly surface infections such as the membrane in diphtheria or the fibrinous exudate in pleuritis or pericarditis similar hyalinization of the fibrin may occur. We have already commented on the hyaline changes which may be seen in epithelium as emphasized by the renal tubule. Likewise in the liver hyaline masses may be found within the cytoplasm of the cells in portal cirrhosis (Fig. 481 and 488) and this is of definite diagnostic significance as this is said to occur only in this condition. In striated muscle, we find hyaline degeneration often spoken of as Zenker's degeneration (Fig. 24) in which the albuminous material of the cell becomes swollen and homogeneous and the striations become lost.

Obviously with such a wide range of conditions in which must be included amyloid disease, which will be discussed separately, there can be no single factor responsible and hyalin itself is obviously merely a gross descriptive term applied to a wide variety of protein substances which have only their glairy appearance and their intense acidophilic staining affinity in common.

PLATE VII
AMYLOID INFILTRATION
CASE 13.—AMYLOIDOSIS

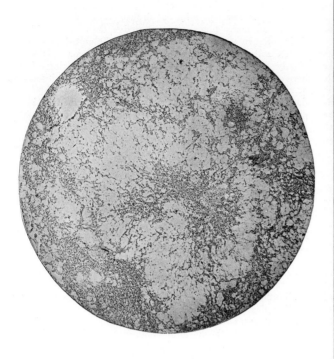

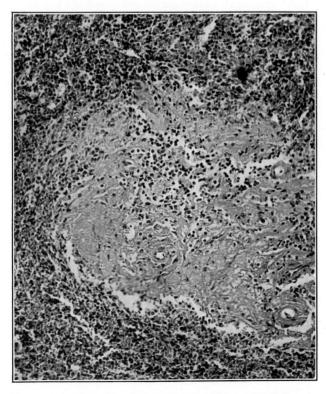

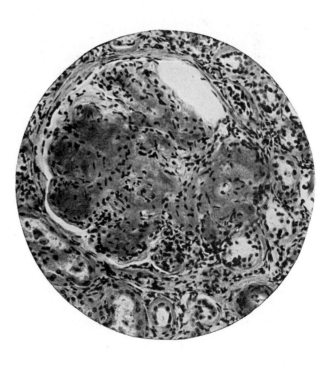

FIG. 27.—LIVER.—Low power photomicrograph to illustrate distribution of amyloid and associated liver damage in a moderately advanced case. App. 30 x.

FIG. 28.—LIVER.—Higher magnification. Observe midzonal distribution of the amyloid; likewise, its position between sinusoidal endothelium and liver cells with their resultant atrophy. (See colored Plate IV, Fig. 17.) App. 150 x.

FIG. 29.—SPLEEN: "SAGO" SPLEEN (See Fig. 505).—Infiltration of a splenic follicle and its eccentrically placed "central" arteriole, with atrophy of lymphoid tissue. App. 150 x.

FIG. 30.—KIDNEY.—Marked involvement of the glomerular tuft with pericapillary infiltration of amyloid producing renal failure. Amyloid stains a characteristic lavender with methyl violet. (See colored Plate IV, Fig. 18.) App. 150 x.

ILLUSTRATIVE CASES

CASE 10. (Ref. #S-101)

Diagnosis.—Uterus—multiple leiomyomata showing hyaline degeneration.

Patient was a Negress of 40 years, admitted to the hospital in coma and bleeding severely from the vagina.

Present Illness.—The history of the patient's illness was obtained from her sister who said that six weeks previously she had apparently been in her usual health. She had complained, however, of a marked menorrhagia for several months with her periods lasting for upwards of two weeks and accompanied by very profuse flow. She awoke to find her sister lying unconscious in bed with the bedding soaked with blood. She called a physician who immediately sent the patient to the hospital.

Past Medical History.—The past history was essentially irrelevant. She had had the usual childhood diseases, according to the patient's sister, but had never been seriously ill in her entire life. A review of her systems added very little except that the patient had had three pregnancies which had all ended in spontaneous miscarriages at approximately three months.

Physical Examination.—The patient was an asthenic adult Negress who was wholly comatose and did not respond to any of the ordinary stimuli. She was of an ashy-gray color and the mucous membranes were almost colorless. She showed a marked Cheyne-Stokes type of respiration. Head otherwise was not remarkable. Nose and throat appeared negative. Chest was symmetrical and well developed. Heart was not enlarged and the sounds were feeble and distant. No murmurs were heard. Lungs seemed clear. Abdomen was negative. Extremities appeared negative. There was a mass of clotted blood on the inner side of both thighs and the genitalia.

Laboratory Findings.—The red cell count was 1,030,-000 with the hemoglobin too low to read by the Talquist method. White blood cells, 14,000 with 78% neutrophiles. Urinalysis was not done as no specimen could be obtained.

Subsequent Course.—The patient was immediately given intravenous fluids and blood donors sent for. Before any transfusion could be given, however, the patient expired.

Autopsy Findings.—The body was that of a fairly well-developed and well-nourished adult Negress who showed marked anemia of her tissues generally. There was no pathology of particular significance except for terminal edema of the lungs and right sided dilatation of the heart. The chief point of interest in respect to the pathology was found in the uterus. This was greatly enlarged and showed numerous myomata, subserous, intramural and submucosal in distribution. One particularly large tumor measuring about 15 cm. (Fig. 590) in diameter was seen as a pedunculated, subserous mass arising from the fundus. On the posterior uterine wall was a submucosal tumor approximately 2 cm. in diameter and from this site the hemorrhage had apparently occurred.

Microscopic Description of a Section Through One of the Tumor Masses.—(Fig. 26) Tissues histologically are seen to present the usual and characteristic appearance of a simple leiomyoma. The cells for the most part are spindle-shaped and represent varying degrees of differentiation of smooth muscle cells. There is some variation in size and appearance. The nuclei are elongated and show rather dense arrangement of their chromatin. These cells occur in more or less parallel bundles which interlace intimately with a diffuse connective tissue stroma. In many places, the connective tissue cells with their collagen are more prominent than the actual smooth muscle cells. They mingle with the actual tumor cells so closely that in many places it is difficult to distinguish between the two except by the use of special Van Gieson, or similar differential stains. Where the collagen is abundant, marked hyaline degeneration has occurred. This is characterized by the fusion of the collagen fibrils to form dense, homogeneous eosin-staining masses.

Under high power, this hyaline degeneration of the stroma seems to result from the swelling and fusing of this collagenous matrix. Where this dense hyalinization has occurred, there is marked atrophy of many of the smooth muscle cells, which is due in part to insufficient nutrition and in part to compression and replacement fibrosis. This appears to be due to an inadequate blood supply. In some of the sections, considerable necrosis, hemorrhage and beginning cystic degeneration may be observed. There is nothing to suggest malignant change.

CASE 11. (Ref. #S-63)

Diagnosis.—Senile atrophic fibrous splenitis with hyaline degeneration of the vessels.

Patient was a 59-year-old colored female, who was admitted to the hospital because of paralysis of her left side, which came on suddenly and was accompanied by loss of consciousness.

Present Illness.—About three months ago the patient developed a slight cold which had more or less persisted. This was followed by a sinusitis and she developed a persistent chronic cough. About two months previously, she lost her ability to speak, although she could understand what was said to her, and she had to answer in writing. This subsided and she had continued in this somewhat invalided state during the interval. Twelve hours before admission, she lost consciousness and her family sent for a physician, who referred her to the hospital.

Past History.—Due to her condition the history was unsatisfactory, because she had lived away most of her life and her family was unfamiliar with her interval history. She was married but had never had any children. Her husband died five years before her admission of an unknown cause. She had had influenza in the 1918 epidemic but no other serious illness so far as the family knew.

Physical Examination.—The head, eyes, ears, nose and throat were negative. Chest was well developed; expansion was good; lungs were clear. Heart was not enlarged. The sounds were of good quality. There was a mitral systolic murmur transmitted to the axilla. The abdomen was negative. Extremities: Weakness of flexion and extension of left leg, with foot drop, and a spastic paralysis of the left arm. The patient was unable to speak.

Laboratory Examination.—Urinalysis was negative. Wassermann test was doubtfully positive. Blood chemistry was negative.

Subsequent Course.—The patient continued steadily downhill, and died one month after admission.

Autopsy Findings.—At autopsy there was evidence of an old rheumatic endocarditis with a terminal bacterial lesion showing several small, pink, friable vegetations 1 to 2 mm. in diameter. The myocardium showed marked degenerative changes and the coronary vessels were sclerosed, although no actual obstruction was noted. The lungs were essentially negative except for terminal edema and congestion. The liver showed some atrophy and presented a picture of cloudy swelling. The kidneys were likewise somewhat smaller than normal. The capsule was thin and stripped with great difficulty leaving a finely granular surface. A few retention cysts were present. The picture was one of combined arterial and arteriolar sclerosis. The spleen was definitely atrophic and weighed 50 gm. The capsule was somewhat thickened and wrinkled, and the spleen cut with slightly increased resistance. In the brain, multiple areas of thrombotic softening on the right and a chronic basilar meningitis were found.

Microscopic Description of Spleen.—(Fig. 25 and 382) Sections microscopically through the spleen present a typical picture of hyaline degeneration of the blood vessels. The most marked lesions are seen in the central arterioles of the lymph follicles. Here in many places the lumen is almost occluded by marked hyaline thickening of the sub-intima and media. In places the differentiation between muscle cells, persistent interstitial connective tissue and degenerating hyalinized collagen is almost impossible to make out. The hyalin, however, is characterized by more intense staining with eosin and by its comparative homogeneity. This form of vascular hyaline degeneration represents one of the most frequently seen forms of the condition, and its effect, as seen in vessels of the brain, heart, kidney or other viscera may easily be surmised from the standpoint of diminished blood supply.

CASE 12. (Ref. #S-213)

Diagnosis.—Zenker's degeneration of striated muscle. Patient was a young white male, aged 26 years, who was admitted to the hospital with a typical picture of lobar pneumonia.

Present Illness.—The onset was sudden, ushered in by a severe chill and followed by a sharp rise in temperature to 103°. Patient had been hunting and had been exposed to extreme cold, having fallen into the icy water several miles from camp. On his return he had felt half frozen and had gone to bed to thaw out. About two hours later he had had a sudden chill, so intense that it had literally shaken the bed, and then developed a high fever. The following morning he had to be taken out of camp on a stretcher and was brought to the hospital.

Past History.—Patient had had an uneventful past medical history, with the usual childhood diseases. He had never had any serious illness previously and had had

no operation. He had never been particularly susceptible to colds or other upper respiratory infections. A review of his cardiovascular, gastro-intestinal and genito-urinary systems proved entirely negative.

Physical Examination.—Patient was a well-developed and well-nourished young male, lying restlessly in bed with an anxious expression. There was a slight suggestion of cyanosis to his lips, mucous membranes and nail beds. His head was normal in shape. His eyes were negative. There was a marked dilatation of his alae nasi with each respiratory effort, and a notable grunting type of respiration. Nose and throat were negative. Chest: Lungs showed marked dullness with increased vocal and tactile fremitus and bronchial breathing over the right lower lobe. Numerous coarse, mucous râles were heard over the rest of the chest, but no signs of consolidation elsewhere were found. Heart was rapid in rate, regular, and no murmurs were heard. Abdomen: Marked abdominal type of respiration was present; no tenderness noted. Extremities negative.

Laboratory Findings.—White blood cells 26,800 with 88% polynuclears. Red blood cells 4,800,000 with 86% hemoglobin. Urine: There was a slight trace of albumin, but it was otherwise negative. Sputum: Pneumococci, Type III, found by Neufeld method.

Subsequent History.—Patient's temperature ranged from 103°-105°, pulse from 110-140 and respirations from 36-50. His white count dropped from an initial 26,800 to 12,600 and the polynuclears fell to 63%, indicative of an overwhelming infection which affected the bone marrow defensive mechanism. He went on steadily downhill, dying the fifth day of his illness.

Autopsy Findings.—At autopsy it was noted with the primary incision that the rectus muscles showed a curious patchy, cloudy, parboiled appearance. Similar involvement of the diaphragm was observed. The heart showed toxic myocardial damage with right-sided dilatation. There was typical early gray hepatization of the right lower lobe and an associated overlying acute fibrinous pleuritis. The liver and kidneys showed marked toxic granular degeneration and the abdominal viscera in general were congested.

Microscopic Examination of the Rectus Muscle.—(Fig. 24) Histologically, a rather striking hyaline degeneration of the cytoplasm of the striated muscle cells may be observed. This varies in degree considerably, some of the cells apparently escaping the degenerative process, while others have lost their striations and the cytoplasm has become swollen, homogeneous and stains intensely with eosin. Some slight hydropic change is also observed with vacuoles of varying size within the cell boundaries. The nuclei all appear intact and the process has not gone on to actual cell death. Considerable interstitial edema, accompanied by some slight cellular infiltration is also present.

AMYLOIDOSIS

Amyloid is a complex hyaline protein substance frequently found in combination with chondroitin-sulphuric acid. In its development it is believed to go through a phase in which the combination with this acid radical is lacking, and indeed it is questioned by some investigators whether it ever actually

exists in such a combined form. Chemically and microscopically amyloid may be identified by its specific staining reactions, and thus differentiated from all other forms of hyalin. Stained with iodine and subsequently acidified with dilute sulphuric acid it characteristically presents a deep mahogany brown tone. With metachromatic stains such as methyl violet or thionin it exhibits its basic qualities by its acidophilic old rose color. It has a strong affinity for Congo Red, one of the vital dyes. This latter characteristic is utilized clinically as a diagnostic test for amyloidosis, a measured amount of the dye being introduced intravenously, and the amount recoverable at the end of an hour being determined. In cases of generalized amyloidosis, 60 per cent or more of the dye is absorbed by the amyloid.

The problem of whether amyloid is a degenerative product or an infiltrative material is still an open question, although the more recent work points suggestively towards its infiltrative nature. The source of amyloid is most uncertain. It may be produced experimentally in animals by such widely diverse substances as coal tar, turpentine, bacterial toxins (especially staphylococcic) and high protein diets. In casein feeding experiments it may be prevented or delayed by the addition of a high fat or carbohydrate content to the diet, and particularly by the use of cholesterol. For these reasons it is believed to be a protein decomposition product, either exogenous or endogenous in origin. Most observers believe that this circulating protein material either is precipitated in the interstitial tissues by some tissue antibody, or that it escapes from the blood stream because of its excessive concentration there, filters into the tissue crevices and there settles out as a "gel" where it may be identified microscopically. On the other hand Mallory believes it to be an abnormal product of the fibroblast and Warren in reporting a case of amyloidosis restricted to the musculature

of the body is inclined to accept this concept, because of the apparent lack of relationship to the blood supply, and the absence of any of the usual associated etiologic factors of chronic disease.

Pathologically amyloidosis may occur in two forms; first, as cases of localized amyloid deposit, usually found at the base of the tongue, in the larynx, bronchi, nasal septum or in relation to the joints where cartilage is normally found, or as extremely rare instances of focal involvement of the heart, muscles or other viscera. In the second or more usual form it is found as a diffuse infiltrative process involving most of the viscera, but almost invariably the spleen, liver and kidneys, where it is deposited just outside the vessels, especially around the central arterioles of the splenic follicles (sago spleen), the sinusoidal endothelium of the hepatic sinuses and the glomerular tufts of the kidney. In these cases we can expect to find a history of long standing chronic wasting disease, notably tuberculosis, syphilis, cancer or chronic suppuration, especially of bone. As the disease condition progresses we find that larger vessels become involved. Amyloid becomes deposited between the smooth muscle cells of the media of arterioles and arteries as well as in the adventitia. Gradually all the viscera become involved and the picture becomes one of diffuse generalized amyloidosis. There is marked enlargement of the abdomen due to the hepatic and splenic involvement; portal obstruction may ensue, respiratory and cardiac embarrassment may occur, and death may result from mechanical interference with normal physiology.

ILLUSTRATIVE CASE

CASE 13. (Ref. #S-38, 66 and 129)
Diagnosis.—Liver, spleen and kidneys: Amyloidosis. Patient was a colored female, aged 30 years, who was admitted to the hospital complaining of a chronic cough, marked weakness and a recent loss of weight.
Present Illness.—Ten years ago the patient developed a cough, which was productive of a moderate amount of sputum. She went to the hospital and was examined thoroughly. Repeated sputum examinations at that time were negative, but the x-ray diagnosis of presumptive tuberculosis was made, and she was recommended to have sanatorium care. She did not return to the hospital because of fear of being sent away. She had had various periods of remission and relapse with times when she became so weak that she had to go to bed for several weeks. However, four years ago she was married and became pregnant. With her pregnancy there was a marked increase in her cough and her other symptoms. She went to another hospital at that time and, because

of her chest condition, had a therapeutic abortion. She refused hospital care for her lung condition and returned home where she stayed in bed for one month. This was followed by a severe hemoptysis and she was forced to return to the hospital and was sent to a tuberculosis sanatorium for one year. During this period she gained fifty pounds in weight and her symptoms largely disappeared. During the past two years she had remained in fairly good health with intermittent attacks of coughing. One month ago she began to show considerable increase in her cough. She developed marked pain in her lumbar region and showed progressive weakness accompanied by considerable weight loss.
Past History.—She had no reliable recollection of her childhood history. So far as she knew neither of her parents suffered from tuberculosis and she assumed that she had had all the usual childhood infections. Up to the time she first developed this cough she had never had any serious illness. A review of her systems was

entirely unsatisfactory as the patient was definitely of a low mental level and her statements were influenced by a marked willingness to please the questioner.

Physical Examination.—Patient was a fairly well developed, emaciated young Negress who looked at least ten years older than her given age. She was extremely weak and dyspneic lying motionless in bed. She had a feeble, hacking cough. Head was normal in contour. Eyes, ears, nose and throat were essentially negative. There was bilateral enlargement of both anterior cervical lymph-node chains. Chest: Expansion was very poor. There was dullness to flatness with increased vocal fremitus over the right lower lobe. There were many râles in both apices. Breath sounds were absent in the right lower lobe. No changes in voice or breath sounds were noted on the left side except at the apex. Heart was normal in size; sounds were of fair quality; there were no murmurs. The abdomen was markedly prominent. The liver edge was a hand's breadth below the costal margin. The spleen was likewise enlarged and palpable two fingers' breadth below the costal margin. There was questionable shifting dullness in both flanks. Gynecologic examination showed a markedly lacerated cervix and a profuse leukorrhea.

Laboratory Examination.—Urinalysis: Albumin was present in moderate amounts. Sediment contained a considerable number of pus cells. Serology: Kahn test 4 plus. Blood chemistry negative. Sputum: All specimens examined showed large numbers of tubercle bacilli.

Subsequent Course.—The patient remained in the hospital about one month going steadily downhill. No active therapy was attempted as the process seemed too advanced to be amenable to any form of treatment although artificial pneumothorax was considered. She died approximately one month after admission.

Autopsy Findings.—The heart appeared normal. Lungs showed diffuse chronic ulcerative and caseous tuberculosis of the entire right side with marked tuberculous bronchial pneumonia and cavitation in the right lower lobe. There was a miliary bronchogenic distribution throughout the entire lung on this side. Extension to the apices and the opposite side was noted. The liver was greatly enlarged weighing 1900 grams. It was rubbery in consistency with rounded edges and presented a typical light brown, glairy picture which on section showed diffuse infiltration of the liver substance with amyloid. The spleen weighed 320 grams. It was considerably enlarged and was somewhat of the same general consistency as the liver. On section it presented a typical picture of a somewhat advanced so-called "sago spleen" with large, grayish-white, glairy areas of amyloid infiltration against a dark, congested background. The kidneys were slightly increased in size. They were pale and the cortices appeared widened. It was difficult to make out grossly whether or not there was amyloid infiltration. The gastro-intestinal tract showed diffuse tuberculous ulceration of the ileum and cecum and a tuberculous appendicitis.

Microscopic Description of Liver.—(Fig. 17, 27 and 28) Microscopic section through the liver presents evidence of diffuse amyloid infiltration which is most marked around the central portions of the lobules. As seen under the low power this anatomical distribution is very striking, although it varies considerably in different portions of the slide. In some areas practically the entire lobule has been replaced by the amyloid material. In others the architectural details are still fairly well preserved. Under high power it will be noted particularly in the peripheral areas of infiltration that the amyloid is laid down between the sinusoidal endothelium and the liver cells. As this substance increases in amount the liver cells have undergone atrophy. Whether as the result of compression or anoxemia it is impossible to tell. Where the amyloid is present in large amounts the liver cells have been completely obliterated and the amyloid occurs in masses separated only by a delicate connective tissue stroma. It will be noted that the amyloid stains intensely with eosin and that it has a homogeneous appearance which is fairly readily differentiated from the other hyaline degenerative changes studied. In one portion of the slide it will be noted that there is a persistent miliary tuberculosis. This is an incidental finding but is of interest in establishing the tuberculous background of the case on histologic grounds.

Microscopic Description of Spleen.—(Fig. 29 and 505) In the spleen the amyloid will be seen microscopically almost completely replacing the lymph follicles, but particularly distributed to the germinal centers of the follicles around the central arterioles. Here, as in the liver, the amyloid has been deposited in such extensive amounts that the normal tissues have been completely replaced by this foreign substance and only occasional connective tissue cells can be seen between the homogeneous masses of amyloid. The pulp spaces are intensely congested and there is a compensatory reticulo-endothelial hyperplasia which some investigators believe to be of significance in this condition.

Microscopic Description of Kidneys.—(Fig. 18 and 30) Microscopic study of the kidney shows the amyloid infiltrative process to be very much less extensive. Indeed at first glance under the low power it is comparatively easy to overlook this process. More careful examination, however, will show that in nearly all of the glomeruli lying between the endothelium of the glomerular capillary and its reflected epithelial covering there is a pinkish homogeneous hyaline material deposited in irregular masses. It does not occur uniformly as a sheath of the vessels but rather as pools as if the material had seeped out through the endothelium and precipitated in the tissue spaces. The extent of infiltration in this particular instance is probably not sufficient to seriously interfere with renal function but it is easy to understand how if this process continues to develop the entire glomerulus will be obliterated in the same manner that the splenic follicles and the liver lobule had been in the tissues studied from those organs.

CHAPTER IV
PATHOLOGICAL PIGMENTATION

Pathological pigmentation of the body is classified on the basis of the source of the pigments as 1. *Exogenous*, including such conditions as anthracosis (carbon), argyria (silver), plumbism (lead) or 2. *Endogenous*. In the endogenous group the cases are further divided into (a) those in which the pigmentation is derived from the breaking down of hemoglobin (*hemoglobinogenous or hematogenous*) including hematin, hemosiderin, hematoidin, hematoporphyrin, hemofuscin and the bile pigments and (b) those cases in which the pigmentation results as a product of actual cell metabolism (*autogenous*), including chiefly the various types of melanin. In addition to these well established groups should also be considered the group of pigmentations spoken of generically under the term "lipochromes." These are the pigments which are normally found in fat, the corpus luteum, the epithelium of seminal vesicles, in the interstitial cells of the testis and ovary, and in the adrenal gland. Pathologically in this group we are accustomed to include so-called brown atrophy and the various forms of xanthomatosis in which there is a deposition of lipoid substances in the tissues. In this latter group should be included the various visceral lesions associated with the diseases of the spleen and reticulo-endothelial system, of which Gaucher's disease, Nieman Pick's disease, and the Hand-Christian-Schueller syndrome are examples. These will be discussed in detail under diseases of the reticulo-endothelial system.

EXOGENOUS PIGMENTS

Of the exogenous pigments, *anthracosis* is the only one of common occurrence. This is one of the group of pneumoconioses of which silicosis, chalicosis and siderosis are the other important forms from the standpoint of industrial medicine, as they all tend to produce chronic fibrous changes in the lungs, which are believed to ultimately render the individual more susceptible to tuberculosis or other chronic pulmonary infection. By *anthracosis* we mean the black pigmentation of the lungs and the regional lymph nodes in the hilar and peribronchial regions, which results from the inhalation of carbon particles and their transportation by the lymphatics to these lymph nodes. Obviously this is seen in its more marked form among coal miners.

Of the other exogenous pigments, those seen following the continued use of certain heavy metals, notably silver and lead, are the most important. In the past the persistent use of silver salts over long periods of time resulted not infrequently in the development of a generalized bluish discoloration of the tissues, which is commonly spoken of as argyria. Even to-day such individuals may occasionally be seen in the sideshows of the circus as "blue men."

In lead poisoning again we may find a curious localized, stippled, blackish pigmentation, the so-called *lead line* along the gingival margins of the teeth. This lead line represents an actual deposit of lead salts in the tissues and is one of the most characteristic diagnostic signs of this condition.

Ochronosis.—Another rare type of pigmentation is one which involves the cartilage, joint capsules and tendons principally. This condition is seen not infrequently associated with long continued use of phenol, usually in the form of dressings to suppurating wounds of a chronic type. It is associated with alkaptonuria in about half the cases and is believed to be due to the effect of tyrosinase upon the aromatic groups in such protein molecules as phenylalanine and tyrosine. Whether this should be classified as endogenous or exogenous in view of the complicated mechanism involved is still a matter of opinion as some cases do not have this antecedent history of what might be termed mild phenol poisoning.

Finally, among the exogenous pigments must be mentioned the artificial introduction of pigments under the skin known as *tattooing*. Under the mi-

PLATE VIII

PATHOLOGIC PIGMENTATION

Hemosiderin

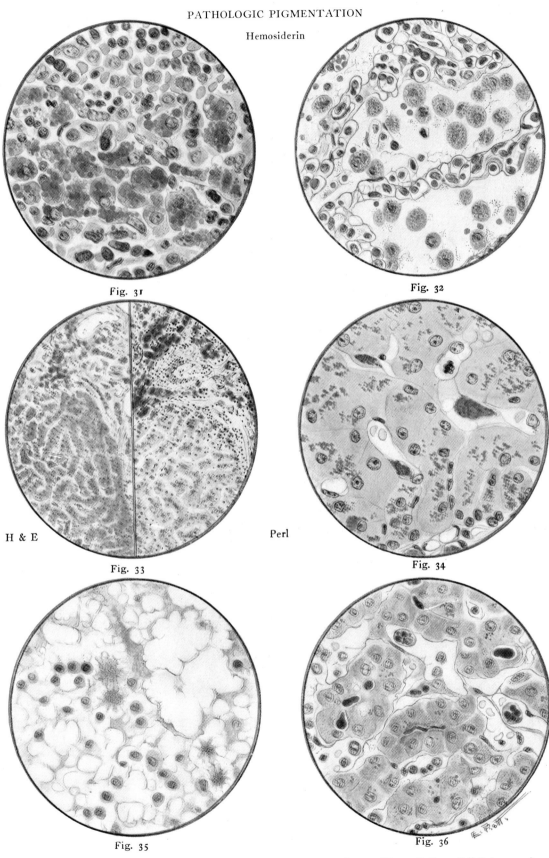

H & E

Perl

Fig. 31

Fig. 32

Fig. 33

Fig. 34

Fig. 35

Fig. 36

Fig. 31—Spleen—Hemosiderosis (case 16)
Fig. 33.—Liver—Hemochromatosis (case 17)
Fig. 35.—Spleen—Infarct-hematoidin (case 2)

Fig. 32.—Lung—"Heart Failure Cells" (case 15)
Fig. 34.—Liver—Hemocromatosis (case 17)
Fig. 36.—Liver—Bile stasis (case 18)

PLATE IX
PATHOLOGICAL PIGMENTATION

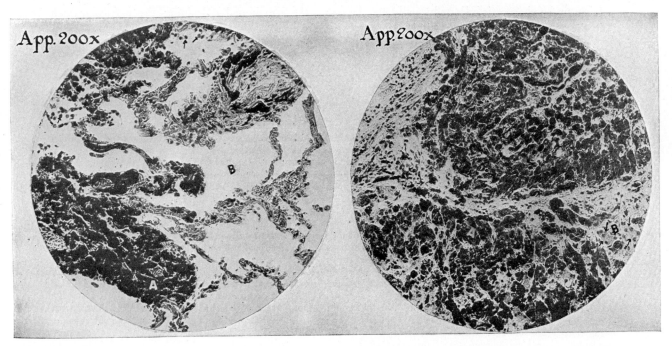

FIG. 37.—LUNG: ANTHRACOSIS.—CASE 14.—Carbon particles in large aggregations are seen within the thickened alveolar walls (A), some within phagocytic mononuclear "dust" cells. Note also associated emphysema (B).

FIG. 38.—LIVER: MELANIN.—CASE 20.—MALIGNANT MELANOMA. Metastatic tumor composed of groups of deeply pigmented cells which give the characteristic "DOPA" reaction for melanin. (See also Plate X, Fig. 42 in color.)

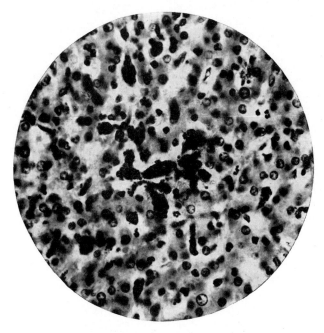

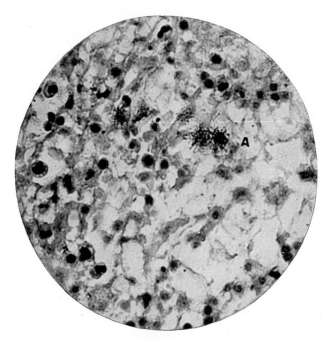

FIG. 39.—LIVER: MALARIA.—cf. CASE 76.—Typical dark, brownish-black, malarial pigment within the Kupffer cells of the liver sinusoids which gives the gross color to the organ at autopsy. App. 400 x.

FIG. 40.—SPLEEN: HEMATOIDIN.—CASE 2.—ANEMIC INFARCTION. Acicular crystals of golden yellow pigment in characteristic burr formation occurring invariably extracellularly. (See also Plate VIII, Fig. 35 in color.) App. 400 x.

croscope it is seen that this foreign pigment is largely taken up by phagocytic cells and usually may be seen in the cytoplasm of these cells within the lymphatics of the corium and not infrequently transported to the lymph nodes draining the particular area involved.

ILLUSTRATIVE CASE

CASE 14. (Ref. #S-188)

Diagnosis.—Lung: Anthracosis.

Patient was a 59-year-old white male who was admitted to the hospital because of vomiting, abdominal pain and the presence of tarry stools.

Present Illness.—Began about one year before admission with anorexia, vague upper abdominal discomfort, occasional attacks of nausea and vomiting. During the course of the year he had shown a steady increase in the severity of these symptoms with the development of definite abdominal pain and tenderness in the epigastric region. He had also shown a loss of some thirty pounds of weight. His vomiting attacks had increased in frequency and had often been associated with brown "coffee ground" material. Intermittently his stools had been deep blackish in color and there had been a tendency toward increased constipation.

Past History.—Patient was born in West Virginia and had worked in the coal mines ever since he was fourteen years of age. He did not recall specifically whether or not he had ever had any of the ordinary childhood diseases. He had always been subject to mild colds and upper respiratory infections which had occasionally kept him from his work for a week or ten days at a time. He had never had any chronic cough or any serious illness which had required hospitalization up to the present time. A review of his systems was uninformative.

Physical Examination.—Patient was a fairly well developed but markedly emaciated white male who appeared fully his given age. Head was essentially negative. Eyes: There was mild catarrhal conjunctivitis but the pupils reacted normally. Mouth was edentulous. Nose and throat were negative. Chest was of the barrel, emphysematous type. Lungs: There were a few scattered coarse râles heard over both sides of the chest. There was neither any dullness nor bronchial breathing present. A suggestion of hyperresonance over both upper lobes was noted. Heart was not enlarged. Sounds were of good quality. There were no murmurs. Blood pressure was 130/84. Abdomen was scaphoid. There was a vague epigastric mass which was tender on deep palpation and through it the aortic pulsation could be felt. The extremities were essentially negative except for the marked muscle and subcutaneous tissue wasting. The reflexes and other central nervous findings were essentially normal.

Laboratory Examinations.—Urine was negative on several occasions. Blood Chemistry: Sugar 130 mgm.; urea 60 mgm.; creatinine 2.2 mgm. Blood: Red blood cells 2,300,000; hemoglobin 58%. White blood cells 12,600 with 72% polynuclears. X-ray examination showed a large filling defect in the cardiac portion of the stomach. The lungs, by x-ray, showed many old calcified areas apparently representing inactive and healed tuberculous foci.

Operative History.—The patient was advised to have an exploratory laparotomy, which was done and a large tumor mass involving most of the cardia was found, which was inoperable. The wound was closed except for a gastrostomy to feed the patient.

Subsequent Course.—The patient went steadily downhill and died three weeks later largely as a result of the emaciation associated with his carcinoma.

Autopsy Findings.—At autopsy the obvious outstanding lesion was a very extensive adenocarcinoma of the cardiac end of the stomach with metastasis to the regional lymph nodes. In addition, the lungs showed an extreme degree of anthracosis. There was associated marked emphysema most prominent in the upper lobes and a practically completely obliterative fibrous pleuritis on the left side. The heart presented a picture of chronic fibrosis of the myocardium. The liver, spleen and pancreas showed no pathology of significance. The kidneys showed a moderate amount of arteriosclerotic nephrosclerosis.

Microscopic Description of a Section of Lung Taken from Near the Hilus to Demonstrate Anthracosis.—(Fig. 37) Under the low power of the microscope, the distribution of the carbon pigment is very striking. The fine carbon particles which have been inhaled into the alveoli have almost entirely disappeared from the alveoli themselves. However, here and there within the alveoli, scattered large mononuclear cells which contain a few small black carbon granules are seen. These are spoken of as *"dust"* cells. For the most part these cells have migrated by amoeboid activity into the alveolar walls and found their way into the lymphatics and perilymphatic tissues. Because of this fact it is usually possible in most cases of anthracosis to actually trace the alveolar outlines through the pleural surface. In the slide under consideration these cells may be seen in large numbers in these areas actually blocking the lymphatics to a considerable extent. The section includes a portion of the hilus lymph node and this under the low power of the microscope appears almost solidly black. Under higher power, it can be observed that the pigment is chiefly intracellular, still within the large mononuclear phagocytes which are packed in masses especially in the peripheral sinuses of the node. Gradually, as the lymph node became filled with these pigment laden cells, the process backed up along the peribronchial lymphatics out to the very periphery of the lung tissue. Apparently all the pigment was originally intracellular, but after a while the phagocytic cells became so distended that many of their cell membranes have ruptured and the pigment may be seen deposited in the interstitial tissues as well. While carbon, as it happens, is largely an inert substance, nevertheless it acts as a foreign body and an irritant. As a result it is seen that there is a very marked secondary connective tissue proliferation in an attempt to wall off this pigment. The nutrition of the tissues has become impaired and later in the sequence of events, the connective tissue has undergone hyaline degeneration so that a combination of fibrosis and thickening of the alveolar walls has interfered with the gaseous interchange in the lung and left the lung a likely target for secondary infection, notably tuberculosis.

ENDOGENOUS PIGMENTATION

HEMATOGENOUS (HEMOGLOBINOGENOUS) PIGMENTATION

Hemosiderin.—Hemosiderin occurs as a golden-brown amorphous or granular pigment. It is the most frequently encountered derivative of blood. It contains an iron radical as may be demonstrated by the familiar Prussian blue reaction in which the tissues are treated with potassium ferrocyanide and dilute hydrochloric acid. Its exact composition otherwise is not fully known and indeed there may be various intermediate forms in the breakdown of hemoglobin which give this reaction. Of one thing, however, we are reasonably certain—that the production of hemosiderin requires the action of cells to produce it. In other words, it is not a simple chemical breakdown of hemoglobin, but is the product of actual biological activity of the cells. It is particularly found where small or large amounts of blood have escaped into the surrounding tissues from the blood vessels. Here the red blood cells break down and the hemoglobin is attacked by the phagocytic cells of the body, notably the tissue histiocytes or large mononuclear phagocytes. Other conditions in which hemosiderin appears under pathological conditions may be seen in the lung in association with venous stasis as a result of cardiac disease, usually of long standing, such as chronic valvulitis. Under such circumstances, again blood cells escape into the alveoli of the lung and there undergo hemolysis with rupture of their protein cell membrane and the liberation of the hemoglobin. This again is taken up as in the tissue spaces in hemorrhage and converted into hemosiderin. Not infrequently such patients will raise sputum which appears rusty in color due to the presence of large enough amounts of this pigment to discolor it. These hemosiderin-laden phagocytic cells may be compared to the "dust" cells of anthracosis and are spoken of commonly as "heart failure cells" (Fig. 32 and 50).

In various forms of infectious disease and in certain types of anemia, particularly in the so-called congenital hemolytic form of anemia, it is extremely common to find that the spleen becomes enormously congested. In typhoid fever among the infectious diseases, this state is most common. Just as in the case of hemorrhage elsewhere the red cells escape into the pulp spaces and gradually break down with a loss of their hemoglobin. Through the action of the mononuclear cells much of this hemoglobin is converted into hemosiderin which may be readily identified miscroscopically and which is found almost entirely still within the cytoplasm of these phagocytic cells although as in the case of anthracosis a certain amount may occur free in the tissue spaces when the phagocytic cells become so distended with pigment as to rupture their cell membranes and discharge their pigment content into the interstitial spaces. This condition of visceral hemosiderin deposition is frequently spoken of as hemosiderosis.

Hemochromatosis.—By hemochromatosis is meant a disease in which we have a fundamental disturbance of iron metabolism with the resultant pigmentation of the tissues generally, particularly the skin and the abdominal viscera. Its etiology is most obscure and various theories have been advanced to explain its occurrence. It is seen not infrequently in conjunction with diabetes and when this occurs the complex has received the name "bronze diabetes." Mallory has suggested the possibility of long continued metallic poisoning, especially copper and phosphorus as contributory factors. In the liver the deposition of the hemosiderin pigment is associated with very marked fibrosis having initially a portal distribution and ending ultimately with a picture of cirrhosis of the liver not unlike the portal cirrhosis of the Laennec type except for the added factor of hemosiderosis. It is a progressive disease ending ultimately fatally, just as Laennec's cirrhosis likewise does (Fig. 33 and 34). See also Fig. 494 in Chapter XLIX relating to liver pathology.

ILLUSTRATIVE CASES

CASE 15. (Ref. #S-15, 40 and 68)

Diagnosis.—Lung—chronic passive congestion with "heart failure cells" (hemosiderin laden).

Patient was a white female 38 years of age admitted to the hospital with the chief complaints of swelling of the feet and shortness of breath.

Present Illness.—The patient's present illness began following the delivery of a normal, full-term baby. She had had a difficult pregnancy having had to remain in bed for the last three months because of the swelling of her lower extremities and her marked dyspnea. Delivery, however, was normal and she was able to return to her home three weeks later, somewhat improved although her dyspnea was still pretty marked on relatively slight exertion. She attempted to attend to her child and do the housework for the next few days but was unable to continue because the dyspnea increased markedly. She noted palpitation of her heart and the edema of her extremities increased progressively. During the last month or so of her pregnancy she had also noticed that she had raised a good deal of phlegm and that it was frequently rusty colored. She attributed this to blood.

Past History.—Patient had a normal childhood with only the ordinary measles and whooping cough as childhood infections. About the age of twenty-five she had a severe quinsy sore throat with bilateral tonsillitis and a retrotonsillar abscess. She apparently recovered from this and did not notice any particular difficulty as a result. She was married at this time but never became pregnant until the past year, and had never been heart conscious until the last few months of her pregnancy when she noticed occasional attacks of palpitation on exertion.

Physical Examination.—The patient was a well developed and well nourished young white woman who appeared to be in acute respiratory distress. Her head was normal in contour. Her eyes, ears, nose and throat were negative. There was marked cyanosis of the lips, mucous membranes and finger nail beds. The chest was symmetrical with well developed lactating breasts. The lungs were resonant throughout but there were numerous coarse râles heard. There was some slight diminution in breath sounds at the base. The heart showed marked enlargement, the left border being 14 cm. to the left of the midsternal line. There was a presystolic murmur heard best over the apex. The rhythm was markedly irregular and the rate was so rapid as to be impossible to count. Electrocardiogram showed marked right axis deviation and the typical picture of auricular fibrillation. The abdomen was moderately prominent. The liver edge was felt 4 cm. below the costal margin. The arms were negative, but the lower extremities practically to the midthigh showed marked edema particularly in the dependent portions.

Laboratory Examination.—Red blood cells 3,200,000 with 73% hemoglobin. White blood cells 8,400 with 52% polynuclear leukocytes, 37% lymphocytes, 9% large mononuclears and 2% eosinophiles. Sedimentation rate was increased. Urine: negative. Blood chemistry: normal. Serology: Kahn test negative.

Subsequent Course.—The patient improved temporarily with bed rest and digitalization. The edema decreased and the patient appeared very much more comfortable in respect to her dyspnea. Suddenly one day, approximately one month after her admission, she developed right hemiplegia, became stuporous and died in the course of a few hours.

Autopsy Findings.—At autopsy there was a markedly enlarged and dilated heart. There was found an old chronic mitral rheumatic type of endocarditis with a terminal acute bacterial vegetative endocarditis. Both stenosis and insufficiency could be demonstrated. The immediate cause of death was found to be an embolus from the heart to the right middle cerebral artery. In addition to the primary cardiac lesion, the secondary manifestations of cardiac insufficiency were seen in a very marked chronic passive congestion and terminal edema of the lungs and a chronic passive congestion of the liver, spleen and kidneys.

Microscopic Description of the Lung.—(Fig. 32 and 50) The microscopic study of the lung shows a very striking capillary distention throughout the lung tissue. There is a definite increase in the thickness of the alveolar walls and in the stroma in general, due to secondary fibrosis. Many of the lung alveoli contain large numbers of mononuclear phagocytic cells which are laden with golden-brown pigment granules. In some of the air-vesicles, red blood cells may still be seen showing beginning hemolysis. In conjunction with the *"heart failure cells"* within the lung alveoli may also be seen similar phagocytic pigment distended cells in the subpleural supporting structures indicative of their amoeboid activity and their migration toward the hilus lymph nodes as in the case of the anthracotic laden cells.

As a part of the picture of chronic passive congestion the outstanding changes which have resulted from the mechanical interference with the pulmonary circulation may be commented upon. In the first place there is the compensatory fibroblastic proliferation which attempts to overcome the persistent dilatation of the alveolar wall capillaries which exists due to back pressure from the damaged heart. In addition there is some dilatation of the alveoli (emphysema) in an attempt to increase the surface area of the lung for gaseous exchange. Like most urban dwellers, who have inhaled city dust for many years, there is also a certain amount of anthracosis present in this lung.

CASE 16. (Ref. #S-67)
Diagnosis.—Spleen—Post-typhoid hemosiderosis.
Patient is a male Negro, aged 25, who was admitted to the hospital because of a suggestive history of typhoid fever with a temperature of 101°, a pulse of 90 and respirations of 24.

Present Illness.—The present illness began about two weeks before admission. The onset was indefinite and characterized by loss of appetite, slight feeling of distention in the abdomen, a feeling of lassitude and weakness and the development of a mild diarrhea. This was accompanied by a slight temperature which had increased slowly until it had reached its admission level.

Past History.—Uneventful. The patient was born in the north and had never had any previous severe illness. He did not know anything regarding his childhood history. A review of his systems was essentially negative. He had always been subject to occasional colds and upper respiratory infections. History of his cardiovascular system was entirely negative. His gastro-intestinal history was one of occasional upsets, usually occasioned by alcohol. His genito-urinary history was apparently negative. He denied venereal infection.

Physical Examination.—A well developed, well nourished, muscular young male Negro was lying quietly in bed in no marked distress. Head was normal in contour. Eyes, ears, nose and throat were negative. There was some bilateral cervical adenopathy. Chest was symmetrical. Lungs were clear throughout. Heart was not enlarged and there were no murmurs. Abdomen was moderately distended and was generally tender on deep palpation. Spleen was definitely felt one finger breadth below the costal margin. Extremities were negative.

Laboratory Findings.—Red blood cells 4,200,000; hemoglobin 85%. White blood cells 5,400 with 38% polynuclears. Urinalysis was negative except for slight opalescence. Cultures revealed the presence of typhoid bacilli. Widal test was strongly positive 1:160 dilution. Wassermann was doubtfully positive. Blood chemistry was negative.

Subsequent Course.—Patient ran a typical typhoid-fever course. The temperature remained between 101 and 103 for approximately two weeks and then showed a slight tendency to drop. The pulse remained low throughout the course of the disease. He became somewhat disoriented at times, but in general did not appear to be acutely ill. His stools continued to be loose and of a pea soup consistency for the entire two weeks. Suddenly during the night the patient developed symptoms of shock with sudden abdominal pain. An emergency laparotomy was done and a ruptured intestine found with marked intra-abdominal hemorrhage. The ulcer was repaired and the patient given a transfusion, but he died the following day as a result of diffuse peritonitis and the marked loss of blood.

Autopsy Findings.—Autopsy presented the usual picture of typhoid fever. The intestine showed diffuse ulceration of most of the Peyer's patches of the terminal ileum. The perforated area was located with the sutures still intact. The spleen showed marked enlargement, weighing 500 gm. The liver was also somewhat enlarged. The heart, lungs and other viscera showed no significant pathology other than very marked anemia.

Microscopic Study of Spleen.—(Fig. 31) Microscopic study of sections through the spleen shows marked congestion of the splenic pulp. The lymph follicles are moderately enlarged and show an unusually wide collar of lymphocytes. The outstanding feature of the slide is the presence of large amounts of golden brown granular pigment, most of which is intracellular within the large mononuclear phagocytic cells. In places, some extracellular pigment is noted where cells have ruptured and pigment become deposited in the interstitial tissue spaces.

CASE 17. (Ref. #S-204 and 205)
Diagnosis.—Liver—Hemachromatosis.

Patient is a white male of 45 years, who was admitted to the hospital because of a steadily increasing pigmentation of his skin, abdominal distention and dyspnea.

Present Illness.—The onset of the patient's present condition could not be well defined as it seemed to have been more or less progressive over a period of about two years. It started with vague abdominal symptoms associated with gastro-intestinal disturbances. There was a moderate amount of flatulence and epigastric distress. There were occasional attacks of vomiting. Bowel movements had varied with what might best be described as intermittent attacks of diarrhea and constipation. For the past six months he had noticed his abdomen steadily increasing in size and he had been tapped by a local physician on three occasions with recurrence within a week or ten days in each instance of the distention. Accompanying this he had experienced marked dyspnea which had been relieved by the abdominal paracenteses. During the past year he noted that his skin had been becoming somewhat bronze in color, particularly in the exposed portions and in the axillae and groins. This was not accompanied by pigmentation of his sclerae and was of a different color from the usual lemon-yellow of jaundice.

Past History.—The patient was not aware of any serious illness in his past history. He had never had any

operations. He believed that he had measles, whooping cough and scarlet fever as a child. A review of his systems was essentially negative. He had never had any heart consciousness. He had not been more than normally subject to upper respiratory infections. Up to the present illness he had had no gastro-intestinal disturbances. Genito-urinary history was negative. He denied venereal infection.

Physical Examination.—Patient was a fairly well developed, middle-aged white male who was about the copper color of the usual concept of the American Indian. It was difficult to estimate the state of his nutrition because of marked distention of his abdomen and a considerable amount of swelling of his lower extremities, but as judged by his facies and upper extremities there had been some relative weight loss. His head, itself, otherwise was not remarkable. His eyes were negative. The pupils reacted normally. The nose, ears and throat were negative. There was no adenopathy. The chest was symmetrical. The lungs were resonant throughout. There were a few crackling râles at both bases. The heart was not enlarged and had no murmurs. Due to the abdominal distention it was impossible to palpate the viscera. The genitalia and extremities were negative.

Laboratory Examination.—Red blood cells 3,100,000 with 70% hemoglobin. White blood cells 7,200 with 69% polynuclears. Blood chemistry: Sugar 180 mgm.; Urea 32 mgm. Repeated laboratory examinations and dietary measures maintained the blood sugar level at about 150 mgm. and the urea remained practically constant around 30 mgm.

Subsequent Course.—The patient was tapped and about 2,000 c.c. of somewhat amber colored fluid were removed from the abdomen. Following this it was found that the liver and spleen were both markedly enlarged, the liver being 3 to 4 finger breadths below the costal margin and the spleen being definitely palpable. The patient's abdomen refilled with fluid within 4 to 5 days and he continued a downhill course with repeated abdominal paracenteses at about ten-day intervals until his death some two months after admission. This was complicated by terminal bronchopneumonia.

Autopsy Findings.—At autopsy, the body was that of a well developed, emaciated male who showed a rather characteristic bronzing of the skin. The heart and lungs were negative except for a terminal bronchopneumonia of both bases. The liver was moderately enlarged. Its surface was coarsely granular and the capsule appeared considerably thickened. Even through the capsule it was a peculiar golden brown color and on section this pigmentation was accentuated. The spleen, likewise, showed marked pigmentation appearing quite definitely copper-colored rather than the usual deep purplish-red. The pancreas was considerably increased in size and was definitely pigmented and very much firmer than usual in consistency. Nothing unusual was noted about the adrenals or the kidneys.

Microscopic Study of the Liver.—(Fig. 33 and 34) Sections were prepared in two ways to bring out the essential nature of the pigment which is present. In general, the architecture of the liver is markedly distorted as the result of a diffuse fibrosis which appears to have had its origin in the portal areas but to have spread without much regard for liver lobule architecture cutting the lobules into varying sized nodules of liver cells. The liver cells themselves are seen to be filled with a granular golden brown pigment. In addition, the Kupffer cells of the persistent liver sinusoids likewise are seen to be distended with similar appearing pigment. In the connective tissue septa of the liver there is considerable pigment, much of which is intracellular within the cytoplasm of large mononuclear phagocytic cells but much of it found lying free in the interstitital spaces between connective tissue fibrils. This much may be made out in the simple hematoxylin and eosin stained preparation. To further identify the pigment, the Perl reaction to demonstrate the presence of iron by the precipitation of Prus-

sian blue was used. A study of such prepared sections shows that the great majority of the pigment does contain iron and for that reason must be considered as being hemosiderin. Here and there some nonstaining masses of pigment may still be seen. These are probably in the nature of hemofuscin. The picture is typical of the condition known as hemochromatosis and shows the widespread diffuse nature of the process, the result of disturbed iron metabolism. A similar picture is found in sections taken from the pancreas, spleen and skin, with the pigment both intra- and extracellularly distributed.

Hematoidin.—The next most common form of pigment encountered pathologically is the iron-free radical hematoidin. This is particularly commonly found in infarctions of the spleen or other organs where the blood supply has been interfered with and the hemoglobin left to break down. Formerly it was believed that hematoidin represented a simple chemical breakdown and was not dependent upon any cell activity. Rich, in recent years, however, has shown fairly conclusively that cell activity is necessary as in the case of hemosiderin formation. Whether hematoidin represents a further breakdown of hemo-

siderin with the release of the iron radical is uncertain or whether it represents a direct product from hematin. At all events, it usually occurs in rather characteristic stellate crystalline form frequently spoken of as burrs. Occasionally before this crystallization takes place it may be seen as amorphous granules. It is commonly considered as an isomer of bilirubin but more recent work suggests that this is not necessarily so, and that it is more probably a complex mixture of pigments, including bilirubin.

ILLUSTRATIVE CASE

(Refer to Case 2, Chapter I, for the clinical abstract.)

Diagnosis.—Spleen—infarction; hematoidin.
Microscopic Description of Spleen.—(Ref. #S-122) (Fig. 35 and 40) This, it will be recalled, represents a case of chronic heart disease terminating with an acute bacterial endocarditis and multiple embolic lesions to various organs producing areas of infarction of which this lesion in the spleen is typical. The section is seen to show a very sharp linear demarcation between the normal splenic pulp and follicles and an area in which practically all cell detail has been lost. This is pale in color, taking very little stain. Only a shadowy outline of the architecture in this area can be made out. Broken down nuclear material is present in considerable amounts. Here and there persistent nuclei and stromal cells, particularly inflammatory cells, can be identified. Along the zone which separates the normal tissue from this dead, necrotic, infarcted area may be seen considerable hemor-

rhage where the blood has seeped into the tissues from the surrounding sinuses and collateral circulation. The infarct as a whole, however, is anemic, as might be expected from the fact that the vessels are endarterioles, and their occlusion shuts off the blood supply.

In the necrotic area may be observed the feature of interest in connection with our study of pigmentation. Clumps of golden brown, acicular crystals arranged in somewhat stellate fashion may be seen completely independent of any cell activity, lying free in the tissue spaces. Were this to have been stained by the Prussian-blue method no iron could have been demonstrated in any of this pigmentary material. No other form of pigment occurs in this particular arrangement so that we are certain of its identity and easy differentiation from hemosiderin or other forms of hemoglobin-derived pigment is possible.

Hematoporphyrin.—In recent years the question of hematoporphyrin has become of considerable interest because of its occurrence in the urine in a variety of diseases and particularly following the use of barbital in its many forms. The presence of any considerable amount of this pigment will give the urine a deep, ruddy color. From the histologic standpoint the demonstration of hematoporphyrin is rather unsatisfactory as it may only be found in minute amounts, usually in the corium of individuals who seem to have a particular sensitivity to this substance.

Hemofuscin.—Hemofuscin is another of the pigments derived from hemoglobin which is of a brownish-yellow color and usually occurs in amorphous form. In the disease hemachromatosis, as has been already noted, a certain amount of the pigment which is found in the tissues is of this variety. Its differentiation from amorphous hematoidin is probably impossible under the microscope as both represent iron-free radicals of the breakdown products of hemoglobin. It is believed to occur normally in the smooth muscle of the intestinal tract and is thought by some investigators to have a very wide range in the body tissues generally. Indeed some investigators have said that the pigment found in the heart and liver in senility is of this nature, although most observers are inclined to include this pigment among the lipochromes. Pathologically the significance of hemofuscin appears to be negligible, only occurring in those conditions where hemosiderin is present in excess and very probably represents merely a further breakdown of hemosiderin itself.

Bile Pigments.—The chief pigmentary constituent of human bile is in the form of bilirubin, which as just commented upon has long been considered as an isomer of hematoidin. The theories regarding the production of bile have undergone many changes in the past few years. Originally the concept of bile-pigment production by the liver was paramount. To-day, with the work of Whipple, Mann and many other investigators, it is recognized that the reticular cells of the body, especially the Kupffer cells of the liver are the active agents in the production of bilirubin and that the actual liver cells play no part except to excrete the pigment into the bile capillaries to be combined with bile salts and cholesterin to form the ultimate bile. Thus bilirubin may, under experimental or pathological conditions, be formed in the spleen, the lymph nodes or even in the bone marrow, be transported to the liver and there re-synthesized as if it had been manufactured by the Kupffer cells. If obstruction to the outflow of bile is interfered with in any way, then the bile backs up into the liver and gains access to the blood stream. If the concentration of the bile in the blood exceeds one part in 50,000 then clinical *jaundice* results. Many such forms of obstruction may occur; from the presence of stone in the bile duct, the presence of tumor outside the biliary tract pressing upon it, the presence of an acute inflammatory process involving bile ducts and capillaries—all may produce such a picture. Further consideration of this problem of jaundice dependent upon other mechanisms will be taken up in relation to the discussion of liver pathology. At the present time we are concerned primarily with the demonstration and appearance of bile as the result of such obstruction to its outflow in the liver and as might be expected, plugs of bile may be seen distending the finer biliary capillaries between the liver cells and cords, as well as in many of the small bile ducts.

ILLUSTRATIVE CASE

CASE 18. (Ref. #S-184 and S-224)

Diagnosis.—Liver—Bile stasis of common bile duct resulting from common bile duct obstruction.

Patient was a 70-year-old white female who was admitted to the hospital because of marked persistent and increasing jaundice associated with diarrhea.

Present Illness.—History began about two months ago when she first noticed a beginning sallowness to her skin. However, she had lost considerable weight in the two or three months preceding that period and had had intermittent attacks of diarrhea off and on for between three and four months. This apparently did not cause her much concern until she developed her jaundice with marked itching of the skin. This had increased steadily in intensity since its onset. She had complete loss of appetite and had had occasional attacks of nausea but no vomiting during this period.

Past History.—Her past history appeared to be entirely irrelevant. She had no recollection of any childhood illness nor of any serious illness during her entire life. Her memory, however, was definitely impaired and she had a "stroke" about two years ago with marked interference with her speech, which had not cleared up satisfactorily. A brother and a sister both died of diabetes. She did not recall of what either her father or mother died. A review of her systems was unsatisfactory because of the patient's lack of sustained attention.

Physical Examination.—Patient was an intensely jaundiced, elderly white female. There was marked cyanosis of the lips and nail beds. She was uncoöperative and resistant to satisfactory physical examination. The head was of normal contour. Eyes: pupils were unequal. There was a cataract in the left eye. The right reacted to light and accommodation. The ears, nose and throat were negative. Chest: Percussion was impaired over the right upper lobe with a definite increase of breath sounds which suggested a beginning bronchopneumonia. The heart was not enlarged but there was a soft, blowing, pulmonic murmur heard. Blood pressure was 120/60. Abdomen: There was a globular mass about 6 cm. below the costal margin on the right, which moved with respiration. Rectal and pelvic examinations were negative.

Laboratory Examination.—Urinalysis showed the presence of a moderate amount of albumin but no sugar. Red blood cells 4,200,000; hemoglobin 85%. White blood cells 11,300 with 77% polynuclear leukocytes. Blood chemistry: Blood sugar 96 mgm., urea nitrogen 15 mgm.

Subsequent Course.—The patient grew progressively weaker and died quietly two weeks after her admission. During this time her jaundice had further increased. There had been marked further weight loss and her bowel movements had remained increased in frequency.

Autopsy Findings.—At autopsy, the body was that of an emaciated elderly white woman, who weighed only 58 pounds. The skin and mucous membranes as well as the sclerae were intensely jaundiced. There was a large tumor mass involving the head of the pancreas, which completely obstructed the common duct through pressure and infiltration. The common bile duct was greatly distended. This distention extended up into the major hepatic branches of the bile duct and involved the cystic duct with secondary dilatation of the gall bladder. Numerous metastatic tumor nodules were seen in the liver which was somewhat atrophied, very firm in consistency and dark green in color due to bile retention. There was a terminal bronchopneumonia involving both bases and the right upper lobe. The heart showed typical senile myocardial degeneration with possible brown atrophy.

Microscopic Description of Liver.—(Fig. 36) Sections microscopically through the liver show the presence of bile pigment within the bile capillaries and smaller branches of the bile ducts. This is evidenced by the presence of amorphous granular, dark brownish staining masses of pigment, which distended these structures. Granular pigment is likewise seen within the cytoplasm of the liver cells representing the unexcreted bilirubin which could not gain access to the plugged bile capillaries. Accompanying this bile stasis is a secondary chronic inflammatory fibrosis and mononuclear cellular infiltration of the surrounding periductile tissues. The liver cells, likewise, show albuminous and fatty degenerative changes as further evidence of their injury.

AUTOGENOUS PIGMENTS

Lipochrome.—Lipochrome pigments are probably largely derived from the carotinoid pigments introduced through the diet. Of these, we may mention carotin, which is apparently identical with the pigment of the corpus luteum. Similarly, xanthophyll, which in recent experimental work is believed to be the coloring matter of the fat cells and is largely derived from the yolk of eggs, should be considered. These substances seem to be a form of pigment in combination apparently with protein material as they occur in the various cells of the body normally. It is only under pathological conditions that they accumulate in sufficient quantities to be of significance. We have already commented upon the condition known as senile or brown atrophy, which is most marked in the heart muscle. This was originally a gross term applied to the curious brownish discoloration of the small, atrophic heart seen in old age. Similar changes have been described as involving other viscera, notably the liver. Microscopically, this pigmentation appears to be the result of the deposition of a golden yellow pigment with a perinuclear distribution, particularly in the heart muscle at the two poles of the nucleus. The muscle fibers themselves are usually reduced in size and the nuclei appear increased in size and number. The significance of this pigmentation is little understood and is probably a normal, physiological, senile manifestation of tissue wear and tear, associated with condensation of the cell protoplasm.

ILLUSTRATIVE CASE

CASE 19. (Ref. #S-226)
Diagnosis.—Heart—brown atrophy; lipochrome pigmentation.

Patient was a white female of 86 years, who was admitted to the hospital because of severe pain in the lower bowel accompanied by increasing constipation finally resulting in complete inability to defecate. This was associated with several attacks of vomiting.

Present Illness.—Patient had been in her usual good health until the relatively sudden onset of her present symptoms. She had been bedridden for the past six years as a result of a fall, with a subluxation of a vertebra and the fracture of the neck of her femur, but had not had any other symptoms during this period.

Past History.—Her past history was essentially negative. She had never had any serious illness or operation. For the past several years, she had had occasional swelling of her ankles toward evening but this had not been noticeable since her accident. She had had nocturia three or four times a night during the past two or three years but had had no other complaints.

Physical Examination.—Patient was a fairly well developed, somewhat underweight, elderly white female. The head was normal in outline and covered with a moderate amount of gray hair. The eyes showed a marked arcus senilis which was bilateral. The ears, nose and throat were negative. The teeth had all been extracted, but there were compensatory dental plates. The neck showed no cervical adenopathy. The chest was negative. The lungs were clear throughout. The heart was not enlarged. There were no murmurs. The sounds were somewhat distant. The abdomen was distended. There was shifting dullness in the flanks. No masses could be felt. Rectal examination showed an obstructive ulcerated annular tumor about six inches above the anal orifice which was causing marked stenosis of the lumen.

Laboratory Findings.—Red blood cells 3,800,000; hemoglobin 76%. White blood cells 12,800 with 84% polynuclear leukocytes. Blood chemistry was negative. Urinalysis showed a trace of albumin but was otherwise negative.

Operative History.—In view of the almost complete stenosis it was felt that palliative colostomy was necessary with the thought of possibly more radical surgery if the patient's condition warranted it. This program was begun with a loop of bowel being brought to the abdominal surface and a colostomy established. The patient suffered marked postoperative shock and her condition appeared critical almost immediately. She survived for a period of two days, but in view of her advanced age it was not surprising that she died quietly at the end of that time.

Autopsy Findings.—Autopsy showed a well developed and fairly well nourished elderly white woman who presented a surgical incision in the left lower quadrant where a loop of bowel was exposed. On opening the abdominal cavity there was noted localized peritonitis around the incisional area. The heart was small, weighing only 180 gm. The myocardium was soft in consistency. The heart was of a deep golden-brownish-red color. The valves appeared extremely atrophied. Numerous atheromatous plaques were found in the arch of the aorta. The coronaries were widely patent, however. There was evidence of terminal cardiac failure as shown by diffuse edema of both lungs and the escape of fluid into the pleural cavities. The liver weighed 940 gm. and likewise showed rather characteristic brown atrophy. The other viscera showed nothing of pathological interest or significance except for a typical ulcerative annular carcinoma of the sigmoid.

Melanins.—By the term melanin is included a group of pigments rather than any one specific substance. Normally, melanin is found in the natural pigments of the skin, hair and the choroid of the eye as well as in the substantia nigra of the brain. Frequently, focal areas of increased pigmentation in the skin may be seen as the so-called "moles." Exposure to sunlight increases this pigmentation physiologically, as a protective mechanism as we see in the case of tan. Freckles represent another instance of increased physiologic pigmentary activity on the part of pigment producing cells or melanoblasts. Such stimulation of these cells may likewise result from nervous and chemical as well as such physical stimuli. The relationship of the nervous system to the melanoblast and pigmentation has been fairly well established in recent years as has the necessity of the presence of an oxidase in the tissues. These facts are best demonstrated in tumors arising from such pigment cells.

All in all, however, the mechanism of melanin production is still far from settled and controversy still rages around the part chromatophores or pigmented cells of the corium play in the picture. From the experimental evidence at hand it would seem that these chromatophores are merely storage cells; that the melanoblasts of the skin contain an oxidizing ferment, dihydroxyphenylalanine, more

Microscopic Description of Heart.—(Fig. 41) A section through the heart muscle presents the typical picture of brown atrophy. The individual muscle fibers seem somewhat decreased in size and more or less separated by interstitial connective tissue. The nuclei of the cells vary considerably in size, many of them appearing small while others show compensatory hypertrophy. Almost every muscle cell is seen to have a mass of bright, golden-yellow pigment arranged with a bipolar distribution in its cytoplasm. Sections which were stained by various methods demonstrated conclusively the absence of any iron fraction in this material. The color appears too light yellow to fall into the usual concept of hemofuscin, and it more closely resembles in its amorphous granular form the picture which one expects to find associated with lipochrome pigment.

commonly spoken of as "dopa," which converts the colorless substance into insoluble melanin.

The melanins are organic, amorphous pigments having certain physical characters which identify them from the other pigments. They are usually dark brown or blackish brown in color, of large molecular size, insoluble in water or most of the usual organic solvents and made up of carbon, nitrogen, hydrogen and oxygen, very commonly having an indol ring and frequently found in combination with sulphur. They are probably derived as an oxidation product from separate protein fractions such as tyrosine in combination with sulphur or some iron-holding constituent. Their relationship to some of the other pigments is at the present time still poorly understood. For example, certain investigators believe that the pigment produced by the malarial parasite is a definite melanin, while others believe it to be a hemoglobinogenous pigment derived from the breakdown of the hemoglobin rather than as a metabolic product of the parasite itself (Fig. 39). Thus, there are these indefinite, indeterminate, intermediate forms of pigment which it is difficult to classify, but for practical purposes our consideration of the melanins will be restricted to those pigments produced by the melanoblast of the body tissues and which are best exemplified by their occurrence in tumors arising from these cells.

ILLUSTRATIVE CASE

CASE 20. (Ref. #S-104)
Diagnosis.—Liver—metastatic malignant melanoma.
Patient was a white female of 38 years, who was admitted to the hospital because of a large, pigmented mass involving the vulva.
Present Illness.—This had been rapidly increasing in size during the past three or four weeks, to the size of about a lemon and had become definitely painful on walk-

ing. She had not noted any other symptomatology in relation to this localized lesion.
Past History.—Patient had always been perfectly normal. She had gone through the usual childhood infections. She was married and had had three normal children, the youngest one being five years of age. A review of her systems was entirely negative. Her respiratory history was not unusual in the amount of upper respiratory in-

fection. Cardiovascular system had been entirely symptomless. Gastro-intestinal: She had presented no more than the usual intestinal upsets. Genito-urinary system was negative. Menstrual history began at 13 and had been regular without undue discomfort.

Physical Examination.—Patient was a well developed, well nourished white female who appeared about 35 years of age. Her head was normal in contour. Her hair was rather coarse and dark. Eyes, ears, nose and throat were negative. Chest was symmetrical. Heart was not enlarged and there were no murmurs. Lungs were clear throughout; there were no râles. Her abdomen was normal in contour. No masses or viscera were palpable. Extremities were negative. Gynecologic examination: A large, infiltrating, firm, deeply-pigmented mass was seen involving the right labium majorus. This showed no definite demarcation from the surrounding tissues and appeared to infiltrate extensively. A presumptive diagnosis of a melanotic tumor was made and radical surgical excision advised in the hope that it might be in time to be effective.

Laboratory Findings.—Red blood cells 4,600,000; 86% hemoglobin. White blood cells 9,400 with 72% polynuclear leukocytes. Urinalysis was negative. Wassermann was negative. Blood chemistry was within normal limits. X-ray examination showed no evidence of any metastatic tumors in the lungs or skeletal system.

Subsequent Course.—Patient had a radical excision of the tumor mass locally. Pathological report came back as a highly malignant melanoma and it was advised to keep the patient under close observation for a period with the thought of possible irradiation. Within three weeks after the operation the patient began to show multiple subcutaneous, pin-sized, bluish discolored areas in the skin pretty generally over the surface of the body. She developed signs of respiratory distress and soon there appeared symptoms related to the central nervous system as if pressure upon the cord about the level of the seventh or eighth dorsal vertebrae had occurred. The patient ran a rapidly downhill course and died less than six weeks after admission.

Autopsy Findings.—At autopsy the entire body was found riddled with metastatic tumor masses. The tumor nodules ranged in size from pin head to large lesions three to four centimeters in diameter found involving the brain, spinal cord, dura, heart muscle, striated musculature, lungs, liver, spleen, kidneys and all the other abdominal viscera. The picture represented a typical, fulminating type of malignant melanoma with generalized metastasis by the blood stream.

Microscopic Description of a Nodule from Liver.— (Fig. 38 and 42) Microscopic description of a representative nodule from the liver presents a similar histologic picture as the tumor from other areas. The tumor is made up of large, irregularly polyhedral or spindle formed cells occurring in clumps and masses supported by a delicate capillary vascular and connective tissue stroma. These tumor cells show many mitotic figures when their nuclei can be identified, but most of the cells are so laden with pigment that it is hard to find the nuclear membrane and outline of the nucleus. Certain of the cells will be seen to be growing so rapidly that they have not had time to produce pigment or at the most only a few small, dark, blackish-brown granules can be seen in the cytoplasm of these cells. The liver tissue is scarcely recognizable except as persistent cords here and there. The tumor has replaced the normal liver structures and only scattered areas can be found in which a suggestion of liver lobulation with the typical portal areas and central veins can be identified. It is of interest to study this slide in relation to those cases in which the pigment is derived from hemoglobin, because in these melanotic lesions the pigment is generally so much deeper brown or black in color that in itself, without further differentiation, the thought of melanin rather than hemosiderin occurs at the first low power examination of the tissue.

CHAPTER V

DISTURBANCES OF CIRCULATION

Disturbances of circulation are the result of many complex factors including mechanical lesions producing dilatation or blocking of the circulatory system, alteration in the chemistry of the blood itself, toxic changes affecting the tissue cells, and lesions affecting the nervous control of the blood and lymphatic vessels. A complete discussion of the mechanism of these various factors is a monumental task in itself and in this condensed presentation only those more striking and significant points will be referred to. The following schematic presentation is given with the hope that the major manifestations of such alterations in the circulatory mechanism may be understood.

OLIGEMIA

By oligemia is meant a decrease in the total amount of the blood in the body. This occurs in such conditions as severe hemorrhage following traumatic amputations or as internal hemorrhage with the rupture of some viscus such as the spleen or liver or the erosion or rupture of a blood vessel, notably the rupture of an aneurysm of the aorta. It may also occur in long wasting diseases, particularly in association with cancer, tuberculosis, the arthritides, and finally, it may be thought of as an almost normal physiological phenomenon in senility. In these latter forms it is of relatively little importance in respect to life. In the form associated with severe hemorrhage, life may be seriously endangered if the blood is not replaced promptly by transfusion or the administration of fluids to at least make up the blood volume loss, the patient presenting the classical picture of shock.

PLETHORA

By plethora is meant the reverse of oligemia, or, an increase in the total amount of blood of *normal* composition within the body. This is seen only in certain types of cardiac disease. Under this term of plethora should be cited two varieties of increased blood volume of abnormal composition.

Polycythemia vera.—This is a condition in which there is an increase in the number of red cells which may reach as high a figure as ten or twelve million per cubic centimeter. The etiology of this condition is unknown. It is a slowly progressive disease which ultimately and invariably ends fatally, although the duration of the condition varies a great deal in individual cases, depending upon the severity of the process. By many this is believed to be a form of malignant tumor involving the red cells of the blood. In this condition the increased volume is due to the increase of red cells which gives a very high viscosity to the blood and tends to slow the circulation so that these patients acquire a curious and practically diagnostic ruddy cyanotic color due to the failure of the red cells to become completely oxygenated.

Serous plethora.—By this term is meant an increased blood volume due to increase of the fluid elements of the blood. This is a transitory process ordinarily and is seen particularly following the intravenous injection of fluids—saline, glucose, etc.—and is of no clinical significance as the normal volume is restored very promptly. In cases where cardiac damage exists and such a serous plethora is induced artificially and too rapidly, it may result in an undue load being placed upon the heart with cardiac failure as a result. For this reason, in many cases, it is often advisable to give small and repeated intravenous fluids rather than the same amount over a shorter period of time.

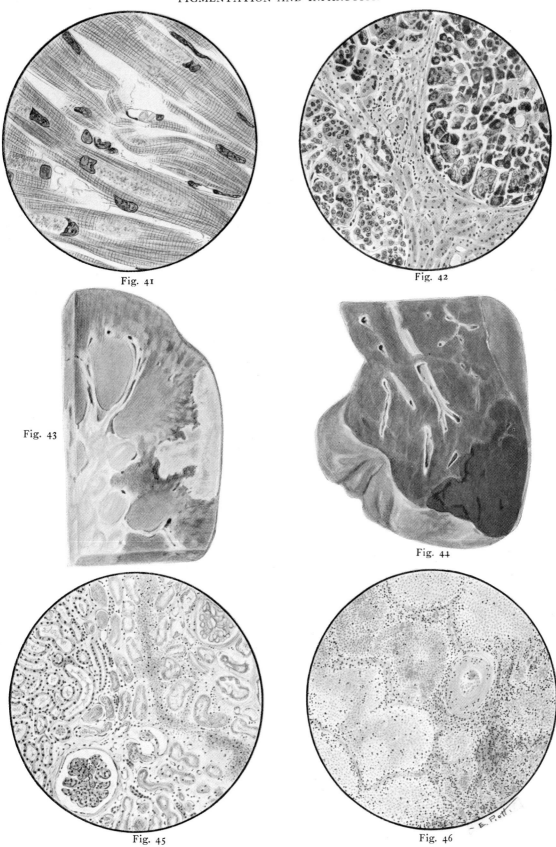

PLATE X

PIGMENTATION AND INFARCTION

Fig. 41

Fig. 42

Fig. 43

Fig. 44

Fig. 45

Fig. 46

Fig. 41.—Heart, Brown Atrophy (Lipochrome), 800 x.
Fig. 43.—Kidney, Anemic Infarct
Fig. 45.—Kidney, Anemic Infarct, 100 x.

Fig. 42.—Liver, Metastatic Malignant Melanoma, 400 x.
Fig. 44.—Lung, Hemorrhagic Infarct
Fig. 46.—Lung, Hemorrhagic Infarct, 100 x.

PLATE XI
CIRCULATORY DISTURBANCES

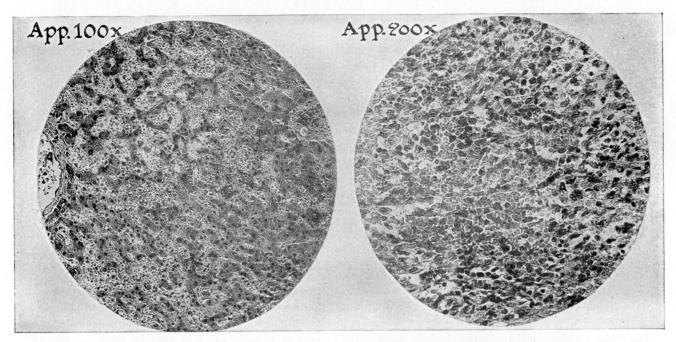

App. 100x

App. 200x

FIG. 47.—LIVER: CHRONIC PASSIVE CONGESTION.—CASE 15.—Typical venous distention of liver sinusoids, most marked around central vein (A), and fading toward periphery of lobule (C), resulting in progressive atrophy of liver cords.

FIG. 48.—SPLEEN: CHRONIC PASSIVE CONGESTION.—CASE 15.—Sinusoids distended with red cells, undergoing hemolysis and conversion into hemosiderin by reticulo-endothelial cells (cf. color Plate VIII, Fig. 31).

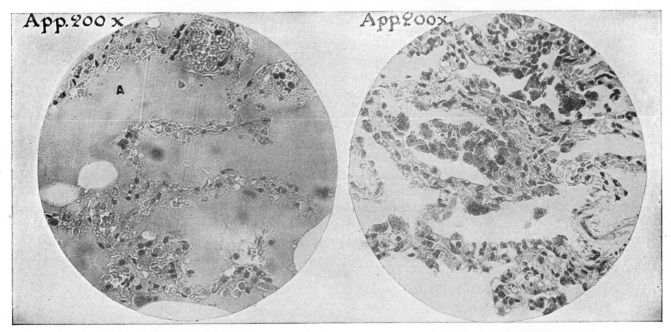

App. 200 x

App. 200x

FIG. 49.—LUNG: EDEMA.—CASE 22.—The alveolar wall capillaries are intensely congested, and the air sacs almost completely filled with a pale, homogeneous, pink-staining material, representing coagulated serum.

FIG. 50.—LUNG: CHRONIC PASSIVE CONGESTION.—CASE 15.—Outstanding feature is presence of hemosiderin-laden "heart failure cells" (A), the result of red cell breakdown through circulatory stasis and diapedesis. (See also color Plate VIII, Fig. 32.)

ISCHEMIA

By ischemia is meant a local diminution in the blood supply due to obstruction of inflow of *arterial* blood. This is frequently spoken of as local anemia. Such obstruction may be the result of some neurogenic vasomotor reaction. The best example of this is seen in the so-called *Raynaud's disease* in which constriction of the arterioles of the fingers and toes occurs, and gradually progresses to the point where trophic disturbances occur, even to the loss of digits. A more familiar and less serious lesion of this type may be seen in the ordinary frost bite or chilblain in which a local ischemia results from the prolonged application of cold to a part. Lesions of this nature may occur from mechanical pressure upon a local arteriole supply or as the result of obstruction from *within* by some foreign material in a small arteriole, as we shall see later in considering diseases of the blood vessels. One might even speak of certain of the degenerative vascular lesions resulting in obstruction to the smaller endarteries known as *endarteritis obliterans* as another type of lesion which might result in local ischemia, although collateral circulation usually maintains the nutrition of the part involved unless it is of such magnitude that actual necrosis and gangrene follow. *Angina pectoris* should be cited as another example associated with such ischemia.

HYPEREMIA

Active.—By the term hyperemia we usually think of a local increase of blood to a part associated with inflammatory or vasomotor dilatation of the arterioles and capillaries. Strictly speaking this term should be called active hyperemia and is essentially a physiological reaction designed to carry an additional nutritional supply to the tissues involved. As an example of such a condition may be cited the physiological dilatation of the blood vessels of the stomach in the process of digestion following the taking of food. Similarly in muscular activity, one finds the same increased blood supply developing as a result of the muscular requirements. Even blushing represents a form of active hyperemia under vasomotor control in response to some emotional stimulus.

Passive hyperemia (chronic passive congestion).— In contrast to this picture of localized active hyperemia may be described another condition of increased blood to a part, which is the result of mechanical obstruction to the *outflow* of blood from the venous side in contradistinction to ischemia and active hyperemia, which are both *arterial* circulatory disturbances. This condition might be called passive hyperemia, but is more commonly known as *chronic passive congestion,* and in general the term congestion as applied to circulatory disturbances implies a venous stasis with a certain amount of cyanotic color change associated with the picture. The most typical example of such chronic passive congestion is seen as the result of chronic valvular disease of the heart such as noted in chronic rheumatic fever with mitral stenosis and regurgitation or in such congenital lesions as pulmonary valve stenosis. Other lesions which might produce a passive hyperemia are comparable to some of those seen in the more active ischemic or hyperemic pictures; namely, local pressure upon the veins in a given area, thrombosis and so forth. Mechanical lesions of various sorts may result in such *local* passive hyperemia. An example of such a lesion is seen in the familiar *varicose veins* where, due to the long continued effect of gravity, the valves of the veins are damaged and blood accumulates in the vessels by gravity until the column of blood becomes so heavy that the vessel is distended and ultimately becomes tortuous. Nutrition of the tissues is interfered with and not infrequently, chronic indolent ulcers occur as a result. In the more generalized type associated with cardiac disease we have already seen the effect of chronic passive congestion in the lung in Fig. 50, as described in Case 15, Chapter IV, where the stagnating blood in the dilated capillaries of the alveolar wall oozed out into the pulmonary alveoli and the hemoglobin became broken down and converted into hemosiderin. In the liver, even more striking mechanical distention of the sinusoids, especially centrally, in the anatomical lobule, occurs, giving rise to a nutmeg appearance to the cut surface of the liver, the atrophied and compressed liver cords standing out in sharp contrast to the deeply cyanotic venous blood in the distended sinusoids (Fig. 47, 477, 478 and 479). In the spleen, the engorgement of the venous sinuses results in an enlarged, fibrotic organ.

PLATE XII

CIRCULATORY DISTURBANCES (Continued)

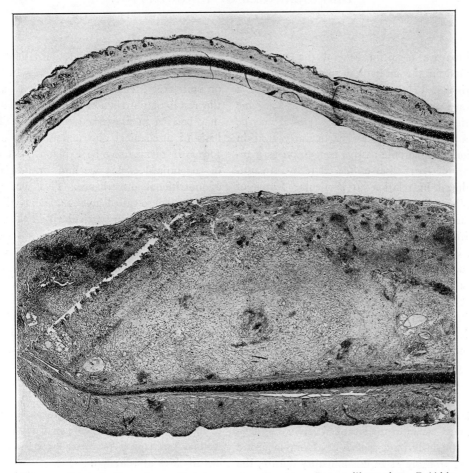

FIG. 51.—RABBIT'S EAR: ACUTE INFLAMMATION.—CASE 21.—Lower illustration.—Rabbit's ear dipped in hot water for two minutes, and sectioned 24 hours later. Note inflammatory edema of interstitial tissues, capillary and lymphatic dilatation, and early perivascular cellular exudation. Upper illustration.—Control ear for comparison. App. 10 x.

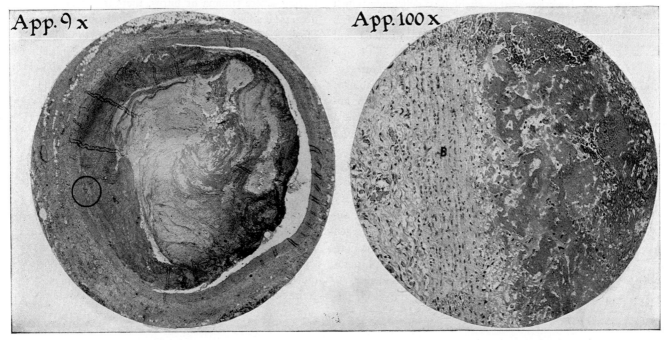

FIG. 52.—PULMONARY ARTERY: THROMBOSIS.—CASE 23.—A large red thrombus arising from the wall of the vessel is seen practically occluding its lumen. App. 9 x.

FIG. 53.—PULMONARY ARTERY-THROMBOSIS.—CASE 23.—High power photomicrograph from area indicated in Fig. 52. Note absence of intimal endothelium and beginning organization of thrombus with its characteristic coral-like, avascular laminae of platelets, red cells and fibrin. App. 100 x.

EDEMA

By edema we mean in general the accumulation of fluid in the interstitial spaces of the supporting tissues. When fluid accumulates within a cell we have seen that this is spoken of as hydropic degeneration. Edema may occur *locally* or it may be part of a *generalized* process particularly seen in conjunction with chronic passive congestion as a result of chronic heart disease. Special terms are usually employed in relation to particular forms of edema. When the accumulation of fluid is generalized throughout the tissues, including the various body cavities the picture is spoken of as generalized *anasarca,* or dropsy as a lay term. When we find localized accumulation of fluid within the peritoneal cavity as a result of obstruction to portal circulation or as part of the generalized picture, this is spoken of as *ascites.* When fluid accumulates in the pleural cavities, it is usually spoken of as *hydrothorax* and when it occurs within the pericardial cavity as a simple transudate in association with cardiac failure and circulatory disturbance it is called *hydropericardium.*

The mechanism of the development of edema is still obscure. Certain of the localized edematous conditions, particularly those spoken of as angioneurotic edemas, are probably of an inflammatory nature, the result of some sensitivity of the patient as a manifestation of allergy. Local edema, as in the scrotum or unilateral edema of an extremity, may often be the result of obstruction to the lymphatics such as may be seen in filariasis (Fig. 203). Thus, on the basis of mechanical obstruction many of the local forms of edema may be explained. In other types of generalized edema we find an associated history of nutritional disturbance. This was particularly seen in the so-called *war edema* as the result of inadequate nutrition particularly in the vitamin content of the food. Increased blood pressure, variations in the colloid composition of the blood, decreased osmotic pressures, injuries which affect the permeability of the vessel wall, tissue changes as the result of toxemias—all these are factors involved in the outpouring of fluid from the circulatory system into the tissue spaces. Thus we find that edema is something which may be readily defined as a pathological process resulting in the interstitial accumulation of fluid either of a local or generalized distribution, but that the mechanism involved in what superficially appears to be a simple process implicates some of the most complex physiological physicochemical as well as mechanical problems of cellular and tissue disturbances of function.

SHOCK

By shock is meant a circulatory deficiency which is not cardiac or vasomotor in origin, and which is characterized by a decreased volume of blood and cardiac output and by hemoconcentration. This definition is suggested by Moon after many years of investigation experimentally in the field and accords in the findings with those of the commission appointed during the World War to study the whole problem of shock. It is included at this time because of its obvious circulatory basis, the mechanism of which, however, is poorly understood. In typical shock we find regularly a lowered blood pressure, a lowered basal metabolic rate, a diminished urinary output, an increased cardiac rate and usually a decrease in the coagulability of the blood, in its oxygen content, in the chlorides and an increase in the nonprotein nitrogen. Numerous other clinical phenomena show marked variability in their incidence. As a rule, in so-called *surgical shock,* or the shock following severe trauma or burns, there is apt to be a decreased alkali reserve and a leukocytosis. In the shock occasioned by intestinal obstruction the alkali reserve is usually increased and there is an initial leukopenia, which is followed by a leukocytosis. Obviously, shock is a picture clinically which may be produced by a large variety of causes. Experimentally it may be induced by the injection of histamine or many other irritant substances. It is particularly commonly seen after severe trauma and even after relatively minor surgical procedures at times. It almost invariably follows severe burns. The pathology of shock may be compared in many respects to the appearance of the organs in chronic passive congestion, but there are certain notable differences. It is perhaps best termed, as Moon expresses it, "acute venous congestion involving particularly the mucous membranes, the lungs, liver and kidneys." It is associated apparently with vascular atony and much of the pathology would seem to be dependent upon increased capillary permeability. The lesions likewise are very comparable to those seen in asphyxia, and indeed the cause of death in asphyxia may well be one manifestation of this condition, which is so poorly understood generally. Unlike chronic passive congestion which represents a chronic condition, we find that the spleen is relatively bloodless whereas in congestion due to circulatory deficiency the spleen takes part in the general congestive picture. The fluids of the blood apparently escape

because of the increased capillary permeability, into the tissues, and edema is apt to follow particularly in the lungs where at times congestion and edema with terminal bronchopneumonia is very prone to occur. Thus, the immediate cause of death in many conditions of apparently totally unrelated etiology may end in this picture of shock in some modified form, best illustrated by the capillary venous congestion of the lungs, the terminal pulmonary edema and the asphyxia so commonly found at the autopsy table.

ILLUSTRATIVE CASES

CASE 15 (Ref. #S-15) for Clinical history, see page 33.
Diagnosis.—Liver—chronic passive congestion; hemosiderosis; central necrosis.

For clinical abstract refer to Case 15, Chapter IV. In the section from the lung in this case, the picture of chronic passive congestion has been described in considerable detail. The outstanding points to recall in this connection are first, the marked congestion of the alveolar wall capillaries due primarily to back pressure of the venous circulation from a damaged mitral valve; second, the marked thickening of the alveolar walls as the result of compensatory fibroblastic proliferation to overcome the capillary dilatation; and third, the mechanical dilatation of the acini in an attempt to increase the surface area to improve the gaseous interchange of oxygen and carbon dioxide. A very complete review of this subject may be seen in the recent report by Parker. As a concomitant of the chronic passive congestive process the escape of red cells into the lung alveoli with the breakdown of hemoglobin and the production of hemosiderin taken up in the "heart failure cells" is also of helpful diagnostic significance.

Microscopic Description of Liver.—(Fig. 47) Sections microscopically present a typical picture of chronic passive congestion. This is evidenced by pressure atrophy of the liver cords around the afferent central vein of the liver lobule. It is accompanied by considerable edema between the sinusoidal endothelium and liver parenchyma in places. Immediately around the central vein the sinusoids appear markedly distended, but in the midzonal and peripheral portion of the lobule the edema just noted may best be observed. In a few areas some actual necrotic changes may be seen in the liver cells around the central portions of the lobules, but for the most part they show only mild degenerative changes. There is a possible slight increase of connective tissue in the portal areas as well. There is some retained hemosiderin, the result of the chronic passive congestion, with stasis and breakdown of the blood pigment which is taken up by the Kupffer cells. Being produced in excess this is still apparent in the liver cells as part of the functional disturbance resulting from the congestion. (See also Fig. 477, 478 and 479.)

CASE 15 (Ref. #S-68) for Clinical history, see page 33.
Diagnosis.—Spleen—chronic passive congestion.
Microscopic Description of Spleen.—(Fig. 48) Sec-

tions through the spleen present evidence of moderate hyperplasia of the germinal centers in the majority of the lymph follicles. More striking, however, are the changes which have resulted from the chronic passive congestion of the organ. There is both a relative and actual increase of connective tissue throughout the organ. This is characterized by an increase in the size of the normal trabeculae as well as by thickening of the perisinusoidal stroma. This, as in the liver and lung, is the result of chronic distention of the sinuses by blood, which has stimulated the connective tissue to grow, in an attempt to produce compensatory functional capacity on the part of the spleen without undue increase in size. The sinusoids and the pulp spaces also show marked congestion. Scattered through the pulp may be noted a certain amount of pigment in the form of amorphous granules. These are mostly of a golden-brown or blackish-brown color and represent hemosiderin, which has been taken up for the most part by mononuclear phagocytic cells. Accompanying the diffuse fibrosis of the spleen may also be seen a diffuse proliferation of the reticuloendothelium. Indeed, the endothelium lining the sinusoids in many places appears almost cuboidal where the cells have undergone compensatory overgrowth. In general it may be seen that in chronic passive congestion of the spleen the outstanding feature is a prominence of the normal sinusoidal architecture due to the diffuse increase of connective tissue and reticulo-endothelium supporting this sinusoidal endothelium.

CASE 21 (Ref. #S-211)
Diagnosis.—Rabbit's ear—acute inflammation and edema. Experimental production of edema in a rabbit's ear. A normal, full grown, white rabbit had its ear dipped in water heated to 60° C. for two minutes and then allowed to let the effect of this mild injury proceed to its greatest height, at the end of twelve hours. By comparison with the normal control ear, it was observed that the injured ear became more and more swollen and that the blood supply obviously was increased as the ear assumed a pinkish color, the result of acute localized hyperemia. As the lesion progressed, the escape of fluid from this increased circulation followed until the entire ear became swollen to three or four times the thickness of the normal ear and as a result of the increased amount of fluid present and from the pain associated with pressure

upon the nerve endings from the distention of the tissues by this fluid, the ear drooped. Part of this was the result of gravity because of the increase in weight. At the end of the experimental period the animal was sacrificed and sections obtained from the injured ear for study. These will be referred to in relation to inflammation in one of the later chapters, but at this time attention should be drawn to the histologic picture of edema.

Microscopic Description of Section of Rabbit Ear.— (Fig. 51) As we look at the section of the ear from the skin to the cartilaginous portion we find that beneath the immediate epithelium the blood vessels of the corium and the lymphatics have become enormously distended. The blood vessel changes will be commented upon in the discussion of inflammation, but may be briefly summarized as showing an increase of leukocytes, which assume a marginal distribution in the vessels and tend to migrate into the surrounding tissue. In addition to these vascular phenomena, the entire subcutaneous tissues will be seen to be increased in thickness, perhaps four or five times over that of a normal ear. This increase in thickness is due almost entirely to the accumulation of fluids between the widely separated strands of collagen which make up the supporting connective tissue stroma of the corium. This is evidenced by a very fine, pink-staining granular precipitate which is almost homogeneous in appearance under the low power of the microscope. At times it may be difficult to differentiate this coagulated fluid from cross sections of the minute collagen fibrils. This is one of the most characteristic pictures of edema, in this instance, of a localized nature produced by a simple physical injury of the tissues.

CASE 22 (Ref. #S-14)

Diagnosis.—Lung—pulmonary edema.

Patient was a white female of 62 years who was admitted to the hospital in a comatose condition.

Present Illness.—The history which was obtained is somewhat unsatisfactory because it was given largely by a daughter of the patient who did not live with her mother and was not familiar with the entire history. However, the patient was in her usual health until about two years ago when she first noticed occasional periods of blindness of a transitory nature. For the two months before admission she had complained of tremors of her left arm and leg, which she could not control and which had been accompanied by a sensation of fear and nervousness. Associated with these nervous manifestations she had noticed occasional swelling of the right side of the face, particularly around the eye. On several occasions these neurologic symptoms reached a point where she had been unable to use the left side of her body. On the day of admission, she had lapsed slowly into unconsciousness.

Past History.—As far as the daughter was aware, her mother had never had any serious illness previously. She had had four children, all of whom were normal in their development. She had never had any operations. Her menstrual history had been entirely normal and she had had her menopause twelve years before admission.

Physical Examination.—Patient was an elderly white female lying in a comatose condition in bed. Her breath was stertorous and she could not be aroused. Her head appeared of normal contour. Pupils reacted very sluggishly to light. There was some apparent edema of the right cheek and around the eye. The ears, nose and throat, as well as they could be examined, appeared negative. Chest: Heart was definitely enlarged. The left border was in the anterior axillary line. There were no murmurs heard. Blood pressure was 160 systolic over 105 diastolic. The lungs showed numerous moist râles at both bases. In the upper lobe, particularly anteriorly, they appeared hyperresonant. No definite dullness was made out on percussion. Abdomen was negative. Extremities: Owing to the comatose condition of the patient it was difficult to make adequate neurologic examination. However, reflexes seemed to be present on the right side but to be absent on the left. Stimulation of the foot resulted in the drawing up of the leg on the right whereas on the left it remained flaccid.

Laboratory Findings.—Urinalysis: Specific gravity 1.010. There was a moderate trace of albumin. Otherwise, nothing of significance was noted. Blood chemistry: Blood urea 100 mgm./100 c.c. Red blood cells 3,100,000; Hemoglobin 65%. White blood cells 14,000 with 82% polynuclear leukocytes.

Subsequent Course.—Patient grew steadily worse. The chest filled up with fluid with resultant dullness at the bases of both lungs and a marked increase in moist râles throughout both sides. She died without regaining consciousness forty-eight hours after admission.

Autopsy Findings.—At autopsy there was what appeared to be an essential hypertensive cardiovascular renal picture. The heart was definitely hypertrophied. This enlargement was particularly marked involving the left ventricle. The kidneys showed a chronic nephrosclerosis with a good deal of scarring suggesting the possibility of coincidental glomerular disease. Lungs: There was marked congestion and terminal pulmonary edema. On section, the lungs were filled with clear, serous fluid which dripped profusely from the cut surface, as from a sponge. The immediate cause of death was felt to be a terminal uremia in conjunction with the chronic cardiorenal vascular picture. Examination of the brain showed a marked arteriosclerosis with thrombosis of the cerebral vessels resulting in several areas of softening.

Microscopic Description of Lung.—(Fig. 49) The lung in this case may serve as an example both of pulmonary edema and as the picture which corresponds to so-called "shock" as the terminal event in so many patients. The alveolar walls of the lungs show moderate thickening with considerable congestion of the capillaries. There is not the striking fibrosis of the alveolar walls noted in the previous case of chronic passive congestion of the lung due to mitral heart disease. More prominent, however, than the actual capillary changes is the picture of edema with the outpouring of serum into the lung alveoli. This is a particular type of edema in which there being no interstitial tissue, the fluid has accumulated in the air sacs rather than between the tissue cells. Microscopically, this serum is recognized as an almost homogeneous, pink-staining coagulant which practically fills all the alveoli. It will be observed that there is relatively little cellular reaction in this picture, only occasional leukocytes, mononuclear phagocytes and desquamated alveolar lining cells being found within the coagulated serum. A very small amount of hemosiderin here and there may be observed within macrophages, but the amount of pigment is negligible.

CHAPTER VI

CIRCULATORY DISTURBANCES

THROMBOSIS, EMBOLISM AND INFARCTION

In a further consideration of circulatory disturbances must be included a very important group which has obstruction of a mechanical nature within the vessel itself as the outstanding factor. Adequate consideration of this group of cases presupposes a thorough knowledge of the normal mechanism of blood coagulation. In this discussion only the simplest outline of the process is given to refresh the memory. Various theories regarding the clotting of blood have been developed in the course of the last century. For practical purposes we are inclined to follow the theory of Howell in respect to its mechanism. In its simplest form the theory requires that normally within the circulating blood fibrinogen, prothrombin and calcium are present. These are the essential factors which play a part in the formation of the clot through activation of the prothrombin by the calcium to form thrombin and the conversion of the soluble fibrinogen into the precipitated insoluble fibrin through the action of the thrombin. However, there is also present in the blood heparin (antithrombin), which acts to prevent the activation of prothrombin except when it, in turn, becomes neutralized by the so-called thromboplastic substance variously named as cephalin, thrombokinase, cytozyme and many other terms. This is derived from the injured tissue cells or, perhaps in part from the blood platelets. When this heparin is thus neutralized and made ineffectual, then the normal clotting process can go on undisturbed. Normally, this process of clotting is a defense mechanism of the body against injury and against the loss of blood through such injuries. Its mechanism results in the sealing of ruptured blood vessels and enables the other processes of repair and cell regeneration to proceed in normal physiological manner to heal the injured area.

Following death we find that the same processes of coagulation proceed in much the same fashion as in life and we find on the postmortem table that the blood within the vessel walls has undergone a type of clotting which is similar to the normal, except that this process is apt to be a slower one than occurs during life. As a result, through gravity, the cells of the blood tend to settle to the dependent portion of the vessels or the chambers of the heart and we have the formation of the typical postmortem "chicken fat" clot, which is characterized by a yellow, edematous, fibrinous clot in its upper portion, and in its dependent portion an accumulation of the red cells. The rate of clotting varies, however, in these cases and in patients who have died with a high fever, and in patients who have died as the result of a severe traumatic injury, we find that the blood clots very much more rapidly due to the liberation of the neutralizing tissue enzymes and the effect of heat, so that the clot appears as of a homogeneous, red color, without the separation, through gravity, into the two or three layers just described. They may still be recognized as postmortem in nature, however, because they are not adherent at any point to the endothelial lining of the circulatory system in contradistinction to the pathological clotting of blood known as thrombosis. At times, however, this process of coagulation, which is basically a defense mechanism, becomes a harmful one through obstruction to the circulation as will be shown in the following paragraphs.

THROMBOSIS

Thrombosis may be briefly defined as the intravascular clotting of blood during life. This requires considerable qualification, however, to give any adequate understanding of the process. It differs from extravascular and postmortem clotting in that there is some point of attachment to the endothelial lining

PLATE XIII
INFARCTION AND GANGRENE

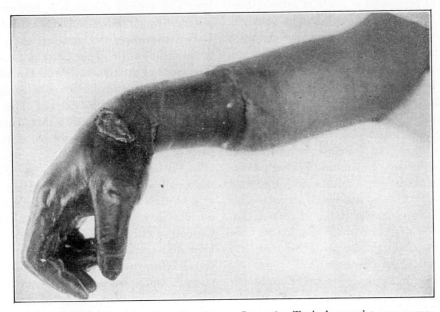

FIG. 54.—RIGHT FOREARM: DRY GANGRENE.—CASE 28.—Typical gauntlet appearance of lesion, the result of arterial embolism secondary to acute ulcerative bacterial endocarditis. The lesion shows the characteristic sharp line of demarcation between the gangrenous and normal tissues.

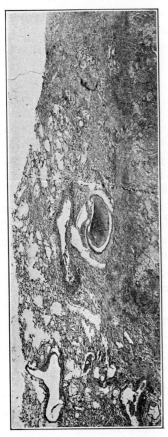

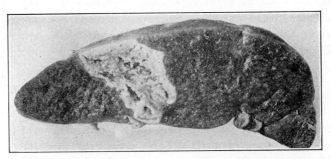

FIG. 55.—SPLEEN: INFARCT, ANEMIC.—CASE 24.—Section of spleen showing wedge-shaped area of infarction in the stage of healing, resulting from arterial embolism. (Cf. color Plate X, Fig. 43.)

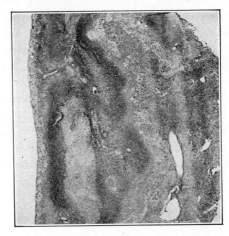

FIG. 56.—LUNG: INFARCTION, HEMORRHAGIC.—CASE 25.—Microtessar photograph showing edge of an hemorrhagic infarct together with the obstructed vessel. App. 10 x.

FIG. 57.—LIVER: INFARCTION, HEMORRHAGIC.—CASE 167.—Microtessar photograph of multiple irregular areas of infarction in acute periarteritis nodosa. App. 10 x.

of the vessel or heart wall at a site of intimal damage, whether traumatic, toxic or infectious in origin. Likewise, there is usually a progressive accretion of platelets derived from the moving blood stream, which produces a characteristic pattern with coral-like laminae instead of the usual simple intermeshing precipitation of fibrin.

Most commonly the process begins in a vein and shows an agglutination of platelets in anastomosing laminae upon the intimal lining of the vessel wall. This, in turn, attracts leukocytes. Through tissue enzymes, the normal clotting mechanism is instituted and fibrin precipitation occurs, which serves to give strength to this intravascular thrombotic blood clot. In the meshes of this fibrin are caught innumerable red cells as the fibrin precipitates. This completes the initial picture, the *red thrombus*.

As the red cells break down and disintegrate, the whole mass of fibrin, platelets, leukocytes and the red cell membranes undergoes hyaline degeneration and becomes a translucent, yellowish-gray, so-called *gray thrombus*. If the vessel is nearly or completely occluded by the primary thrombus formation the stagnant blood column beyond coagulates and becomes adherent to the original thrombus mass, again largely through the accretion of agglutinated plate-

lets. This type of thrombus is frequently termed a *propagating thrombus* and may extend all the way from the vessels of the lower extremity continuously to the right auricle of the heart in the extreme case. The point of attachment of this thrombus is spoken of as the *head,* and the free portion of clot within the blood vessel is called the *tail*. This is important in that part or all of such a thrombus may become detached and be carried in the blood stream to other parts of the body as emboli.

In the healing of a thrombus the endothelium of the vessel attempts to grow over the surface just as epithelium does in a denuded area of skin, to re-establish its continuity, and maintain the blood flow. Connective tissue likewise grows out from the sub-intimal layer to organize the mass of clot and convert it ultimately into adult connective tissue. In many instances when the thrombus has completely occluded the lumen, cords of endothelium will grow in from either end, fuse and form lumina from the pressure of the blood stream, just as in embryonic life, so that a certain amount of circulation may be reëstablished directly, as well as by the development of a collateral blood supply. This process is spoken of as *canalization* and will be studied again more specifically under the diseases of blood vessels.

EMBOLISM

Embolism may be defined as the obstruction of some part of the arterial system through impaction of any undissolved material brought there by the blood current. The commonest source of embolism is obviously a thrombus which becomes detached in part or in whole. In addition, bacteria, tumor cells, parasites and other substances introduced from without may act as emboli. In traumatic injuries, notably fractures of the long bones, fat globules or even air bubbles may cause death by blocking the blood supply to the vital centers in the brain stem.

The distribution of emboli naturally relates directly to their source. Those arising from the venous side of the circulation, the right auricle, the tricuspid and pulmonic valves obviously occur in the lung (unless there is a patent foramen which permits the passage of particles from the right to the left side of the heart). Those arising from the pulmo-

nary veins, the left auricle, mitral and aortic valves get into the systemic aorta and are carried to the extremities, the brain, spleen, kidney or other viscera depending on their size and the eddying of the blood current at the ostia of the branches of the aorta.

The importance of embolism varies directly with the location of the embolus in respect to the maintenance of circulation to the part supplied by the particular vessel involved. Where there is adequate anastomosis or a double blood supply as in the case of the liver or lung, such embolism is rarely permanently serious unless it involves a major vessel, as not infrequently occurs in pulmonary embolism. Practically it is only when non-anastomosing terminal vessels are involved that the process goes on to its full development, infarction. This is a direct result of anoxemia of the tissues, from interference with the arterial circulation.

ILLUSTRATIVE CASE

CASE 23. (Ref. #S-132)

Diagnosis.—Lung—pulmonary artery with embolus and organizing thrombus.

Patient was a 54 year old white male admitted to the hospital complaining of precordial pain and indigestion.

Present Illness.—Patient stated that he felt perfectly well up until the morning of his hospital admission. Following a rather hearty breakfast and having had to hurry to catch a train, he suddenly developed a severe pain in the epigastric region, which spread over the entire precordium. This was followed by nausea and vomiting, and his breathing became definitely impaired with a rapid, shallow type of respiration. He was rushed to the hospital by ambulance and at the time of admission was in such a state of acute distress that he was unable to talk.

Past History.—His father and mother both died at an age over seventy. No member of the family was known to have suffered from carcinoma, heart disease, Bright's disease or any form of central nervous disease.

Physical Examination.—Patient was a well developed, well nourished, middle-aged male lying in bed in acute distress. There was marked cyanosis around the neck and face. There was a suggestion of right facial weakness. The peripheral skin temperatures were lowered. The pupils were pin point in size but reacted normally to light and distance. His nose, ears and throat were negative. The chest was of the barrel type with equal expansion of both lungs. There was no dullness and, in fact, there was generalized hyperresonance. No râles were heard. Heart was not enlarged on percussion. The sounds were distant. There were no murmurs heard. Abdomen was negative. Extremities were negative.

Laboratory Findings.—Red blood cells 4,690,000 with 12.5 gm. (90%) hemoglobin. White blood cells 10,000 with 90% polynuclear leukocytes of which 20% were of the non-filamented form. Urinalysis: Specific gravity was 1.012 and there was a slight trace of albumin. Blood chemistry was negative. Wassermann was also negative.

Subsequent History.—On the day of admission, the patient's blood pressure was 116/86. The pain in the epigastric and precordial regions radiated during the course of the day down the left arm. This pain was relieved by morphine. During his stay in the hospital of nearly two months he developed a systolic murmur at the apex. His fluid intake was unsatisfactory and to maintain his fluid balance he was given intravenous glucose. This resulted in a thrombosis of the veins in both antecubital fossae. The patient had several minor repetitions of this picture of precordial pain with referred pain down the left arm and died during a similar severe attack.

Autopsy Findings.—At autopsy the chief points of importance were an old and a recent infarct of the heart, the result of coronary occlusion in the left anterior descending branch. The heart, itself, showed moderate enlargement. Within the right ventricle was found a large, coiled embolus measuring 8 cm. in length. One end appeared to be smooth while the other was rough and ragged and seemed to have broken away from some point of attachment. The lungs showed several areas of embolism with subsequent thrombosis and infarction. No other infarcts were noted. Examination of the veins in the antecubital fossae showed the presence of practically obliterating thrombi, one of which had a rough surface corresponding closely to the surface of the clot found within the left ventricle. The cause of death in this case was primarily the acute myocardial infarction, but it was complicated by the presence of multiple pulmonary areas of thrombosis and secondary infarction.

Microscopic Description of Lung.—(Fig. 52 and 53) The section includes a large sized branch of the pulmonary artery with considerable surrounding lung tissue. The lumen of the vessel is completely occluded by a thrombus. This is easily recognized by the characteristic, curiously laminated arrangement of the clot. The picture suggests a combined lesion representing an original embolic phenomenon with the thrombus having arisen from some other source and being carried by the blood stream to the lung. This is borne out by the appearance of the thrombus itself, which shows a central gray portion which is of older duration, whereas around the periphery and at its point of attachment to the pulmonary arterial wall the more recent red picture is paramount. Under high power, the coral-like laminae of hyalinized platelets and fibrin are clearly observed. At the point of attachment it can be seen that the endothelium of the intima has completely disappeared. The lesion has been present at that point for some little time as there is marked subintimal connective tissue proliferation, which is beginning to grow out into the thrombus in an attempt at organizing the lesion. Microscopically, the histology confirms the clinical history and autopsy findings. It points to an embolic origin for the lesion, with the secondary development of a slowly growing thrombosis in this branch of the pulmonary artery.

INFARCTION

By this term, we mean the resultant death of the tissues which have been deprived of their blood supply through *arterial* obstruction. The commonest cause of infarction is embolism, which occurs suddenly and, in general, does not permit of the establishment of a collateral blood supply to maintain the nourishment of the tissues. A literal translation of the word embolism indicates a "stuffing" with blood. This is, theoretically at least, what occurs in the infarcted area, but in those organs in which there is a terminal arterial blood supply such as the kidney, spleen, heart and brain, this picture of an increased amount of blood is not apparent except around the edges of the lesion. In organs such as the lungs or liver, this "stuffing" with red cells is usually a very prominent feature of the lesion due to the extraordinary extent of the anastomotic or supplementary blood supply as in the case of the hepatic artery and the portal circulation, or the pulmonary and bronchial double vascular supply.

Infarcts are classified on the basis of their gross appearance as either *red* or *white;* in other words, as *hemorrhagic* or *anemic.* As has been suggested from the above discussion, infarction occurring in the lung (Fig. 44, 46 and 56) or liver (Fig. 57) is usually of the red or hemorrhagic type due to the double blood supply, while those of the kidney (Fig. 43 and 45) are usually of the white, or anemic type. In the spleen it is very common to find an initial red infarct which gradually becomes anemic (Fig. 55) as the process goes on. This is dependent upon the diffuse blood supply of the pulp with its freely anastomosing vascular channels.

In infarction we find that the cells, through the loss of their blood supply and a persistent anoxemia, undergo all the degenerative changes which we have thus far studied; viz.: fatty, granular and hydropic. These degenerative features, however, are carried far beyond the simple reversible phase which we have seen to date. In addition to the cytoplasmic changes the nuclei likewise undergo degeneration and with the loss of nuclear function the cells actually die and disintegrate. Where this occurs the architecture of the normal structures gradually becomes lost and the entire area involved, particularly if supplied by an endartery such as we find in the spleen, presents a wedge-shaped area of necrosis. The edges of these areas at the outset usually show the presence of many red cells and an influx of polymorphonuclear leukocytes, which take part in the reaction in an attempt to clear up the necrotic tissue. Gradually connective tissue grows in from the sides of the infarcted area accompanied by the formation of new capillaries and the end picture of such an infarcted area, if it does not affect a vital structure such as the brain stem, is a fibrous scar comparable to the familiar scar seen in the skin following a cut or other injury.

ILLUSTRATIVE CASES

CASE 24. (Ref. #S-82)

Diagnosis.—Kidney—infarction, anemic.

Patient was a white woman of 55 years, who was admitted to the hospital complaining of severe headache and weakness, which came on suddenly while sitting at the breakfast table.

Present Illness.—The present illness really dated back to a period about six months before when she complained of a sharp pain in the lumbar region. This was so severe that she nearly fainted and had to go to bed for several days. The pain gradually subsided and she was able to get around the house and do her ordinary work. During this period she had symptoms pointing definitely to impaired cardiac function with dyspnea and periods of palpitation. Bed rest, however, seemed to improve her condition so that she had never called a physician to take care of her during any of these attacks. She had several similar episodes during the six months' interval up to the acute cerebral accident which brought her to the hospital. Even at that time she did not lose consciousness and did not call a physician until a neighbor insisted.

Past History.—The past history was apparently irrelevant as far as her present illness was concerned. Both her father and mother lived to old age and there was no history of cardiorenal vascular disease in any of the members of her family. She was one of nine brothers and three sisters, seven of whom were older than she and had died of various causes. She had had high blood pressure for several years and had been unable to work except around the house. A review of her systems was essentially negative. She had never been heart conscious until the past six months. She had had no serious upper respiratory infections and did not think that she ever suffered from rheumatic fever. Her gastro-intestinal history had been uneventful. Genito-urinary history was likewise normal. Menstrual history did not enter into this picture as she had had her menopause eight years before admission.

Physical Examination.—On admission, the patient seemed dizzy and confused. She was somewhat irrational at times and had difficulty in expressing herself. Her head was of normal contour. Eyes, ears, nose and throat showed nothing abnormal. Chest was symmetrical. Lungs showed numerous râles at both bases but no impairment of resonance or any change in breath sounds. Heart was definitely enlarged to the left. Heart sounds were of poor quality. The auricular rate was impossible to count and it was felt that the patient had auricular fibrillation.

Laboratory Findings.—Blood count on admission showed 3,600,000 red blood cells with 70% hemoglobin and 16,000 white blood cells with 87% polynuclear leukocytes. Urinalysis showed a trace of albumin and a high specific gravity of 1.022. Blood urea was 45 mgm.

Subsequent Course.—The patient grew rapidly worse in the hospital, losing consciousness and going into a deep coma from which she failed to awaken, dying twenty-four hours after admission.

Autopsy Findings.—At autopsy the outstanding features noted were first of all a cerebral thrombosis, a markedly enlarged heart with a large auricular appendiceal thrombus, and old anemic infarcts of the spleen and kidney. There was a rather striking generalized arteriosclerosis.

Microscopic Description of the Infarcted Area in the Right Kidney.—(Fig. 43 and 45) Examination of the area of infarction in the kidney shows a typical anemic picture. It is possible to determine three distinct zones in examining this tissue. At the periphery of the area of infarction the essentially normal kidney tissue is identified. There is, however, evidence of marked arteriosclerosis present with narrowing of the lumina of the larger blood vessels and considerable interstitial connective tissue increase. It will also be noted that there is compensatory dilatation of the smaller blood vessels which represent the anastomosing branches of the smaller arteries and arterioles. In the area at the very edge of the infarct, there is a zone of frank hemorrhage and leukocytic infiltration. This is the result of the outpouring of blood cells from the anastomosing branches. Centrally, we find the actual infarcted tissue with necrosis. This infarct is still comparatively recent and as a result the necrosis has not gone on to completion, nor has fibrous tissue replacement scarring become a prominent feature. Under high-power examination of the tissue, it can be seen that the nuclear and cytoplasmic details of the individual cells have become lost and in many places have faded out altogether so that cell outlines have completely disappeared. The area of infarction is obviously non-functioning renal tissue, but the renal structures may still be faintly observed. It is of interest further to see how definitely outlined this wedge-shaped lesion is with a narrow zone of persistent, relatively normal renal tissue overlying the cortical portion of the infarct. This narrow zone has a blood supply from the capsular vessels and for that reason fails to be included in the infarct, which resulted from occlusion of the renal vessel within the substance of the kidney itself.

Case 25. (Ref. #S-18)
Diagnosis.—Lung—pulmonary infarct, hemorrhagic.
Patient was a white male of 44 years, who was admitted to the hospital with the chief complaint of dyspnea.

Present Illness.—The onset of the present illness began ten months before admission when he first noticed dyspnea on exertion with inability to climb two flights of stairs without stopping to rest half way up. By the end of three months this dyspnea had increased to such a point that it necessitated his stopping work and he was in bed off and on for the next six months until his present admission. He had a sense of constriction in his chest with occasional attacks of substernal pain. He had lost thirty pounds in weight during this illness, and he had noticed definite nocturia two to three times a night and an associated polydipsia.

Past History.—The patient's past history was difficult to evaluate. He did not recall any serious illness, even as a child, except for an attack of influenza in 1918 during the epidemic, when he was confined to bed for about six weeks. He had not had any other illness or operation. His family history was also negative. His occupational history was of no significance in respect to his illness. He had always worked as a clerk and had not done any heavy physical work for many years.

Physical Examination.—The patient was a middle-aged white male who was extremely dyspneic and apprehensive. His head was normal. Eyes, ears, nose and throat were negative except for the fact that he had very poorly cared for teeth with marked caries. Lungs were clear throughout with no râles. Heart was greatly enlarged. The left border was percussed in the anterior axillary line. There was a loud systolic murmur heard at the mitral area. There was a gallop rhythm with numerous extra-systoles. Blood pressure was 210/130.

Abdomen: Liver was moderately enlarged being three finger breadths below the costal margin in the anterior axillary line. The genitalia were negative. Extremities showed a small amount of ankle edema.

Laboratory Findings.—Urinalysis showed constant albuminuria of rather marked grade accompanied by occasional granular casts. Blood count was 4,300,000 red blood cells with 15 gm. (97%) hemoglobin. White blood cells 9,700 with 68% lymphocytes. Wassermann was negative. Blood chemistry: Urea nitrogen 21 mgm. Electrocardiogram showed an auricular flutter with right bundle branch block.

Subsequent Course.—The patient improved temporarily under digitalis and bed rest, but this was only temporary in its effect. His dyspnea returned with greater severity and was accompanied by an increase of the edema in the feet and ankles. He developed terminal auricular fibrillation and a generalized anasarca with cardiac failure and died approximately one month after admission.

Autopsy Findings.—At autopsy there was found a very markedly hypertrophied heart with a very striking rheumatic endocarditis involving principally the pulmonary artery, although to a very much more limited extent the other three valves. There was an associated right auricular mural thrombosis and a left ventricular mural thrombus. There was marked hypertrophy of the muscle wall, particularly on the right side of the heart. Multiple infarcts were found in the lungs, spleen and kidneys, and there was a picture of rather marked chronic vascular nephrosclerosis of the so-called essential hypertensive arteriolar type.

Microscopic Description of Section from the Lung Showing an Infarct.—(Fig. 44, 46 and 56) Microscopically, sections are taken through the marginal zone of one of the infarcted areas of the lung. They show a similar process to that noted in the preceding renal infarct except that the picture is much more hemorrhagic in nature. The lung alveolar outlines are faintly identified, but as in the preceding case, the cell detail has been lost and only a shadowy network of tissue remains to identify it as lung. Filling all the alveolar spaces and actually replacing apparently many of the alveolar walls which have become completely destroyed is a mass of hemorrhage which shows varying degrees of disintegration. Here and there some pigment formation may be observed with the presence of mononuclear phagocytes in the peripheral portion of the infarct. This enormously hemorrhagic picture is the result of the combined anastomotic blood supply from interlacing, overlapping pulmonary arterioles coupled with a bronchial arterial extravasation of blood as well. That the process has been present for some time is seen by the amount of disruption of the red cells and the beginning fibrosis observed in part of the periphery of the tissue.

May we refer back at this time to Case 2, Chapter 1 (Fig. 35 and 40) showing a late anemic infarct of the spleen. This tissue was previously studied for the presence of hematoidin, but represents an identical process to that in the two cases just presented.

CHAPTER VII
PART I
NECROSIS AND GANGRENE

NECROSIS

By necrosis is meant the death of localized collections of cells within the living body as, for example, an abscess. This may be the result of many different factors. Among the most important are those relating to the circulatory apparatus as has been brought out in the preceding chapter under a consideration of infarction, which represents a very definite type of necrosis. The dead tissue in such localized areas of necrosis is spoken of as a *sphacelus* when it involves soft tissues, and as a *sequestrum* when it involves bone. Necrosis has been divided into various forms dependent chiefly upon the causative factors involved. Among the more characteristic and specific types of necrosis should be included the following.

Coagulation Necrosis.—(Fig. 40, 43, 45 and 55) By coagulation necrosis is meant that type of necrosis seen particularly as the result of anemic infarction, where the entire blood supply is cut off, usually suddenly, by an embolus. Typically, within the infarcted area, the cytoplasm of the cells undergoes coagulation through the action of the liberated intracellular enzymes. This results, as has been observed in the discussion of infarction, in the temporary preservation of the underlying architectural detail of the tissues until such time as they completely disintegrate. Grossly, such an area of coagulation necrosis, whether the result of infarction or some other cause, appears dry and opaque.

Liquefaction Necrosis.—(Fig. 61) By this term is meant that type of necrosis in which the necrotic material becomes softened and liquefied. Gradually it will even become absorbed often leaving cystic areas. This is the usual type of necrosis seen in the central nervous system, but is also found in the marginal areas of infarcts, particularly in the more hemorrhagic type of infarction as well as in many inflammatory exudates. Here the causative

bacteria with their exotoxins or endotoxins as well as the proteolytic enzymes of the leukocytes are factors in the production of this liquefaction picture. An example of such liquefaction necrosis may be seen in the simple staphylococcic abscess as represented by the familiar furuncle or boil.

Caseation or Caseous Necrosis.—(Fig. 58 and 59) By this term is meant a peculiar type of focal, avascular, slow coagulation necrosis especially associated with tuberculosis and syphilis. In this form, the necrotic tissue presents a soft, dry, cheesy appearance similar to that of coagulated casein, as the curd of cottage cheese. This curious appearance is due largely to the high fat content of the lesion as a result both of the lipoid material surrounding the bacteria and of the character of the inflammatory exudate, which is largely composed of mononuclear cells rather than the polynuclear leukocytes with their liquefying proteolytic enzymes. This monocytic series of inflammatory cells possesses other characteristic functions largely being related to phagocytosis or the absorption of foreign material rather than to its dissolution by enzymic action. Gradually this lipoid material breaks down, saponifies and ultimately undergoes calcification or fibrosis.

Fat Necrosis.—(Fig. 60) By fat necrosis is ordinarily meant that process which develops as the result of liberation of pancreatic lipase following injury to the pancreas. Such injury may result from occlusion of the pancreatic duct by stone or other extraneous pressure with the backing up of bile to activate the fat-splitting enzyme. This pancreatic lipase, escaping from the normal duct system, acts upon those fat cells with which it comes in contact to produce a characteristic type of necrosis. The necrosis appears in the pancreatic interstitial fat, in the subperitoneal fat and in the omentum, as opaque white, chalky lesions. In the pancreas these

PLATE XIV

NECROSIS

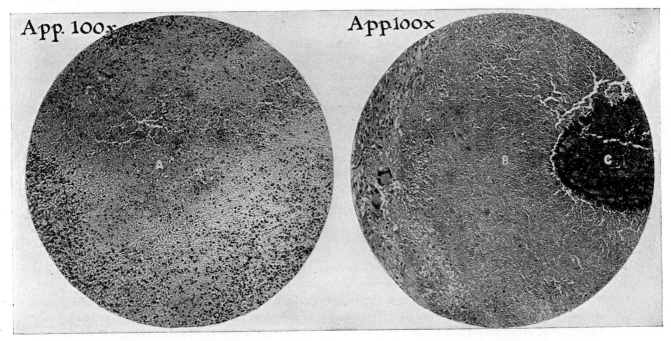

FIG. 58.—LUNG: CASEOUS NECROSIS (CASEATION).—CASE 30.—
TUBERCULOSIS.—Caseous necrosis (A) in rapidly spreading tuberculosis, with but slight cellular response and absence of giant
cells. App. 100 x.

FIG. 59.—LYMPH NODE: CALCIFICATION IN CASEOUS TUBERCULOSIS.
—CASE 30.—Caseous tubercle (B) with central area of calcification (C) and peripheral cellular reaction and giant cell formation (A). App. 100 x.

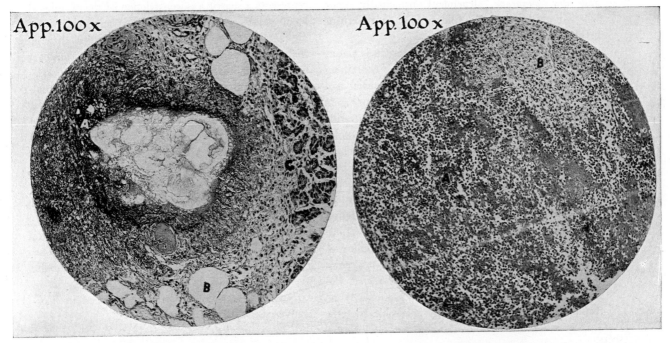

FIG. 60.—PANCREAS: FAT NECROSIS.—CASE 27.—A central mass of
typical fat necrosis with peripheral zone of hemorrhage (A)
surrounded by uninvolved fat cells (B) and pancreatic parenchyma (C). App. 100 x.

FIG. 61.—LUNG: ABSCESS.—LIQUEFACTION NECROSIS.—CASE 26.—
Wall of abscess cavity showing coagulation necrosis at B;
liquefaction necrosis with pus formation at A. App. 100 x.

lesions are apt to be surrounded by a zone of acute inflammation with marked secondary polymorphonuclear leukocytic infiltration so that they become complicated by liquefaction necrosis. Just as in the case of caseation where the lesion is not too extensive in the pancreas to cause the death of the patient, the lesion ultimately shows a type of healing. The fat is split into fatty acids and glycerol, undergoes saponification and ultimately either becomes calcified or replaced by connective scar tissue.

In addition to the fat necrosis just described above in relation to pancreatic injury, we may also have fat necrosis involving any of the adipose tissue, particularly appearing in the subcutaneous regions and the breast as the result of trauma. These cases usually present a picture more of acute and chronic inflammation than they do of simple fat necrosis. This is the result of the extensive injury to the surrounding structures, associated with hemorrhage and leukocytic invasion. Basically, however, the actual destruction of the fat cells may proceed in the same manner, by liberation of the fat, through its subsequent breakdown, and saponification to its ultimate calcification.

GANGRENE

The term *gangrene* covers a variety of lesions which makes its definition particularly difficult and complex. In its simplest form, gangrene may be defined as necrosis plus putrefaction. However, ordinarily by gangrene we mean either first, the rather specialized type of cell death seen in an extremity as the result of an inadequate blood supply; or second, the liquefaction necrosis of some organ or part of an organ such as the appendix or the lung due to the action of putrefactive bacteria. Gangrene, accordingly, may occur in two types, *moist gangrene* and *dry gangrene,* dependent principally upon whether or not there is fluid present in the tissue involved.

Moist Gangrene.—By moist gangrene is meant that type of gangrene occurring in tissues containing fluid, particularly in areas where both arterial and venous injury are present. Such conditions as a strangulated hernia, volvulus of the small intestine or compound fracture of an extremity are examples in which moist gangrene is usually observed. There is rapid autolysis of the dead tissues with the production of indol, skatol, sulfide of iron and other chemical products which result in a marked discoloration of the area and an associated foul, putrefactive odor. Death of the individual is very apt to follow as the result of the absorption of the complicated toxins which are elaborated.

Gas Gangrene.—By gas gangrene is meant the special type of moist gangrene seen particularly in traumatic wounds and caused by anaerobic bacteria such as the *Clostridium Welchii.* This was a very important type of gangrene seen in war injuries as the result of deep wounds from shell fragments and the like.

Dry Gangrene.—By this term is meant that type of gangrene usually seen in an extremity particularly in old age where the vascular supply is slowly shut off through obliteration of the lumen of the vessels by atherosclerosis and in which no collateral circulation exists. This type of lesion may be seen in such trophic disturbances as Raynaud's Disease, which represents a spastic vasoconstriction of the peripheral blood vessels resulting essentially in gangrene of the digits. The tissues are dry so that bacteria develop their putrefactive changes very slowly. The part becomes dry, black and mummified. The discoloration results from the bacterial action on the hemolyzed hemoglobin to form iron sulfide. There is a sharp line of demarcation between the devitalized and the living tissue (see Fig. 54). The lives of cases suffering from this type of gangrene may very frequently be saved by the amputation of the extremity well above the gangrenous line so that maintenance of the vitality of the tissues may be preserved and absorption of the necrotic, gangrenous by-products may not result in profound toxemia and death. Such gangrene is often associated with diabetes or with simple senility, or may be the result of embolic phenomena involving the terminal arteries of an extremity as is unusually well exemplified in illustrative case #28.

NECROBIOSIS

The histologic criteria to determine whether or not cell death has occurred may well be considered at this point. The death of a single cell is spoken of as *necrobiosis,* whereas the death of a tissue in part or in whole is spoken of as *necrosis.* Thus far, we have observed the numerous metabolic degenerative changes which may affect the cytoplasm of the cell principally. These consist of fatty, hydropic and granular degenerations, and these changes may be reversible up to a certain point. That point is established when we find microscopic evidence of nuclear degenerative changes which are irreversible. Of these changes, the following are the most significant.

Karyolysis (Chromatolysis).—By this term is meant the gradual swelling of the nucleus with a loss of the normal chromatin granules and rods. These appear first to become concentrated around the nuclear membrane. Gradually, even this chromatin material disintegrates and apparently dissolves. The final stage of this type of nuclear degeneration is seen with the slow disintegration of the nuclear membrane or of its rupture and subsequent disappearance. At times, such karolytic changes may cause the nucleus of the cell to completely fill the entire cell substance with the cytoplasm condensed around the cell membrane. Usually accompanying these nuclear changes are such extensive degenerative changes affecting the cytoplasm that the cell membrane likewise becomes disrupted and the entire cell disintegrates and disappears.

Pyknosis.—By this term is meant roughly the reverse of karyolysis. The nucleus shrinks in size with condensation of its chromatin until it appears as a solid mass without any nuclear detail. Accompanying this frequently the cell cytoplasm likewise undergoes either condensation with extensive granular degeneration or it may show any of the other fatty or hydropic changes previously described.

Karyorrhexis.—By this term is meant a form of pyknosis in which chromatin, after undergoing this curious condensation, breaks up into minute, deeply staining, formless granules. These are gradually extruded from the cytoplasm of the cell and appear in the tissue spaces as formless masses of pyknotic chromatin, which are attacked by phagocytic cells and are dissolved by the action of the proteolytic enzymes.

These various changes, karyolytic or karyorrhectic in nature, represent obviously definite physico-chemical changes within the cell and are dependent in their development upon alterations in cell membrane permeability, in hydrogen-ion concentration and in differences in concentration of colloids and electrolytes in the surrounding tissues. From the histopathological standpoint, however, the important point to remember is that when these degenerative changes affect the nucleus of a cell, that cell has undergone or is undergoing cell death, or necrobiosis. The predominance of one or the other of these various nuclear degenerative changes may influence us in our interpretation of the particular mechanism involved in any given case and on that account give us some opportunity of making an etiologic diagnosis. However, whether or not we are able to interpret these changes from a differential diagnostic standpoint, the fact remains that we are dealing here with a very fundamental biological process, the whole mechanism of cell death.

ILLUSTRATIVE CASES

As examples of coagulation necrosis, CASE 2, Chapter I, Fig. 40, 43, 45 and 55, and CASE 24, Chapter VI, of infarction of the spleen and kidney respectively serve admirably to illustrate the features of coagulation necrosis.

CASE 26. (Ref. #S-32)

Diagnosis.—Lung—multiple abscesses.

Patient was a 28 year old colored male admitted to the hospital because of severe sore throat.

Present Illness.—The present illness began ten days before admission as an ordinary sore throat. This became much worse with enormous swelling of the throat so that the patient had difficulty in swallowing and talking. A local physician diagnosed it as a retrotonsillar abscess and seventy-two hours after its onset, he lanced it.

Forty-eight hours later, the patient developed high fever with chills and sweating and was so ill that he was referred to the hospital on the following day.

Past History.—The past history is irrelevant. The patient had never been particularly susceptible to sore throats or upper respiratory infections. He had the usual childhood diseases, including scarlet fever, measles and whooping cough. A review of his systems otherwise added nothing of value in respect to his current illness.

Physical Examination.—Patient was a young colored male, who could swallow and talk only with great difficulty. He was in a clammy perspiration and during the examination had a definite chill. His head was normal in outline. Eyes and ears were negative. Examination of his nose and throat showed a markedly enlarged left tonsil with pus exuding from the crypts. The right tonsil was also enlarged, but was considerably smaller than the left as the result of two incisions which were draining freely apparently from a peritonsillar or retrotonsillar abscess. There was a moderate bilateral cervical adenopathy with the glands somewhat tender on palpation. The chest was symmetrical. Lungs showed no dullness. There were a few scattered râles most marked at the right apex. The heart was not enlarged. The sounds were normal. There were no murmurs. Blood pressure was 110/70. The abdomen was negative. The extremities were negative.

Laboratory Findings.—Urinalysis showed a specific gravity of 1.010, a trace of albumin but no sugar. There were a few granular casts and leukocytes. The blood picture showed a red count of 4,600,000 with hemoglobin of 92%. White blood cells 11,500 with 78% polynuclear leukocytes. Throat cultures yielded a predominance of Streptococcus viridans and hemolytic Influenza bacillus. Blood culture was negative at the end of forty-eight hours.

Subsequent Course.—During the following twenty-four hours, the patient developed signs of definite infection of the lung, more marked at the right base. Here, dullness developed with increased tactile and vocal fremitus. Breath sounds became bronchial in character. There was a normal Queckenstedt on the right, but none on the left. A diagnosis of thrombosis of the left internal jugular vein was made. This was exposed under local anesthesia and tied off. The patient was given several immune serum transfusions but died a week after admission with a typical septic picture and a suggestion of lung abscess.

Autopsy Findings.—At autopsy, the body was that of a small, emaciated young colored male. There was a hemolytic jaundice present in the sclerae. The scar of the left internal jugular operation was still open. The heart was negative. The lungs showed many sharply circumscribed yellowish areas of necrosis with pus formation ranging from one to three centimeters in diameter. These were spread throughout the right lung and several similar small lesions found in the opposite lung. There was associated terminal edema, congestion and bronchopneumonia around the multiple abscesses. The abdominal viscera showed several acute beginning areas of infarction. They were markedly congested and presented a picture of generalized sepsis.

Microscopic Description of Section from Lung.—(Fig. 61) Section from lung shows a typical picture of multiple abscess formation. This is the result of an upper respiratory infection with inhalation of the infected material. The organisms have obviously landed in the terminal bronchioles or atria and have there set up their characteristic acute inflammatory reaction. The nature of the inflammatory process with extensive liquefaction necrosis suggests strongly a secondary Staphylococcus infection, as these organisms are most prone to produce this type of lesion. It will be noted that there is in each of the characteristic abscessed areas a central zone of complete liquefaction necrosis where no viable cells can be identified, the whole material consisting of broken down necrotic cellular detritus undergoing dissolution. Around the edges of the abscess cavity recognizable polymorphonuclear leukocytes and large mononuclear phagocytic cells can be seen. The bronchial mucosa or lung tissue in each instance as the case may be has been likewise

completely destroyed by the reactive process, and the proteolytic enzymes have broken down these structures. Surrounding the immediate zone of abscess formation may be seen a secondary acute inflammatory exudative pneumonia with the lung alveoli filled with leukocytes, fibrin and red cells. There is an attempt at connective tissue proliferation to wall off the local abscess formation, but due to the acute nature of the process, this has not had time to progress to a very marked degree.

CASE 27. (Ref. #S-73 and 78)
Diagnosis.—Pancreas—acute hemorrhagic pancreatitis with fat necrosis.

Patient was a white woman of 62 years, who was admitted to the hospital because of acute upper abdominal pain associated with persistent vomiting.

Present Illness.—The present illness began forty-eight hours before admission with a sudden attack of vomiting and pain in the upper abdomen. This was most marked in the upper left quadrant. The vomitus was composed of bile stained material. The pain had been of a colic-like variety and had not radiated in any particular direction.

Past History.—As a child the patient had the usual childhood illnesses but was rather indefinite as to detail. She had always been in reasonably good health and had never been hospitalized before. A review of her systems brought out a few points of possible suggestive significance. She had never been subject to upper respiratory infections to any extent. She had not been aware of any cardiovascular disturbances. She had had a history of qualitative dyspepsia for many years associated with marked constipation which had required the use of radical catharsis (Epsom salts) at about three or four day intervals. Her appetite had been variable and she had developed a cautiousness regarding fatty and fried foods, which seemed to bring on her dyspeptic attacks. Her genito-urinary history had been normal up to the last few months when she had noticed an increased frequency and rather scanty urine with considerable burning sensation. Her menstrual history was always normal and she had had her menopause about eight years before admission.

Physical Examination.—The patient was an elderly appearing white female lying in bed in obvious discomfort and with marked apprehension on her facies. She appeared acutely ill although she had a normal temperature, but an elevated pulse rate. Her head was negative. Eyes, ears, nose and throat were normal. She had an upper artificial denture. Her tongue was badly coated. Chest was symmetrical with some suggestion of senile emphysema. Lungs were clear. Heart was not enlarged. Heart sounds seemed of poor quality and were distant. There were no murmurs. Abdomen was markedly distended. There was a definite suggestion of fluid and dullness in both flanks with tympany above and with pain and tenderness throughout the abdomen, but particularly marked in the left upper quadrant. There were no masses palpable because of the tenderness. Extremities: There was a rheumatoid arthritis of the small joints of the hands. The extremities otherwise were negative.

Laboratory Findings.—Red blood cells 5,120,000; hemoglobin 88%. White blood cells 19,450 with 95% polynuclear leukocytes of which 42% were nonfilamented forms. Urinalysis showed a slight trace of albumin but was otherwise negative.

Subsequent Course.—A tentative diagnosis of acute pancreatitis was made and an emergency exploratory laparotomy was done. At operation there was found to be a recurrent cholecystitis superimposed upon an old, chronic lesion with marked thickening of the gallbladder wall. The gallbladder was opened and drained and seventeen small gallstones were removed. The common duct likewise was opened and a large stone approximately 1 cm. in diameter was found in the ampulla where it had acted in ball-valve fashion so that no jaundice had developed. There were scattered areas of fat necrosis noted in the omentum and around the peritoneum in the vicinity of the pancreas. The pancreas itself appeared considerably thickened and showed diffuse hemorrhage into its substance. The patient went downhill very rapidly and died during the same night.

Autopsy Findings.—The outstanding pathology was found to be an acute hemorrhagic pancreatitis with extensive fat necrosis of the mesentery, omentum and retroperitoneal fat. There was generalized arteriosclerosis noted. The heart and lungs appeared essentially normal except for a terminal edema and congestion representing the picture of postoperative shock. The abdominal viscera otherwise showed no significant changes except for the gallbladder, which has already been described in the operative procedure.

Microscopic Description of Pancreas and Surrounding Retroperitoneal Fat Tissue.—(Fig. 60) Microscopic examination of the pancreas reveals a diffuse necrotic picture associated with extensive hemorrhage. In places, the pancreatic acinar structure is completely lost and the tissue has undergone what amounts almost to liquefaction necrosis. More characteristic and typical of the process, however, is the picture seen in the interstitial fat between the pancreatic lobules and in the retroperitoneal and mesenteric fat. Here, as a result of the breakdown of the pancreatic duct system through the backing up of the bile into the duct with the activation of the pancreatic lipase, the characteristic picture of fat necrosis has resulted. Pancreatic lipase has escaped into the surrounding tissue and there has acted upon the normal fat cells to cause beginning digestive changes. This consists essentially of the breakdown of the fat into fatty acids and the release of the glycerol fraction. This has been followed by the saponification of the fatty acids through the deposition of soluble mineral salts. The result is seen in the opaque appearance of the fat with the degeneration of the fat cells as such. The nuclei have disappeared. The cell membranes for the most part have been ruptured and undergone secondary degeneration so that only here and there may they be identified. The mass of free fat is seen then, as rather blackish granular staining material, which represents the necrotic, saponified material. These areas of fat necrosis vary in size and extent considerably, but in their essential histology are the same in their microscopic appearance.

CASE 28. (Ref. #S-301)
Diagnosis.—Hand—dry gangrene.
Patient was a 25-year-old colored female who was admitted to the hospital because of a sudden, sharp pain in her right arm associated with numbness and tingling of the fingers and subsequent loss of sensation with beginning discoloration of the hand.

Past History.—The patient, as a child, had been subject to repeated attacks of tonsillitis. This was accompanied at the age of about five with a marked chorea, which persisted for over a year and then spontaneously subsided, although it had required bed care most of the time. She was not aware of any definite heart disease following the chorea but had noticed in the past few years that she had had some dyspnea on exertion. She had had no other serious illness requiring hospitalization and had not had any operation other than the removal of her tonsils. A review of her systems gave no additional information. Her menstrual history was normal, having begun at the age of twelve and having been regular without any dysmenorrhea.

Physical Examination.—Patient was a well-developed, well-nourished, young, light-colored Negress, who was lying in bed without any apparent discomfort. Her head was normal in contour. Eyes, ears, nose and throat were negative. Her teeth were in good condition. There was no appreciable adenopathy. Chest was symmetrical with well developed breasts. Lungs were clear throughout. There were no râles heard. There was no dullness or change in voice or breath sounds. Heart was definitely enlarged, the left border being at the anterior axillary line in the fifth interspace. There was a blowing systolic murmur best heard over the mitral area and transmitted to the axilla. The abdomen was moderately protuberant, and the liver edge was felt two fingers' breadth below the costal margin. It was not tender. The spleen could not be felt. No pathology was noted in the lower extremities. The left arm appeared normal. The right arm showed a definite beginning blackish discoloration of the fingers and the skin of the back of the hand. There was a sharp line of demarcation at the wrist level. Below this point no pulse could be felt. Above this point, the pulse was perceptible but was markedly diminished in volume.

Laboratory Findings.—Red blood cells 4,600,000; hemoglobin 83%. White blood cells 12,600 with 86% polynuclear leukocytes. Urinalysis was negative. Blood chemistry was within normal limits. Wassermann was negative.

Subsequent Course.—During the course of the next few days there developed a complete dry gangrene of the right hand and wrist with a typical gauntlet appearance. There was a sharp line of demarcation between the normal and gangrenous tissues. The patient refused amputation and was treated conservatively during this period. She died suddenly with evidence of cerebral pathology.

Autopsy Findings.—At autopsy there was found an old chronic rheumatic valvulitis involving the mitral valve exclusively. Superimposed upon this was a terminal acute bacterial endocarditis with chronic ulcerative vegetations. This acute endocarditic process extended to involve the wall of the right auricle and there was an extensive auricular appendiceal thrombus. The immediate cause of death was found to be an embolus involving the brain stem. The lungs, liver, spleen and kidneys all showed rather marked chronic passive congestion as a result of the long continued rheumatic mitral lesion. An anemic infarct in the kidney was also found at autopsy. The vessels of the right arm were dissected and an embolus with subsequent thrombosis was found at the bifurcation of the brachial artery with a large, saddle-like embolus blocking both major branches. This accounted for the marked gangrenous process involving the entire hand and lower arm (Fig. 54).

CALCIFICATION

Calcium metabolism is one of the extremely complex metabolic mechanisms of the body as yet poorly understood. The parathyroids and the vitamins both seem to have some regulating mechanism to help maintain a constant blood calcium content. This normal level is maintained even by withdrawing calcium from the bones if there is a deficient intake to maintain the regular balance. Excess calcium in the diet seems to be of little effect in elevating the blood calcium except in a transient fashion. Excess parathyroid activity or the injection of its active principle, parathormone, results in hypercalcemia by excess withdrawal of calcium from the bones and the subsequent deposition of this calcium pathologically in abnormal situations. This is spoken of as metastatic calcification and such lesions may occur in any of the viscera or body tissues.

The normal process of calcification, as applied to bone formation, should be termed *ossification* in contradistinction to the abnormal deposition of calcium in other places which is more accurately spoken of as calcification. The calcium ratio of nine parts phosphate to one part carbonate is maintained, however, no matter where the deposition of calcium occurs either physiologically as in bone formation or pathologically as in metastatic lesions.

Whether the physical factors or the chemical factors are the more significant in determining localization of such calcification is still a source of controversy. Probably both physical and chemical actions are equally important. It is certain that localization of pathological calcium deposition is dependent upon severe injury or death of cells and it appears to be this effect which determines its localization and distribution. It is not believed that pathological calcification ever occurs in normal, healthy cells. Necrosis, particularly caseous necrosis and hyaline degeneration are the usual precursors of calcification.

In the case of calcification of a caseous tuberculous lesion, it is easier to interpret the picture (see Fig. 59) as being the result of the breakdown of the lipoid material in the necrotic area into fatty acids with their subsequent insoluble calcium salt saponification. This is ultimately followed by the deposition of calcium phosphate and carbonate in the usual ratio of nine to one. It is more difficult to attribute any specific physical equation such as a lowered local carbon dioxide tension as the basis of the calcification as some investigators hold. It is quite possible, however, that the physical structure of the tissue does seem, perhaps, to determine the localization of such calcium deposits. A further discussion of this problem will be found in the sections relating to bone pathology, especially in respect to vitamin and parathyroid pathology. At this time, this brief outline of the problem serves to call attention to the general features of the process, which are exemplified by a study of tissues removed from such abnormal areas of calcification.

Illustrative Cases

CASE 29. (Ref. #S-208)

Diagnosis.—Heart—papillary muscle with calcification.

Patient was an 80-year-old white male first admitted to the hospital because of a lump in his left mandible.

Present Illness.—The patient had been in his usual health up to the time of admission except for this small lump in his left mandibular region, which was slowly increasing in size. He had had an increased blood pressure for many years and occasionally had attacks of palpitation and dyspnea on exertion, but these he credited to the infirmities of old age and did not pay any undue attention to them.

Past History.—Past history was essentially negative and was irrelevant as far as his present illness was concerned. He had had no history of rheumatic fever or rheumatism, nor any other acute infectious disease which might account for any cardiac pathology. It was felt that most of his health problems were related to a generalized arteriosclerosis which was steadily increasing in degree.

Physical Examination.—The patient was a fairly well developed, somewhat undernourished, elderly white male. His head was normal in shape except for a palpable mass at the angle of the left jaw about the size of a walnut, which was attached to the mandible. He had a bilateral arcus senilis but his pupils reacted normally to light and accommodation. His ears, nose and throat were negative. He was edentulous, but had artificial dentures. Chest was symmetrical but somewhat barrel shaped. Lungs were clear throughout with hyperresonance in the upper lobes. Heart was slightly enlarged. Rhythm was regular. There were no murmurs heard. Abdomen was negative. Extremities were negative.

Laboratory Findings.—Red blood cells 4,100,000; hemoglobin 83%. White blood cells 6,800 with 72% polynuclear leukocytes. Urinalysis showed a slight trace of albumin but was otherwise negative. X-ray examination showed a metastatic neoplastic process.

Subsequent Course.—He was given a pre-operative series of x-ray treatments and was then operated upon with removal of the tumor mass. Following this the patient showed recurrence of the tumor in about two months after the surgical treatment, and was given another series of x-ray treatments which showed very little effect upon the neoplasm. He began to have pain in the region of his left ear and the left upper eyelid. This was accompanied by headache and a slowly increasing loss of vision on the left side. He continued to progress steadily downhill and gradually lapsed into coma. Blood chemistry at this time showed a urea nitrogen of 160 mgm. Terminally, he developed pulmonary edema at the bases of both lungs and died of bronchopneumonia.

Autopsy Findings.—At autopsy, the heart presented the typical picture of arteriosclerotic hypertrophy. It weighed 445 gm. The musculature, particularly of the left ventricle, showed diffuse fibrosis. In the posterior papillary bundles the tips presented a marked calcification. The valves showed some sclerotic thickening, particularly in the aortic. There was generalized arteriosclerosis of the aorta which became more progressive in extent toward the bifurcation of the iliacs. The kidneys showed an old chronic arteriosclerotic type of nephrosclerosis. The prostate was moderately enlarged with a small, firm nodule measuring 0.5 cm. in the middle lobe suggesting carcinoma. The jaw bone had been removed on the left side and there was a mass of necrotic tissue, which it was hard to identify, replacing the normal structures. Whether any tumor was present was hard to tell without microscopic study.

Microscopic Description of a Papillary Muscle of the Heart.—A study of the papillary muscle microscopically shows the presence of very extensive fatty and hyaline degenerative changes involving the muscle fibers. There is diffuse interstitial fibrosis present. Muscle fibers show attempted hypertrophy with increase in size of the nuclei. Scattered through the muscle fibers where fatty and hyaline degenerative changes have occurred may be seen a sprinkling of blue-staining calcific granules, which have been deposited in the tissues as part of the usual picture of calcification following extensive degenerative changes.

CASE 30. (Ref. #S-187)

Diagnosis.—Lymph node—caseous tuberculosis with beginning calcification.

Patient was a Negress of 30 years who was admitted to the hospital because of a cough of a month's duration.

Present Illness.—As far as the patient knew, she had been in her usual good health until one month before admission. At that time she developed a cold and slight cough. She stayed in bed for one week but did not seem to improve. Her cough continued and she had occasional night sweats. She returned to work but developed a feeling of easy fatigability, lassitude and a loss of appetite. For this reason she was sent by her employer to a physician who made a tentative diagnosis of possible tuberculosis. She was sent to the hospital for study.

Past History.—The patient had had mumps, measles and scarlet fever as a child. At the age of twelve she had a severe attack of pneumonia. Since that time, however, she had been in good health as far as she was aware. A review of her systems was essentially negative. She had had no more than the usual upper respiratory infections. Her cardio-vascular system had been negative. She had always had a good appetite and her bowel movements had been regular. Her genito-urinary history was

negative. Her menstrual cycle began at the age of twelve and had been regular.

Physical Examination.—The patient was a well developed adult Negress, who stated that she felt perfectly well except for a cough. Her head was normal in shape. Eyes were negative. Ears, nose and throat were negative. Her gums showed a moderate pyorrhea. Chest was well developed and symmetrical. Expansion seemed equal. Percussion of the chest, however, revealed an area of cavitation at the left apex with some consolidation at the right apex. Numerous crackling râles were heard on the right. At both bases there was some suggestion of fluid with distant voice sounds. The heart was not enlarged and there were no murmurs. Abdomen: the liver edge was palpable just below the costal margin. Extremities were negative.

Laboratory Findings.—Urinalysis showed a high specific gravity (1.029) and a trace of albumin. There was also a trace of sugar. Wassermann was negative. Blood chemistry showed a sugar of 125 to 130 mgm. per 100 c.c. Sputum was positive for tubercle bacilli with myriads of organisms in each field. X-ray examination confirmed the diagnosis of bilateral pulmonary tuberculosis with left apical cavitation.

Subsequent Course.—The patient presented a curious euphoria in spite of the marked physical signs. She complained of nothing but her cough which was annoying in its frequency. She developed a rise in temperature in the afternoons and a progressive loss of weight. Pneumothorax was attempted unsuccessfully twice. The patient went steadily downhill and died six months after the onset of her illness.

Autopsy Findings.—At autopsy a diffuse bilateral chronic ulcerative fibrocaseous tuberculosis of both lungs was found with a large cavity involving most of the left upper lobe. There was a terminal generalized miliary tuberculosis. There was an obliterative bilateral adhesive pleuritis. This was more marked on the left. The mediastinal lymph nodes showed marked fibrocaseous tuberculosis with some calcification. There was a terminal ulcerative tuberculous process involving the terminal ileum, cecum and appendix, and there was an associated bilateral tuberculous salpingitis.

Microscopic Description of a Hilus Lymph Node.—(Fig. 59) The lymph node may be identified by its capsule and the persistence of a few lymph follicles. There is an attempted reticulo-endothelial hyperplasia of the stroma. The peripheral sinuses are packed with lymphocytes and large mononuclear phagocytes. The bulk of the node shows a typical caseous necrosis. In the periphery of the lesion may be vaguely seen a suggestion of the original architectural detail of the node, but for the most part the process has gone on to the point where tissue identification is impossible. Most of the lesion is made up of a granular, pink-staining necrotic debris which, however, shows no liquefaction. There is found in an eccentrically located part of the caseous area a mass of blue-staining granular material representing calcific deposit. This occupies perhaps one-fourth of the lesion and represents an attempt at reparative calcification. Around the edges of the tuberculous area may be seen the characteristic palisading, radially arranged, so-called "epithelioid" cells. Merging with this zone of cellular proliferation may be seen marked lymphocytic infiltration and reparative fibrosis attempting to localize and wall off the inflammatory process.

CHAPTER VIII

THE AVITAMINOSES

THE VITAMINS

No subject perhaps in medicine has offered more speculation and research in the past fifteen years than the vitamins, those curious supplementary food factors, the absence of which lead to some of the most profound metabolic disturbances, even to death. Gradually they are being isolated chemically, so that today certain of them can even be produced synthetically and used successfully therapeutically and prophylactically. There are at least six known vitamins, with several other less certain ones still to be identified. They may be listed either alphabetically in relation to the disease which they produce, or on the basis of their lipoid or aqueous solubility. Vitamins A, D and E are fat soluble; B (B_1), C and G (B_2) are water soluble.

Vitamin A.—This is found chiefly in cod liver oil; also in small amounts in butter, egg yolk, and green vegetables. Its source is from the carotins, notably Beta carotin (provitamin A) which is the standard unit in medical use today. Its absence produces the condition known as *xerophthalmia* or *keratomalacia.* This is characterized by the drying up of the lacrimal gland and cornea with subsequent ulceration and infection. In mild form it is seen as night-blindness due to depletion of the visual purple. In the severe experimental disease it goes on to death, associated with a metaplasia of the epithelium of the respiratory, alimentary and genito-urinary tract to a keratinizing squamous type, approaching neoplasia. It is thought to have some value as an anti-infectious agent, though as yet unestablished.

Vitamin B (B_1).—This is the antineuritic vitamin, found especially in brewer's yeast, but present in all green stuffs, and especially in germinating grains. Its absence produces the clinical disease *beriberi,* a curious condition following the prolonged use of a diet of polished rice (China) or of white bread, tea and salt cod-fish (Labrador). It is characterized clinically by (1) peripheral neuritis, (2) edema and (3) cardiac failure, an almost specific triad. In the experimental disease in birds (rice disease), the polyneuritis is present, but the edema and heart failure are lacking, and an added anemia, lymphopenia and hyperglycemia are present which are not seen in human beri-beri. It is believed that an added infective factor is necessary in true beri-beri.

Perla, in a recent review, comments upon the apparent relationship of vitamin "B" to resistance against infection. This is evidenced by much experimental data in which mice, rats, guinea pigs, pigeons, and dogs, all show a marked increased susceptibility to various infections when fed on diets deficient in vitamin "B." Attention is further drawn to the fact that leprosy occurs endemically in those areas where the diet of the population is particularly deficient in this vitamin. In fractionating vitamin "B," it has been shown that "B_1" is essential in the process of oxidation in brain and nerve tissue, that it is important in maintaining the normal rate of growth, and that it is further necessary for normal gastrointestinal peristalsis and gastric secretion.

Vitamin C.—Synonyms: hexuronic acid, l. ascorbic acid, cevitamic acid. It can be synthesized from l. sorbose and is a strong reducing agent. Its chief source from the practical standpoint is *orange juice,* but it occurs generously in milk, in most fruits, vegetables and to a limited extent in fresh meat, especially liver. It is easily destroyed by heat, so cooking reduces the available amount. Recent experimental work on chicks has shown that there are apparently two fractions concerned in the development of the clinical pictures associated with deficiency of this vitamin. Whether they should be separately classified remains to be confirmed. At all events the hemorrhagic factor can be definitely split off from the factor responsible for the skeletal changes in the experimental disease, and it has been tentatively called Vitamin K.

Clinically the absence of the vitamin C complex produces the disease known as scurvy (scorbutus—

PLATE XV
AVITAMINOSES—SCURVY AND RICKETS

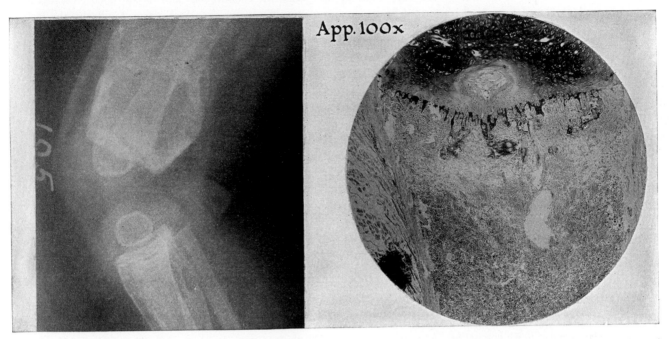

App. 100x

FIG. 62.—ROENTGENOGRAM.—KNEE JOINT: SCURVY.—CASE 31.—
Extreme subperiosteal hemorrhage with elevation of periosteum
of ends of long bones, epiphyseal displacement, condensation of
bones at epiphyseal line and demineralization of adjacent
diaphyses.

FIG. 63.—RIB: SCURVY (Experimental).—Typical widening of
epiphyseal line of costochondral junction with cessation of osteogenesis, and resultant abnormal calcification, and "Trömmerfeld" zone of demineralization. App. 100 x.

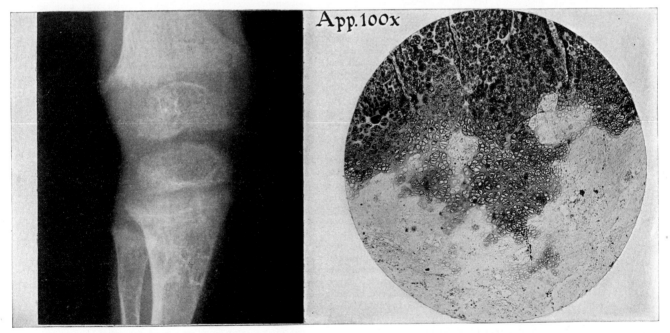

App. 100x

FIG. 64.—ROENTGENOGRAM.—KNEE JOINT: RICKETS.—CASE 32.—
Demineralization, especially of epiphyses, widening (flaring)
and irregularity of epiphyseal ends of the diaphyses, thickening
of cortices on concave aspect, and beginning deformities from
weight bearing.

FIG. 65.—RIB: RICKETS.—cf. CASE 32.—Apparent proliferation of
cartilage and osteoid tissue of widened epiphyseal line of costochondral junction, which fail to ossify properly, thus producing
thickening of epiphyseal area (cf. rachitic rosary). App. 100 x.

in infancy, Moeller-Barlow's disease). This, in its well developed form is characterized by two major sets of clinical features: First, an anemia and a series of hemorrhagic lesions, including bleeding and infection of the gums, hemorrhages into the skin and mucous membranes, the orbits, the joints and particularly under the periosteum of the long bones. The second group of changes are those associated with skeletal disturbances, particularly seen in infants and young children, and involving the epiphyses of the long bones, interfering with growth. In the experimental animal where the disease can be pushed to an extreme, it is found that the changes are by no means limited to the bones, but involve all the connective tissue derivatives. There appears to be a reversion of the intercellular matrix of the fibroblast, the chondroblast and the osteoblast towards a myxomatous or even "sol" state. Similarly, the history of scurvy can be traced in the tooth changes.

In the infant the basic lesion of scurvy appears to be a cessation of osteogenesis at the epiphyseal line especially. Resorption of bone goes on, however, so the bone becomes rarefied. At the epiphyseal line the cartilage cells lose their orderly appearance and a line of calcified cartilage appears instead of the usual ossification. The marrow becomes edematous and hematopoiesis diminished in the adjacent areas. Hemorrhage into the marrow cavity and under the periosteum occurs. No disturbance of calcium metabolism appears to develop to explain these profound bony changes, nor can any evidence of parathyroid dysfunction be demonstrated.

ILLUSTRATIVE CASE

CASE 31. (Ref. #S-302)

Diagnosis.—Costochondral junction scorbutus.

Patient was a white male infant of 11 months, who was admitted to the hospital because of severe attacks of crying and screaming at night, with failure to move his legs, and hemorrhages into the gums.

Present Illness.—The child's illness began eight weeks before admission when the mother noted that the child was becoming very irritable and seemed to wish to be left alone. She noted that he screamed when he was picked up. He developed a cold in the head at this time for which he was treated locally. His condition, however, failed to improve and his symptoms were becoming much more marked during the two weeks prior to admission. He had practically remained motionless in bed and had seemed unable to move his lower extremities, and only to move his upper ones with obvious pain. There had been some hemorrhage noted into the conjunctivae, and there had been marked bleeding from the gums. His legs became markedly swollen and had shown increasing tenderness.

Past History.—The child was a full-term, normally delivered baby, who was breast fed only for the first two weeks of life, as the mother's supply gave out. He was put on a cow's milk formula of one-half milk and one-half water with a tablespoonful of molasses, and the mixture boiled. The amount had been increased at intervals until at the time of admission the child was upon thirty ounces of milk, ten ounces of water and three tablespoonfuls of molasses. Up until approximately one month before admission his appetite had been good and his bowel movements regular, but in the last month his appetite had been very poor and he had scarcely taken half of his formula at a time. The child cut his first tooth at four and one-half months and began to creep at eight and one-half months of age. He had been given cod liver oil daily from the time he was started on his artificial formula, but had never been given any orange or tomato juice.

Physical Examination.—The child appeared to be a well nourished but somewhat pale male infant, who appeared his given age. He was lying in bed crying and turning his head from side to side. His legs were held in a position of marked eversion and it was noted that both legs were badly swollen. The child could move his toes but did not move the legs. Head was of normal contour. Fontanels were normal in respect to his age. There was no prominence of his parietal or frontal bosses. No discharge from his ears. Conjunctivae were pale except for a few hemorrhagic spots. Extra-ocular movements were normal. Nose: Mucosa was pale and dry. Mouth: The two lower incisors were both erupted. The four upper incisors were erupted. There was evidence of an acute ulcerative, hemorrhagic process around the gums in relation to the teeth. This was of a deep, cyanotic purplish red color and pressure produced bleeding very readily. The hard palate also appeared of this spongy, purplish red color. The throat was not particularly inflamed. Chest was symmetrical. Expansion seemed equal and regular. Lungs were clear throughout. Heart was normal in size. The rate seemed somewhat rapid. There were no murmurs. There was a definite nodular enlargement of the costochondral junctions. This was particularly marked in the middle tier of ribs. Abdomen: No masses were felt. No areas of tenderness noted, but the child cried on deep palpation. Extremities: Both lower extremities were held everted and in partial flexion. The legs were markedly swollen, with shiny tense skin. The child screamed whenever the legs were manipulated. It was impossible to evaluate the reflexes.

Laboratory Findings.—Examination of the blood showed an initial admission red cell count of 2,540,000 with 4.5 gm. of hemoglobin (27%); a white count of 13,000 cells with 57% polynuclear leukocytes. The blood smear showed marked anisocytosis, poikilocytosis and achromia. Occasional normoblasts were seen. Blood chemistry gave a urea of 14 mgm., creatinine of 1.5 mgm., uric acid of 2.5 mgm., and sugar of 118 mgm. per 100 c.c. Tuberculin tests were negative. Kidney function tests were normal. Urinalyses were essentially negative except for a very slight trace of albumin on several examinations.

X-ray Examination.—(Fig. 62) (Courtesy of Dr. W. Edward Chamberlain). This is a beautiful textbook picture of the x-ray appearance of scurvy. Tremendous subperiosteal hemorrhages have occurred over the distal and proximal thirds of the shafts of all of the long bones of the lower extremities. As a result of these subperiosteal hemorrhages, the epiphyses, together with a dense layer of bone from the epiphyseal end of the diaphysis, have been floated away with actual displacement amounting to actual pathological fracture. The abnormal density of this layer of bone at the epiphyseal end of each diaphysis, and the extensive demineralization of the bone immediately on the diaphyseal side of the condensed layer, are also typical.

The diagnosis of acute scorbutus was made, and the patient was put on a high vitamin diet, especially of vitamin "C."

Subsequent Course.—Within a week after the institution of proper treatment the appearance of the child had improved phenomenally. He was able to use his extremities and to play normally with the other children in the ward. His appetite improved immediately, as did his color. By the end of two weeks the red count and hemoglobin had increased to 4,180,000 red blood cells with 7 grams or 42% hemoglobin. The white count had dropped to 9,100 cells with 45% polynuclear leukocytes and the changes in the red cells had markedly improved. The blood calcium at this time showed 10.8 mgm. per 100 c.c. X-ray examinations were made at intervals and showed progressive calcification of the subperiosteal hemorrhages. The child remained under observation for a total period of two months until he appeared to be completely recovered from his avitaminosis and was discharged to his home, cured.

Microscopic Description of the Costochondral Junction of a Guinea Pig in which Acute Scurvy had been Induced by a Diet Deficient in Vitamin "C."—(Fig. 63) It is obvious that scurvy as a pathological condition is almost never encountered today at the autopsy table. Our only opportunity of studying the advanced changes is in the experimentally induced disease in the lower animals. For this purpose a rib from a guinea pig suffering from this condition is presented for histologic consideration. There is unevenness of the junction of the bone and cartilage with marked disorganization of the rows of cartilage cells. There is a shortening of these rows with a decrease in the number of trabeculae and a relative increase of blood in the marrow cavity. The marrow space has become filled with a mass of connective tissue, the so-called "Trömmerfeld zone." There is some cystic degeneration in the marrow spaces. There is marked abnormal calcification of the cartilaginous trabeculae with apparent cessation in active bone formation. It will be noted that the cortical portion of the bone has become extremely thinned and that there is characteristic broadening of the costochondral junction, which corresponds to the nodular rosary formation noted grossly, and is to be differentiated from the rachitic lesion.

Vitamin D.—This is the fat soluble vitamin whose absence produces the disease *rickets (rachitis)*. This is a very complex substance thought probably to be an *isomer of ergosterol* (provitamin D) with the chemical formula ($C_{27}H_{41}OH$), as it may be produced synthetically by the irradiation of ergosterol. Over-irradiation may break this into two or more fractions, one the true D or D_1 vitamin; the other, tentatively called D_2 or toxisterin (more recently calciferol). This latter is not antirachitic and may produce marked toxic effects, often with an associated hypercalcemia. The principal practical source of vitamin D is still from cod or halibut liver oil, although it is also present in moderate amounts in egg yolk, butter, etc. It can be separated from the vitamin A factor by oxidation of the latter. It can also be developed similarly in human tissues from the sterols of the subcutaneous fat by ultraviolet irradiation ($300 \pm \mu\mu$ waves).

The interest in vitamin D lies in its relationship to calcium and phosphorus metabolism in the development of rickets and osteomalacia clinically. Rickets is a disease of infants developing usually before the sixth month of life and rarely remaining active beyond two years, although the deformities may persist permanently in extreme instances. It is dependent upon an unbalance in the calcium-phosphorus ratio, the latter always being low, the former usually so. It results in a defective calcification of the bones, especially the long bones, at the epiphyseal ends, and of an utter disorder of cartilaginous proliferation in these areas which appears as irregular tongue-like processes producing an enormously thickened, but soft, zone of false bone where the normal line of ossification should occur, in contrast to the abnormal calcification of this area in scorbutus.

ILLUSTRATIVE CASE

CASE 32. (Ref. #S-160)

Diagnosis.—Rib—rachitis (costochondral junction).

Patient was a 4-year-old male child admitted to the hospital with the chief complaint of bowing of the legs, which was first noted when the child started to walk at the age of 13 months.

Past History.—The child was a full-term, normally delivered child who was breast fed for over a year. Cod liver oil and orange juice were added to its diet when it was weaned. At two years of age the child was taking sixty drops of Viosterol. For one year prior to hospital entry, the patient had been taking 1 teaspoonful of Squibb's Super D Vitamin extract and one tablespoonful of cod liver oil daily.

Physical Examination.—At the time of admission the child appeared to be a well-developed and well-nourished male, who appeared his given age. His head showed some increase in its circumference with rather marked prominence of the parietal and frontal bosses. The chest was symmetrical and the lungs appeared clear with no alteration in breath sounds. The heart was not enlarged, and there were no murmurs. The abdomen was markedly protuberant. This prominence of the abdomen seemed to be due to a ptosis of the stomach and viscera with marked distention of the bowel with gas. Neither the liver nor spleen were palpable. The genitalia were negative. The legs showed marked bowing.

Laboratory Findings.—Red blood count showed 3,200,-000 cells with hemoglobin of 58%. White blood cells numbered 10,200 with 46% polynuclear leukocytes. The smear showed a mild degree of secondary hypochromic anemia. Blood chemistry: Serum calcium 7.7 mgm., serum phosphorus 3.8 mgm. per 100 c.c.

X-ray Findings.—(Fig. 64) (Courtesy of Dr. W. Edward Chamberlain)

The x-ray findings in rickets, all of which are emphasized to a greater or less degree in this case are:

1. Demineralization, more marked at the epiphyses and epiphyseal ends of the diaphyses;

2. Irregularity in the pattern of bone as laid down at the surfaces of the ossification center of the epiphyses, as well as at the epiphyseal end of the diaphyses;

3. Deformity due to softening plus weight bearing or other stresses;

4. Increase of thickness of cortex of deformed bone on the concave side (important in the differentiation from inflammatory deformities, such as are found in lues, where the thickened cortex is on the convex side of the deformity, or bowed long bone);

5. Widening of the epiphyseal ends of the diaphyses (so-called flaring); and

6. Periosteal bone formation (a laying down of bone under elevated periosteum).

Subsequent Course.—In view of the unusual history of the child having taken cod liver oil since approximately one year of age, with the development of such marked rachitic changes in the bones, it was thought advisable to take a biopsy specimen from the femur to definitely establish the histologic diagnosis. This was done and examination of the tissue removed from the left femur in the epiphyseal region was interpreted as typically rachitic in etiology. At the end of four years, the x-ray findings were reported as still showing marked rickets in the stage of well advanced healing. The question arose in this case as to whether or not this might not well represent one of those instances in which the healing had been delayed by an excess of the vitamin in Viosterol. The patient clinically showed marked improvement and ran an uneventful course with clinical recovery, and when last seen appeared to be normal in all respects except as commented upon above by x-ray examination of his long bones.

Microscopic Description of a Comparable Costochondral Junction from an Eighteen Months' Old Child Showing Marked Rickets, Who Died of Bronchopneumonia Associated with Measles.—(Fig. 65) The picture microscopically seems to be essentially the reverse of the process as seen in scorbutus. Here there is tremendous proliferation of the cartilaginous trabeculae as irregular cords and strands of cartilage cells. The line of ossification is definitely impaired as in the case of scurvy. In this instance, however, it is the result of the cartilaginous overgrowth rather than the result of premature calcification of imperfectly developed cartilage. As a result of this proliferative reaction, there likewise develops a nodular thickening of the costochondral junction because of this excess tissue. Where bone exists, it will be seen to be apparently normal and all the changes taking place in this picture are found at the epiphyseal end of the long bones, as in this case.

Vitamin E.—A fat soluble complex higher alcohol isolated by Evans from green leaves and seeds. Practically, it is found in greatest amount in wheat germ, so its principal dietary source is whole wheat bread. This is the so-called "anti-sterility vitamin," because its lack produces degeneration of the spermatozoa in the male, and changes in the placenta in the female resulting in miscarriage early in pregnancy.

Vitamin G.—Synonyms: B_2 (because also antineuritic as B_1); P-P (pellagra preventing). This is found in greatest concentration in yeast, but also is found in liver, and green vegetables. It can easily be separated from the B_1 fraction. Its absence is associated with the disease *pellagra*, but here as with beri-beri, secondary infection seems to be an important related factor. This is a severe disease, occurring chiefly in the south among the poorer people living largely on a diet of corn (often spoiled), salt pork and molasses. It is characterized by a curious symmetrical pigmentation of the exposed parts of the skin, marked digestive and mental disturbances and profound muscular weakness.

In Perla's recent review of vitamin "B," he has further brought out the fact that "B_2" may be further split into a considerable number of fractions which have variously been termed "B_3," "B_4," "B_5" and "B_6." In addition, it has been shown that one of the essential constituents of vitamin "B" is riboflavin. This substance seems to be essential in the metabolism and nutrition of epithelial structures. Its absence causes the development of cataracts and cutaneous lesions, particularly alopecia, in rats. Another factor commented upon in the preceding paragraph, the pellagra-preventing "P-P" fraction, seems in the light of recent investigation to have nicotinic acid as its active principle. This seems to have been well established experimentally in preventing or curing the disease both in animals and in actual clinical cases. It is further suggested that some one of these "B" fractions is further important in the formation of the anti-anemic principle and in the stimulation of active hematopoiesis. Thus, the importance of an adequate dietary intake of whole vitamin "B," becomes apparent.

CHAPTER IX

ACUTE INFLAMMATION

Definition.—In its simplest form, the definition of inflammation may be described as the local reaction of the body to injury or irritation. In a rather more extended form it may be said that "inflammation is the sum total of action and reactions of the body against an irritant introduced from without or generated within, with the purpose of destroying, neutralizing or removing the injurious agent and paving the way for restitution to normal regeneration or repair." By this comprehensive definition we find then, in the broader sense, that inflammation includes (1) the complicated vascular and cellular response locally at the site of the injury (2) the systemic reaction of the body with fever and immunity development and (3) the reparative efforts of the body both locally and generally. Many pathologists prefer to limit their conception of inflammation to the local, immediate, protective defense mechanism as indicated under (1) above, but the majority tend to lean towards the larger point of view.

Causes.—As suggested by its definition the causes of inflammation must be legion. They include such widely diverse agents as chemical substances, physical agents, bacteria, animal parasites and many autogenous metabolic products which express themselves as alterations in function of the organism.

CHEMICAL AGENTS.—Among the chemical agents, there is enormous range which covers many aspects of the whole field of industrial medicine. We are, perhaps, more particularly concerned with the acute inflammatory changes induced by the administration, either accidentally or with suicidal intent, of strong acids, alkalies or other poisons. In the industrial field, there are many substances, among them the volatile chemicals, which gain access to the lungs by inhalation or may be absorbed through the skin, which will produce violent, acute inflammatory response. Many of these will be considered in the section devoted to the specific organ systems under systemic pathology.

PHYSICAL AGENTS.—Among the more obviously physical agents which produce acute inflammatory changes, we must think of heat in its many forms as a cause of burns. Cold, likewise, is a source of acute inflammation at times as seen in typical frost bite or chilblains. Pressure may result in destruction of tissue with accompanying inflammatory changes. Traumatic injuries of all sorts may produce very marked inflammatory response. The presence of a foreign body in the eye or trachea is an example of acute irritation, which brings forth the usual inflammatory tissue response. Electricity may similarly cause tissue injury through accidental electrocution; and light rays, including particularly the ultraviolet rays of the sun and the gamma rays of x-ray therapy, will produce definite burns with their corresponding tissue changes. We are all familiar with the commonest of this type of inflammation as seen in the usual picture of sunburn. It must be remembered that such inflammatory changes may proceed to a point where the absorption from the inflammatory reaction may interfere with normal waste excretion to an extent where the kidney is not able to maintain adequate elimination of these toxic products and death may result.

Cardinal Symptoms

The symptoms of acute inflammation have been recognized for many centuries. They consist of 1. redness; 2. swelling; 3. increased heat, and 4. pain. These are the familiar rubor, tumor, calor and dolor of the ancients. These symptoms may be explained on the basis of the complicated vascular and cellular response of the tissue as will be shown in the following paragraphs.

74

PLATE XVI
ACUTE INFLAMMATION

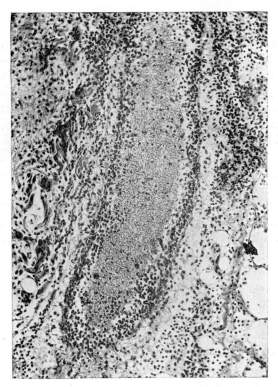

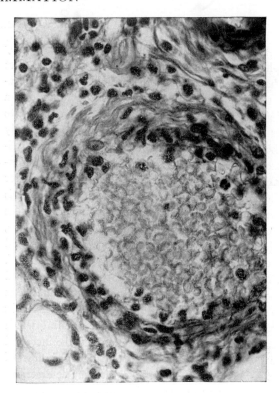

FIG. 66.—SKIN: INFLAMMATION.—VASCULAR PHE-NOMENA.—CASE 34.—ERYSIPELAS.—Tangential section of widely dilated blood vessel in acute inflammatory zone, showing characteristic margination of white cells (leukocytes) and perivascular cellular infiltration. App. 100 x.

FIG. 67.—APPENDIX: INFLAMMATION.—VASCULAR PHE-NOMENA.—CASE 33.—ACUTE APPENDICITIS.—Diapedesis of leukocytes through the wall of a markedly dilated arteriole. App. 400 x.

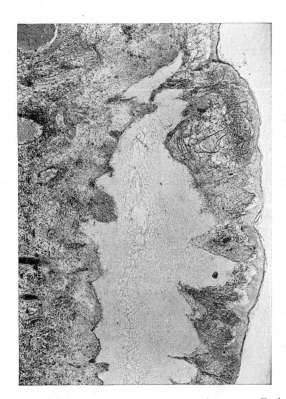

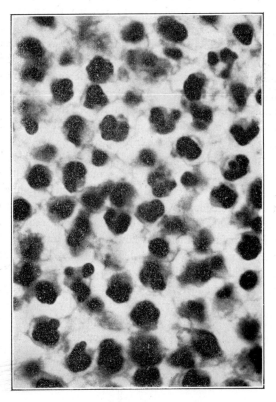

FIG. 68.—SKIN: INFLAMMATION.—ANTHRAX.—Early cutaneous lesion characterized by extreme serosanguineous inflammatory exudation separating the superficial layers of the skin to form ultimately the "malignant pustule." App. 15 x.

FIG. 69.—ACUTE INFLAMMATION: ACUTE LEUKOCYTIC EXUDATE.—CASE 34.—Inflammatory exudate made up almost entirely of polymorphonuclear leukocytes, many showing degenerative changes of cytoplasm. App. 1200 x.

Vascular Changes in Inflammation

1. Following the initial injury or irritation by whatever etiologic agent, we find that the first change which occurs in the injured area is a paralytic dilatation of the blood vessels. This follows a definite sequence, occurring first in the small arteries or arterioles, then involves the veins and finally there is capillary dilatation at the site of the irritation. This follows an initial transitory vasoconstriction, which is usually not observed except under elaborate experimental circumstances. The picture is the result of the action of the irritant on the tissues locally. This causes the production of histamine, which in turn acts on the nervous mechanism and probably on the musculature of the vessel wall itself. This dilatation of the vascular bed in the inflamed zone explains the cardinal symptom of redness due to the increased amount of blood in the vessels. It likewise explains in part at least the swelling which occurs in the area of inflammation and the increased heat which are both due to the increased flow of blood to the injured area. The pain may be described as a corollary to these findings as the result of pressure on the nerve endings.

2. Following the dilatation of the vascular system in the inflamed area, there is a temporary acceleration of the blood flow in the attempt to bring more blood to the injured part to remove the noxious agent. This is followed by a slowing of the blood stream due to the widening of the capillary bed as may be easily explained on simple physical laws. If this paralytic dilatation becomes extreme, the slowing of the blood flow may even go on to complete stasis with thrombosis, particularly if the injurious agent has acted directly upon the intimal lining of any of the vessels in the injured area.

3. Accompanying this slowing of the blood stream, there is a very striking margination of the leukocytes (Fig. 66 and 67). The explanation of this phenomenon is still a matter of conjecture to some extent. There is a central core of red cells which maintain the blood flow unless or until actual thrombosis occurs, but the leukocytes slowly wander from this slow blood stream to the vessel walls where they adhere, due to their amoeboid activity. Ultimately they may be seen actually migrating (Fig. 67) by direct amoeboid motion through the vessel walls out into the perivascular tissues. This is explained on the basis of positive chemotaxis, which in its last analysis probably may best be interpreted in the light of physicochemical alteration in hydrogen-ion concentration, surface tension, capillary permeability, and differences in osmotic tension as has been brought out so well by the work of Mudd and his associates.

4. A passive escape of the blood plasma and the red cells follows this active migratory leukocytic invasion. This is definitely believed to be due to the capillary permeability with the mechanical forcing of the substances into the surrounding tissue spaces. With the escape of the plasma the normal process of coagulation takes place with the development of a delicate fibrinous coagulum between the cells. The passage of red cells and leukocytes between the intact, but permeable vessel-wall is spoken of as *diapedesis*. If the escape of red cells is associated with rupture of the vessel wall as in the case of actual traumatic inflammation, it is spoken of as *rhexis*. This secondary infiltration of the tissues by the fluid portion of the blood accounts for much of the cardinal symptom of swelling. This obviously represents a localized type of edema on the basis of our earlier discussion.

5. The extent of these latter phenomena of diapedesis and interstitial edema depends largely upon the severity of the injury to the capillary and venous endothelium, which renders the vessel walls more readily permeable. The severity of the injury depends obviously upon the nature of the injurious agent. The evidence for injury to the endothelial lining of the vessel walls is seen in typical degenerative changes affecting these cells. These are manifested by granular changes, by hydropic swelling of the cell and even by fatty vacuolization of these cells. Where the injury is not too intense to cause nuclear degeneration it will be noted that the lining cells proliferate. This we may as well recognize at this time as almost a general precept in biology: the effect of a substance depends very largely upon its concentration. In minimal amounts many injurious agents produce cell stimulation, whereas in larger amounts they produce cell destruction. In part, the degenerative changes affecting this vascular lining endothelium are the result of a local anoxemia due to the stagnant blood flow.

PLATE XVII

PHAGOCYTOSIS

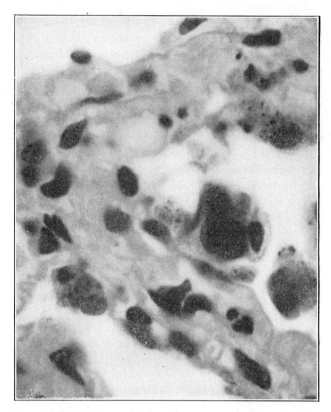

FIG. 70.—LUNG: CHRONIC PASSIVE CONGESTION.—CASE 15.—High power photomicrograph illustrating the phagocytosis of hemosiderin granules by large mononuclear "heart failure cells" within a lung alveolus. App. 1000 x.

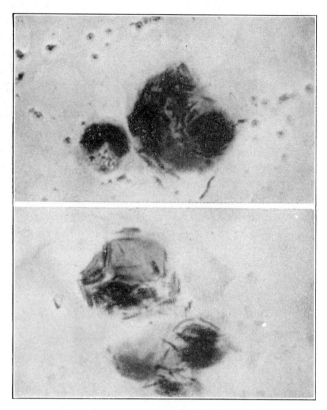

FIG. 71.—NASAL MUCOSAL SCRAPINGS: LEPROSY.—CASE 62.— Typical large mononuclear phagocytic "lepra" cells containing myriads of leprosy bacilli in characteristic "jackstraw" pattern. App. 1500 x.

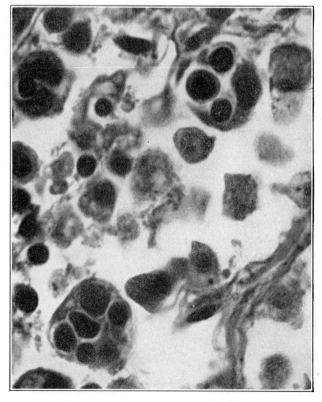

FIG. 72.—LYMPH NODE: TYPHOID FEVER.—CASE 53.—Tissue macrophages engulfing red cells, lymphocytes, bacteria and cell debris, as seen in peripheral sinus of lymph node. App. 1000 x.

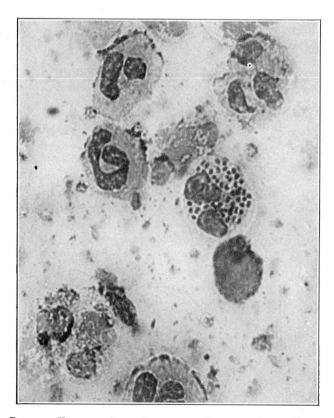

FIG. 73.—URETHRAL PUS: GONORRHEA.—CASE 35.—Smear illustrating the diagnostic mass phagocytosis of gonococci by polymorphonuclear leukocytes. Note degeneration of the cells. App. 1500 x.

6. The phenomenon of *phagocytosis* follows the perivascular accumulation of leukocytes and wandering tissue phagocytes at the site of injury. By phagocytosis is meant a vital function of certain types of cells. This consists of the ability of the cell to engulf solid particles (Figs. 70 and 72). These particles are then either digested and dissolved by the enzyme action of the cell or if the cell is not capable of digesting the foreign material, it becomes extruded. This important function of the cells which take part in the inflammatory process is one of the most important vital processes of the body. In itself, it has been the subject of many monographs and an enormous amount of work. More recent studies, particularly those of Mudd and his associates, have brought out the essential simplicity of the process as explained by basic physicochemical laws depending very largely upon differences in surface tension. A similar function termed "pinocytosis" has been applied to the engulfing of liquid particles.

The mechanism of phagocytosis may be observed in tissue cultures or in hanging drop preparations kept at body temperatures under the microscope. The phagocytic cell, due to the differences in surface tension of the foreign body and its own cell membrane, results in the throwing out of pseudopodia, which spread around the foreign material until the pseudopod fuses with its own body and the foreign material becomes entirely incorporated in the cytoplasm of the phagocytic cell. This is of particular importance in those inflammatory processes associated with bacterial diseases, which make up one of the largest and most important group of human diseases. This is because phagocytosis is probably the principal method of the body of removing and destroying the organisms responsible for the infection. This process represents one of the major mechanisms in the development of immunity, as phagocytosis is one of the chief activities induced by the immune tissues (Figs. 71 and 73). Recent experimental studies suggest that chemotherapy may increase this function.

Cells of the Inflammatory Exudate

To familiarize ourselves with the cells which take part in the inflammatory picture, we need to review briefly the appearance of the normal cells of the peripheral blood as these are the principal cells which take part in this process, with the addition of the fixed and wandering tissue cells. As we have just seen, the initial response, however, in any acute inflammatory reaction is the vascular one characterized by the perivascular infiltration of the tissues by the cells of the blood. A review of their morphology is important at this time so that they may be identified in subsequent slides, no matter at what tangential angle they may be cut.

Normally the peripheral blood contains six varieties of white corpuscles, in addition to the adult red cells, and all of these six types may be identified in the inflammatory tissue cellular response although their differentiation is at times difficult. Normally we find the following proportion of cells within relatively narrow limits (Fig. 74):

1. Neutrophilic polymorphonuclear leukocytes   58 -68%
2. Eosinophilic polymorphonuclear leukocytes   1 - 2%
3. Basophilic polymorphonuclear leukocytes..   0.5- 1%
4. Large lymphocytes....................   5 - 7%
5. Small lymphocytes....................   25 -35%
6. Large mononuclears (monocytes) ....   3 - 5%

The principal differential identifying features of these cells are indicated below. With the various polychrome stains such as Wright's, Jenner's and so forth, their identification is comparatively simple. With the routine hematoxylin and eosin tissue stain, these differences are less readily made out, especially in the cells of the lymphocytic series in which the cytoplasm stains with eosin instead of with the characteristic blue of the tri-acid polychrome stains. (Cf. Figures 74 and 75, colored plate XVIII.)

Leukocytes

The polymorphonuclear leukocytes are cells which range from 10 to 12 micra in diameter and are of the three types indicated above.

Neutrophiles.—(Fig. 69) The neutrophiles may be seen to have a very faint, grayish-pink staining cytoplasm in the eosin-hematoxylin preparation in which it is difficult frequently to identify any of the characteristic neutrophilic granules as seen in the ordinary trichrome stained blood film. They may be recognized readily, however, by their deep staining segmented and lobed nuclei. Under certain pathological conditions involving the bone marrow, abnormal cells of the myeloid series may likewise appear in any inflammatory reaction, but where these are found the presence of this underlying hematopoietic disorder may be suspected and discounted in the interpretation of the immediate acute inflammatory reaction.

Eosinophiles.—The adult eosinophile usually is seen to have a two-lobed (occasionally 3-lobed) nucleus. These are characterized by a rather broad band between the lobes and resemble closely the immature "stab" form of the neutrophilic leukocyte except for the difference in the cytoplasm. Typically the cytoplasm of the eosinophile contains rather coarse, intensely red, eosin-staining granules. These retain their eosin-staining characteristics both in the usual trichrome blood stain and in the eosin-hematoxylin tissue preparations so that they are usually comparatively easy to recognize.

Basophiles.—In tissue preparations stained by the usual hematoxylin-eosin method, the basophiles are relatively more difficult to recognize. However, only in rare instances is a basophilic infiltration of the tissues in any inflammatory reaction of any diagnostic significance. Basophiles present a morphologic picture so similar to that of the eosinophile that it is at times impossible to tell them apart. In general, it may be said that the granules of the basophile are larger and they tend to be distributed more generally through the cytoplasm of the cell so that they overlie the nuclei at times and are usually not as numerous as are the eosinophilic granules. With the trichrome stains they stain an intense bluish purple. In the eosin-hematoxylin preparations, they take the eosin dye.

Lymphocytes

The lymphocytes, both large and small, may be identified fairly readily by their nuclei. In tissue inflammatory exudates, the nucleus in the two types usually appears almost identical. In some of the larger cells it may be proportionally increased in size, but regardless of the size of the cell, the characteristic arrangement of the nuclear chromatin serves as a means of recognition. The small cells measure from 8 to 10 micra, the large from 12 to 15 micra. The nucleus, in each instance is small, round, and tends to be centrally placed. The chromatin stains intensely with the hematoxylin and tends to have a peripheral distribution around the nuclear membrane, which gives the typical so-called "cart wheel" appearance. The cytoplasm, which is barely visible in the small lymphocytes, but more prominent in the large form, stains rather clear bright pink with the eosin-hematoxylin method. This is in contrast to the characteristic blue color of the cytoplasm seen in the trichrome blood stains, and with the usual blood stains the nuclei show a more typical vesicular arrangement of their chromatin granules than in the tissue preparation. (See color plates XVIII and LXVII.)

Monocytes

These cells, which are relatively few in number in the peripheral blood under normal circumstances, are larger than lymphocytes, measuring anywhere from 15 to 20 micra. They may usually be identified by their nucleus, which varies considerably in shape. In the younger forms it may be ovoid or almost round. As the cell matures, it becomes indented and in its adult form it has a typical horseshoe arrangement. The cell is likely to contain a moderate number of small, neutrophilic staining granules, and for this reason the cell in the earlier days of hematology was considered as a developmental form somewhere between the early myeloid and adult neutrophilic cell. For this reason it was frequently spoken of as the transitional cell. This term is best forgotten to-day as the origin of the cell is now definitely recognized as coming from the reticulo-endothelial apparatus of the bone marrow rather than from the myeloid series. In the eosin-hematoxylin stained preparation the cytoplasm stains a similar grayish-pink to that of the neutrophile and similarly the granules may be ill defined. In the trichrome blood stains these granules are more definitive in their appearance having a definite neutrophilic purplish color and the cytoplasm being on the blue-gray side. (See Fig. 74, 75, 512 and 513.)

At this time it should be mentioned that there are two other important cells which take part in many inflammatory reactions, the plasma cell and the large mononuclear phagocyte or histiocyte. These cells will be discussed in the following chapter in relation to the chronic types of inflammation, as it is in this group of inflammatory conditions that they play their greatest role.

Illustrative Cases

Case 33. (Ref. #S-225)

Diagnosis.—Appendix—acute inflammation.

Patient was a young white male of eighteen, who was admitted to the hospital complaining of rather vague generalized abdominal discomfort of three days' duration.

Present Illness.—The onset of the present illness was rather indefinite. It began as noted above, as generalized abdominal distress, during the course of the evening following a rather heavy meal. Accompanying this, during the next three days before admission, there developed considerable nausea. The abdominal discomfort became definitely a painful sensation, which seemed to localize in the right lower quadrant of the abdomen. At that time he went to a physician and was found to have a temperature of 100.5°. His white blood count showed 10,200 cells with 78% polymorphonuclear leukocytes. There was a suggestion of tenderness on palpation in the right lower quadrant. The diagnosis of acute appendicitis was made, but it was hoped that the attack might be aborted, and the patient was advised to remain in bed using an ice bag constantly over the appendix area for the next twenty-four hours. The following morning, however, he developed exquisite pain and tenderness associated with muscle spasm over the right lower quadrant. His temperature rose to 102.5°, pulse to 120 and his white blood count to 24,800 cells with 94% polymorphonuclear leukocytes. He was profoundly toxic and was sent to the hospital as an emergency with the diagnosis of ruptured appendix.

Past History.—His past history was entirely irrelevant in respect to his present illness. A review of his systems showed nothing of importance.

Physical Examination.—At the time of admission the patient was so profoundly sick that no physical examination was made other than to listen to his heart and lungs which were found to be within normal limits.

Subsequent Course.—The patient was sent immediately to the operating room and a ruptured appendix was found with localized abscess formation, retrocecal in position. He had a prolonged convalescence complicated by localized peritonitis in the right lower quadrant, and the development of subsequent adhesions which required a secondary operation. However, ultimately he recovered completely.

Pathological Report.—*Gross Description.*—The operative specimen consisted of an appendix which measured 6 cm. in length by 1.5 cm. in diameter. At the distal portion the entire appendix was buried in a mass of hemorrhagic, necrotic-appearing tissue. A definite point of rupture was noted in the middle of this necrotic area. There was a thick, fibrinous exudate over the entire surface of the appendix and meso-appendix.

Microscopic Description of Appendix.—(Fig. 77) The section which is studied consists of an irregularly hemispherical piece of tissue representing half a cross section of the appendix. On the flat base at the right may be identified a narrow edge, which is appendiceal mucosa. Most of the mucosa has been destroyed and the lumen filled with acute inflammatory exudate. The subserosa is enormously thickened and on the peritoneal surface may be seen a thin layer of fibrous exudate.

The persistent mucosa shows an increased mucous secretion. In the submucosa, there is marked edema, congestion and even hemorrhage. Centrally, there is a mass of necrotic, inflammatory exudate made up of broken down polymorphonuclear leukocytes showing liquefaction necrosis and the production of pus. The special interest in the study of this tissue lies in the thickened subserosal layer. The musculature, it will be noted, is largely destroyed and necrotic. Scarcely enough remains for identification. In the edematous tissue outside the musculature lies the whole picture of inflammation. All the features mentioned in the above discussion of acute inflammation may be observed: first, acute hyperemia with dilated capillaries and lymphatics; second, margination of the leukocytes within the blood vessels; third, perivascular leukocytic emigration and infiltration. Indeed, actual migration of leukocytes through vessel walls may be observed (see Fig. 67). Fourth, edema, which even separates the collagen fibers of the supportive connective tissue cells is striking. Fifth, phagocytosis of cellular debris of all sorts by the leukocytes and mononuclear cells is present; and finally, sixth, proliferation of young connective tissue cells as part of the secondary phase of restitution and repair may be noted. These vary from young fibroblasts with oval nuclei and little collagen to adult, well developed, twisted, elongated, condensed nuclei and fibroglia and collagen fibers (Fig. 76 and 82). Careful study of this inflammatory exudate reveals the presence of all the various cells which we have discussed —polymorphonuclear leukocytes, eosinophilic leukocytes, lymphocytes, plasma cells, large mononuclear phagocytes and red cells—all embedded in a mass of serum representing the fluid portion of the blood, which makes up the final element necessary for the complete exudate.

PLATE XVIII

INFLAMMATORY CELLS

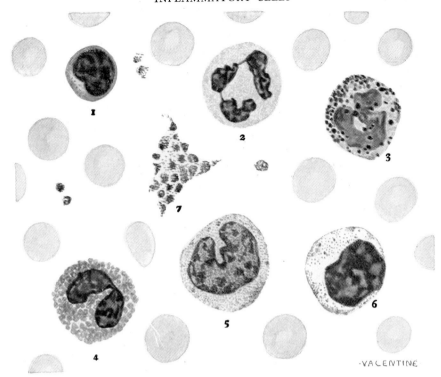

Fig. 74.—Normal White Cells of the Blood: These are the cells taking part in *acute* inflammatory exudation: 2, neutrophilic polymorphonuclear leukocyte; 1, small lymphocyte; 6, large lymphocyte; 4, eosinophile; 3, basophile; 5, large mononuclear (Wright's blood stain); 7, thrombocytes. App. 1200 x.

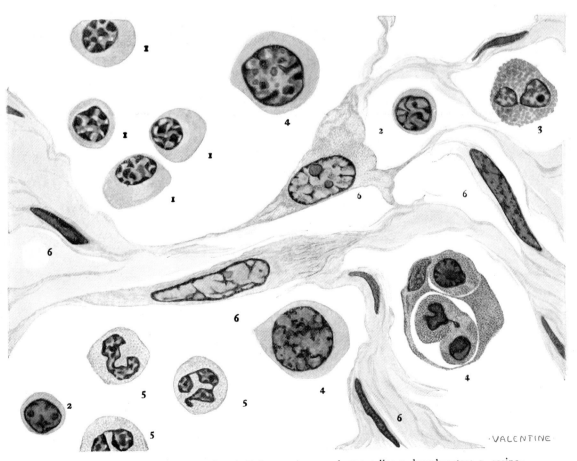

Fig. 75.—Tissue Cells in Chronic Inflammation: 1, plasma cells; 2, lymphocytes; 3, eosinophile 4, large mononuclear phagocyte (histiocytes, macrophages); 5, segmented neutrophiles; 6, developmental forms of the fibroblast (hematoxylin and eosin stain). App. 1200 x.

CASE 34. (Ref. #S-212 and 147)

Diagnosis—Skin—erysipelas; acute inflammation.

Patient was a white woman of seventy, who was admitted to the hospital with a history of having injured her ankle against a rocking chair forty-eight hours earlier. This was followed by swelling and severe pain accompanied by a chill and a fever of 103.5°.

Present Illness.—Patient had been in her usual health up until the accident which preceded her hospitalization. She had paid no particular attention to this injury, which she had felt was a very insignificant and trivial superficial abrasion, but during the course of the forty-eight hours following, it had become markedly reddened and swollen and was accompanied by stiffness of the whole lower leg. She likewise complained of transient attacks of dizziness following the chill and fever.

Past History.—Her past history was entirely irrelevant in respect to the present illness. She had never had any serious sickness previously and never had been operated upon. A review of her systems presented only the usual minor upper respiratory and digestive disturbances.

Physical Examination.—The patient was a well developed, well nourished elderly white female of apparently fully her given age. Head was normal in contour. There was a sparse amount of gray hair. There was a bilateral arcus senilis. Pupils reacted normally to light and accommodation. The ears, nose and throat were negative. She had two complete artificial dentures. There was no cervical adenopathy. The thyroid was not palpable. Chest was symmetrical. Breasts were atrophic. Lungs were clear throughout. Heart was not enlarged. The rate was rapid. There were no murmurs. Blood pressure 150/86. Abdomen was soft. No masses were felt. There was no tenderness. Extremities: The upper extremities were normal except for a rather marked arteriosclerosis of the lower extremities. The left leg was normal. The right leg was involved in a diffuse inflammatory process. Over the external malleolus, there was a small, superficial area of ulceration. Surrounding this, there was a rather brownish-red faded inflammatory process measuring about 4 to 5 cm. in diameter. Beyond this rather dull red area was noted a marked flaming red edematous zone, which extended completely around the ankle and up the leg to about the midportion. Associated with this acute inflammatory picture was generalized edema of the deeper tissues. There was a sharp zone of demarcation from this acute red area to the normal tissue above the area of inflammation. Red streaks, however, along the inner aspect of the thigh were noted, representing an extension of the inflammation by way of the lymphatics with a secondary acute lymphangitis. The regional lymph nodes in the right groin were enlarged and tender on palpation.

Laboratory Findings.—Red blood count was normal with 4,100,000 cells and 83% hemoglobin. White blood cells 18,400 with 95% polynuclear leukocytes. Urinalysis showed a moderate trace of albumin; otherwise, negative.

Subsequent Course.—The patient appeared extremely toxic and became more and more mentally confused as time went on. The lesion spread progressively up the leg, still maintaining a rather sharp line between the active area of inflammation and the normal tissues. As the lesion spread, the fiery red color faded out below the line of extension and became the same deep mottled red noted in the original area. The white count increased to 30,000 with 96% polynuclear leukocytes. The lesion continued to spread until it involved the entire leg and spread over the buttocks and vulva. Temperature became septic and ranged from 99.4° to 104.5° daily. The patient was treated by being given injections of erysipelas streptococci anti-serum and two small transfusions, as well as the usual supportive treatment. None of this therapy apparently affected the course of the disease and she progressively became weaker. There was a terminal edema and congestion of the lungs with what was thought to be probably a beginning terminal bronchopneumonia.

Autopsy Findings.—At autopsy, the only pathology of significance was the local inflammatory picture of erysipelas, which had covered the lower abdomen as well as the buttocks and vulva. In addition, there was generalized arteriosclerosis and marked toxic granular degeneration of the viscera, especially the heart, liver and kidneys. There was a terminal edema and congestion of the lungs, but no definite pneumonic consolidation could be demonstrated.

Microscopic Description of Section of Skin from the Inflammatory Zone.—(Fig. 66) The whole picture of the complex vascular and cellular phenomenon of acute inflammation can be made out with little difficulty. Just beneath the superficial epithelium, extreme dilatation of the vessels, especially the capillaries and small venules is noted. The lymphatics likewise show marked dilatation and are filled with almost homogeneous coagulum containing considerable numbers of inflammatory cells. Around the blood vessels there is definite perivascular infiltration of the tissues as the result of migration of the leukocytes. The margination of the leukocytes within the blood vessel walls is particularly well illustrated in these tissues. An enormous amount of edema of the interstitial tissues is perhaps the most characteristic feature of the inflammatory process. As the result of the outpouring of so much of the fluid element of the blood, fibrin has precipitated as a delicate network of interlacing strands. Where these are in contact with one another they have fused and a slightly nodular thickening spoken of as *"nodal"* points can be observed. In addition to these acute exudative phenomena, the process has gone on to a certain amount of liquefaction necrosis as the result of the toxic action of the bacteria and the proteolytic leukocytic enzymes. From the histology alone, it would not be difficult to suspect a streptococcus as the etiologic agent in the production of this particular serous type of inflammation, but without bacterial confirmation, it would be impossible to make a positive diagnosis in this respect as many other causes could be effective in the production of a similar serous type of exudation. This is not unlike, in many respects, the picture seen in the rabbit's ear as the result of simple thermal injury, and perhaps this teaches the lesson that one should be purely objective in a histologic diagnosis, unless the specific etiologic agent in the production of the lesion can be demonstrated.

CASE 35 (Ref. #S-233)

Diagnosis.—Acute gonorrhea; to illustrate phagocytosis.

Patient was a young white male 21 years of age, who came to the out-patient clinic because of a purulent discharge from the penis.

Past History.—The patient admitted exposure to possible infection from gonorrhea forty-eight hours before the onset of his present symptoms. These began as a painful, burning sensation at the meatus, which was followed by a catarrhal, glairy mucous secretion, which tended to close the meatus and make micturition difficult. About twelve hours before his coming to the clinic, a thick, creamy pus-like discharge appeared in the urethral orifice.

Physical Examination.—The patient was a well developed and nourished, normal appearing young white male. His head appeared negative. Eyes, ears, nose and throat were normal. Chest was well developed and symmetrical. Lungs were negative. Heart was not enlarged. There were no murmurs. Abdomen was normal. Extremities were negative. Genito-urinary examination.—There was considerable swelling and redness of the foreskin and around the urethral meatus from which a thick, pus-like exudate could be expressed. Rectal examination was negative. Examination of the testes showed no involvement at that time.

Laboratory Findings.—Blood count: Red blood cells 4,800,000; hemoglobin 93%. White blood cells 9,600 with 78% polynuclears. Bacteriological examination of the urethral pus (Fig. 73 and 156) showed the presence of countless gram-negative diplococci, most of which were contained within the cytoplasm of polymorphonuclear leukocytes. Some of the leukocytes had ruptured and the bacteria could be seen lying freely in the exudate in the smear preparation.

CHAPTER X

SUBACUTE AND CHRONIC INFLAMMATION

The problem of inflammation cannot be simply dismissed by a consideration of the acute exudative vascular phenomena because it merges so frequently into a subacute or chronic stage, which in turn presents so many features associated with repair that they must be considered as a whole. In the last chapter, we have seen that the acute inflammatory process consists of an exudative reaction associated with hyperemia and the outpouring of cells into the tissues. This reaction is spoken of as an *exudate,* and exudates are classified on the basis of the predominance of one or the other of the vascular components in response to various types of irritants:

Hemorrhagic, when red cells outnumber the fibrin, serum and leukocytes;

Serous, when the edema is the most outstanding feature;

Fibrinous, usually applied to surface lesions (trachea, peritoneum, etc.) where fibrin is the most obvious element of the exudate, and

Purulent, when leukocytes predominate and liquefaction necrosis (suppuration) is present.

If inflammation were restricted to this acute exudative manifestation it would be entirely satisfactory to limit our conception of inflammation to this part of the picture, but as has been commented upon, the tissue response to this acute inflammatory process results in regeneration of the various types of cell which are injured and the proliferation of the fixed and wandering tissue cells.

CHRONIC INFLAMMATION

By chronic inflammation is meant that form of inflammation in which connective tissue proliferation as part of the inflammatory process is the most striking feature. This is spoken of as *proliferative* or *productive* inflammation. It is seen from the outset in certain types of infectious lesions, notably tuberculosis, syphilis and those diseases caused by the higher bacteria and fungi. It is also seen as a later stage of an acute inflammatory process in which the irritating agent is not removed by the exudative process, and a transition to the chronic productive inflammatory picture ensues. Associated with this connective tissue reaction, we find a chronic type of cellular infiltration consisting principally of mononuclear cells, especially lymphocytes, plasma cells and the large, wandering tissue macrophages (Fig. 75). To this latter type of cell many terms have been given, of which the more familiar are large mononuclear cells, endothelial leukocytes, histiocytes, clasmatocytes and so forth. This mononuclear cellular infiltration gradually replaces the leukocytic polynuclear exudate as the acute inflammatory picture becomes one of chronic inflammation. Such cells appear early in those chronic granulomatous inflammatory processes caused by organisms of low virulence, which do not call out the more striking acute vascular reaction, as emphasized in the preceding chapter.

SUBACUTE INFLAMMATION

To further complicate the conception of inflammation as a whole clinically, we must recognize an intermediate type of reaction, the so-called *subacute inflammation.* We must recognize that transition from the acute to the chronic may at times only represent stages in the same process as the result of the irritant having lost its virulence. An example of this may be seen in chronic staphylococcic inflammation of the bone (chronic osteomyelitis). From the pathologist's standpoint, the recognition of subacute inflammation on a histologic basis is unsatisfactory. From the histologic standpoint, as soon

PLATE XIX
CHRONIC INFLAMMATION—REPAIR

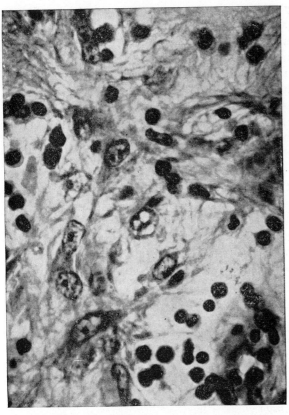

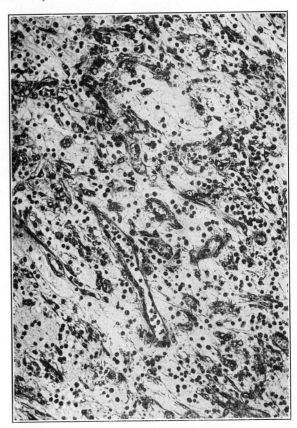

FIG. 76.—GRANULATION TISSUE.—CASE 38.—Young proliferating fibroblasts in chronic inflammation. Observe particularly the large ovoid, vesicular nuclei with prominent nucleoli and the relatively few collagen fibers present. App. 400 x.

FIG. 77.—GRANULATION TISSUE.—CASE 37.—Typical fibroblastic proliferation and new capillary vessel formation are striking. Persistent inflammatory cellular exudation is likewise present. App. 50 x.

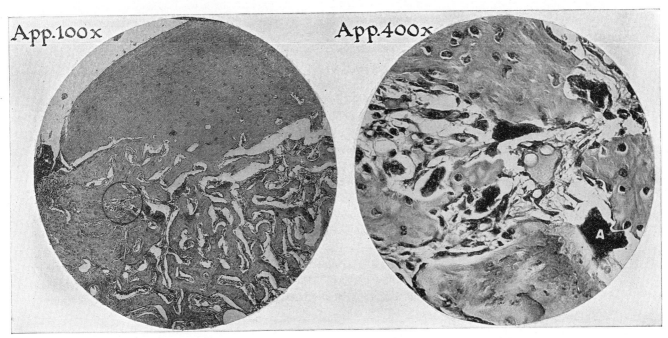

FIG. 78.—BONE REPAIR.—CASE 39.—Lower power photomicrograph of rabbit femur with callus formation. Note part played by both periosteal and endosteal cells in the repair process. App. 100 x.

FIG. 79.—High power of Fig. 78.—Osteoblasts, new bone trabeculae (B) osteoid tissue and osteoclast activity (C) are all significant features of the reaction. App. 400 x.

as productive fibrosis has begun, then the lesion is more strictly speaking past the acute stage and entering a chronic form. The term "chronic" is, after all, a relative term and on the basis of exact criteria it is difficult to admit the existence of an intermediate type of picture. Perhaps this is best illustrated in the problem of appendicitis. The surgeon recognizes various degrees of inflammatory reaction ranging from the acute gangrenous on the one hand to the chronic fibrous obliterative on the other. Between these two extremes lies a vast number of cases which the clinician thinks of in terms of subacute. By this he clinically means that the patient is not as sick as he would be if the lesion were more violent in its manifestations. Such patients often go on to spontaneous recovery, but the condition is apt to recur at irregular intervals. Histologically, such appendices present evidence of a mild, acute inflammatory reaction. They show all the usual vascular phenomena, but in a minimal degree. There is usually evidence of reparative fibrosis and at times the persistence of a small amount of leukocytic infiltration of the tissues. The pathologist is more likely to think of such cases as representing acute inflammation with repair and healing rather than as subacute. Where cellular infiltration and productive fibrosis exist, then strictly speaking, the lesion should be considered as a chronic inflammatory reaction. But chronic inflammation, beyond the simple histologic evidence of cellular infiltration and productive fibrosis, must include the concept of continued irritation so that such a lesion in its truly chronic form persists. When the irritant is removed, then healing replaces the productive inflammatory fibrosis. Such fibrous tissue repair may best be termed replacement fibrosis in contradistinction to the chronic inflammatory productive form, although no essential histologic difference is apparent in the actual cells involved.

The Inflammatory Cells of Chronic Inflammation

Plasma Cells.—(Fig. 75 and 80) For practical purposes the plasma cell may be considered as a modified lymphocyte. A great deal of argument and discussion regarding the origin of these cells may be found in the literature. This cell was first described and recognized by Unna. It is apparently a normal tissue cell in the intestinal mucosa and elsewhere but appears in greatest numbers in any chronic inflammatory process. Perhaps in syphilis is the outpouring of these cells more prominent than in any other condition. The cell itself is ovoid in outline and measures approximately 10 to 12 micra in diameter. It is capable of a somewhat limited amoeboid motion, but in fixed preparations it appears in its characteristic oval form. The nucleus is always eccentrically placed and is usually found at one pole of the cell. The cells may be identified easily in tissue when cut in their long axis by several characteristic features. The nucleus itself is identical in appearance to that of the normal lymphocyte with the same cartwheel arrangement of the chromatin in the usual hematoxylin-eosin preparation. It is surrounded, however, by a pale zone, which appears crescentic, and tends to stain rather more with the eosin than does the remainder of the cytoplasm of the cell. Unlike the adult lymphocyte the cytoplasm itself stains a rather deep purplish red. Opinions seem to vary regarding the function of the plasma cell. In general, it is held that it probably produces a proteolytic enzyme. Whether or not it is capable of phagocytosis is likewise unsettled, but it may be said without fear of contradiction that phagocytosis is a rare function of these cells. The proteolytic activity of the cell has been demonstrated by Opie, who believes that the mononuclear cells in general, in the presence of a weakly acid reaction in the tissues are capable of producing a ferment, which is more or less like pepsin in its nature, and which he has termed lymphoprotease.

Large Mononuclear Wandering Cells.—(Fig. 75 and 81) Of all the cells of the body, perhaps the large mononuclear phagocytic wandering cell has occasioned more dispute as to its origin than has any other. These cells are somewhat similar in appearance to the monocytes of the blood and for that reason it has been held by some that they are identical. Maximow, in tracing the source of these cells felt that they could be ascribed to developmental forms of the lymphocyte and proposed the term "polyblast." Mallory was able in typhoid fever to trace the source of the large mononuclear phagocytic cells of the exudate from the lining endothelium of the blood vessels. Ranvier proposed the name "clasmatocyte" as a means of identification. Marchand

PLATE XX
THE CELLS IN CHRONIC INFLAMMATION

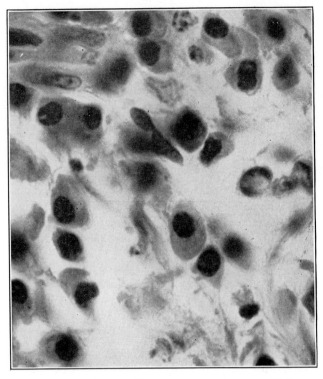

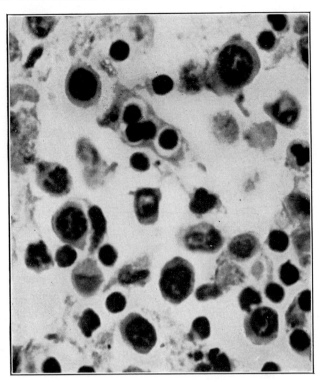

FIG. 80.—PENIS: CHRONIC INFLAMMATION.—SYPHILIS.—CASE 54.—
Inflammatory cells in primary lesion. Note the preponderance of
plasma cells with their characteristic eccentric lymphoid type
nucleus and deep staining cytoplasm. App. 1000 x.

FIG. 81.—MOUTH: CHRONIC INFLAMMATION.—ULCERATIVE STOMA-
TITIS.—CASE 36.—In this instance large mononuclear cells (macrophages) predominate. Observe their large size, vesicular
nuclei, pale cytoplasm and phagocytic capacities. App. 1000 x.

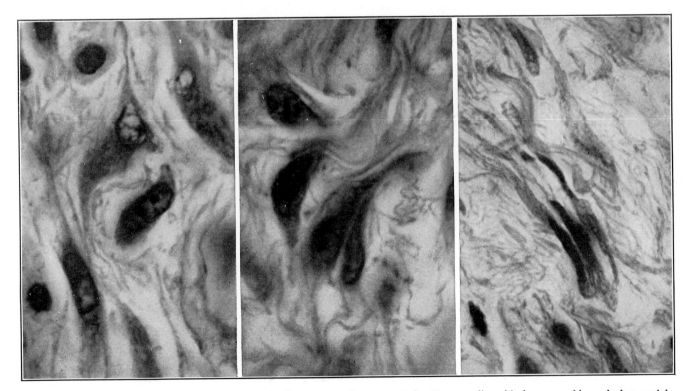

FIG. 82.—APPENDIX: DEVELOPMENTAL STAGES OF THE FIBROBLAST.—CASE 33.—*Left:* Young cells with large, ovoid, vesicular nuclei,
prominent nucleoli, beginning fibroglia but little collagen formation; *Middle:* Nuclei elongated, denser staining, well developed
fibroglia and moderate amount of wavy collagen; *Right:* Adult connective tissue cells densely staining spindled nuclei, dense fibroglia and collagen. App. 1000 x.

believed that they arose from the adventitial cells of the blood vessels and for that reason he gave them the name of "adventitial cells." Metchnikoff, likewise, in his studies on inflammation, coined the term "macrophage," particularly descriptive of the appearance and function of the cell. It was Aschoff who first ascribed the now familiar reticulo-endothelial system as the fountain head of these cells, and to differentiate them he proposed the name "histiocyte," which is perhaps the most familiar of the terms applied to these cells by pathologists generally today.

It is quite possible that these wandering mononuclear phagocytic cells may arise from a variety of primitive cell types and that some of them may remain as fixed tissue cells such as those we find within the framework of the lymph nodes of the spleen, whereas others are free to migrate where the demand for their activity calls them. In general, the three terms, large mononuclear wandering cells, histiocytes and macrophages are used synonymously. For practical purposes it seems more satisfactory to hold this universal concept of their identity than to try to create minute differences in their appearance and function as a result of differences of opinion as to origin.

They are readily identified in the tissues as large mononuclear cells measuring from 15 to 20 micra in diameter. They tend to be round or slightly irregular in outline with a sharply defined cell membrane. Their nucleus is variable in form ranging from round to ovoid or indented and kidney-shaped. It is usually eccentrically placed. The nucleus has a delicate, vesicular appearance with small, scattered granules of chromatin. The cytoplasm tends to be rather deeply staining as we see the cells in most of the inflammatory reactions. They are so commonly engaged in their phagocytic capacity that it is perhaps more common to find their cytoplasm distended with ingested dead cells, bacteria, cell debris or other foreign material. Under such circumstances these cells may become enormously increased in size, measuring as much as 40 or 50 micra in diameter. They may be confused at times, because of their similarity in appearance, with the parasitic amoebae. These are the scavenger cells which come into almost every inflammatory picture as the vanguard of the initial acute leukocytic response. It is they which phagocytize and digest the dead and wounded polynuclears

and lymphocytes. They may even be seen engulfing red cells. We have seen the part they played in the development of the blood pigments, notably hemosiderin. Perhaps no cell has a wider range of activity than does this useful scavenger, which acts as a choreman, taking care of all the odd jobs which follow any damage to the organism.

Foreign Body Giant Cells.—(Fig. 83, 85 and 86) In addition, in chronic inflammatory lesions, we also often find large multinucleated cells, which it is believed represent the fusion of several or many of the large mononuclear phagocytic wandering cells. These are spoken of as *foreign body giant cells* and serve in a functional capacity to surround and engulf larger foreign particles than the individual cell can do. Typically, these nuclei tend to be arranged in somewhat radial fashion around the periphery of the cell. The nuclei may number anywhere from three or four up to fifty or sixty. They are rather characteristic ovoid nuclei, with a loose, basket-like arrangement of their chromatin and without any apparent nucleoli. The cytoplasm is in the form of a syncytial mass, but with a well defined cell membrane as a rule. It tends to stain a rather intense red with a slightly basophilic purplish cast, not unlike the staining reaction of the plasma cell.

By comparison we find what are spoken of as tumor giant cells in contradistinction to the foreign body giant cell. An illustration of one of these (Fig. 84) is presented. The nucleus in the tumor giant cell is atypical. It is larger than normal and is often multinucleated. It presents irregular division of the chromosomes so that incomplete nuclear division occurs, resulting in this apparent lobulation of the nucleus. Chromatin material is much more dense than in the normal nucleus, and the nuclear membrane likewise tends to be much thicker and deeper staining. The cytoplasm of the cell, also, frequently shows rather striking degenerative changes. As an intermediate type of giant cell may be cited the form which is found principally in the so-called benign giant cell tumors of bone. Essentially, these are the same in their makeup as are the foreign body giant cells previously described. However, there is a very striking tendency for the nuclei to be centrally placed in the cell rather than around the periphery as in the typical Langhans' giant cell. The nuclei, themselves, however, cannot usually be differentiated from those of the more familiar cell. Additional

PLATE XXI
GIANT CELLS

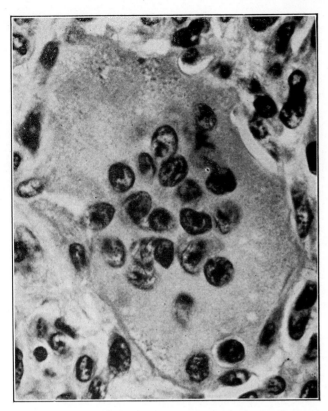

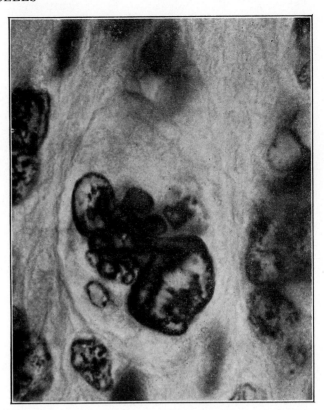

FIG. 83.—FOREIGN BODY GIANT CELL OF TYPE SEEN IN BE-
NIGN GIANT CELL TUMOR OF BONE.—CASE 96.—Multinucleated
syncytial mass of cytoplasm with tendency toward irregular
scalloping of edges and indefinite cell membrane. Nuclei are
round or ovoid, centrally placed and somewhat hyperchromatic.
App. 1000 x.

FIG. 84.—TUMOR GIANT CELL OF TYPE SEEN IN MALIGNANT
SARCOMA.—CASE 93.—Characteristic anaplastic, atypic malignant
cell. Ill-defined cell outline, enormous multilobulated, hyperchromatic nucleus resulting from incomplete nuclear division through
abnormal chromosome distribution in mitosis. App. 1000 x.

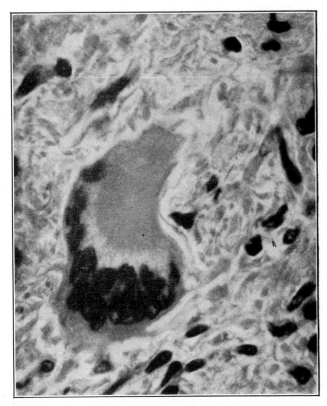

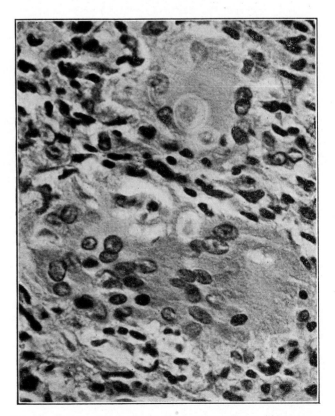

FIG. 85.—FOREIGN BODY GIANT CELL OF THE LANGHANS' TYPE
SEEN IN TUBERCULOSIS.—CASE 56.—The cell is irregular in outline; the nuclei are ovoid, and radially arranged, several layers
deep, at the periphery of cell in horseshoe fashion; cytoplasm
contains phagocytosed material. App. 1000 x.

FIG. 86.—FOREIGN BODY GIANT CELL OF THE USUAL TYPE SEEN
IN CHRONIC INFLAMMATION.—CF. CASE 64.—BLASTOMYCOSIS.—
Large multinucleated cell with normal appearing, diffusely distributed nuclei; cytoplasm containing phagocytosed material, in
this instance blastomyces; cell membrane poorly defined. App.
800 x.

examples of these tumor giant cells, both of the foreign body giant cell tumor of bone and in various other neoplastic conditions, will be discussed in the section, ONCOLOGY. This illustration is merely inserted at this point for comparison with the inflammatory type of giant cell.

ILLUSTRATIVE CASE

CASE 36 (Ref. #S-300)

Diagnosis.—Ulcerative stomatitis; chronic inflammation; large mononuclear cellular infiltration.

Patient was a colored female of 56 years, who was admitted to the hospital because of pain in the left side of her chest with difficulty in breathing.

Present Illness.—The onset of her present condition was rather gradual over a period of a few days. The pain was knife-like in character radiating toward the shoulder. It was accompanied by marked expiratory difficulty and by the development of a fever of a moderate degree.

Past Medical History.—Patient was a known diabetic and had been treated in the hospital four years previously. She had required about one month's hospitalization in order to get her carbohydrate metabolism under adequate control. She then attended the metabolic clinic for her diabetes at biweekly intervals for the next year, but because she felt nothing symptomatic gave up any further observation. During the interval she had been in her usual health but had noted an increase of both frequency and amount of urination.

As a child she believed she had most of the ordinary contagious diseases including diphtheria. She had pneumonia eighteen years ago with no apparent aftermath. She had an operation on her stomach, which she thought was for the removal of a tumor six years before admission. Due to frequent and recurrent attacks of tonsillitis, she had her tonsils out about twelve years ago. A review of her systems otherwise revealed nothing apparently relevant. She had occasional gastro-intestinal disturbances until the time of her operation, but other than moderate constipation since that time she had not been bothered by her stomach. Her cardiovascular system had not caused her any symptoms. Her genito-urinary history was probably unreliable. She disclaimed venereal infection. Her menstrual history had been normal in character and she had had her climacteric eight years previous to this admission.

Physical Examination.—Patient was a well developed and nourished elderly appearing Negress, who was extremely dyspneic. Her head was normal in shape. Facies showed a suggestive partial left-sided paralysis, although this was by no means complete. The sclerae suggested some hemolytic jaundice. There was ptosis of the left lid. Pupils reacted normally and were equal and regular. Ears were negative. Nose: There was a perforation in the posterior part of the septum. Chest was symmetrical. Expansion was diminished on both sides. Breath sounds were well heard on the right, but were distant on the left. There were no râles heard and there was no definite alteration in breath sounds. Heart was markedly enlarged to the right and left, with a systolic aortic murmur. Blood pressure was 240/140. Abdomen was obese. There was a large midline scar, the site of her previous operation. Neurologic examination showed

no gross loss of motor or sensory function other than the facial weakness already noted.

Laboratory Findings.—Red blood cells 4,200,000; hemoglobin 78%; white blood cells 14,000 with 71% polynuclears. Serology: Wassermann and Kahn tests both four plus. Kidney function test gave a total urea clearance of 39%. Blood urea 18 mgm./100 c.c. Spinal fluid was negative.

Nose and throat consultation showed very marked subglottic stenosis which was interpreted as probably syphilitic in origin.

Subsequent Course.—This subglottic stenosis increased in severity accompanied by marked edema, until an emergency tracheotomy became necessary following an unsuccessful attempt at intubation. Following this, the symptoms improved, but the patient developed very marked ulcerative stomatitis. This apparently gave rise to a blood stream infection caused by hemolytic streptococci. The patient went on to develop terminal bronchopneumonia and after a very stormy period with a septic temperature ranging from 99 to 107° daily, died in profound toxemia.

Autopsy Findings.—There was a very extensive acute hemorrhagic ulcerative stomatitis, acute ulcerative laryngitis, acute edema of the epiglottic and periglottic tissue with a marked fibrosis, which produced complete stenosis. There was a tracheotomy wound which appeared clean. There was an old aortic valvulitis with some linear striations of the aorta suggesting luetic aortitis. There was a terminal bilateral basal bronchopneumonia. As contributory factors, a benign vascular nephrosclerosis was present. All the viscera showed evidence of marked toxic granular degeneration.

Microscopic Description of the Tissue Removed from the Ulcerative Stomatitis.—(Fig. 81) Microscopic examination of the tissues removed from the ulcerative stomatitis presents evidence of a combined inflammatory process. Most striking in this lesion is the mononuclear cellular predominance in spite of the acute nature of the clinical course. That this represents a long standing chronic inflammatory process, presumably syphilitic in etiology, is borne out by the history and particularly the laboratory findings of a four plus Wassermann. The histology shows a diffuse productive fibrosis with a very marked cellular infiltration. There is considerable accompanying edema of the tissues. Large mononuclear wandering cells are found in profusion, particularly in the loose, edematous interstitial tissue. In addition, occasional plasma cells and many lymphocytes are found as part of the accompanying chronic inflammatory reaction. Occasional polynuclear cells are seen adding evidence of the superimposed acute terminal picture. The mononuclear cells may be recognized by their large size, their eccentrically placed nuclei and the fact that many of them are actively engaged in phagocytosis, their cytoplasm being distended with engulfed cellular debris.

Diagnosis.—Lung—miliary tubercle with foreign body giant cell production.

Microscopic Description of the Foreign Body Giant Cell Reaction in a Miliary Tubercle.—(Fig. 85). (For clinical history, see CASE 59 (Ref. #S-28), Chapter XVI). Careful study of one of the miliary tubercles in this case emphasizes the importance of the foreign body giant cell in its development. In examining the lung under low power, the presence of these large, multinucleated cells is one of the outstanding features of the pathology. In almost every tubercle, whether of a submiliary beginning variety or in some of the larger, conglomerate lesions made up of several fused tubercles, these giant cells stand out prominently. In examining them under the high power, it will be observed that in general the cells are anywhere from 10 to 20 times the size of any single other cell in the picture. The cytoplasm of these cells is made up of a syncytial mass of rather deep purplish-red-staining cytoplasm. The nuclei tend to be arranged in horseshoe fashion radially around the periphery of the major portion of the cell. In general, these are a single layer deep. In places, however, it will be noted that they may occur in two or three parallel rows. The nuclei are all well formed and adult in appearance. They are ovoid with a definite nuclear membrane, and have a vesicular appearance with small scattered chromatin rods and granules. Nucleoli are rarely to be seen. There is no distortion of these nuclei as is so characteristic of the nuclei of tumor giant cells in which multilobed arrangement of the nuclear material is so prominent, nor is there any hyperchromatism to these cells. They merely seem to represent the fusion of a number of large mononuclear phagocytes which have joined together in the attempt to remove the tubercle bacilli and other lipoid material or cell debris which has not been dissolved by the proteolytic action of the earlier polynuclear leukocytes in the development of the lesion. By staining these cells appropriately with carbol fuchsin it is possible in many instances to actually demonstrate the presence of the tubercle bacillus within their cytoplasm. Indeed, in certain cases, whole clumps of tubercle bacilli can be seen. Due to their protective waxy capsule the organism is extremely resistant to phagocytosis and to digestion, even when taken into the cytoplasm of the cell. Due to the ameboid motion of the cell they may be carried to the periphery of the lesion. In many instances, the organism may kill the cell rather than the cell destroy the organism. In this way the cell breaks down and the organisms are again released to migrate further into the tissues and thus extend the lesion from its original focus.

Diagnosis.—Penis—syphilitic chancre; chronic inflammation—plasma cell infiltration.

Microscopic Description of the Inflammatory Cells in a Primary Syphilitic Lesion.—(Fig. 75 and 80) (For clinical history, see CASE 54 (Ref. #S-296), Chapter XV). Examination of the tissue from the primary chancre presents an unusually excellent place to study the cells of a chronic inflammatory process, and particularly for the recognition of plasma cells. The lesion briefly may be described as showing a superficial ulceration of the epithelium with the chronic granulomatous inflammatory reaction in the deeper tissues. There is moderate dilatation of the capillaries and, indeed, a rather marked tendency toward capillary proliferation as granulation tissue toward the ulcerated surface. Between these rather prominent vessels there is an accompanying fibrosis and cellular reaction. Especially characteristic is the perivascular mononuclear cellular infiltration seen as "streamers" under the low power of the microscope as the vessels radiate from the focus of infection. Examination of this inflammatory cellular exudate under higher magnifications shows a large preponderance of plasma cells. These, as has been described in the section above, consist of large ovoid cells with the characteristic crescentic appearance of the cytoplasm around their eccentrically placed lymphoid type of nucleus. The tendency for these cells is to stain rather more intensely and to show rather more basophilic affinity in their cytoplasm than does the typical small lymphocyte. The point to be stressed in the present study of these cells is the marked variation in their appearance as seen in the cut section. When they are observed cut in their long axis they are easy of identification, but when they are cut tangentially or in cross section, it is often extremely difficult to be sure that one is not dealing with a simple small lymphocyte or even an unusual large mononuclear cell. It will be observed that there is a very considerable fibrous tissue proliferation seen in conjunction with this particular picture. While it is true that one of the important differential criteria microscopically in recognizing syphilitic lesions is this tendency toward productive fibrosis, yet it must be commented upon that almost invariably in tissue other than the central nervous system that this productive fibrosis is commonly seen in relation to plasma cells. It is believed by many, therefore, that the cell itself is an important factor in the development of this fibrous tissue reaction.

CHAPTER XI
REPAIR AND REGENERATION
ATROPHY, HYPERTROPHY AND HYPERPLASIA

REPAIR

In the recovery from any inflammatory reaction, the tissues have to go through a reparative phase which varies considerably in degree dependent upon many factors. The basis of this repair process consists in the first place of the elimination of the irritant. As we have seen, the etiologic agents which may produce the initial inflammatory processes are legion, but in general may be thought of as toxins either endogenous or exogenous in origin. In this latter group must be included all the bacteria with their endo and exo toxins. In addition to these toxic substances we must consider the physical agents such as trauma, heat, cold and so forth.

The elimination of the respective irritant, therefore, depends in the first place upon its character. The principal mechanism of defense of the body is found in the acute inflammatory reaction by which an increased blood flow develops to carry away toxic products for their final elimination by the respiration or the kidneys. At the same time, we have seen that serum from the blood stream pours out into the tissues in an effort to dilute the injurious agent if it has any miscible properties following which it may then be reabsorbed and carried away by the blood or lymph streams. We have seen that solid particles are engulfed by phagocytes of various kinds and either digested or rendered harmless by this policy of isolation within the cytoplasm of the cell and finally, we find that if there has been any actual loss of tissue through abscess formation, sloughing, or necrosis of any other kind, that connective tissue is stimulated to proliferate and thus fill in the area of destroyed tissue. This fibroblastic proliferation is termed *replacement fibrosis.*

If the irritant is not completely removed by any of the above indicated methods of destruction, digestion and absorption, then we find that the connective tissue still proliferates, but in this case in an attempt to wall off the site of injury from the rest of the body. This reaction is spoken of as *productive fibrosis.* Here we see one of the most fundamental biological principles at work, and yet while we recognize the effect and the rationale of the mechanism, we are still at a loss to explain how or why these changes take place and by what physical or biological laws they are controlled from a functional standpoint. The best explanation for this phenomenon is based on the experimental discovery that injured tissue, especially dying cells, liberate a growth stimulating enzyme commonly spoken of as a *trephone.* This is further borne out by tissue culture experimental evidence. Another theory which has been advanced is that there is normally a growth inhibiting factor present in tissue which becomes lost with the death or injury of the cells. Thus the regeneration or proliferation of cells is renewed as in embryonic life. This balance of growth stimulating and growth inhibiting factors is one of very fundamental significance and about which not only pathologists and physiologists, but biologists in general have devoted years of experimental study, only to leave us with the problem still unsolved and largely based on hypothesis. This balance of power between growth restraint and growth stimulation is of particular interest in considering the development of tumors. It represents in a modified form one of the older theories regarding the origin of tumors, the so-called tissue tension theory of Ribbert, which will be discussed at greater length in the chapter on the causation of tumors.

This process of repair is best seen probably in its simplest form in the healing of a simple surgical wound in which infection has not occurred. On the other hand, even in infected wounds or in inflammatory processes anywhere within the body, the basic principles of repair are the same in every instance,

94

modified chiefly by the nature of the infectious or other responsible agent and by the nature of the tissues involved.

Wound Repair (Healing by First Intention) Primary Union.—By these terms are meant the process by which any uncomplicated surgical incision undergoes healing. This is perhaps best illustrated by any incision through the skin such as results following any exploratory laparotomy. In this instance the surgeon's knife is the injurious agent which produces the inflammatory reaction. It does a minimal amount of damage. Those cells directly in the path of the knife are severed and undergo necrosis. Following the operative procedure the edges of this incision are brought in as close apposition to one another as possible and sewed together. This leaves only a fine linear area in which the usual inflammatory reaction can take place. A small amount of exudate (serum, fibrin, red blood cells and leukocytes) is found in this area of injury. Necrotic cells may be identified by the loss of nuclear detail by karyolysis and karyorrhexis of the nuclei. Cellular debris is found in the interstitial tissues. Polynuclear leukocytes are attracted through positive chemotaxis by the presence of this necrotic tissue. They, in turn, liberate their proteolytic enzymes and aid in the dissolution of this small amount of necrotic and injured tissue.

With the inflammatory process, trephones are presumably liberated or the inhibiting factor against cell growth is lost and within a few hours (usually from six to twelve) young fibroblasts may be seen growing across the exudative field. Accompanying this fibroblastic proliferation we note, in addition, that capillary endothelium is likewise stimulated to proliferate. New endothelial buds may be identified growing out from the vessel walls and accompanying the connective tissue cells. By this means a new blood supply is carried to the inflammatory zone. After this area is safely bridged by the new young fibroblasts, which usually takes from two to three days, the epithelium similarly bridges the surface area. However, in respect to epithelium, none of the specialized skin derivatives, including the hair follicles, sudoriferous or sebaceous glands are ever reformed in the healing of the wound.

Although initial repair begins almost as soon as the injury has taken place, nevertheless it takes from two to three weeks for these young fibroblasts to develop into their adult connective tissue cell form with the production of sufficient intercellular collagen to give complete support to the tissues. This new formed vascular connective tissue covered by epithelium is spoken of as a *cicatrix* or *scar*. At first, such a scar is *red* due to increased vascularity or hyperemia of the tissues as the result of the enormous number of new formed capillary vessels and because the new formed epithelial layer is still only two or three cells deep and remains transparent. Gradually as the epithelium thickens and the collagen increases the need for such a generous blood supply is lost and these new formed vessels are slowly obliterated by pressure of the collagen, which becomes compact and dense as compared with its original loose, wavy, fibrillar appearance. As an end picture there develops a fine, linear, *white scar*. This process, however, is a matter of several months and in any extensive skin wound the development of the final cicatrix may take nearly a year before the red color disappears and leaves the final scar. This, then, is the story of the repair of a wound in its simplest form and its bare essentials.

Repair by Second Intention.—By contrast with the picture just presented by a simple uncomplicated sterile surgical skin wound, unfortunately we have many wounds which become infected. This may be the result of the initial injury through accidental trauma of some type or as the result of having to open an abscess or an abdominal cavity in which peritonitis is present as the result of a ruptured appendix, for example. In such skin wounds, the process becomes much more complicated in the development of the final repair picture. Basically, however, it is very similar in its character.

It is one of the elementary principles of surgery that healing of an infected wound must take place from the base. Thus, at times it may be necessary to cut away dead tissue from the surface to leave a wide, gaping wound which will fill in from the base. However, just as in the case of a simple, uncomplicated wound, fibroblasts grow out into the exudate which fills this gaping area, these fibroblasts grow in from the bottom and the sides along with newly formed capillary vessels just as in primary union repair. In this case, however, capillaries tend to form minute loops, which viewed from the surface appear as red, punctate areas embedded in a granular, grayish background made up of the new connective tissue. From this gross appearance the term *granulation tissue* arose to describe this type of repair associated with low grade or chronic infections.

Such a layer of granulation tissue may at times become tremendously thickened with both replacement and productive fibrosis. The process will continue with more and more connective tissue and capillary endothelial hyperplasia until such a time as the surface infection has almost entirely subsided. However, if the lesion becomes completely sterile, with a loss of all bacterial activity, it apparently prevents the surface epithelium from growing over this newly-formed connective scar tissue. A slightly moist serous exudate on the surface containing the necessary growth stimulating factor, probably as the result of the continued injury to the cells as they proliferate, is much more effective in the ultimate healing of such a lesion.

If the original irritating organism persists, such granulations may become exuberant and rise several millimeters or more above the epithelial surface. This usually occurs on skin wounds and is spoken of as "proud flesh." When this exuberant overgrowth of granulation tissue forms, epithelialization is impossible until this newly-formed granulation has been removed by the knife or cautery. Gradually, as in the case of primary union, dense fibrous scar tissue replaces the earlier granulation tissue. This goes through the same clinical red and white stages, but naturally because of the greater surface area involved the development of the final white cicatrix takes much longer and may not develop in its entirety for as long as ten to twelve months. It is of interest to know that in respect to the trephone theory of cell growth stimulation that if such granulation tissue is rendered completely aseptic chemically with the destruction of all bacteria that the repair process stops. As has been commented upon it is necessary for some slight serous exudate to be present to produce the necessary growth stimulant and permit organization and regeneration to proceed at a normal rate. This surface exudate has been spoken of by the clinicians of a past generation as "laudable pus," and it is interesting to note how appropriate the term remains even to this day.

Repair of Bone.—Basically the principles involved in bone repair are identical with those which we have seen in the simpler repair by primary union or by the development of granulation tissue in infected surface wounds. It is complicated by the presence of the highly specialized bone tissue. When a bone becomes fractured or even if only the periosteum is injured by some trauma, obviously cell injury with resultant necrosis of cells takes place, and an exudate develops in the injured area just as it would in the soft tissues except that it is restricted by the bone cortex. In the case of a fracture, we may have a simple "green stick" fracture occur when the injury is minimal and takes place in the soft, growing bones of an infant or young child. In this instance there is no displacement of the bone fragments, which are still held within their periostal membrane. The repair of such a crack in a bone might well be compared to the healing of a simple surgical sterile incision and be termed repair by primary union. On the other hand a bone may be much more severely fractured, with many fragments of bone displaced into the soft tissues and even if the injury has been severe enough, the ends of the broken bone may be forced through the soft tissues and the skin to produce a so-called compound comminuted fracture. In such an instance the repair process might be again compared to the more complicated mechanism as seen in the development of granulation tissue.

In either instance there is the initial outpouring of red cells, serum, fibrin and leukocytes. In the same way, by the presence of the necessary growth stimulating factors, connective tissue and endothelium are stimulated to grow. In addition, however, there exists in the bone the osteoblasts and chondroblasts which are specialized connective tissue derivatives. These cells, occurring chiefly in relation to the endosteum and periosteum, are likewise stimulated to proliferate. They maintain their normal ability to produce new trabeculae of bone-like tissue. At the outset, however, this is lacking in calcium. It appears as normal trabeculae which stain with eosin, but is apt to show considerable irregularity in its staining reaction due to the beginning calcification. This newly-formed reparative bone is spoken of as *osteoid* tissue and because of its lack of ossification it is produced in excess to provide functional strength. This overgrowth of osteoid tissue is spoken of as a *callus*. Gradually calcification takes place and osteoclasts enter the picture to resorb any excess bone until the normal structural arrangement of the bone is accomplished. Where displacement has taken place and the ends of the bones override, there may always exist a certain amount of deformity, but it is amazing how the callus forms in such a way as to provide the maximum strength to the bone and to replace as nearly as possible its normal architectural arrangement. If the periosteum and endosteum are removed experimentally from an animal or are destroyed in a fracture for any considerable distance from the site of the injury, then new bone formation is either delayed or completely prevented. In the treatment of fractures, it is often advisable to pack the site of the fracture with bone chips from the fractured ends of the bone because each of these bone chips which still has any endosteal or periosteal osteoblasts adherent to its surface will serve as new centers of bone formation and thus render the repair process more rapid. Such fragments of bone as lack this osteoblastic activity undergo necrosis and absorption just as any other soft tissue does. As has already been commented upon, such necrotic fragments of bone are spoken of as sequestra. At times these may act as foreign bodies and prevent satisfactory union of the injured bone if they fail to be absorbed, in which case it is at times necessary to remove them surgically.

REGENERATION

Thus far, in considering the repair of injury, we have noted that it involves the growth of the reparative cells of the body, fibroblasts and the vascular endothelium. In addition, we have seen that where special tissues are involved, their cells likewise regenerate in an effort to reëstablish function. This process of regeneration is a variable one depending upon the individual type of cell involved. Roughly speaking, the more highly differentiated the tissue, the less regeneration takes place. A very hasty survey of some examples of these differences may serve to bring out this point. Striated muscle is, to all intents and purposes, incapable of actual regeneration. When injury occurs involving the muscle cells, there is an abortive attempt on the part of the sarcolemma to proliferate. At times, one may even see the nuclei of the muscle undergoing nuclear differentiation with the formation of club-like thickenings on the ends of the severed or injured muscle cells. In cross section, such reparative attempts simulate the appearance of foreign body giant cells not infrequently and may be mistaken for these scavenger phagocytic cells.

If nerve cells are destroyed, no regeneration is possible, and once retrograde changes have affected the nerve cell nucleus, then function of the part supplied by that cell becomes lost. On the other hand, severance of the nerve axones or dendrites may result in very profound degenerative changes of the cell, but this is not an irreversible reaction unless the nerve cell itself is destroyed, and new axones and dendrites will ultimately grow to replace the injured members. Similarly, glomeruli within the kidney are incapable of actual regeneration. Where damage has affected a renal glomerulus we find proliferative attempts on the part of both the lining capillary endothelium and the capsular epithelium to compensate for this damage but the result is usually a mass of scar tissue with the obliteration of the function of that particular glomerulus. On the other hand, when an entire kidney has become destroyed, the other kidney enlarges and its component parts increase in size in an attempt to compensate functionally for the loss of the one kidney.

The liver is probably one of the most easily injured organs in the body. Almost every mild toxemia associated with infections elsewhere, with digestive disturbances, with exogenous substances may cause definite necrosis of liver cells. In experimental chloroform poisoning more than half of the liver cells may easily be destroyed, and yet at the end of a comparatively short period of time, no evidence of liver damage may be detected histologically, so great is the capacity of the liver cell to regenerate. Similarly the tubular epithelium of the kidney, especially the cells lining the convoluted tubules, which are likewise particularly susceptible to injury, are also capable of amazing regenerative powers. On the other hand, the lung is almost incapable of any real regeneration. Compensatory dilatation of the alveoli with an increase of the number of lining alveolar cells may take place, but where lung is destroyed, it is usually permanently replaced by scar tissues. Similarly, heart muscle is incapable of regeneration to any significant degree. Likewise, injuries which affect the reproductive organs tend to be permanent in their nature and regeneration of these cells is impossible; while on the other hand, destruction of any of the reticulo-endothelial organs may take place with a compensatory regeneration of these cells to maintain their function, even if such new cell growth occurs in a distant organ.

For example, in the case of the surgical removal of the spleen, for any cause, one finds hyperplasia of the reticulo-endothelial cells of the lymph nodes and bone marrow.

HYPERTROPHY AND HYPERPLASIA

We have seen in relation to this discussion of the repair of tissue with the regeneration of cells that at times a marked increase in the size of the cells or of the organ may take place as a compensatory mechanism. This increase in size of an organ may be the result of increase in the size of the individual cells or in the number of the cells.

By *hypertrophy* is meant an increase in the size of the cells making up the component parts of an organ, which in turn produce hypertrophy of the organ. Such an hypertrophy is seen in the enlargement of the heart as a result of valvular disease or other injury. Similarly, such hypertrophy is seen in the uterus during pregnancy. In both these instances, there is no increase in the number of cells, but merely one of increase in size to maintain the functional activity of the organ.

On the other hand, we have seen in the repair of many injuries that there is an actual increase in the number of cells. This is spoken of as *hyperplasia*. Under normal circumstances, hyperplasia as part of the picture of repair goes on only to such a point where physiological functional activity of the involved organ or tissue is produced. When that point is reached, a state of equilibrium between cell growth and cell destruction takes place and the normal rate of growth to take care of the usual wear and tear of cells reëstablishes itself. In cases where prolonged irritation and injury exists, correspondingly increased proliferation of cells continues. This we have seen in the production of exuberant granulation tissue which serves no useful functional capacity. As a source of chronic irritation such persistent hyperplasia is but a step removed from the more significant and serious neoplasia of malignancy with its associated high mortality.

ATROPHY

By atrophy is meant the decrease in size of an organ or of the correspondent cellular elements thereof. Atrophy may occur as the result of many conditions. In the first place, we may speak of what might well be termed a normal physiological atrophy as part of the picture of senility. Likewise, the normal physiological atrophy of the reproductive organs following the active sexual phase of life may also be cited as another example of this type. We have seen the appearance of organs in an elderly individual where the lipochrome pigments have accumulated with a diminution in the size of the cells in the familiar "brown atrophy" of the heart, liver and other viscera.

In the last analysis, perhaps atrophy might always be considered the end result of disuse. Where nerve injury has occurred and no longer do we receive stimuli to a part, there also we find atrophy of the structures involved. Perhaps this is best seen in the condition known as infantile paralysis or anterior poliomyelitis where the motor nerve cells in the spinal cord are destroyed in a haphazard pattern and there is resultant atrophy of the muscles supplied by those nerve cells. In the same way, we speak of pressure atrophy as the result of localized pressure upon structures. This is particularly noticed in relation to impaired circulation and atrophy of the liver cells around the central vein as the result of long standing uncomplicated chronic passive congestion from cardiac disease, which represents an excellent example. Another example of such pressure atrophy is seen in the small, contracted kidney, the result of occlusion of the ureter with the back pressure gradually causing atrophic degeneration of the entire renal structure. Such examples could be multiplied almost indefinitely. More difficult to explain are those forms of atrophy seen following an initial extraordinary degree of hypertrophy. Here we find a loss in functional capacity which may well have a neutrotrophic background in its development. This is particularly seen in people who use their muscles to excess. It is not uncommon to find in the forearms of musicians.

In general, however, all cases of atrophy are the

result of some interference with functional capacity either as the result of physiological developmental change, of interference with nutrition or of inter-ference with the nerve supply, resulting in disuse and gradual regression in size of the organ because of atrophy of its individual cells.

ILLUSTRATIVE CASES

CASE 37. (Ref. #S-7)

Diagnosis.—Appendix—Acute inflammation; suppura-tive necrosis; productive inflammatory repair of a peri-appendiceal abscess.

Patient was a white female of 58 years, who was admitted to the hospital with a history of right lower quadrant pain of about one week's duration.

Present Illness.—Onset was gradual and without much gastro-intestinal disturbance. She had not consid-ered it serious enough to require medical attention until the day of admission. She had had a little vague ab-dominal distress, but no nausea or vomiting until just before her admission. She did not think she had had any fever during this interval and had been able to do her regular housework.

Past History.—The past history was irrelevant in respect to her present illness. She had had the usual childhood diseases but had never been seriously enough sick during her adult life to require hospitalization. She suffered from occasional upper respiratory infections. She had no gastro-intestinal disturbances other than rather marked and persistent constipation of many years' duration. Her genito-urinary and catamenic histories were normal. She had had her menopause ten years ago.

Physical Examination.—Patient was a well developed and nourished elderly white woman who was lying in bed and appeared to be in acute pain. Her head was negative. Eyes, ears, nose and throat were normal. Chest was symmetrical. Lungs were clear. Heart was not en-larged and there were no murmurs. Abdomen was mod-erately distended. There was board-like rigidity of the right rectus and right lower quadrant muscles so that deep palpation was impossible. The entire abdomen was tense and sore on palpation. No masses could be made out. Rectal examination revealed a mass in the right lower quadrant which was extremely sensitive on pres-sure.

Laboratory Findings.—Temperature 102.5°. White blood cells 18,000 with 94% polynuclears. Urinalysis showed a slight trace of albumin but was otherwise negative.

Subsequent History.—A diagnosis of ruptured appen-dix was made and an emergency appendectomy done. A retrocecal periappendiceal abscess was found in which the stump of the appendix was identified. This was cov-ered with thick, plastic exudate and showed considerable organization. There was a localized peritonitis where the infection had spread from the localized abscess cavity. The abdomen was closed with a deep drain and the patient made a relatively uneventful recovery.

Pathological Report.—*Gross Description.*—Pathologi-cal specimen consisted of an irregularly shaped, some-what ovoidal mass of tissue which measured 4 cm. in thickness by 4.5 cm. in length. It was covered by a thick, plastic, fibrinous exudate, firmly adherent to the under-lying structures and showed evidence of definite organi-zation. On section, a lumen could be made out represent-ing the appendix and surrounding this, the thickened appendiceal wall could be identified.

Microscopic Examination of the Periappendiceal Tissue.—(Fig. 77) Study of the tissue in relation to the appendiceal wall shows evidence of an unusually beauti-ful example of fibroblastic proliferation and the forma-tion of new capillaries. The appendiceal mucosa is largely necrotic, only occasional acinar structures persist-ing by which it can be identified. Overlying this is an acute purulent exudate with extensive necrosis beneath a layer of polynuclears. Repair of this acute necrotic process has also begun and new formed capillaries can be seen growing out into this exudate. Here, also, fibro-blasts may be identified in varying stages of develop-ment. Throughout the peri-appendiceal tissue, one has opportunity to study the development of connective tissue from the very earliest fibroblast with a large, almost round nucleus and beginning fibroglia fiber development to the adult cell with its elongated, contracted nucleus and its abundant collagen. This picture of productive fibrosis and vascular proliferation represents the typical picture of repair and serves better than any amount of description can do to illustrate the nature of this process.

CASE 38. (Ref. #S-133)

Diagnosis.—Rectal fistula—chronic inflammation; granulation tissue; tuberculosis.

Patient was a white male of 54 years who was ad-mitted to the hospital because of pain and redness in the perineal area accompanied by marked pruritus ani.

Present Illness.—The present illness began two weeks before admission in its acute form. However, his history dated back two years when he had the beginning of a gastro-intestinal history which resulted in a cholecystec-tomy one and one-half years before the present illness, and in a partial subtotal gastrectomy six months before the present illness because of an ulcer which did not re-spond to medical treatment. Since that time he had been badly constipated and required considerable radical catharsis.

The local discomfort in the perineal region grew stead-ily worse over the two weeks' period until it became so extreme that the least motion caused him exquisite pain. He had considered it as a simple boil and had been at-tempting self-medication with the application of heat, but the abscess never apparently "came to a head," so that he returned to the hospital for relief.

Past History.—Patient had had a rather long and stormy medical history. He apparently had a normal childhood with only the usual mild diseases. He was a carpenter and plasterer by occupation and had several minor accidents, one about ten years ago resulting in a blood stream infection which required hospitalization of about six weeks. Subsequently he had an appendectomy and had had an almost constant history of gastro-in-testinal disturbances over the last ten years, which re-sulted in the various operative procedures commented upon in the present illness. His family history was apparently negative in respect to tuberculosis, cancer, diabetes and Bright's disease.

Physical Examination.—On admission the patient seemed to be a fairly well developed, middle aged white male in a poor state of nutrition. His head was not remarkable. Eyes, ears, nose and throat were essentially negative. There were scars noted, one six inches long in the right side of his abdomen just below the costal margin, and another over the right lower quadrant where he had had his appendectomy. His chest was symmetrical and somewhat emphysematous in appearance. Lungs were clear. Heart was normal in size. The rate was regular and there were no murmurs heard. The abdomen, other than for the scars, appeared negative. There was marked swelling, redness and tenderness in the perineal region. Rectal examination showed marked tenderness around the anal ring. No hemorrhoids were demonstrated. A diagnosis of perirectal abscess was made and the abscess was incised and drained.

Laboratory Findings.—Red blood cells 3,200,000; hemoglobin 76%. White blood cells 9,400 with 68% polynuclear leukocytes. Urinalysis showed an occasional trace of albumin, but nothing else of significance.

Subsequent Course.—The lesion developed into a fistula, which persisted for a year at which time he was operated upon with the idea of trying to remove the fistulous tract. This resulted in temporary healing. At the present time, the lesion is known to have broken down again and the fistula to have reëstablished itself as a draining sinus, which extends to the rectum.

Pathological Report.—*Gross Description.*—Specimen consisted of a mass of fatty fibrous tissue with a small piece of rectal mucosa on one end of the specimen and what appeared to be an elliptical skin fragment on the other.

Microscopic Description.—(Fig. 76) Sections through the sinus tract microscopically are seen to present evidence of a marked chronic inflammatory process. The picture is one of both reparative fibrosis with the formation of granulation tissue and of chronic productive inflammation. The granular reparative factor is evidenced by new capillary vessel proliferation which is growing toward the surface as capillary loops. Supporting these are found fibroblasts tending to be arranged in parallel fashion at right angles to the new-formed vessels. Embedded in this entire mass of granulation tissue are found all varieties of chronic inflammatory cells of which lymphocytes and large mononuclear phagocytes predominate. Occasional eosinophilic leukocytes are found and also a moderate number of plasma cells. Careful search through the tissue reveals the presence of occasional rather typical Langhans' giant cells arranged in relation to a small area of caseous necrosis, which are surrounded by large mononuclear cells arranged in rather palisading or radial fashion. This arrangement strongly suggests a tuberculous etiology for this particular inflammatory process, but it is obviously complicated by secondary bacterial invasion from without.

CASE 39. (Ref. #S-210)

Diagnosis.—Femur (rabbit)—bone repair.

For the demonstration of bone repair it was felt that the entire process could be best exemplified by the study of sections from an animal bone in which bone destruction had been produced. The object of this selection of material was that the entire cross section of the bone could be studied as a whole, thus showing the relationships of periosteum and endosteum to the reparative process. The experimental animal was a young rabbit in whom bone repair might be expected to proceed rapidly. The femur of the rabbit was exposed under sterile surgical precautions and a narrow gutter made for a distance of approximately 1 cm. on one side of the bone, cutting through the cortex only. The wound was closed surgically and repair allowed to proceed for two weeks. At the end of this time the animal was sacrificed and the bone removed for histologic study.

Pathological Description.—Grossly, it was observed that at the point of operation there was marked thickening of the bone over the injured area. This merged with the normal periosteum laterally at both ends of the wound. Likewise the soft tissues showed extensive reparative fibrosis.

Microscopic Description.—(Fig. 78 and 79) Sections microscopically taken through the bone in cross section show a rim of normal cortical bone which occupies about three-fourths of the total diameter. In the gap between the two portions of normal cortex may be seen a wildly proliferating mass of new-formed osteoid tissue. This is arising both from the endosteum and from the periosteum and likewise appears to arise from the osteoblasts covering the various bone fragments which had been forced into the marrow cavity by the operative procedure. Wherever periosteal or endosteal osteoblasts persist, this proliferation with the development of interlacing osteoid trabeculae is going on. Under the microscope it is noted that this osteoid tissue lacks the density and calcification of adult bone. This is observed in its staining reaction in particular, taking a rather bluish or pinkish color as compared to the usual rather intense eosin-staining picture. Likewise, the normal haversian systems of bone are lacking. This phenomenon of osteogenesis with the production of an initial osteoid tissue is obviously in excess of the normal functional requirements. This excessive bone-like tissue is spoken of as a "callus." Gradually, calcification occurs and osteoclastic activity proceeds at a greater rate than osteogenesis until a new balance of bone formation and bone destruction is reached with the return to normal in the appearance both grossly and microscopically of the injured bone.

In the development of such newly-formed bone, particularly in young, rapidly growing animals, it is not uncommon to find, as in this case, a preliminary phase in which cartilage as well as osteoid tissue is produced. In other words, newly-formed bone in its reparative phase may go through a developmental change comparable to the development of membranous bone as well as by the usual picture of adult bone formation.

CHAPTER XII

TYPES OF INFLAMMATION

*SEROSITIS, MUCOSITIS (CATARRHAL INFLAMMATION),
ULCERATION, SUPPURATION, PHLEGMONOUS
INFLAMMATION*

In the preceding chapters we have discussed the general biologic nature of the inflammatory process. We have seen that inflammation, occurring as it does as the result of so many and such varied etiologic agents, may present extraordinary differences in its histologic and morphologic aspects. And yet the underlying reaction is similar in each instance, dependent in the last analysis upon the same vascular and fixed tissue elements. It is comparable perhaps to the contractor or builder, who with the same stone, lumber, glass and mortar can create an entire community of homes, no two of which are identical in appearance. For convenience we have come to classify the acute inflammatory lesions on the basis of the predominance of one or more of the constituents of the blood in the exudate, as hemorrhagic, serous, fibrinous or purulent, just as we speak of a house as being stone, brick, stucco, clapboard or shingle, although obviously all the fundamental materials must be present in the final product to some extent. Similarly in the subacute and chronic inflammatory processes we find the same variation in response of the fixed and wandering tissue cells, so that the picture which results is in the great majority of instances recognizable as of a fairly definitely specific etiology.

While this strictly morphologic classification of inflammation is obviously the most nearly exact biologic method, we find that from the clinicopathologic standpoint it is more generally useful to designate the type of inflammation upon the basis of the tissue or organ involved, and upon the extent or degree of the inflammatory process.

Thus, inflammation which involves a serous surface is spoken of as *serositis;* one involving a mucous surface, as *mucositis.* In mild inflammatory processes in which the irritant is usually not sufficient to produce actual necrosis of cells, we find that the earliest signs of inflammation are those of hypersecretion on the part of these various surface types of cells. In the case of such an irritant involving a serous surface such as the pleura, we find an outpouring of the serous secretion of the pleural serosal cells, and the accumulation of a clear or slightly cloudy fluid in the pleural cavity. Chemical examination of this fluid will show that its specific gravity is higher than similar appearing fluid which would accumulate as the result of cardiac failure, for example. This latter would be a simple *transudate.* The fluid of inflammatory origin will show a higher protein content, and on centrifugization the sediment will be found to contain a variable number of inflammatory cells; leukocytes, lymphocytes and desquamated serosa, so that it has to be considered as a true *serous* exudate.

In the same way, when a mucous membrane is irritated mildly we find that the goblet cells in particular are stimulated to an oversecretion of mucus. This may be seen typically in mild infections of the nose and throat, or in irritation of the gastric or intestinal mucosa as the result of mild food poisonings, of alcohol, of irritation from the presence of a tumor, etc. Grossly in such cases one sees an excess of glairy, tenacious mucus on the surface of the mucosa. Microscopically, this mucus will be found arising from the deep mucous glands, the cells of which are increased in size. In the meshes of this mucinous material will be found variable numbers of leukocytes and often, bacteria. The reaction is obviously a protective mechanism on the part of the body to produce an almost impenetrable layer of mucus on the surface of the mucosa to prevent further injury by the irritant. Such an inflammation is spoken of as *catarrhal* (Fig. 87, 88, 89, 90, 91, 92, 93 and 94).

In both the serositis and mucositis pictures we find

PLATE XXII
ACUTE MUCOSITIS (CATARRHAL)

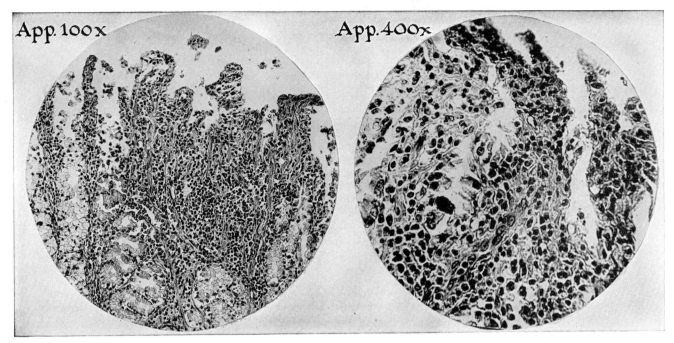

F<small>IG</small>. 87 and 88.—S<small>TOMACH</small>: C<small>ATARRHAL</small> I<small>NFLAMMATION</small>.—C<small>ASE</small> 40.—High and low power photomicrographs of an area of gastric mucosa showing cellular infiltration of tunica propria, increased mucus production and glandular epithelial degeneration and desquamation. Approx. 100 and 400 x.

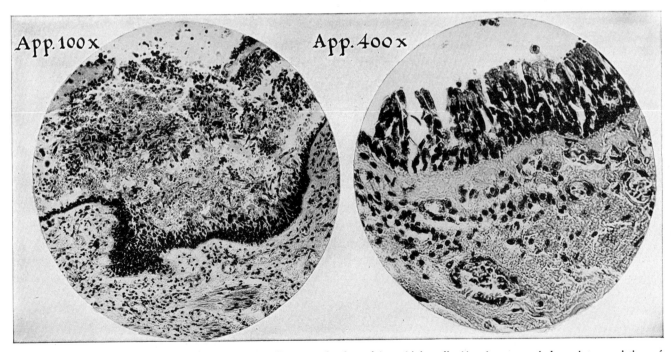

F<small>IG</small>. 89 and 90.—B<small>RONCHUS</small>: C<small>ATARRHAL</small> B<small>RONCHITIS</small>.—C<small>ASE</small> 41.—Section of bronchial wall. Abundant catarrhal exudate consisting of mucin, leukocytes and desquamated epithelium, in lumen. Capillary dilatation, edema and leukocytic infiltration of submucosa. Approx. 100 and 400 x.

other evidence, as a rule, that the process is a true inflammatory one, in that *hyperemia* is present, producing reddening of the surface. Likewise usually some edema is demonstrable, especially in the mucosal lesions. Often some diapedesis of leukocytes or red cells has occurred microscopically as well.

From the standpoint of nomenclature, we find, as the severity of the injury increases, and the inflammatory picture correspondingly increases in degree, that additional clinical terms are applied to differen-tiate these various gradations. As a clinical means of estimating prognosis, such terminology is unquestionably of value. It tends, unfortunately, to confuse the problem from the strictly morphologic basis. It involves the modifying of our simple concept of inflammation as based on the hemorrhagic, serous, fibrinous or leukocytic (purulent) nature of the exudate in the acute picture, or the productive fibrosis of the chronic form by the addition of appropriate descriptive adjectives.

Necrotic Inflammation

Thus, we find that a mucositis may become complicated by extensive submucosal involvement. Vascular damage may occur. Thrombosis of vessels in the area may ensue, with necrosis of the area involved, as in infarction. The vessel walls may rupture and diffuse hemorrhage result. Such a picture might well follow the ingestion of strong poisons such as bichloride of mercury, caustic soda and the like. In such a case coagulation necrosis of the tissues would result from the direct action of the toxin, as well as by the secondary interference with the blood supply. When such necrosis of any considerable amount of tissue occurs, it is spoken of as *necrotic inflammation*. If hemorrhage is a prominent feature of the lesion then it becomes *hemorrhagic necrosis* (Fig. 107 and 108). In the simpler forms, especially when produced by chemical poisons, the lesion may remain free of bacteria. Under such circumstances the leukocytes, which accumulate through chemotaxis, slowly liquefy the necrotic tissue, especially at the base of the lesion where they are found in greatest numbers as they migrate from the capillaries. A line of separation, or cleavage forms, and mechanically the whole mass of dead tissue *sloughs* away, leaving an *ulcerated* mucosal surface varying in extent.

Septic and Gangrenous Inflammation

If bacterial infection complicate such a process it it spoken of as a *septic necrotic inflammation* and designated by the name of the specific organism in addition if identified. If the bacteria are of the putrefactive variety, as has been already discussed in Chapter VII, the inflammatory process is spoken of as *gangrenous* (Fig. 109). This is obviously commonly seen in the lesions of the intestinal tract.

Ulceration

In considering this end result of such necrotic inflammation mention was made of the development of an ulcer. By *ulcer* is meant a break in the continuity of any surface or lining epithelium, whether skin or mucous membrane as the result of such a necrotic inflammatory process. The term goes beyond the concept of mere loss of epithelium. A superficial erosion of the skin might easily be the result of mild trauma, as frequently results from scraping of the skin. This superficial type of injury is spoken of as an *abrasion*. True ulceration implies a lesion which has extended to involve the deeper structures of the skin or mucous membranes as well, so that in healing, a permanent cicatrix results from the replacement fibrosis which develops. In the great majority of cases infection plays a rôle in the picture.

Suppuration

When the inflammation extends beyond the surface mucosa or serosa and involves the deeper tissues, we find still other terms in use. Indeed it is not uncommon to find infections spreading by way of lymphatics or the blood stream to the regional lymph nodes or to distant parts of the body. This process of

PLATE XXIII
CHRONIC MUCOSITIS (Catarrhal)

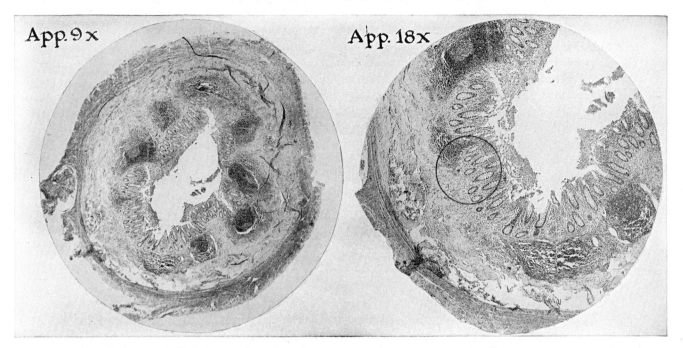

FIG. 91.   FIG. 92.

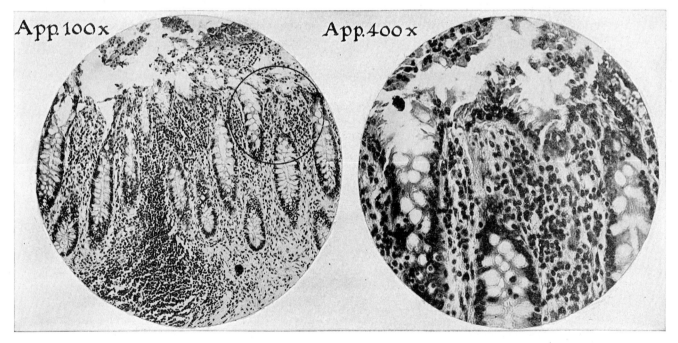

FIG. 93. APP. 100 X   FIG. 94. APP. 400 X

APPENDIX.—CATARRHAL APPENDICITIS.—CASE 42.—Marked thickening of submucosa due to fibrosis from previous inflammation is prominent in Fig. 91 and 92. The more typical catarrhal inflammatory changes are seen in the mucosa, consisting of mononuclear cellular infiltration of the tunica, hyperactive glandular "goblet" cells, and characteristic catarrhal exudate in the lumen (Fig. 93 and 94).

humoral distribution with the development of secondary lesions is spoken of as *metastasis*. This term we shall encounter in more common usage in respect to malignant tumors, but is equally accurately employed in respect to such secondary bacterial lesions. Many visceral or deep skeletal tissue inflammatory changes may accordingly be encountered clinically or at the postmortem table which duplicate in their basic reactions, the primary or mother lesion, except as modified by the architectural details of the tissues involved. Such inflammatory reactions are apt to be bacterial in origin, and therefore specific in nature in their cellular response, but even under such conditions certain general terms will be found in use. Among these is the term "suppuration." By this is meant a leukocytic exudate associated with liquefaction necrosis and the localized production of pus.

It may be induced experimentally by the intramuscular injection of strong irritants such as turpentine, croton oil, or even a 50% glucose solution. Clinically it is seen as a complication in the intravenous or intramuscular use of some of the more toxic drugs or antisera. Probably the most typical and most familiar example of suppuration is seen in the development of an *abscess* caused by the Staphylococcus aureus. This organism has a powerful, nondiffusible lytic toxin and has a strong positive chemotactic attraction for polymorphonuclear leukocytes. As a result of this intense concentration of two highly active proteolytic agents we have rapid *suppurative necrosis* develop. Similar suppuration may obviously take place in relation to ulcerated lesions of the skin, mucous membranes or other tissues such as the meninges. (Fig. 110.)

PHLEGMONOUS INFLAMMATION

In like manner we may find a diffuse serous, or seropurulent infiltration of the tissues without resulting liquefaction necrosis. Such a reaction is commonly associated with infections produced by the hemolytic streptococci. Extension of the initial streptococcic throat infection of septic sore throat, for example, to the deep tissues of the neck is quite common. In this instance we find the streptococcus has a weakly lytic, but strongly diffusible toxin which stimulates a marked serous outpouring in the infected area. Such a picture is frequently described as *"phlegmonous" inflammation*. It may be seen frequently accompanying scarlet fever, diphtheria, so-called Ludwig's angina, agranulocytic angina and other similar acute infections of the throat. Similarly it may occur in any part of the body as an extension or complication of an initial infection such as a wound of the hand or foot, or even in the wall of the appendix for example, before suppuration or gangrene supervene. Again, phlegmonous lesions of the pelvis make up a large group of gynecologic cases.

To summarize; in its broadest sense, inflammation is the reaction of the body to injury. Every inflammatory process is characterized by some combination of vascular and cellular response to the injury, dependent upon the nature of the injurious agent.

Inflammation may be characterized as being either acute or chronic.

In acute inflammation the exudative picture is predominant. The exudate in acute inflammation is characterized as serous, fibrinous, hemorrhagic, leukocytic (purulent) or some combination of these, as serofibrinous, fibrinopurulent, etc. dependent upon the predominating element. Inflammation involving a serous surface is called serositis; involving a mucous surface, mucositis. Degrees of inflammation of surface injuries are indicated by modifying adjectives in the following progressive fashion: catarrhal (mucositis) or serous (serositis); pseudo-diphtheritic or membranous (fibrinous mucositis); diphtheritic or necrotic (mucositis); gangrenous (usually mucositis). Acute inflammation involving deeper tissues is apt to be spoken of as *phlegmonous* when serum predominates; as *suppurative,* when liquefaction necrosis associated with pus formation occurs.

Chronic inflammation may follow acute inflammation if the irritant is not removed by any of these cellular reactions. Or, it may exist from the very outset, if the injurious agent is of a low degree of toxicity. The histologic picture of chronic inflammation is one of mononuclear cellular infiltration, accompanied by productive fibrosis.

ILLUSTRATIVE CASES

CASE 40. (Ref. #S-8)

Diagnosis.—Stomach—acute and chronic catarrhal gastritis (mucositis).

Patient was a white female fifty years of age, admitted to the hospital semistuporous and critically ill with cardiac decompensation.

Present Illness.—Her present illness began several weeks before admission with progressive dyspnea and edema of the lower extremities. She was known to have had heart disease for several years and had had two other periods of acute decompensation from which she had recovered with bed rest, and had been able to carry on her ordinary household duties. The present attack, however, had been much more severe in character. She had noted marked cyanosis of her face in addition to the dyspnea and progressive edema of the feet and ankles.

Past History.—The patient had had a normal childhood with the usual mild infections. She was married and had had three normal children. At the age of twenty-four, she had had what was thought to be a mild attack of acute rheumatic fever, which subsided spontaneously and she was not aware of any cardiac sequelae until about six years ago. At that time she had palpitation and dyspnea on exertion. As a result of this cardiac picture she had led a very quiet existence since that time. For the past several years, she has suffered from vague gastro-intestinal disturbances which she had thought of as dyspepsia. She had had occasional attacks of vomiting accompanied by nausea, and she had a history of chronic constipation. Her respiratory system was essentially negative except for the dyspnea. Her genito-urinary and menstrual histories were negative.

Physical Examination.—Patient was a well developed, somewhat obese middle-aged woman lying in bed in a semistuporous condition. She could be aroused only with great difficulty and her attention could be held only momentarily. Her head was normal in contour. Her eyes reacted to light. Ears, nose and throat were negative. Chest was symmetrical. There was a moderate suggestion of emphysema with a tendency toward a barrel shaped chest. Lungs showed numerous crackling râles, mostly at the bases. There was no definite dullness detected. The heart was greatly enlarged, the left border being in the midaxillary line. There was a soft, blowing systolic murmur transmitted to the axilla, best heard over the mitral area. Blood pressure was 180/100. Heart sounds were distant. There was marked irregularity. The pulse varied from 60 to 120. Abdomen was moderately protuberant. The liver edge could be felt two fingers' breadth below the costal margin. The lower extremities were enormously swollen to the point where the skin showed several areas of rupture with serum oozing from these cracks. The edema had extended above the legs to the trunk in the dependent portions.

Laboratory Findings.—Urinalysis showed a moderate amount of albumin and a high specific gravity (1.027). The red blood count showed 4,800,000 cells with 89% hemoglobin. White blood cells 14,000 with 86% polynuclears. Blood chemistry showed an increase of urea to 46 mgm.

Subsequent Course.—The patient developed a terminal bronchopneumonia with respirations rising to 50.

Temperature, however, remained low ranging between 97 and 100°. She developed definite auricular fibrillation and grew rapidly worse, dying only 48 hours after admission.

Autopsy Findings.—At autopsy, a marked chronic myocarditis was found with myocardial fibrosis. There was an old rheumatic mitral valvulitis with both insufficiency and partial stenosis present with marked dilatation of the heart, particularly on the right side. Chronic passive congestion of the viscera was prominent. This was particularly prominent in the mucosa of the entire gastro-intestinal tract. There was a thrombosis of the superior mesenteric artery with terminal gangrene of the bowel and secondary peritonitis. A definite terminal bronchopneumonia in the right base was found. The stomach was markedly distended. It contained over two liters of mucoid, somewhat bile tinged fluid. The normal rugae were absent. The mucous membrane, itself, was thickened and grayish-brown in color, with diffuse cyanosis of the entire mucosal surface. Follicular erosions of the mucosa were noted throughout the stomach, but especially in the region of the pylorus.

Microscopic Description of Section of Stomach.— (Fig. 87 and 88) Microscopic section of the stomach shows a hyperplastic, thickened mucosa with a marked papilliform appearance of the surface, associated with chronic inflammatory changes in the stroma. The individual papillae are thickened and edematous. There is marked hyperemia with some perivascular diapedesis. Considerable secondary lymphocytic infiltration is to be noted. The surface epithelial cells appear increased both in number and in size. There is a considerable increase in the amount of mucous secretion, with the mucus found extending into the glands, as well as on the surface of the mucosa. Considerable desquamation of the surface epithelium has occurred and this cellular debris is seen admixed with the mucous exudate.

The etiology of this particular picture may well be attributed to the chronic passive congestion of the organ as a result of the cardiac history, plus a more recent irritation very probably set up by swallowing infected sputum coughed up from the lung.

CASE 41. (Ref. #S-26)

Diagnosis.—Bronchus—acute catarrhal bronchitis (mucositis).

Patient was a young adult white male, who was admitted to the hospital with a history of a severe cold of about one week's duration, which he described as having gone down on his chest.

Present Illness.—Patient was too ill to question further in respect to his history, so that his previous history was not possible to obtain.

Physical Examination.—Owing to the extremely critical condition of the patient, it was impossible to make more than a cursory examination. His head was normal in contour. Pupils reacted normally to light and distance. Eyes, ears, nose and throat appeared normal. Examination of his chest revealed a diffuse bilateral bronchopneumonia involving all five lobes. This was characterized by an almost complete solidification of the lung with marked dullness and bronchial breathing.

Breath sounds were increased in intensity. The chest was filled with moist, crackling and mucous râles. The heart was moderately enlarged. There were no murmurs heard. Pulse rate was 140. Abdomen was negative as were his extremities.

Subsequent Course.—The patient died within a few hours of his admission of the diffuse pneumonic process. Attempts at bacteriologic typing of the causative organism revealed the presence of Streptococcus in the sputum, which was subsequently proved to be of the hemolytic variety.

Autopsy Findings.—At autopsy there was a marked acute catarrhal laryngeal tracheobronchitis with diffuse confluent bilateral bronchopneumonia. There was an associated toxic granular degeneration of the myocardium, liver and kidneys.

Microscopic Description of Section from the Bronchus.—(Fig. 89 and 90) Identification of the cartilaginous rings serves to orient the observer. On the inner side of the cartilage is seen the hyperemic submucosa showing many of the deeper bronchial glands which are distended in many instances with mucus. The stroma is moderately edematous and shows some slight cellular infiltration—chiefly lymphocytic. The mucosa itself presents a varying picture. At one side it shows marked inflammatory hyperplasia and thickening; at the other side the epithelium is largely desquamated except for a single layer of rather distorted epithelium. In places, adherent to the mucosa or free in the lumen, a considerable amount of mucus admixed with inflammatory cells, both mononuclear and polynuclear, may be seen. These reactions establish our diagnosis of acute catarrhal mucositis.

In addition, at the edge of the slide is found a lymphnode showing rather marked acute inflammatory changes. There is marked congestion, even to the point of hemorrhage, considerable edema, definite lymphocytic hyperplasia and some slight leukocytic infiltration.

Under high power, it is of interest to note the marked divergence from normal of the ciliated lining epithelial cells. These are hypertrophied and swollen. Many of them show a great increase of mucus within their cytoplasm. There is a loss of the cilia and many of the cells show karyolytic and karyorrhectic necrotic changes affecting the nuclei.

Case 42. (Ref. #S-6)
Diagnosis.—Appendix—chronic catarrhal appendicitis (mucositis).
The patient was a white male sixty years of age, who was admitted to the hospital because of a history of intermittent, vague abdominal pains, tending to be most marked in the right lower quadrant.

Present Illness.—The patient went to his physician because of one of these recurrent attacks of abdominal pain, which was a little more severe in character than formerly. It had been accompanied by some nausea, which had been relieved by alkalies.

Past History.—The patient's past history was unimportant except in respect to his gastro-intestinal tract. He had never had any serious illness which had required hospitalization. He had a number of mild upper respiratory attacks and had had influenza in the 1918 epidemic. His cardiovascular system seemed negative. His genitourinary history was normal. For about the past five or six years the patient had complained of intermittent attacks of epigastric pain, which were relieved by food and alkalies. He had never noted any jaundice with these attacks. The last two or three of them had shown a certain tendency to localize in the right lower quadrant. He had never had any definite nausea with any attack until the present illness, but had had marked flatulence.

Laboratory Findings.—Red blood cells 4,300,000 with 87% hemoglobin. White blood cells 9,800 with 72% polynuclear leukocytes. Urinalysis was negative.

Subsequent Course.—On the basis of these vague gastro-intestinal symptoms, exploratory laparotomy was advised with the thought that his condition was probably the result of a chronic gallbladder or chronic appendicitis. Accordingly, a high rectus incision was made and the abdomen explored. A chronic cholecystitis with cholesterol stones was found and a markedly thickened appendix. These were both removed and the patient had an uneventful recovery and was discharged cured.

Pathological Report.—*Gross Description.*—Specimen consisted of an appendix measuring 4 cm. in length by 1 cm. in diameter. There was moderate thickening of the entire wall of the appendix. The serosa appeared smooth and covered by a normal, glistening serosal membrane. The mucosa was intact.

Microscopic Description.—(Fig. 91, 92, 93 and 94) Section microscopically shows a ring of tissue lined on the inside by mucous membrane, and covered on the outside by peritoneal serosa except at one point where the mesoappendix has been cut. Beginning from within, the following features may be noted: (1) within the lumen may be seen considerable mucus admixed with both polynuclear and mononuclear cells; (2) this mucus in places is adherent to the mucosa and may be seen as tenacious strands deep in the glands and even extending from the goblet cells; (3) marked hypertrophy of the mucous epithelial cells with most of them distended with secreted mucus; (4) edema, congestion and lymphocytic infiltration of the submucosa; (5) persistent lymph-follicles; (6) submucous fibrosis; (7) some interstitial fibrosis of the muscular wall; and (8) fibrous thickening of the adventitia.

CHAPTER XIII

TYPES OF INFLAMMATION (*Continued*)

PART I

FIBRINOUS, SERO-FIBRINOUS AND FIBRINOPURULENT SEROSITIS AND MUCOSITIS

In the preceding chapter we have discussed inflammation from the standpoint of the clinical terminology as affecting the surface epithelium of the skin or mucosa, those involving the serous coats under the generic heading of serositis and those inflammations which tend to occur in the deeper tissues where phlegmonous or serous exudation or suppuration are particularly prone to occur. In the present discussion we wish to carry this study a step further with the emphasis being laid upon the pathologcal process rather than upon the anatomical distribution of the lesion. Theoretically, it is possible to have an inflammatory picture in which one of the four major elements of the inflammatory exudate predominates almost to the exclusion of the others. The division of this inflammatory reaction into hemorrhagic, serous, fibrinous and purulent inflammation has already been commented upon. Very few examples of pure hemorrhagic inflammation exist. Perhaps the two most nearly approaching this picture are seen in the two infections, anthrax and influenza. In the serous type of inflammation, we have seen that streptococci, particularly the hemolytic streptococcus, tend to be the most common cause of this particular type of reaction. Similarly, we have found that the staphylococcus is most representative of the pure suppurative or purulent type of acute inflammation. In the same way, it may be said that diphtheria in its local reaction on the mucous surface of the pharyngeal and upper respiratory mucosa comes closest to representing a pure fibrinous exudate.

More commonly, however, we find that a combination of these inflammatory pictures is apt to result from infection by the great majority of the pathogenic organisms of man. In this discussion we wish to emphasize this more complicated mechanism and il-lustrate it with cases showing the range of variation in the picture from the relatively straightforward fibrinous exudate of diphtheria (see Chapter XIX) through the serofibrinous and fibrinopurulent inflammations which particularly involve the serous membranes of the body. In addition should be included in this group of lesions certain of those infections which produce the same general type of reaction in the meninges, notably epidemic cerebrospinal meningitis caused by the meningococcus.

In any discussion of bacteria, it will be noted that the organisms are apt to be classified upon the basis of the inflammatory reaction which they produce. Thus we speak of the pyogenic (pus producing) cocci which include particularly the staphylococcus aureus, the meningococcus, the gonococcus and the pneumococcus. This classification, however, is somewhat inexact for, in general, these organisms as well as many of the bacillary forms, including such a generally harmless bacterium as the colon bacillus, may at times when they invade the tissues set up a purulent reaction but one in which fibrin is particularly prominent. In general, it may be said that fibrinous exudates, either in their simpler forms or in their more complex varieties are found in relation to surface lesions. Thus we find a fibrinous exudate may fill the lung alveoli in pneumonia. After all, the lung may be thought of simply as a complicated sheet of cells arranged in the particular pattern in which it is to provide the maximum surface area for the exchange of oxygen and carbon dioxide. Similarly, the meninges may best be considered as a covering membrane, even although they in turn are enclosed within the cranial vault. Likewise, the pleurae, the pericardium, the peritoneum and the serosal lining of the various joints and bursae represent surface structures which, because of this fact,

PLATE XXIV
ACUTE SEROSITIS (Fibrinopurulent)

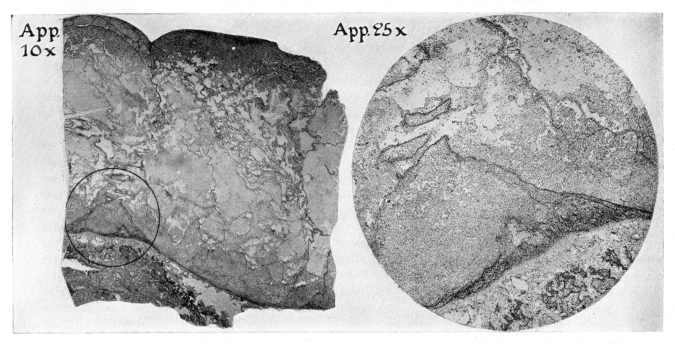

FIG. 95 and 96.—Pleura: Acute Fibrinopurulent Pleuritis.—Case 44.—Edematous, hyperemic pleura, covered by a thick, plastic exudate consisting of fibrin, leukocytes and serum.

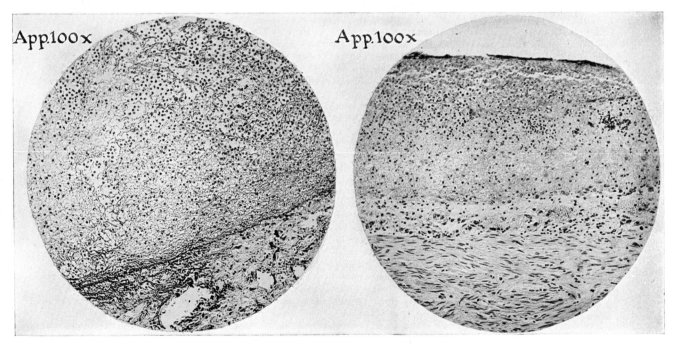

FIG. 97.—Pleura.—High power photomicrograph of hyperemic pleura and exudate from Case 44, above. Note loss of serosal cells of pleura.

FIG. 98.—Peritoneum: Acute Fibrinopurulent Peritonitis.—Case 46.—Section through peritoneal surface of stomach wall which includes muscular layer, thickened serosa, and fibrinous exudate undergoing liquefaction necrosis.

are usually found to present fairly characteristic types of inflammatory response when infection occurs. Thus, we see that it is not the organism alone which is responsible for the type of reaction which occurs in the tissues, but that the inflammatory response is dependent to a very considerable extent upon the character of the tissue which is infected. Accordingly, it is not surprising to find that many bacteria may produce relatively comparable changes when they invade a given structure such as the pleura. But even when this general reaction occurs there still are differences in the gross and microscopic picture of the inflammatory process by which, in the great majority of cases, a differential diagnosis may well be made.

In general, any infection or injury of any extent to a serosal surface results in the outpouring on the surface of the serosa of the fluid element of the blood, plasma. From this plasma the fibrin is precipitated, presumably by the same mechanism by which normal clotting takes place. This fibrin is laid down in irregularly parallel layers as a protective membrane on the surface of the serosa to prevent further extension of the injury. If the offending organism happens to be a hemolytic streptococcus, then we find that serum continues to be poured forth into the exudate and the fibrinous layer is composed of a thick, edematous layer of relatively fine strands of fibrin. On the other hand, if we have a pneumococcus infection, we find that the fibrin is likely to be laid down in much heavier bands and because of the inherent positive chemotactic nature of the pneumococcus for leukocytes they accumulate in enormous numbers and their proteolytic enzymes in turn tend to break down and dissolve the fibrin, which is, after all, a protein substance. These differences can perhaps best be brought out by a series of illustrative cases which tend to emphasize the primary similarity of the process, a fibrinous exudate laid down as a protective membrane on the infected surface. The individual variations which result from the differences in response to the various bacteria make up one of the important chapters in our concept of histologic differential diagnosis.

ILLUSTRATIVE CASES

Simple Acute Fibrinous Inflammation.—Probably the best example of an almost pure fibrinous exudate as seen in any of the infectious diseases is the local lesion in response to the presence of the diphtheria bacillus in that disease. It seems preferable to consider diphtheria as a disease entity at a later date, but the reader is referred at this time to the discussion of the local condition as it affects the trachea or bronchi (see Chapter XIX, Fig. 183, 184, 185, 186 and 187).

A similar picture may be observed in the thrombosis of a blood vessel. In such a lesion the element of infection is usually lacking so that the complication of the presence of bacteria does not enter into the pathological process. On the other hand, this lesion being intravascular is somewhat confused by the presence of large numbers of red cells between the strands of fibrin. Curiously this condition is not commonly thought of clinically as an inflammatory one unless it is complicated by the presence of infection (see Chapter VI, Case 23, Fig. 52 and 53).

Finally, as another example of relatively pure fibrinous inflammation should be cited the early stage of lobar pneumonia, in which the initial response of the lung to the presence of the pneumococcus is an extremely heavy fibrin deposition upon the surface of the lung alveoli.

CASE 43. (Ref. #S-23 and S-27)
Diagnosis.—Lung—lobar pneumonia, stage of red hepatization.

Patient was a colored female of 45 years, who was admitted to the hospital complaining of cough, chills and fever, and pain in the chest.

Present Illness.—The onset of the present illness dated back approximately a week or ten days before admission when the patient developed a severe cold in the head. Three days before admission, she had a severe chill followed by high fever with pain in the right side of her chest, which was aggravated by deep respiration. This was accompanied by a racking cough which increased in severity. She also noted shortness of breath, which was also progressive in character, and for the past twenty-four hours she had been raising a small amount of rusty-colored sputum.

Past History.—Her past history was essentially irrelevant except for the fact that for several years she had had dyspnea on exertion and transitory periods of ankle edema. She had been treated for high blood pressure for the past three or four years and was supposed to have had an essential hypertensive cardiovascular condition. She had had diphtheria, malaria and typhoid fever as well as the usual childhood diseases. Her menstrual history had been normal.

Physical Examination.—Physical examination revealed an adult colored female lying in bed apparently suffering from marked dyspnea and prostration with some evidence of cyanosis. Her head was negative. Eyes, ears and nose were normal. The mouth showed marked furring of the tongue with sordes of the lips. The throat was markedly congested. Chest expansion was limited on the right side. There was dullness over the entire right chest with increased tactile fremitus and bronchial breathing. The left lung was clear. The heart was not enlarged. The sounds were of good quality with a rate of 90 to 130 and an occasional dropped beat.

PLATE XXV

ACUTE SEROSITIS (Fibrinopurulent)

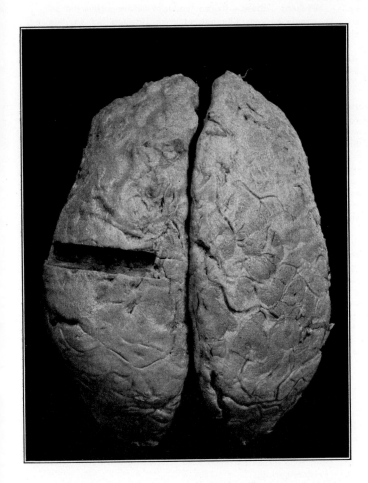

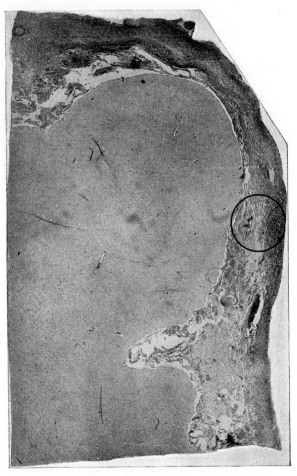

Fig. 99.—Brain: Acute Epidemic Cerebrospinal Meningitis (Meningococcic.).—Case 45.—Gross photograph to show abundant, plastic, fibrinopurulent exudate in subarachnoid, flattening the cerebral convolutions.

Fig. 100.—Low power microtessar photograph showing distribution of exudate in relation to the brain surface. App. 10 x.

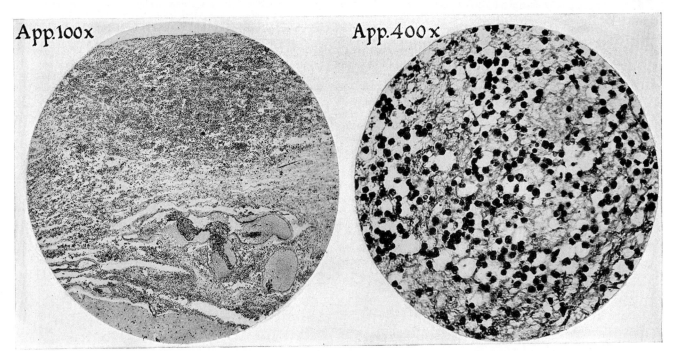

App.100x

App.400x

Fig. 101.—Low power area from indicated area in Fig. 100 better revealing the hyperemia of arachnoid vessels, the character of the exudate and the absence of cerebral involvement.

Fig. 102.—High power detail of exudate. Note degenerative changes of the inflammatory cells with beginning liquefaction necrosis and suppuration.

Blood pressure 160/80. The liver edge was palpable below the costal margin and somewhat tender. The abdomen was otherwise negative. There was a slight amount of pitting edema of the feet and ankles.

Laboratory Findings.—Red blood cells, 3,800,000 with 75% hemoglobin. White blood cells 6,800 with 84% polynuclears. Sputum examination revealed a type IV pneumococcus.

Subsequent Course.—The patient grew progressively worse, with increasing dyspnea and cyanosis, and died.

Autopsy Findings.—The pericardium showed acute fibrinous pericarditis. There was marked myocardosis of the heart. There was an acute fibrinous pleuritis of the right pleura. The right lung revealed lobar pneumonia with late hepatization. The left lung showed compensatory emphysema, congestion, and pulmonary edema. There was parenchymatous degeneration of the liver and nephrosis of the kidneys. The spleen showed toxic splenitis.

The right lung filled the right chest completely. The upper and lower lobes were consolidated and airless throughout. Over their surface, a thick fibrinous exudate was present. On section, the cut surface was dry and pale reddish gray in color. The surface was slightly rough and granular. The middle lobe showed emphysema.

Microscopic Description of Section of Lung.—(Fig. 411) Microscopic study of the tissue shows that all the air vesicles are distended with a fibrinous exudate in the meshes of which are found many red cells and a few large mononuclears and polymorphonuclear leukocytes. The alveolar walls are thickened and distended with a serofibrinous exudate. There is beginning perivascular leukocytic invasion of the alveolar walls with escape of some of the leukocytes into the air sacs. The tissue has been stained by the phosphotungstic acid-hematoxylin method, which stains fibrin intensely. This emphasizes the prominence of the fibrin in this early pneumonic exudate. Fibrin is seen to be laid down for the most part upon the lining surface of the alveoli. Strands of fibrin may be seen passing through the pores of Cohn to spread out in fan-like fashion upon the surface of the alveoli. The tissue includes a portion of the pleura, and it will be noted that there is an extension of the acute inflammatory process to the pleura as well. The subserosal connective tissue shows marked serous infiltration and dilatation of the capillaries. Around these, beginning leukocytic diapedesis may be observed. The serosal cells are still present and easily identified. Upon their surface lies a fine fibrillar layer of fibrin containing a few inflammatory cells.

Within the alveoli some of the large mononuclear cells which are present will be seen to be distended with yellowish-brown granular pigment representing hemosiderin, which has formed as the result of the breaking down of the red cells in the early exudate. These hemosiderin laden cells, in addition to occasional actual red cells, account for the rusty color of the sputum in pneumonia.

CASE 44. (Ref. #S-1)

Diagnosis.—Lung (pleura)—pleuritis (acute fibrino-purulent serositis).

Patient was a white male of 64 years, who was admitted to the hospital because of a severe cold on his chest.

Present Illness.—Began ten days before admission as a simple coryza. The patient went through the various stages in the development of a cold with first a marked serous watery discharge from his nose, which in turn was followed by the development of a mucopurulent exudate. The infection and inflammatory process spread down the respiratory tree with the development of a hacking cough. He became feverish and went to bed for two or three days before calling a physician. He became much sicker and had marked difficulty in respiration so that he called in a doctor, who found a diffuse bronchopneumonia, and sent him to the hospital.

Past History.—The previous history was essentially irrelevant in this case. The patient had a normal childhood. He had never been seriously ill in his entire life. A review of his systems was negative except for very minor qualitative digestive upsets, usually the result of indiscretions in diet. Genito-urinary history was negative. He had no more than the usual quota of mild upper respiratory infections.

Physical Examination.—Patient was a well developed white male, who appeared acutely ill, lying propped up in bed. He appeared somewhat cyanotic and had a grunting type of respiration. His facies were flushed and moist. Pupils were regular and equal. Eyes and ears were negative. There was still a mucopurulent discharge from his nose. Examination of his throat showed a marked reddening of the entire pharynx and a postnasal discharge of similar mucopurulent material. Examination of his chest showed a diffuse bilateral bronchopneumonia involving both lower lobes. Heart was not perceptibly enlarged. The rate was somewhat rapid. There were no murmurs. Abdomen was negative. Extremities were negative.

Laboratory Findings.—Red blood cells 4,300,000 with 86% hemoglobin. White blood cells 18,600 with 92% polynuclears. Urinalysis negative. Sputum examination showed a mixed bacterial flora with hemolytic streptococci predominating.

Subsequent Course.—The pneumococcic consolidation in both bases began to shown signs of resolution and it was thought that the patient was beginning to improve. However, he developed a septic temperature with daily ranges from 96° to 104°, and while the left chest continued to improve, the right chest in its lower half became more and more dull with a loss of breath sounds.

X-ray examination of the patient at this time revealed a suggestive pleural effusion, and a diagnosis of acute pleuritis with possible beginning empyema formation was made. Before operation was deemed advisable, the patient died with a rapid progression of his toxic symptoms.

Autopsy Findings.—At autopsy, a resolving pneumonia in the left lower lobe of the lung was found and an atelectatic right lower lobe was present. There was a marked serofibrinous exudate with effusion of about 500 c.c. of turbid, fibrin-flecked fluid. Cultures of this fluid yielded hemolytic streptococcus.

Microscopic Description of Section from Pleural Surface of Lung.—(Fig. 95, 96 and 97) At one side of the specimen there is a deep reddish area noted which is found to consist of lung tissue. The alveoli are compressed and considerable hemorrhage has occurred. It may be identified as lung tissue by the presence of a distorted bronchus, by anthracotic pigmentation and by the presence of alveolar walls. There is a pneumonia present

PLATE XXVI

ACUTE SEROSITIS (Fibrinous)

Pericardium—Organizing Fibrinous Pericarditis.—Case 47

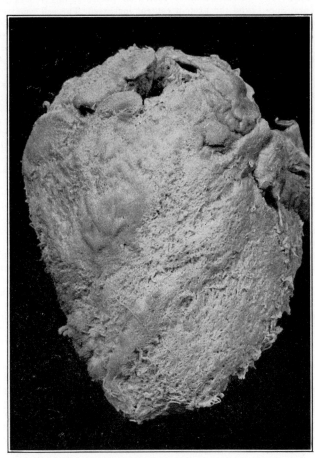

Fig. 103.—Gross photograph of heart covered with thick, shaggy, plastic, fibrinous exudate (so-called "bread and butter" exudate).

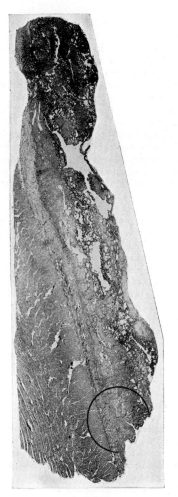

Fig. 104.—Microtessar photograph of the distribution and extent of the fibrinous exudate covering the thickened epicardium. App. 10 x.

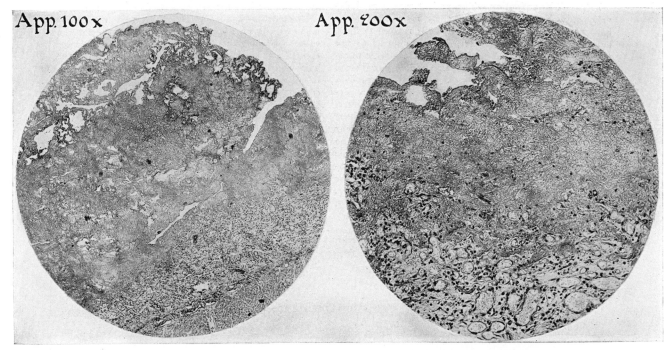

Fig. 105.—Higher magnification of area indicated in Fig. 104 emphasizing the almost exclusive fibrinous composition of the exudate, with but few inflammatory cells, and these chiefly mononuclear.

Fig. 106.—High power photomicrograph showing organization of exudate by fibroblasts and new capillaries because of failure of its absorption through cytolytic liquefaction necrosis. App. 200 x.

evidenced by cellular exudate in the lung alveoli. The pleural serosa has been destroyed and the subserosa shows marked inflammatory change. On the pleural surface there is a thick exudate which can be recognized as being made up of strands of fibrin separated by a pale pink granular substance (serum) and many inflammatory cells. These cells are more numerous near the surface of the exudate and the fibrin is more prominent at the base.

Under high power or oil immersion, fully 95% of the inflammatory cells are seen to be polymorphonuclear leukocytes. These vary in their staining reaction due to degenerative changes or actual cell death. There is evidence of phagocytosis with bacteria or deep staining cell debris in the cytoplasm of the cells. The fibrin is characteristic—straight or angulated strands of homogeneous pink-staining material with "nodal" points of fusion where strands cross one another. The serum is easily identified by its fine granular, almost homogeneous appearance.

The picture, as a whole, then, is one of acute inflammation of a serous surface (acute serositis). The exudate is of a mixed type with serum and fibrin predominating. There are many pus cells present, however. This is termed serofibrinopurulent pleuritis. Because of some liquefaction of the leukocytes we recognize beginning suppuration. Clinically, this would be called a beginning *empyema,* a complication and extension of a pneumonic process.

CASE 45. (Ref. #S-4)
Diagnosis.—Brain (cortex)—epidemic cerebrospinal meningococcic meningitis.

Patient was a young male Negro, twenty-four years of age, admitted to the hospital with a history of sudden onset of a chill accompanied by fever, headache, nausea, vomiting and painful stiffness of the neck.

Present Illness.—These symptoms began twenty-four hours before admission and were accompanied by fever. He had been perfectly well previously.

Past History.—On admission, the patient was in a somewhat disoriented state so that it was difficult to obtain any reliable data concerning his previous history. Apparently he had never had any serious illness nor any operations.

Physical Examination.—The patient was a well developed, well nourished young adult male Negro. His head was normal in contour. His pupils reacted to light, but because of his semistupor, it was difficult to tell whether they reacted to accommodation. Ears were negative. There was no evidence of any middle ear disease nor of any mastoid tenderness. Nose was negative. Throat showed slight congestion. Tonsils were hypertrophied. The neck was definitely rigid and the slightest attempt to bend his head caused obvious pain. Chest was symmetrical and well developed. Lungs were clear throughout. Heart was not enlarged. There were no murmurs. Blood pressure was somewhat low with the systolic 108 and the diastolic 76. Abdomen was negative. There was nothing abnormal noted about the genitalia or extremities except in respect to the reflexes. The knee jerks were grossly exaggerated symmetrically. There was a bilateral Kernig and Babinski reflex present. The temperature on admission was 102°.

Laboratory Findings.—Red blood cells 5,100,000 with 90% hemoglobin. White blood cells 18,000 with 86%

polynuclear leukocytes. Spinal fluid was cloudy and under definitely increased pressure. Sugar was reduced and the protein content increased. The cell count showed 12,000 per c.mm., with 96% polynuclear leukocytes. Intra- and extracellular gram-negative diplococci were present in large number in smear preparations. On the basis of these findings, a diagnosis of epidemic cerebrospinal meningococcic meningitis was made.

Subsequent Course.—The patient was given antimeningococcic serum intraspinally twice daily for the next three days. He was likewise given an intravenous injection of serum at the time of admission. He developed marked internal strabismus and became definitely stuporous. The muscles of his back became rigid with resulting opisthotonus. The temperature remained elevated during his three days in the hospital. He gradually sank into profound coma and died.

Autopsy Findings.—At autopsy the only findings of significance were the presence of an acute fibrinopurulent diffuse meningitis, most marked at the base of the brain, and generalized secondary toxic changes of the parenchymatous organs.

Microscopic Description of a Section Through the Cortex.—(Fig. 99, 100, 101 and 102) The section microscopically shows a moderate edema and congestion of the brain tissue. No degenerative changes affecting the nerve cells are noted. The chief interest lies in a study of the exudate on the surface of the brain, involving the arachnoid and pia. The dura has been removed, as the exudate is all subdural in distribution. The picture as a whole is one of a delicate lace-like network of fibrin strands. The capillary vessels of the membranes are easily identified because of their dilatation and perivascular leukocytic infiltration. Scattered through the fibrinous exudate may be found considerable fine pink-staining granular material representing serum, as well as many inflammatory cells. A differential count of these cells show them to be about 98% polynuclears. Towards the surface of the exudate considerable liquefaction necrosis has occurred with the leukocytes showing marked fragmentation and disintegration.

Here and there it is possible to identify the typical biscuit-shaped diplococci, both within the leukocytes and lying free in the inflammatory exudate. With a special Gram stain to bring out the organisms, they could be found with much greater ease and in large numbers.

Discussion.—Epidemic cerebrospinal meningococcic meningitis is an acute infection caused by the meningococcus, of which there are several types. It may occur in epidemic form, but more often as a sporadic infection. The organisms gain entrance to the body through the nasal mucosa usually and enter the blood stream (in severe cases producing capillary thrombi—"spotted fever") before localizing in the meninges, for which they have some poorly understood selective affinity. Specific serum therapy is thought to have reduced the mortality from about 75% to 10 or 15% if used early. Recently doubt has been cast on the specificity of this therapy. (For a more detailed discussion, refer to Chapter LXIII).

CASE 46. (Ref. #S-134)
Diagnosis.—Peritoneum—acute fibrinopurulent peritonitis (serositis).

Patient was a white male, fifty-seven years of age,

PLATE XXVII
ACUTE MUCOSITIS

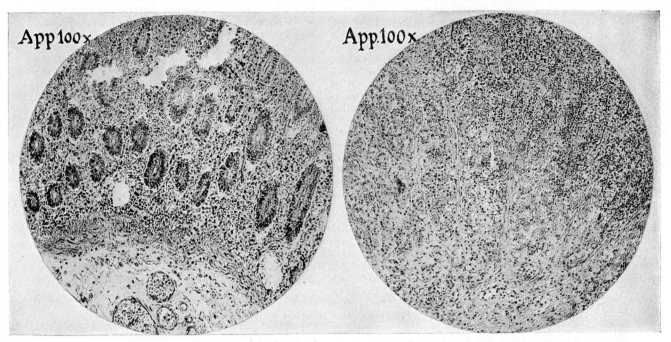

FIG. 107.—COLON: ACUTE HEMORRHAGIC COLITIS.—CASE 49.—Section from colon in HgCl₂ poisoning. Diffuse hemorrhagic exudation into mucosa with necrosis of superficial layer. App. 100 x.

FIG. 108.—STOMACH: ACUTE HEMORRHAGIC GASTRITIS.—CASE 50.—An area of gastric mucosa showing extensive hemorrhage into tunica propria and beginning coagulation necrosis. App. 100 x.

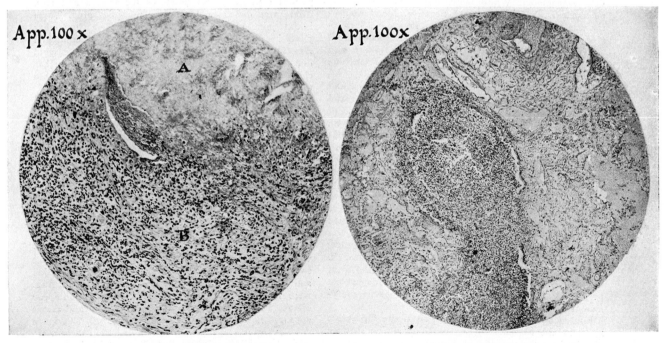

FIG. 109.—UTERUS: ACUTE GANGRENOUS ENDOMETRITIS.—CASE 51.—Line of demarcation is shown between gangrenous area at (A) and the still viable myometrium at (B), with acute cellular infiltration. App. 100 x.

FIG. 110.—LUNG: BRONCHIECTATIC ABSCESS; SUPPURATION.—CASE 48.—Dilated bronchus distended with pus. Persistent bronchial mucosa may be observed at one side.

who entered the hospital with a history of postprandial epigastric pain of three months' duration.

Present Illness.—The patient had suffered from several severe attacks of pain during this interval, but in general, the onset had been gradual over a period of probably considerably more time than the three months, which he felt represented the first severe attack which he had. This pain was usually associated with the taking of food and was accompanied by marked gaseous eructations. With this, he had associated constipation. During this three months' period he lost 18 pounds in weight.

Past History.—The patient had never had any serious illness previously. He had had the usual childhood infections and had had his share of the ordinary upper respiratory infections. He had never had any cardiovascular symptoms. His gastro-intestinal history was negative except for occasional qualitative attacks of indigestion following dietary excesses. Genito-urinary history was negative. He denied venereal infection.

Physical Examination.—Patient was a well developed elderly white male. His head was negative. The scalp was partially bald. His eyes, ears, nose and throat were essentially negative. His chest was somewhat emphysematous in form. His lungs were clear throughout with possibly some hyperresonance in the apices. His heart was not enlarged. The rhythm was regular. There were no murmurs. Blood pressure 138/94. Abdomen was moderately distended and there was a general feeling of discomfort rather than any actual pain or tenderness on palpation. No masses were definitely felt, but there was difficulty in palpating deeply because of the distention and general discomfort. The extremities were negative. Reflexes were normal.

Laboratory Findings.—Red blood cells 2,800,000 with 63% hemoglobin. White blood cells 8,400 with 62% polynuclears. Wassermann was negative. Blood chemistry was negative. Examination of the stool on a protein-free diet gave a positive benzidine test for occult blood.

X-ray examination showed a huge gastric residue with an irregularly outlined narrowing of the pyloric antrum. This was thought to be carcinoma.

Subsequent Course.—Gastroscopy was performed and the diagnosis of carcinoma established by biopsy and histologic examination. It was recommended, because of the localization of the carcinoma in the pyloric region, that partial gastrectomy might be curative in effect. He was operated upon and the lower two-thirds of his stomach resected. The cardiac portion was then joined with the jejunum. He had a very stormy immediate postoperative history; the gastrojejunostomy wound apparently broke down and allowed the escape of stomach contents into the peritoneal cavity. This set up a very severe, diffuse peritonitis of which the patient died ninety-six hours after operation.

Autopsy Findings.—At autopsy, the gastrojejunostomy was exposed and a marked autolytic sloughing area in the anterior portion was found, which was the source of the infection in a very diffuse generalized fibrinopurulent peritonitis. Toxic granular degeneration of the parenchymatous organs was also present.

Microscopic Study of a Section from the Operative Field in the Stomach.—(Fig. 98) The section may be identified by the presence of smooth muscle tissue from the stomach wall. The mucosal surface has been destroyed by autolysis by the gastric juices. The peritoneal surface of the tissue is covered by an acute fibrino-

purulent exudate. On the surface of this exudate under high power may be observed liquefaction necrosis. In this hematoxylin and eosin stained preparation, bacteria may be identified, although poorly defined by this staining technique. Phagocytosis by polynuclears can be made out. The suppurative process is characteristic of the proteolytic action of the leukocytes on the fibrin of the exudate. The massing of the leukocytes on the surface is typical of the positive chemotaxis of the bacteria for them. In the deeper layers of the exudate, the typical fibrinous network is easily made out. The peritoneal serosal cells have been destroyed entirely and cannot be identified, and the inflammatory reaction has extended into the omental fat tissue which is invaded by various types of cell. Hyperemia, edema, perivascular infiltration and all the other characteristics of acute inflammation are prominent features of the picture.

Discussion.—In this case we see one of the major risks which accompany almost any surgical operative procedure involving the gastro-intestinal tract, *viz.*, the danger of autolysis and of secondary infection from escaped gastro-intestinal contents. This is perhaps especially true of gastric surgery, but may even follow a simple appendectomy, in the hands of the most skillful surgeon.

CASE 47. (Ref. #S-2)

Diagnosis.—Pericardium—organizing fibrinous pericarditis.

Patient was a child of thirteen years, who was admitted to the hospital with a history of acute rheumatic fever with cardiac involvement of only four weeks' duration.

Present Illness.—The onset of the present illness was painful swelling of the joints of the fingers and toes. There was definite redness over the joint area. These initial joint symptoms subsided somewhat, but other joints became involved, including the shoulder and hip. Associated with this diffuse arthritic picture, the child developed marked shortness of breath with pain in her chest and was taken to a physician, who referred her to the hospital.

Past History.—The child was a normally delivered and breast-fed baby up to ten months of age. As a young child, during the first three or four years of life, she developed measles, whooping cough and chickenpox. Her tonsils were markedly enlarged, for which she was operated upon at the age of ten. She had had several mild attacks of tonsillitis previous to this operative procedure, but since that time had not noted any throat infections. Her nutritional history had always been satisfactory. She seemed particularly susceptible to colds. She had had a rather severe coryza just before the development of the present illness.

Physical Examination.—The patient was a well developed, well nourished white female child of about twelve. Head was normal in shape. Eyes were negative and reacted normally to light and accommodation. Ears were negative. There was no evidence of middle ear disease and no mastoid tenderness. The nose and throat appeared normal. The chest was symmetrical. The lungs were negative to percussion. On auscultation there were a few crackling râles at both bases. The heart was markedly enlarged to the left, reaching the midaxillary line. There was a soft, blowing systolic murmur transmitted to the axilla. The pulse rate was increased to

130. The abdomen was somewhat prominent and the liver edge could be felt just below the costal margin. The extremities were negative. On admission, the child had a temperature of 103° and respirations of 20.

Laboratory Findings.—Red blood cells, 4,100,000 with 78% hemoglobin. White blood cells 4,000 with 76% polynuclear leukocytes. Blood sedimentation rate was almost doubled. Blood cultures were negative.

Subsequent Course.—During the child's two weeks' stay in the hospital, repeated blood cultures remained negative. She developed a friction rub over the apex of the heart with a characteristic leather-like to and fro sound. The child became more and more dyspneic and died of congestive heart failure.

Autopsy Findings.—At autopsy there was a generalized pancarditis with a typical fibrinopurulent pericarditis and a generalized mitral, aortic and tricuspid rheumatic valvulitis. There was a terminal bronchopneumonia, which it was thought might be rheumatic in type. The other viscera showed only evidence of congestion and toxic granular degeneration.

Microscopic Study of a Section from the Heart and Pericardium.—(Fig. 103, 104, 105 and 106) The tissue can be identified as heart muscle by the branching bundles of striated cardiac muscle fibers, but the greater part of the tissue is made up of the epicardium and overlying dense fibrinous exudate. In this exudate are found many inflammatory cells with mononuclears, including lymphocytes, plasma cells and large mononuclear leukocytes predominating, although many polynuclear leukocytes are still present. This is a comparatively old lesion as evidenced by the hyalinization and compactness of the fibrin, and by the fact that newly formed capillary vessels can be seen growing into this dense fibrin. Also, the epicardium itself is greatly thickened as the result of a diffuse proliferation of connective tissue. This can be easily identified by the large amount of collagen and the characteristic appearance of the nuclei. In this epicardial tissue likewise are seen many inflammatory cells with mononuclears predominating.

With close search, under high power, endothelial "buds" may be seen growing from the existing vessels, becoming distended with blood, and thus forming new capillaries. Connective tissue cells may likewise be studied to advantage in this section, presenting as they do all stages from undifferentiated fibroblasts to adult cells with elongated nuclei and considerable intercellular collagen formation.

Discussion.—This process of replacement of a fibrinous exudate by fibrous tissue is spoken of as the *organization of fibrin*. It may be seen in many conditions, the simplest example of which is the organization of a sterile fibrinous thrombus in a blood vessel. Under such circumstances no capillary production is seen, and the process is spoken of as *avascular* organization. Where infection has taken place the other signs of inflammation are seen as in this slide, and the organization requires vascularization in addition.

PART II

SUPPURATIVE, NECROTIC, HEMORRHAGIC, PSEUDO-MEMBRANOUS, MEMBRANOUS (DIPHTHERITIC), SEPTIC, AND GANGRENOUS INFLAMMATION

Under these various terms are found the great majority of the lesions which affect mucous membranes in contradistinction to the group which we have been discussing in the previous chapter, which predominantly involve serosal surfaces. Naturally, as might be expected, there is considerable overlapping of these groups, for the histologic classification of inflammation does not necessarily conform to the clinical nomenclature. As we have seen, however, as the inflammatory process becomes more and more severe, the descriptive terminology is employed clinically as a means of recognizing these differences in degree and their concomitant prognoses. In this group of inflammatory conditions, again illustrative case histories serve perhaps better than any amount of general discussion to emphasize these differences. We must include those cases of leukocytic or purulent inflammation which result in liquefaction necrosis and pus formation to produce the clinical picture of suppuration. This type of inflammation may be caused by a wide variety of bacteria, as well as in its simpler manifestations, by chemical or physical agents. For our purpose, to illustrate the more usual forms of suppurative inflammation, it is perhaps best to start with the lesions produced by the staphylococcus aureus.

Staphylococcic Infections

The Staphylococcus pyogenes aureus is the foremost of the pyogenic cocci. It is a gram-positive organism occurring in grape-like clumps when seen in smear preparations. It is a ubiquitous organism found almost universally. It is a common contaminant of the skin, and is not infrequently found as an inhabitant of the nasopharynx. Normally it is a harmless organism which causes no particular difficulty. Its bacteriologic characteristics are of importance in relation to the lesions which it produces. It grows readily on most culture media. It is preferably an aerobe, but will grow under partial anaerobic conditions. It has a strongly lytic, nondiffusible toxin, which is the important factor in the localization of the characteristic abscess which it forms. Culturally, it grows as a compact colony of smooth, creamy consistency with a rounded edge, and gradually produces the characteristic golden pigment by which it is so readily identified.

When this organism enters the body through any break in continuity of the epithelium of the skin or mucous membrane as a direct infection or secondarily as the result of some other inflammatory process as occurs at times in the lungs particularly, it sets up its characteristic inflammatory reaction wherever it localizes. It does not produce a specific disease as many bacteria do, and for that reason it is being considered at this time as a type of infection rather than as a specific disease process. In its simplest manifestation, we find the infection of a single hair follicle with the development of a *furuncle* or "boil." If the infection spreads through the base of the follicle to the deeper tissues and wanders in the subcutaneous structures to break out again to the skin surface in multiple points, then the lesion is spoken of as a *carbuncle*. If it is inhaled into the lung, it may set up a pneumonia or it may localize with the development of a lung abscess. If, as not infrequently occurs, it gains access to the blood stream, it may be carried to distant organs of the body and set up metastatic abscesses. Perhaps most commonly the cortex of the kidney is the site of such metastatic lesions, although in overwhelming blood stream infections multiple abscesses of every structure of the body are by no means uncommon, including even the heart and brain.

Thus we see that while the staphylococcus is in itself a harmless inhabitant of the nasopharynx or of the skin, yet with lowered resistance on the part of the individual, or with a strain of bacteria whose virulence is greater than normal, and an opportunity to gain access to the tissues even this organism may become one of the most significant infectious agents of any of the bacteria. With blood stream infections there has been an almost assured fatal outcome except in those cases, occurring in childhood, particularly, in which the infection became localized in the

marrow of one or more of the long bones to produce a localized acute osteomyelitis. This, not infrequently, with surgical intervention and drainage might be cured. With modern immunologic and chemotherapeutic methods, particularly with the use of bacteriophage, the outlook of staphylococcic septicemia has steadily improved, although it still remains a very serious infection with an extremely high mortality.

Just as the staphylococcus is the commonest organism which produces the more nearly typical purulent suppurative inflammatory lesion, so other bacteria may produce a somewhat similar picture. For example, the colon bacillus, which we have already seen may be instrumental in the development of a fibrinopurulent exudate in the peritoneal cavity, may, when it has gained access to the pelvis of the kidney, produce a suppurative infection which may result ultimately in the complete destruction of the kidney substance. Again, if it gains access to the blood stream, it may give rise to many bizarre inflammatory lesions, not the least striking of which may be a purulent meningitis.

In many of these more severe types of inflammation, the suppurative or necrotic part of the picture is dependent upon secondary bacterial invasion. It is not uncommon to find, for example, an intestine which has undergone extensive injury as the result of mercury poisoning, which in itself produces an acute hemorrhagic necrosis, but which becomes complicated by a secondary bacterial invasion of this necrotic tissue. In such a case we may find the development of a true diphtheritic membranous exudate on the surface of the underlying primary inflammatory process only to be followed by sloughing as the result of suppurative necrosis of these deeper tissues. From our pathological standpoint, therefore, these terms are descriptive rather than fundamental in their concept. They represent a combination of the several basic inflammatory exudative and vascular phenomena which we have already studied. It is in the character of these secondary changes that the wide variety of pictures results. Examples in the form of illustrative cases ranging from the staphylococcic suppurative abscess lesion as it occurs in the lung or in an appendix, up to the hemorrhagic necrosis of the intestine in mercury poisoning, or the gangrenous necrosis of the endometrium in a case of criminal abortion and secondary putrefactive bacterial infection of the uterus will serve to illustrate the wide range of such inflammatory processes.

One further point regarding the nomenclature of these more severe inflammatory exudates should be clarified at this time; namely, the difference between the pseudomembranous type of inflammation seen in diphtheria and the true membranous, or so-called diphtheritic type of inflammation. By the term *pseudomembranous* is meant an acute fibrinous exudate predominantly, which is relatively loosely attached to the mucosal surface. Typically the basement membrane of the mucosal epithelium is not destroyed by such an inflammatory process. However, a certain amount of integration of the surface exudate with the inflammatory response in the submucosal tissues must of necessity exist. This is the type of exudate seen in uncomplicated diphtheria. Such a membrane may comparatively easily be stripped away from the overlying mucosa, leaving a raw surface with occasional bleeding points but in the repair following this picture, reepithelialization of the surface takes place and no ultimate damage to the mucous membrane occurs.

On the other hand, by true membranous inflammation is meant an acute necrotic process with extensive destruction of the mucosa, including the basal layer of the surface epithelium. It is true there is usually a dense fibrinous exudate on the surface of such a lesion and that this membranous exudate resembles grossly the appearance of the exudate in diphtheria. It is for this reason that the term *diphtheritic* has been applied to this more severe, necrotic membranous type of inflammatory reaction. Such a reaction is more likely to be the result of infection by other bacteria than the diphtheria bacillus. Not infrequently, such a lesion may occur in the throat or trachea as the result of streptococcic invasion. In the intestinal tract such lesions may follow infection by certain of the dysentery bacilli or, as has been already mentioned, by such severe chemical injury as mercury poisoning. Such exudates are diphtheritic, but not diphtheria, and this essential difference between the pseudomembranous inflammation of diphtheria and the diphtheritic picture of more severe necrotic ulcerative membranous inflammation of mucous surfaces is one which should be carefully borne in mind.

ILLUSTRATIVE CASES

Case 48. (Ref. #S-128)

Diagnosis.—Lung—multiple abscesses (Staphylococcus aureus).

Patient was a white female, thirty years of age, who was admitted to the hospital with a clinical diagnosis of "influenza."

Present Illness.—The patient's illness started with a severe coryza three days before admission. She became acutely ill the following day, with a sharp rise in temperature, and on examination was found to have diffuse bilateral pneumonia and was sent into the hospital for treatment.

Past History.—The patient's previous history was irrelevant. She had had the usual childhood diseases. She had not been particularly susceptible to colds or upper respiratory infection. Her cardiovascular system was negative. Her gastro-intestinal history showed only qualitative digestive disturbances of no apparent significance. She was married and had had one child. Her menstrual history had been entirely negative.

Physical Examination.—The patient was an acutely ill young white woman. She had an anxious facies with rather marked cyanosis of her mucous membranes and nail beds. Her eyes were negative. Ears were negative. There was no evidence of middle ear involvement. There was no mastoid tenderness. The throat was edematous and had a dusky, cyanotic red color. Examination of her chest showed a diffuse bilateral bronchopneumonia with increased breath sounds, bronchial breathing, and innumerable fine and coarse crackling râles. The patient

was semistuporous as a result of profound toxemia. Her heart was rapid but otherwise negative. Abdomen was normal. Extremities were negative.

Laboratory Findings.—Red blood cells 4,100,000 with 83% hemoglobin. White blood cells 4,000 with 20% polynuclear leukocytes. (A low white count, leukopenia, is often seen in influenza, but the percentage of polynuclears is usually not disproportionate as in this case. A low white count of this type during the course of severe infection, especially in pneumonia, is a poor prognostic sign, indicative of hematopoietic paralysis and a poor resistance.)

Subsequent Course.—The patient went rapidly downhill, the pneumonia spreading throughout the lungs, and she died the third day following her admission to the hospital.

Autopsy Findings.—Pathology, other than general evidence of toxemia with cardiac dilatation, was restricted to the lungs. About 300 c.c. of thin, bloody exudate were found in the left pleural cavity. There was no fluid on the right side. There was a plastic fibrinous exudate over both left and right lower lobes. Each lung weighed about 430 gm. Both lower lobes were the site of a diffuse serosanguineous pneumonia. In addition, multiple foci of suppurative necrosis (abscesses) were found throughout these lobes. Many of these were associated with the bronchi. There was a diffuse fibrinopurulent tracheitis and bronchitis in addition.

Bacteriology.—Cultures from heart's blood and from both lower lobes yielded hemolytic staphylococci (aureus).

Microscopic Description of Tissue from the Lung.—(Fig. 110) This includes a portion of the pleural surface on one side, which may be identified by the swollen, degenerated serosal cells. As in most infections of the lung, there is an extension of the inflammatory process in the lung to the pleura, and a dense hyalinized fibrinous exudate is present on the pleural surface.

The general microscopic picture is one of a diffuse hemorrhagic type of pneumonic exudation. The histology varies from place to place. In some areas hemorrhage predominates; in others a serous exudate is more prominent. Variable amounts of fibrin are seen within the alveolar exudate and an extremely scanty leukocytic reaction can be made out in these areas.

Outstanding, however, are five or six irregularly spherical foci of liquefaction suppurative necrosis. Some of these are seen as being definitely related to the smaller bronchioles as the bronchial mucosa can still be identified in places, although most of it has been destroyed. Others of these abscesses are more extensive and are irregularly outlined by lung parenchyma. The lesion is too acute and rapid in its development for any suggestion of fibrous tissue proliferation to have occurred in an attempt to wall off and localize the abscesses by the formation of the so-called pyogenic membrane. This necrotic tissue, under high power, is seen to consist chiefly of polynuclears, most of them so degenerated as to be hardly recognizable. The necrotic tissue stains very lightly. Numerous bluish granular masses can be seen which, under oil immersion, may be identified as developing colonies of staphylococci.

CASE 49. (Ref. #S-84 and S-85)

Diagnosis.—Intestine—acute mercury bichloride poisoning; acute hemorrhagic, diphtheritic, necrotic inflammation.

Patient was a young woman of twenty-eight, who was admitted to the hospital about three hours after having taken 30 grams of mercury bichloride with suicidal intent.

Present Illness.—The onset of the symptoms began just before the patient's admission and was characterized by severe abdominal pain and uncontrollable vomiting. This was followed by very marked diarrhea. The stools consisted chiefly of fluid admixed with blood and mucus.

Past History.—It was impossible to obtain the past history because the patient was in a state of collapse and unable to give any information.

Physical Examination.—Physical examination revealed a well-developed, somewhat undernourished young white woman. Head was negative. Eyes, ears, nose and throat were within normal limits. Her chest was symmetrical. Lungs were clear. Heart was not enlarged. Pulse was small, thready and irregular. Blood pressure was 90/70. Abdomen was negative. Extremities were negative.

Subsequent Course.—Gastric lavage was done repeatedly along with colonic irrigations. This resulted in temporary improvement with diminution in the amount and severity of the vomiting and in the diarrhea. However, the following day intense salivation was noted, which is one of the cardinal symptoms of mercury poisoning. There was also a progressive diminution in urinary output, which resulted in complete anuria on the

fifth day. Following this, as a result of the renal shutdown, she went rapidly downhill and developed the picture of uremia with coma and convulsions, dying on the seventh day.

NOTE: Mercury, when taken by mouth, is absorbed by the stomach and is eliminated, not only by the kidney, but by the gastro-intestinal tract as well. The most striking lesions are those found in the colon, where apparently concentration of the metal occurs and results in a very severe hemorrhagic, necrotic inflammatory process with secondary infection and a diphtheritic or membranous exudate forming on the mucosal surface.

Autopsy Findings.—At autopsy, the outstanding lesions were those involving the kidney and the colon. These consisted of an acute tubular nephritis or nephrosis and a hemorrhagic, ulcerative necrotic inflammation of the colon with a diphtheritic membrane on its mucosal surface. In addition, there was marked edema and congestion of the brain and toxic changes affecting the other parenchymatous organs.

Microscopic Description of Section from the Colon.—(Fig. 107) There is a rather typical acute diphtheritic necrotic type of inflammation involving the superficial mucosa. This is complicated by diffuse hemorrhage which extends well into the submucosa. The deeper glands are readily identified, but their cells show extensive degenerative changes. Many of them have already reached the point of necrosis with the nuclear changes of karyorrhexis predominating. The entire mucosa and submucosa is extensively infiltrated with inflammatory cells, with polynuclear leukocytes predominating.

On the mucosal surface a thick layer of fibrin is observed, which is undergoing proteolytic breakdown as the result of the leukocytic enzyme action. In the submucosa there is very marked edema with dilatation of the capillaries and lymphatics. This lymphatic distention is particularly prominent and they may be seen engorged with fine pink-staining granular lymph and many inflammatory cells, predominantly lymphocytes, which are being carried away from the involved area. Vascular and lymphatic capillaries may be differentiated only by the presence of red cells in the former. All the evidence of acute inflammation is here: hyperemia, distended vessels, margination of leukocytes, migration of leukocytes, and perivascular cellular infiltration. Even minute capillary thrombi may be noted in places.

The muscular layer, and the adventitia show similar but less extensive evidence of injury and subsequent inflammation.

CASE 50. (Ref. #S-243)

Diagnosis.—Stomach (dog)—food poisoning; acute hemorrhagic necrosis.

In this instance we have opportunity to realize that these lesions are not necessarily restricted to human beings, but are general pathologic processes which may occur in any living animal tissue. The clinical history in this particular case relates to the activities of a young setter puppy who, in characteristic puppy fashion, had been on an exploring expedition of several hours' duration much to the consternation of his owner. It was with relief that they welcomed his return, but an hour or so later he became more and more apathetic and began to have attacks of vomiting. These increased in frequency and severity and the vomitus became blood tinged. It was difficult to tell whether the blood came from the stomach itself or whether it was mechanical bleeding, the result of the severe retching, with rupture of small capillary vessels. Enemata, purging and gastric lavage failed to control the situation to any extent. The dog was given every medical attention, with the use of intravenous, subcutaneous and rectal administration of fluid as supportive measures, but to no avail. He died forty-eight hours later.

Autopsy Findings.—The only significant lesion found at autopsy was an almost uniform, diffuse, acute, hemorrhagic, necrotic inflammation of practically the entire gastric mucosa. This was fiery red in color, with many small follicular areas of ulceration on the surface of the thickened, swollen rugae.

Microscopic Description of Section Through the Stomach Wall.—(Fig. 108) The histologic picture in this case is in many respects comparable to that noted in the previous history. There is an intense hemorrhagic, necrotic (diphtheritic) inflammatory process involving the superficial mucosa. In the deeper layers, easily recognizable chief and parietal cells are seen which are still viable, and by the presence of which a tissue diagnosis can be established. Acute inflammatory changes are seen in the submucosa, as in the preceding case. Edema and cellular infiltration are present in this area, but to a lesser extent. The case seems to represent one of food poisoning and strongly suggests a caustic substance of some type.

CASE 51. (Ref. #S-5)

Diagnosis.—Uterus—septic abortion; acute gangrenous endometritis.

Patient was a married woman of thirty years, who was admitted to the hospital because of a sudden chill and fever following a criminal abortion.

Present Illness.—For economic reasons, the patient and her husband decided that they could not afford any more children and, upon her becoming pregnant for the third time, they consulted a midwife, who agreed to abort her. This was done, apparently with no attempt at surgical asepsis, and twelve hours following the emptying of her uterus, she developed the acute symptoms for which she was admitted.

Past History.—Her past history was entirely irrelevant in respect to the present situation. She had had an entirely normal background with no particular derangement of any of her systems. Her menstrual history had been entirely negative up to the present illness.

Physical Examination.—The patient was a well developed, well nourished young white woman, who appeared profoundly toxic. Her head was essentially negative. Eyes, ears, nose and throat were normal. Chest was symmetrical and well developed. Lungs were clear throughout. Heart was not enlarged. The rate was rapid. There were no murmurs. Abdomen was moderately dis-

tended. There was marked tenderness over the lower abdomen which precluded any very satisfactory examination. There was a foul smelling vaginal discharge. Extremities were negative.

Laboratory Findings.—Red blood cells, 3,200,000 with 70% hemoglobin. White blood cells, 26,800 with 92% polynuclear leukocytes. Urinalysis showed the presence of a marked trace of albumin. Blood chemistry was negative. Blood culture yielded a hemolytic streptococcus at the end of forty-eight hours.

Subsequent Course.—The patient presented a picture of acute sepsis with a temperature ranging from 97 to 104° daily. She was profoundly toxic and did not respond well to any form of therapy. Her uterus was drained as best it could be, and everything humanly possible was done to maintain her strength with the hope that she might overcome the infection. Bacteriophage was used without any marked improvement, and various chemotherapeutic agents were attempted intravenously, likewise without success. The patient went progressively downhill, dying of her toxemia and septicemia on the fifth day after admission.

Autopsy Findings.—At autopsy there was found a general toxic cloudy swelling of the heart muscle, liver and kidneys. The uterus was large, soft and boggy with very little evidence of involution. On opening it, a thick, foul smelling, greenish-gray colored, shaggy, membranous exudate was seen adherent to the entire endometrial surface.

Microscopic Description of Section of Uterus.—(Fig. 109) Microscopic study of the tissue from the uterus includes a portion of the endometrial surface. The great bulk of the slide is made up of a solid staining area of irregularly interlacing bundles of hypertrophied smooth muscle cells with a somewhat edematous connective tissue stroma. This arrangement of the muscle fibers marks it as uterus almost unmistakably. Furthermore, tongues of tissue extend toward the inflammatory zone merging with what must once have been the base of the endometrium, and many large decidual-like cells can be seen, which indicate the diagnosis of pregnancy as well. No actually recognizable endometrial tissue is found, but huge vascular sinusoids are seen, suggesting the relationship to the placental attachment. Many of these are thrombosed. Other similar bays are filled with a fibrinous exudate.

The entire endometrial surface is replaced by a sloughing, grayish, gangrenous exudate (A) in which bluish granular masses can be seen representing bacteria. There is very little remaining cellular detail to be made out in this zone. Beneath this gangrenous material is a zone of acute inflammatory cellular infiltration (B). Due to the architecturally dense arrangement of the muscle cells, involvement of the deeper layers and extension through the uterine wall directly have been held in check to a large extent.

CHAPTER XIV

TYPES OF INFLAMMATION (*Continued*)

SUBACUTE INFLAMMATION, SPECIFIC BACTERIAL INFECTIONS

TYPHOID FEVER

Typhoid fever is a specific bacterial infection caused by the Bacillus typhosus. It is a systemic infection involving particularly the reticulo-endothelial tissues of the body with the most marked lesions being found in the small intestine, restricted to the Peyer's patches and lymph follicles, the spleen, mesenteric and retroperitoneal lymph nodes, the bone marrow, the liver, the gallbladder and less regularly, the lungs and periosteum.

The disease is characterized by a gradual onset with the initial symptoms usually a fever, headache, malaise and lassitude, which are followed by mental disturbances. Clinically, on physical examination we find "rose spots" on the abdominal wall which are the result of minute emboli of typhoid bacilli in the superficial capillaries, followed by an enlargement of the spleen and usually by tenderness of the entire abdomen with demonstrable peristalsis. Examination of the blood shows a leukopenia, the white cell count often being in the vicinity of 3,000 cells with a diminution in the polymorphonuclears. This is the result of diffuse infiltration of the bone marrow by large mononuclear cells, the result of reticulo-endothelial proliferation, which crowd out the normal blood cells.

As the disease progresses, we see a steady increase of these aforementioned symptoms over a period of about two weeks. They then reach a fastigium with a temperature of 102 to 103° and a disproportionately slow pulse, rarely exceeding 100. The patient becomes disoriented and often actually requires restraint. There is a curious, involuntary twitching of the muscles known as "subsultus tendinum," and an almost choreiform plucking at the bed clothes, termed "carphologia." This fastigium lasts for approximately an additional two weeks during which period the patient may die of the toxemia associated with the disease, or at the latter part of this period

may die of one of the two more common complications of the infection, namely perforation of the ileum with resultant secondary peritonitis or erosion of a blood vessel in the ileum at the base of one of the typical ulcers with resultant fatal hemorrhage. These two complications may occur concomitantly so that the hemorrhage is intra-abdominal.

There follows a period of convalescence of an additional two to three weeks and these briefly described complications of perforation and hemorrhage may occur during the earlier stages of this phase of the infection.

Pathology.—The pathology of the gastro-intestinal tract is one of a preliminary hyperplasia of the reticulo-endothelial system of the Peyer's patches with secondary sloughing of this tissue leaving shallow ulcers (Fig. 112). These ulcers are always parallel to the long axis of the intestine in contradistinction to the ulcers of tuberculosis which are at right angles to the axis. The ulcers heal with regeneration of the lymphoid tissue and mucosa leaving no evidence of scarring in the uncomplicated case. The splenic enlargement is due to the same reticulo-endothelial hyperplasia which results in occlusion of the vascular channels so that red cells accumulate in enormous numbers presenting the typical acute red type of splenic tumor; a picture of acute congestion. Similar changes occur as areas of focal necrosis in the liver and may result in inflammatory changes in the meninges and of the periosteum giving rise to typhoid meningitis, and typhoid periostitis, especially of the tibia and spine.

A certain number of cases following the subsidence of symptoms continue to harbor the bacteria either in the kidney or the gallbladder. There the organisms adapt themselves to their environment and may persist for many years. Such individuals act as potential carriers of the disease.

PLATE XXVIII

SUBACUTE INFLAMMATION

TYPHOID FEVER—CASES 52 AND 53

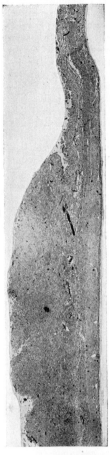

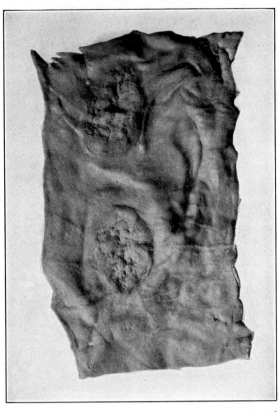

FIG. 112.—ILEUM.—CASE 52.—Gross photograph of typical early ulcerative lesions involving Peyer's patches.

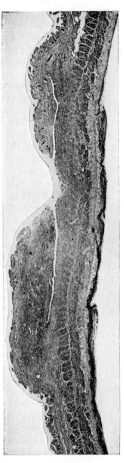

FIG. 111.—ILEUM.—CASE 52.—Hyperplastic Peyer's patch (pre-ulcerative). App. 10 x.

FIG. 113.—ILEUM.—CASE 53.—Peyer's patch with typical ulceration. App. 10 x

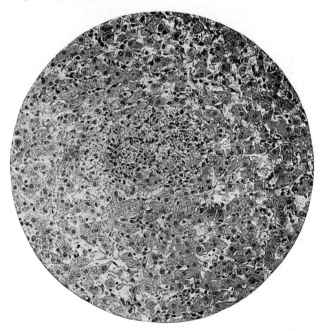

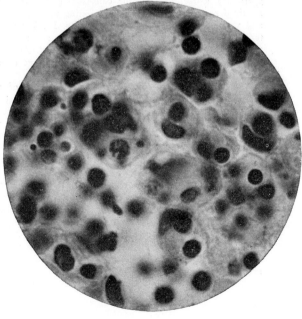

FIG. 114.—LIVER.—CASE 52.—Focal necrosis in liver parenchyma, the result of lodgment of bacteria and the accumulation of an exudate composed almost exclusively of large mononuclear cells. App. 100 x.

FIG. 115.—LYMPH NODE.—CASE 53.—Peripheral sinus containing large mononuclear phagocytes filled with ingested red cells, lymphocytes and cell detritus. App. 900 x.

ILLUSTRATIVE CASES

CASE 52. (Ref. #S-124 and S-125)

Diagnosis.—Ileum—Peyer's patch; pre-ulcerative stage (9th day of disease). Liver—focal necrosis.

Patient was an Italian girl nineteen years of age, who entered the hospital on the fourth day after the onset of her symptoms.

Present Illness.—These symptoms consisted of the gradual development of malaise, pain in the lower back region, a moderately high fever reaching 102° and a watery diarrhea of twenty to twenty-five bowel movements daily. This diarrhea had improved slightly during the preceding day or two. The fever had persisted, however, and a diagnosis by the family physician of typhoid fever was made tentatively, and she was referred to the hospital.

Past History.—Patient had never had any previous serious illness. She had had the usual measles, whooping cough and chicken pox as a child. She had had her tonsils removed when she was five years of age. She had had only occasional colds. She had no symptoms pointing to her cardiovascular system, gastro-intestinal system nor to her genito-urinary system. Menses began at eleven and had been regular since that time.

Physical Examination.—Patient was a well developed, well nourished young Italian girl. Her head was normal in contour. Eyes, ears, nose and throat were negative. Her chest was symmetrical and well developed. No râles were heard in the lungs. Heart was not enlarged. Her pulse was relatively slow, being only 96, in respect to her temperature, which was 102°. There was moderate distention of the abdomen with generalized tenderness. There was visible peristalsis. The patient showed prostration and weakness. Extremities were negative.

Laboratory Findings.—Red blood cells 4,200,000 with 84% hemoglobin. White blood cells 6,900 with 76% polynuclear leukocytes and 23% lymphocytes. Widal test positive, 1—64 dilution. Urinalysis negative. Blood cultures positive for Bacillus typhosus.

Subsequent Course.—Patient became rapidly and progressively worse. She became confused, disoriented and required restraint. She insisted on getting up to go home, and was kept in bed only with difficulty. During an interval while the nurse's back was turned, she managed to get out of bed and fell, striking her head. As a result, she died of a massive subdural hemorrhage on the ninth day of her illness.

Autopsy Findings.—There was a hematoma of the occipital region with marked subdural hemorrhage over the brain surface. Heart showed toxic myocarditis. Spleen was greatly enlarged to more than twice the normal size and presented the typical picture of acute "red" splenic tumor. There was marked hyperplasia of the mesenteric and retroperitoneal lymph nodes, which had a grayish, gelatinoid appearance on section.

Microscopic Description of Section Through Peyer's Patch in the Ileum.—(Fig. 111) By following the mucosal surface of the ileum from the normal glandular portion, it is apparent that the mucosa overlying the Peyer's patch is intact and shows no evidence of ulceration. Under low power, it is noted that there is a marked inflammatory hyperplasia of the lymphoid tissues which are at least doubled in amount. Evidence of inflammation is seen in the dilated blood vessels and lymphatics. The germinal centers appear particularly hyperplastic and show varying degrees of toxic degenerative changes even to the point of beginning necrosis. The process is by no means restricted to the mucosal surface of the intestine but extends as a serous and mononuclear infiltration between the muscle bundles and even to involve the serosa, which is considerably thickened.

It is under high power that the diagnostic features of Bacillus typhosus infection can best be recognized. There is a marked proliferation of the reticulo-endothelial cells of the body, and the characteristic lesion is one of extreme infiltration of the tissues by these large mononuclear cells. It is in connection with this reaction that much of the argument regarding the origin of the mononuclear cells has arisen, for the vessels become packed with them so that the blood supply actually appears to become shut off. For this reason Mallory developed the theory that these cells are of vascular endothelial origin. At all events the vascular endothelium in these lesions does proliferate and apparently blocks the capillaries at times, whether or not the cells actually migrate as mononuclear phagocytes into the tissues. Essentially then, the pathology of this early lesion of typhoid fever is one of large mononuclear invasion of the tissues, associated with reticulo-endothelial hyperplasia. This is seen in the bone marrow, spleen, mesenteric lymph nodes, even the lungs and the liver, as well as in the intestine, although obviously the portal of entry must be the intestine.

Microscopic Description of Section from Liver.—(Fig. 114) Moderate granular and fatty parenchymatous degeneration of the liver cells generally is seen. Typical small focal areas of necrosis are also noted. This is characterized by hyperplasia of the Küpfer cells of the sinusoids and the packing of the sinusoids with large mononuclear cells in response to the presence of the bacteria. Either bacterial toxins or anoxemia of the liver cells from this vascular obstruction, or both, results in these minute necrotic lesions with secondary leukocytic invasion. They heal by regeneration of liver cells without scar formation.

CASE 53. (Ref. #S-246 and S-247)

Diagnosis.—Typhoid fever—late ulcerative (28th day); ileum—Peyer's patch; late ulceration; spleen and lymph node—splenitis and adenitis.

Patient was a white boy of 16 years, admitted to the hospital one week after the onset of rather vague gastro-intestinal symptoms.

Present Illness.—This onset was characterized by a gradual loss of appetite, lassitude, malaise, the development of bilateral frontal headache and some dizziness. It was hard for him to be sure of the exact time that these symptoms began, and he dated the active recognition of his illness to forty-eight hours before admission, when he had such a severe nosebleed that he went to a doctor to stop it. The nose was packed to control the bleeding, and the physician told the patient that he had a fever and should remain in bed. With the removal of the packing the following day he again had a severe nosebleed and showed such increasing weakness that it was suggested he should go to the hospital. He had had no history of diarrhea during this period.

Past History.—The past history is irrelevant. As far as his mother recalled, he had all the usual childhood diseases. As he was one of twelve children, it is highly probable that this was the case in spite of the mother's inability to recall in detail the individual medical histories of her children. He apparently never had any serious illness, however, and a brief review of his respiratory, vascular, gastro-intestinal and genito-urinary systems yielded nothing of significance.

Physical Examination.—Patient was a well developed, well nourished young boy lying in bed with a flushed face, clammy skin and perspiring profusely. He appeared acutely ill. There was slight photophobia. There was dried blood in the nares. The tongue was dry and coated. Heart and lungs were negative. Abdomen was slightly distended and generally tender on deep palpation. Rose spots were noted on the abdomen. The spleen was palpable. Extremities were negative.

Laboratory Findings.—Urinalysis negative. Red blood cells, 4,600,000 with 89% hemoglobin. White blood cells, 4,000 with 19% polynuclears and 78% lymphocytes. Widal test positive in the 1—160 dilution. Blood cultures were positive for Bacillus typhosus.

Subsequent Course.—The patient ran a relatively uneventful course for the next two weeks. He had apparently reached his fastigium and continued with his blood count remaining low, temperature ranging from 101 to 103°, and the pulse, dicrotic at times, varying from 80 to 110 (note the disproportion of pulse and temperature as compared to other acute infectious diseases). Suddenly in the middle of the night, he awoke with a severe chill and a temperature which rose to 106°, and a blood count of 9,150 cells of which 84% were polymorphonuclears. There was marked abdominal rigidity. An emergency laparotomy was done, and a perforation of the ileum 25 cm. above the ileocecal junction was found and sutured. The abdomen was closed with a drain. He developed peritonitis and terminal pulmonary edema, dying on the twenty-eighth day of his illness.

Autopsy Findings.—There was generalized peritonitis and *Cl. welchii* septicemia. The heart showed marked toxic myocarditis with cardiac dilatation. There was terminal bronchopneumonia of the right lower lobe. The spleen showed acute splenomegaly, and there was hyperplasia of the mesenteric and retroperitoneal lymph nodes. There was ulceration of Peyer's patches and the lymph

follicles of the intestine. There was a repaired perforation of the ileum, focal necrosis and parenchymatous degeneration of the liver and toxic nephrosis.

Microscopic Description of a Section Through the Ileum.—(Fig. 113) The same basic pathological changes described in the preceding case may be demonstrated in this section. In this instance, however, occurring at the end of the fourth week of the disease, the lymphoid tissues have largely sloughed away leaving a shallow, depressed ulcer. At the base of this ulcer may be found the same evidence of inflammation noted previously; namely, hyperemia, reticulo-endothelial hyperplasia and diffuse infiltraton of the tissues by large mononuclear cells. Many of these large cells will be found acting as phagocytes and may be seen to contain red cells, lymphocytes and broken down, necrotic polynuclears which have infiltrated the tissue superficially as the result of the secondary ulceration. The edges of this ulcer will be seen as sloping and comparatively smooth, with no undermining of the tissues as is characteristic of other infections such as tuberculosis.

Microscopic Description of Spleen and Mesenteric Lymph Node.—(Fig. 115) The microscopic appearance of these two reticulo-endothelial organs is so similar that the findings can be described together. The only essential difference in the two tissues is found in the normal architecture. The lymph node may easily be identified by its capsule and peripheral sinuses, which are filled with mononuclear cells and by the absence of vascular pulp which identifies the spleen. The splenic sinuses are easily distinguishable from the lymphoid sinuses of the node. In addition, in the spleen, considerable hemosiderosis is present as the result of the breaking down of the red cells and the conversion of the hemoglobin into hemosiderin by the large mononuclear phagocytic cells. Because of the complication of the blood and blood pigment in the spleen, the lesion is more easily analyzed in the lymph node. The outstanding feature of histologic interest and diagnosis is the presence of large numbers of enormous macrophages, which crowd the peripheral sinuses and are filled with broken down red cells, lymphocytes and polynuclear leukocytes. Indeed, typhoid fever represents one of the best opportunities for the study of phagocytosis by large mononuclear cells. In addition, there is a diffuse reticulo-endothelial hyperplasia of the entire gland. Many areas of actual necrosis are noted. The germinal centers in particular show definite degeneration.

CHAPTER XV

TYPES OF INFLAMMATION (*Continued*)

CHRONIC PRODUCTIVE INFLAMMATION, SPECIFIC BACTERIAL INFECTIONS

SYPHILIS

Syphilis is a specific infection of man produced by the *Treponema pallidum* (*spirochaeta pallida*), a spirochetal organism which enters the body through an abrasion of the skin or mucous membranes and spreads throughout the body by the lymphatics and blood stream long before the primary lesion is demonstrable. Clinically it is divided into three (or four) stages, dependent upon the development of different tissue sensitivities.

First stage.—*Primary lesion—chancre.*—This appears at the site of inoculation (95% are genital) as a hard nodule from two to six weeks after exposure (Figs. 116 and 120). This soon ulcerates and the diagnosis may be made by the demonstration of the spirochete in large numbers by the darkfield in the serous exudate from this ulcerated surface (Fig. 127). This primary lesion is usually painless and heals spontaneously in the course of a few weeks. The pathology consists of a dense, diffuse perivascular and perilymphatic cellular infiltration of the tissues which is predominantly made up of plasma cells, lymphocytes and large mononuclears with secondary polynuclear invasion as ulceration takes place. This perivascular distribution is striking, appearing as typical "streamers" fading away from the main body of the lesion (Figs. 117, 118 and 119). It is also usually accompanied by enlargement of the nearest lymph node draining the area, known as the "satellite bubo." The histology of this secondary lesion is a similar lymphoid and mononuclear packing of the tissues accompanied by productive fibrosis, and by appropriate staining methods, spirochetes may be seen in large numbers.

Several methods have been devised to demonstrate spirochetes in the tissues. They are notoriously difficult to stain, and by the usual hematoxylin and eosin method, it is impossible to bring them out. By over-staining with some of the triacid blood stains, particularly by Giemsa's method, it is possible in a fairly high percentage of cases, especially in primary lesions where the organisms are present in large numbers, to identify them by the fact that they take a deep purplish-red color. More satisfactory, in general, for the demonstration of the spirochete is some modification of the original Levaditi silver nitrate method. The best results are obtained by fixing the tissues in formalin, then impregnating them with silver nitrate for at least several days or an indefinite length of time and subsequently developing the silver in the same manner as with a photographic plate, by the use of pyrogallic acid. The silver is precipitated on the surface of the organism, which then appears as a dark brown or black spiral against a yellowish-brown background. Warthin's modification of this method is applicable to cut sections as well. The organism, itself, varies considerably in length but has a typically tightly coiled corkscrew appearance with a flagella-like tip at either end (Fig. 121 and 127).

Second stage.—The secondary lesions appear after a latent period of several weeks or months. These consist of changes affecting particularly the ectodermal tissues. This results in localized thickening of the mucous membranes, especially in the buccal cavity, and in lesions involving the skin in the form of a macular rash. These mucous membrane lesions are spoken of as "mucous patches." Histologically, the same changes are seen as in the primary lesion; namely, plasma cells, lymphocytic and large mononuclear cell infiltration of the tissues accompanied by inflammatory hyperplasia of the specific tissue cell involved, and a secondary productive fibrosis. In addition to the above mentioned lesions, the loss of hair (alopecia) of a patchy, moth-eaten type may occur as the hair follicle epithelium

PLATE XXIX

CHRONIC INFLAMMATION

Syphilis—Primary Chancre.—Case 54

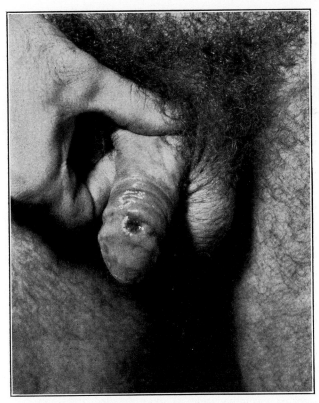

FIG. 116.—PENIS: CHANCRE (HUNTERIAN).—Typical, superficial, indurated, ulcerative lesion involving chiefly the corona.

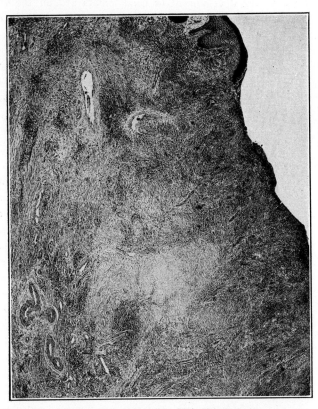

FIG. 117.—Microtessar photograph. This demonstrates one margin of the ulcerated area with the typical diffuse cellular reaction and tendency toward perivascular "streamer" formation. App. 10 x.

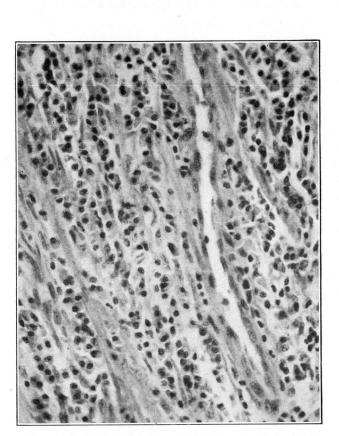

FIG. 118.—Photomicrograph from deeper layer to emphasize the parallelism of the inflammatory cells going to make up the perivascular "streamers." App. 200 x.

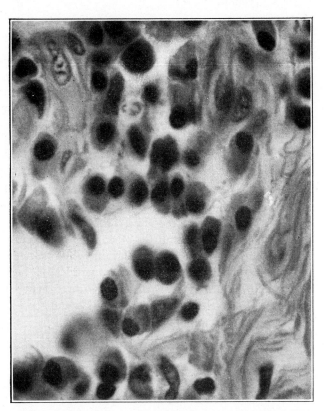

FIG. 119.—High power detail of cellular reaction, consisting almost exclusively of plasma cells. Note typical cell shape and nuclear structure. App. 900 x. (See also Fig. 75 and 80.)

becomes involved. In more advanced lesions we find the development of condylomata around the vulva or anal region. These are of the flat type in contradistinction to the pointed form of other nonspecific infections.

Third stage.—The later characteristic lesion of syphilis is spoken of as a "gumma" (Fig. 122). This is usually found in the viscera. The most common sites for the localization of this lesion are found in the liver, the spleen, the testis, the brain and in the soft or hard palate. A diffuse involvement of the rectal mucosa may result in stricture. Superficial gummata may occur in the skin leaving rather characteristic ulcers. Gummata of the lung may occur as well. The appearance of the gumma is rather characteristic. There is a central area of tough, cheesy, yellowish-white, necrotic material surrounded by a zone of dense, chronic productive inflammatory fibrosis almost in the form of a capsule. Under the microscope, this is seen to be an avascular necrosis with a marked chronic inflammatory reaction around the periphery of the lesion. This inflammatory reaction consists of marked fibroblastic proliferation, diffuse plasma cell, lymphocyte and large mononuclear infiltration. Unlike tuberculosis, rarely do the large macrophages fuse to form foreign body giant cells, and this is a point of considerable help from the practical standpoint in making a differential diagnosis between tuberculosis and syphilis.

Fourth stage.—The fourth stage of syphilis appears at a long interval after the initial infection, sometimes as late as twenty years. It affects particularly either the vascular system or the central nervous system. The commonest lesion to develop is an aortitis (Fig. 123, 124, 125 and 126) in which the media of the aorta particularly becomes involved with resulting weakening of the wall. These lesions are curiously restricted for the most part to the arch of the aorta and are not infrequently followed by aneurysmal dilatation. The lesions are likewise restricted to the arterial side of the circulation when they extend beyond the aorta. They are seen most frequently in the smaller, terminal arterioles, especially in those of the brain and cord.

The central nervous manifestations of syphilis other than the gumma already commented upon occur in two forms. One of these affects the brain substance itself and is known as general *paresis;* the other is largely restricted to the posterior columns of the spinal cord with resultant sensory disturbances. This condition is known as *tabes dorsalis* or *locomotor ataxia.* It is characterized clinically by the shuffling gait, by the loss of many reflexes and the presence of the so-called Argyll-Robertson pupil, which is incapable of responding to light or accommodation. A more detailed discussion of the central nervous type of syphilis will be found in the chapter devoted to the degenerative diseases of that system (see Fig. 659).

Congenital Syphilis

Strictly speaking, in spite of the clinical terminology, syphilis cannot be classified as an hereditary disease, for it is inconceivable that an ovum or sperm infected by treponemata would be capable of fertilization and subsequent development as an embryo, so that actually while the newborn child is infected with syphilis, it is as a result of a direct infection from the placenta of the infected mother. Such infections should better be termed "congenital."

Obviously one never finds a primary lesion of syphilis in the congenital form of the disease. It is possible to find all the other lesions other than the chancre, however, in this intra-uterine-contracted form of the disease. Characteristically, however, there are rather definite differences between the lesions of the congenital syphilitic and those of the acquired form of the disease.

The outstanding picture, which is self-diagnostic, is seen in the newborn infant, who develops, either at birth or shortly after, a mucopurulent discharge from the nares most aptly described as the "snuffles." This symptom is the result of diffuse spirochetal infection of the mucous membranes of the nose and pharynx and may be compared in a rough way to the mucous patches of the secondary stage of acquired syphilis. Also, we see in this newborn infant, typical fissures at the mucocutaneous junctures, particularly in the corner of the mouth and at the nose and around the anal orifice. These mucocutaneous lesions are likewise accompanied by a very striking exfoliating type of dermatitis, particularly involving the palms of the hands and soles of the feet, although at times involving almost the entire skin. Supplementing these specific changes, the infant has

PLATE XXX
CHRONIC INFLAMMATION
SYPHILIS

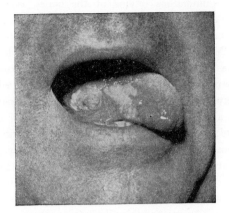

FIG. 120.—TONGUE: CHANCRE.

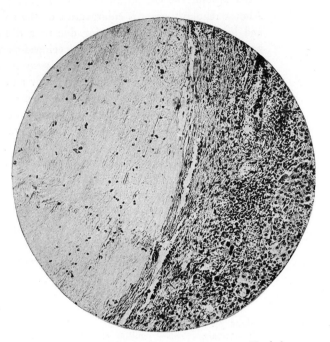

FIG. 122.—LIVER: HEALED GUMMA.—CASE 55.—Healed gummatous lesion at left with marked hyalinization, liver parenchyma at right and intermediate inflammatory zone. App. 100 x.

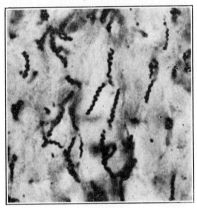

FIG. 121.—LUNG: CONGENITAL SYPHILIS. —CASE 58.—Treponema pallidum demonstrated by Levaditi method. App. 1600 x.

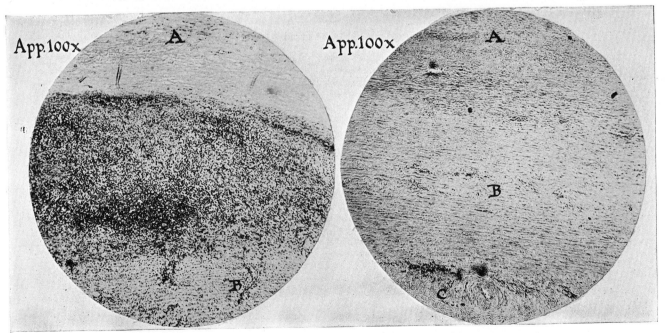

FIG. 123.—AORTA: SYPHILITIC AORTITIS, ACTIVE.—CASE 56.— Thickened, hyalinized intima at (A); multiple, confluent miliary gummata with extensive destruction of media at (B). App. 100 x.

FIG. 124.—AORTA: SYPHILITIC AORTITIS, LATE.—CASE 57.— Similar thickening of intima at (A) as in Fig. 123; residual perivascular cellular infiltration and fibrous scarring of media and adventitia at (B) and (C). App. 100 x.

a dry, wizened up appearance, often spoken of as an "old man look."

Certain children may appear free of these stigmata at the time of birth but develop their lesions later, often around the end of the first or second year. Almost regularly there is enlargement of the spleen and liver, this enlargement being due to a diffuse, patchy sclerosis with incompletely developed parenchymatous cell function. This is also seen in the pancreas. If it occurs, as it may, at birth and involves the lungs, we have the development of the so-called *pneumonia alba* in which, because of the diffuse interstitial fibrosis of the alveolar walls, the lung is not capable of expansion (Fig. 121).

Still other instances of congenital syphilis are seen in a considerably older group of children at the time when they are beginning to develop their second teeth. In this group we find the formation of the so-called hutchinsonian or peg incisor teeth and involvement of the sense organs, especially the VIII nerve with marked deafness and the development

of an interstitial keratitis. Not infrequently we also see gummatous lesions of the bones, especially in the bridge of the nose, which is destroyed leaving the so-called "saddle nose."

More striking, perhaps, even than these lesions are the bone lesions seen in the young age group at or shortly after birth. Here, we find a dense white line between the epiphysis and diaphysis, corresponding in a general way to the diffuse fibrosis of the liver and spleen and other organs already described. This dense zone of scarring interferes seriously with nutrition of the growing bone and results in failure of the bone to develop normally. Not infrequently an associated periostitis and diffuse osteitis are likewise seen. The most striking lesions are those of the long bones of arms and legs. The ribs, likewise, may show involvement and not infrequently a somewhat similar lesion may be found in the cranial bones producing the so-called *cranio-tabes* (Fig. 128, 129, 130 and 131). A more detailed discussion of these bone lesions may be found in Chapter LXV.

ILLUSTRATIVE CASES

CASE 54. (Ref. #S-296)
Diagnosis.—Penis—syphilitic chancre.
Patient was a twenty-eight year old Negro male, who came to the hospital because of painful micturition and sores on his penis.
Present Illness.—The patient was in his usual good health until approximately one month ago. At that time he noticed swelling of the prepuce, which gradually increased in size until two weeks later when it broke down and ulcerated, with a serosanguineous discharge. The lesion was not particularly painful, but because of the associated edema, the patient was unable to retract the prepuce. Micturition was painful and accompanied by vague abdominal distress. The patient had never previously had any medical care.
Past Medical History.—Patient was not married. He was of a low grade of intelligence so that details of his past history were difficult to obtain and probably were not reliable. His father was dead of unknown cause. His mother was still living and he had one brother living. There was no history of familial disease as far as he knew. He had no knowledge of any childhood diseases and did not remember any serious illness. He had had no operations. He drank moderately but disclaimed the use of drugs. A review of his systems gave no added information.
Physical Examination.—Patient was a young, asthenic, well developed Negro male, who did not appear acutely ill. He presented no abnormalities of gait. Head was normal in shape. Hair was normal in appearance. Eyes, ears, nose and throat were essentially negative. Pupils were regular and equal and reacted normally. He had several carious teeth, but otherwise nothing of significance was found. Chest was symmetrical. Lungs were

clear throughout. Heart was not enlarged and there were no murmurs. Blood pressure 118/75. Abdomen was scaphoid. There was no tenderness and no evidence of fluid. No hernia; no lumbar tenderness. There was bilateral inguinal adenopathy. Genito-urinary tract: There were five eroded areas upon the mucocutaneous junctional region of the prepuce. They were superficial in nature, firm, with slightly raised borders, irregular and had yellowish-white areas present in the crater from which a serosanguineous, foul smelling discharge was obtained. There was marked paraphimosis. There was no pain or tenderness of the scrotum or testes. Extremities were negative. (Fig. 116)
Laboratory Findings.—Darkfield examination revealed occasional spirochetal organisms with the morphology of *Treponema pallidum*. The Kline test was weakly positive. Urethral smear was negative for gonococci. Urinalysis was essentially negative, except for a good many leukocytes. Blood examination: Red blood cells, 4,500,000 with 77% hemoglobin. White blood cells, 9,250 with 46% polynuclear leukocytes and 44% lymphocytes, 5% large mononuclears, 3% eosinophiles and 2% basophiles.
Subsequent History.—Because of the phimosis and paraphimosis it was deemed advisable to do a circumcision on this patient in spite of the presence of the chancre and in this way the specimen was obtained.
Pathological Specimen.—*Gross Description.*—Specimen consisted of a piece of the prepuce with several superficially ulcerated areas at the mucocutaneous margin. One of these particularly was extremely firm in consistency, especially at the base, and gave the suggestion of a button-like lesion. There was a moderate serosanguineous discharge from the granulating surface.

PLATE XXXI
CHRONIC INFLAMMATION
SYPHILIS

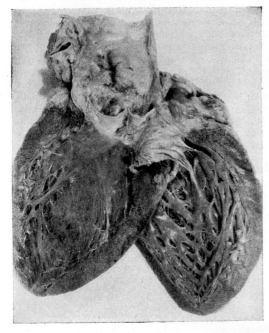

FIG. 125.—HEART: SYPHILITIC VAL-
VULITIS AND AORITIS.—CASE 57.—
Cord-like thickening of valve edge,
widening of commissures and aortic
scarring.

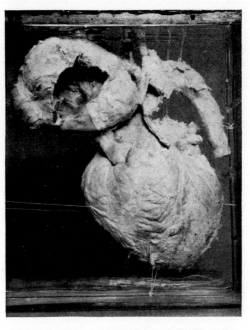

FIG. 126.—HEART AND AORTIC ARCH: RUPTURED
SYPHILITIC SACCULAR ANEURYSM.—Cf. CASE 56.

FIG. 127. — TREPO-
NEMA PALLIDUM—
DARK FIELD.—CASE
54.

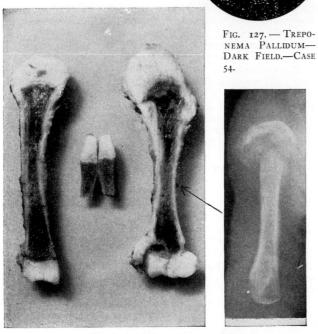

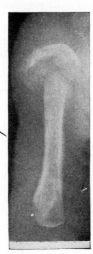

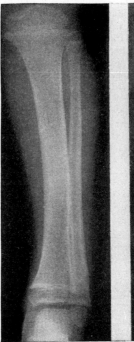

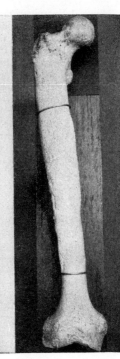

FIG. 128.—LONG BONES: CONGENITAL
SYPHILIS.—CF. CASE 54.—Note particularly epiphyseal changes.

FIG. 129. — X-
RAY OF FIG. 128.

FIG. 130.—X-RAY OF
TIBIA: SYPHILITIC OS-
TEITIS.

FIG. 131.—FEMUR:
CHRONIC SYPHILITIC
PERIOSTITIS.

Microscopic Description.—(Fig. 117, 118 and 119) Sections microscopically present a picture very typical of a primary syphilitic chancre. The epithelium on the edge of the ulcerated area shows a moderate hyperplasia. The ulcer crater is superficial in nature and covered with a thin exudate of fibrin and leukocytes. Deeper in the tissue, there is noted considerable fibrosis. More striking, however, is the extraordinary degree of mononuclear cellular infiltration in which plasma cells predominate in the ratio of pretty nearly five to one. This reaction is notably perivascular in distribution and the blood vessels themselves show a rather characteristic endarteritic thickening strongly suggestive of lues. From the base of the ulcer, long, perivascular streamers may be seen extending into the deeper tissue. These consist of perivascular aggregations of plasma cells, lymphocytes and large mononuclears.

CASE 55. (Ref. #S-47)

Diagnosis.—Liver—hepar lobatum and healed syphilitic gumma.

Patient was a Negro male of 50 years, who was admitted to the hospital with a high fever and marked shortness of breath.

Present Illness.—The onset of the patient's illness was sudden, with a severe chill and a rise in temperature to 103.5°. This was followed by pain in the right side of his chest and marked shortness of breath. He was seen by a local physician who made a diagnosis of lobar pneumonia and sent him to the hospital.

Past History.—The patient's past history was unreliable. He never had had any serious illness as far as he could remember. A review of his systems was not particularly enlightening except that he vaguely recalled as a young man having had a penile sore which lasted for several weeks, and he also admitted several attacks of gonorrhea.

Physical Examination.—Patient was a well developed, somewhat emaciated middle-aged Negro. His head was normal in shape. Eyes were negative. Pupils responded to light and accommodation. Ears were negative. Nose and throat showed moderate congestion of the mucosa and a mucopurulent discharge from the nares. The tongue was coated. The chest was well developed. There was definite restriction of respiration on the right side. There were signs of consolidation with increased breath sounds, bronchial breathing and many coarse, crackling râles. Heart was not enlarged and there were no murmurs. Abdomen was negative. Extremities were negative. There was a questionable penile scar on the corona.

Laboratory Findings.—Red blood cells, 4,100,000 with 85% hemoglobin. White blood cells, 26,000 with 92% polynuclear leukocytes. Wassermann was four plus. Sputum examination yielded a type IV pneumococcus by the Neufeld method.

Subsequent Course.—He went downhill rapidly. He developed more pronounced dyspnea and marked cyanosis. His heart rate increased and he became profoundly toxic, dying on the seventh day of his disease in a semistupor.

Autopsy Findings.—Heart showed diffuse toxic myocardial degeneration. The aorta showed some linear striation and wrinkling in the arch suggestive of syphilis. Lungs showed typical gray hepatization of the right lower lobe with associated acute fibrinopurulent pleuritis. The liver was diffusely scarred and irregularly lobular. On section, multiple healed fibrous scars suggesting healed gummata were evident. There was toxic hepatitis and nephrosis with fibrosis of the spleen.

Microscopic Examination of Section from the Liver. (Fig. 122) In examining this tissue we find evidence of a focal scarred area which, in view of the other findings of syphilis, it seems reasonable to assume represents a healed gumma. It stands out as a pink-staining area made up of dense hyalinized connective tissue not unlike a keloid in appearance. This mass of scar tissue is surrounded by a condensation zone of fibrous tissue, which might be described as a pseudocapsule. Into this area a marked chronic mononuclear inflammatory cellular infiltration may be observed. Prominent among these inflammatory cells are plasma cells and lymphocytes. The picture suggests the end result of avascularization of the area as the result of the obliteration of the capillary vessels and the further shutting off of the blood supply by the extraordinary extent of the cellular infiltration of the tissues. This is also heightened by the mild toxic action of the spirochetes. It is rare to find a syphilitic gumma in its active stage today because of the effectiveness of antisyphilitic treatment and the intensive campaign aimed at the early diagnosis and treatment of the syphilitic infection.

CASE 56. (Ref. #S-64)

Diagnosis.—Aorta—acute miliary gummata; syphilitic aortitis; aneurysmal wall.

Patient was a fifty-three year old colored woman, who was admitted to the hospital complaining of extreme dyspnea.

Present Illness.—It was impossible to assign a definite time interval to the patient's illness. She had had a long history of asthmatic attacks, the current one being more severe than any previously. It was usually accompanied by an unproductive, "brassy" cough. There was no edema of the feet or ankles. She had had occasional attacks of pain over the precordium in conjunction with her so-called "asthma."

Past History.—The patient's past history was totally unreliable and did not help in the establishment of a diagnosis. As far as could be determined, she had had all the usual illnesses of childhood. She had had numerous attacks of upper respiratory infection and influenza in 1918. She had had qualitative digestive disturbances. She disclaimed any genito-urinary symptoms and any knowledge of venereal infection.

Physical Examination.—The patient was a fairly well developed but rather emaciated middle-aged colored woman lying propped up in bed and showing marked cyanosis of her face and neck, accompanied by severe dyspnea. The head, itself, in other respects showed no abnormalities. Pupils reacted sluggishly to light and accommodation. Ears, nose and throat were negative. Examination of the chest revealed a heart which was enlarged to the left with the apex beat in the 6th interspace, three centimeters outside the mid-clavicular line. No murmurs were heard. The patient had a blood pressure of 210/100. There was dullness over the mediastinal region so that it was difficult to outline the right heart margin. Lungs showed numerous crackling râles, but there was no definite dullness or alteration in the breath or voice sounds. Abdomen was negative. Extremities were negative. Gynecologic examination revealed a lacerated cervix with a mucoid discharge.

Laboratory Findings.—No laboratory findings were obtained because the patient died suddenly three hours after admission, before any studies could be made.

Autopsy Findings.—The pericardium was filled with clotted blood. The heart, itself, was small weighing 250 grams, but showed evidence of myocardial degeneration. There was an aneurysm measuring 9 x 8 x 6 cm. in the anterior mediastinum arising from the innominate artery which had ruptured into the pericardial sac. This started as a fusiform dilatation of the innominate, but gave rise to a large sacculated aneurysm about 5 cm. above its origin from the aortic arch. This caused pressure upon the trachea, esophagus and showed beginning erosion of the sternum. Other findings were not significant, except for four fibrotic areas in the spleen, probably representing healed gummata. The aorta, itself, showed numerous greyish, elevated plaques with characteristic linear puckering. The coronaries were moderately sclerotic.

Microscopic Description of Section from the Wall of the Aorta.—(Fig. 123) Study of the tissue reveals an intimal surface, which shows some atheromatous thickening. There is beginning accumulation of large mononuclear cells, which are distended with lipoid material. This is accompanied by some fibrous tissue increase. The most striking feature of the lesion is the presence of a marked cellular infiltration of the media of the aorta. This is characterized by a diffuse perivascular infiltration by plasma cells, lymphocytes and large mononuclear cells. This perivascular infiltration follows the course of the vasa vasorum, which accounts for the distribution of the inflammatory reaction. Intimal thickening of these small vessels is present to such a degree as to produce obliteration of the lumen in places. The lesion is by no means restricted to the media, but extends to involve the adventitia as well. Again, the most marked histologic changes are seen around the small vessels of the adventitia. This produces a somewhat similar streamerlike appearance of the tissues, as is seen in the primary lesion or chancre. This particular case represents an unusually severe and relatively acute type of lesion with the production of multiple miliary gummata. The gummatous nature of this process is seen by the beginning caseous necrosis focally in the inflammatory zone immediately around the medial vessels. In this instance the lesions are so numerous and so large as to represent almost a continuous confluent process. Another feature of significance is the breaking up of the elastic tissue fibers in the wall of the aorta.

Case 57. (Ref. #S-65)

Diagnosis.—Aorta—syphilitic aortitis (late).

Patient was a married Negro male, 39 years of age, admitted to the hospital complaining of dyspnea.

Present Illness.—The patient's present illness began indefinitely about four months ago when he first noticed blood streaked sputum in the morning. This recurred at irregular intervals, but was never severe enough to cause him much concern. It was accompanied, however, by palpitation of his heart and progressive dyspnea, which were the symptoms which sent him to a physician, who referred him to the hospital for diagnosis and treatment.

Past History.—The patient did not recall any childhood diseases. He had a chancre twenty years ago, which healed spontaneously after several weeks. He never had any treatment for it and did not recall the development of any secondary lesions. A review of his systems otherwise was irrelevant.

Physical Examination.—Patient was a well developed, well nourished, middle-aged Negro male, who did not appear acutely ill. His head was normal in appearance. Eyes showed marked sluggishness in their reaction to light and accommodation. Ears, nose and throat were negative. Chest: lungs were clear with no alteration in voice or breath sounds. Heart was definitely enlarged with the apex in the sixth interspace in the anterior axillary line. There was a systolic thrill present and a diastolic murmur over the aortic, and a double murmur at the mitral area. Blood pressure was 170/60. There was definite Corrigan and capillary pulse. Abdomen was negative. Genitalia showed no definite penile scar. Extremities were negative.

Laboratory Findings.—Red blood cells, 3,600,000 with 72% hemoglobin. White blood cells, 8,200 with 68% polynuclear leukocytes. Urinalysis was negative. Wassermann was four plus. Electrocardiogram suggested a definite left preponderance. X-ray examination showed enlargement of the heart and dilatation of the aorta, which was felt to be syphilitic in nature.

Subsequent Course.—The patient was started on antisyphilitic treatment. His cardiac picture, however, was so advanced that he showed no improvement. His dyspnea became progressively worse and was accompanied by marked cyanosis. He developed terminal pulmonary edema and died six weeks after admission.

Autopsy Findings.—Pericardial sac contained 300 c.c. of clear fluid. There was a marked syphilitic aortitis and syphilitic involvement of the aortic valve. The heart weighed 695 gm. (normal is 350 gm.) There was marked hypertrophy of the myocardium—mostly left-sided—accompanied by diffuse myosclerosis and myocardial degeneration. The myocardium also showed considerable fibrosis. The aorta, throughout its length showed a few elevated gray plaques and a moderate amount of longitudinal linear puckering. The lungs were edematous. Both pleural cavities were filled with clear fluid. There was chronic passive congestion of the viscera.

Microscopic Description of Section Through the Aorta.—(Fig. 124) Examination of the aorta shows a late, almost healed stage of syphilitic aortitis. The small branches of the vasa vasorum are thickened or even obliterated in places. About them are still seen some inflammatory mononuclear cells, plasma cells and lymphocytes. There is an increase of connective tissue in these areas which for the most part is adult in type with a great deal of collagen. This connective tissue may be seen replacing a considerable portion of the media. Elastic tissue fibers have been extensively destroyed and the contraction of the scar tissue has resulted in the wrinkling of the intima as noted grossly. It is of interest in such cases to use special stains to demonstrate the degeneration and splitting of the elastic laminae, which is almost pathognomonic of syphilitic infection—not only in the aorta, but in the smaller arterioles. Incidentally, syphilitic lesions are almost exclusively restricted to the arterial tree, the venous side remaining usually uninvolved from the histologic point of view, and further, the great majority of the lesions are localized in or about the arch of the aorta, the major aortic branches remaining uninvolved even a centimeter or so from their origin. The intima in these cases shows marked fibrotic thickening to compensate for the loss of media, just as the most marked fibrosis is seen in the adventitia as a protective strengthening of the wall at the damaged site.

CASE 58. (Ref. #S-33 and S-34)

Diagnosis.—Lung—pneumonia alba; congenital syphilis.

Patient was a white male infant of three months referred to the hospital because of a persistent nasal discharge and a dry, unproductive cough. His nutritional history was unsatisfactory. The baby was weaned at six weeks and had not gained appreciably since. On admission, the chest examination showed impaired resonance, an increase of breath sounds and many râles. Respirations were very rapid, fifty to sixty. He developed intense cyanosis. X-ray showed a diffuse bronchopneumonia, and evidence of a very acute syphilitic osteitis. There was ulceration of the roof of the hard palate. The spleen and liver were both enlarged. There were mucous patches and an anal fissure.

Laboratory Findings.—Red blood cells, 2,300,000 with 56% hemoglobin. White blood cells, 46,800 with 39% polynuclear leukocytes, 43% lymphocytes and 18% other cells. Spinal fluid and blood Wassermann tests were both positive (four plus).

Subsequent Course.—The patient's pneumonic picture became progressively worse and he died a few days after admission. In this connection, it was interesting to note that the mother had had three previous pregnancies; the first child died at six weeks of age, the second was born prematurely and died at birth, and the third terminated by a spontaneous miscarriage. At that time she learned that she had syphilis and was given a partial course of antisyphilitic treatment.

Microscopic Description of Sections from the Lung, One Prepared by the Usual, Hematoxylin and Eosin Staining Method, and the Other by Levaditi's Method to Demonstrate the Organisms.—(Fig. 121) The microscopic appearance of the lung tissue with the usual technique shows such extensive avascular necrosis that it is difficult to recognize the tissue as being lung. There is a diffuse exudative pneumonic consolidation of almost nonaerated, congenitally atelectatic lung. Such cellular reaction as can be made out is found to consist chiefly of plasma cells and lymphocytes.

In the Levaditi preparation the general tissue staining reaction is a brownish-yellow. Cell detail is largely lost. Nuclei may be identified by their rather sharp delineation of a darker brown color. The same is true of the nuclear chromatin. The chief point of interest in this specimen is the recognition of the teeming myriads of treponemata. These appear as black twisted spiral threads between the cells. They are not to be confused with straight strands of fibrin or wavy fibers of the stromal tissues, which are apt to stain a rather dark brownish-black as well.

The spirochetes are always present in the syphilitic lesion but are most readily demonstrated in the tissues from the syphilitic fetus because of their great numbers. It must be recognized that the organisms appear much larger than they actually are by this technique, because the reaction involved is precipitation of silver on their surface rather than a staining of their substance.

CHAPTER XVI

TYPES OF INFLAMMATION (*Continued*)

CHRONIC PRODUCTIVE INFLAMMATION, SPECIFIC BACTERIAL INFECTION

TUBERCULOSIS

Tuberculosis is a chronic inflammation produced by the tubercle bacillus. The infection is not confined to man but is found in many species of the animal kingdom. The organism (Fig. 134 and 154), the tubercle bacillus, is a medium sized, straight or slightly bent rod, nonspore-bearing, growing slowly on artificial media, acid-fast, multiplying only in the tissues of man and animals, but capable of existing for considerable time outside of the body due to its waxy covering. A number of types of the organism have been described in respect to the various types of mammalia—human, bovine, avian, piscine and reptilian. Only the human and bovine varieties are pathogenic for man. The disease, as the name implies, is characterized by the formation of nodules or tubercles. The earliest gross tubercles seen in the tissues are known as miliary tubercles. The smallest diagnostic microscopic lesion is the histologic submiliary tubercle.

Modes of Infection.—*Inhalation.*—Inhalation of dust containing the organism; inhalation of droplets from sneezing and coughing of tuberculous individuals; inhalation of ingested organisms from the mouth.

Ingestion.—The organism may be ingested in milk or milk products.

Cutaneous inoculation.—Rarely the organism may be inoculated directly through cuts and abrasions of the skin (butcher's and pathologist's tubercle).

Congenital tuberculosis.—A few cases of tuberculosis of this type are said to have resulted through tuberculous lesions of the placenta.

The reaction of the body to the entrance and growth of the tubercle bacillus depends upon: 1. the virulence of the organism; 2. the dose; 3. the resistance or immunity of the tissues; 4. the degree of allergy to the tubercle toxin.

Primary Reaction (childhood tuberculosis). —When the tubercle bacillus enters the tissues of a child (or an adult) for the first time the organism meets with little or no resistance, progressing usually to the peripheral portion of the lung where the primary lesion is most frequently found. Here the organisms multiply and produce necrosis. The tissues respond by the proliferation and accumulation of both large and small mononuclear cells ("epithelioid" cells and lymphocytes). As the organisms multiply, some enter the lymphatics and are drained to the peribronchial lymph nodes, which enlarge, show a similar reaction and later caseate. The primary lesion, in the majority of cases will become limited by a thin fibrous tissue capsule and the caseous central portion usually undergoes calcification. This, not infrequently, is followed by actual ossification. This primary lesion is usually spoken of as the *Ghon tubercle* (Fig. 142). A similar fate will overtake the lesion in the lymph node in the great majority of instances. On the other hand, if the virulence of the organism be great or the dose excessive, or if the child develops a marked allergy to the toxin the organism will not be destroyed and the tuberculous process will spread. The caseous lymph node may soften and ulcerate into a bronchus. Myriads of organisms will be inspired into the adjacent lobe with resultant rapidly spreading fatal tuberculous bronchopneumonia. The blood stream may be invaded with generalized miliary tuberculosis resulting. The outcome, therefore, of the primary invasion is either the healed Ghon tubercle or the death of the child by a rapidly spreading process.

Secondary Reaction (adult tuberculosis).— If the individual survives the primary invasion, there is produced a resistance or immunity together

PLATE XXXII
CHRONIC INFLAMMATION (Continued)
Tuberculosis

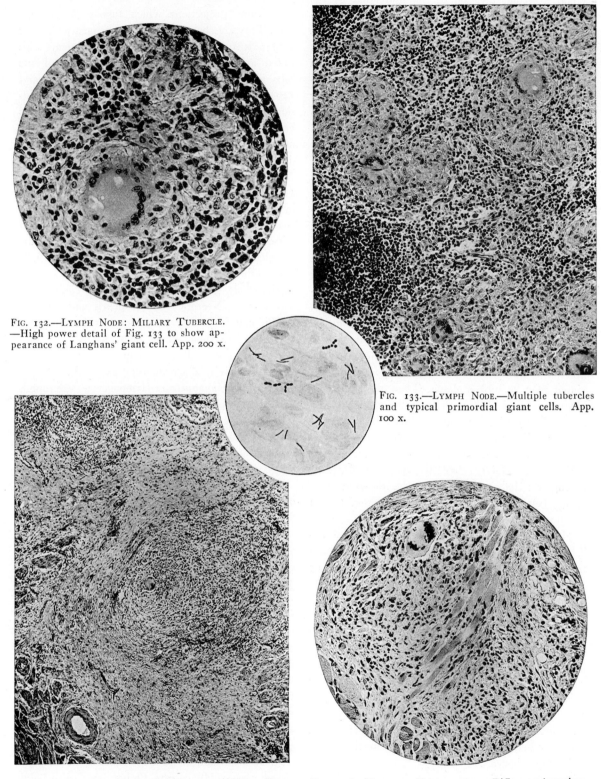

FIG. 132.—LYMPH NODE: MILIARY TUBERCLE. —High power detail of Fig. 133 to show appearance of Langhans' giant cell. App. 200 x.

FIG. 133.—LYMPH NODE.—Multiple tubercles and typical primordial giant cells. App. 100 x.

FIG. 135.—FALLOPIAN TUBE: TUBERCULOSIS.—With miliary tubercle formation and chronic productive inflammatory fibrosis. App. 15 x.

FIG. 136.—TONGUE.—TUBERCULOSIS.—Diffuse tuberculous reaction with destruction of muscle. App. 100 x.

FIG. 134.—TUBERCLE BACILLI IN SPUTUM. App. 1000 x.

with a variable degree of allergy of the tissues. Upon a second invasion of the individual by the organism, the resultant inflammatory reaction prevents the progress of the organism through the tissues, tending to localize the infection. The regional lymph nodes of such a tuberculous area show little or no involvement. From animal experimentation it has been shown that within a few hours after the entrance of the tubercle bacillus into the tissues, a considerable exudate of serum and leukocytes occurs. This is spoken of as an allergic response. The initial reaction gradually subsides and is followed after several days by the productive inflammatory reaction. Caseous necrosis usually occurs early and is a prominent feature of the picture. In addition to the formation of individual tubercles, there is an attempt to wall off the process by proliferation of fibrous tissue. If the resistance of the patient be good, the virulence and dose of the organism not too great, the infection *will* become walled off or healed by the abundant fibrous tissue reaction. Such lesions are encountered in the great majority of adults in the apex of the lung.

If the dosage or virulence of the organism be great, the resistance or the immunity of the individual may be broken down. Then the process is likely to spread rapidly through the tissues in the same way that it occurs in a primary or childhood type of infection. The organism may even get into the blood stream causing a hematogenous dissemination, and miliary tubercles may be scattered throughout the organs of the body. Between these two extremes, varying degrees of reaction to the organism are seen.

Histopathology of the Miliary Tubercle.— The earliest histologic lesions of tuberculosis are not visible to the naked eye. They are composed of roughly concentric masses of cells and are rather sharply demarcated from the surrounding tissues. Three more or less distinct areas may be recognized in the lesion: 1. a central area usually showing coagulation or caseation necrosis in which the organism may be demonstrated (Fig. 132, 133, 135, 136, 137, 138 and 139); 2. a pale zone surrounding this area resulting from the proliferation of large phagocytic mononuclear cells ("epithelioid" cells). Within this zone giant cells may be seen; and 3. an outer marginal zone of small mononuclear cells, chiefly lymphocytes.

The *epithelioid cells* are pale with vesicular,

elongated nuclei, poor in chromatin. They are irregularly elongated in shape and frequently show cytoplasmic projections which fuse with adjacent cells. They are characteristically arranged with their long axis toward the center of the lesion. This radial arrangement, with the heaping up of the cells is spoken of as "palisading" (Fig. 148 and 149). The origin of these cells is a point of considerable debate. From a practical standpoint it seems best to consider them as histiocytes or so-called large mononuclear phagocytes, which have already been described.

The *giant cells* are of the foreign body type (Fig. 85, 132, 133, 136 and 141) and are formed by the fusion of "epithelioid" cells, as a rule. The characteristic arrangement of the nuclei in radial horseshoe fashion has come to be known as the Langhans' type of foreign body giant cell, which is quite different in its appearance from the so-called foreign body giant cell, as seen in an epulis or a bone tumor. Necrotic cellular debris and tubercle bacilli may frequently be demonstrated within the cytoplasm of these giant cells. In very young tubercles, a giant cell may occupy a central position. This is spoken of as a primordial giant cell.

The *small mononuclears* (lymphocytes) are round, and have deeply staining nuclei which fill the cell. They migrate into the area from adjacent lymphoid tissue of the part. A delicate reticulum can be demonstrated by special staining within the tubercle and is most abundant when the resistance is high.

Progress of the Histologic Lesions.—1. If the organisms be destroyed promptly, the histologic miliary tubercles may completely resolve.

2. If the organisms continue to grow, the central area of caseation extends. Additional "epithelioid" cells accumulate and lymphocytes continue to migrate to the outer portion of the lesions. Several such expanding miliary tubercles may coalesce to form the conglomerate tubercle. As has already been described, this extension of the lesion results from the fact that the tubercle bacillus is so difficult to destroy and because of the amoeboid activity of the "epithelioid" cells. With the migration of the cell to the periphery of the lesion, not infrequently it is destroyed by the tubercle bacilli. Its cell membrane ruptures and the organisms are liberated in the peripheral portion of the lesion.

3. If the tempo of the infection is speeded up the tissues may rapidly caseate. Only a few "epithelioid"

PLATE XXXIII

CHRONIC INFLAMMATION

MILLIARY TUBERCULOSIS.—CASE 59

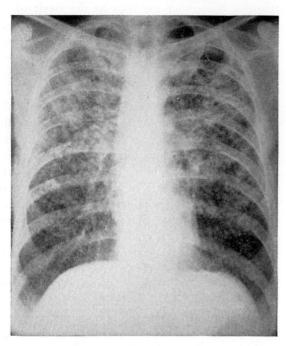

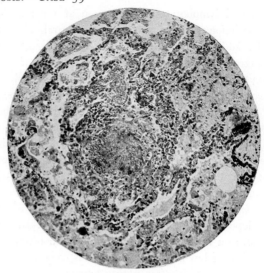

FIG. 138.—LUNG: ACUTE MILIARY TUBERCLE. App. 100 x.

FIG. 137.—X-RAY.—CHEST.—Typical miliary tuberculosis with fine mottling of the lung fields.

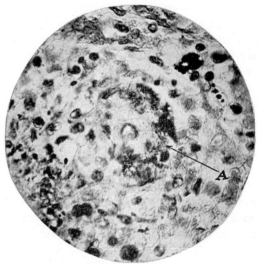

FIG. 139.—DETAIL OF TUBERCLE showing Tubercle bacilli within lesion. App. 400 x.

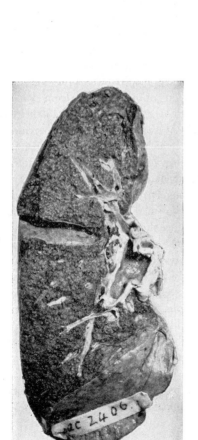

FIG. 140.—LUNG.—Gross photograph of cut surface to show uniform size and distribution of the miliary lesions.

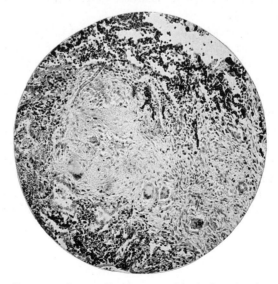

FIG. 141.—LUNG: Conglomerate histologic tubercle. App. 100 x.

cells and lymphocytes may be seen at the margin of the lesion, and giant cells may be entirely absent.

In addition to the proliferative and exudative changes described above, varying degrees of attempted healing with the production of tuberculous granulation tissue are seen. These attempts to heal or wall off the lesion succeed in proportion to the resistance of the individual to the infection.

The classification of tuberculous lesions depends upon the characteristics of the tissue reactions. There are five more or less generally accepted forms of tuberculosis:

Fibroid Tuberculosis.—This represents a slow developing type of lesion, the result of marked resistance on the part of the individual and often an organism of low-grade virulence. It is characterized by marked fibrosis, often with complete replacement of the tuberculous areas of infection. Likewise, calcification is a common associated reparative process in this type of the disease. There is an absence of the acute necrotic picture. Miliary tubercles are rarely found, and giant cells are incidental to the diagnosis.

Fibrocaseous Tuberculosis.—In this most common type of tuberculosis, we find a more extensive and typical picture. It represents the result which one expects to find in an individual of average resistance and an organism of average virulence. It is characterized by the production of large amounts of tuberculous granulation tissue. There are many well-formed tubercles with a moderate amount of caseous necrosis and usually very prominent giant cell formation. In the lung, it not infrequently goes on to the development of cavities, which show attempts at fibrous tissue walling off, but which rarely go on to the point of replacement fibrosis as in the fibroid type of the disease (Fig. 144, 145, 146 and 147).

Caseous tuberculosis.—By this type of tuberculosis is meant a form in which the resistance of the individual is obviously almost negligible, and the virulence of the organism is very marked. There is very extensive caseation. In the lung, this may practically involve the entire lung as an almost uniform, diffuse process. There is very little fibrous tissue reaction. The lesion is apt to be too acute for the development of giant cells, and "epithelioid" cells are only few in number (Fig. 143).

Acute miliary tuberculosis.—By miliary tuberculosis is meant the development of multiple miliary tubercles throughout the body as the result of a hematogenous dissemination of the tubercle bacillus. These gain entrance to the blood stream usually from a primary focus in the lung or elsewhere by erosion of the wall of a blood vessel (Fig. 137, 138, 139 and 140).

Hyperplastic tuberculosis.—This is a comparatively rare form characterized by the continued production of tuberculous granulation tissue without the development of characteristic caseation necrosis and tubercle formation to any extent. Scattered giant cells are not infrequently encountered. This is particularly seen in the cervical lymph nodes of children in bovine infections, and also in the cecum as another common site (Fig. 132 and 133).

Methods of Spread.—In this discussion of tuberculosis, only the general features of the process have been described. Tuberculosis may be primary in the respiratory system or in the gastro-intestinal system. Not infrequently, however, the primary lesion clinically may occur, particularly in children, in the regional lymph nodes in relation to the histologic primary lesion. Thus, infection of the mediastinal nodes or of the mesenteric nodes is by no means uncommon. It is generally assumed that tuberculosis elsewhere in the body, notably tuberculosis of the bones, tuberculosis of the kidney and tuberculosis of the reproductive system, which represent the three most common sites, as well as tuberculous meningitis, are secondary manifestations of the disease with some hidden primary lesion from which the organisms are derived and carried to their new focus of activity. Occasional cases of tuberculosis are observed in which no demonstrable primary lesions elsewhere can be found clinically, roentgenologically or even at autopsy, but these are very rare and probably merely represent cases in which the primary lesion was so small that it was overlooked.

To produce the secondary lesions then, the tubercle bacillus must be disseminated. This may occur as the result of *direct extension,* as we have already seen, particularly through the activity of the mononuclear phagocytic cells; *by extension along natural passages;* for example, a focus of tuberculosis in the lung may spread by bronchogenic extension to distant parts of the lung, or tubercle bacilli may be raised in the sputum and swallowed to produce tuberculous enteritis; *by lymphatic extension;* this has been emphasized particularly in the development of the lymphadenopathy of childhood tuberculosis in which

PLATE XXXIV
CHRONIC INFLAMMATION
TUBERCULOSIS (Continued)

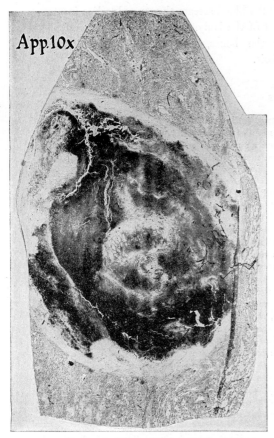

FIG. 142.—LUNG: GHON TUBERCLE.—CASE 60.—
Note walling off of lesion by dense fibrous pseudocapsule, and central calcification. App. 10 x.

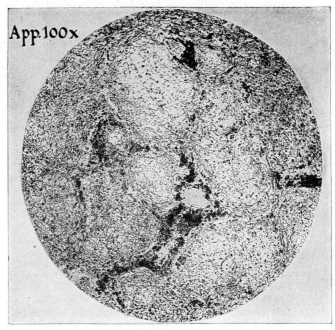

FIG. 143.—LUNG: CASEOUS TUBERCULOUS PNEUMONIA.—Massive
caseous necrosis with architectural structure still visible. App.
100 x.

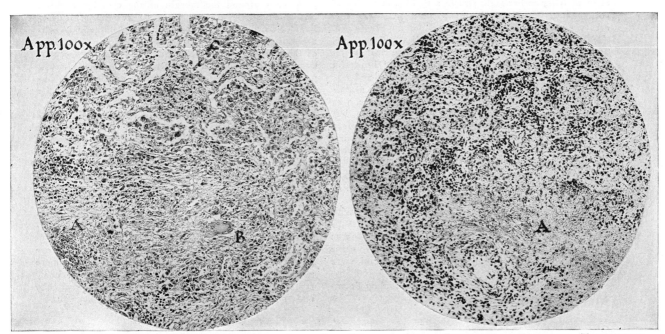

FIG. 144.—LUNG: TUBERCULOUS BRONCHOPNEUMONIA.—Area of
caseous tuberculosis (A) surrounded by alveoli filled with typical mononuclear exudate (C). Giant cell at (B). App. 100 x.

FIG. 145.—LUNG: FIBROCASEOUS, ULCERATIVE TUBERCULOSIS.—
CASE 61.—Central area of caseation at (A) surrounded by
epithelioid cells and lymphocytes and accompanied by fibrous
tissue proliferation at right. App. 100 x.

the primary lesion is often minimal, and the lymphatic tissue involvement much more prominent; and finally, *by the blood stream;* under these circumstances we may have either a very diffuse generalized miliary tuberculosis often fatal in its

outcome, or with the dissemination of only a few bacilli by the blood stream they may localize in some other part of the body, such as the kidney, fallopian tube or the bones, to produce local forms of tuberculosis.

ILLUSTRATIVE CASES

CASE 59. (Ref. #S-28, S-136, and S-164)
Diagnosis.—Lung—miliary tuberculosis, acute.

Patient was an eighteen months old female Negro child, who was admitted to the hospital because of a history of persistent projectile vomiting.

Present Illness.—The onset of the child's illness was gradual with what seemed to be a cold, which began five days before admission accompanied by a persistent cough. This was followed by intermittent attacks of vomiting, which increased in frequency and severity and became of the projectile type. She gradually developed a rigidity of the body with opisthotonos. The day before admission she had several convulsions. It was following such a convulsion that she was finally brought to the hospital, with a temperature of 102°, a pulse which averaged about 160 and respirations of around 40 per minute.

Past History.—The child was a six-pound, normally delivered baby. She had been artifically fed from birth because the mother had no milk. She developed normally so far as her aunt knew up to the end of her first year. At that time she developed a severe cold with a persistent cough for two or three months. This then improved and she had been fairly well during the interval until the onset of the present illness. She had not gained satisfactorily, however, and was slow in walking and talking. The mother had developed a frank pulmonary tuberculosis and had been sent away for sanatorium care, dying two months before the child's admission.

Physical Examination.—The child was fairly well developed, but definitely undernourished in appearance. She was lying on her right side in a position of moderate opisthotonos. The head itself appeared negative. The eyes were staring and the child did not appear to see. Ears were negative. Nose and throat were negative. There was moderate enlargement of the cervical lymph nodes bilaterally. The chest showed definite bronchial breathing over the left base with diffuse coarse and fine scattered râles throughout both lungs. The breath sounds generally were increased in intensity and there was definite impairment of resonance over the entire left chest. The heart was not enlarged. Pulse rate was very rapid reaching 180 at times. There were no murmurs. Abdomen was protuberant. The extremities showed marked exaggeration of the knee jerks and the ankle clonus. Kernig was positive on both sides. There was marked rigidity of the extremities, of the back and of the neck. There was a definite nystagmus.

Laboratory Findings.—Red blood cells 2,800,000 with 63% hemoglobin; white blood cells 21,000 with 69% polynuclears and 31% lymphocytes. Spinal fluid was under increased pressure. Cell count was 160 per cubic millimeter with 85% lymphocytes. Tubercle bacilli were found.

Subsequent Course.—The patient went rapidly downhill dying 48 hours after admission.

Autopsy Findings.—Lungs: palpation revealed many shot-like nodules throughout both lungs; the apex of the left showed an area of consolidation 1.5 cm. in diameter. On section, many small grayish, semitranslucent tubercles and an area of grayish-yellow consolidation at the apex were seen. The peribronchial lymph nodes were enlarged and apparently caseous. The bronchi showed a considerable quantity of mucoid and pus-like exudate. Tiny miliary tubercles were found in the spleen, liver and kidneys as well. The brain was wet (edematous); the pia arachnoid at the base was semitranslucent and numerous tubercles were seen.

Microscopic Description of Section from the Lung.—(Fig. 138, 139 and 141) The lung tissue may be identified by the alveolar arrangement and the presence of typical bronchial mucosa. Scattered throughout the lung substance, however, are seen many miliary tubercles which show a rather intensely eosin-staining central caseous necrotic area and a zone of proliferating cellular activity around them, which sharply demarcates the lesions from the unaffected lung tissue.

The lesions vary considerably in size, ranging from submiliary aggregations of "epithelioid" cells up to fairly large conglomerate tubercles. The smaller submiliary lesions are found to be made up of "epithelioid" cells arranged more or less concentrically and showing a few polynuclears around them. Some of these cells have fused to form typical Langhans' giant cells. More typically, the lesion is somewhat larger and shows a central area of caseation with one or more characteristic giant cells around the margin of the caseous material. Accompanying this caseation is a proliferation of "epithelioid" cells and connective tissue. The "epithelioid" cells are rather irregularly arranged at the periphery, many of them with their long axis directed toward the center. Others tend to show a concentric arrangement. In this peripheral zone of inflammatory cells, numerous lymphocytes have accumulated as well. These are chiefly of the small, adult variety.

The entire lesion tends to be relatively avascular without the marked hyperemia and perivascular infiltration of acute inflammation. There is, however, some inflammatory edema of the tissues. In some of the giant cells, particles of foreign material may be identified representing broken down cellular debris in the lung alveoli. By appropriate staining of one of these lesions, the presence of tubercle bacilli may be made out. This is done by the usual Ziehl-Neelsen carbol fuchsin method, which stains tubercle bacilli, because of their acid-fast nature, an intense red.

Some of the lesions, as has already been noted, are larger conglomerate tubercles showing much more marked proliferative fibrosis. These lesions probably represent earlier hematogenous foci, which have gradually undergone the typical chronic granulomatous productive

PLATE XXXV
CHRONIC INFLAMMATION
TUBERCULOSIS

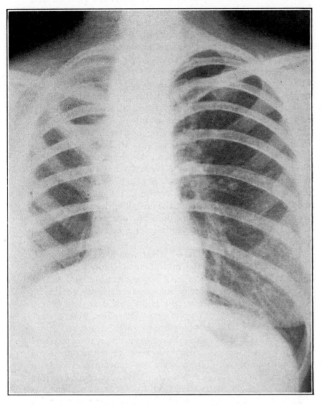

FIG. 146.—X-RAY.—CHEST.—Increased hilar density; diffuse clouding of right lung field especially upper lobe (tuberculosis) with apical cavitation (cf. CASE 61).

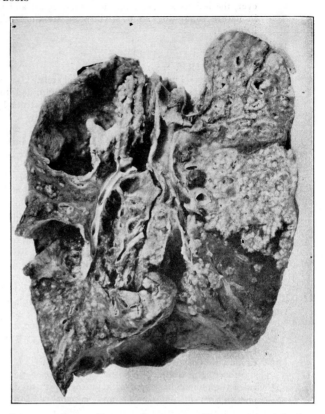

FIG. 147.—LUNG: CHRONIC PULMONARY TUBERCULOSIS (cf. CASE 61).—Postmortem section showing advanced cavitation at right apex and terminal rapid tuberculous bronchopneumonia in left lower lobe.

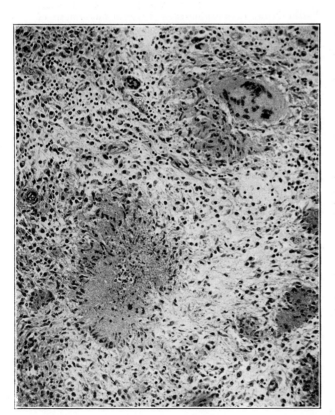

FIG. 148.—UTERUS: TUBERCULOUS ENDOMETRITIS.—Typical miliary tubercles, showing central caseation, palisading of marginal epithelioid cells, mononuclear cellular reaction and productive fibrosis. App. 200 x.

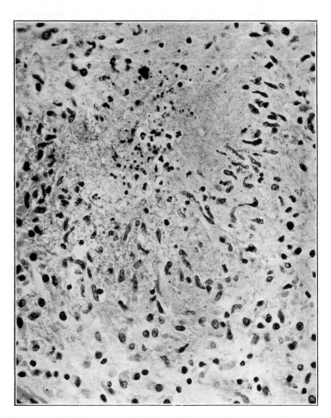

FIG. 149.—High power field from Fig. 148, better showing the arrangement and character of the cells taking part in the tuberculous reaction. App. 400 x.

fibrous tissue changes, in some instances proceeding to almost fibrous scar formation. For the most part, however, the lesions are relatively uniformly small and acute in nature suggesting an overwhelming terminal miliary infection.

CASE 60. (Ref. #S-189)

Diagnosis.—Lung—calcified Ghon tubercle.

Patient was a white male, aged 34, admitted to the accident ward with a history of having been struck by an automobile.

Past History.—It was impossible to obtain any history from the patient as he was admitted in an unconscious state and remained unidentified during his stay in the hospital.

Physical Examination.—Patient was a well developed, well nourished white male of the asthenic type of build. There were numerous abrasions of the scalp. On palpation there appeared to be a fracture line over the right temporoparietal area. Eyes showed an internal strabismus. There was hemorrhage from his nose and from his right ear. The left ear appeared negative. Nose and throat showed some hemorrhage in the posterior pharynx. The heart and lungs were negative. Abdomen was negative. Genitalia appeared normal. Extremities were negative except for several abrasions, the result of his accident.

Laboratory Findings.—Red blood cells 4,800,000 with 92% hemoglobin. White blood cells 9,600 with 73% polynuclear leukocytes. Urinalysis was negative. X-ray examination showed a fracture of his skull.

Subsequent Course.—The patient developed numerous râles throughout his chest with patchy areas of dullness, particularly at both bases and succumbed forty-eight hours after admission without regaining consciousness.

Autopsy Findings.—Autopsy examination revealed a fracture of the skull with subdural hemorrhage. The lungs showed pulmonary edema, hypostatic congestion and terminal pneumonia. At the periphery of the upper lobe of the left lung near the base, a discrete calcified nodule about 1 cm. in diameter (a typical Ghon lesion) was found. The peribronchial lymph nodes at the hilus were small and firm, one showing a central area of calcification.

Microscopic Description.—(Fig. 142) Specimen consists of a section of lung containing a large purple-staining lesion approximately 1 cm. in diameter. The lung tissue surrounding this lesion shows considerable edema, congestion and some beginning exudate into the alveoli. The lesion, itself, consists of a central mass of necrotic and largely calcified caseous material surrounded by a dense fibrous tissue capsule. This fibrous tissue capsule shows extensive hyalinization. There is a very moderate amount of chronic mononuclear cellular infiltration consisting chiefly of lymphocytes. No giant cells are seen. No ossification of this particular Ghon lesion has occurred.

CASE 61. (Ref. #S-140)

Diagnosis.—Lung—fibrocaseous tuberculosis with secondary tuberculous bronchopneumonia.

Patient was a forty-three year old colored male, who was admitted to the hospital complaining of a cough and a "bad stomach."

Present Illness.—The patient was apparently well until two months ago when he began to have a productive cough with occasional blood spitting. He said he had lost considerable weight, about fifteen pounds. He had a poor appetite, occasional nausea and vomiting, but no diarrhea. The patient had noticed recently afternoon fever, and he had severe night sweats.

Past History.—His past history was essentially negative, except that at the age of twenty-four he had an attack of pneumonia which had kept him in bed for nearly a month. His father and mother were both dead, and the patient did not know from what cause. He had one sister, who had died at a tuberculosis sanatorium. He had two brothers both living and well as far as he knew. A review of his systems was of little help in interpreting his present condition. He had no idea what childhood diseases he might have had. Other than the attack of pneumonia, he had never been seriously sick and had never had any operations. He had occasional qualitative attacks of stomach trouble, but they never were severe enough to cause him any concern. His genitourinary system was essentially negative. He denied venereal infection.

Physical Examination.—Patient was a well developed, somewhat undernourished middle-aged colored male. His head was normal in shape. Eyes, ears, nose and throat were negative. Chest was somewhat asymmetrical with diminished expansion over the right apical region. There was dullness over both apices on percussion. There were numerous subcrepitant râles heard in these areas. There was definite bronchial breathing over the right apex and whispered pectoriloquy over the right upper chest. Heart was not enlarged. There were no murmurs. Abdomen was negative. Genitalia were negative. Extremities were normal.

Laboratory Findings.—Red blood cells, 3,500,000 with 75% hemoglobin. White blood cells, 7,800 with 71% polynuclear leukocytes. Urinalysis negative. Sputum examination: There was a moderate amount of mucopurulent, greenish sputum, which was positive for tubercle bacilli. X-ray examination showed typical tuberculosis of the lungs with marked cavitation of the right upper lobe.

Subsequent Course.—The patient followed a progressive downhill course with extension of the process to the lower lobes, and he died one month later.

Autopsy Findings.—Autopsy examination revealed the lungs adherent to the chest wall, particularly at the right apex. The lungs crepitated to a diminished degree and numerous irregular areas of consolidation could be palpated. When sectioned, a small cavity 3 cm. in diameter was seen in the upper right lobe, which was serpiginous in character. The wall contained some fibrous tissue. Scattered throughout the remainder of the lobe were conglomerate grayish and yellowish areas. The rest of the lung was studded with tiny grayish tubercles. Considerable frothy blood tinged fluid could be expressed from the dependent portions of the lungs. The peribronchial lymph nodes were enlarged, but no evidence of caseation was present. The spleen and liver showed a few grayish tubercles about 2 mm. in diameter.

Microscopic Description of Section from Lung.—(Fig. 145) Sections from various portions of the lung present a somewhat variable picture. In general, the histopathology may be described as representing a rather characteristic fibrocaseous type of tuberculosis with secondary tuberculous bronchopneumonia. There are numerous miliary tubercles seen which are much larger than those noted in the preceding case. These show extensive areas of caseation centrally and only moderate proliferative reaction of epithelioid cells about their periphery. Occasional giant cells are found. The surrounding alveoli are filled with catarrhal, gelatinous exudate made up of mucoid and coagulated serum in which many large mononuclear cells may be identified. In many areas, the lung is atelectatic due to the compression of the alveolar walls because of the presence of the rather large areas of tuberculosis with intervening areas of exudate, which have cut off the air way.

In reviewing this case, it seems as if the lesion at the apex of the right lung was probably the original site of the infection. Due to lowered resistance, rapid spread by continuity, by lymphatic and bronchogenic pathways took place, resulting in a diffuse secondary bronchopneumonia throughout the lung. These characteristics are well brought out in a study of the tissues. The typical caseation, giant cell formation and secondary catarrhal inflammatory exudate in the alveoli are all prominent features of the picture. It is possible to note the actual ulcerative process in one corner of the tissue. This represents the wall of a tuberculous cavity lined by typical tuberculous granulation tissue. The characteristic features of granulation tissue in general are evidenced by the proliferation of young capillaries and the associated productive fibrosis. As happens so frequently in such active tuberculous lesions, beginning caseation of this newly formed reparative tissue also occurs and is due to the persistence of the bacteria in the lesion. It is this mechanism which explains the direct extension of the process.

CHAPTER XVII

TYPES OF INFLAMMATION (*Continued*)

CHRONIC INFECTIOUS GRANULOMATA OTHER THAN TUBERCULOSIS AND SYPHILIS

The term *"infectious granulomata"* applies to a large group of infectious diseases characterized by productive inflammation and the development of a granulation type of inflammatory tissue. These infections are legion. Their classification becomes a somewhat difficult problem because of the wide variety of etiologic agents which are involved in their production. In this discussion of the granulomata, an etiological classification, so far as possible, will be followed. In general, with the exception of two or three specific infectious diseases caused by well-recognized bacteria, the great majority of the infectious granulomata result from infections by the higher bacteria and particularly the fungi. These infections all present many features in common, most of them starting as infections of the skin or mucous membranes clinically. Many of them remain localized; others may become generalized, or at least show secondary metastatic lesions in other instances. Among the most important of the infectious granulomata in man may be mentioned leprosy, actinomycosis, blastomycosis, yaws and lymphogranuloma inguinale. However, a whole host of other diseases have been recognized in the last decade or so with the development of more exact methods of laboratory diagnosis, especially bacteriology, and brief mention of some of these other less common infections will be made in the discussion of each etiologic group. It is obvious that a complete review of these granulomata is impossible in such a condensed presentation.

PART I

DISEASES CAUSED BY SPECIFIC BACTERIA

Leprosy.—Leprosy is a specific, chronic, systemic, infectious disease caused by the *Bacillus leprae*. This organism is, like the tubercle bacillus, an acid-fast, rod-shaped bacterium, which was first described by Hansen in 1874 in Norway. It has proved resistant to any of the usual methods of cultivation until recent years, when this aspect of the problem seems to have been overcome by McKinley and his group. The disease produced by this organism occurs in two forms: 1. the more familiar tubercular or nodular form, and 2. the other, anesthetic form, in which trophic disturbances of the extremities take place. The two forms may be combined. The mode of transmission is still uncertain, although contact is the most probable. The incubation period is extremely variable and may be as long as twenty years, according to some authorities. The recognition of the disease clinically may not be made for several years after the infection has actually begun.

The basic pathology of the common nodular form of leprosy depends upon the infiltration of the tissues by the lepra bacilli, which are taken up by large mononuclear phagocytic cells in the cytoplasm of which they grow in coil-like fashion. Many of these cells are destroyed and the lepra bacilli dispersed in the tissues. In response to their presence, a rather characteristic chronic productive fibrosis of a loose structure develops in which many blood vessels and lymphatics are found. There is little or no necrosis, but there is a heaping up of this chronic granulomatous tissue beneath the epithelium with resultant changes in the surface epithelium. Either inflammatory hyperplasia of the epithelial cells occurs or, more often, the epithelium undergoes a thinning with a loss of the hair follicles, sweat and coil glands. It is interesting to note that unlike tuberculosis or most of the other infectious granulomata, when ulceration through trauma or secondary in-

PLATE XXXVI
CHRONIC GRANULOMATOUS DISEASES

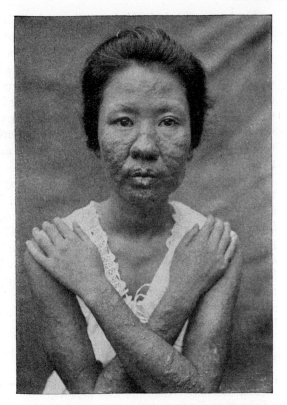

FIG. 150.—Gross photograph of patient showing typical tubercular skin lesions involving face and upper extremities.

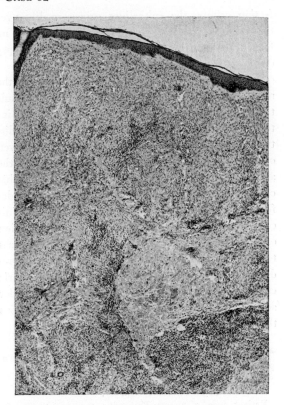

FIG. 151.—Low power photomicrograph through cutaneous leproma. Diffuse chronic granulomatous productive fibrosis, well vascularized, replacing corium. App. 15 x.

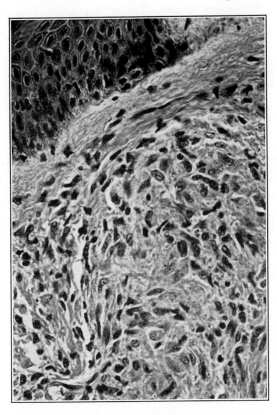

FIG. 152.—Higher power showing flattening of epithelium with loss of rete pegs and characteristic whorllike arrangement of fibroblasts with infiltration by large mononuclear cells, some containing bacteria (Fig. 153). App. 200 x.

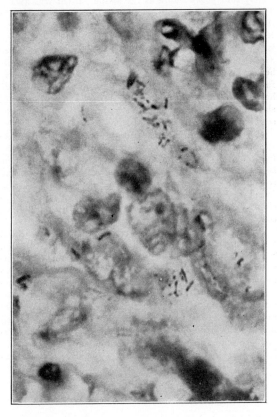

FIG. 153.—Oil immersion photomicrograph with several typical lepra ("foam") cells in which the beaded organisms may be recognized (cf. Figs. 71 and 155). App. 1000 x.

fection occurs, the epithelium grows readily over this well vascularized leprous tissue. There is no fear of chronic ulceration as the result of biopsy diagnosis from a typical lepra nodule.

In the anesthetic form, there is invasion of the nerve trunk by the lepra bacillus with the result that the nerve becomes destroyed and its function interfered with. This is followed by the trophic disturbances mentioned with the loss of digits or even of whole hands or feet, which are seen in the advanced stage as mere stumps. Similar trophic changes affect the nasal septum with marked deformities resulting. The diagnosis of leprosy clinically is usually made or substantiated by examination of scrapings from the nasal mucosa, which appears to be either the portal of entry or the site of predilection for the organism. It is here that the bacteria can usually be first demonstrated, and in cases under adequate treatment, it is from these nasal lesions that the bacteria last disappear.

The lepra cell is in itself almost diagnostic. It is a large mononuclear phagocytic cell characteristically distended with pale fat droplets, which by the usual tissue preparation appear as vacuoles. This is in addition to the presence of the bacteria, which occur so characteristically. This lepra "foam" cell may be carried in the lymphatics and the blood stream to distant organs, and typically, aggregations of such cells in the liver, in the spleen and lymph nodes are prone to occur.

It should be remembered that leprosy is a systemic infection, not a skin disease. Furthermore, it might be noted that leprosy by itself probably rarely is the actual cause of death of an individual. The person suffering from leprosy, however, is peculiarly susceptible to other infection, and the cause of death is usually some intercurrent infection, particularly tuberculosis. For this reason it is well to bear in mind the essential differential features of tuberculosis and leprosy histologically.

ILLUSTRATIVE CASE

CASE 62. (Ref. #S-264 and S-265)
Diagnosis.—Skin nodule—leprosy.
Patient was a young Philippine woman, twenty-six years of age, who was admitted to the leprosarium because of typical nodular leprosy.
Present Illness.—The present illness began approximately four years before as far as the patient was aware. This occurred as slight brawny reddened thickenings of the skin over the maxillae and in the lobes of the ears. It was accompanied by a rather indefinite rash, particularly over the back and shoulders, although scattered areas were noted on the forearms. These did not cause her any trouble at the time and, in characteristic native fashion, she had recognized the onset of the disease and had remained in as complete seclusion as possible until she was finally found by the district health officer, who sent her to the hospital for diagnosis.
Past History.—Her past history was irrelevant in respect to the source of her infection. Her mother and father were both living and well and neither of them had suffered from leprosy. She was married and had two small children. There was no evidence of leprosy found in any of the other members of her family, including the husband and children. She had had no known contact with any lepers.
Physical Examination.—Physical examination showed a well developed, fairly well nourished young Filipina. There was a typical nodular leprosy present, which involved particularly the face and upper extremities. No definite areas of anesthesia were noted. The head otherwise was normal in shape. Eyes were negative and reacted normally to light and distance. Ears showed definite nodules particularly involving the lobes. The nose showed marked thickening of the mucous membrane with catarrhal exudate. The throat appeared negative. Heart and lungs were normal. Abdomen was negative. Upper ex-

tremities, as previously noted, showed typical leprous nodules. The lower extremities were negative.
Laboratory Findings.—The diagnosis of this case was confirmed by biopsy specimen from one of the skin nodules, and by scrapings from the nasal mucosa. These both showed the presence of large numbers of typical lepra bacilli.
Subsequent Course.—Patient was admitted to the leprosarium and was put under treatment with one of the Chaulmoogra oil derivatives. There was a definite improvement in her picture over a period of a year or more. Whether or not she has been included in the group of arrested cases, we are unable to report at this time.
Microscopic Description of Section from the Biopsy of a Lepra Skin Nodule.—(Fig. 150, 151, 152 and 153) The epithelium overlying the nodule is seen to be markedly thinned. There are very few rete pegs, which can be made out. The basal layer shows marked pigmentation due to the racial characteristic. There is some slight superficial keratinization and scaling of the epithelium. Beneath this thinned epithelium is found a mass of typical chronic leprous granulation tissue. This is made up of whorls of connective tissue with loose, interlacing bundles of collagen fibers. Scattered throughout the tissue are found numerous large lepra cells. Some of these show multilobulated nuclei. Others show two or more nuclei. Their cytoplasm is filled with vacuoles giving an almost foam-like appearance to the cell structure. In a corresponding section from the same nodule, which is stained by the Ziehl-Neelsen method (Fig. 155 and 71) for the demonstration of the bacteria, lepra bacilli in myriads are found both in the interstitial tissue spaces and particularly within the lepra cells. Here the organism seems to grow by transverse fission and occurs in clumps, often spoken of as resembling a pile of "Jack

PLATE XXXVIII

CHRONIC GRANULOMATA (Continued)

DISEASES CAUSED BY FUNGI

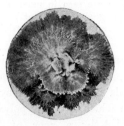

FIG. 160.—MONILIA ALBICANS.—30-day giant culture.—CASE 65.—Reduced ½.

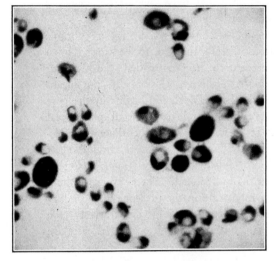

FIG. 161.—*M. ALBICANS.*—Smear preparation from culture (Heidenhain's iron hematoxylin). Yeast-like forms with prominent vacuoles predominate, but a few organisms showing primitive hyphal tendencies are present. App. 600 x.

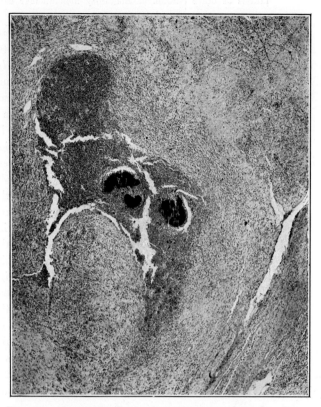

FIG. 162.—FALLOPIAN TUBE: ACTINOMYCOSIS.—CASE 63.—Lumen filled with purulent exudate and containing several colonies of actinomyces. Epithelial lining cells destroyed; wall enormously thickened by chronic productive fibrosis and inflammatory cellular infiltration. App. 25 x.

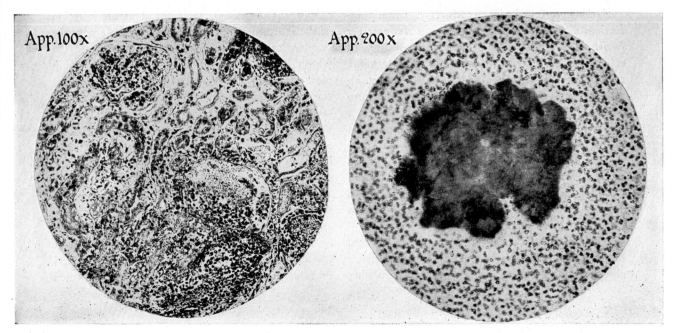

FIG. 163.—KIDNEY: MULTIPLE ABSCESSES.—*M. Albicans.*—CASE 65.—Widespread involvement of glomeruli, tubules and interstitial tissues with areas of liquefaction necrosis containing typical yeast and primitive hyphal forms of the organism. App. 100 x.

FIG. 164.—CASE 63.—High power detail (from Fig. 162) of a single colony of actinomyces, showing tendency toward "clubbing" of organisms peripherally, giving fuzzy appearance to edge. App. 200 x.

straws" within the cytoplasm of the cells between the fatty vacuoles. The whole tissue shows a very marked vascularity and many dilated lymphatics. In addition to the typical lepra cells are found accumulations of other chronic inflammatory mononuclear cells, including some plasma cells, but chiefly adult lymphocytes. There is no evidence of caseation, and no typical foreign body giant cells, as are seen in tuberculosis, are noted. The relatively healthy appearance of the tissues, with the absence of degenerative changes is striking.

Glanders.—Glanders is another specific chronic infectious granulomatous lesion which is transmitted from animal to man. It is caused by the *Bacillus mallei,* a gram-negative bacillus. The organism may be identified by its characteristic yellow, creamy growth on potato medium. Diagnosis of the disease is either made by the recovery of the organism or by the intraperitoneal injection of material from a lesion into a male guinea pig. This is followed by a severe acute inflammatory reaction in the tunica vaginalis within twelve to twenty-four hours, known as the Strauss reaction. The disease in the horse is often spoken of as "farcy." It is apt to occur as an infection of mucous membranes and to spread by the lymphatics where nodular swellings occur. The histology is nonspecific. There is a chronic productive fibrosis with a diffuse mononuclear infiltration. Lesions rarely show the formation of giant cells, and for that reason without the demonstration of the bacteria, it may be extremely difficult to make an accurate histologic diagnosis. The disease runs a chronic course as a rule of several months to years, and has a very high mortality rate. It may gain access to the blood stream and be carried particularly to the lungs where it produces an acute pneumonic picture. This pneumonia is characterized by small central foci of exudate which is chiefly polynuclear in character, surrounded by a zone of intense hemorrhage. If the patient lives long enough, beginning productive fibrosis follows, but these patients tend to die of generalized metastatic abscesses within a comparatively short time.

Rhinoscleroma.—Rhinoscleroma is a chronic granulomatous disease thought to be caused by a small gram-negative bacillus called the *Bacillus rhinoscleromatis,* although this is by no means definitely established. The lesion begins in the nose and may spread to the laryngeal and pharyngeal structures. It is relatively easily diagnosed histologically by the presence of large, round, clear cells which are filled with a gelatinous material, the so-called Mikulicz cell. These are sometimes difficult to demonstrate in the presence of secondary ulceration and infection. It is a comparatively rare disease in this country, although occasional cases are seen.

PART II

DISEASES CAUSED BY FUNGI

Actinomycosis.—Actinomycosis is a chronic infectious disease produced by the fungus *Actinomyces bovis*. It is characterized by the production of colonies of closely packed mycelium with terminal radiating spores which become covered with an eosin-staining substance resembling a capsule and producing a clubbed effect. These colonies vary from yellow to almost black in color and may be identified in the material from the lesion and diagnosis established in this way. The mode of transmission is obscure as no direct infection from animal to man has been proved. It is thought that the organism gains entrance to the body through some break in the skin or mucous membrane.

This organism produces rather more acute changes than most of the other fungi and develops a definite abscess cavity immediately surrounding the growing colonies of organisms. It is found as an infection of the face and neck region most commonly where it develops as a chronic granulomatous abscess in the jaw with marked secondary inflammatory thickening of the surrounding tissue. The next most common site is in the intestinal tract as an infection of the cecum and appendix. It may spread to the liver, if untreated, where it forms typical multiple liver abscesses. Each of these abscesses is surrounded by a layer of granulation tissue which is characteristic of all this group of infections. The organism is extremely resistant to any bactericidal or chemotherapeutic agents and for this reason therapy consists of the complete removal of the infected tissue by wide excision. Occasionally primary infection of the lungs occurs and rarely, as in the case presented for your study, an infection of the fallopian tubes

PLATE XXXIX
CHRONIC GRANULOMATA (Continued)
BLASTOMYCOSIS

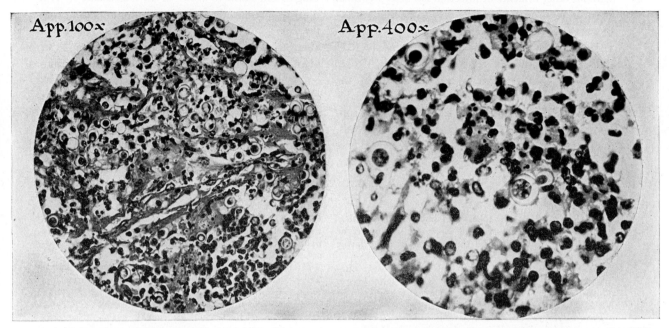

App.100x

App.400x

FIG. 165.—LUNG: BLASTOMYCOSIS.—CASE 64.—Characteristic mixed inflammatory exudate within pulmonary alveoli; necrosis of lung parenchyma. Organisms identified by their highly refractile capsules are present in great profusion. App. 100 x.

FIG. 166.—BLASTOMYCOSIS.—CASE 64.—High power photomicrograph from another area. This illustrates the characteristic reproduction of the blastomyces by lateral budding with suggestion of figure "8" formation. App. 400 x.

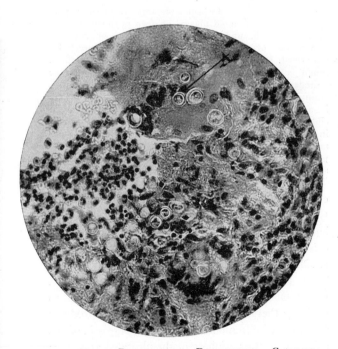

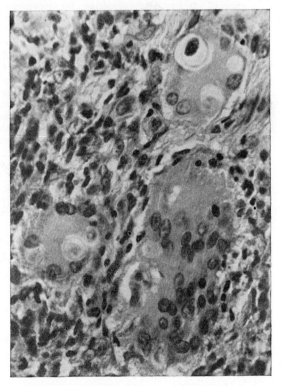

FIG. 167.—SKIN: BLASTOMYCOSIS DERMATITIDIS.—Cutaneous lesion. Organisms with their doubly refractile capsules stand out prominently in the midst of the chronic inflammatory exudate. App. 200 x.

FIG. 168.—High power detail from another area: Characteristic foreign body giant cell reaction with phagocytosis of the blastomyces is striking (cf. Fig. 86). App. 400 x.

without other evidence of infection has been recorded.

MADURA FOOT.—Madura foot is another variety of fungus infection, spoken of also as *"mycetoma."* It is seen most commonly as an infection of the foot. This is chiefly encountered in India, although there have been cases reported from other parts of the world. The lesions appear as relatively small, painless nodules which gradually break down and suppurate, and just as in the case of actinomycosis, minute granules may be found in the pus. These range from black to white or various shades of red. These represent the colonies of the organism, and the color is in part due to the presence of blood pigment. The colonies are made up of a tangle of mycelium showing the same tendency toward peripheral clubbing, which is seen in the more familiar actinomycotic picture, although as a rule it is not as prominent a morphologic feature. This organism is usually considered as a subspecies of the Actinomyces and is called *Actinomyces mycetoma.*

ILLUSTRATIVE CASE

CASE 63. (Ref. #S-250)

Diagnosis.—Fallopian tube—actinomycotic salpingitis.

Patient was a white married woman, thirty years of age, admitted to the hospital complaining of acute lower abdominal pain.

Present Illness.—Her health had been excellent during the past three months until twenty-four hours before admission, when she had a very severe attack of pain in her left lower abdomen.

Past History.—She had a normal childhood. She was married and had one living and well child. Her health had been good until three months before the present admission, when she had a similar acute attack of lower abdominal pain, for which she was referred to the hospital. A diagnosis of pelvic abscess was made and drainage by colopotomy was done. She was discharged improved to her local physician for treatment of this draining sinus. A review of her systems added nothing of significance.

Physical Examination.—Patient was extremely toxic and in acute pain. Her head, eyes, ears, nose and throat were normal. Heart was not enlarged. The rate was regular and there were no murmurs. Lungs were clear throughout. Abdomen was somewhat tender generally, but markedly so in the lower portion and particularly in the left lower quadrant. Vaginal and rectal manual examinations showed a large mass in the pelvis, which was extremely tender. A diagnosis of pelvic abscess was made.

Laboratory Findings.—White blood cells 12,600 with 84% polynuclears. Urinalysis showed a trace of albumin.

Subsequent Course.—Drainage of this pelvic abscess was made by colopotomy, and a subsequent exploratory laparotomy was done. The left tube and ovary were involved in what grossly appeared to be a chronic tuberculosis. The case followed the anticipated course with the development of multiple liver abscesses, and the patient died two years after the original operative procedure.

Microscopic Description of Section from Fallopian Tube.—(Fig. 162 and 164) It is almost impossible to identify the source of this tissue without knowing its origin from the fallopian tube. By careful search one may find a small amount of smooth muscle tissue arranged in somewhat circular fashion representing the wall of the tube. None of the villi can be made out. The entire contents of the tube have been replaced by a mass of chronic granulation tissue in which extensive fibrosis and chronic mononuclear cellular infiltration has taken place. In addition, in the central areas of these chronic granulomatous lesions are found foci of suppurative necrosis which represent abscess cavities filled with polymorphonuclears in all stages of preservation and degeneration. In some of these abscess cavities will also be found the typical colonies of *Actinomyces*. These appear as irregularly lobulated masses of deep purplish staining material which, under oil immersion, can be resolved into masses of twisted mycelium which can scarcely be unraveled. Peripherally in each of these colonies will be found a zone of stellate arranged radiating thicker strands of material which stain more intensely with the eosin than does the main mass of the colonies. There is a suggestion of clubbing to this material, although clubbing is never as prominent in human infection as it is in infection in the cow where the lesion occurs most commonly in the udder. This udder infection is probably the principal source of the disease in man through transmission by infected milk.

Blastomycosis (American).—In blastomycosis we are dealing with a group of yeast-like fungi, which have many features in common and which require very exacting cultural study for their differentiation. The organisms usually reproduce by budding and develop mycelium only in culture. There are two fairly well recognized forms of the disease, both produced by the Blastomyces dermatitidis (Gilchrist and Stokes). [This should not be confused with the so-called European blastomycosis, which will be discussed under the heading of Torula.] The cutaneous type is the more common, making up the great bulk of the clinical cases. The lesions are found chiefly on the face and hands. They grow as localized papular lesions, which soon suppurate and ulcerate. They tend to be indolent and to spread over a considerable area. They are extremely resistant to ordinary therapy. The lesion is one which produces very marked chronic inflammatory hyperplasia of the skin around the periphery of the ulcerated area. It is

PLATE XL

CHRONIC GRANULOMATA
Diseases Caused by Spirochetes
Yaws—Frambesia.—Case 66

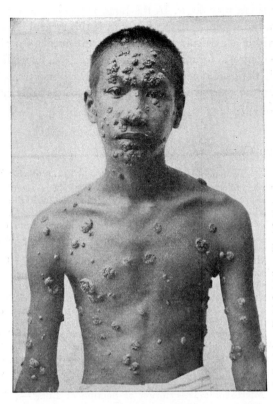

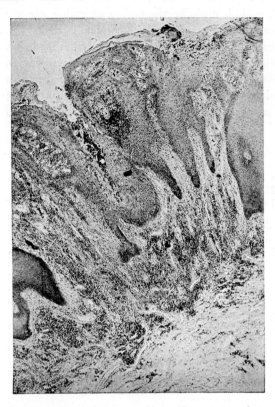

FIG. 169.—YAWS: FRAMBESIA.—Typical diffuse distribution of the secondary cutaneous yaws. Individual lesions present the characteristic localized papillary proliferation of the epithelium.

FIG. 170.—SKIN: SECONDARY YAW.—Low power photomicrograph through a typical secondary skin lesion. This emphasizes the hyperplasia of the epithelium and the extensive cellular infiltration of the corium. App. 15 x.

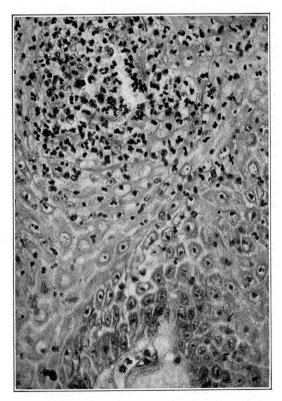

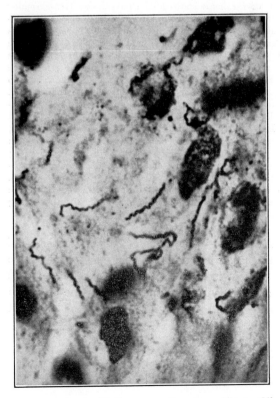

FIG. 171.—SKIN: SECONDARY YAW.—High power photomicrograph from Fig. 170. Proliferation of the epithelium is marked. Note mitotic figures. Acute secondary leukocytic infiltration is present. App. 200 x.

FIG. 172.—SKIN.—T. Pertenue.—SECONDARY YAW.—Oil immersion photomicrograph stained by Levaditi's method. Organisms appear as irregularly twisted spirals lacking the tight corkscrew appearance of the Treponema pallidum (cf. Fig. 121). App. 1500 x.

said that it may even go on to actual tumor formation, although this must be extremely rare. The diagnosis is made by the finding of such a chronic ulcerative lesion and the demonstration of the typical organism in scrapings or biopsy tissue from the lesion (Fig. 167 and 168). In the tissue, these occur as spherical, highly refractile, encapsulated structures and typically may be found in budding form. In the other form of the disease we are more likely to develop systemic lesions. The lung is the usual primary site, but metastatic lesions in any of the viscera may occur. In the lung, the organism seems to grow unusually profusely as if this structure provided a particularly suitable culture media. In the cutaneous form, there is no appreciable mortality if the condition is properly recognized and treated. In the systemic form, the cases almost invariably end fatally.

ILLUSTRATIVE CASE

CASE 64. (Ref. #S-288)

Diagnosis.—Lung—blastomycosis.

Patient was a colored male adult, twenty-four years of age, who was admitted to the hospital because of a cough, which had persisted over a period of several months and had been increasing in severity.

Present Illness.—The patient complained of raising a moderate amount of mucoid, greenish discolored sputum, particularly in the morning on arising. His local physician had examined him and felt that while the findings were not positive, there was a very great likelihood of an incipient pulmonary tuberculosis.

Past History.—Nothing relevant to his present illness was found in his past history. He had had numerous mild upper respiratory infections, but had never had pneumonia. His mother and father were both living and well. There was no history of tuberculosis in the family as far as he was aware. A review of his systems was completely negative.

Physical Examination.—The patient was a well-developed, fairly well-nourished young adult Negro who showed evidence of some recent weight loss. The skin was somewhat loose and had rather poor turgor. The mucous membranes were relatively pale. Chest: Examination of the heart showed no enlargement. Heart sounds were normal but somewhat distant. There were no murmurs. Lungs: Over the right apex the breath sounds were somewhat diminished and there were many fine crepitant râles. Percussion revealed a slight impairment of the note but no actual dullness. Scattered râles were heard throughout the remainder of both lungs, but no other areas of suspected consolidation were identified. The remainder of the physical examination was essentially negative.

Laboratory Examinations.—Blood: Red blood cells, 3,230,000; white blood cells, 12,400. Differential count: Polymorphonuclear neutrophiles 81%; lymphocytes 16%; large monocytes 2% and eosinophiles 1%. Sputum examinations were repeatedly negative for tubercle bacilli. However, on the second examination, characteristic *Blastomyces* were identified, many of them showing peripheral budding.

X-ray examination showed a haziness of the right upper lobe of the lung which lacked the characteristic features of tuberculosis. It suggested an interstitial and peribronchial type of pneumonitis. No cavitation was observed. The hilus lymph nodes showed moderate enlargement, particularly on the same side as the lung lesion.

Subsequent Course.—Patient pursued a steadily but slowly progressive downhill course with the pulmonary lesion extending to involve practically the entire lung on the right side with some questionable areas of similar involvement on the opposite side. The patient died of generalized diffuse blastomycosis of the lungs.

Autopsy Findings.—Autopsy examination revealed a diffuse chronic granulomatous type of bronchopneumonia involving the entire right lung and the major portion of the left upper lobe. The other findings were those of emaciation and secondary anemia.

Microscopic Description of Section of Lung.—(Fig. 165 and 166) There is what appears to be a rather ordinary diffuse bronchopneumonic exudate seen filling the alveoli. It is patchy in distribution. It is accompanied by considerable interstitial fibrosis and peribronchial thickening. There is a mucopurulent catarrhal exudate noted in the bronchioles. High power examination, however, readily demonstrates the presence of large numbers of characteristic *Blastomyces*. These, as is very commonly the case in tissue infections, are seen almost entirely in the form of yeast-like bodies, namely large, round or ovoid structures having a highly refractile capsule with a well defined nucleolus and scattered nuclear chromatin material. Here and there, typical budding will be seen illustrating the method of reproduction of the cells. Giant cells are numerous and they will be found to be acting as phagocytes, many of them containing organisms. The exudate otherwise will be found to be a mixed one with polynuclears predominating. However, many large monocytes and even lymphocytes are seen and there is some tendency toward pseudotubercle formation in places. It lacks, however, the radial arrangement of the cells usually seen in tuberculosis.

Moniliasis.—The *Monilia albicans* is the chief pathogenic member of this group, the common cause of thrush in infants and young children. This is an infection of the mucous membrane on which plaques of these fungi grow, chiefly by budding, but also by mycelial proliferation. In malnourished infants, this organism may extend down the gastrointestinal tract producing extensive moniliasis of the entire mucosa. Occasionally it gains entrance to the blood stream and multiple granulomatous abscesses may develop in all tissues of the body including the meninges, as in the case presented here.

Sprue is likewise an infection in which the monilia plays a very important part in the production of the symptoms. This is particularly seen in the tropics, but may occur elsewhere, even in the temperate zones. It is a chronic gastro-intestinal disturbance characterized by enormous frothy bowel movements, which have a strong odor of yeast. This is frequently associated with qualitative dyspeptic symptoms which go on to a severe gastro-intestinal derangement. It is felt that other factors may be

important in the development of the clinical picture serving to lower the resistance of the individual to such a point that the *Monilia* is capable of becoming pathogenic. Among such etiologic factors may be cited climate and diet, notably a diet deficient in vitamins. The condition is accompanied by very severe anemia, at times even to be confused with the pernicious macrocytic form, although quite as frequently being of a very striking microcytic, hypochromic type. Ashford's many years' work in Puerto Rico did more than anything else to give us our present understanding of this disease.

ILLUSTRATIVE CASE

CASE 65. (Ref. #S-155)
Diagnosis.—Kidney (rabbit)—experimental moniliasis (culture obtained from a case of thrush with secondary monilial meningitis).

Patient was a white infant of 22 months, admitted to the hospital with a history of two weeks' illness.

Present Illness.—The present illness was characterized by fever, cough and respiratory distress.

Physical Examination.—Physical examination reveals a loose, patchy *white* membrane covering the buccal mucosa, the uvula and pharynx. There was a bilateral bronchopneumonia with impaired resonance, bronchial breathing and râles. Moderate rickets was present. Neurologic examination showed a curious plantar flexion and absence of deep and superficial reflexes.

Laboratory Examination.—Spinal fluid was under increased pressure, but clear. Forty-eight hour cultures yielded *M. albicans*. Cell count was only 2 lymphocytes per c.mm.

Subsequent Course.—Temporary improvement followed the removal of the membrane by suction. This was followed by otitis media and meningitis characterized by nuchal tenderness, right strabismus and terminal convulsions. The white blood count averaged 16,000 cells with 80% polynuclears. Cultures from the membrane showed typical *M. albicans*.

Autopsy Findings.—Lungs showed a diffuse chronic bronchitis, peribronchitis and peribronchial bronchopneumonia of a gray patchy and unusually firm type of consolidation suggesting organization. Sections confirmed the monilial basis of this process. Examination of the brain

showed marked congestion of the overlying vessels with a whitish yellow exudate over the entire surface. The ears both showed acute purulent otitis media.

Cultures from all organs, including ear, meninges, heart's blood, spinal fluid and gastro-intestinal tract yielded predominantly or exclusively *M. albicans* (Fig. 160 and 161).

For identification of the type of monilia, pure cultures were grown in various media and inoculated into rabbits. This produced extensive miliary abscesses throughout the viscera, as well as a definite meningitis.

Microscopic Description of Section of Kidney from Rabbit, Which Had Been Infected Experimentally With a Culture of Monilia from the Above Case.—(Fig. 161 and 163) Examination of the tissue shows it to consist of kidney with well defined glomeruli and tubules. The tissue has been stained by Heidenhain's iron hematoxylin method to demonstrate to better advantage the organisms. Under low power the entire tissue is found to be studded with innumerable foci of necrosis and degeneration. Many of these appear in relation to the glomeruli. Others are seen in the interstitial tissue and have extended to involve tubules. All gradations of degeneration of tubular epithelium may be encountered. Within these necrotic areas will be found the organism in large numbers. In places they may be identified as ovoid or almost spherical bodies. In other places definite mycelial development may be made out. The lesion is so overwhelming that the typical granulomatous productive fibrosis has not as yet had time to appear, and the process is essentially one of multiple abscess formation.

Torula Infections.—The organism responsible for these infections is variously classified as a cryptococcus, as an oidium or as a blastomyces. It would seem best to belong in one of the two former categories as, so far as we are aware, it never forms mycelium. This is the organism, however, which has for many years been classified as the European form of blastomycosis, although Busse and Buschke originally described the organism as a saccharomyces. From the standpoint of priority, it is

probably best to use the more preferred nomenclature of *Cryptococcus hominis,* although the term *Torula* in American literature has become so firmly implanted that it would be difficult to eliminate it.

It has a specific affinity for the central nervous system where it produces a rather characteristic meningo-encephalitis. The differential diagnosis usually lies between a tuberculous meningitis or the so-called benign lymphocytic meningitis. In its slow onset and low cell count, the lesions likewise are difficult to differentiate from a relatively hyperplastic type of tuberculosis except for the demonstration of the large, cyst-like organisms. It is probable that some of the cases of so-called Torula meningitis should better be thought of as instances of moniliasis with meningeal involvement rather than Torula, which appears to be a very rare infection.

Coccidioidal Granuloma.—In similar fashion, there is a disease most frequently involving the lungs; less often the bones and the skin, which is caused by another organism, the classification of which is still in confusion. The organism is another round, highly refractile encapsulated body, which is called variously *Oidium coccidioides* and *Coccidioides immitis.* Unlike Blastomyces, with which it is at times confused, it reproduces by the production of endospores and by the formation in culture of a mycelium. Budding has never been observed. It is the cause of a disease which was first described in California and became known as the "California Disease" until it was recognized that it may be found throughout the United States. In infections caused by enormous doses in individuals who are particularly reactive to its presence, recovery may be expected whereas in those individuals in which the infection is either less in amount or slower in development, it is prone to go on through a prolonged chronic course to a fatal outcome. It is extremely difficult to differentiate even histologically from tuberculosis because of the presence of pseudotubercles, "epithelioid" cells, giant cells and the usual productive fibrosis, except that the organisms are easily recognized in the lesion and frequently within the giant cells.

Sporotrichosis.—Sporotrichosis is again closely related to this group of infections. In appearance the organism is not unlike the Blastomyces, but it is hard to demonstrate in material from the lesions and it is usually necessary to establish diagnosis by culture. The infection is usually found on the skin and runs a long, chronic course. It develops as a local abscess, not unlike the lesions of actinomycosis, which breaks down and suppurates, leaving a chronic granulating surface. The lesion spreads by way of the lymphatics so that very frequently a series of nodular lesions, which in turn break down like the initial lesion, may be found.

Streptothricosis.—Streptothricosis is one of the more recently recognized groups of infection which involve the lung. These cases produce a chronic granulomatous type of reaction in the lung tissue very similar to that of tuberculosis. By culture, and occasionally by smear, an organism has been cultivated which has a delicately branching, filamentous appearance, and which has been grouped by some investigators with the actinomyces. The lesion may not always remain in this chronic form, but as in the case of glanders, may assume an acute hemorrhagic or even gangrenous picture, and the organism may gain access to the blood stream and produce distant visceral lesions in a similar way. Microscopically, the difficulty of differential diagnosis from tuberculosis in the characteristic case of streptothrix infection is more difficult than in the case of any of the other fungus infections. This is because the histology is so similar in its composition, even to the point of pseudo-tubercle and giant cell formation, and for the fact that the organisms are so difficult to demonstrate in the tissues.

Aspergillosis.—Another group of fungi may likewise at times be the cause of chronic pulmonary disease, which might be mistaken clinically for tuberculosis. The lesions vary a great deal in the individual case and depend upon the particular species responsible for the picture. Conveniently many of the Aspergilli produce pigment in their growth, and the presence of the rather characteristic dark brown, green or black pigment is helpful in the differential diagnosis.

PART III

DISEASES CAUSED BY SPIROCHETES

Yaws (Framboesia).—Yaws is a specific infectious disease caused by the *Treponema pertenue.* Some uncertainty still remains in the minds of certain investigators as to whether or not yaws may be an atypical manifestation of syphilis. This is occasioned chiefly by the fact that both conditions are caused by spirochetes, that they tend to run somewhat parallel courses with the same convenient division into three or four stages and that they both give positive serologic tests, and that they respond to similar therapy. There are certain outstanding differences, however, which seem to separate them in clear-cut fashion. In the first place, yaws is not a venereal disease, and it is extremely rare to find primary genital lesions. In the second place, and more convincing, is the fact that both diseases may occur simultaneously in that a patient with yaws may develop a primary penile chancre during the course of the first disease. The primary lesion in yaws usually occurs on the site of an ulcer or abrasion over some bony prominence and particularly in the adult, of the lower extremity. Thus the ankle, over one or the other of the malleoli, or the knee, are perhaps three of the most common sites for the spirochete to gain access to the body and produce its characteristic proliferative lesion. A brief incubation period is followed by the development of the primary nodule, which consists of epithelial hyperplasia and productive fibrosis in the corium with chronic mononuclear cellular infiltration very similar to that which makes up the picture in syphilis.

A generalized systemic invasion occurs and the second stage follows in the course of a few weeks or months, with the development of multiple lesions all over the skin, which are identical in appearance with the initial lesion, except that until they subsequently ulcerate, they lack the complicating factors of the infection usually seen in the primary lesion. These secondary lesions persist almost indefinitely without treatment and ultimately break down, ulcerate and are replaced by chronic granulation and scar tissue.

Late lesions occur affecting the bones and less frequently the central nervous system. Particularly characteristic are the lesions of the soles of the feet and palms of the hands, which might be compared to subcutaneous gummata. These are extremely resistant to healing and interfere seriously with the individual's ability to work. Many indolent ulcers follow some of these primary or secondary lesions and likewise should be thought of in terms of late lesions.

Outstanding, however, is the relative lack of blood vessel involvement as compared to the vascular picture in syphilis. There may at times be a certain amount of endarteritis, but the striking medial involvement of the aorta and larger arterial lesions is conspicuously absent.

In no condition is there a more dramatic recovery with proper therapy. The administration of arsenicals, especially as neoarsphenamine, results in a rapid diminution in the size of the lesions and their gradual and ultimate disappearance within a matter of a few weeks, save for such scars as remain, the result of secondary ulceration and infection.

A recent study by Ferris and Turner of tissues taken from typical lesions has emphasized the similarity of the histopathology of the two conditions, syphilis and yaws. For the most part, in yaws, the spirochetes are found in the dermis with relatively few in the corium. In syphilis, on the other hand, their distribution in the corium is much more striking. The epithelial proliferation in yaws is ordinarily much more prominent than in syphilis, although, at times, as seen in the form of mucous patches or condylomata, it may be an outstanding feature of the picture in syphilis. The productive fibrosis and the perivascular mononuclear cellular infiltration, particularly with plasma cells, are likewise a prominent part of the pathology in yaws.

ILLUSTRATIVE CASE

CASE 66. (Ref. #S-299)
Diagnosis.—Skin—yaw.
Patient was a Filipino of 18 years, who contrary to the usual story, developed a primary penile lesion. This persisted as a slow, ulcerated lesion with hyperplastic epithelial changes accompanied by considerable pain and discomfort for several weeks. This was followed by a crop of cutaneous, discrete, secondary lesions. These appeared as epithelial overgrowths, almost as verruca-like papillomatous masses. They involved the skin from the scalp to the feet and numbered over five hundred. They had the characteristic raspberry-like surface with a rather dusky, congested appearance, which has given rise to the name of the disease, framboesia. With the consent of the patient, a biopsy from one of these nodules was taken for histologic study.

Microscopic Description of a Section Through a Secondary Yaw.—(Fig. 169, 170, 171 and 172) The section of tissue shows an epithelial surface which is normal at one side of the block. It rises sharply, almost as a mushroom-like overgrowth of epithelium, above the skin level nearly 1 cm. in height. Two or three superficial areas of beginning ulceration with secondary serofibrinous and leukocytic infiltration are seen on the surface. For the most part, however, the lesion is made up of enormously hyperplastic masses of epithelium with prominence of the rete pegs, which dip deep into the corium. Between the rete pegs in the corium, the vessels are surrounded by inflammatory cells, chiefly mononuclear. There is marked fibrosis between the epithelial pegs. In the deeper tissue, marked lymphocytic and plasma cell infiltration is seen. Likewise, it has a perivascular distribution and almost forms "streamers" toward the deeper portions.

Sections which have been stained by the Warthin method for the demonstration of spirochetes show the presence of the organisms for the most part between the epithelial cells of the epidermis itself, with very few in the corium. Many of these cells show degenerative changes and some evidence of actual cell division with mitotic figures. No striking vascular changes other than capillary dilatation and proliferation are observed.

PART IV

DISEASES CAUSED BY FILTRABLE VIRUSES

Lymphogranuloma Inguinale.—This disease has frequently been spoken of as the fourth venereal disease. It is a specific infectious disease caused by a filtrable virus. The primary lesion usually is found as a penile one in the male and as a vaginal or cervical one in the female. It appears as a small papule, which is accompanied by marked enlargement of the regional lymph nodes. These go on to break down as a chronic granulomatous ulcerated lesion. The process spreads by way of the lymphatics and accordingly, in the female, the extension is apt to be perirectal rather than to the inguinal nodes. This results in a chronic granulomatous stricture of the rectum in the female, which has not infrequently been confused with syphilis. Histologically, the picture of lymphogranuloma is one which might best be described as pseudotuberculous in appearance. There are frequently giant cells with a proliferation of "epithelioid" cells and a central area of broken down material which is rather more purulent than caseous as seen in tuberculosis. In the rectum there is a tendency toward superficial ulceration with the mucosa replaced by typical chronic granulomatous tissues.

Diagnosis of the disease is readily made by the intracutaneous injection of sterile pus from a lesion as originally described by Frei. A modification of this test has been devised, utilizing an extract of a mouse brain, which has been previously injected with the virus as the antigen. The mouse appears to be susceptible to the disease, the virus producing a very severe encephalomyelitis when injected directly into the brain substance. The virus is not strictly neurotropic, however, because the cerebral picture does not follow if the virus is injected intravenously or subcutaneously into the animal unless the brain is previously traumatized. The disease runs a prolonged and chronic course, but there is no mortality attributed to it directly.

The name proposed for this disease, unfortunately, has occasioned a great deal of confusion because of the fact that this term is used in European literature frequently to apply to the disease known in this country as Hodgkin's disease. Moreover, there is another infection known as *granuloma inguinale,* which is in no way related to this infection, except as it produces lesions of a granulomatous type in relation to the genitals and the regional lymph nodes draining the area.

PART V

DISEASES CAUSED BY UNKNOWN OR UNCLASSIFIED AGENTS

Granuloma Inguinale.—As has just been commented upon, the disease known as granuloma inguinale is another specific infectious disease, usually considered as one of the venereal infections. The etiology of this disease is still obscure. Histologically, it is very common to find numerous intracellular, rod-like bodies in the phagocytic, large mononuclear cells. These are frequently called Donovan bodies, but should be distinguished from the more familiar Leishman-Donovan bodies of kala-azar. In addition, very commonly, a bacillary organism has been recovered culturally, which has been variously named. It is most frequently termed the *Bacillus venereogranulomatosis.* Whether this condition requires the symbiotic action of these two organisms or whether they are incidental in the production of the disease is uncertain. It is even possible that this disease is due to some filtrable virus, as yet undetermined.

CHAPTER XVIII

VIRUS DISEASES

GENERAL DISCUSSION

Many of the more common infections are now attributed to various specific viruses. This group of infectious diseases includes an enormous range of conditions, which affect not only man and other mammalia, but find their counterpart in infections of insects and plants. Among the more familiar diseases now considered as of almost undisputed virus origin may be cited the common cold, measles, influenza, small-pox and chicken-pox, molluscum contagiosum, yellow-fever, rabies, poliomyelitis and epidemic encephalitis as well as both herpes simplex and herpes zoster, and possibly whooping cough. In addition to these familiar infections of man might be mentioned the contagious epithelioma of fowl (fowl pox), foot and mouth disease of cattle, infectious papillomatosis of rabbits (Shope), sac-brood disease of bees and innumerable infections of plants of which tobacco mosaic disease has more recently been brought to our attention. Indeed, Rous and other investigators go so far as to believe that filtrable viruses may be responsible for certain malignant tumors, notably among them the fowl sarcoma which bears his name.

Virus infection in general is characterized by being produced by an infectious substance which will pass the pores of the finest Berkefeld or similar earthen filter which holds back all visible forms of bacteria. Certain of these viruses appear to be specific in nature. Others, such as those associated with the common cold and whooping cough and influenza apparently require the symbiotic relation of some secondary bacteria. Others are specific in themselves in such diseases as poliomyelitis and epidemic encephalitis. The pathology of this group of infections is so diverse as to make an adequate discussion impossible in the space available. In general, it may be said that viruses are likely to produce inclusion bodies either intranuclear or intracellular in distribution and where these are found it is fairly definite evidence of the virus nature of the disease. This has been appreciated for many years, ever since the papers of Councilman and Ewing in respect to small-pox in which disease the importance of the so-called Guarnieri bodies was first emphasized. Such inclusion bodies have even been described in poliomyelitis and whooping cough, but with much less regularity. In many of the virus infections they have not been successfully demonstrated as yet. Among these may be cited the common cold, measles and epidemic encephalitis.

In a group as divergent as this, very few generalities can be drawn. In the group of diseases of the respiratory tract which might be spoken of as a triad: measles, pertussis and influenza, we have the development of a curious interstitial type of pneumonitis in contradistinction to the usual exudative pneumonia which fills the lung alveoli. A secondary streptococcic pneumonia is apt to supervene and be the effective factor in breaking down the individual's resistance and causing death.

In the group of central nervous diseases, we find viruses which apparently are specifically neurotropic, or at least largely neurotropic in their affinity and distribution. Among these, particularly, may be cited poliomyelitis, epidemic encephalitis and herpes simplex (simple cold sore). The similarity of poliomyelitis and epidemic encephalitis has been brought out by many observers, the pathology histologically being quite comparable, but with the distribution of the lesions being restricted largely to the cerebrum in the case of encephalitis and to the spinal cord and brain stem in poliomyelitis. As an example of the various types of virus infections, we have selected poliomyelitis as illustrative of the neurotropic type of virus disease. A brief description of the pathology follows.

PLATE XLI

DISEASES CAUSED BY FILTRABLE VIRUSES
ACUTE ANTERIOR POLIOMYELITIS.—CASE 67

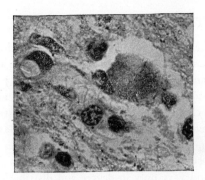

FIG. 173.—ANTERIOR HORN: MOTOR NEURONE. — NEURONOPHAGIA. App. 1200 x.

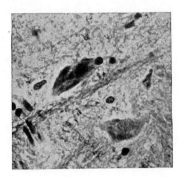

FIG. 174.—NERVE CELLS showing degeneration and chromatolysis. App. 800 x.

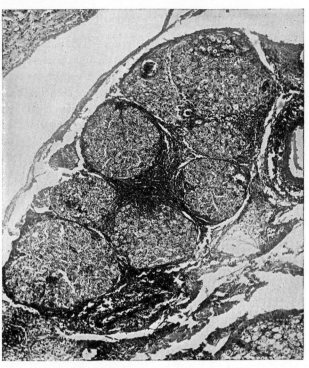

FIG. 178.—NERVE ROOT.—Observe marked inflammatory mononuclear cellular infiltration of arachnoid about the nerve roots, one of the earliest findings pathologically.

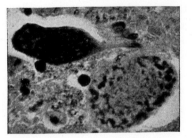

FIG. 175.—MOTOR NERVE CELLS showing degeneration of Nissl granules. App. 1200 x.

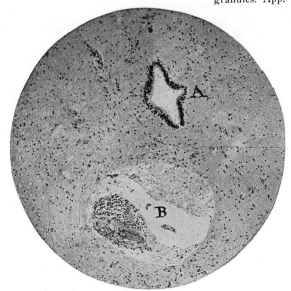

FIG. 176.—SPINAL CORD.—Low power photomicrograph showing early changes; central canal may be identified at "A"; Virchow-Robin space (B) is shown distended with fluid; perivascular "cuffing" of vessels by round cells, chiefly lymphocytes is marked. App. 100 x.

FIG. 177.—SPINAL CORD.—Portion of anterior horn; nerve cell degenerative changes may be observed at (A) Aggregations of cells represent scavenger, ("Gitter") microglial phagocytes at site of previous motor nerve cells (B), which have undergone destruction. App. 100 x.

NEUROTROPIC VIRUS INFECTIONS

Poliomyelitis (Infantile Paralysis).—The pathology of poliomyelitis presents two distinct phases: One of these which appears early in the course of the disease in humans affects the reticulo-endothelial system. This is not pathognomonic but is similar to the toxic changes seen in other acute infectious diseases. It is characterized by marked hyperplasia of the reticulo-endothelial apparatus notably affecting the lymphoid tissues of the intestine, the mesenteric lymph nodes, the spleen, the tonsils to a less marked degree and regularly the thymus. The weight of the thymus in poliomyelitis averages 15 to 20% more than it does in any of the other acute infectious diseases of childhood. The visceral pathology is one of mild toxic degeneration with cardiac dilatation and myocardial changes of a mild grade. Toxic hepatitis and nephrosis are observed. The liver, grossly, has an almost characteristic old rose discoloration as viewed through the capsule. Another feature of the general pathology of poliomyelitis is the presence of petechial hemorrhage in the gastric mucosa in over a third of the cases. This we attribute to toxic injury of the vascular endothelium and believe that the hemorrhages in the central nervous system might possibly be explained on the same basis.

The other major phase of the pathology is seen in the central nervous system where the virus has a specific neurotropic effect. The portal of entry would appear to be particularly the olfactory bulbs as evidenced by the changes found in these organs at times in the human cases and fairly regularly in the experimental animal. This does not preclude the passage of the virus along any other nerve tracts and the earliest changes in the central nervous system are those involving the pia arachnoid, particularly around the nerve roots (Fig. 178). The changes in the nervous system histologically are identical in development and vary only in degree and distribution. There is an initial edema and congestion of the entire central nervous system, but most marked from the brain stem down. This is followed in many instances by petechial hemorrhage. There is a curiously selective involvement of the anterior horn motor neurons. These nerve cell changes are one of two types, either karyolytic or karyorrhectic. This is accompanied by the accumulation of microglia cells which become transformed into typical scavenger "Gitter" cells which phagocytize the necrotic ganglion cells (Fig. 174 and 175). This is entirely apart from the perivascular lymphocytic inflammatory infiltration which is so characteristic of the disease. The neuronophagia (Fig. 173) by these microglia cells is one of the outstanding diagnostic features. In the extreme cases, actual liquefaction necrosis of considerable areas of the cord may occur. In healing, in late cases, a definite gliosis has been observed.

ILLUSTRATIVE CASES

CASE 67. (Ref. #S-157)
Diagnosis.—Spinal cord—acute poliomyelitis.

Patient was a boy of 8 years, admitted to the hospital with a history of a mild gastro-intestinal upset of forty-eight hours' duration, associated with diarrhea and nausea, but no vomiting. There was a slight fever, and a mild coryza. These symptoms seemed improved when suddenly he developed nuchal tenderness, headache and a rapidly progressive paralysis, more marked at the outset in the lower extremities, but soon involving the upper extremities, intercostals and muscles of deglutition.

Laboratory Findings.—Spinal puncture yielded a slightly opalescent fluid under moderate pressure. A specimen, from which 260 cells were counted, yielded 12% polynuclears and 88% lymphocytes.

Subsequent Course.—He died on the fourth day of his disease of respiratory failure, in spite of efforts to maintain life by placing him in a respirator.

Autopsy Findings.—Visceral pathology: There was moderate cardiac dilatation and toxic myocarditis, cloudy swelling of the liver, toxic splenitis, hyperplasia and follicular necrosis of lymphoid tissues of the ileum, mesentery and spleen. There was hypertrophy of the thymus, toxic nephrosis and petechial hemorrhage in the stomach. Central nervous pathology: Grossly there was marked generalized edema and congestion of the meninges and of the brain, brain stem and cord. On section there was marked mushrooming of the cord over the meninges. Softening and petechial hemorrhages were observed.

Microscopic Description of Section through Lumbar Cord.—(Fig. 176) Section microscopically through the lumbar cord presents all the features of the pathology as described under the general discussion of poliomyelitis. Here we see, particularly involving the anterior horns, considerabe congestion and edema with a varying amount of perivascular lymphocytic "cuffing." In addition, focal aggregations of microglial cells may be seen, each collection of which represents the site of a former nerve cell. In these clumps of neuronophagic microglial scavenger cells (Gitter cells) may be found the remnants of the motor nerve cells. Some of these are still identifiable but for the most part they show only fragments of their cytoplasm. Some of the cells may be identified with karolytic swelling of their nuclei, the

PLATE XLII
DISEASES CAUSED BY FILTRABLE VIRUSES AND RICKETTSIA-LIKE ORGANISMS

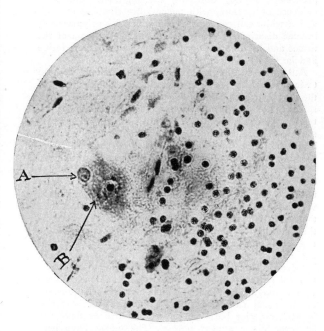

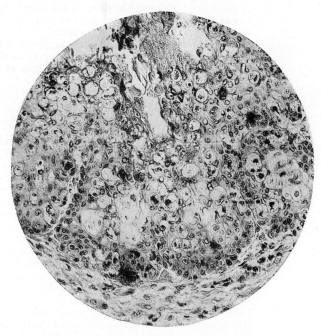

FIG. 179.—BRAIN: RABIES.—cf. CASE 69.—Photomicrograph of a section from the brain of an infected dog, showing a large nerve cell undergoing degeneration. Negri inclusion body is seen at (A) not to be confused with nucleolus at (B). App. 400 x. (See also Fig. 159.)

FIG. 180.—RABBIT.—SKIN.—INFECTIOUS PAPILLOMATOSIS.—cf. CASE 70.—Note marked epithelial proliferation and presence of intra-cellular inclusion bodies of varying size. App. 200 x.

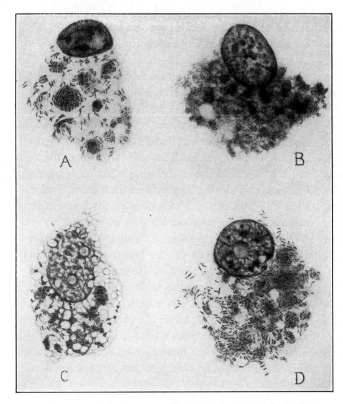

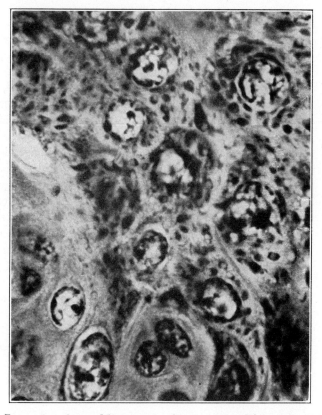

FIG. 181.—CARRION'S DISEASE.—BARTONELLIASIS.—A & B: intra-cytoplasmic bartonellae from blood of Oroya fever patient; C & D: ditto from Verruga peruana nodule, grown artificially in guinea pig tunica cells in Maitland medium. Giemsa stain. (Reproduced through courtesy of the authors, Pinkerton and Weiman, and of the Soc. for Exp. Biol. & Med. from an article entitled "Carrion's Disease," appearing in Vol. 37, Dec. 1937.) App. 1000 x.

FIG. 182.—SKIN.—MOLLUSCUM CONTAGIOSUM.—High power photomicrograph to show the characteristic intracellular inclusion bodies of the disease. Note their varying size, distribution and frequent vacuolated appearance (cf. Fig. 180 from Infect. papillomatosis). App. 1200 x.

accumulation of the Nissl granules around the periphery
of the cell cytoplasm and swelling of the cytoplasm with
loss of the cell membrane and gradual disintegration of
the cell. Several areas of actual necrosis will also be
seen. Many of these Gitter cells show varying degrees of
vacuolization and degeneration. Were they to be stained
with fat stain, they would show the presence of much
neutral fat.

CASE 68. (Ref. #S-158)
Diagnosis.—Spinal   cord—poliomyelitis,   late   (270
days).

Patient was a boy of 19 years who originally entered
the hospital nine months before his present admission
with a typical picture of poliomyelitis. This had been
ushered in by a mild upper respiratory infection and
fever of 48 hours' duration, which was followed by complete paralysis of his lower extremities and partial paralysis of his arms. Spinal fluid showed 80 cells, all
lymphocytes. The disease ran an uneventful course with
the upper extremity paralysis improving considerably but
almost no change in the legs. He was sent home and kept
under orthopedic care during the interval, but remained
in about the same condition until three days before the
present hospitalization. At that time he developed a sore
throat and fever of 102°. This was followed 48 hours
later by a diffuse punctiform, scarlatinal type rash.
There was no known possible exposure to scarlatina, but
a hemolytic streptococcus was obtained in culture from
the throat. Accompanying the development of the rash
there was evidence of meningeal irritation with headache, drowsiness and some stiffness of the neck. Spinal
fluid at this time was clear but under increased pressure; the sugar and protein content were normal; the

cell count showed 38 lymphocytes per c.mm. The patient
progressed rapidly downhill, showing more and more
evidence of toxemia, with temperature climbing to 105°,
and a white cell count of 18,000 with 84% polynuclears;
became disoriented and stuporous. Marked edema of the
throat and larynx developed. Heart sounds became feeble
and he finally died on the 8th day of his illness.

Autopsy Findings.—Autopsy examination showed
toxic myocarditis, cardiac dilatation, terminal edema of
the lungs, parenchymatous degeneration of the liver, toxic
splenitis, toxic nephrosis, and acute inflammation of the
tonsils, pharynx, glottis, epiglottis, larynx, etc. Brain
showed moderate edema and congestion of meninges and
brain substance. Cord showed marked edema with mushrooming on section. There was no evidence of meningitis.

**Microscopic Description of a Section of the Lumbar
Cord.**—(Fig. 177) A section of the lumbar cord from
this late case of poliomyelitis microscopically presents a
very interesting picture. There are still some remnants of
the active inflammatory process present as evidenced by
the presence of some perivascular lymphocytic reaction
and occasional areas where microglial scavenger cells
are still present in small clumps. For the most part,
however, the acute inflammatory picture has disappeared.
Careful search through the anterior horn areas will reveal scarcely any remaining motor nerve cells. Instead
of the usual twenty or more nerve cells to be found
in each anterior horn, not more than two or three can
be seen. These appear normal. The others have been
destroyed by the previous acute stage of the disease and
it is interesting to note that there has been a replacement
gliosis which corresponds to the replacement fibrosis seen
in inflammatory processes affecting the skeletal tissue
other than the central nervous system.

Epidemic Encephalitis (Sleeping Sickness).—For
the past twenty years or more, a disease first described by Von Economo in 1917 has been a problem which has not yet been satisfactorily solved.
It spread much as the influenza epidemic did, as a
pandemic, throughout the world, and has persisted
in sporadic fashion since. Clinically the original epidemic was ushered in by an acute febrile attack accompanied by sensory disturbances, changes in the
reflexes and somnolence. However, wide variations
from this picture were found as the disease spread,
and myoclonic varieties accompanied by marked delirium were not uncommon. More serious, perhaps,
than the immediate disease itself have been the
sequelae, with the development of the parkinsonian
syndrome, simulating paralysis agitans several years
after the original illness.

The etiology of this disease, with its pleomorphic
manifestations, is firmly believed to be a filtrable
virus similar to that which causes poliomyelitis. As
has been commented above, the histologic lesions are
very similar except restricted for the most part to
the brain rather than the spinal cord. For a more

complete discussion of encephalitis, the reader is referred to Chapter LXIII on the inflammatory diseases of the central nervous system.

Rabies (Hydrophobia).—Rabies is a specific infection by another of the neurotropic viruses. The
clinical manifestations of this disease are so well
known that they need no particular comment. The
virus enters the tissues through the local wound and
spreads along the axis cylinders of the nerves to the
central nervous system. There, it seems to multiply
until it becomes an overwhelming infection resulting
ultimately in death. There is an incubation period
of usually not less than ten days to three weeks or
more before symptoms occur.

The pathology of rabies is comparatively simple.
In the ganglion cells of the brain, particularly in
the Ammon horn cells of the hippocampus, are found
peculiar, strongly staining acidophilic bodies within
the cytoplasm of the nerve cells. These vary tremendously in size from small granules up to large
masses almost filling the cell body. Not infrequently
a basophilic, granular mass may be observed within
this inclusion body. Various interpretations have

been given as to the nature of these structures. It is generally held that they represent some degenerative product, the result of invasion of the cell by the virus rather than a visible form of the virus, because they will not pass through the Berkefeld filter and are not, in themselves, infectious. Fortunately, we are able to treat the disease successfully from the prophylactic standpoint after an individual has become infected by the bite of a rabid animal. It should be mentioned that many animals, including cats as well as dogs, may carry the virus. It was

Pasteur's brilliant work in attenuating the virus of rabies by drying the spinal cords of rabbits which had been previously infected and by injecting this material into human beings who had been bitten which has saved thousands of lives since that time. More recently, the use of formalinized virus as derived from such rabbit cords has been used with apparently equal success and has eliminated the possibility of the occasional susceptible individual acquiring the disease from the inoculation of the living, although attenuated virus.

ILLUSTRATIVE CASE

CASE 69. (Ref. #S-159)
Diagnosis.—Brain (dog)—rabies. (Stained for Negri bodies).

Patient was a four year old child, who came home crying, saying she had been bitten by a dog. Three small wounds were found on her face; one on her cheek, one on the bridge of her nose and one near the chin. She was taken to a doctor, who cauterized and sutured the wounds. The child was given tetanus antitoxin. The wounds healed uneventfully. Four weeks later the patient vomited, had marked loss of appetite and became irritable. She developed choking attacks which increased in frequency and severity. She was taken to the hospital where she rapidly developed nervous symptoms of extreme motor excitability, attempting to bite doctors and nurses. She became completely maniacal and had to be placed in a restraint jacket. Her cardiac action became weaker and weaker, finally stopping. There was a terminal hyperpyrexia of 107°.

The animal presumably responsible (as checked up subsequently because it was found in the neighborhood) had been apprehended in the interval and destroyed. Tissues were sent to the laboratory to establish the diagnosis, which was readily done microscopically.

Autopsy Findings.—The postmortem examination of the body was entirely negative except for a rather marked rigor mortis, postmortem lividity in the dependent portions and generalized venous congestion. The

findings in the central nervous system were similarly disappointing and non-specific in character, consisting solely of moderate edema and congestion. There were no hemorrhages noted grossly. (Similar negative findings were observed in the dog).

Microscopic Description of a Section from the Brain of the Dog, Stained with Phloxine and Methylene Blue to Demonstrate the Negri Bodies.—(Fig. 159 and 179) (Animal tissues are used because the Negri Bodies are much more numerous and easier to demonstrate). Sections microscopically show a portion of cerebellum which may be identified by the characteristic arrangement of the nerve tissue with the characteristic convolution of the cerebellum. By careful search of the Purkinje cells, it will be noted that fully one-third to one-half of them contain parasitic inclusion bodies which tend to stain more intensely with the phloxine than does the surrounding cytoplasm or the nucleolus. These inclusion bodies vary in size considerably. Some of the cells may be found to contain as many as three to four. Others may contain a single very large inclusion body. Secondary degeneration of these cells has taken place as evidenced by karolysis of the nuclei at times with degeneration of the Nissl granules and of the typical nerve cell nucleolus. In studying these slides it is well to remember that the nucleoli of the nerve cells likewise stain intensely with phloxine and should not be mistaken for Negri inclusion bodies.

Herpes.—Both *herpes simplex* (*fever blisters*) and *herpes zoster* (*shingles*) have been shown conclusively to be caused by specific viruses. They may remain for long periods of time latent within the tissues and only develop their characteristic lesion as the result of some other tissue insult, particularly associated with the febrile diseases. Under such circumstances the characteristic vesicles develop in the skin or mucous membranes and tend to either appear in relation to nerve endings or along the course of nerve trunks. The virus apparently is neurotropic in that it extends along the nerves to the posterior ganglia, and intranuclear inclusion bodies may commonly be demonstrated in the ganglion cells in these

areas. One more or less striking difference occurs in the two conditions. In *herpes zoster*, apparently a more or less lasting immunity is conferred on the individual; in *herpes simplex*, if anything, the individual appears more sensitized and is liable to recurrent attacks.

These viruses are of particular interest in relation to some of the other virus infections, both experimentally and in man. It is thought highly possible by some investigators that one variety at least of epidemic encephalitis, the St. Louis type, may result from an attack of herpes simplex. It is certain that many cases of experimental encephalitis in rabbits are of this nature, and more recently experimental data in respect to an encephalitis with a species specificity for monkeys, the so-called "Virus B," likewise seems definitely associated with such a herpes etiology.

EPITHELIAL VIRUS DISEASES

Of the epithelial forms of virus disease, smallpox, chickenpox and molluscum contagiosum seem to represent the most characteristic examples of such infection in man. In animals, we have corresponding conditions, notably infectious papillomatosis of rabbits and the contagious epithelioma of chickens. A discussion of the pathology of varicella will be found in the succeeding chapter in relation to the so-called "contagious" diseases.

As an example of this group of epithelial lesions, which are characterized by the apparent localization of the virus in the surface epithelial cells, we have selected the infectious papillomatosis of rabbits as described by Shope as one of the most typical forms. This is strictly comparable in many respects to molluscum contagiosum, the counterpart of the disease as seen in man. It apparently, however, produces greater cell proliferation and has less lytic action on the tissues than has the virus of molluscum contagiosum (Fig. 182), so that the histology is somewhat more readily interpreted. The microscopic description is given in the appended case history.

ILLUSTRATIVE CASE

CASE 70. (Ref. #S-215 and S-244)
Diagnosis.—Skin (rabbit)—Shope virus disease.

Animal was a wild cottontail rabbit sent to the laboratory for the diagnosis of several elevated plaques in the skin varying in size from 1.0 to 3.0 cm. These were for the most part irregularly oval in outline, averaging from 0.5 to 1.0 cm. in thickness with a relatively verrucous-like surface. They were freely movable over the underlying structures. They were restricted to the hair-bearing area, stopping abruptly about 1 millimeter from the mucocutaneous junction. The hair over these masses had either absent or poorly developed. On palpation they had a rather elastic feeling and did not pit on pressure. On section there was noted a somewhat papillary-surfaced, thickened epithelium and a gelatinoid appearance to the underlying tissues, which were grayish-white in color and suggested myxomatous connective tissue grossly. The masses were sharply demarcated by a pseudocapsule of condensed corium from the underlying tissues.

This condition in recent years has been recognized and established as one of three curiously specific virus infections (Shope virus) of rabbits, especially the cottontail and certain strains of domestic animals. It is not transmissible to any other laboratory animal or even necessarily to all other strains of rabbits.

Microscopic Description of a Section from the Skin Lesion.—(Fig. 180) There are two main features in the histopathology of the lesion. In the first place there is an enormous overgrowth of the superficial epithelium with distortion of the usual pegs. Keratinization is incomplete as the great majority of the cells are swollen. Most of them contain eosinophilic staining globoid masses, the so-called intracellular inclusion bodies. Some of these have been extruded into the tissue spaces between the cells. In some cells multiple such inclusions are seen, varying considerably in size. This slide is presented primarily for the opportunity to study the appearance of such inclusions as they are representative of the entire group of allied virus infections, although exaggerated in extent. Such inclusion bodies today are practically universally accepted as prima facie evidence of a virus disease. This particular tumor, when emulsified and filtered, will reproduce the condition in other rabbits if rubbed into the scarified skin, or injected subcutaneously. Curiously it does not seem to be infectious by contact, other rabbits never developing the condition when penned together.

The other phase of the histopathology is the suggestive neoplastic overgrowth of the underlying connective tissue. In areas a myxomatous degeneration of the collagen may be seen; in other areas a suggestion of neural tissue is found. The exact classification of the lesion is difficult because of its involvement of both ectodermal and mesodermal derivatives. Various terms have been applied. Infectious neurofibromatosis, infectious fibromyxomatosis, infectious fibropapillomatosis have all been suggested.

MISCELLANEOUS VIRUS INFECTIONS

Yellow Fever.—This is a specific infectious disease caused by a virus which is transmitted by the bite of an infected mosquito, the *Aedes aegypti.* However, the virus apparently requires at least ten days to two weeks within the body of the mosquito to increase sufficiently in amount or to go through some developmental phase to render it infective to the second individual. The virus produces a very serious infection associated with vomiting of blood, petechial hemorrhages in the skin and mucous membranes, and marked destruction of the liver and kidneys accompanied by a severe jaundice. This particular virus seems to have a more toxic effect than most any other of the known viruses producing such extensive tissue changes as it does. It has been shown to have a moderately marked neurotropic character in that in the experimental animal the virus will localize in the brain after previous injury to the central nervous system has been produced. Immunity can be produced in individuals by the use of such an antigen from the infected brain tissue from mice. This is best done in conjunction with the injection of immune serum from a patient who has recently had the disease, much in the same way that the toxin antitoxin mixtures of diphtheria have been used to immunize against that infection.

Coryza (Common Cold).—The work of Dochez and his associates has established the common cold among those diseases produced by a specific filtrable virus. This virus can be maintained alive in tissue culture or in media containing embryonic tissues and can be successfully transplanted almost indefinitely. The virus appears to be responsible for the initial onset of the infection with the associated early catarrhal symptoms and serous outpouring from the mucous membranes. In rare instances, this initial coryzal picture is of short duration and is the only evidence of inflammation which develops. More often, however, the initial infection is complicated by some secondary contaminant from the usual naso-pharyngeal bacterial flora. Upon the nature of the secondary invader depends the usual train of symptoms which accounts for the wide difference in the clinical picture which follows the initial infection.

Psittacosis (Parrot Fever).—Psittacosis is an acute infectious disease now believed to be due to another of the filtrable viruses. It, like whooping cough, influenza and other infections, is usually complicated by the presence of a secondary bacterial invader, in this instance the *Bacillus nocardi.* It is fairly readily transmitted from parrots, which are the usual source of the infection, to man. It is characterized usually by rather high fever, malaise going on to prostration, and frequently delirium. In the more marked cases, there is a secondary and complicating bronchopneumonia, which results in a rather high mortality. In epidemic form, this may reach twenty to twenty-five per cent. In the sporadic cases, the figure usually drops to ten or twelve per cent. The pathology is not unlike the interstitial pneumonitis of measles, influenza and pertussis, and the encephalomyelitis which occurs at times is likewise comparable to that condition seen as a complication of measles and pertussis.

Dengue (Break Bone Fever).—Dengue is another of the acute infections produced by a filtrable virus. Its mortality is negligible. It is transmitted by the bite of a mosquito, usually the *Aedes aegypti.* It is usually ushered in by a moderate fever and a feeling of general malaise, with severe aching pains of the muscles, bones and joints. This slowly subsides over the course of two or three days when there is usually a recurrent rise in temperature and the development of a diffuse, macular rash which gradually fades and may desquamate much as do measles and scarlatinal rashes. The duration of the disease is usually somewhere between ten days and two weeks, and leaves the patient for some little time with a marked feeling of weakness and easy fatigability. The nature of this virus is unknown. It produces no immunity, and recurrent attacks are very prone to occur in areas where the virus is endemic.

Tobacco Mosaic Disease.—Recent work on a virus infection affecting the tobacco plant has suggested that the virus is not a viable substance itself, but something in the nature of an enzyme. Stanley, in a brilliant series of articles, has demonstrated that the activating agent which produces tobacco mosaic disease may be obtained in fairly pure crystalline inert form. Similar work suggests that the Shope virus may be of a similar enzymic nature and this brings up the possibility as to whether all virus diseases should be considered in this light or whether the enzyme which these investigators have obtained in these particular diseases is merely a catalytic agent which activates virus already present but in a quiescent state.

More will be said regarding the part played by viruses in the development of tumors in the section devoted to their consideration. Nothing is to be gained by any further discussion of the many other forms of virus infections which occur in the lower animals. Goodpasture's and River's work, particularly, in this field should be mentioned, and for the student interested in delving further into this fascinating part of experimental medicine the reader is referred to their original contributions. Aside from those diseases which have been discussed in the preceding paragraphs, it must be remembered that several of the common infectious diseases likewise are of presumptive virus origin. Among these must be mentioned measles and influenza. These will be discussed in their respective sections, the former in the chapter on the contagious diseases; influenza in the chapters on lung pathology.

CHAPTER XIX

MISCELLANEOUS SPECIFIC INFECTIOUS DISEASES

PART I

CONTAGIOUS DISEASES

Diphtheria.—Diphtheria is a specific, acute infectious disease caused by the *Corynebacterium diphtheriae*. This is a gram-positive rod characterized by the presence of metachromatic granules and the tendency to develop involution forms (see Fig. 183), when grown on Loeffler's blood serum medium. The organism is further characterized by being one of the few bacteria to produce a true exotoxin. This is of significance in interpreting its pathology. It causes a dual reaction in the body, one phase being due to its typical involvement of mucous surfaces locally; the other to its systemic toxic manifestations.

The local lesion is usually found involving the mucosa of the naso-pharynx, tonsils and in the more severe cases the larynx, trachea and bronchi. Diphtheria may be primary elsewhere, as an infection of the vaginal or rectal mucosa, as an infection of the skin, but always a superficial surface infection. The local reaction consists of the laying down of a typical dense fibrinous exudate on the infected surface. In the respiratory tract it is of significance to note that while the surface epithelium is destroyed, the basement membrane usually remains intact.

Hence the term "pseudomembrane" as applied to the true diphtheria lesion in contradistinction to the more extensive necrotic lesion of the streptococcus or dysentery bacillus in which the membrane is continuous with the deep tissue reaction, the so-called diphtheritic, necrotic, true membranous inflammation.

The secondary manifestations of diphtheria are seen in all the viscera, but especially involving the heart, and as a neurotropic toxin, producing paralysis of the muscles of deglutition and degeneration of the vagi. The systemic lesions are noted in all the lymphoid tissues with marked toxic degeneration of the germinal centers of the follicles and an associated reticulo-endothelial hyperplasia. In the liver and kidney, fatty and granular degeneration occur. Occasionally true glomerular nephritis follows. In the heart all gradations of toxic myocarditis from mild fatty and granular changes down to extensive interstitial myocarditis are found. In the fatal cases there is usually bundle branch block, which may be shown by electrocardiogram. This is the result of diffuse involvement of the heart wall, including the neuromuscular element.

ILLUSTRATIVE CASE

CASE 71. (Ref. #S-11)

Diagnosis.—Trachea—diphtheria; pseudomembranous fibrinous exudate.

Patient was a white male child five years of age admitted to the hospital on the fifth day of his illness.

Present Illness.—This had begun as a sore throat which the mother disregarded for the first three days. On the fourth day, a local physician was called who diagnosed it as a streptococcus infection, but took cultures which were reported the following day as diphtheria, and the child was rushed to the hospital. He was given 40,000 units of antitoxin intravenously and an additional 40,000 units intramuscularly.

Physical Examination.—Physical examination revealed an almost moribund child, gasping for breath,

cyanotic and in a stupor. There was evidence of pneumonic consolidation with impaired resonance, altered breath sounds and rāles. Exact information regarding the extent of the pneumonia was impossible because the child was too sick to examine in detail. Heart sounds were distant and irregular.

Laboratory Findings.—Red blood cells, 4,100,000 with 80% hemoglobin. White blood cells, 22,600 with 84% polynuclear leukocytes. Urinalysis showed a moderate amount of albumin of a high specific gravity and occasional red cells.

Subsequent Course.—An emergency tracheotomy was performed with temporary relief, but the child failed rapidly, dying within twenty-four hours of admission, apparently of cardiac failure.

PLATE XLIII

THE "CONTAGIOUS" DISEASES

DIPHTHERIA.—CASE 71

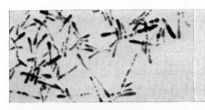 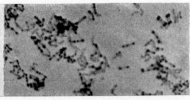 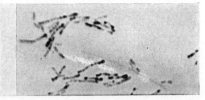

FIG. 183.—VARIANTS OF THE CORYNEBACTERIUM DIPHTHERIA.—Note "clubbing," metachromatic granules and parallelism. App. 1500 x.

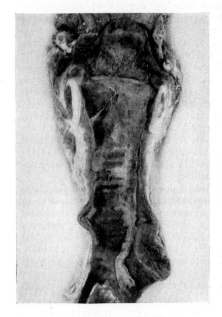

FIG. 184.—LARYNX AND TRACHEA.—Typical pseudomembranous, fibrinous exudate extending into bronchus on right side. It has become loosened in part following antitoxin administration. (Slightly reduced.)

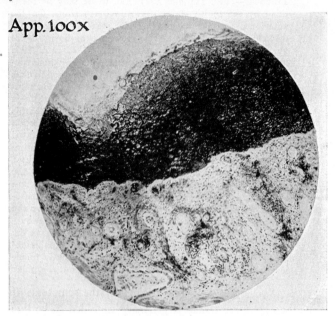

FIG. 185.—TRACHEA—"STAG-HORN" ACUTE FIBRINOUS PSEUDO-MEMBRANOUS EXUDATE.—Note how superficial the position of the dense, fibrinous exudate is; the preservation of the basement membrane of the mucosa and the submucosal hyperemia, edema and acute inflammatory reaction. App. 100 x.

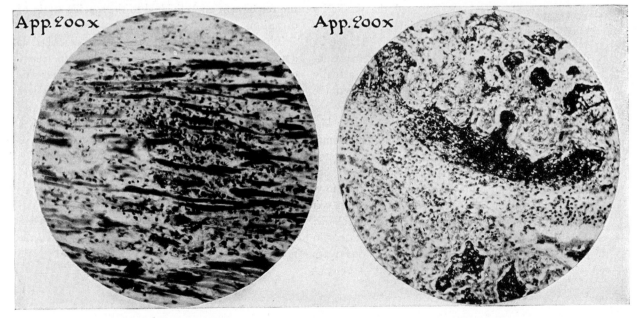

FIG. 186.—HEART—ACUTE INTERSTITIAL MYOCARDITIS.—Unusually marked toxic degeneration of musculature with leukocytic infiltration and beginning actual liquefaction necrosis.

FIG. 187.—LUNG—DIPHTHERITIC PNEUMONIA.—Note extension of typical fibrinous exudate from the terminal bronchiole into the pulmonary alveoli.

Autopsy Findings.—Autopsy examination revealed a typical cyanotic purplish red injection of the pharynx and buccal mucosa. The membrane had been stripped from this region, but fragments still adhered to the tonsils, uvula and posterior pharynx. The trachea, larynx and major bronchi were nearly plugged with a dirty, grayish-white membrane partially loosened from the mucosa. There was an underlying acute tracheo-bronchitis. There was secondary bilateral bronchopneumonia. Heart showed acute dilatation and extreme toxic myocarditis. There was acute toxic nephrosis, hepatitis and splenitis present.

Microscopic Description of Section from the Trachea.—(Fig. 184 and 185) The tissue may be identified by the bluish staining cartilaginous rings. On the anterior aspect the mucosa may be seen to be markedly thickened and hyperemic. The typical "stag-horn" dense fibrinous exudate is seen on the mucosal surface. This has torn off in part, following serum therapy and suction. It will be noted that although the epithelial cells have disappeared, the basement membrane for the most part is still demonstrable. This explains the readiness with which the membrane can be detached. Beneath this the submucosa shows evidence of acute inflammation with hyperemia, edema, a small amount of precipitated fibrin and a perivascular leukocytic reaction migrating to the surface. No bacteria can be demonstrated in these deeper structures as a rule. The bacteria are on the surface of the exudate in the greatest numbers, as are also the polynuclears. Some superficial liquefaction necrosis of the exudate may be observed, as a result of the proteolytic enzyme action of the leukocytes. These bacteria are best demonstrated by using a stain such as the Gram stain, or with Zenker-fixed tissue, phloxine-methylene blue, both of which stain the diphtheria bacillus a dark blue or purple and tend to bring out the polar

granules, which are so characteristic of these organisms. Extension of the pseudo-membranous exudate into the pulmonary alveoli is also noted (Fig. 187).

CASE 71. (Ref. #S-153)
Diagnosis.—Heart—acute (diphtheritic) myocarditis.
Microscopic Description of a Section from the Heart.—(Fig. 186) The cardiac musculature is easily recognized by the characteristic interlacing bundles of striated muscle fibers. There is a very marked interstitial edema with congestion of the small nutrient vessels of the heart musculature. Leukocytic infiltration of the interstitial tissue is prominent. Even the muscle fibers show varying degrees of degenerative change. Fatty degeneration, granular degeneration and even hydrops of many of the muscle fibers may be seen. This is evidenced by a loss of striation, marked fragmentation, hyaline changes of the cytoplasm, karyolytic and karyorrhectic nuclear changes and actual necrosis of some of the cells. This necrotic muscular parenchymatous material is seen infiltrated by the leukocytes which are attempting phagocytosis and lysis through their proteolytic enzyme action. This acute degenerative lesion appears to be the result of the direct action of the toxin upon the muscle fibers. As such lesions progress the usual fibrous tissue response takes place and we find essentially a replacement fibrosis with marked fibrous scarring of the heart muscle.

In one case studied, which did not die until the sixty-first day of illness, the fibrous scarring appeared as marked as in many cases of advanced vascular disease of the heart in older individuals, and it is felt that such severe diphtheritic infections may well be an occasional cause of subsequent cardiac pathology, although it is probably true that this is most unusual.

Scarlet Fever.—The etiology of the symptoms of scarlet fever to-day is generally conceded to be due to a hemolytic streptococcus. Whether this is a specific organism, or whether the picture is the result of individual susceptibility to the action of hemolytic streptococci is one aspect of the problem still under study and is still open to question. Likewise, various investigators have suggested the possibility of there being an initial virus infection necessary before characteristic secondary symbiotic invasion by the streptococcus can occur. These differences of opinion only go to show how little is still actually established as facts in our knowledge of even the common contagious diseases of childhood.

At all events, the pathology of scarlet fever histologically is dependent upon the toxin of the hemolytic streptococcus. This has been demonstrated conclusively by the Dicks, Dochez and many other subsequent investigators. In this respect, therefore, the changes produced by this circulating toxin can scarcely be considered specific or pathognomonic. Practically, however, such tissue changes as occur in scarlet fever are not seen in any of the other types

of contagious diseases except rarely in conjunction with a secondary hemolytic streptococcic infection accompanying measles, pertussis or diphtheria. Thus, it seems reasonable to assume that there is some specificity of bacterial types, and we are inclined to believe that such streptococcic manifestations in other conditions than scarlatina very likely represent the response of an individual to the specific strain of organism.

The characteristic lesion may best be described as a toxic injury of the vascular endothelium, chiefly of the venous side of the circulation. Whether this is direct, or allergic in nature is not known. There results a proliferation of the lining endothelium, an outpouring of serum and the development of a perivascular mononuclear infiltration consisting of lymphocytes predominantly, with some plasma cells and large mononuclears. These lesions are found generally distributed all over the body. They are present almost regularly in the liver, heart and kidney, and demonstrable frequently in other viscera, particularly the adrenal, spleen, lung, and even the pituitary and testis.

PLATE XLIV
THE "CONTAGIOUS" DISEASES
SCARLET FEVER (SCARLATINA).—CASE 72

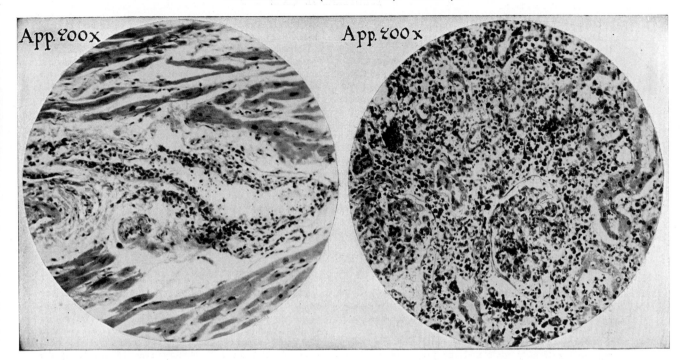

FIG. 188.—HEART.—Typical intimal endothelial proliferation, sub-intimal and perivascular monocytic cellular infiltration with slight interstitial edema.

FIG. 189.—KIDNEY.—Marked non-suppurative, interstitial
inflammatory reaction arising as a vascular lesion similar
to that observed in Fig. 188 in the heart.

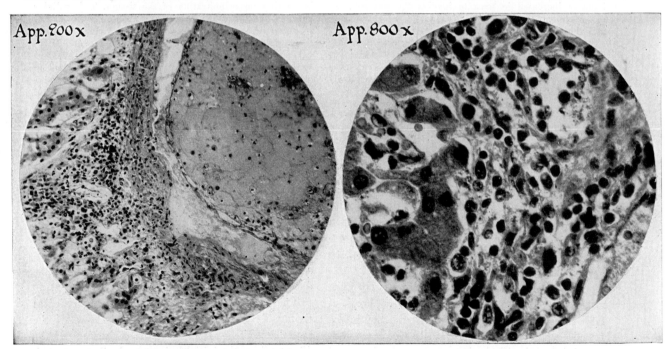

FIG. 190.—ADRENAL.—Identical type of vascular lesion,
with thrombosis, resulting from intimal endothelial injury
by scarlatinal toxin. Note perivascular monocytic infiltration.

FIG. 191.—LIVER.—High power detail photomicrograph to
show the essential vascular nature of the lesion with
marked intimal proliferation.

(Reproduced by courtesy of the *Am. Jour. of Pathol.* from an article entitled "The Visceral Pathology in Scarlet Fever" in the May
1936 number, by Brody, H., & Smith, L. W.)

ILLUSTRATIVE CASE

CASE 72. (Ref. #S-150)

Diagnosis.—Heart—acute toxic myocarditis (scarlatina).

Patient was a white female, twenty-four years of age, who entered the hospital on the third day of her illness.

Present Illness.—This began as a severe sore throat, accompanied by dysphagia. She became utterly prostrate, ran a high fever, 104.5° on admission, and on the day of admission developed a typical punctiform scarlatinal rash over her entire body, but with more marked involvement of the face, neck, axillae and groins.

Physical Examination.—Physical examination showed a well developed, fairly well nourished white female lying in bed. Her head was of normal contour. Eyes, ears and nose were negative. Her throat was of a flaming scarlet color with marked hypertrophy of the papillae of the tongue ("strawberry" tongue). The skin rash was typical in appearance. Her lungs showed impaired resonance óf both bases with altered breath sounds and the presence of numerous râles. Her heart was not enlarged. The rate was rapid. There was a soft, systolic murmur in the mitral area.

Laboratory Findings.—Red blood cells, 3,600,000 with 78% hemoglobin. White blood cells, 26,800 with 88% polynuclears. Urinalysis showed a moderate amount of albumin.

Subsequent Course.—Even on admission the patient appeared extremely toxic and the prognosis was poor. She developed jaundice on the fifth day, which progressively increased until her death on the eighth. The lung findings were considered as bronchopneumonia, which likewise increased in area to involve the greater part of both lungs. Terminally the heart sounds became febrile and she apparently died of cardiac failure.

Autopsy Findings.—At autopsy there was a fading punctiform rash with a beginning furfuraceous desquamation of the skin and an intense jaundice. Heart was markedly dilated, yellowish-brown in color, extremely friable in consistency, showing evidence of toxic myocarditis. Lungs both showed a diffuse grayish-red patchy consolidation. The liver was enlarged, weighing 2,200 grams, yellowish-brown in color, friable and evidently markedly degenerated. The spleen was enlarged, congested, and showed toxic splenitis. Adrenals were engorged in their medullae; granular in their cortices. Kidneys were a mottled reddish-yellow in color and showed marked toxic degeneration.

Microscopic Description of Section from Heart.—(Fig. 188) There is a very extensive picture of myocardial inflammation seen throughout numerous areas of the heart. This is more marked than is seen in the average case. The myocardium itself shows marked interstitial edema and congestion. Nearly all the blood vessels show marked endothelial proliferation with perivascular mononuclear infiltration about them. Nothing resembling an Aschoff body can be identified. Very few polynuclear cells are seen in this vascular reaction. Muscle cells are undergoing secondary degeneration with swelling of their cytoplasm, loss of striations, a moderate amount of fragmentation and definite granular and fatty changes. The inflammatory process has spread in this instance to the pericardium, which shows similar lesions in the epicardial tissues and an acute terminal fibrinopurulent exudate on the surface.

CASE 72. (Ref. #S-151)

Diagnosis.—Liver—acute toxic hepatitis.

Microscopic Description of Section from the Liver of the Same Case.—(Fig. 191) Study of the liver microscopically confirms our impression of the vascular nature of this reaction. The most striking changes are seen in the portal areas around the small blood vessels. It is definitely not an inflammatory reaction involving the bile ducts or canaliculae. The lesion obviously starts in the vascular endothelium in the same way as has been noted in the heart, and is characterized by diffuse cellular perivascular infiltration of the tissues. This cellular reaction is chiefly mononuclear in nature with a few scattered polymorphonuclears. In this particular instance, the reaction is unusually marked and very acute. It involves not only the hepatic vessels, but the sinusoidal endothelium as well. This has resulted in considerable liver necrosis in this particular instance, which apparently accounts for the jaundice. More necrosis is found in this case than is usually true, but the basic picture is similar in its nature to that seen in the heart.

By way of additional comment, tissues from the kidney and adrenal in this case again show very marked inflammatory changes of a comparable nature. These may be observed in Fig. 189 and 190.

Measles.—Measles is another specific, acute infectious disease which is believed to be due to a filtrable virus as the result of rather extensive experimental studies over the past two decades. In itself, measles is probably rarely a fatal disease, except in communities where the disease has not been rampant for many generations. Such an outbreak of fatal measles has been described in the South Sea Islands where entire populations have been decimated. More familiarly, however, measles is a mild infectious process characterized by coryza, sore throat and followed by a macular rash of a rather confluent nature, which usually starts in the head and neck region and spreads down the body. In infants under two years of age, the disease is a very serious one because of the complicating and associated secondary streptococcic pneumonia which produces a very high mortality.

The pathology of measles has not been studied as thoroughly as many other diseases because of the fact that so few cases die in the early stage of the disease where the initial lesion may be demonstrated. Even studies of the mucous membrane and skin lesions have been comparatively few in number. The

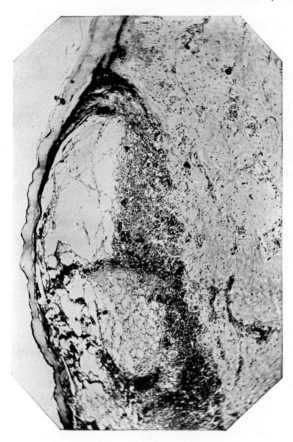

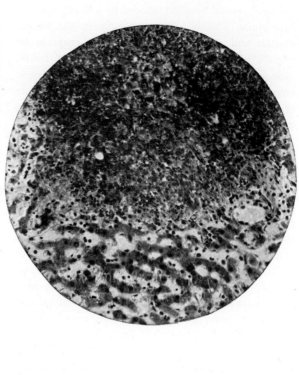

FIG. 192.—CUTANEOUS LESION.—Typical vesicle between basal and cornifying layers of epiderm, filled with serum and beginning leukocytic exudate. App. 50 x.

FIG. 193.—LIVER.—Focal area of liquefaction necrosis, comparable to cutaneous lesion. Note peripheral zone of leukocytes. App. 200 x.

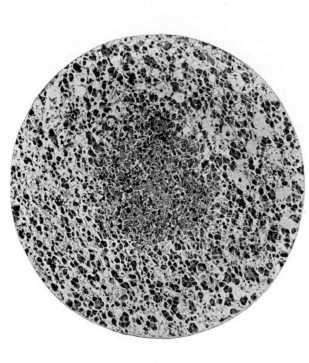

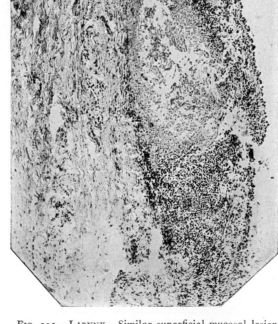

FIG. 194.—ADRENAL.—Marked toxic degenerative changes of parenchymatous cells surrounding focal area of necrosis. App. 100 x.

FIG. 195.—LARYNX.—Similar superficial mucosal lesion as that observed in the skin, but arising in deeper tissues, breaking through to the surface. App. 50 x.

characteristic mucous membrane lesion is spoken of as the Koplik spot and consists of a bluish white, pin-head central area surrounded by a dusky zone of hyperemia. This occurs particularly in the buccal mucosa and usually precedes the skin eruption by anywhere from twenty-four to forty-eight hours. Histologic studies of these lesions suggest an allergic type of reaction, although it may well be the direct reaction to the presence of virus locally. It consists of acute hyperemia with perivascular cellular infiltration in which particularly large mononuclear cells predominate. The skin rash is similar in its histologic appearance. There is rarely any true hemorrhage into the tissues and the rash can be blanched by pressure. There is, however, marked congestion, perivascular edema and cellular infiltration, predominantly mononuclears. It has been noted that appendicitis is one of the complications of measles occurring with a relatively greater incidence than should be expected and in the appendices of such cases, amazing hyperplasia of the lymph follicles and lymphoid tissues generally has been noted. More characteristic, however, has been the presence of enormous large mononuclear cells approaching the giant cell type seen in Hodgkin's disease and other conditions. So far as is known, this curious reaction of the lymphoid tissue, which has also been described in the tonsils in cases of measles, is not found in any other condition.

As a complication of the initial infection, we find that bronchopneumonia, due to a hemolytic streptococcus, as a rule, although at times produced by other bacteria, presents certain features which are fairly characteristic and of differential diagnostic significance. In this connection, the diplococcus of Tunnicliff has been suggested as a probable agent or the etiologic factor in the disease. More recent work, however, by Broadhurst further substantiates the theory regarding the viral nature of the etiologic agent. She and her coworkers seem irrefutably to have demonstrated the virus by special nigrosin staining methods.

The basic pathology in the lungs of the measles patient appears to be an interstitial pneumonitis. This is evidenced by marked thickening of the peribronchial and peribronchiolar structures and of the alveolar walls. This is due to edema and interstitial mononuclear cellular infiltration, hyperemia and even beginning fibrous tissue proliferation. In its uncomplicated form, little or no inflammatory exudate is found in the lung alveoli. In the fatal cases, however, a secondary hemolytic streptococcic serofibrinous pneumonic exudation occurs with all the usual reactive picture to the presence of the secondary invader. This initial interstitial inflammatory process is of great significance in relation to the interpretation of the virus nature of the infection as it is seen in only two other types of pulmonary infection, early, fulminating cases of influenza and to a less extent in pertussis.

ILLUSTRATIVE CASE

CASE 73. (Ref. #S-191)

Diagnosis.—Lung—interstitial pneumonitis (measles); hemolytic streptococci.

Patient was a child, five years of age, who was admitted to the hospital with a history of having had what appeared to be a progressive cold for three or four days preceding the development of a typical macular measles rash. This was accompanied by some photophobia, a catarrhal conjunctivitis, a typical short, soft cough and a fever which rose to 104°. Koplik's spots were observed the day before admission.

Physical Examination.—On admission, the patient appeared almost stuporous. Head was normal in contour. The eyes showed marked lacrimation and considerable reddening of the conjunctivae. Ears were negative. Nose was negative. The throat showed rather marked bright red congestion which involved the tonsils particularly. The chest was symmetrical. Lungs showed no dullness on percussion. There was no modification of the breath sounds, but there were numerous moist crackling râles throughout both sides. There was a typical macular rash over the face, chest and upper extremities. The heart was rapid but otherwise appeared normal. Abdomen was somewhat distended. Extremities were negative.

Laboratory Findings.—The red cells were normal with a count of 4,500,000. Hemoglobin 82%. White blood cells, 4,200 with 84% polynuclears. (This leukopenia is one of the typical and characteristic diagnostic features of measles, particularly in its early stage. Ordinarily, however, the differential count should show a more relatively proportionate decrease of the various types of cells. The increase of polynuclears here is suggestive of secondary infection.) Urinalysis: Dark amber, Sp. Gr., 1.028; albumin present in large amount.

Subsequent Course.—During the next forty-eight hours, the white count rose to 18,600 with 92% polynuclears. Signs of consolidation in the right lower lobe developed. The heart sounds became distant and the child went downhill rapidly, dying 72 hours after admission.

Autopsy Findings.—At autopsy there was still evidence of a fading measles rash with beginning furfuraceous desquamation over the neck and chest. Heart was dilated, pale and flabby (toxic myocardosis). Lungs:

the right lower lobe showed a diffuse, confluent broncho-pneumonia with a sero-sanguineous exudate from which hemolytic streptococci were recovered. There was a marked mucopurulent tracheobroncho-bronchiolitis with peribronchial thickening involving the rest of the lungs. Liver and kidneys showed toxic, granular degeneration. The spleen showed toxic splenitis.

Microscopic Description of a Section of Lung.— (Fig. 423) Low power study of the tissue shows that the inflammatory process is confined chiefly to the bronchioles. This is characterized by marked catarrhal inflammation of the wall and extension of the process to the adjacent alveoli where some inflammatory exudation is seen. The peribronchial connective tissue shows marked thickening. This is the result of edema and large mononuclear cellular infiltration. In addition, occasional lymphocytes, plasma cells and even eosinophiles may be seen. This peribronchial inflammatory reaction has extended to the alveolar walls for a considerable distance from the bronchi.

These findings just described represent the basic viral portion of the picture. In addition, we find a secondary inflammatory process characterized by marked serofibrinous exudation within the alveoli. This is accompanied by considerable leukocytic exudate within the terminal bronchioles and atria. By appropriate staining methods, the presence of streptococci in long chains may be observed. This was confirmed by bacteriologic study.

*Chickenpox (Varicella).—*Varicella is another specific infectious disease believed due to a filtrable virus although the evidence for this latter statement is not fully established. Clinically, it is characterized by a variable incubation period ranging from about seventeen days to four weeks. It is highly communicable and it is unusual for an individual to escape infection during childhood. If the disease occurs in later life, it may be particularly severe. Ordinarily, varicella is not considered a serious infection, but occasionally rare examples of fatal cases have been recorded.

The basic lesion appears to be intracutaneous or mucous membrane in location. The virus affects cells between the basal membrane and the surface. With good fortune one may at times be able to make out the typical Paschen-cell inclusion bodies comparable to the Guarnieri bodies of smallpox (Fig. 157). For the most part, however, we find that the cells become swollen, degenerated and gradually break down to become a mass of necrotic tissue. This necrotic tissue tends to accumulate fluid by absorption and the lesion produces the characteristic bleb on the surface. This ulcerates and the lesion becomes secondarily infected with healing taking place from the lower layers of the epithelium as in any other superficial wound. Ordinarily, this lesion being so superficial in its distribution leaves no permanent scar. If, through scratching or particularly extensive necrosis the underlying corium is involved, then permanent pitted scars, so-called pox, persist through fibrosis of the deeper tissues. In a very severe form of chickenpox known as varicella gangrenosa, the virus has a generalized hematogenous distribution with similar focal necrotic lesions occurring in practically all the viscera. This is accompanied by deep infection of the skin, usually over the thigh and buttocks with foul, sloughing, ulcerated areas, which are very extensive. Death results probably as a combination of absorption of proteolytic tissue toxins as well as the result of the direct toxic action of the virus itself.

ILLUSTRATIVE CASE

CASE 74. (Ref. #S-303)
Diagnosis.—Liver—varicella gangrenosa.

Patient was a thirty year old male, who was admitted to the hospital because of the development of a vesicular rash all over his body, but more particularly seen around the face, neck and shoulders. This resulted from exposure to infection from his own child. There was the usual incubation period of three weeks preceding the development of this eruption. He was referred to the hospital by the district health officer with the question of smallpox being raised as a differential diagnosis, and because home conditions made it impossible to care for him there.

Physical Examination.—Physical examination was essentially negative at the time of his admission, except for this unusually heavy, typical chickenpox eruption. The vesicles were unusually large. They presented the typical umbilication, and gradually dried with the formation of superficial scabs.

Laboratory Findings.—Laboratory findings were entirely negative on admission, and it was thought that he would run an uneventful course.

Subsequent History.—After the first five days in the hospital, successive crops of Varicella lesions began to develop (Fig. 192) and progressively involve the trunk and lower extremities as well as the shoulders and upper extremities. These caused the patient a great deal of discomfort associated with severe itching, and in spite of actual restraint he produced secondary infection of several of these lesions with a resulting furunculosis. Over the left buttock area these vesicles became almost confluent and an area of gangrene began to form over the bony prominence of the trochanter. This spread to involve practically the entire left buttock and upper thigh. It was accompanied by profound toxemia with delirium, high fever and a white blood count rising to 30,000. The patient went on and died ten days after admission of this profound toxemia.

Autopsy Findings.—An extensive area of gangrene over the left thigh and buttocks was noted. Vesicles involving the esophagus and mucous membrane of the gastro-intestinal tract were seen (Fig. 195). Vesicles on the peritoneal surface of the liver and spleen were readily demonstrated. Sections of the viscera showed acute hemorrhagic, punctate lesions scattered through the substance of the parenchymatous organs, including the adrenals (Fig. 194).

Microscopic Description of a Focal Lesion in the Liver.—(Fig. 193) The tissue microscopically shows a central area of acute hemorrhagic necrosis. Here practi-cally no cells can be identified. It is a mass of necrotic cell debris. Around the edges of this hemorrhagic mass of necrotic material degenerating cells can be made out. There is a localized, acute, cellular exudate in which polymorphonuclear leukocytes predominate. The liver cells show all degrees of degeneration with karyorrhexis predominating as the terminal event. The lesions are obviously of only brief duration as they are so discrete and acute in nature. There is little or no attempt at repair around the periphery. The picture is one of lique-faction necrosis accompanied by secondary hemorrhage into the necrotic tissues.

Smallpox (variola).—Smallpox to-day is such an unusual clinical condition that very little need be said regarding it. It is again a specific infection caused by a filtrable virus. The history of smallpox is practically the history of modern preventive medicine. Since the recognition by Jenner in 1796, of the value of vaccination, the disease has gradually become more and more under control. Wherever compulsory vaccination is enforced, smallpox is a disease of the past. Where vaccination does not exist, occasional sporadic outbursts of the disease occur.

Pathologically, the picture of the vesicle in small-pox is almost indistinguishable from that of varicella, save in degree. As a rule the variola vesicle is larger, and more often destroys the basal layer of epithelium and involves the corium than does the lesion of varicella, thus resulting in more marked scarring. Likewise, it more often involves the mucous membranes of the mouth and throat than does its milder relation, chicken pox. The establishment of its virus nature has been confirmed by many investigators. The presence of inclusion bodies, so-called Guarnieri bodies, has been demonstrated for many years (Fig. 158). The work of Councilman and Ewing in this field, before the recognition of the significance of the possibility of virus disease, is of the greatest interest in this connection. Goodpasture's more recent work in establishing that these virus inclusion bodies are probably composed of aggregates of the minute elementary bodies seen in vaccinia and first described by Paschen is of particular significance. He has recently proposed the term *Borreliota* as the generic name to be applied to these various inclusion bodies and in the case of smallpox has suggested that they might well be called *Borreliota variolae hominis.*

Pertussis (whooping cough).—Pertussis is still another of the acute infectious diseases, usually of childhood. Its etiology is somewhat under question, but the presence of the Bordet-Gengou or pertussis bacillus is necessary for the development of the clinical picture. Whether or not this is preceded by a virus invasion of the tissues is still open to proof. The work of McCordock and Muckenfuss suggests that this may be true, for they have been able to demonstrate in a considerable number of cases the presence of an intracellular nuclear inclusion body in the bronchial mucosa. The more recent work of Goodpasture in inoculating the embryonic membrane of fertile eggs with the pertussis bacillus alone and the subsequent production of fetal pulmonary pathology comparable to that seen in the human case would point to the fact that the pertussis bacillus alone is responsible for the disease. The organism is a small gram-negative coccobacillus similar in appearance to the influenza bacillus, but grown on artificial media with much greater difficulty and doing best on a medium containing partially reduced hemoglobin and with a pH as low as 4.5.

The disease clinically begins slowly after approximately a ten-day incubation period and the diagnosis is usually not established until the characteristic "whoop" is heard, except in the case of multiple infection in a family, or in epidemics, particularly in a contagious disease hospital. The early diagnosis is obtained by the "cough plate" method, the patient coughing on to a specially prepared blood agar plate. The organism is rarely found in the buccal cavity or pharynx, but only below the larynx in the trachea and primary bronchi. It may be the only organism found in some of the secondary bronchopneumonias which complicate the disease, but more often the cause of death in the secondary infections is again the hemolytic streptococcus as in the case of measles. Pertussis has a higher infant mortality rate than any two other of the contagious diseases.

The pathology of pertussis may be briefly described as a simple catarrhal inflammation of the trachea and bronchi. The organism may be found in myriads tangled in the cilia of the epithelium. It is associated with a marked peribronchial infiltration, in this instance, almost exclusively of lymphocytes. Following this initial tracheobronchial involvement, the lesion spreads as an interstitial pneumonitis, with marked thickening of the alveolar walls by a diffuse mononuclear exudate. In the fatal case, a secondary streptococcic serofibrinous pneumonic exudate is seen within the lung alveoli. The pertussis bacillus is capable of producing a mild toxin, which apparently has a specific lymphoid stimulating effect, with the development of a marked lymphocytosis, which in some instances may exceed 100,000 lymphocytes per c.mm. of blood and be confused clinically with leukemia. Likewise, the toxin tends to have a neurotropic affinity and acute encephalitis with hemorrhage and lymphocytic infiltration, associated with nerve cell degeneration is by no means a rare com-plication of the disease. [See case 180 (Ref. #S-152) Chapter XLIII.]

Mumps.—Mumps is a specific infectious disease caused by a virus which is found in the saliva of infected individuals. Its source, except as it is passed from one individual to another, is not known. It produces an acute inflammation of the parotid or submaxillary glands. It may, and usually is unilateral, but bilateral involvement is fairly common. It is associated with painful deglutition. Complications of this infection are seen in curious predilection of the virus to produce an acute hemorrhagic inflammation of the testis, and less frequently of the ovary. In the testis this assumes the appearance of a hemorrhagic interstitial orchitis. It may lead to actual sterility. It likewise has a tendency to invade the central nervous system and may produce deafness, involvement of the optic nerve and even encephalomyelitis.

PART II

SPECIFIC INFECTIONS TRANSMITTED FROM ANIMAL TO MAN

Anthrax.—Anthrax is a specific infectious disease caused by the anthrax bacillus, a large, gram-positive bacillus with characteristic square ends. It is primarily a disease of cattle and sheep, and is usually found in man as an industrial problem affecting workers with such hides. As a result, it is frequently spoken of as "wool sorter's disease."

The characteristic lesion produced by this organism is the so-called "malignant pustule" (Fig. 68). This is a localized infection of the skin with the development of a vesicle, which forms between the layers of the skin, much as occurs in smallpox. It is characterized, however, by marked hemorrhage so that the picture is a serosanguineous one for the most part. Around the base of the lesion, the other evidence of acute inflammation is observed with hyperemia, edema and leukocytic infiltration. Grossly, the lesion tends to dry centrally and to have a dark purplish red crust with the peripheral zone of erythema and edema. The lesion may remain localized and heal spontaneously. Formerly, it was considered better therapeutically to excise the lesion, but it has since been shown that the mortality is much lower when these cases are treated expectantly. From such a local lesion, the blood stream may be-come infected and a diffuse septicemia with generalized hemorrhagic lesions of all the viscera may follow. At other times, the organism may gain entrance to the body by way of the respiratory tract where it sets up an acute bronchopneumonia, which probably is invariably fatal. One of the outstanding features of the disease is the enormous numbers of organisms present in the lesions or in the blood stream, and other organs, when generalized septicemia occurs. In fact, the diagnosis can usually be made by the examination of a single drop of blood which will be found teeming with myriads of these enormous bacilli.

Bubonic Plague.—Plague is another specific infection caused by the *Bacillus pestis*. It is most often transmitted by the bite of a flea, acting as the intermediate vector. The disease occurs in two major forms; first, the so-called pneumonic form in which the organism probably gains access to the respiratory tract by inhalation. This particular form of the disease is the most virulent and is usually seen in epidemic form. The lesions are those of a hemorrhagic pneumonia with a secondary hyperemia and generalized infection of the viscera. The second form, the bubonic, is the more common type of the disease. This is characterized by painful swelling of the lymph nodes usually in the groin. These are tremendously swollen and on examination are found to present an acute hemorrhagic type of necrotic inflammation. Polynuclear and large mononuclear phagocytes filled with bacteria are present in large numbers. The process is very acute and the lymph nodes commonly break down to form abscesses, which may rupture.

The histopathology is not specific, and the diagnosis is made bacteriologically.

Tularemia.—Tularemia is a specific infection caused by the *Bacterium tularense*. The organism is a small, gram-negative, nonmotile, aerobic one which grows best on a medium containing coagulated egg yolk, or a piece of fresh tissue. It has a pleomorphic appearance with coccoid and bacillary forms. The disease is an interesting one from the standpoint of public health. It is endemic in animals, particularly of the rodent group. It was first described by Francis as occurring in the ground squirrels in Tulare County, but it has been found since to be universal in distribution. The chief source of the infection is the ordinary jack rabbit. The infection may be transmitted to man by direct contact with infected material, so that butchers, hunters and food handlers are particularly liable to the infection. It may also be carried by a variety of insects, including particularly certain ticks, bedbugs and the deer fly. The disease, again, is seen in two forms from the clinical standpoint. In the one, glandular involvement is predominant. In the other, there is no apparent primary lesion, and the picture is one which is clinically confused with typhoid. The diagnosis in this latter form is more often made by serologic agglutination tests. In the glandular type, the patient is taken acutely ill with marked prostration and a relatively high fever. The lymph nodes are greatly enlarged and painful. The lymph nodes often appear before the lesion can be detected. They go on to suppuration and secondary ulceration. In rare fatal cases, septicemic lesions with multiple semigranulomatous areas of necrosis are found in the lungs and viscera. In the milder forms the disease is sometimes mistaken for tuberculosis. It is not a frequent infection, but is one which should be borne in mind in cases of uncertain diagnosis.

Undulant Fever (Brucellosis).—Undulant fever (Malta fever) is a specific infectious disease caused by a small Gram-negative organism now called the *Brucella melitensis*. It is closely related to two other organisms of this group known as the *Brucella abortus* of cattle, and the *Brucella suis* of hogs. The melitensis form is transmitted to man chiefly by the milk obtained from goats, who are highly susceptible to this form of the disease. It is characterized by a rather characteristic temperature curve and by its chronicity. It has a very low mortality rate. In those few fatal human cases which have been reported, a rather granulomatous lesion involving chiefly the reticulo-endothelial system has been described. Meningeal involvement and periosteal lesions have likewise been found. Its diagnosis is made by serological agglutination with a known strain of the organism.

Relapsing Fever.—This a specific infectious disease caused by a spirochete called the *Spirochaeta obermeieri*. It is transmitted by the bite of insects, particularly lice. The organisms penetrate the skin and gain entrance to the blood stream. Most of the cases have been reported in the tropics or in semitropical countries, but with modern travel they are found on occasion widely disseminated. The mortality is very low. The pathology is not specific. It consists for the most part of a hemorrhagic involvement of the mucous membranes and serosal surfaces. The diagnosis is made by the finding of the organism in the blood stream.

Weil's Disease (Spirochetosis Icterohaemorrhagica).—This is a somewhat closely related spirochetal infection characterized by a rather sudden onset accompanied by marked jaundice, a high fever, submucosal and subcutaneous hemorrhages and acute nephritis. The source of the infection is the rat. Its transmission from the rat to man is problematical. It is probably most frequently carried by fleas, but it is believed possible for the spirochete to enter the body through the intact skin, and the disease was seen frequently among soldiers in the rat-infested, wet trenches during the World War.

The pathology of the disease is that of an acute, hemorrhagic septicemia with a very marked toxic hepatitis and tubular nephrosis. Material stained by the Warthin modification of the Levaditi method shows the presence of large numbers of spirochetes within the tissues.

Carrion's Disease (Bartonelliasis).—By the term Carrion's Disease, it is believed two separate clinical conditions should be included: first, *Oroya fever*, and second, *Verruga peruana*. In the light of recent studies by Pinkerton and Weinman, it has been shown rather conclusively that these are merely different manifestations of the same disease, an infection due to the small pleomorphic organism known as the *Bartonella bacilliformis*. The infection is restricted geographically very sharply to an area in Peru. The first stage of the infection may apparently frequently be asymptomatic, and as a result is overlooked clinically. In the more severe forms, which probably merely mean a more massive infection, the clinical picture is one of a severe progressive anemia accompanied by fever and with a very high mortality rate. Strong, and others, in recent years have shown that the association of a paratyphoid B infection simultaneously with the Bartonella infection is of particularly grave significance from the mortality standpoint (Fig. 181).

The pathology of this stage of the disease consists of the invasion of the red corpuscles by the organism, which destroys the red cells rapidly. In the fatal cases it is usually accompanied by severe secondary toxic lesions of the viscera.

Verruga peruana, as distinct clinically from the more malignant *Oroya fever,* is characterized by the presence of cutaneous nodules, which are angiomatous histologically. In the recent work by Pinkerton and Weinman, it has been shown that the same organism is present in these cutaneous lesions as are usually seen in the red cells of *Oroya fever,* and in such instances, occasional red cells could be found containing the specific infectious agent. The organism is found as an intracellular parasite, particularly in the endothelial cells of the lymph nodes, liver and intestine, and has been successfully cultivated in tissue culture from guinea pig and rat tissues. The organism grows as a mass of small, coccoid, granular or even bacillary forms, which it is believed represent merely pleomorphism rather than successive stages in the development of the organism. There is a very striking similarity in the appearance of these clumps of organisms to that of the intracellular Rickettsia of typhus, and Rocky Mountain spotted fever.

The results of this study show that the most important reservoir for the infectious agent is in the group of subclinical human cases, and that the Peruvian guinea pigs in the endemic area were likewise infected in a considerable proportion of cases, although it is questionable whether this organism is identical with the human type. This organism is entirely different from the *Bartonella muris,* which is found in rats, and *Bartonella muris*-free rats could not be successfully inoculated with the *Bartonella bacilliformis*.

In the cutaneous nodules of *Verruga peruana,* the histopathology is perhaps best described as a chronic granulomatous type of lesion, but complicated by the extreme vascularity and angiomatous development previously commented upon.

THE RICKETTSIA DISEASES

Typhus Fever.—This is an acute infectious fever believed to be caused by the *Rickettsia prowazeki.* The disease is found chiefly in the central European and Balkan States, and also in Mexico. The clinical picture is one of sudden onset with a high fever, marked prostration, the development of a bronchopneumonia and a rather characteristic petechial rash which may go on to actual necrosis. The pathology of the disease grossly is one of petechial hemorrhage generally accompanied by marked toxic changes in the viscera, with severe granular degeneration.

The microscopic pathology, which has best been described by Wolbach, is found to consist of a proliferation of the vascular endothelium, particularly that of the peripheral capillaries. This is associated with thrombosis of these minute vessels. In properly prepared specimens (sections should be cut not over two micra in thickness and overstained by Giemsa's method), the Rickettsia bodies may be seen within the cytoplasm of the lining endothelial cells.

The source of the infection seems to be the body louse. The reservoir is not definitely known. In the louse, the organism can be demonstrated within epithelial cells of the gastro-intestinal tract, to which tissue they appear restricted. It requires a period of seven days after infection for the organisms to multiply to a sufficient number for the louse to be infectious. It is not necessary that the individual be bitten as the organisms are present in the excreta of the lice and may pass through the skin through scratches or abrasions. The diagnosis of the disease is fairly well established clinically by the characteristic syndrome associated with the macular rash. From the laboratory standpoint, the Weil-Felix heterologous antibody reaction with the *Bacillus proteus,* for some poorly understood reason, gives a positive reaction in over 90 per cent of the cases, and for that reason is a great diagnostic aid.

Rocky Mountain Spotted Fever.—This is another specific infectious Rickettsia disease caused in this case by the *Dermacentroxenus rickettsii,* as named by Wolbach. This disease is largely restricted to the Rocky Mountain district of the United States, although it has spread considerably beyond the original geographical area. It is an acute disease associated with high and prolonged fever, marked muscular pain, neurologic symptoms, particularly headache, and a macular eruption similar to the lesions of typhus. It is because of its original localization to the Rocky Mountain area and because of the petechial eruption that the disease acquired its name. The Rickettsia are transmitted by a tick, the *Dermacentor venustus.* The disease can be transmitted to most of the laboratory animals, including the monkey, rabbit and guinea pig. In the male guinea pig, particularly, there is a curious predilection for localization within the genitalia accompanied by marked necrosis. The organism has even been demonstrated within spermatozoa and ova, and been transmitted from an infected to a noninfected animal in this manner.

The pathology is similar to that of Typhus fever. There is an endothelial proliferative reaction in the blood vessels, with their cytoplasm filled with minute coccal bacillary Rickettsia bodies. These vascular lesions are commonly associated with thrombosis, hemorrhage and necrosis.

Trench Fever.—Trench fever is another of the specific Rickettsia diseases believed to be caused by the *Rickettsia quintana.* The infectious agent is carried in this instance again by the body louse, and its importance was first recognized during the war. It is characterized clinically by a high temperature, marked prostration and severe pain in the bones and joints similar to the pain seen in dengue or break bone fever. In many instances it is associated with a red, macular rash which may show focal hemorrhage. There is no mortality associated with this particular disease. The disease may be transmitted by the injection of red cells from one individual to another, but not by the injection of serum alone. After the acute phase of the disease, the organisms remain dormant within the individual for many months and recurrences have followed at intervals of more than a year.

One other disease is sometimes included in this series of Rickettsia infections, although the basis for this is not so definite as yet from the experimental standpoint. The so-called tsutsugamushi disease occurring around that district in Japan presents so many features in comman that it is usually believed to be of the same etiology.

PART III

ANAEROBIC BACTERIAL INFECTIONS

Of the anaerobic bacterial diseases, tetanus and the group of gas-producing organisms are the only ones of importance. Their pathology is not pathognomonic, and the diagnosis is made only in conjunction with the bacterial and clinical diagnosis.

Tetanus (Lockjaw).—Tetanus is a specific infectious disease caused by the anaerobic bacillus, *Clostridium tetani.* It results as a rule from some deep penetrating wound, particularly from such wounds as result from the stepping on a rusty nail and the like. It grows best in symbiosis with aerobic contaminants superficially and is, therefore, usually found as a complication of other infection. The organism lives normally in the gastro-intestinal tract of domestic animals, particularly horses, so that this infection is perhaps more often seen in rural districts than in urban communities. There is no specific pathology which can be demonstrated. Organisms multiply in the wound and produce their toxin, which is neurotropic in its affinity. It is carried to the central nervous system by way of the peripheral nerves, chiefly directly along the axis cylinders. The incubation period varies from about two or three days up to two weeks or more. The shorter incubation period is usually seen in relation to wounds of the face, as the nerve trunks are shorter. This tendency for the development of muscle spasm in the jaw muscles accounts for its common name, lockjaw. Congestion of the viscera and of the central nervous system are about the only gross demonstrable changes.

Gas Bacillus Infections.—*Clostridium Welchii (Aerogenes Capsulatus).*—There are three anaerobic gas bacilli, which are frequently found as the cause of death in infected wounds. These include *Clostridium welchii,* the *Vibrion septique* and the *Clostridium edematiens.* These are all gas-producing because of their strong fermentive action upon the various carbohydrates of the tissues. They all go on to produce the condition known as gas gangrene, a type of injury which is particularly seen in warfare, but is encountered to a considerable extent in civil life in association with severe traumatic injuries such as traumatic amputations and the like. The tissues break down rapidly and gas bubbles form which infiltrate the loose connective tissue stroma so that on palpation of the skin even at some little distance from the point of injury, a crepitation may be produced as the gas bubbles are compressed. In addition, Welch's bacillus particularly produces a strong toxin which probably plays a part in the death of the patient. The blood stream is apt to be invaded relatively early, and a generalized septicemia may result. Such patients, following death, unless the bodies are immediately put in the ice box, are liable to become tremendously blown up so that their features even may not be recognizable. At autopsy, all tissues are found infiltrated with the bacteria and to be accompanied by putrefactive necrosis. The liver, particularly, has been described as characteristic. It presents the picture of the so-called "foamy" liver, a spongelike mass of necrotic liver tissue shot through with thousands of small, spherical gas bubbles with the characteristic foul, putrefactive odor of gas bacillus infection.

This should be differentiated from the changes which occur as the result of postmortem invasion of the blood stream and body tissues by intestinal bacteria, especially *B. coli* and others of the colon, carbohydrate-splitting group. The porous appearance of the cut surface of the various viscera is frequently referred to as a "foam" liver, spleen or brain for example. Such a picture is found only in bodies which have not been properly refrigerated and thus encourage the growth of these carbohydrate-splitting, gas-producing organisms.

CHAPTER XX
DISEASES CAUSED BY ANIMAL PARASITES

The importance of animal parasites as a cause of disease has long been recognized, particularly in tropical countries, where they probably rank equal with bacteria in producing pathology. However, with the advent of the mechanical age, and the speeding up of methods of transportation, parasitic diseases once confined almost exclusively to restricted sections of the world, are now being seen as sporadic cases in the temperate portions of the United States and throughout the civilized portions of the world in general. It seems not improbable, therefore, that in the future physicians generally will require an ever-increasing knowledge of such diseases.

The animal parasites of man are rather widely distributed throughout the lower animal kingdom. The great majority, however, belong to the protozoa and helminthes. A few species of arthropoda may be associated also with human disease.

The life cycle of most animal parasites is quite complex, frequently requiring one or two intermediate hosts. When animal parasites enter the body of man, the condition is spoken of as an "infestation," the word "infection" being more correctly applied to a bacterial disease.

"Host" is the name applied to the animal, insect or human being suffering with an infestation. When the adult or sexual stage is present the term "definitive host" or "ultimate host" is used. "Intermediate host" is applied to the host in which the development of the embryo takes place (asexual cycle). The term "vector" or "carrier" is applied to the conveyor of parasites to a new host. Frequently the vector may also be a host for the parasite, in whose body a portion of the life cycle takes place.

The pathology of the more important parasites and parasitic diseases is briefly discussed, with a brief consideration of the life cycles and methods of transportation. The structural details of the parasites, however, have not been included. For these, the reader is referred to textbooks on parasitology.

The following is a table showing the biologic position of the more important protozoa and helminthes infesting man:

CLASSIFICATION OF PROTOZOA PARASITIC TO MAN

SPECIES IN ITALICS ARE DEFINITELY PATHOGENIC TO MAN

CLASS	GENUS	SPECIES
Sarcodine	Entamoeba	E. coli
		E. gingivalis
		E. *histolytica*
	Endolimax	E. nana
	Iodamoeba	I. butschlii
	Dientamoeba	D. fragilis
Infusoria	Balantidium	B. *coli*
	Nyctotherus	N. faba
Mastigophora	Giardia	G. intestinalis
	Trichomonas	T. hominis
		T. vaginalis
		T. buccalis
	Chilomastix	C. mesnili
	Embadomonas	E. intestinalis
	Enteromonas	E. hominis
	Trypanosoma	T. *gambiense*
		T. *rhodesiense*
		T. *cruzi*
	Leishmania	L. *donovani*
		L. *tropica*
		L. *braziliensis*

PLATE XLVI

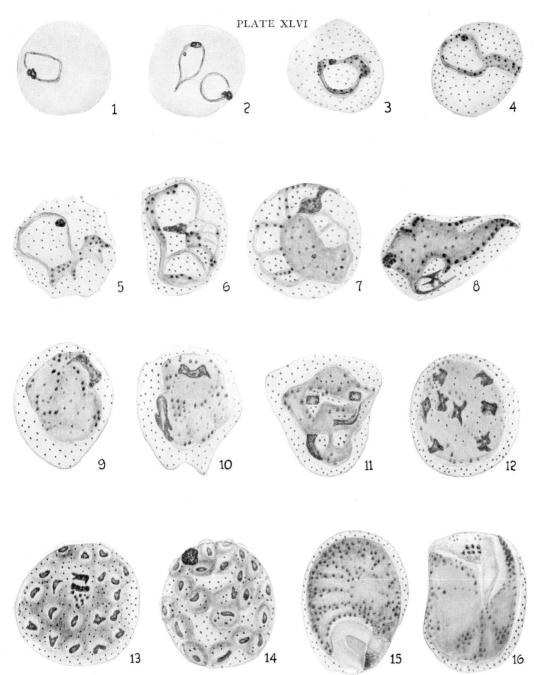

Fig. 196.—PLASMODIUM VIVAX.—Sexual and asexual developmental forms of the parasite within the red cells of man from a case of benign tertian malaria. *Plasmodium vivax,* the parasite of benign tertian malaria of man, as seen in dried blood-films stained with Romanowsky stain. 1-2, Young ring forms, 3-8, Growth of schizont—enlargement of red cell, formation of Schüffner's dots, and development of pigment in cytoplasm of parasite; 9-14, Nuclear multiplication and schizogony; 15, Female gametocyte (macrogametocyte); 16, Male gametocyte (microgametocyte). (From Wenyon, Protozoology, Baillière, Tindal and Cox, London.)

PLATE XLVII
PARASITIC INFESTATIONS

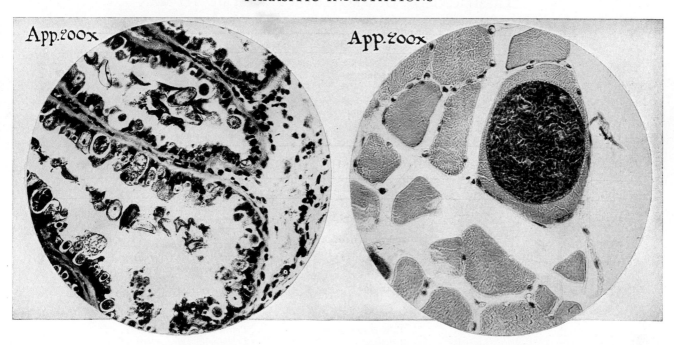

FIG. 197.—LIVER (RABBIT)—COCCIDIOSIS.—Low power photomicrograph from an area showing proliferation of the bile ducts, many cells of which contain coccidia (Eimeria stiedae) in various phases of development.

FIG. 198.—STRIATED MUSCLE (PIG)—SARCOCYSTIS MIESCHERIANA.—CASE 77.—Photomicrograph showing a cross section of "Miescher tube" in which a large number of sickle-shaped spore bodies are seen.

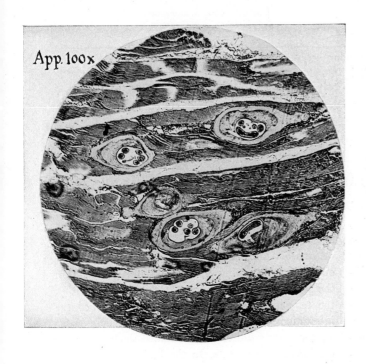

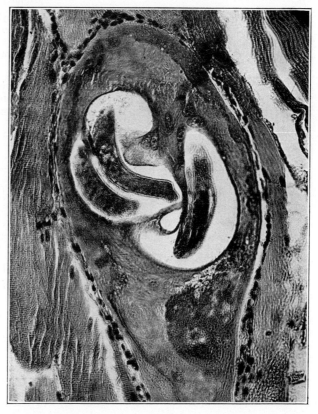

FIG. 199.—STRIATED MUSCLE (GUINEA PIG)—TRICHINIASIS.—CASE 81.—Low power photomicrograph showing several encysted coiled larvae of the Trichinella spiralis.

FIG. 200.—STRIATED MUSCLE—TRICHINIASIS.—CASE 81.—High magnification of a Trichinella spiralis cyst containing the coiled larva surrounded by its capsule and a layer of fibrous tissue in which a few round cells and eosinophiles may be seen.

CLASSIFICATION OF PROTOZOA PARASITIC TO MAN

SPECIES IN ITALICS ARE DEFINITELY PATHOGENIC TO MAN

CLASS	GENUS	SPECIES
Sporozoa	Eimeria	E. wenyoni E. oxyspora E. snijdersi
	Plasmodium	*P. vivax* *P. malariae* *P. falciparum*
	Sarcocystis	S. miescheriana

CLASSIFICATION OF HELMINTHES PARASITIC TO MAN

CLASS	FAMILY	SPECIES
Nematoda	Ascaridae	*Ascaris lumbricoides*
	Oxyuridae	*Enterobius vermicularis*
	Ankylostomatidae	*Ankylostoma duodenale* *Necator americanus*
	Rhabdiasidae	*Strongyloides stercoralis*
	Filariidae	*Wuchereria bancrofti* *Loa loa* *Acanthocheilonema perstans* *Onchocerca volvulus*
	Fuelleborniidae	*Fuellebornius medinensis*
	Trichocephalidae	*Trichocephalus trichiurus*
	Trichinellidae	*Trichinella spiralis*
	Gigantorhynchidae	*Macracanthorynchus hirudinaceus*
Trematoda	Fasciolidae	*Fasciola hepatica* *Fasciolopsis buskii*
	Opisthorchidae	*Clonorchis sinensis* *Opisthorchis felineus*
	Heterophyidae	*Heterophyes heterophyes*
	Troglotrematidae	*Paragonimus westermani*
	Schistosomatidae	*Schistosoma hematobium* *Schistosoma mansoni* *Schistosoma japonicum*
Cestoda	Diphyllobothriidae	*Diphyllobothrium latum*
	Dipylidiidae	*Dipylidium caninum*
	Hymenolepididae	*Hymenolepsis nana*
	Taeniidae	*Taenia solium* *Taenia saginata* *Taenia echococcus* (*Echinococus granulosus*)

PROTOZOAN PARASITES OF MAN

Amoebae.—A number of amoebae may be found infesting the intestine of man. *Endamoeba histolytica, Endamoeba coli* and *Endamoeba nana* are the three most common. Rarely the *Iodamoeba butschlii* or *Dientamoeba fragilis* are present. *Endamoeba histolytica* alone is pathogenic to man. The others live a saprophytic existence as commensals of the intestinal tract.

Amoebiasis or amoebic dysentery is the term applied to infestations by *Endamoeba histolytica*. Clin-

ically, three varieties of the infestation are recognized, acute amoebic dysentery, subacute or chronic amoebic dysentery and a carrier state.

Amoebic infestations are very common throughout the world, being somewhat more prevalent in the subtropics. It is an important infestation within the temperate zone. The highest incidence of the infestation probably occurs in China, where about 14 per cent of individuals examined show either the carrier or disease state. In the United States, varying geographically, from 3 to 10 per cent are said to show the infestation.

No intermediate host is required in this infestation. The disease is spread by the ingestion of the cysts of the parasite, which are produced in chronic and carrier stages. The ingestion of the cysts is usually accomplished by the eating of uncooked foods which have been contaminated by carriers, or even washed in polluted water. The cyst may also be ingested by the drinking of contaminated water. The motile trophozoite cannot spread the disease since it dies out rapidly in the stool. On ingestion, the cysts become active trophozoites in the intestine, invading the mucosa of the large bowel, usually first producing lesions in the cecum, the flexures of the colon and in the sigmoid. (See Chapter XLVI.)

Due to a cytolytic enzyme the amoebae produce necrosis of tissue within the submucosa eventually resulting in the characteristic bottle neck ulceration of the intestine (Fig. 456 and 458). The organisms may enter the venous radicals of the portal circulation and be conveyed to the liver, where, in about 20 per cent of the cases, they produce usually a solitary abscess. (See Fig. 457.) The organism may rarely reach other organs, such as the brain, with the production of like areas of necrosis. Infrequently, an amoebic abscess of the liver may perforate the diaphragm and produce an amoebic abscess in the base of the lungs.

Flagellates.—A number of flagellates are commonly found in the feces of man. The most frequent are *Trichomonas hominis, Chilomastix mesnili, Giardia intestinalis (Lamblia intestinalis), Embadomonas intestinalis, Enteromonas hominis (Tricercomas intestinalis).* Their life-cycle consists of a vegetative, motile form, and a cyst stage.

They are somewhat smaller than the amoebae, and are rapidly motile due to special organs such as flagellae or undulating membranes, or both. For description of the anatomical features of the individual parasite, the student is referred to a textbook on parasitology.

Like the amoebae, the trophozoite rapidly disappears on leaving the body, but the cyst may exist for some considerable time in the stool. It is questionable if any of the group of parasites are truly pathogenic. The *Giardia intestinalis,* which particularly inhabits the upper small intestine, and may be found at times in the gallbladder, is thought by some to produce subacute and chronic duodenitis together with chronic inflammatory changes in the gallbladder. The motile organisms are frequently recovered from duodenal drainage in such cases. The other intestinal flagellates are frequently found without evidence of pathology.

Intestinal Ciliates, Balantidium Coli.—Although several species of ciliates have been described as found in the intestine of man, only one, *Balantidium coli,* has been shown to be definitely pathogenic.

The organisms are from 60 to 100 microns long and 50 to 70 microns wide, oval in shape, slightly more pointed at the anterior end, where a funnel-shaped mouth is present. The surface is covered with fine cilia which enable the organism to move rapidly. In stained specimens, near the mid-portion of the body, is a kidney-shaped nucleus, usually accompanied by a small micronucleus.

The cytoplasm contains vacuoles and granules. The cyst is 50 to 60 microns in diameter, is surrounded by a thick cyst wall, possesses a kidney-shaped nucleus and granular cytoplasm.

The infestation is infrequent in man, but is very common among hogs, where it exists as a commensal organism of the intestine without producing symptoms. It is probably from this animal that the organism is introduced into man.

The life-cycle is similar to that of the amoebae, the trophozoite or active stage occurring in the large intestine, the resistant cysts passing out in the feces.

Pathology. After the ingestion of the cysts, the active trophozoites emerge in the intestine. In the large intestine they invade the mucous membrane, producing necrosis, and eventually ulcerations, which result in a form of ulcerative colitis, simulating amoebic ulcerations. The ulcers are usually oval or rounded, with undermined edges. The necrosis may extend below the mucosa.

On histologic examination, groups of organisms are seen within the mucosa and submucosa together with areas of necrosis (Fig. 460). The exudate is made up mainly of mononuclear cells, with macrophages predominating.

Sporozoa.—INTESTINAL SPOROZOA, COCCIDIA.—Practically all coccidia are true tissue parasites. They infest, however, tne intestine of lower animals, being found commonly in vertebrate and invertebrate hosts. Two species, *Isospora hominis* and *Isospora belli,* have been described as appearing in man, although there is much doubt as to whether even these are pathogenic.

The life-cycle of the organism is passed in one host. The resistant forms are passed out in the feces, where they are capable of existing for some little time. When they are ingested by susceptible hosts, the small oval organism or sporozoite enters a cell, where it is known as a trophozoite. The trophozoite enlarges until it practically fills the cell. This mature trophozoite or schizont, by multiple division of the nucleus and segmentation of the protoplasm, divides into a number of small forms known as merozoites. These break out of the cell, completing the asexual cycle known as *schizogony*. The merozoites attack other cells and repeat the asexual cycle.

Certain trophozoites, instead of developing merozoites, develop within the cell, sexual forms (1) female known as macrogametocyte, and (2) male known as microgametocyte. From these male and female gametocytes, adult gametes will arise.

After maturation, male and female gametes unite forming the so-called zygote. This body enlarges, passes out of the cell, becomes surrounded with a thick cyst wall, and is known as the *oöcyst*. Within the oöcyst several spores are formed. Usually this part of the sexual stage takes place outside the body in the feces. When the oöcysts are ingested the spores formed within produce the sporozoites which invade the cells of the host, thus beginning the repetition of the life-cycle. The formation of the sex cells, cysts, etc., constitute what is known as *sporogony*.

Coccidia have been found associated with symptoms of diarrhea in a number of cases reported in man, and attempts have been made to associate them with ulcerations of the colon. At present, however, no definite proof has been brought forth to establish pathogenicity. In lower animals, however, they constitute a very important source of pathology, especially in the rabbit, where infestation in the liver occurs frequently, with marked proliferation of the duct epithelium, such changes often interfering with the experimental work (Fig. 197).

ILLUSTRATIVE CASE

CASE 75. (Ref. #S-248)
Diagnosis.—Liver (rabbit)—coccidiosis.
In this case, the lesions were found at autopsy in one of the laboratory rabbits, which had been used as a test animal for the Friedman modification of the Ascheim-Zondek reaction for pregnancy.
Autopsy Findings.—The liver was found to be studded with small white nodules 2 to 5 mm. in diameter. Many of these appeared slightly cystic. No other gross demonstrable pathology was found.
Microscopic Description of a Section of Rabbit's Liver.—(Fig. 197) The tissue under the low power appears to be almost honeycombed with cystic areas. These cystic areas are found to be lined by a layer of epithelium which shows very extraordinary papillary hyperplasia. The lesions apparently arise in the bile ducts, and it is the bile duct epithelium which takes part in this almost neoplastic appearing reaction. The point

of interest in the study of this tissue is the recognition of the intracellular coccidia showing almost every possible stage of differentiation from the sporozoites up to the gametocytes. The mechanism appears to be invasion of the epithelial cell by the sporozoite with gradual increase in size and the development of a large nucleus and karyosome. The nucleus apparently divides by repeated fission and forms a variable number of merozoites, which are liberated with the rupture of the schizont. These, in turn, either go through the same cycle and develop into other schizonts or into gametocytes. The sexual cycle, likewise, occurs with the ultimate formation of oöcysts. These later must pass out with the feces and be swallowed by a new host before further development can take place. The tissue has been stained by Heidenhain's iron hematoxylin method as this brings out the histologic details of the parasites more satisfactorily.

MALARIA.—Malaria is another sporozoan disease. The more important varieties are *Plasmodium vivax* (tertian malaria); *Plasmodium malariae* (quartan malaria) and *Plasmodium falciparum* (estivo-autumnal or malignant tertian malaria).

The disease is widespread throughout the world between 60 degrees north and 40 degrees south latitude, its prevalence depending upon the presence of the specific vector, the *anopheles* mosquito, and a reservoir of the organisms in clinically active cases of the disease or in carriers.

The disease is characterized by paroxysms of chills and fever having a definite periodicity. In the benign tertian variety forty-eight hours intervene between attacks. In the quartan type, the paroxysms occur every third day; whereas in the estivo-autumnal, the attacks occur less regularly every 48 hours, and are prolonged.

The life cycle of the plasmodium, part of which takes place in the body of a mosquito, is complex. The asexual cycle is seen in man, the sexual cycle in the mosquito. In other respects it follows rather closely the same phases as described under the intestinal sporozoa, the coccidia.

The sporozoites invade the red cells of man after the bite of an infected mosquito. The trophozoite enlarges until it practically fills the cell and is known as a schizont. By multiple division of the nucleus and cytoplasm it gives rise to small forms known as merozoites. At this time the red cell ruptures, and the merozoites are freed into the blood stream, where each attacks another red cell and repeats the asexual cycle (*schizogony*).

The paroxysmal chill clinically results from the liberation of large numbers of merozoites simultaneously into the blood stream, together with certain toxic products produced by the parasite itself, including large amounts of malarial pigment, the result of cell hemolysis, and the metabolic digestive capacity of the parasite. As has been commented upon in the chapter on pathological pigmentation, the exact nature of the pigment is uncertain.

In addition to the formation of merozoites, some trophozoites develop into sexual forms known as macrogametocytes and microgametocytes. These remain quiescent as long as they stay within the body of man. However, upon entering the gastro-intestinal tract of a mosquito, following the biting of a malarial patient or carrier, the macro and microgametocytes develop and fuse, forming a zygote, which rapidly enlarges, becomes motile (oökinete), and burrows through the wall of the stomach. Here it greatly increases in size and is called an oöcyst. By multiple nuclear and cytoplasmic division spindle-shaped soporozoites are formed within in large numbers. These break out of the cyst and penetrate the venosalivary gland of the mosquito. The cycle of the parasite within the mosquito requires about nineteen days.

If such an infested mosquito bite man, the sporozoite will penetrate the red cells of the peripheral blood and repeat the asexual cycle.

The important species of malaria may be identified by the appearance of the parasite within the red cells of the peripheral blood. In the description that follows, the appearance of the organism is as seen after blood smears have been stained with Wright's or Giemsa's stain.

With this method, the chromatic material of the parasite stains a ruby-red color, the cytoplasm a delicate pale blue (sky blue), the pigment of the parasite black or dark brown, the red cells pale salmon red, and the platelets and nuclei of leukocytes a reddish purple.

Plasmodium Vivax (Tertian Malaria).—The erythrocytes are larger than normal and pale staining. The young parasite, when first seen within the red cell, somewhat resembles a signet ring in shape, the ring being one-third the diameter of the infested cell. The signet portion of the ring consists of a small mass of chromatic material staining red, the rest of the ring being made up of a band of cytoplasm (blue staining). In the center of the ring is a clear, unstained vacuole.

The growing parasite (trophozoite) is irregular in shape, shows one or more chromatic masses with several vacuoles, and some scattered malarial pigment. A number of tiny pale-pink dots (Schuffner's dots) may be seen within the red cell outside the parasite. The segmenting parasite (schizont) practically fills the cell and is made up of 15 to 20 chromatic masses, each surrounded by a blue cytoplasm. When fully developed these are called merozoites. Their arrangement is irregular within the cell with a considerable mass of malarial pigment near the center.

The macro- and microgametocytes (sexual forms) have deep blue cytoplasm. They are round or oval in shape, have a large mass of chromatin and considerable scattered pigment, the pigment in the female being coarser.

In the examination of a malarial slide, any or all of the above forms may be present in the smears of peripheral blood, although usually one will predominate (Fig. 196).

Plasmodium Malariae (Quartan Malaria).—The erythrocytes in this type are normal in size and staining reaction. The young trophozoite occupies about one-third of the diameter of the red cell, and is similar in form to that of tertian malaria. The ring of protoplasm is somewhat heavier, and the chromatic mass is larger.

The growing trophozoite tends to be elongated or band-like, the bluish cytoplasm extending as a band across the cell. Through the cytoplasm numerous irregular elongated red-staining chromatic masses are seen, together with coarse, scattered pigment. Schuffner's dots are not present. The mature parasite (schizont) shows 6 to 10 chromatic masses surrounded by blue cytoplasm arranged as a rosette. Coarse brown or black pigment is seen near the center. The sex forms resemble *Plasmodium vivax,* but the pigment is coarser in texture.

In tertian malaria any or all of the above forms may be seen in the smear from the peripheral blood with one type usually predominating.

Plasmodium Falciparum (Estivo-Autumnal Malaria).—The erythrocytes are smaller than normal and may show distortion. The ring forms (trophozoites) are quite delicate and about one-fifth of the diameter of the red cell. The chromatic mass is small, and the cytoplasmic ring narrow. It is common to see more than one ring in a single cell, which is quite unusual with *Plasmodium vivax* and *Plasmodium malariae*.

The growing parasite (trophozoite) and the division forms (schizont) are rarely seen in the peripheral blood. They may be found in smears from the spleen. The schizont resembles that of *Plasmodium malariae*.

The sexual forms are important and characteristic in this type of malaria. They are sausage-shaped and bring about distortion of the red cell. The male (microgametocyte) is bluish-gray in color, and contains a chromatic mass near the center, which is made up of loosely-arranged chromatic material, intermingled with scattered malarial pigment. The female (macrogametocyte) is thinner, more crescent-shaped, pale bluish in color, and the ends tend to be slightly more pointed. The central chromatic mass and pigment are much more compactly arranged than in the male form. At times the parasite seems to be free, although careful examination shows the deformed red cell which is practically colorless, taking the stain very lightly.

In estivo-autumnal malaria, only the ring forms and crescents are ordinarily found in the peripheral blood smears. However, in overwhelming infestations the growing trophozoite and schizont may be found.

Pathology.—The pathology of malaria is principally due to the destruction of red cells by the parasite, the liberation and disintegration of products of hemoglobin, together with malarial pigment produced by the parasite itself. There results pigmentary infiltration in various organs, imparting to them a slatish-gray color, which is the prominent feature of cases of prolonged infestation coming to autopsy.

In addition to the pigmentation, the destruction of red cells leads to a secondary form of anemia. The cachexia of malaria is partially due to this factor and to other toxic products, which are possibly produced by the organism. Another pathological feature is the result of the actual presence of parasites in such large numbers as to bring about obstruction to capillaries in the intestine, spleen, liver, and particularly in the brain.

Spleen.—In both acute and chronic forms of the disease, the spleen is enlarged. In the acute form, the organ is pultaceous, and on section presents a reddish surface, in which the pulp is greatly congested and soft in consistency. Histologically, innumerable parasites are found in the splenic sinuses, and the reticulo-endothelial cells are loaded with dark brownish or black pigment.

In the chronic form, the spleen becomes enormously enlarged and may weigh over 1000 gm. It is slatish-gray in color, the capsule is thickened, and shows hyalinization. The organ is firm. On section, there is a marked increase of the fibrous tissue. The splenic follicles are apt to be more prominent than normal. The cut surface is dark, reddish in color. Histologically, in addition to large quantities of pigment within the reticulo-endothelial cells, and phagocytic mononuclears, often numerous parasites may be seen. Adhesions commonly exist between the spleen and adjacent viscera.

Liver.—In acute malaria, the liver is usually not grossly enlarged, but in the chronic form the organ may be somewhat increased in size. On section its color is usually darker than normal. Through the capsule it is apt to appear of a rather typical slatish-gray. This is due to the presence of large amounts of pigment (Fig. 39).

Histologically, this pigment is found to lie chiefly in the Küpffer cells. Occasionally, small areas of focal necrosis may be seen in the parenchyma in relation to the sinusoids.

Brain.—The membranes of the brain may likewise impart a pale slatish-gray color to the organ, due to the presence of pigment within phagocytic mononuclears in the meninges, particularly about the capillaries. Within the brain itself pigment is deposited within phagocytic cells adjacent to the tiny capillaries and occasionally these vessels are occluded by aggregations of the parasites themselves giving rise to tiny areas of softening.

Intestine.—In the intestine, a similar slatish-gray color may be seen, due to inclusion of pigment within phagocytic mononuclears within the mucosa.

Bone Marrow.—Within the bone marrow in severe cases a dark color is produced by like pigmentary infiltration of numerous mononuclear phagocytes.

ILLUSTRATIVE CASE

CASE 76. (Ref. #S-305)

Diagnosis.—Acute benign tertian malaria.

(Fig. 196) Patient was a white male, aged 24, admitted with a history for the past ten days of chills, fever and sweating, coming on at intervals of forty-eight hours. He recently had moved from Louisiana, where he had resided for ten years. He was a laborer by occupation.

A typical paroxysm, as observed in the hospital, came on about three o'clock in the afternoon with a severe chill, and rapid rise in temperature to 105. The skin was cold and slightly cyanotic. Pulse was 110 to 120. At the end of about an hour, the patient complained of feeling very hot, the temperature, however, remaining approximately the same. The face and hands were flushed; pulse was 90. The patient remained in this stage four to five hours. This stage was followed by profuse sweating,

with extreme relaxation, with a feeling of comfort and relief of the symptoms. The patient usually fell asleep from exhaustion during the sweating stage. The complete paroxysm usually required not more than ten hours.

Physical Examination revealed enlargement of the spleen.

Laboratory Examination.—Blood count: Red blood cells, 3,100,000. The erythrocytes contain numerous parasites (*Plasmodium vivax*) in various stages of development. Anisocytosis of red cells is present. Hemoglobin 62%. White blood cells, 7,200. Polymorphonuclears 70%; lymphocytes 23%; mononuclears 6% and eosinophiles 1%. Some mononuclear leukocytes contain pigment. Urinalysis revealed a trace of albumin.

Subsequent Course.—The patient improved under treatment, and has remained free from symptoms for some months.

TRYPANOSOMES.—Many species of Trypanosomes have been found in the blood of lower animals and man. In the lower animals, in most instances, the organism produces no symptoms. In man, they may be associated with very serious clinical symptomatology and an extremely high mortality.

The adult parasites are actively motile, have a fusiform body, pointed at each end and flattened from side to side, 15 to 30 microns in length. In the central part is a large nucleus. In the posterior end is a small chromatic mass called the parabasal body. Immediately adjacent is a second small chromatic body, the blepharoplast from which undulating membranes and marginal flagellae arise. The membrane extends along one side of the organism to the anterior end, and the flagella continues beyond for a variable distance.

The life-cycle is complex, the organisms varying considerably in morphology in the course of their development, as for example the intracellular forms, which are amotile, oval and possess neither undulating membrane nor flagellae, and resemble Leishmania bodies.

The parasites require an insect vector in which part of the life-cycle takes place. It has been shown that these vectors can spread the organism mechanically for a few hours after ingestion of infected blood, and likewise after the life-cycle has taken place, which usually requires about 2 to 3 weeks. In epidemics it is probable that the mechanical spread is of great importance. The reservoir of the parasite in human trypanosomiasis is probably in man himself, although certain wild animals (arma-

dillo, bat, opossum, antelope, etc.) have been shown to harbor the parasite.

The three species of importance as disease-producers in man are: (1) *Trypanosoma gambiense,* producing African sleeping sickness, with the vector an insect host, the tsetse fly (Glossina palpalis); (2) *Trypanosoma rhodesiens,* producing Rhodesian sleeping sickness, the vector being another tsetse fly (Glossina morsitans); and (3) *Trypanosoma cruzi,* producing Chaga's disease in Central and South America, spread by the kissing bug (Triatoma megista).

Sleeping Sickness.—Sleeping sickness is a disease characterized by a remittent, irregular type of fever usually accompanied with glandular enlargement. After the febrile period of the disease, the patient gradually progresses into a final stage in which somnolence and apathy are prominent symptoms. Death usually results from coma or intercurrent infection.

The disease as produced by the gambiense variety is less acute, whereas the rhodesian type is more rapid, and the patient may reach the final stage within a few months of the first symptoms.

Pathology.—The organism is found in the peripheral blood in small numbers early. The lymph nodes are enlarged and show congestion with lymphoid hyperplasia. The lesions late in the disease are seen chiefly in the brain, where an extensive meningo-encephalitis is the main feature. Trypanosomes may be recovered from the spinal fluid at times.

Chaga's Disease.—Chaga's disease occurs particularly in infancy, although it may persist in later life. It is characterized by diarrhea, enlargement of the spleen, lymph nodes, thyroid, and frequently accompanied by nervous manifestations.

Pathology.—In this disease there is marked enlargement of the spleen. The liver and mesenteric lymph nodes show moderate enlargement. The brain and cord show numerous small hemorrhages in the rapidly fatal cases. Histologically, the heart and various other muscles may show small colonies of parasites within the cells. These parasites are oval in shape, have a slightly eccentrically placed nucleus with a small basal granule adjacent (Leishmania forms).

LEISHMANIA.—Three important species are recorded in man: (1) *Leishmania donovani,* producing *kala-azar* in India, China and North Africa, and infantile kala-azar in the Mediterranean basin; (2) *Leishmania tropica,* producing *oriental sore* about the Mediterranean basin; and (3) *Leishmania braziliensis,* producing *espundia* in South and Central America.

The life-cycle is rather complex and requires an intermediate insect host, which may be one of the biting sand flies (Phlebotomus argentipes); also, certain bedbugs (Cimex hemiptera). In the insect host, motile forms somewhat similar to trypanosomes occur. In man, the organism is chiefly found within large mononuclear cells as an amotile, oval parasite 2 to 4.5 microns in diameter, having a large nucleus with a smaller chromatic mass adjacent. These are known as Leishmania forms or Leishman-Donovan bodies. They are present in large numbers in the reticulo-endothelial cells of the spleen, liver, kidneys, bone marrow, etc. They result from rapid division of a single phagocytosed parasite. When fully matured the parasites rupture the cell, escape into the blood stream and are immediately picked up by other phagocytic mononuclears. When insects bite such a patient a few of the parasites may be ingested, thus completing the life-cycle. The carriers may transmit the disease both directly and after the life-cycle is complete.

Kala-azar.—Kala-azar is a disease characterized by chronic irregular fever and enlargement of the spleen and liver. Infantile kala-azar runs a more acute course.

Pathology.—At autopsy the spleen is found greatly enlarged with a thickening of the capsule and frequently adhesions. There is a considerable increase in the fibrous tissue of the organ, and many parasites are seen in enlarged mononuclears and reticulo-endothelial cells. In various other tissues of the body, especially the liver and lymph nodes, small groups of parasites are seen histologically for the most part intracellularly.

Oriental sore.—Oriental sore is a cutaneous lesion in the form of a particularly chronic ulcerative granuloma which only heals after many months. Histologically, sections reveal, in addition to the chronic granulomatous inflammatory reaction, phagocytic mononuclears containing the parasite.

Espundia (American Leishmaniasis).—This disease produces lesions somewhat similar to those seen in oriental sore. The Leishmania bodies may be found in the tissues of the chronic ulcerative granuloma.

SARCOSPORIDIA.—The Sarcosporidia are parasites of considerable importance in birds, some reptiles and many species of mammals. They are commonly seen in mice where the organism is the *Sarcocystis muris.*

The infestation is acquired by the ingestion of the organism from the feces or tissues of the infested animal. The sickle-shaped spore body penetrates the epithelial cells of the digestive tract soon after ingestion. They soon reach the muscles by the lymphatics and blood vessels, where they develop sporocysts. These are elongated cysts with numerous trabeculae filled with sickle-shaped spores.

They form in the fibrous tissue between the muscle fibers and are surrounded by round-celled exudate with some fibrous tissue. Grossly, they are elongated, and spoken of as "Miescher's tubes" (Fig. 198).

Man is very rarely the host for this parasite, but several cases have been reported. The organism is known as the *Sporocystic miescheriana.* The muscles of the heart, the laryngeal and skeletal muscles are involved. Cases on record have been reported from India, Sudan and Barbadoes. The infestation seems not to particularly harm the host. This statement is true with most of the animal infestations, although the infestation in the mouse is particularly fatal.

ILLUSTRATIVE CASE

CASE 77. (Ref. #S-249)

Diagnosis.—Striated muscle (pig)—sarcosporidiosis.

As in the case of the coccidiosis, this example of sarcosporidiosis was found accidentally in the routine collecting of anatomical material from the slaughter house.

Microscopic Description of a Section of Striated Muscle from a Pig.—(Fig. 198) Microscopic examination of the tissue shows a number of the encysted parasites. These appear as elongated, sausage-shaped bodies, which on cross section appear almost round. They have a dense, hyalinized cuticle which encloses a large number of smaller sausage-shaped structures known as Miescher's tubules. In these, the typical falciform spores develop. The parasite is capable of producing a strong toxin known as sarcocystine, which accounts for the marked inflammatory reaction which occurs in the surrounding tissues at times. It is not unlike the appearance of trichina in the inflammatory cellular response. There is a moderate mononuclear infiltration of the tissues accompanied by beginning fibrosis.

CHAPTER XXI

DISEASES CAUSED BY ANIMAL PARASITES (*Continued*)

HELMINTHES

Nematoda, Round-worms.—Many species of round-worms infest the alimentary tract and at times the tissues of lower animals, and in a few cases those of man. These worms are multicellular, highly complex parasites, whose general form is cylindrical and nonsegmented. The sexes are separate, and the various organ-systems are well developed, particularly the reproductive and intestinal.

ASCARIS LUMBRICOIDES, THE COMMON ROUNDWORM OF MAN.—This infestation is found rather generally throughout the world, being more abundant in tropical countries. The female has a cylindrical body about 23 cm. in length and 0.5 cm. in diameter. The male is slightly smaller. The infestation is seen in man, in hogs and other domestic animals.

The ova are passed out in the feces. They are 60 by 45 micra, dark brownish in color, and are covered by coarsely mammillated albuminous covering. Beneath this, a clear transparent shell encloses an unsegmented protoplasm (Fig. 213).

The infestation is acquired by the ingestion of the fertilized eggs, which reach the duodenum and hatch. Before the larvae can pass into the adult stage, an extra-intestinal migration is necessary. They penetrate the lymphatics, enter the blood and from thence to the lungs. Here they escape into the air spaces and are coughed up in the sputum. Many are lost fortunately during this period, but some of the larvae are swallowed, and in the intestine reach maturity. About eight weeks are required to complete the cycle. After copulation, the mature female may produce a large number of eggs, which pass out in the feces (200,000 daily). The adults wander about the intestinal tract. Occasionally they may get into the stomach and have been known to be vomited. At other times, they pass into the colon and are excreted with the feces. They occasionally invade the bile ducts and may give rise to obstructive symptoms (Fig. 209). They also may obstruct the appendix. When large numbers of the parasites are present they may produce intestinal obstruction. In the lungs occasionally, petechial hemorrhages result from the migration of the larvae.

ILLUSTRATIVE CASE

CASE 78. (Ref. #S-306)

Diagnosis.—Liver.—Obstructive jaundice due to *Ascaris lumbricoides* infestation with terminal cholemia.

(Fig. 211) Patient was a young Filipina, 12 years of age. She was admitted to the hospital in a state of delirium, with rapid pulse, a temperature of 104°, and icteric tinge to the skin and sclerae.

Present Illness.—For the past six months the child had suffered attacks of jaundice, in which a definite yellowish hue was imparted to the skin, and the patient became depressed. Gastric disturbances with occasional vomiting accompanied the attacks. After ten days or two weeks, the jaundice gradually cleared up and other symptoms disappeared.

About ten days before admission the patient was taken with a similar attack, with fever, jaundice and depression. The condition grew progressively worse and the patient became delirious twenty-four hours after admission.

Physical Examination.—Physical examination revealed moderate jaundice of the skin, with definite icteric tinting of the sclerae. The mucous membrane of the mouth showed a similar discoloration. The liver was slightly enlarged and tender. The gallbladder could not be palpated. The stool was pale in color.

Laboratory Findings.—Urine: greenish-tinted; contained a trace of albumin and an occasional bile-stained hyaline cast. Blood count: white blood cells 10,200. Polymorphonuclear leukocytes 75%; lymphocytes 15%; monocytes 2% and eosinophiles 8%. Icteric index 30; van den Bergh, biphasic. Feces examination showed ova of Ascaris lumbricoides and diminution in bile pigment. Patient failed to respond and died 24 hours after admission.

Autopsy Findings.—The tissues, particularly the serous membranes throughout the body, showed bile-staining. The most interesting feature of pathology was found in the liver. This organ was enlarged slightly and greenish-yellow in color. Some obstruction was apparent in the common bile duct, it being impossible to express bile by pressure upon the gallbladder. The gallbladder was moderately distended. On opening the liver and bile ducts, seven adult round-worms (*Ascaris lumbricoides*) were

PLATE XLVIII
PARASITIC INFESTATIONS

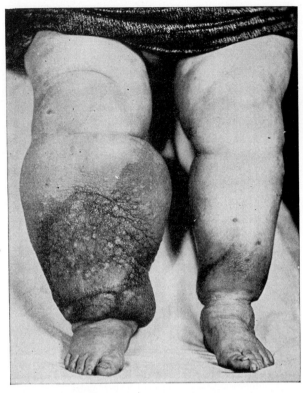

FIG. 201.—EXTREMITY: ELEPHANTIASIS (cf. CASE 80).—Resulting from obstruction to lymphatic circulation by filarial infestation of the regional lymph nodes.

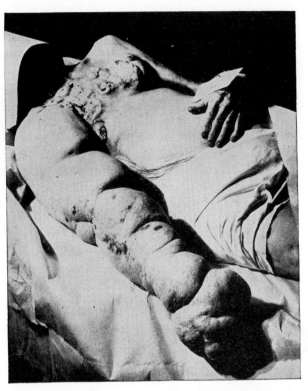

FIG. 202.—ARM: LYMPHEDEMA (cf. CASE 145).—Lymphedema secondary to carcinoma of breast with metastatic involvement of axillary lymph nodes and postoperative fibrous scar tissue formation.

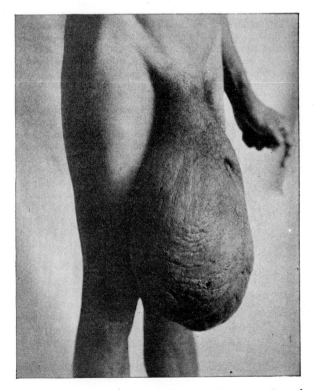

FIG. 203.—FILARIASIS, SCROTAL TYPE.—CASE 80.—Scrotal elephantiasis in a case of infestation by the Wuchereria bancrofti. The scrotal enlargement is rather firm and elastic, not pitting on pressure, as in simple edema.

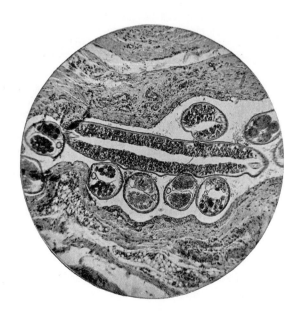

FIG. 204.—LYMPH NODE: FILARIASIS.—Low power photomicrograph showing the Wuchereria bancrofti lying within the lymph vessels. Note the perilymphatic fibrosis. App. 50 x.

found, the largest measuring 25 cm. in length. One of the worms occluded the common duct. The mucous membrane at this portion was swollen and reddish-gray in color. The bile in the ducts and gallbladder was rather thick and stringy, containing considerable mucus.
Microscopic Description of a Section of the Liver.

(Fig. 209) Histologic examination of the liver reveals the picture of biliary stasis with considerable pigmentation and degeneration of the liver parenchyma. There is some slight proliferation of the bile duct epithelium. The kidneys, spleen and heart show parenchymatous degeneration together with bile staining.

ENTEROBIUS VERMICULARIS, THE PINWORM.— This parasitic infestation is very common throughout the world. The female is about 5 to 12 mm. in length, the male somewhat smaller. The worm is cylindrical in shape, with tapering extremities.

The ova are pale, ovoid and flattened at one side (plano-convex), 50 to 25 microns in size. Within this shell the developing embryo is seen folded upon itself (Fig. 213).

The infestation is acquired by the ingestion of fertilized eggs, which in the duodenum hatch, and in about two months, after several moults, the sexually-mature adult stage is reached. After copulation in the upper small intestine, the gravid females descend to the rectum, and during sleep pass out of the rectum and lay their eggs in the perianal region.

The adult females, while inhabiting the lower colon, produce injury by sucking on the intestinal mucosa with resulting petechial hemorrhagic areas. Like lesions in the rectum and perianal region produce irritation and intense itching. Occasionally, the adult parasites may migrate to the appendix, producing irritation, inflammation and obstruction of that organ (Fig. 212). Females may migrate into the vagina and produce marked irritation with itching. The infestation is most frequently found in children, but is probably more prevalent in the adult than is usually thought.

ILLUSTRATIVE CASE

CASE 79. (Ref. #S-307)
Diagnosis.—Appendix—acute gangrenous appendicitis with associated *Enterobius vermicularis* infestation.

(Fig. 212) Patient was a white female of 13 years, who was admitted to the hospital with the chief complaint of pain in the abdomen.
Present Illness.—The illness began four days before with diffuse abdominal pain and vomiting. The patient was given a laxative. The pain continued for two days and then localized in the right lower quadrant. Vomiting persisted and increased in frequency. Bowels had not been moved for two days.
Past History.—The patient's past medical history was negative. Menses were irregular and associated with some pain, lasting from four to six days. Her last period ended on the day of admission.
Physical Examination.—Abdomen was flat and symmetrical. Tenderness and rigidity were noted in the right lower quadrant. Rebound present. Peristalsis was active throughout the abdomen except in this region. No masses were palpated.
Laboratory Findings.—Red blood cells numbered 3,800,000 with 78% hemoglobin. White cells 10,800. Differential count showed 81% polynuclear, 16% lymphocytes and 4% eosinophiles. Urinalysis was negative.

ANKYLOSTOMA DUODENALE (NECATOR AMERICANUS), HOOKWORM DISEASE.—Infestations by hookworm are common in tropical and subtropical countries throughout the world. It is an important infestation of the Southern United States, where it is chiefly due to the *Necator americanus*. In the old world, the *Ankylostoma duodenale* is most commonly found.

Operative Procedure.—The patient was operated under general anesthesia, and the appendix found walled off by fibrous adhesions and the tip surrounded by a small amount of foul-smelling pus. The distal 2.5 cm. of the appendix were apparently gangrenous. From this area a small fecal concretion extruded through an area of perforation as the appendix was removed. The incision was partly closed and a drain inserted.
Subsequent Course.—The postoperative course was rapid and satisfactory. The patient was discharged after fourteen days from the time of admission.
Pathological Specimen.—Gross Description.—The appendix measured 7 x 3 cm. The distal portion was somewhat larger in diameter and had a dark yellowish, seminecrotic appearance. Immediately adjacent was the point of rupture with yellowish, purulent material escaping.
Microscopic Description of a Section of the Appendix.—(Fig. 212) The appendix shows gangrenous inflammation of the distal portion with necrosis of the entire wall. In the proximal part, the mucous membrane shows considerable desquamation with diffuse infiltration of exudate, chiefly polymorphonuclear leukocytes, throughout the submucosa and muscular coat. In the lumen, bodies of several Enterobius vermicularis could easily be identified by the ova and other structural details (Fig. 211).

The parasites are about 1 cm. in length, the anterior end of which is bent dorsally to give the appearance of a hook; thus the name. The mouth is characterized by a buccal armature of chitinous plates or teeth.

The ova are oval in shape, practically colorless, 65 by 30 microns in size. One, two, four or occasionally eight cells are seen within. The shell is wide

PLATE XLIX

PARASITIC INFESTATIONS

Clonorchiasis—Liver Fluke Disease.—Case 82

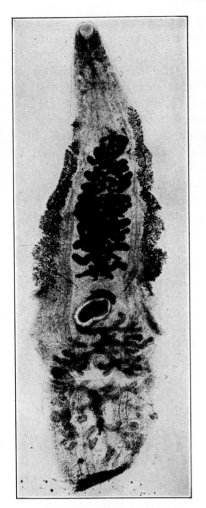

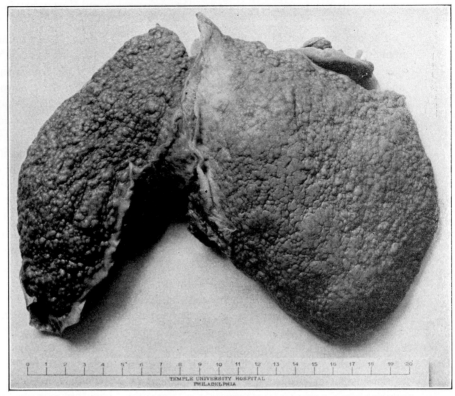

FIG. 206.—LIVER: CIRRHOSIS.—In this liver a number of adult flukes (Clonorchis sinensis) were found. Histologic study reveals marked periductile fibrosis with hyperplasia of the bile duct epithelium (cf. Fig. 492).

FIG. 205.—ADULT FLUKE—CLONORCHIS SINENSIS. App. 10 x.

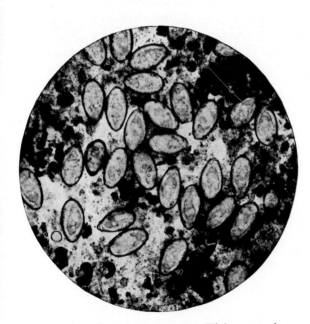

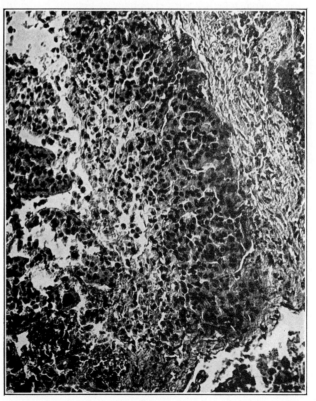

FIG 207.—OVA—CLONORCHIS SINENSIS.—High power photomicrograph of ova within material from biliary drainage. Note the typical operculated eggs in which an ill-defined miracidium may be made out. The terminal tiny hook is not well defined. App. 400 x.

FIG. 208.—LIVER CELL CARCINOMA. (Cf. CASE 82).—High power photomicrograph showing typical liver cell carcinoma apparently resulting from irritation brought about by infestation by Clonorchis sinensis. These were found in the ducts together with large numbers of ova. App. 100 x.

(Courtesy of Am. J. Digest. Dis. & Nutrition (1938) IV, 789. "Primary Liver Carcinoma in Liver Fluke Disease,"
W. A. Swalm, E. S. Gault and L. Morrison.)

and transparent. In freshly-passed feces, rarely more than 4 cells are found, and the hatching embryos never (Fig. 213).

The ova are passed in the feces, and if deposited in moist soil with a temperature of from 25 to 30° C. hatch in about forty-eight hours. The larvae grow, and after about five days are infectious to man. They penetrate the skin usually between the toes, although they may enter between the fingers. At the site of entrance, a local inflammatory reaction results (ground itch). They gain entrance to venules of the subcutaneous tissue, pass through the lung, and to the small intestine by the trachea and esophagus, where they reach sexual maturity in about five weeks. They attach themselves to the wall of the duodenum by means of the chitinous mouth parts.

Pathology.—The small intestine shows numerous bleeding spots, the result of injury produced by the mouth parts of the parasite. Many hookworms are seen protruded from the villi, their head end deeply buried in the mucosa. They secrete a toxic substance which tends to delay coagulation and which apparently also has an effect upon the hematopoietic organs since the degree of anemia is out of proportion to the amount of blood lost through the injury. In severe cases, the anemia is extreme and is frequently accompanied by eosinophilia, sometimes as high as 14 per cent. There are numerous nervous phenomena, together with symptoms of general intoxication, apparently due to the toxic products absorbed from the parasites. In children, growth and sexual maturity are delayed and mental development retarded. In fatal cases, the heart, liver and kidney may show extensive parenchymatous and fatty degeneration.

STRONGYLOIDES STERCORALIS.—This is a small round-worm frequently found as an infestation in tropical and subtropical countries. The life-cycle is somewhat similar to that of the hookworm, except that the eggs usually hatch in the intestine of man and the larvae are passed in the feces. The eggs are 55 by 32 micra, oval, almost transparent, and resemble those of the hookworm, except that they have more cells within, 16, 32, etc. The embryos are found in the feces and are 250 by 500 microns in length, 15 to 24 microns in width. The adults in-

habit the intestine, and with the exception of possibly a mild catarrhal inflammation, give rise to no pathology.

FILARIA.—A number of filaria have been described as parasitic to man. The more important species are: (1) *Wunchereria bancrofti* (*Filaria bancrofti*), (2) *Loa loa,* the eye worm; (3) *Onchocerca volvulus;* (4) *Acanthocheilonema perstans* (*Filaria perstans*); and (5) *Fuellebornius medinensis* (*Dracunculus medinensis*) guinea worm.

They are found in tropical and subtropical countries, particularly in Africa and the East. The adults inhabit the lymph vessels of man. They are filiform organisms from 4 to 8 cm. in length. After copulation, microfilaria, about 250 microns by 8 microns, are produced which are present in the peripheral blood at some time during the day or night. The microfilaria are ingested on the bite of a mosquito (*Culex fatigans, Aedes variegatus,* etc.). Here a developmental stage takes place, after which the mosquito becomes infectious.

Chills and fever, associated with recurrent lymphangitis and slowly-developing elephantiasis, are the main clinical features.

Pathology.—The pathology of filariasis is due to lymphatic obstruction and lymphangitis produced by the adult parasite within the vessels of the abdominal lymphatics (Fig. 204). The inflammatory lymphangitis results in marked perilymphatic fibrosis, together with thrombosis of many of the vessels. As a result, depending upon the group of lymphatics involved, elephantiasis will appear after the infestation has persisted for some months or years (Fig. 201).

The embryos may be demonstrated in the peripheral blood. If the lymph drainage to the extremities is obstructed, marked varicosity of lymph vessels and elephantiasis of the extremities will ensue. At times the thoracic duct may be obstructed in its lower portion and marked varicosity of the abdominal lymphatics result. If rupture occurs chylous ascites may be present. If the lymphatics about the bladder or elsewhere in the urinary tract are affected, varicosities, and sometimes by rupture, chyluria may appear. Elephantiasis of the scrotum may also ensue (Fig. 203), and cause marked incapacity.

PLATE L
PARASITIC INFESTATIONS

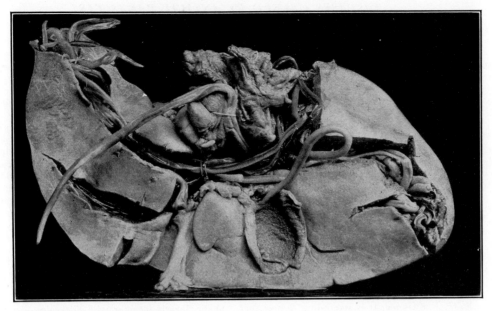

FIG. 209.—LIVER: ASCARIS LUMBRICOIDES INFESTATION.—CASE 78.—Gross photograph showing adult parasites within dilated intrahepatic bile ducts, thereby producing biliary stasis and cholemia.

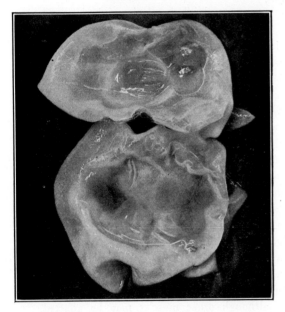

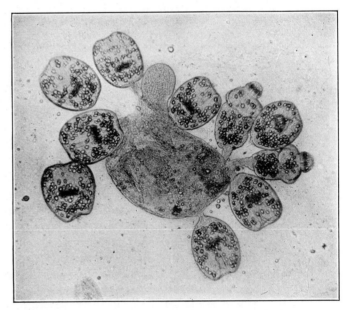

FIG. 210.—HYDATID (ECHINOCOCCUS) CYST.—CASE 83.—A large, hydatid cyst, which before opening measured 12 cm. in diameter. The wall is composed of a pearly white, smooth translucent membrane. Cyst contained a quantity of clear fluid and a number of daughter cysts.

FIG. 211.—HYDATID DISEASE—SCOLICES.—CASE 83.—Brood capsule showing typical developing scolices. The rostellum and crown of hooklets are seen near the centre of the rounded heads. App. 75 x.

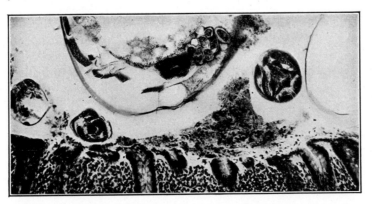

FIG. 212.—APPENDIX: ENTEROBIUS VERMICULARIS INFESTATION.—CASE 79.—Lumen of appendix containing several pinworms shown in longitudinal, and transverse section. Note typical plano-convex ova. Mucosal surface of appendix covered by muco-purulent exudate. App. 100 x.

ILLUSTRATIVE CASE

CASE 80. (Ref. #S-308)

Diagnosis.—Scrotum: Filariasis and elephantiasis.

Patient was a male, forty years of age, who had resided in the Philippines most of his life, but occasionally had traveled in the United States and Canada. He gave a history of having had a number of attacks of "elephantoid fever" over a period of ten years.

During the paroxysms the inguinal lymph nodes were greatly enlarged and painful; and the spermatic cord was enlarged and tender, with gradual increase in the size of the scrotum. The paroxysms lasted for several days, accompanied by headache, occasional vomiting, irregular fever, and finally profuse sweating, after which the patient quickly recovered.

During the last two years the scrotal enlargement persisted and increased until it measured about 30 cm. Lately, the attacks became more frequent; the patient noticed fullness in the abdomen and also a milkiness of the urine.

Microfilaria were found nocturnally in the blood in a previous hospital admission. It is interesting to note that while the patient sojourned in cold climates, such as Canada and Northern United States, the paroxysms did not occur.

The patient was admitted to the hospital for observation and subsequently developed a pulmonary complication with evidence of a patchy consolidation, apparently bronchopneumonia. He did not respond to treatment and died.

Autopsy Findings.—Pericardium was negative. Heart showed parenchymatous degeneration of the myocardium. There was bronchopneumonia of the lungs with pulmonary edema. Spleen showed acute congestion; liver parenchymatous degeneration and the kidneys, toxic nephrosis with moderate bilateral hydronephrosis. The peritoneum showed chylous ascites, the bladder chyluria, and the scrotum elephantiasis. There was chronic lymphangitis with thrombosis of numerous branches of the lymph vessels of the scrotum, bladder and abdominal lymphatics. There was thickening of the thoracic duct. Adult filaria were demonstrated in some of the lymph vessels (Fig. 204).

Microscopic Description of a Section from an Involved Lymphatic.—(Fig. 203) Histologic examination of tissue taken from the area of involved lymphatics revealed marked thickening of the wall due to perilymphatic fibrosis together with thickening of the wall itself. Within one of the vessels illustrated, the coiled filaria are seen in cross section. Other vessels show occlusion or thrombosis.

Note: Very commonly the lymphatics of the lower extremities are involved with associated elephantiasis.

TRICHINELLA SPIRALIS, TRICHINIASIS.—Trichiniasis is a disease due to the infestation by the *Trichinella spiralis,* and characterized in the early state by fever, diarrhea, nausea, abdominal pain, and later with symptoms of acute myositis. It is almost invariably associated with a very marked eosinophilia, although the total leukocyte count may not be unduly high. Differential counts as high as 40 per cent or 50 per cent are by no means uncommon. This infestation is quite widespread in its distribution, being more prevalent where pork is consumed improperly cooked or raw. The infestation is common in man, in hogs, rats, cats and dogs. Many other animals may be infested. Rats about slaughter houses show a very high incidence of the infestation. About 4 to 6 per cent of hogs going to slaughter are infested. Both the larval and adult stage are seen in a single host.

Life cycle.—Man acquires the disease by the ingestion of partially cooked or raw pork containing encysted larvae in the muscle. In about twenty-four hours, the encysted larvae are freed in the small intestine. In forty-eight hours they have reached sexual maturity and copulation takes place. The gravid females burrow into the wall of the intestine and deposit embryos, about 100 microns in length and 5 to 6 in diameter, within the lymph spaces. From eight to nine days are required from the ingestion of the infected meat to the production of embryos. Embryos continue to be produced by the gravid females for several weeks. Many embryos pass out into the intestine and in the feces; others may be found within the blood where they are carried passively to various organs. They penetrate the capillary walls and become encysted within the connective tissue of the muscle.

Pathology.—The gastro-intestinal and toxic manifestations are apparently due to the invasion of the parasites and the liberation of embryos into the circulation. The penetration of the muscle and encystment is accompanied by an acute interstitial myositis with swelling, tenderness and pain of the affected muscles. The heaviest infestation is usually seen in the diaphragm, pharynx, tongue and intercostal muscles, although other muscles may be affected. Histologic examination of the affected muscle reveals numerous encysted embryos coiled within a cyst-wall secreted by the embryo, which in turn is surrounded by a reactionary exudate of round cells, fibroblasts, mononuclears, and occasional polynuclear and eosinophilic leukocytes. This exudate later is replaced by fibrous tissue (Fig. 199) and the embryo itself becomes calcified. The cyst measures about 400 microns in length by 250 microns in width, and contains within, the embryo, measuring about 750 microns, and coiled upon itself (Fig. 200).

PLATE LI
PARASITIC DISEASES

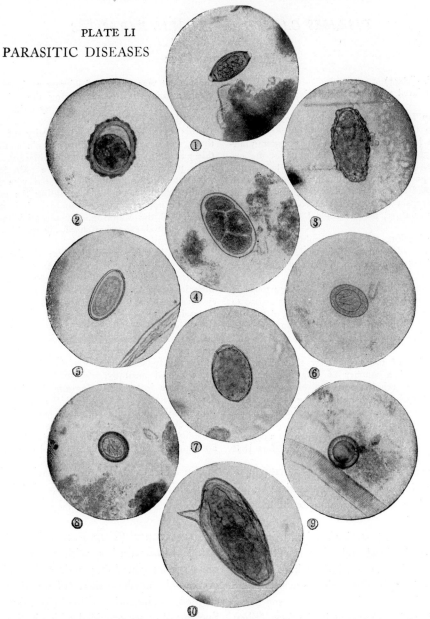

Fig. 213.—Ova which may be found in the feces, showing comparative size (photographs, x 250): 1. *Trichuris trichuria* (whipworm); 2. *Ascaris lumbricoides* (roundworm), fertilized; 3. *Ascaris lumbricoides,* unfertilized; 4. *Necator americanus* (hookworm), four-cell stage; 5. *Oxyuris vermicularis* (pinworm); 6. *Hymenolepsis nana* (dwarf tapeworm); 7. *Diphyllobothrium latum* (fish tapeworm), the edge of the lid being out of focus; 8. *Taenia saginata* (beef tapeworm); 9. *Taenia solium* (pork tapeworm) lying beside a striated muscle-fiber; 10. *Schistosoma mansoni* (blood fluke).

(From Todd & Sanford, *Clinical Diagnosis by Laboratory Methods,* W. B. Saunders Co., Philadelphia.)

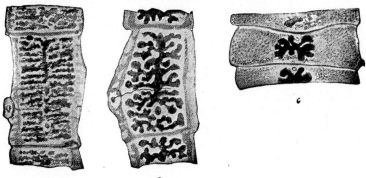

Fig. 214.—Segments of the three large tapeworms of man, showing arrangement of uterus. (a) *Taenia saginata;* (b) *Taenia solium;* (c) *Diphyllobothrium latum* (x 5).

(From Kolmer & Boerner—*Approved Laboratory Technic,* 2 ed. D. Appleton-Century.)

ILLUSTRATIVE CASE

CASE 81. (Ref. #S-53)

Diagnosis.—Striated muscle—trichiniasis; encysted trichinae.

Patient was an Italian woman, 44 years of age, who was admitted to the hospital because of fever, nausea and pain, which had localized in the right upper quadrant, of forty-eight hours' duration, although at the onset there had been generalized pains in all her bones. She had had several previous attacks similar in nature, which had been diagnosed as chronic cholecystitis, and she had a qualitative dyspepsia relating to fried foods. Pain was of an intermittent nature, nonradiating, but very severe, like labor pains.

Physical Examination.—Physical examination revealed an obese, middle-aged woman with tenderness in the upper right quadrant on palpation. Heart and lungs were negative. Blood pressure was 112/68.

Laboratory Findings.—Red blood cells, 4,300,000; hemoglobin, 10 grams (63%). White blood cells 10,000 to 20,000, with 33 to 42% polynuclear leukocytes, 6 to 13% lymphocytes, 1 to 2% monocytes and 40 to 60% eosinophiles. Stool examination was negative for parasites and ova.

X-ray examination of the gallbladder showed a low dye concentration and a number of ring-like shadows suggesting nonopaque (cholesterol) gallstones.

Operative History.—On the basis of the high eosinophilia, a muscle biopsy was done, and the diagnosis of trichiniasis was established histologically.

Subsequent Course.—Subsequent history from a daughter, who spoke more English, brought out the fact that the patient was very fond of raw pork sausage and had eaten a good deal of it during the winter. No other members of the family showed any evidence of trichinal infestation.

This case illustrates the difficulty of diagnosis, at times, when some underlying chronic condition such as this patient had, a chronic gallbladder, masks the actual acute picture. The original diffuse pain in this patient was not given sufficient weight and was thought to be a mild "grippy" condition initiating the gallbladder attack. The upper right quadrant pain is best explained as invasion of the diaphragm by the trichinae. It is likely that no actual exacerbation of the gallbladder condition existed at all.

The patient improved slowly and was discharged at the end of three weeks on the road to recovery.

Microscopic Description of Section of Striated Muscle.—(Fig. 199 and 200) The tissue shows the encysted larvae cut in various planes as they have embedded themselves in the connective tissue stroma of the muscle. There is a moderate mononuclear cellular reaction about the parasites associated with some fibrosis. The dense, almost hyalinized cyst wall is easily identified and the coiled and twisted larvae may be readily recognized and reconstructed mentally.

This case is too early for any definite calcification to have occurred but has passed the most acute phase in which the cellular infiltration is particularly prominent. In this particular instance, the inflammatory response has subsided to a large mononuclear and lymphocytic one accompanied by a considerable number of eosinophiles.

TRICHOCEPHALUS TRICHIURUS, THE WHIPWORM.—The organism inhabits the cecum and colon of man. It is found as a common parasite in tropical and subtropical regions.

The adult has a thick posterior portion, being thin and whip-like at the head end, thus resembling a whip. It measures about 4 cm. in length. The slender anterior portion penetrates the mucosa of the intestine.

A large number of ova pass out in the feces. They measure 50 by 23 microns. They are brownish in color, having an inner and outer shell, with a transparent area between, and two knob-like structures at either pole (Fig. 213).

If the ova fall in moist soil, the embryos develop in a varying period of time. On ingestion of the eggs, the larvae grow to adult size and attach themselves to the intestine. No intermediate host is required.

Pathology.—Few, if any, symptoms result from the infestation of the whipworm, though occasionally, due to the injury of the intestinal wall, secondary infection may occur. At times large numbers of the worms have been found in the appendix, and may produce catarrhal inflammations of this organ. This infestation is not accompanied by any eosinophilia.

TREMATODES (THE FLUKES).—The flukes are flat, leaf-like parasites, with a nonsegmented body, most species containing both male and female sex organs (hermaphroditic). The cuticle is specially adapted for absorption of food from the environment. Sucking discs are provided which enable the parasite to adhere. A number of species infest man. The most important are: *Fasciolopsis buskii, Fasciola hepatica* and *Clonorchis sinensis.*

Their life cycle is extremely complex, the adult state taking place in man with developmental phases in one or two other hosts. The life cycle is well illustrated by *Clonorchis sinensis,* the Chinese liver fluke. The operculated ova, containing a ciliated miracidium pass out in the feces of infested man. If the environment is suitable the eggs hatch and the miracidium seeks out a fresh water snail. It penetrates the lymph spaces and undergoes development (sporocyst, redia, cercaria) and leaves the body to swim about in the water, penetrating the gills of fresh water fish (carp family), in the muscle of which it encysts. The infestation is acquired by eating the partially cooked or raw fish containing the cysts. In the intestine the encysted cercaria are liberated, the young flukes enter the bile ducts and grow to adult sexual maturity, where they produce large numbers of eggs, which may be recovered from the gallbladder, or duodenum, and are also found in the feces. The ova of the flukes are oval, usually dark in color, and have a lid or operculum at one end, which facilitates the escape of the embryo. They usually contain, when passed in the feces, a well-developed miracidium.

FASCIOLOPSIS BUSKII, THE INTESTINAL FLUKE.—It is about 7 cm. in length and 1 cm. in width, inhabiting the upper small intestine, where it may produce stasis and injuries resulting in small hemorrhages or even infections of the mucous membrane.

The life cycle is similar to that previously described. The ova, which are 135 by 80 micra, are brownish in color, oval in shape, with a delicate operculum at one end, passing out with the feces. It is particularly found in oriental regions, especially in China where it is spread by the peeling of infested caltrops and water chestnuts by the teeth. These plants contain the encysted cercaria. The intermediate host is a form of fresh water snail.

FASCIOLA HEPATICA.—This is an important fluke of sheep, rarely of man. It is 3 cm. in length, and produces "liver rot" in animals, due to the presence of the organism in the biliary tract. The intermediate host is a form of snail. The cercaria encyst themselves upon grasses and aquatic vegetation, thus grazing animals are infested. The ova are passed out with the feces, and measure 140 by 80 micra, are operculated, and similar to *Fasciolopsis buskii*.

CLONORCHIS SINENSIS, CHINESE LIVER FLUKE.—The infestation is confined to China and the East, where it is common in provinces in which raw or partly cooked fish is an article of diet. Occasional cases are found in this country in patients coming from the Orient. The infestation is not confined to man, but animal reservoirs are found. The life cycle has already been given. Two intermediate hosts, one a mollusk and the other a fresh water fish, are required to complete the life cycle.

The ova are 29 by 16 micra, shaped like an old-fashioned electric light bulb with a tiny curved spine and flattened at the other end. They are light brown in color and contain a well-developed miracidium (Fig. 207).

Pathology.—The adult flukes infest the bile ducts of the liver (Fig. 205). Here, due to their mechanical presence and by irritating secretions, they produce proliferation of the duct epithelium together with obstruction. In heavy infestations, small areas of necrosis of 1 to 3 cm. in diameter may occur, containing large numbers of the flukes. There is also a marked increase in the interlobular and periductile fibrous tissue of the liver. In the more chronic cases the liver thus presents a picture of cirrhosis (Fig. 206). The parasites may persist for a number of years, as long as twenty. Occasionally the irritation, in addition to producing proliferative changes in the duct epithelium, may result in the development of carcinoma of the liver either of the liver cell or bile duct epithelial type, which may spread and eventually destroy the patient (Fig. 208).

ILLUSTRATIVE CASE

CASE 82. (Ref. #S-309).

Diagnosis.—Atrophic portal cirrhosis with ascites due to infestation of the bile ducts by *Clonorchis sinensis*.

(Fig. 208) Patient was a Chinese male, aged 39. His occupation was that of a laundryman. He was admitted to the hospital complaining of swelling of the feet, legs, scrotum and abdomen, which had persisted for the past four months.

The patient's attention was called to the swelling of his feet by the fact that his shoes seemed too small. A few weeks later, the scrotum seemed to enlarge. He was born in China and came to the United States from South China in 1910. He returned to China and remained there for two years, 1924-26.

Physical Examination.—Blood pressure 140/74. Temperature, pulse and respirations were within normal limits. There was slight jaundice of the sclerae. Pupils reacted to light and accommodation. Chest examination revealed generalized râles throughout with some dullness at the left base. Heart was enlarged to the left. Abdomen: some ascites were apparently present. The abdominal wall was edematous. The scrotum was markedly edematous. Liver was two fingers below the costal margin and was tender. Extremities showed marked subcutaneous edema.

Laboratory Findings.—Blood count: Red blood cells 4,400,000 with 12.5 grams of hemoglobin. White blood cells 5,700 with 67% polymorphonuclear leukocytes and 23% lymphocytes. Urinalysis was negative. Serology was negative. Blood chemistry: nonprotein nitrogen, 33. Total protein, 6.8 grams. Albumin, 3.2. Globulin, 3.6, with albumin/globulin ratio of 0.88. Icterus index, 20 units.

Van den Bergh, delayed direct reaction. Indirect, 1.8 mgm. per 100 c.c. Cholesterol, 200. Serum calcium, 9.5. Serum phosphorus inorganic, 4.06. Phosphatase, 6.86. There is a trace of urobilinogen. Stool negative for ova and parasites. Takata ara, positive. Ascitic fluid, negative for malignant cells; and sterile. Eye ground normal except arteriosclerosis, grade I, hypertensive type. X-ray: G.I., negative.

Subsequent Course.—A few days after admission, paracentesis abdominis was done and four quarts of pink fluid withdrawn. Again, two weeks later, two and one-half quarts of fluid were removed. Patient became progressively weaker, ascites more severe and he became comatose and died without recovering consciousness.

Autopsy Findings.—There were 700 c.c. of faintly hemorrhagic fluid in the peritoneum. The liver weighed 825 gm. and was markedly contracted, shrunken and fibrotic, presenting a typical hobnail appearance. (Fig. 206). The liver was pale in color. The hobnailing was quite regular. A few vascular adhesions were present between the adjacent peritoneum and diaphragm

in the capsule of the liver. The individual knobs were about 2 to 8 mm. in diameter. There was no evidence of malignancy. The liver seemed not to be bile-stained. Gallbladder was normal in size and contained 10 c.c. of brownish-black bile, which was rather viscid. No stones were present.

Examination of this bile microscopically revealed the presence of numerous ova of *Clonorchis sinensis*. Careful dissection of the ducts of the liver resulted in the recovery of five adult flukes. The spleen was enlarged, firm, slatish-gray in color and presented a congested surface in which the trabeculae and follicles were prominent. Kidneys showed nephrosclerosis. Varicosities of the esophageal and gastric veins were noted. Abdominal varicosities were not demonstrated.

Microscopic Description of a Section of the Liver. —(Fig. 492) Examination of the liver reveals a diffuse perilobular and interlobular fibrosis consisting of mature fibrous tissue together with considerable bile duct proliferation. The process is quite diffuse. No definite areas of necrosis are seen. An occasional round cell and plasma cell may be seen in connection with the extensive fibrosis.

Note: In another case coming to the attention of the authors, with somewhat similar history, autopsy revealed, in addition to the presence of a diffuse cirrhosis, papillomatous-like proliferation of the larger bile duct epithelium, and in the right lobe of the liver a large primary liver cell carcinoma (malignant hepatoma), and several areas of necrosis 1 to 3 cm. in diameter containing a number of adult flukes were present. The antemortem diagnosis of this case was directly made by the finding of the eggs from bile obtained from nonsurgical biliary drainage (Fig. 208).

OPISTHORCHIS FILINEUS.—This is a fluke common to the bile ducts of cats and dogs, occasionally found in man. The life cycle, pathology and transmission are similar to that of Clonorchis sinensis. The ova measure 30 by 12 micra, and resemble those of Clonorchis sinensis.

PARAGONIMUS WESTERMANI, THE LUNG FLUKE. —This fluke is of some importance in the East and also in Central and South America. The flesh-colored fluke is small, about 1 cm. in length. Its life cycle requires two intermediate hosts, a snail and a crayfish or crab. Certain wild animals also act as host reservoirs. The disease is acquired by the eating of partially cooked crab or crayfish. In Korea the uncooked juice of the crayfish is used by the natives as a medicine in certain fever and diarrheal states.

The ova are found in the sputum, and also may appear in the feces, having been swallowed. They are 95 by 55 micra in size, brownish in color and operculated.

Pathology.—The parasite, on reaching the lung,

forms burrows, particularly in the lower lobes, with occasional cyst-like nodules. All the lesions are surrounded by a thick fibrous wall. The burrows frequently connect with bronchi, and the eggs, which are produced in large numbers, are discharged with the sputum. In some cases hemorrhage of the lung may occur.

SCHISTOSOMA, SCHISTOSOMIASIS, BLOOD FLUKES. —Three Schistosoma are found infesting man (1) *Schistosoma hematobium*, in Africa and about the Mediterranean basin; (2) *Schistosoma mansoni*, in South America, parts of Africa and the West Indies; and (3) *Schistosoma japonicum*, in the Orient.

The Schistosoma are somewhat cylindrical, and the sexes are separate. The life cycle requires a snail as an intermediate host. The infection is acquired by the motile cercaria penetrating the skin of man while working or swimming in water. In certain parts of the East and in the Nile Valley, crops are planted and cultivated in flooded fields, thus exposing the laborer to infestations of this type.

Pathology.—The adults take up their residence in small veins about the bladder, rectum, etc. The ova work their way through the wall and appear in the urine and feces. Considerable inflammatory reaction takes place, together with necrosis, ulceration of the mucosa, and hemorrhage, with bleeding into the bladder or rectum. There thus results a rather marked anemia. Eosinophilia is irregularly present.

In *Schistosoma hematobium* infestations, the veins about the bladder are particularly affected, so that hematuria is an important symptom. In addition to the lesions mentioned, malignancy of the bladder may arise, as a result of the irritation produced by the ova.

The ova may be found in the urine, are 140 by 55 micra, oval in shape, and contain a well-developed miracidium. There is a definite terminal spine at one end. They are nonoperculated.

In *Schistosoma mansoni* infestation, the veins of the lower intestine are usually predilected; and in addition to ulcerations, hemorrhage, and papillomatous proliferation of the mucosa occur.

The ova are passed in the feces, measure 150 by 60 micra, are nonoperculated, and contain a well-developed miracidium. There is a characteristic large lateral spine (Fig. 213).

In *Schistosoma japonicum* infestation, the intestinal veins contain the adult; the eggs are passed into the feces. They are 85 by 60 microns in size, oval in shape, and contain a well-developed miracidium. They are nonoperculated. The pathology is somewhat similar to that produced by Schistosoma mansoni.

Cestodes, Tapeworms.—Tapeworm infestations are very common throughout the world in both animals and man. The parasites are flat, tape-like worms with a minute head provided with suckers and hooklets, from which a segmented body develops. They are hermaphroditic, and have a special cuticle through which nutrition is absorbed from the surrounding environment. Their mature segments are sexually complete, so that each may produce large numbers of eggs.

Man is the ultimate host in most tapeworm infestations and harbors an adult sexually-mature parasite. An intermediate host is required, in which the larval forms are developed. Occasionally man may be the intermediate host (somatic tineasis).

TAENIA SAGINATA, THE BEEF TAPEWORM.—It has a tiny pyriform head, 1 to 2 mm. in diameter, with 4 lateral suckers. The body consists of from 1000 to 2000 segments, and the worm is from 10 to 25 feet long. The mature segments are longer than they are wide and contain a uterus with 18 to 30 lateral branches (Fig. 214).

The ova are passed out in the feces in large numbers. They are round in shape, 35 micra in diameter. The outer covering is radially striated. Within, a hexacanth embryo with hooklets can be seen (Fig. 213).

The worm attaches itself to the upper part of the intestine, the body extending for a number of feet

free in the intestinal lumen. The symptoms are due to their large size and absorption of food from the intestine, together with production of a certain degree of irritation. The larval stage is not seen in man.

Life cycle and transmission of disease.—The ova pass out in the feces, and the eggs are ingested by animals, especially cattle. In the gastro-intestinal tract the embryo (hexacanth embryo) reaches the muscle by way of the lymph and blood stream. Here it becomes encysted (*Cysticercus bovis*) as an elliptical, pearly gray area 9 by 5 mm., visible grossly in the muscle. The cysts are ingested by man in the eating of raw or partially cooked ground beef or improperly cooked sausage containing the cysts.

TAENIA SOLIUM, PORK TAPEWORM.—The head is globular about 1 to 2 mm. in diameter with 4 sucking disks and a number of hooklets. It is about 8 to 12 feet long with approximately 1000 segments. These are characterized by a uterus with 8 to 10 branches (Fig. 214).

The ova are passed out in the feces and appear almost identical with those of *Taenia saginata* (Fig. 213). The adult parasite attaches itself to the upper intestine and produces symptoms much the same as *Taenia saginata*.

The life cycle is similar to that of *Taenia saginata,* except the intermediate host usually is a hog. The encysted larvae (*Cysticercus cellulosa*) may be seen as oval, pearly bodies in the muscle of infested pork (measly pork). If this pork be ingested insufficiently cooked or raw, the infestation may result. Very rarely man may act as intermediate host, and the larval encysted stage may occur. *Taenia solium* infestations are rare in the United States, but much more common in Europe. *Taenia saginata* is the most common greater tapeworm infestation in the United States.

TAENIA DIBOTHRIOCEPHALUS, DIPHYLLOBOTHRIUM LATUM, FISH TAPEWORM.—This infestation is of importance, particularly in the Orient, although a few cases have occurred about the Great Lake region of the United States and Canada.

Man is the ultimate host and harbors the adult worm. The parasite is 10 to 34 feet in length. The head is almond-shaped, about 2 to 3 mm. in length, and has two lateral sucking grooves. No hooklets are present. The body is made up of about 4000 segments. The mature segments are broader than they are long and are characterized by a rosette-shaped uterus (Fig. 214). The ova are oval, about 70 by 45 micra, and are operculated. No embryo is seen within (Fig. 213). The intermediate host requires a larval stage in a cyclops and finally an encysted stage in one of the fresh water fishes (pike, perch, trout, etc.). The infestation is acquired in man from the eating of raw or insufficiently cooked fish. The pathology is the same as in *Taenia solium* and *Taenia saginata* infestations.

TAENIA ECHINOCOCCUS, HYDATID DISEASE, DOG TAPEWORM.—In this worm, man acts as intermediate host, the adult stage being passed in the dog. The adult *Taenia echinococcus* is small, 3 to 5 mm. in length, consisting only of a head and three segments. The head is equipped with four sucking disks and a number of hooklets.

When ova are ingested by man the embryos develop in various organs of the body, particularly the liver, producing hydatid cysts. When the embryos penetrate the tissues, the body of the embryo gradually develops into a cyst of varying size, from 2 to 3 cm. up to 15 or 20 cm. Secondary cysts are formed by invagination of the inner wall. From secondary cysts tertiary cysts may develop, and finally tiny heads or scolices are produced by evagination of portions of the cyst wall. These scolices become detached in the cyst fluid (Fig. 210). In the fluid the tiny scolices are seen to be equipped with hooklets and sucking disks. Ordinarily, the head is invaginated into the body cavity. Thus chitinous hooklets appear as if in the middle portion (Fig. 211).

After a period of months, the heads degenerate, but the chitinous hooklets persist in the fluid. This fluid is very toxic and may produce grave symptoms if spontaneous rupture of the cyst occurs, or if the fluid is spilled during surgical removal. In the various organs the cyst is surrounded by a zone of fibrous tissue, in which may be seen numerous mononuclears, phagocytes, eosinophiles, etc. The spontaneous rupture of the cysts lead to implantation of daughter cysts in other locations, which develop in a similar manner as the parent cyst.

ILLUSTRATIVE CASE

CASE 83. (Ref. #S-310)

Diagnosis.—Taenia echinococcic cysts of the liver; infestation with *Taenia echinoccocus*.

(Fig. 210 and 211) Patient was a white male, 22 years of age, admitted to the hospital with a history for the past nine years of paroxysms characterized by a numb feeling in the abdomen, lasting for two to three days. During the attack there were also nervous depression and irritability. No digestive disturbances had been noticed. His appetite was good but he had lost weight steadily (20 pounds in the last three years).

Physical Examination.—Physical examination revealed a rounded mass about the position of the gallbladder. Exploratory laparotomy revealed the presence of a cyst 12 cm. in diameter, pearly-white in color, attached to the undersurface of the liver and pressing against the gallbladder and cystic and common ducts. The gallbladder was somewhat distended. A second cyst was discovered attached to the large intestine near the splenic flexure, and a third about 5 cm. in diameter was discovered attached to the surface of the bladder. The cysts were removed surgically without rupture.

Subsequent Course.—The patient made an uneventful recovery and has had no recurrence of the symptoms to date (8 years).

Gross Pathology.—The specimens consisted of three cysts, measuring 12, 6 and 5 cm. respectively (Fig. 210). They were smooth-walled except for the area of attachment. They contained an almost clear fluid which on centrifugation revealed numerous brood capsules with scolices of the Taenia echinococcus (Fig. 211).

These heads are formed from evagination of projections from the cyst wall which become detached and constitute brood capsules. The head is equipped with a rostellum, about which are surrounded a number of hooklets. These can be readily seen in the figure. Usually, the rostellum and hooklets are invaginated into the body or main portion of the scolex, so that the hooklets appear near the centre. Upon irritation or pressure the rostellum pops out. The scolex measures 175 microns in diameter.

On opening the cyst, daughter cysts are seen, some attached to the wall, others floating free in the fluid, the largest measuring 3 cm. in diameter. The pathology of the other two cysts is essentially the same as that described.

Note: In old cysts the fluid does not contain the scolices, these having undergone degeneration. The chitinous hooklets, however, persist, and diagnosis can sometimes be made by recovering them in the fluid.

HYMENOLEPSIS NANA, DWARF TAPEWORM.—This infestation is very common, particularly in children in the United States and elsewhere. Man is the ultimate and intermediate host, the adult and larval stage both occurring in the intestine. The adult worm inhabits the intestine, is 2 to 4 cm. in length, and possesses about 200 segments. The head has four sucking disks and a number of small hooklets. The eggs pass into the intestine, some of which penetrate the mucosa and develop encysted embryos which, after a period, emerge as larvae and develop into adult worms.

Their ova pass out in the feces. They are 40 micra in diameter and very transparent, easily overlooked. They contain an embryo with hooklets and surrounded by three membranes (Fig. 213). The infestation is spread to other animals and man by ingestion of ova. A mild chronic, catarrhal enteritis constitutes the pathology. The symptoms may be slight or indefinite. Moderate eosinophilia is present.

DIPYLIDIUM CANINUM.—This is the common infestation of domestic animals, cats and dogs. Occasionally it is seen as an infestation of man. The symptoms are indefinite or absent, and little or no pathological changes are seen in the infestation. The ova are similar to *H. nana,* but larger.

CHAPTER XXII

ONCOLOGY

CLASSIFICATION OF TUMORS

A tumor is an autonomous new growth of tissue. By the use of this single term, "autonomous," we cover all the salient features of the more elaborate descriptive definitions of lawless, purposeless, and the like.

No system of classification of tumors has as yet been devised which is entirely satisfactory, primarily because the classification of any morbid process which is not based on etiology is at best a makeshift procedure designed only as a matter of practical convenience. In the absence of any possible etiological classification in our present state of knowledge, our next most useful approach to the problem is from the histologic and histogenetic basis. Theoretically, an embryologic classification should be desirable. Practically, it has served no useful purpose, because tumors histogenetically, as a rule, do not retrace their embryologic steps nor behave as embryonic tissues, being influenced apparently more by environment and by their acquired differentiated characteristics. The most satisfactory and complete embryologic classification thus far developed is that of Adami which is given below in its simplest form—shorn of verbiage and descriptive discussion.

I. *Lepidomata* (Membrane tumors)	A. Primary	1. Epilepidomata (from epiblast) 2. Hypolepidomata (from hypoblast)
	B. Secondary	1. Mesolepidomata (from mesothelium) 2. Endothelial lepidomata (from endothelium)
II. *Hyalomata* (Pulp tumors)	A. Epihyalomata (neuroma—glioma, etc.)	
	B. Hypohyalomata (chordoma)	
	C. Mesohyalomata (mesenchymal tumors) a. Mesothelial hyalomata (rhabdomyoma)	

From the practical standpoint we find that as a matter of usage, many tumors are actually classified on a regional, topographical basis. This is especially true of certain tumors which are almost invariably found in definite anatomical positions, regardless of their potential histogenesis. Thus, tumors of the brain are apt to be considered together as a group without particular regard to histogenesis. Similarly, tumors of bone are grouped clinically, although they may cover a rather diverse histogenic ancestry. The special tumors as adamantinomata or hypernephromata present such typical features that they become characterized on an anatomical basis almost exclusively. Likewise, tumors of uncertain ancestry have acquired an anatomical, topographical or descriptive histologic nomenclature entirely apart from their actual histogenesis. Thus, meningioma, psammoma, and synovioma are examples of our complaisancy rather than of our purism of terminology.

The most generally used method of nomenclature of tumors to-day is scarcely worthy of the term classification, as it is merely a system of cataloging on the basis of morphologic resemblance to the theoretical tissue or cell of incidence or origin. The system is based, in general, on the theory that specific type tumors may arise from each of the differentiated blast forms of cell, and that more complex mixed or teratoid tumors may result from the neoplastic development of undifferentiated cells such as particularly are seen in the ovary or testis.

Certain generalities may well be introduced at this point in respect to nomenclature. The suffix "oma" signifies tumor, as derived from the Greek, and means neoplasia of cells, rather than the generic idea of swelling which the name itself implies. Tumors of epithelial cells, whether of epiblastic or hypoblastic origin, if malignant in character, are known as *carcinomata.* This term, meaning crablike tumor, arose from the appearance of cancer of the breast as it invaded in claw-fashion the surrounding tissues. If the malignant tumor be of mesoblastic origin it is called a *sarcoma;* viz., fibrosarcoma, lymphosarcoma, etc. From the lay standpoint, *all* malignant tumors are generically classified as *can-*

PLATE LII

TUMOR GIANT CELLS

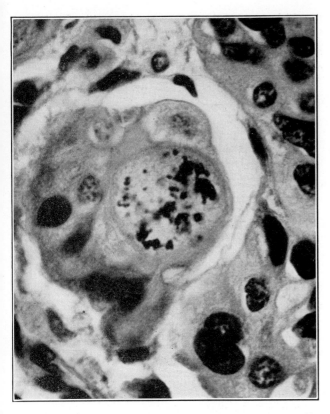

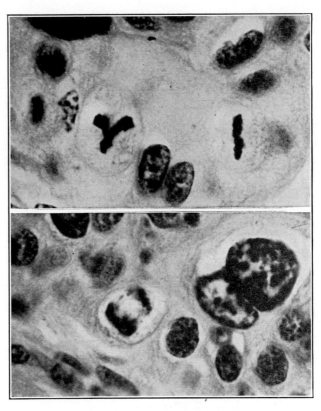

FIG. 215.—ESOPHAGUS: EPIDERMOID CARCINOMA.—CASE 141.—Illustrating an atypic mitotic figure with chromosomes dividing unequally in six or more directions to result in a multilobulated tumor giant cell such as Fig. 84, 216 and 218. App. 1000 x.

FIG. 216.—CASE 141.—Composite photomicrograph to show variation in chromosomal division. Note triad arrangement (upper left), unbalanced diaster (lower left) and typical multilobulated giant cell (lower right). App. 1000 x.

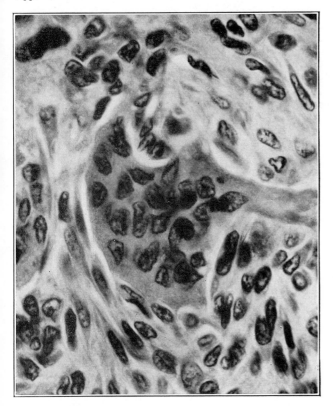

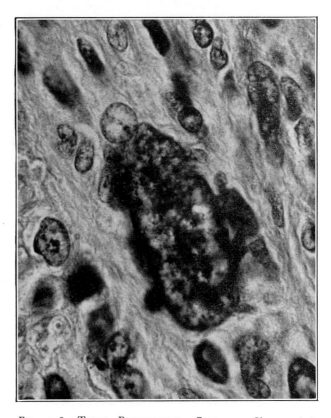

FIG. 217.—BONE—GIANT CELL TUMOR.—CASE 96.—By contrast, note this giant cell with its serrated cytoplasm and its multiple centrally placed nuclei, all showing complete nuclear division. App. 800 x.

FIG. 218.—THIGH—FIBROSARCOMA.—CASE 93.—Characteristic abortive cell reproduction in malignant sarcoma. Observe enormous size, lobulated appearance, and intense hyperchromatism of nucleus App. 1000 x.

cer. This is a scientific misnomer, but a term of practical value in discussing malignant diseases.

For the sake of simplicity, the following arrangement is suggested to serve as a skeletal framework, to which most of the tumors can be readily fitted. This represents a combination of the various text and reference volumes' classifications, being based on regional, histologic and histogenetic grounds.

CLASSIFICATION OF TUMORS

TISSUE OR CELL TYPE	BENIGN	MALIGNANT
I. Tumors of connective tissue origin		
1. Fibroblast	Fibroma	Fibrosarcoma
2. Lipoblast	Lipoma	Liposarcoma
3. Myxoblast	Myxoma	Myxosarcoma
4. Chondroblast	Chondroma	Chondrosarcoma } Osteogenic sarcoma
5. Osteoblast	Osteoma	Osteosarcoma
II. Tumors of muscle		
1. Leiomyoblast	Leiomyoma	Leiomyosarcoma
2. Rhabdomyoblast	No benign forms found	Rhabdomyosarcoma
III. Tumors of hematopoietic and reticuloendothelial system		

1. Lymphoblast (lymphocyte)	Lymphoma	1. Lymphosarcoma
		  a. Small cell type
		  b. Large cell type
		2. Lymphoid leukemia
		  (lymphoadenosis)
		3. Hodgkin's disease (?)

2. Myeloblast (myelocyte)	No benign forms found	Myeloid leukemia (Myelosis)
a. Plasma cell myeloblast (?)	" " " "	Plasma cell myeloma (multiple myeloma)
b. Endothelial myeloblast (?)	" " " "	Endothelial myeloma (Ewing's tumor of bone)
3. Erythroblast	" " " "	Erythroblastosis
IV. Tumors of pigment cells		
1. Melanoblast	Melanoma (naevus)	Malignant melanoma
V. Tumors of nervous system		
1. Neuroblast { a. neuro-epithelium	Neurocytoma	Neuroblastoma (retinoblastoma)
{ b. nerve fibers	Neuroma	Neurosarcoma
2. Glioblast	Glioma { astrocytoma oligodendroglioma spongioblastoma, etc.	Malignant glioma (gliosarcoma or glioblastoma multiforme)
VI. Tumors of endothelium		
1. Endothelioblast	1. Hemangioma 2. Lymphangioma	Angiosarcoma
2. Dural endothelium (?)	Dural endothelioma (meningioma)	
VII. Tumors of epithelium		

1. Pavement cell type epitheliomata (epiblast)	Papilloma	Squamous carcinoma
		  (epidermoid)
		Basal cell "carcinoma"
		  (Usually benign clinically)

2. Glandular cell type (hypoblast)	Adenoma Polyp	Adenocarcinoma

VIII. Complex tumors—mixed tumors, teratomata, embryomata.
    1. *Simple mixed tumors*—composed of two or more differentiated cell types each being neoplastic in its own right, and named according to its composition: adenosarcoma, lympho-epithelioma, etc.
    2. *Teratoid tumors*—composed of cells derived from more than one germinal layer in varying degrees of differentiation, in an attempt to develop a new individual within the tissues of the host. These may be conveniently divided into two types:
        a. *Embryoma*—a tumor derived from primitive germinal cells (totipotential cells), theoretically capable of complete differentiation into a new offspring, including the development of fetal membranes, but often showing simple cell proliferation (embryonal carcinoma).
        b. *Teratoma*—a tumor derived from a segregated somatic blastomere containing a jumble of tissues of two or three germ layers in varying degrees of differentiation. Basically benign, any tissue within such a tumor may become malignant, as a carcinoma or sarcoma.

INTRODUCTION TO ONCOLOGY

Oncology is that science relating to the study of tumors. In starting our investigation of tumors it is well to bear in mind that cancer to-day stands second only to heart disease as the principal cause of death in man, having climbed from tenth place in scarcely more than two decades. For that reason it becomes more and more important for us to learn all that we can concerning the origin, the natural history and the control of the various manifestations of this extraordinary biologic process.

In the first place, let us recognize from the out-set that *cancer* is not a single disease, but a generic term applied to a variety of conditions of different etiology, running typical specific courses affecting particular organs or tissues, and having but one property in common—the autonomous new growth of cells. We use the generic term *infection* in the same way, to cover an enormous group of diseases, each having its specific etiological agent, running its characteristic course, showing selective tissue involvement and having but one property in common, that of reaction to the specific infecting agent.

GENERAL CHARACTERISTICS OF TUMORS

Tumors are parasitic growths derived from the tissues of the host. Many tumors are benign in character throughout their life history. Others are malignant from the very outset of their existence. Certain benign tumors may take on malignant characteristics after many years of existing in a dormant, unchanged form.

The most important characteristic of tumors is their autonomy. Tumors do not obey any of the ordinary laws of growth for normal tissues. This, even more than their increased energy of growth, is the significant factor. Normal cell growth is under some definite restraint and control. Even inflammatory proliferation and regeneration of tissues normally stops when the repair process is completed. Tumor proliferation transcends these usual controlling factors and proceeds at its own pace.

Tumors, as a result of this lawless growth, are without function. Glandular tumors do not have a duct by which to discharge their secretions. Only in the case of ductless gland tumors is this functional capacity ever exhibited, and then only rarely, probably inadvertently, and usually harmfully.

Tumors are not only lawless, functionless, and parasitic, but they are able to maintain their rate of growth and existence on an extraordinarily inadequate blood supply as compared to normal tissues. For example, a lipoma will maintain its fat content even though the host may become emaciated.

On the other hand, many tumor cells are much more sensitive to the action of radiation by x-ray or radium than their normal counterparts. This has served as one of our most effective weapons in the control of cancer, as a result. In general, the more undifferentiated a tumor cell appears, the more sensitive to radiation it is. Tumors with a dense stroma of connective tissue, cartilage or bone are particularly resistant to radiation, as are the great majority of the slow-growing benign tumors composed of well differentiated, adult-appearing types of cells, whereas lymphosarcoma and surface epithelial tumors are often very sensitive to irradiation.

Tumors grow by multiplication of their own cells, usually by mitotic division. They grow either (1) by expansion, with compression atrophy of the tissue of the host locally (benign tumors), or (2) by infiltration, penetrating between the cells of the tissue in which they arise (malignant tumors). As the extension of tumor cell growth proceeds in the case of malignant tumors, we find that invasion of lymphatic channels or even blood vessels may occur. Tumor tissue may continue growing as a cord within such a channel, or cells may be transported by the lymph or blood streams to regional lymph nodes or to distant parts of the body as emboli. This process is spoken of as *metastasis*. The distribution of such metastases may fairly well be foretold from our knowledge of the anatomy of the part involved. In the case of vascular invasion the process is usually venous so that pulmonary metastases are the usual order. Certain tumors further tend to show a selective distribution of their secondary metastatic nodules, much as certain infectious diseases tend to have specific affinities. Thus, for example, tumors of epithelium more frequently extend by lymphatics; tumors of mesodermal origin by the blood stream. Carcinoma of the prostate is apt to have its metastatic lesions restricted to bone, etc.

Differentiation of Benign and Malignant Tumors. —Tumors may be histologically benign but cause death because of their location. Certain tumors of the brain and mediastinum fall into this class. Pathologically, a tumor is considered malignant only if it is (1) invasive, (2) produces metastasis and (3) if untreated it will kill the patient regardless of its location. Ordinarily, it is relatively rapidly growing. It shows many mitotic figures, and these are frequently atypical in appearance with the development of multilobulated nuclei, the so-called "tumor giant cell," in contradistinction to the usual foreign body giant cell (Fig. 215, 216, 217, 218, 83, 84, 85 and 86). It tends to recur if removed surgically. It fails to reproduce the structure of the tissue of origin. The less differentiated the cells appear, the more malignant the tumor. This loss of differentiation is spoken of as *anaplasia*. A benign tumor, on the other hand, is slow growing, and encapsulated. The cells are adult in type and well differentiated. Mitoses are absent or rare. It never metastasizes, and it does not kill except because of location. Furthermore, in malignancy the development of a profound myelophthisic anemia, weight loss, cachexia, etc., are an essential clinical part of the picture.

Many other features aid us in differentiating malignant from benign tumors with experience. The consistency is often helpful. In rapidly growing tumors the consistency is apt to be soft due to the failure to develop any appreciable connective tissue stroma. This is especially true of sarcomata. On the other hand, certain slow growing, but no less ultimately fatal epithelial tumors, especially cancer of the breast, are apt to have a very dense, almost cartilaginous texture due to extreme development of the stroma. This type of tumor is spoken of as *scirrhous* (hard). This overstimulation of the connective tissue stroma in such tumors is spoken of as a *desmoplastic* reaction. If this desmoplastic process is lacking we may have a rather soft, grayish-appearing tumor which, from its supposed resemblance to brain substance grossly, is termed *encephaloid* descriptively. Such tumors are always of a higher grade of malignancy.

Again, the color of a tumor may be of help grossly in estimating the relative degree of malignancy. More rapidly growing tumors, especially the sarcomata, are apt to be very vascular, so they present a reddish color. With rapid growth, necrosis is frequent; so areas of soft, yellowish, gray or white, almost caseous material may be seen, into which often extensive hemorrhage occurs.

Inflammatory Versus Neoplastic Hyperplasia.—One of the most difficult problems facing the pathologist microscopically is the differentiation of malignancy from excessive inflammatory hyperplasia. At times the processes seem to merge, the inflammatory tissues ultimately undergoing malignant change if the normal growth restraint factor becomes lost. Roughly speaking, productive inflammation is a diffuse process involving a whole area and all the cells of a tissue or organ, while a tumor is localized to one cell type and to a circumscribed area. Tumor cells show anaplasia, loss of polarity, variation in size, hyperchromatism of their nuclei, atypical mitosis with tumor giant cell formation. In some conditions such as chronic mastitis or Hodgkin's disease, which is believed by some to be infectious in origin, there is an insensible transition from this apparent inflammatory reaction to a true neoplastic picture. Such a picture is spoken of as *precancerous,* and is of great prognostic significance at times.

Attempts have been made in recent years to estimate the degree of malignancy of a tumor histologically on a graded basis, on a scale running from Grade 1 (lowest grade) to Grade 4 (highest grade). In the case of tumors of skin and mucous membranes, this system has been of great help from the prognostic standpoint. In other tumors it is of little practical value. It is based on the relative incidence of neoplastic cells and the histologic criteria of the degree of malignancy of these cells. This is estimated by the amount of nuclear hyperchromatism, the number and type of mitotic figures and the degree of anaplasia. If less than one-fourth of the cells in a given lesion are of the neoplastic variety, then this tumor may be considered as of Grade 1 malignancy. If from 25 to 50 per cent of the cells are malignant, it is graded as 2; 50 to 75 per cent as Grade 3 and 75 to 100 per cent as Grade 4. Personally, in our experience, the appearance of the cells in respect to their embryonal appearance as compared to the adult differentiation and the evidence of stromal or tissue invasion have proven of more value in estimating the degree of malignancy than a purely quantitative counting of the number of malignant cells. Likewise, it has been our experience that, with very few exceptions, three grades of malignancy, perhaps best expressed as low, medium and high, are more satisfactory in estimating the prognosis of a given case than the more exact numerical method outlined above.

CAUSATION OF TUMORS

Theories regarding the causation of cancer are age-old in the history of medicine. References may be found dating back to the prechristian era attributing humoral disorders, dietary indiscretions and a variety of similar things to the production of tumors. Our real knowledge concerning the etiology of tumors has developed, however, only in the last comparatively few years. Several theories have been evolved, some of which still have features of value in the light of modern interpretation; others of which have fallen by the wayside for lack of scientific support.

In the first place it may be said, with no fear of contradiction, that the basic intrinsic factor which induces malignant degeneration of cells is as yet a totally unknown one. Most of our knowledge is based on the interpretation of the extrinsic or tumor stimulating factors. The view that unrestrained and malignant proliferation is a universal cell property must be accepted in the light of the enormous amount of knowledge accumulated through many centuries, but that this growth factor must have a similar universal cause is utterly untenable. It is obvious that cancer is not a single disease any more than inflammation is a single disease, but a biological reaction of tissues produced by as many etiologic agents as are the numerous bacterial, spirochaetal, viral and parasitic.

INTRINSIC FACTORS

As far as intrinsic factors are concerned, the most significant one is that relating to heredity.

Heredity.—In the recent cancer symposium held at the University of Wisconsin, the importance of heredity was brought out by Mecklin. The work of Slye, Little, and a host of other animal experimentalists in the field have shown that malignancy in cells behaves as a recessive mendelian characteristic. The frequency of multiple familial cases is now believed to be of real statistical significance rather than a coincidental occurrence as was formerly taught.

Implantation Tumors.—The great volume of experimental work in cancer relates to the study of various forms of animal tumors which have been transplanted. In the case of mice, this has been successfully carried on over hundreds of generations with the development of specific cancer-producing strains and cancer-resistant strains. Maude Slye in her work has decided that in such transplantable tumors, malignancy is a recessive characteristic and behaves according to mendelian law.

Organ Susceptibility.—Investigators recently have insisted that tumor growth could be explained only on the assumption of some profound change in the character of the cells of the organ in which it occurs.

Altered cell metabolism.—Warburg has commented that the cells of cancer differ from normal cells in that they have much greater power of glycolysis associated with enormous energy production manifested by cell growth.

EXTRINSIC FACTORS

Parasitic Theory.—This theory is revived from time to time, especially by the various pseudoscientific investigators in the field of cancer. It has long been felt that some universal parasite should be the factor which incites cells to neoplastic overgrowth. This is supported in the case of one type of tumor, a tumor occurring in the stomach of rats in association with the presence of a worm known as the *Spiroptera neoplastica*. This was observed by Fibiger in 1907, who noted that rats in whose stomachs these parasitic worms were found showed the presence of an actual gastric cancer. However, he was unable to reproduce the disease in rats until he discovered that in order to induce these changes it was necessary for the rat to eat the cockroach which harbored the parasite during its encysted stage and that it was in the development of the parasite in the stomach that the condition occurred.

Tissue Tension Theory.—Waldeyer, Thiersch and Ribbert all have held that the principal inciting cause of cancer was the loss of equilibrium between the normal connective tissue and the epithelium. This was induced usually by an inflammatory reaction of the connective tissue which relieved the tissue tension permitting the unrestrained growth and infiltration of the epithelium. Today the lymphocytic inflammatory reaction has been shown to be an effective barrier to the extension of the tumor so that this theory, while having many convenient phases, has been largely discarded.

Cohnheim's Theory.—The most important theory regarding the development of tumors is that proposed by Cohnheim, who suggested that at some stage of embryonic life, cells of blastomeres might become isolated or displaced. Such cells still possessed potential growth factors, but lay dormant in this foreign soil until some reaction caused their activity and their capacity to grow at a rate comparable to their embryonic state. This theory is of importance particularly from the standpoint of explaining the location and character of many tumors. It is of little value in explaining the exciting cause of the overgrowth of these displaced cells.

Chronic Irritation.—The most generally accepted theory of the cause of cancer to-day is that of chronic irritation. Innumerable examples of this might be cited of which a few are given.

CHEMICALS.—Yamagiwa, in 1915, showed that the application of tar daily to the ears of rabbits would in the course of six to twelve months produce typical carcinoma of the skin. Similar tumors may be reproduced in man and the mouse, but to date it has been impossible to cause this lesion in dogs, guinea pigs or rats. An enormous amount of literature has resulted from these original experiments and the understanding of this type of carcinogenic agent is proceeding rapidly. Among other related substances may be mentioned 1.2.benzathracene, plenanthrene, aniline, miscellaneous coal tar products, Sudan III, arsenic, zinc chloride, etc.

TRAUMA, PARTICULARLY REPEATED.—In general, it is doubtful whether a single traumatic injury is of great significance in the induction of the carcinomatous process. However, a considerable number of medicolegal compensation cases have been settled for the plaintiff on the basis of such injury. More often, however, it is found in the history of the patient that repeated trauma of lesser magnitude is more often followed by malignant disease than results from the single, more severe injury.

PHYSICAL AGENTS, such as x-rays, radium or even sunlight. Cancers arising from these physical agents are much less frequently seen to-day than formerly, with the improvement in the method of using these agents therapeutically and in the protection of the operator.

ORGANIC CELL PRODUCTS, including several of the hormones: folliculin, estrin and decomposition products of bile. It thus appears that the scope of these chronic inflammatory producing agents is most extensive and almost identical with the excitants of simple inflammation. This fact compels the conclusion that both inflammation and neoplasia are the expression of universal cell properties and are correlative.

FILTRABLE VIRUSES.—Finally, in respect to the current investigative work in the etiology of cancer must be cited the theory that cancer is a virus disease. Because of certain transplantable tumors, notably the fowl sarcoma of Rous, the Shope papillomatosis of rabbits, and the renal tumors in frogs described by Lucké, in which filtrates of the tumors have been used for their transmission, the theory has been evolved that these are virus diseases. Critical analysis by Ewing and others of this problem in a wholly impartial fashion suggests that this activating substance may not be a true virus, but is a cell product of the tumor in the nature of an enzyme. The weight of the evidence seems to be in favor of this latter view, although it is still too soon to have any final judgment in this matter. In this connection, the fact that Stanley has recovered a crystalline substance in tobacco mosaic disease, a condition believed to be viral in origin, is another suggestive point in favor of the enzyme nature of the activating substance. There seems to be little doubt that some filtrable substance obtained from an extract of tumor, or even in certain instances, serum alone from such an animal is capable of activating a neoplastic growth of cells. This is particularly true in certain of the transplantable fowl tumors. Much further study will be required to prove the exact nature of this activating factor.

BIOLOGIC METHODS OF DIAGNOSIS

The diagnosis of malignancy by serologic methods has long been the aim of the investigator in oncology since it is evident that one of the chief problems with which we are concerned is reducing the mortality of cancer. This requires early diagnosis. Unfortunately, up to the present time many cases of visceral malignancy escape recognition until they are in an advanced stage, often beyond the help of surgery or radiation therapy. Even in instances of tumor in organs which can be visualized, a serious doubt often exists in the mind of the physician as to whether or not a given tumor is benign or malignant. It is common practice under such circumstances for the physician to advise the patient to keep the suspected lesion under observation and if it shows any signs of increase in size, then to perform a diagnostic biopsy and use more radical therapy if need be.

Over the past quarter of a century, a large number of laboratory tests have been devised in an attempt to remedy this serious situation. These have largely been based upon the usual complement fixation and precipitin reactions, and in general have not proved of any great value in the early case, although many such tests have shown fairly high figures in respect to the advanced forms of malignancy. Unfortunately by the time such tests become of significance, the clinical diagnosis is usually thoroughly established.

More recently, a new method has been proposed by Gruskin, which seems to be of definite promise in respect to the early diagnosis of tumors. By this method, the intracutaneous inoculation of an antigen prepared from fetal ectodermal or mesodermal tissues is used respectively for the recognition of carcinoma and sarcoma. For the carcinoma antigen, an extract of the fetal tissue from human liver, pancreas and salivary gland is used and the Wharton's jelly from the umbilical cord is correspondingly employed as the antigen for those malignant tumors arising from the mesenchymal tissues. The intracutaneous inoculation of an extract of these substances in positive cases results in the development of a char-

acteristic urticarial wheal with pseudopodia. In the hands of various investigators, this procedure has resulted in an extremely high degree of accuracy as checked by subsequent clinical and pathological observations. Its particular value in the early case of malignancy cannot be overestimated. The chief difficulties which are encountered in its use are seen in individuals whose skin is not in good condition. Thus, in the late stages of malignancy where cachexia and dehydration of the skin exist, the test may fail to give a positive reaction, but the clinical picture is usually sufficiently established so that this is not a serious criticism of the method. On the other hand, there are instances associated with endocrine disturbances, dermatoses of one sort or another and instances where the patient has jaundice or his picture is complicated by some toxemia such as might be found in association with high fevers or with renal impairment and uremia, where the skin test does not give reliable resutls. Under such circumstances a serologic flocculation test may be used, employing the same antigen. This is likewise of great value in those doubtful cases in which the skin test cannot be satisfactorily utilized.

In reviewing the cases which have been tested by these methods, it appears that well over ninety per cent accuracy has been established. It is our hope that the further development of this method may prove to be of the great importance which these preliminary studies indicate. The thought is presented at this time in reviewing the problem of malignancy as a whole with the idea of stimulating interest in the development of a means of increasing the early diagnosis and recognition of malignancy rather than with the thought that this particular method is in its final form.

CHAPTER XXIII

PSEUDOTUMORS

The material under consideration in this chapter consists of a group of lesions which resembles, in certain respects, true tumors. This resemblance ceases on microscopic study when the histologic evidence of neoplastic change of the cells is found to be lacking. The cells in such pseudotumors will show evidence of inflammatory hyperplasia. They may show actual hypertrophy, but the nuclei remain normal, without characteristic hyperchromatism and without evidence of abnormal mitosis. In fact, mitosis of any sort in such lesions is relatively infrequently found. There is no anaplasia of the cells. The stroma of such lesions likewise presents none of the characteristic degenerative changes associated with true neoplasm. Their chief resemblance to true tumors consists in the fact that they represent localized enlargements of tissues, which on analysis will be found to have an inflammatory basis for their background.

Nasal polyps.—These are comparatively common lesions found in the practice of the nose and throat specialist. Their exact nature and etiology are under considerable dispute. It is generally conceded, however, that the polyp is basically an inflammatory lesion, most commonly the result of some local allergy of the nasal mucosa. Such cases are found very frequently in individuals presenting other manifestations of allergy. The lesion is dependent upon the local edema of the submucosa with a chronic inflammatory cellular infiltration consisting chiefly of lymphocytes, large mononuclears, plasma cells, and commonly, eosinophiles in large numbers. This latter feature is explained on the basis of allergy as being one of the common cellular reactions seen in such allergic conditions as asthma, hay fever and urticaria. The accumulation of fluid acts mechanically to cause the mucosa to become dependent, and gradually there develops a pedunculated mass of loose, edematous, submucous connective tissue covered by a somewhat thickened inflammatory mucosa. This, in turn, frequently undergoes ulceration with secondary infection and other evidence of inflammatory change with leukocytic infiltration. Such lesions, when removed surgically, are prone to recur because the underlying cause is not altered by the surgical procedure. However, many cases do remain either cured or improved for long periods of time, and surgical removal of such polypi as a palliative procedure, with the reëstablishment of normal nasal breathing is of great comfort to the patient.

ILLUSTRATIVE CASE

CASE 84. (Ref. #S-95)

Diagnosis.—Nose—nasal polyp.

Patient was a twenty-eight year old single, white, American woman, who was admitted to the hospital complaining of pain in the left cheek, associated with headaches and a pain in the left ear, with a purulent discharge from the ear.

Present Illness.—Present illness began about six weeks before admission with a cold. This was followed by marked obstruction to the nose and the development of diffuse frontal headaches. Gradually there developed a tenderness over the left antrum region and the patient became deaf in the left ear. This was followed by excruciating pain in the ear, with the development of an abscess, that apparently ruptured spontaneously and had been draining since that time. The patient's local physician finally referred her to the hospital for more radical treatment than he was able to give.

Past Medical History.—Patient had the usual childhood diseases. She had always suffered from recurrent and frequent colds, which had been accompanied as a rule by marked obstruction to her breathing on the left side of her nose. This had been much more marked with the present illness than previously. The rest of her past history was irrelevant. She had had no serious illnesses nor operations. A review of her systems other than her upper respiratory tract appeared to be negative.

Physical Examination.—Patient was a well-developed young woman who presented evidence of more or less acute discomfort in her facial expression. Physical examination was essentially negative except for the local condition involving her nasopharynx. There was a moderate injection of the entire nasopharynx. The tonsils were enlarged and congested. There was considerable peritonsillar edema, which encroached upon the eustachian tube on the left. Mirror examination of the nasopharynx showed the presence of a fair sized polypoid lesion, which was apparently the cause of the obstruction.

PLATE LIII
PSEUDOTUMORS

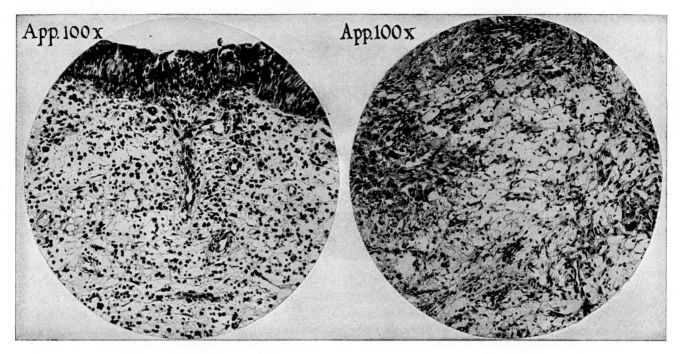

FIG. 219.—NOSE: POLYP.—CASE 84.—Loose, edematous stroma filled with chronic inflammatory cellular exudate, the whole pedunculated lesion covered by hyperplastic but typical pseudostratified epithelium. App. 100 x.

FIG. 220.—EYELID: XANTHOMA.—CASE 86.—Clumps of typical lipoid-laden, vacuolated reticulo-endothelial cells embedded in dense fibrous stroma of corium. App. 100 x.

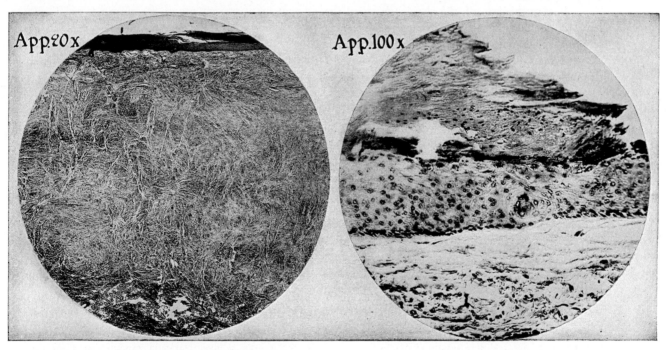

FIG. 221.—SKIN: KELOID.—CASE 88.—Thinned epidermis with absence of rete pegs and appendages, pseudoneoplastic overproduction of dense hyalinized collagen with marked thickening of corium. App. 20 x.

FIG. 222.—SKIN: SEBACEOUS CYST.—CASE 87.—Pseudostratified epithelial cells lining cyst wall, lumen of cyst containing broken-down sebaceous material. App. 100 x.

This was accompanied by considerable postnasal drip. Examination through the nares was less satisfactory, although the polyp could be visualized.

Laboratory Examinations.—These were essentially negative. The bleeding and coagulation times were within normal limits.

Operative Procedure.—On the basis of these findings, the antrum was drained and the polyp removed surgically. There was considerable bone necrosis involving the antrum, which was filled with pus and lined by chronic granulation tissue. The polypoid mass was pseudopedunculated and hung down in pear-like fashion from the mucosal surface.

Gross Description of Pathological Specimen.—Gross specimen consisted of several ragged, hemorrhagic fragments of what appeared to be infected granulomatous tissue, one of which was somewhat ovoid in shape with a narrow, pedunculated base. This measured 1 cm. in its greatest diameter.

Microscopic Description of Section from Nasal Polyp.—(Fig. 219) Microscopically, the typical ciliated, cylindrical epithelium may be identified covering the tissue. In places, persistent cilia may be seen. The underlying tissue consists of an extremely edematous, loosely arranged connective tissue stroma in which the individual collagen fibrils are widely separated. There is evidence of an inflammatory reaction characterized by dilatation of the vessels and a rather extensive cellular infiltration. This is made up of a mixed cellular exudate in which mononuclear cells predominate. As is quite common, lesions of this type are apt to be of a chronic nature. There are many eosinophiles seen. Plasma cells, large mononuclear phagocytes and lymphocytes make up the bulk of the cellular exudate. However, a good many polymorphonuclears may also be identified. The blood supply in this lesion consists only of the dilated capillary bed of the submucosa, which distinguishes it from a true neoplasm with its independent vascular development.

Condylomata.—As has been commented upon in the chapter discussing syphilis, one of the important secondary lesions is the so-called *condyloma*. This represents a marked chronic inflammatory hyperplasia of the skin and subcutaneous tissues, particularly found in the moist skin folds around the anus and genitalia. It is the result of definite spirochetal invasion of the tissues with productive fibrosis. The overlying epithelium is stimulated to inflammatory hyperplasia and may become considerably thickened, even to a point where it suggests papillary proliferation. The mechanism of the development of the lesion is, therefore, not unlike the polypoid picture seen in the nasal mucosa, resulting in a pedunculated, elevated mass of tissue covered by epithelium. In this instance, however, the activating agent is a specific infectious organism rather than an allergic one.

Sections through such a lesion show a marked increase in the amount of subcutaneous connective tissue. The overlying epithelium shows very little suggestion of rete peg formation and is usually considerably thickened with a marked increase in the number of cells. The underlying stroma is diffusely infiltrated by plasma cells, lymphocytes and large mononuclears. As in the case of the nasal polyp, no evidence of neoplastic change of any of the cells is seen. The nuclei are normal. Mitotic figures are absent, or if present are of the normal type. There is no nuclear hyperchromatism and no anaplasia of the cells. The histologic picture is one of simple inflammatory hyperplasia rather than a transitional picture approaching inflammatory neoplasia.

ILLUSTRATIVE CASE

CASE 85. (Ref. #S-96)

Diagnosis.—Skin—condyloma latum (syphilis).

Patient was a white female twenty-three years of age, who was admitted to the gynecologic service because of a profuse vaginal discharge.

Present Illness.—The present symptoms began about three weeks before admission. This was accompanied by a generalized, diffuse, maculopapular eruption of a dull red color. At about the same time, the patient noticed marked pruritus about the anus and vulva.

Past History.—Her past history was entirely unsatisfactory. The patient was uncooperative and of a low grade mentality. As far as she could recall, she had never had any serious illness. She had had one miscarriage and one stillborn child three years before admission. She denied any knowledge of venereal disease. A review of her systems other than the genito-urinary was negative. She had had intermittent attacks of leukorrhea ever since her first pregnancy, but these had never been marked enough to cause her to seek medical advice until the present time.

Physical Examination.—Physical examination showed a well developed and somewhat undernourished young white woman. There was a generalized maculopapular eruption over the entire trunk and extremities. Numerous mucous patches on the soft palate and buccal mucosa were present. There were numerous characteristic condylomata lati of the labia and around the anal orifice. The perineum was markedly relaxed. The uterus appeared normal in position. The cervix was eroded and showed a marked mucopurulent discharge. No adnexal pathology was determined clinically.

Laboratory Findings.—Red blood cells 3,100,000; hemoglobin 70%. White blood cells 9,400 with 73% polynuclear leukocytes. Urinalysis: specimen was markedly turbid as contaminated from the vaginal discharge. In itself, it was negative except for the presence of considerable numbers of *Trichomonas vaginalis*. Blood Wassermann was 4 plus. Darkfield examination from the mucous patches in the mouth was positive for spirochetes.

Subsequent Course.—A diagnosis of secondary lues was made and intensive antisyphilitic therapy instituted.

The Trichomonas infestation of the cervix was likewise treated energetically with marked improvement in the condition within a period of two to three weeks. Several of the condylomata were removed surgically after it was found that they failed to regress materially under the antisyphilitic treatment. This was done for the comfort of the patient, and to aid in the establishment of a histologic diagnosis.

Pathological Specimen.—Biopsy specimen consisted of two pieces of dense fibrous tissue covered with somewhat thickened epithelium, except at their bases at the point of attachment.

Microscopic Description of a Section of Condyloma. —Microscopic examination of this tissue shows a marked inflammatory hyperplasia of the overlying epithelium.

There is considerable acanthosis. The epithelium is of the pavement type and shows a definite increase in the number of cells. In places, it is thinned out and shows very little evidence of rete peg formation. In other areas the rete pegs are elongated and broadened. There is leukocytic infiltration of the superficial layers. The underlying stroma is made up of dense fibrous tissue in which marked mononuclear cellular infiltration has occurred. In this lesion, plasma cells and lymphocytes predominate. There is a tendency for perivascular mantling to be present. Some endarteritic thickening of the smaller vessels is noted. There is no hyperchromatism and no anaplasia, and the picture is simply one of inflammatory hyperplasia rather than the transitional type of inflammatory neoplasia.

Xanthoma.—This lesion is one which is particularly confusing in respect to classification. It is held by most pathologists to represent a non-neoplastic process. It appears to be related to some poorly understood disturbance of lipoid metabolism and has no specific etiologic basis.

The pathology of the process consists of a localized aggregation of lipoid laden, large mononuclear phagocytic cells within the subcutaneous tissues. These are not sharply demarcated from the surrounding structures by a capsule, but do not suggest invasion as would be expected if they were neoplastic in nature. The lesion is seen particularly around the eyelids, although it may occur anywhere in the body. It is very frequently multiple. It is usually small in

size, rarely exceeding 1 to 2 cm. in diameter. It appears as a yellowish, elevated mass just beneath the skin, which is freely movable over the lesion, unless inflammatory changes have proceeded to such a degree that there is fixation.

Microscopically, no evidence of neoplastic change in any of the cells can be detected. It is rare to find mitotic figures, and there is an absence of hyperchromatism and anaplasia. Recurrences of these lesions may occur following their surgical removal because the underlying etiological factor has not been altered. The great majority of cases, however, remain free from such recurrence. For a more complete discussion of xanthomatosis see Chapter LII relating to the spleen and reticulo-endothelial system.

ILLUSTRATIVE CASE

CASE 86. (Ref. #S-120)

Diagnosis.—Skin—xanthoma tuberosum.

Patient was a white female of 44 years, who came to the hospital because of a burning sensation of the eyes, especially on the left side. Her eyeballs seemed to be tender on pressure through the lids.

Past History.—The patient's past history was one of varying medical complaints, but in reference to the present condition, of very little significance. She had worn glasses for a number of years. The last time she had her eyes examined was approximately four to five years before the present trouble. She was given glasses at that time, which improved her sight. For the past two years she had had occasional scotomata, with intermittent transitory twitching of the lower lids. There had been a small, elevated, yellowish plaque in the upper lid of the left eye for at least ten years. This grew slowly in size for the first several years, but had shown no further increase during the last three or four years.

Physical Examination.—The patient was a well developed, well nourished, middle-aged white woman, who showed no external evidence of any serious illness. Examination of her head was essentially negative except for the presence of a small, discrete xanthomatous nodule in the left upper lid. Eye examination otherwise was

relatively negative. Pupils were regular and equal and reacted normally. Visual fields were normal. Fundi showed slight hypertensive vascular spasm.

Subsequent History.—The refractive error was corrected and it was advised to have the xanthoma removed for the patient's comfort. This was done under local anaesthesia and the lid healed satisfactorily. The patient was discharged.

Pathological Specimen.—Biopsy specimen consisted of a small, pea-sized, yellowish nodule with an elliptical skin fragment overlying it.

Microscopic Description of a Section of Xanthoma. —(Fig. 220) The overlying epithelium shows moderate atrophy with thinning of the superficial layers. Many of the deeper cells appear somewhat pyknotic and degenerated. In the underlying connective tissue are found clumps of enormous polyhedral cells having a foamy cytoplasm. The nuclei of these cells are typically of the large mononuclear variety. With frozen section technique, the vacuolated cytoplasm of these cells is found to be filled with lipoid material. These masses of cells are embedded in a relatively dense connective tissue stroma and are rather sharply demarcated from the surrounding tissues, although no definite capsule can be recognized microscopically. This histologic picture suggests the characteristic histology of the so-called "xanthoma."

Sebaceous Cyst.—Sebaceous cysts are relatively common lesions, which are found most frequently in the scalp area in relation to cystic dilatation and degeneration of the sebaceous glands associated with certain of the hair follicles as the result of inflammatory obstruction to the discharge of sebaceous material. They may also arise as the result of embryonal displacement of surface epithelium beneath the skin level. Such lesions frequently simulate tumors and are often removed surgically for this reason.

They consist typically of an epithelial lined cyst in which varying degrees of differentiation of the epithelium toward the sebaceous glandular type may be observed. The contents of such a cyst is composed of grumous, sebaceous material. Not infrequently this breaks down with the production of fatty acids and cholesterol. This latter may be identified by the rhombic clefts in the sebaceous material by the usual methods of fixation which dissolve the cholesterin. Frequently, secondary calcification follows, as it does elsewhere in the body with the breakdown of fatty material. These pseudotumors vary in size from small lesions half a centimeter or so in diameter to large, nodular masses 8 or 10 cm. in size. The familiar "wen" falls in this group of sebaceous cysts. At times, these cysts are so distended with their secretion as to create an impression of a solid tumor rather than a cyst. They are benign lesions, which are of no clinical significance except for cosmetic reasons, and because of localized pain, on occasion, as the result of their location.

ILLUSTRATIVE CASE

CASE 87 (Ref. #S-217)
Diagnosis.—Skin: sebaceous cyst.

Patient was a married white female of 26 years, who was admitted to the hospital because of a bloody diarrhea of six months' duration and a loss of weight of thirty pounds.

Present Illness.—The patient stated that she was well until six months before admission. At that time, she suddenly developed a diarrhea with almost constant bowel movements, twelve to twenty per day. She was treated by a physician with indifferent results, the symptoms improving somewhat at times, but recurring with greater severity at others. About one month before admission, she began to note bright blood in the bowel movements, and their frequency increased. She consulted another physician and was examined by x-ray for the first time. Barium enema revealed marked deformity of the colon and sigmoidoscopy established the diagnosis of multiple polypi clinically. She had pronounced anorexia and had lost about thirty pounds during this period and her symptoms had continued unabated. She was referred to the hospital for operative treatment.

Past History.—The patient had measles, whooping cough and diphtheria as a child before the age of ten. Ever since she was six years of age, she had had a series of painless subcutaneous swellings over her face, trunk and extremities. These increased slowly in size at first and then remained stationary with no further growth. Up to the time of the present admission she had had ten or twelve of these nodules removed for cosmetic reasons. A review of her systems showed that she had never had any significant upper respiratory infections. Her gastro-intestinal history was negative except that she developed moderate nocturia with the current diarrhea. Her menstrual history began at the age of thirteen and was fairly regular until the past year. She was married and had had two normal children, the youngest being one and one-half years of age.

Her family history was essentially negative. Her father died of an automobile accident. Her mother was living and well. She had one brother who was believed to have had epilepsy, but had died of pneumonia.

Physical Examination.—The patient was a fairly well developed, emaciated young white woman. Her head and scalp showed numerous small rounded, firm swellings. None of these showed any evidence of active inflammation. They were painless on pressure. They were subcutaneous in location with the skin freely movable for the most part over them. Her eyes, ears, nose and throat were negative. There was a small scar on the right side of the neck where one of these subcutaneous nodules had been removed. Mouth showed poor dental hygiene with a severe pyorrhea. Tonsils were hypertrophied and showed definite chronic inflammatory changes. Her chest was symmetrical. Breasts were moderately well developed and likewise contained several of these small subcutaneous nodules. Her heart and lungs appeared negative. Abdomen showed typical linea striae. There were no definite intra-abdominal masses palpated. The liver did not appear enlarged. Extremities were negative except for some twenty or thirty similar subcutaneous firm nodules one to two centimeters in diameter. Reflexes were negative. Rectal examination: There were no masses felt on rectal examination, but the examining glove was covered with bright blood on its removal and there was no evidence of hemorrhoids.

Laboratory Examination.—Red blood cells 3,900,000 with 74% hemoglobin. White blood cells 7,550 with 63% polymorphonuclear leukocytes, 29% lymphocytes, 3% monocytes and 5% eosinophiles. Urinalysis was negative. Stool examination showed a normal intestinal bacterial flora.

On the basis of the previous x-ray examination, the films of which were brought to the hospital by the patient, an exploratory laparotomy was advised with the thought in mind of a combined abdominal perineal proctosigmoidectomy.

Operative Procedure.—An 18 cm. vertical, lower left transrectus incision was made and the entire rectum, with a portion of the sigmoid was removed. The remainder of the sigmoid was anastomosed to the terminal portion of the rectum.

Subsequent History.—The patient did well for the first forty-eight hours and then developed a peritonitis of which she died the following day.

Autopsy Findings.—At autopsy, the body was noted to be covered with numerous subcutaneous nodules which varied in size from that of a pea up to the size of a large orange. These nodules were freely movable except that they appeared attached to the undersurface of the skin. The largest of these masses were found in the buttocks and thigh region. Several of these were removed for histologic study. They were definitely encapsulated and on section found to be filled with a white, cheesy-like sebaceous material. The walls of the cysts measured 2 to 4 mm. in thickness and had the general appearance of the wall of a typical sebaceous cyst.

The immediate cause of death was seen in the diffuse peritonitis which was present and had resulted from sloughing of the surgical anastomosis.

Examination of the original sigmoidorectal specimen and of the remainder of the large intestine showed a diffuse polyposis (Fig. 315) of several dozen pedunculated polypi varying considerably in size. Some of these were almost large enough to cause partial obstruction.

Keloid.—A keloid represents an atypical repair process of the skin. This is seen particularly following certain types of injury, particularly after severe burns. It is, for some unexplained reason, particularly common in the Negro race, although by no means restricted to it. In the Negro, it may result following very minor injuries and is particularly seen in the scar of an operative incision. Keloids represent one of those border-line conditions, which represent a simple inflammatory hyperplasia as a rule, but at times simulate true tumor production very closely both in the overgrowth of the tissue and the striking tendency for recurrence when such scars are removed.

The remainder of the organs were negative on gross examination.

Microscopic Description of One of the Sebaceous Cysts.—(Fig. 222) Examination of the tissue microscopically shows a thick fibrous tissue capsule which sharply demarcates the cystic cavity from the surrounding corium. There is a moderate amount of chronic inflammatory lymphocytic infiltration in the surrounding tissues. Lining the cyst is found a pseudo-stratified epithelium with a variable amount of submucosal connective and lymphoid tissue. Here and there a suggestion of glandular epithelium persists. The lumen of the cyst is filled with caseous material in which a few cholesterin crystals and large foreign body giant cells may be identified. The picture is typical microscopically of a simple sebaceous cyst. In this instance we seem to be dealing with a congenital condition which is somewhat unusual. At first, it was thought these tumors probably represented lipomata, but on more careful examination, particularly histologically, no doubt as to their nature could be raised.

For a description of the gastro-intestinal pathology, see Chapter XLVII.

Microscopically, the pathology is characterized by dense overgrowth of the connective tissue intercellular collagen. This results in the compression atrophy of the nuclei so that the mass appears almost as solid collagen, often with nuclei which are scarcely identifiable and are exceedingly few in number in relation to the amount of interstitial stroma. Commonly, hyaline degeneration accompanies the picture so that the collagen loses its characteristic, wavy arrangement and appears as an almost homogeneous mass of pink, hyaline-staining material. The epithelium overlying the scar is usually thin and, as might be expected, shows none of the skin appendages relating to hair follicle production.

ILLUSTRATIVE CASE

CASE 88 (Ref. #S-227)
Diagnosis.—Skin—keloid.
Patient was a forty year old colored female, who was admitted to the hospital because of marked contracture scars of the neck and wrists, resulting from an old, second degree burn.
Present Illness.—Four months before the present admission, the patient was severely burned about the neck and wrists as the result of her clothing catching on fire from some cleaning fluid, which ignited. She was so severely burned that she required hospitalization for about one month. Following this, scars developed, which were of the keloid, hyperplastic type, elevated considerably above the rest of the skin surface. As time went on, these scars tended to contract to the point that the patient's head had to be held in marked flexion. The neck line was completely distorted with the chin drawn down to the chest wall. Similar hyperplastic scars occurred over both wrist areas. These were covered by a thin, shiny skin and were lacking in pigment.

Past History.—The patient had been well up to the time of her injury. She did not recall whether or not she had had any of the usual childhood diseases. She had, however, had her tonsils removed as a child. She also had her appendix removed fifteen years before the present admission, and five years ago had had a hysterectomy because of fibroids. A review of her systems was of no significance in respect to the present situation. She had always been bothered with moderate constipation. Her respiratory system was unusually free from the ordinary infections. Menstrual history had always been irregular with only about seven or eight periods yearly up to the time she had had her hysterectomy.
Physical Examination.—Physical examination other than the local lesions relating to the contracture scars was essentially negative. Pupils were regular and equal and reacted normally. Nose and throat were negative. Chest was symmetrical. Heart and lungs were negative. Abdomen was moderately prominent. Extremities were negative. The scars extended from the lobes of both

auricles down to a point just below the clavicles, including both sides of the neck and the chin. Over these areas the skin was shiny and pinkish gray in color. The scars were elevated, thick, unyielding in consistency and showed numerous ridges. This mass of scar tissue had obliterated the neck line from the mental process to the manubrium. Similar elevated scars over the radial aspect of both wrists were noted. They were rather sensitive and tender on pressure and were associated with severe pruritis.

Laboratory Findings.—Blood Count: Red blood cells, 4,700,000 with 78% hemoglobin. White blood cells, 7,450 with 46% polynuclears, 43% lymphocytes, 9% monocytes, 1% eosinophiles and 1% basophiles. Urinalysis was negative.

Subsequent History.—A plastic repair of the scarred areas was attempted with excision of the scar, and skin grafts obtained from the abdominal wall. The wrist lesions healed promptly. The neck scar was slower in its repair and the central area sloughed its grafts twice before complete epithelialization of the scarred area was obtained. Six months later, the patient was readmitted because of recurrent keloid proliferation of the scarred

areas along the edges of the repair. These were likewise excised, the skin freed by subcutaneous incision, and the edges drawn together. At the time of this report, eight months later, only very slight thickening of the scars is to be noted.

Pathological Report.—Gross Description.—Specimen grossly consists of several pieces of scar tissue covered by a thin, shiny epithelium and with adipose tissue on their undersurface.

Microscopic Description of a Section of Keloid.—(Fig. 221) Microscopic study of the tissue shows marked connective tissue overgrowth of the deeper structures. The surface is covered by a thin, atrophic layer of stratified squamous epithelium. The rete pegs are atrophic and the epithelium appears simply as a thin layer over the surface. No sweat glands, sebaceous glands or hair follicles are present. The bulk of the tissue consists of hyalinized collagen in which scattered nuclei can be identified. Most of these are atrophic, somewhat pyknotic, distorted fibroblasts. There is accompanying secondary round cell infiltration. Blood vessels, even of a capillary nature, are conspicuous by their absence. The underlying adipose tissue is within normal limits.

CHAPTER XXIV

TUMORS OF CONNECTIVE TISSUE ORIGIN

As may be noted in the general classification, there are a considerable number of tumors which arise histogenetically from derivatives of connective tissue. The largest number of these are of actual fibroblastic origin. Others, however, are derived from specialized derivatives of the fibroblast, including particularly the fat cells, bone and cartilage. Because of the wide variation in the character of the tissue of origin, including such diverse structures as tendons, fascia, dermis, ovarian stroma and the like, and because of the amazing divergence of tumor tissue from the normal, such tumors may be expected to show an almost infinite variation individually in their histology. This is, of course, particularly true of the more malignant forms of these tumors. In their benign form, the differentiation of the cell toward the normal adult cell of origin is apt to be maintained, and at times it may be difficult to decide whether a particular lesion is actually neoplastic rather than inflammatory in origin.

In addition to these complicating factors, it must be recognized that connective tissue plays an extremely important rôle in relation to most tumors. In some tumors such as those involving peripheral nerves and smooth muscle, notably in the uterus, it is difficult to decide whether the connective tissue is the tissue primarily involved or whether it is the result of stimulation from the neoplastic activity of the other tissue. Thus, in the group of tumors spoken of as "neurofibromata," it is quite uncertain whether the primary tumor cell is not the connective tissue sheath cell rather than the actual nerve fiber. Similarly in the uterus, the familiar "fibroid" is so frequently composed of connective tissue in excess of the smooth muscle that again the question as to the cell of origin has been raised as an issue. In general, it is our concept that a tumor should be classified on the basis of the type of tissue in which the tumor arises and that the connective tissue reaction may be considered as a desmoplastic process in the development of a supporting stroma. Therefore, such tumors as the neurofibromata belong more properly in the group of neurogenic tumors, and the tumors of the uterus should more accurately be termed "leiomyomata" than the familiar "fibromyomata" which is a term of very general usage. By this concept, then, only tumors composed exclusively of connective tissue or its derivatives should be included in this group. As far as possible, this is the plan which is followed in this presentation.

PART I

Benign Forms

Fibromata.—The true fibromata are benign tumors arising directly from connective tissue. They present a wide range of histologic differences ranging from the edematous, soft type of tumor, the so-called *fibroma molle,* up to the hard fibroma of almost cartilaginous density, the so-called *fibroma durum.* All gradations of such connective tissue between these two extremes exist.

The microscopic picture varies so tremendously that generalization in this regard is difficult and somewhat unsatisfactory. Typically, however, the benign fibroma is made up of adult connective tissue cells with their characteristic, elongated nuclei and the presence of typical fibroglia fibers and a variable amount of collagen. Whether they are soft or hard in character depends largely upon their location and their blood supply, and upon the relative amount of collagen which the cells produce. In the soft fibroma we find usually that there is a wide separation of the individual collagen fibers by edema, which is usually the result of interference with the blood supply. In the fibroma durum, on the other hand, we find the collagen densely packed. Histologically, such tumors may simulate the appearance of a

PLATE LIV
BENIGN TUMORS OF CONNECTIVE TISSUE CELL ORIGIN

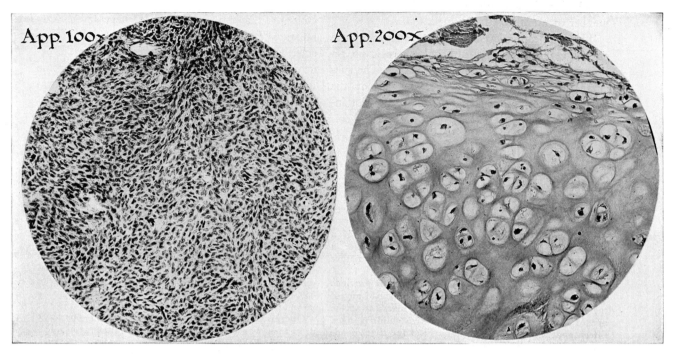

FIG. 223.—OVARY: FIBROMA.—CASE 89.—Uniformly differentiated spindle cells with purposeless interlacing appearance—no mitotic figures, anaplasia or other evidence of malignancy. App. 100 x.

FIG. 224.—ULNA: CHONDROMA.—CASE 91.—Benign, neoplastic overgrowth of cartilage cells showing some irregularity in size and distribution.

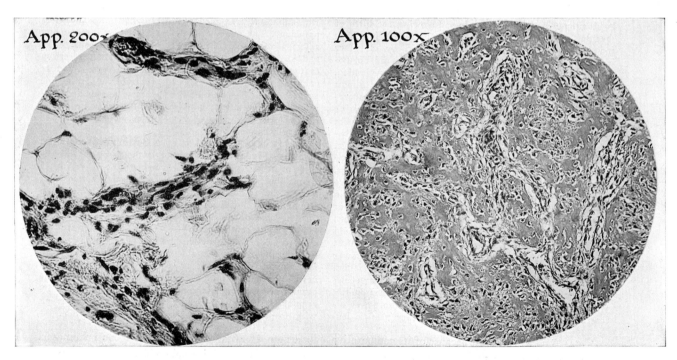

FIG. 225.—BROAD LIGAMENT: FIBROLIPOMA.—CASE 90.—Normal appearing adult fat cells with moderate connective tissue stroma. Section includes part of capsule at lower left. App. 200 x.

FIG. 226.—SCAPULA: OSTEOMA.—CASE 92.—Irregular new bone formation with increased osteoblastic activity and less normal maturation than seen in simple bone repair. App. 100 x.

keloid when the amount of collagen is great and the number of nuclei relatively small.

There are certain predilections as to site for these connective tissue tumors, although there is no restriction anatomically as to their location. The subcutaneous tissue is, perhaps, the location of the greatest number of these tumors. They are not infrequently multiple, tend to be small, definitely circumscribed, spherical or ovoid in shape and sharply separated from the surrounding structures by a capsule. The ovary, also, is a common site for the development of a rather specialized type of fibroma durum derived from the typical differentiated ovarian stromal connective tissue.

ILLUSTRATIVE CASE

CASE 89. (Ref. #S-252)

Diagnosis.—Ovary—fibroma.

Patient was a white female of 41 years, who was admitted to the hospital complaining of low back pain, a moderate leukorrhea and dull pain in the right lower quadrant.

Present Illness.—Her admission was the result of a slowly progressive increase of these symptoms over a period of a number of years. Nothing of an acute nature had occurred to necessitate hospitalization.

Past History.—The patient did not recall any previous illness of significance. She denied ever having had any of the usual childhood diseases. She was married at the age of eighteen years and had had two children, aged fifteen and thirteen years respectively at the time of admission. A review of her systems was essentially negative. She had the usual quota of mild upper respiratory infection. She never had any gastro-intestinal disturbances. She never was heart conscious. Her catamenia began at the age of fourteen and was regular at twenty-one day intervals. She had no dysmenorrhea, metrorrhagia or menorrhagia of any degree.

About ten or twelve years ago, following the birth of her last child, she noticed a rather persistent low back pain. This was irregularly accompanied by a rather profuse leukorrhea between her periods. She did not notice any particular frequency or unusual constipation. For the past five years, the leukorrhea had been almost persistent and the low back pain had increased in severity. She had been to a physician who advised operative intervention with the hope of relieving symptoms, but she postponed this month after month until the pain became so constant as to cause her a good deal of insomnia.

Physical Examination.—Patient was a well developed, well nourished female about forty years of age. Her eyes, ears, nose and throat were essentially negative except that the tonsils were definitely the site of a chronic inflammatory process. She had an artificial upper denture. Her heart and lungs were negative. Abdomen was moderately protuberant. No palpable masses could be felt, but there was a sensation of definite discomfort approaching pain on deep palpation of the right lower quadrant. There was no rebound phenomenon found. There was no dullness in the flanks. Motion was somewhat limited in the right sacroiliac joint. Extremities were negative. Gynecologic Examination: There was bilateral laceration of the cervix with rather profuse leukorrhea. There was marked retroversion of the uterus present and beginning rectocele and cystocele. The right ovary could be palpated, and it was definitely enlarged and tender.

Exploratory operation was advised with a plastic repair of the perineum, a uterine suspension and possible oophorectomy.

Laboratory Findings.—Urinalysis: Catheter specimen was within normal limits. The noncatheter specimen showed large amounts of pus as a result of the vaginal discharge. Blood count: Red blood cells 4,400,000 with 90% hemoglobin. White blood cells 9,450 with 71% polymorphonuclears and 25% lymphocytes.

Operative History.—The above outlined operative procedure was carried out, and in addition, appendectomy and right salpingo-oophorectomy were performed. The laceration of the cervix was repaired and a plastic repair of the cystocele and rectocele was done.

Subsequent Course.—The patient made an uneventful recovery and was discharged home, cured.

Pathological Report.—Gross Description.—Specimen consisted of an ovary, tube and appendix. The appendix was apparently removed routinely as it showed no gross pathology. The ovary was definitely enlarged, measuring 15 x 12 x 10 cm. The tube was adherent to the ovary and showed considerable fibrous thickening. On section of the ovary, there was a corpus lutem cyst noted at one pole with several smaller follicular cysts in this general area. The bulk of the specimen was made up of rather soft, succulent, pinkish-gray tumor tissue which showed several areas of hemorrhage. It had a rather rubbery consistency.

Microscopic Description of a Section Through the Ovary.—(Fig. 223) Examination of the tissue microscopically presents a rather uniform hyperplasia of relatively young, but fairly differentiated connective tissue cells having the rather characteristic appearance of ovarian stroma. The nuclei are ovoid for the most part, although some of them are somewhat elongated and resemble adult connective tissue cells. The nuclei tend to show considerable hyperchromatism. The tumor is relatively cellular and the amount of collagen varies considerably in different parts of the neoplasm. Occasional normal appearing mitotic figures may be identified. The connective tissue tumor cells are found arranged in irregular fasiculae interlacing in their architecture but with no possible regard for any purposeful function.

Note: A case of interest because of its comparative rarity is mentioned at this point, of a simple benign fibroma of the right auricular wall of the heart (see Fig. 227). This was an incidental finding at autopsy in a man of 46 who had died of lobar pneumonia. The tumor was a dense spheroid mass about 3.5 cm. in diameter embedded in the myocardium grossly. On section it showed coarse interlacing bundles of

PLATE LV
BENIGN TUMORS OF MESENCHYMAL ORIGIN

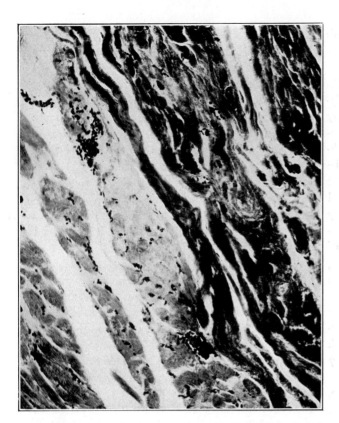

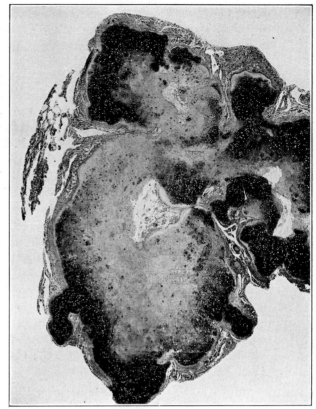

FIG. 227.—HEART: FIBROMA.—(Masson's Trichrome Stain) Heart muscle, identified by its striations at left; bands of dense, hyalinized fibrous tissue representing the tumor at right. App. 100 x.

FIG. 228.—LUNG: CHONDROMA.—Irregularly nodular mass of cartilage ranging from young proliferating cells peripherally, to adult tissue with degenerative changes, centrally, embedded in lung substance. App. 10 x.

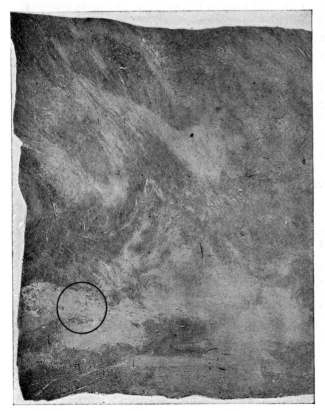

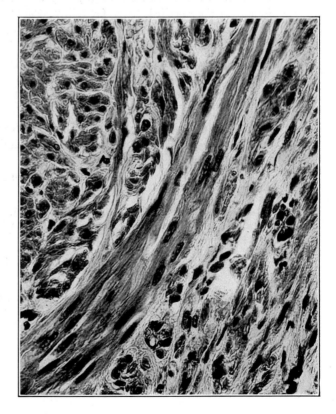

FIG. 229.—UTERUS: LEIOMYOMA.—CASE 99.—Microtessar photograph to emphasize the purposeless arrangement of bundles of muscle cells embedded in their fibrous tissue stroma, both showing extensive hyaline and myxomatous degenerative changes. App. 10 x.

FIG. 230.—UTERUS: LEIOMYOMA.—cf. CASE 99.—High power area illustrating the typical appearance of the smooth muscle cells and stroma as seen in longitudinal, tangential and cross sections. App. 400 x.

white fibers which under the microscope were confirmed by special connective tissue stains—Masson's trichrome, Mallory's aniline blue, and Van Gieson's —to be densely packed collagen.

Myxomata.—The question of whether a true tumor of myxoblastic origin ever exists is still debatable. In the development of the fetus, the only place where true myxoblasts are found is in the umbilical cord in the so-called "Wharton's jelly". Obviously, tumors arising from these cells must be extremely rare, but from the theoretical standpoint it is possible for them to occur. From the practical standpoint, myxomata are diagnosed not infrequently which are probably best interpreted as being fibromata with extensive myxomatous degeneration of their collagenous stroma. Not infrequently, such, large, bulky, soft, edematous retroperitoneal tumors are included in this group of myxomata. We believe that these are best interpreted as representing rather extreme examples of the soft fibroma with corresponding myxomatous change of the collagen. Such a tumor has been described in (Fig. 22); Case 7 (Ref. #S-239), Chapter II.

Lipomata.—In the development of the embryo, the fat cells are derived directly by differentiation from the original mesenchyme and are, therefore, believed to represent a variety of connective tissue embryologically and histogenetically. In the course of the differentiation of these cells, they appear in islands as the so-called "fetal fat cells," which are large, ovoid cells with rather ovoid nuclei and a finely vacuolated cytoplasm, which is pale staining. These do not look unlike aggregations of large mononuclear phagocytic cells except that the nucleus is likely to be more characteristic. As the body develops further, these cells go through a transitional stage, developing into the adult type of fat cell. In this process, the neutral fats accumulate within the cytoplasm of these cells as droplets, which gradually coalesce to form a single large mass of fat. This distends the cytoplasm of the cell to such an extent that the nucleus is compressed and pushed to one side to produce the characteristic "signet ring" appearance. Both from the fetal and the adult types of cell, tumors may arise. These are more readily diagnosed grossly than they are microscopically because histologically the tumor is found to be composed wholly of normal-appearing cells. It is only by the separation of these cells from the surrounding adipose tissue by a thin, often almost membraneous connective tissue capsule that they may be grossly identified and distinguished from normal supportive body fat.

There is a striking tendency for these tumors to occur in certain locations. In the male, they are particularly common around the neck region; in the female, they are frequently encountered in the breast. Likewise, such tumors are apt to be located in the subcutaneous fat of the back and buttocks. They are very frequently multiple and ordinarily remain as benign tumors. Cases exist on record in which as many as two and three hundred such small subcutaneous nodules have been found. They tend to grow very slowly and to reach a phase of equilibrium with no further increase in size, sometimes for many years. They vary greatly in size from small, ill-defined nodules one centimeter or so in diameter up to huge tumor masses which hang as pedunculated tumors from the skin, particularly on the back. One such tumor which we have seen weighed forty-six pounds and measured nearly two feet in diameter. Rarely, such tumors may be of serious importance from location. Particularly is this true of those rare instances of mediastinal involvement where from pressure upon the nerves and great vessels, even a fatal outcome may ensue.

ILLUSTRATIVE CASE

CASE 90. (Ref. #S-245)
Diagnosis.—Broad ligament—lipoma (fibrolipoma).
Patient was a white married woman of 41 years, who was admitted to the hospital because of lower abdominal pain of about four months' duration.
Present Illness.—The onset of the present illness began by the patient's complaining of a vague feeling of soreness in her lower abdomen associated with frequent attacks of sharp pain on the right side, which tended to radiate toward the vulva. This tenderness and these attacks of pain continued irregularly for about a week. There was a remission of symptoms for nearly a month and since that time, there have been several recurrent attacks of the same nature but with greater frequency and severity. The abdominal soreness had become constant during this period. There had been no other symptoms except a rather marked urinary frequency, which also manifested itself as a nocturia which required the patient's getting up four to five times per night.
Past History.—The patient's past history was of considerable interest in regard to the present illness. As a child, nothing occurred of significance. At the age of twenty-two, the patient had two serious abdominal operations, which she believed were for an appendix and

PLATE LVI
MALIGNANT TUMORS OF MESENCHYMAL ORIGIN

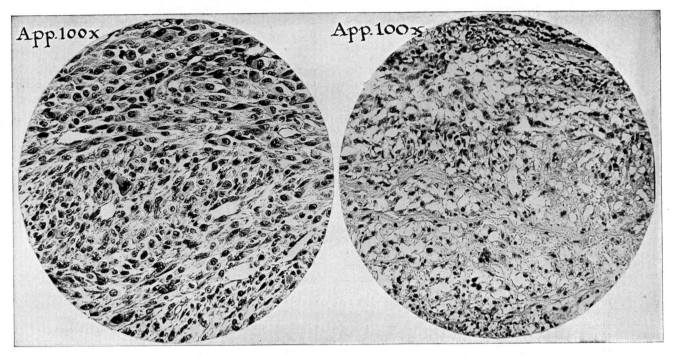

FIG. 231.—THIGH: FIBROSARCOMA.—CASE 93.—Observe evidence of rapid growth, extreme cellularity, relative absence of collagen, nuclear hyperchromatism, mitotic figures and tumor giant cells (see Fig. 84 and 218). App. 100 x.

FIG. 232.—SUBCUTANEOUS TISSUE: LIPOSARCOMA.—CASE 94.—Malignant tumor derived from potential fat cells in varying stages of differentiation; less differentiated areas closely resemble fibrosarcoma. App. 100 x.

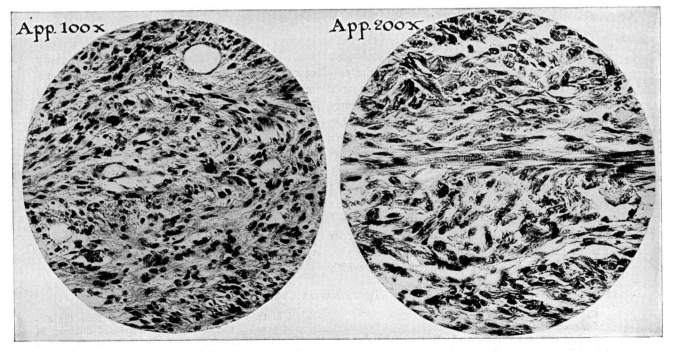

FIG. 233.—UTERUS: LEIOMYOSARCOMA.—CASE 100.—Disorderly cell growth, absence of differentiation of muscle cells, presence of tumor giant cells, marked hyperchromatism and increased vascularity. App. 100 x.

FIG. 234.—KIDNEY: RHABDOMYOSARCOMA.—CASE 101.—Observe again the wild, purposeless cell growth and other features of malignancy. Tumor may be identified by the striations seen in the better differentiated cells. App. 200 x.

for the removal of her uterus. She had always been rather sickly with various complaints relating to her several organ systems. She had been subject to upper respiratory infection, particularly sinusitis, and had had a submucous resection of her nose, a tonsillectomy and drainage of her maxillary antrum. She had been married since she was twenty, but had no children before her hysterectomy. Eight years ago she had a large abscess of the breast which required surgical drainage and took several weeks to clear up. Her gastro-intestinal history had been fairly uneventful until the present illness. During the preceding four months she had had a marked loss of appetite and some twenty pounds in weight. This was accompanied by a feeling of general easy fatigability, lassitude and weakness. Her catamenic history was negative following her second abdominal operation. Because of these various complaints, the patient consulted a physician, who found a mass in the pelvis and referred the patient to the hospital for exploratory laparotomy.

Physical Examination.—The patient was a fairly well developed and nourished middle-aged white woman lying fairly comfortably in bed. The head was negative. The eyes, ears, nose and throat showed nothing of significance. She was edentulous, but had two compensating plates. Her heart and lungs appeared negative. Blood pressure, 120/80. Abdomen was slightly prominent. There were two lower abdominal scars. On palpation, the whole abdomen was relatively tender. This was most marked in the right lower quadrant. There was no rigidity. The extremities were negative. Gynecologic examination revealed a firm mass, somewhat irregular in outline, which appeared fixed, lying to the right of the cervix in the pelvis.

The patient was advised to have an exploratory operation with the hope of being able to remove the mass and relieve her symptoms.

Chondromata.—Chondromata arise for the most part from areas where cartilage is found normally. Thus, they are seen particularly around the epiphyseal ends of the long bones, in relation to the cartilage of the ears and nose, and less frequently of the larynx and bronchi. At times they may occur as a metaplasia of connective tissue in most any part of the body. Grossly, their location and the fact that they are apt to be bulky, irregular nodular masses arising often as pedunculated lesions (as in the larynx) is of practical diagnostic value. Histologically, they are composed of fairly well differentiated cartilage cells that are hard to differentiate from normal cartilage.

One group of particular interest is that which

Laboratory Findings.—Red blood cells, 4,070,000; hemoglobin, 76%. White blood cells, 8,250 with 54% polynuclears and 41% lymphocytes. Urinalysis was essentially negative, there being present only a trace of albumin.

Operative Procedure.—A low, midline incision was made and the old scars excised. A mass was found in the right side of the pelvis attached to the stump of the uterus, but within the broad ligament. This mass was easily shelled out. It had no well-defined pedicle but apparently derived its blood supply wholly from the peripheral vessels.

Pathological Report.—Gross Description.—The specimen consisted of a large mass of fatty fibrous tissue. The tumor measured approximately 12 x 8 x 7 cm. On one side it appeared to be covered with serosa. On the other, it had a delicate connective tissue membrane which could be considered as a capsule. On section, it was found to be made up of normal appearing fatty fibrous tissue having the usual color of fat. The cut surface gave a suggestion of lobulation. One small area of beginning cystic degeneration was found. This contained a small amount of brownish fluid.

Microscopic Description of a Section of the Tumor. —(Fig. 225) Microscopic examination of the tissue reveals what appear to be normal fat cells for the most part. These are embedded in a rather diffuse, septate connective tissue stroma which has a very delicate capillary blood supply. The histology confirms the gross diagnosis of the lesion as representing a tumor of fat cell origin, the so-called "lipoma." Were it not, however, for the gross findings, it would be impossible to differentiate this from normal fat tissue. Because of the relative prominence of the connective tissue stroma, it is legitimate to designate this particular tumor as a fibrolipoma.

involves the intervertebral disks of the vertebral column. Three conditions occur here which are a source of confusion in differential diagnosis. The true tumor is the least frequently seen. More often, we find a chronic inflammatory hyperplasia of the cartilage, which is spoken of as *enchondrosis;* and finally, there is a lesion which in recent years has been better recognized than formerly. This is a traumatic rupture of the intervertebral disk or nucleus pulposa with protrusion of the cartilage into the spinal canal. The differential diagnosis is better made from the gross and radiologic findings than from the histology. All three varieties of such lesions may produce pressure symptoms and require operative intervention.

ILLUSTRATIVE CASE

CASE 91. (Ref. #S-98)
Diagnosis.—Chondroma.
Patient was a white male of 38 years, who was admitted to the hospital because of difficulty in moving his left elbow.
Present Illness.—The patient's difficulties began about one year ago following an injury to his elbow. This re-

sulted in the breaking off of a bone chip from the olecranon process. Gradually, there developed difficulty in moving the elbow. The patient described the sensation as if there were a point of obstruction over which the joint would suddenly move with a sharp sensation of pain and a clicking sound.
Past History.—The patient's previous history was en-

tirely irrelevant. He had the usual mild childhood diseases and scarlet fever. A review of his systems was negative.

Physical Examination.—The patient was a well-developed, well-nourished and rather muscularly built white male, who appeared around thirty-five years of age. His head was negative. Eyes, ears, nose and throat were within normal limits. There was no adenopathy. Heart and lungs were negative. Abdomen was flat, with no masses or tenderness. Extremities were negative except for the elbow joint. This, on palpation showed some distortion of the normal bony outline with a rather nodular, irregular feeling. On bending the elbow, a definite clicking sound could be heard, which was associated with sharp pain.

Laboratory Findings.—Laboratory findings were negative.

Operative History.—A semilunar incision was made along the anterior border of the brachio-radialis muscle. The extensor muscles were retracted laterally. The an-terior capsule of the elbow joint was exposed and opened in its long axis. Eleven small chondromata were removed and the arm put up in a sling.

Subsequent Course.—The patient made an uneventful recovery.

Pathological Report.—Gross Description.—Specimen consisted of eleven irregularly-shaped nodular, round, cartilaginous bodies. These were dense in consistency, covered by a smooth, glistening tissue and on section presented a bluish-white, cartilaginous matrix.

Microscopic Description of One of These Cartilaginous Masses.—(Fig. 224) Histologically, the tissue consists of a hyaline matrix, which here and there shows a suggestion of fibrillar structure. This varies in its staining reaction somewhat, but for the most part shows the rather characteristic bluish, basophilic reaction of chondromucin. There are numerous small empty spaces scattered irregularly throughout the tissue containing shrunken cartilage cells.

Note: A similar lesion is presented (Fig. 228) from a case of a young woman who came to autopsy because of a meningitis. A small, discrete, irregularly nodular, cartilaginous mass was found in relation to one of the small bronchi in the lung. This measured approximately 1.5 cm. in diameter. In view of the absence of any evidence of tuberculosis in this patient, it was felt that this represented a true cartilaginous tumor arising from misplaced cartilaginous cells in the development of the bronchial tree rather than a somewhat atypical Ghon tubercle. The latter more commonly is seen as a calcified or ossified lesion, which lends further weight to the presumptive diagnosis of chondroma in this instance.

Osteomata.—True tumors of bone of a benign nature are comparatively rare. They are seen especially around the bones of the face and skull and other flat bones such as the Scapula although they may occur in relation to the periosteum anywhere.

Histologically, they appear essentially as bone callus, being composed of normal appearing bone trabeculae, and are often difficult to differentiate without a clinical history and radiologic examination. As in the case of the chrondromata, such lesions may at times occur in relation to other bones, including the bodies of the vertebrae. With vertebral involvement, the same problem of differential diagnosis from inflammatory hyperplasia occurs. In particular they are to be differentiated from the various forms of arthritis which result in hyperplastic deformities of the vertebrae. Such inflammatory overgrowths of bone are spoken of as exostoses, corresponding to the enchondroses of cartilaginous origin. As a rule, the osteomata are of no serious significance except from pressure, and rarely if ever undergo malignant change.

ILLUSTRATIVE CASE

CASE 92. (Ref. #S-304)

Diagnosis.—Bone (scapula)—osteoma.

Patient was a school girl of 15 years, who was admitted to the hospital because of a lump in the right scapular region.

Present Illness.—The child's mother first noticed this lump four days previously. She believed that it must have appeared suddenly because she could not understand how she could have avoided noticing it earlier otherwise. It had not increased in size, however, during this interval. The child had not had any pain or discomfort from it and it had given no symptoms whatever.

Past History.—The patient had measles and scarlet fever before the age of five. She had her tonsils removed at the age of eight because of recurrent attacks of tonsillitis. A review of her systems was entirely negative.

Physical Examination.—Patient was a well developed, fairly well nourished girl of about fifteen years. Her head was negative. Eyes, ears, nose and throat were essentially negative. She presented a mild herpes simplex infection of the lips. Heart and lungs were negative. Abdomen was negative. No masses or viscera were palpable. Genitalia and extremities were negative. There was a bony, hard tumor about the size of a hen's egg attached to the angle of the right scapula. A tentative diagnosis of osteoma was made with the recommendation that it be removed surgically.

Laboratory Findings.—Red blood cells, 4,600,000 with 78% hemoglobin. White blood cells, 9,250 with 56% polymorphonuclear leukocytes and 35% lymphocytes. Bleeding and coagulation times were normal. Urinalysis was essentially negative.

Operative Procedure.—A transverse incision over the tumor mass was made and the lesion removed as completely as possible.

Subsequent Course.—The patient made an uneventful recovery, but there was a recurrence of the mass approximately one year later. This was again removed and up to the present time, no further recurrence has taken place.

Pathological Report.—Gross Description.—The specimen consisted of an irregularly nodular mass approximately 7 cm. in its greatest diameter. It was more or less spheroid in outline, but at one side there was a rough, hemorrhagic, bony surface representing the point of attachment. The tumor was extremely dense in con-

sistency and could not be sectioned except with a saw. Thin sections from this tumor were prepared by decalcification in weak nitric acid for histologic study.

Microscopic Description of the Tumor Tissue.—(Fig. 226) Specimen microscopically is made up of normal appearing bony trabeculae which are individually covered by typical osteoblasts. There is no particular arrangement of these trabeculae but so far as can be made out microscopically nothing abnormal regarding their appearance can be noted. There is a tendency toward some slight hyperplasia of the cells such as one might see in callous formation. There are no mitotic figures observed, and the nuclei are within normal limits. Occasional osteoclasts are observed.

PART II

Malignant Forms

Just as we may have specific tumors arising from the individual cell types as benign neoplasms, so may we have their malignant counterparts arising from the same cell types. Here, however, the variation in morphology is much greater as the tumors may present varying degrees of malignancy. All malignant tumors arising from the connective tissue cell derivatives may be spoken of generically as *sarcomata*, with the modifying prefix to describe the type of cell from which they seem to arise. The tumors may be said to occur in the same relative ratio in respect to the different types as is true of the benign forms, the fibrosarcoma far outnumbering the others.

No particular advantages are obtained by any further generalization regarding this extremely important group of tumors. In general, it may be said, however, that they are prone to occur in the younger age group and to present a rather high degree of malignancy, with an extremely high mortality. Indeed, a permanent cure from any one of these tumors is the exception rather than the rule. Fortunately, however, with our greater knowledge regarding the life history of these tumors and their relative response to surgery and irradiation, much better results should be obtained as time goes on.

In view of the importance of the malignant forms of the cartilaginous and bone cell tumors, these will be considered separately in the following chapter under the heading "Tumors of Bone."

Fibrosarcomata.—The fibrosarcoma is a malignant tumor arising from the fibroblast. It may be seen at

all ages from infancy to old age. The peak, however, usually occurs somewhere between the fifteenth and thirtieth year, which is in contradistinction to the age group of the carcinomata, occurring in the next two decades. The tumors range all the way from neoplasms which scarcely can be recognized as malignant histologically up to rapidly growing, anaplastic tumors filled with multinucleated tumor giant cells, atypical mitoses and all the other earmarks of malignancy. Indeed, at times these more malignant forms of tumor can scarcely be identified as of connective tissue origin, so undifferentiated and anaplastic have the cells become. Unfortunately, these tumors tend to invade the blood vessels relatively early in their development and to become distributed by the blood stream to all parts of the body as metastatic tumor masses. This is, of course, particularly true in the lung where the tumor cells are likely to be enmeshed in the delicate alveolar capillaries, there to become engrafted, and to grow in even more malignant and rapid fashion.

Location is of great importance in respect to prognosis. The histologic gradation of such tumors is of comparatively little value because it is so impossible to tell whether or not metastasis has already occurred regardless of the complexion of the histologic architecture. Such tumors are not infrequently found arising in the extremities as well as in the trunk, and when this occurs and amputation can be performed early enough, then recovery may occur. Likewise, many of these tumors are relatively sensitive to irradiation; and fortunately, the more highly undifferentiated and anaplastic the tumor is, the more likelihood there is of its responding to irradiation. A single example of this type of tumor is presented as illustrating the more malignant form and emphasizing the significant histologic criteria of diagnosis.

ILLUSTRATIVE CASE

CASE 93. (Ref. #S-219)

Diagnosis.—Thigh—fibrosarcoma.

Patient was a white male of 47 years, admitted to the hospital because of a mass in the anterior portion of his right thigh.

Present Illness.—The patient first noticed a lump in his thigh approximately one year before the present admission. This gradually increased in size over a few weeks until it reached the size of a small lemon. The patient went to a physician who recommended irradiation therapy. He was given thirty-five x-ray treatments at another hospital, with no change in the size of the mass. Two months later, he noticed another subcutaneous lump about the size of an acorn over the great trochanter. This was removed surgically as a biopsy specimen. The diagnosis at that time was not certain, but a sarcoma was suspected. He was then treated with a series of intramuscular injections of some "antitumor" serum. The tumor failed to respond to this treatment and, indeed, started to grow more rapidly. He had another series of X-ray treatments with the result that the tissues broke down and he developed secondary infection of the wound superficially. This cleared up under local therapy. About that time, he began to develop severe pain, which tended to radiate down his leg. The mass continued to increase in size and the patient, who had become dissatisfied with the results of his treatment decided to try another hospital. At the time of admission to this hospital, his thigh was about one and one-half times the normal diameter.

Past Medical History.—The patient did not recall anything about his childhood. Twenty years ago he was in a tuberculosis sanatarium for two years but had had no recurrence of pulmonary symptoms since. Because of this tuberculous history, he had felt that the mass in his leg was probably related to his old infection. About fifteen years ago, he had an attack of acute appendicitis and his appendix was removed. A review of his systems otherwise was of very little help in respect to his present condition. The patient believed that his trouble started about six weeks before he first noticed the lump in his leg, as the result of a relatively mild traumatic injury to his thigh.

Physical Examination.—The patient was a fairly well developed, somewhat emaciated middle-aged white male, who appeared extremely apprehensive. His head was normal in contour. His eyes, ears, nose and throat were negative. His chest expansion was somewhat decreased. This was most marked in the right apical region. There was decreased resonance over this area and the breath sounds were distant, as if heard through a markedly thickened pleura. The heart was negative clinically. Abdomen was somewhat prominent. The liver was three fingers' breadth below the costal margin. There was a small scar in the right lower quadrant (appendectomy). The examination of the extremities showed the right thigh about one and one-half times the size of the corresponding member. There was a linear incision about eight inches long over the anterior surface. This was filled with fungating, granulating tissue. There was superficial infection with a foul odor to the exudate on the surface. A tentative diagnosis of fibrosarcoma was made and the patient was advised to have an amputation.

Laboratory Findings.—Red blood cells, 3,800,000 with hemoglobin 56%. White blood cells, 10,500 with 67% polymorphonuclear leukocytes, 23% lymphocytes and 8% monocytes. Urinalysis was negative. Blood chemistry was within normal limits with the urea showing 15 mgm. per 100 c.c. Serology was negative.

Operative Procedure.—A radical iliac abdominal amputation of the left leg was done. The entire left leg, half of the ilium, acetabulum and half of the ischium were removed.

Postoperative History.—The immediate postoperative condition of the patient was poor. He was given several transfusions and intravenous saline and glucose hypodermoclysis. He improved steadily and was discharged one month after his admission with a granulating area in the operative wound approximately the size of a twenty-five cent piece.

Pathological Specimen.—Gross Description.—Specimen consisted of the entire right leg with a portion of the ischium, ilium and the acetabulum at the posterior middle border of the thigh. About 5 cm. below the groin was a large ulcerating, granulomatous lesion approximately 10 cm. in diameter. There was a fungating overgrowth of tumor tissue which made up the base of the ulcer. On splitting the leg longitudinally, this tumor mass was found to measure approximately 25 cm. in length. It apparently arose from the deep fascial tissues and had no definite relation to the periosteum. The tumor as a whole was a pinkish gray in color, but there were many areas of necrosis and hemorrhage.

Microscopic Description of Tissue from the Tumor. (Fig. 231) The tumor is made up of cells of all shapes and sizes. Many of them are multinucleated, tumor giant cells. Numerous atypical mitoses are seen. The general character of the cells, however, can be recognized as definitely of a spindle type, and in places where cell differentiation has proceeded to any extent, intercellular collagen has been laid down in variable amounts. In these more differentiated areas, the cells tend to be arranged in irregular fasciculi, which are interlacing in appearance. Here, the nuclei are relatively ovoid with some of them definitely becoming elongated, with blunt ends. Some actual fibroglia fibers may be identified. The tumor as a whole, however, shows an extreme degree of anaplasia with a wild overgrowth of tissue which shows all the classical features of extreme malignancy.

Myxosarcomata.—The myxosarcoma is like its benign counterpart, a speculative neoplasm. In general, it is probable that no such true tumor is encountered clinically, but that the neoplasms which usually are diagnosed by this term represent again fibrosarcomata with extensive myxomatous degeneration.

Liposarcomata.—Liposarcoma is a variety of tumor about which there is considerable debate. Opinions vary greatly as to its frequency. The obvious difficulties encountered in histologic examination of a tumor of connective tissue origin which is invading fat or one which is differentiating into fat cells are apparent at once. It is unquestionably true that a certain number of such fat cell sarcomata actually do occur and these usually show reversion from fetal and adult fat cell forms to relatively undifferentiated cells resembling primitive fibroblasts. As a rule, these tumors are of a relatively lower grade malignancy than the more characteristic simple fibrosarcomata already described, but should be considered from a prognostic standpoint, in this former group of cases. Because of the higher degree of cell differentiation as a rule, and likewise because of the lipoid content of these tumors, they are generally found to be much more resistant to irradiation. An illustration of a tumor believed to fit best into this classification is presented.

ILLUSTRATIVE CASE

CASE 94. (Ref. #S-240)

Diagnosis.—Thigh—liposarcoma.

Patient was a white male of 36 years, admitted to the hospital because of a painful lump in the left thigh, which had been increasing in size.

Present Illness.—The patient's history was of interest in that about eighteen years ago he began to develop multiple small nodules all over the body. These grew slowly in size, the largest becoming not larger than a walnut. They were not painful and caused him no symptoms. He had two of these removed for cosmetic reasons from his neck, and a diagnosis of lipomata was made at that time, twelve years ago. One of these tumors had started to increase in size during the four or five months before his present admission, and had become moderately painful. It was for that reason that the patient sought medical aid.

Past History.—Patient did not recall ever having had any of the childhood diseases. Indeed, he had never been ill so far as he could remember other than a very occasional cold. His appetite and digestion were unusually good and he had always been able to eat any and everything without distress of any sort. His genito-urinary history was entirely negative. He denied venereal disease.

Physical Examination.—The patient was a well-developed, somewhat obese, middle-aged white male. His head was normal in contour. Eyes, ears, nose and throat were negative. Neck: There were several small subcutaneous, elastic-feeling nodules two to three centimeters in diameter felt over the back of the neck. Several similar nodules, none of them over 2 to 3 cm. were felt in the subcutaneous tissues of the trunk and thighs. Chest was symmetrical. Heart and lungs were negative. Abdomen was obese. Extremities were negative except for the presence of a mass about 12 cm. in diameter in the midthigh region. This was freely movable in the subcutaneous tissues. It was regular in outline. It was not tender on palpation but he complained of pain radiating to the knee at times in association with this mass. A diagnosis of multiple lipomata was made and excision of this larger mass advised.

Laboratory Findings.—Urinalysis was negative. Red blood cells, 5,020,000 with 83% hemoglobin. White blood cells, 9,300 with 82% polymorphonuclears and 16% lymphocytes.

Operative History.—Under local anesthesia a large fatty tumor mass was removed from the thigh. In addition two of the larger masses from the neck were removed for the comfort of the patient.

Pathological Report.—GROSS DESCRIPTION.—Specimen consisted of an ovoidal mass 12 cm. in diameter except as modified by the presence of a few soft lobules. This was completely covered by a smooth capsule. The capsular surface was a pale pinkish-gray. On section the cut surface was moderately yellow. The mass was somewhat cheesy in consistency with numerous soft areas of complete necrosis. Around the periphery, there were firmer nodules, almost white in color and translucent in appearance. In some of the necrotic areas, hemorrhage had occurred.

Microscopic Description of the Tumor.—(Fig. 232) Examination of the tissue shows a curious combination of adult fat cells intimately related to irregular bundles of elongated spindled cells with nuclei which are rather difficult to identify. Many of them tend to show almost pointed ends. In other areas, the nuclei appear rounded. Many of these cells show no apparent definitive cytoplasm. Others, however, do show a fairly sharp nuclear membrane. These somewhat spindled cells with definite cytoplasm show marked fatty vacuolization. Here and there, masses of these cells, cut in cross section, can be identified. Occasional mitotic figures are found. These appear to be normal. Many of the nuclei are hyperchromatic; others show karyolytic degeneration. There is considerable pleomorphism of the cells. Around the necrotic areas, the tumor appears relatively vascular, and in these areas the tumor cells are preserved in the immediate vicinity of the blood vessels.

Frozen section of the tissue stained by Scharlach R confirms the fatty nature of the tissue. In the more mature cells there is a great deal of fat. It is believed that this does not represent fatty degeneration of tissue but that it represents the differentiation of the fibroblasts toward the adult fat cell and that, therefore, the diagnosis of this tumor should be liposarcoma in view of the histologic evidence of malignancy.

CHAPTER XXV

TUMORS OF BONE

Tumors which involve bone make up such an important group of neoplasms that they merit separate consideration. We are accustomed to speak generically of these tumors as "bone tumors." Histogenetically, however, the tumors which involve bone are derived from several different cell types and strictly speaking should be correspondingly classified. From the practical consideration, however, as we indicated in the outline of the tentatively proposed classification, this is one group of tumors which it is more customary to consider from a regional or anatomical basis than from a histogenetic one.

There are four major varieties of tumor which are ordinarily included in this group: (1) the true bone-producing tumors derived from the osteo- and chondroblasts, (2) the so-called benign giant cell tumor of bone, (3) the plasma cell myeloma which is usually seen as multiple lesions, and (4) the endothelial myeloma or Ewing's tumor as it is more familiarly known. These will be considered separately. For a more complete presentation of the entire problem of bone tumors, the reader is referred to the classical monograph of Geschichter and Copeland, entitled "Tumors of Bone."

OSTEOGENIC SARCOMA

In the preceding chapter we have already discussed the benign forms of tumors arising from cartilaginous and bone-producing cells, the chondroblast and osteoblast. These are correspondingly designated as simple chondroma and osteoma, and remain as pure cell type tumors.

When we turn to the consideration of the malignant tumors of these cells, we find that they are best classified, generically, under the heading of osteogenic or bone-producing tumors. This broad terminology includes a wide variety of tumors as listed in the older textbooks, in which the more minute differential features of these tumors were emphasized. It is still true that we may, on occasion, find malignant tumors arising from cartilage or from pre-existing benign cartilaginous tumors which maintain for long periods of time their essential cartilaginous character and might, from a strict standpoint, be labeled as chondrosarcomata. More often, however, we find that the connective tissue cell, in its differentiation toward these specialized cartilaginous and bone-producing cells, does not maintain this differentiation between cartilage and bone formation too closely. As a result, most tumors, even although cartilage-like cells predominate, will be found to include areas of atypical ossification and osteoblast activity. For purposes of prognostic differentiation, it is convenient at

times to add in parenthesis to the diagnosis of osteogenic sarcoma, the modifying terms which designate the preponderance of one or another of these various cell differences. Thus, we still employ such cumbersome terminology as chondromyxosarcoma, fibrochondrosarcoma, osteochondrosarcoma, and any combination of these various terms. These, as noted above, are merely variants of the basic bone-forming cells and are so termed depending upon the relative histological predominance of one or another of the cell types (Fig. 239 and 242).

In addition, there is a tumor which arises specifically from the periosteum of the bone, apparently from cells which have not as yet differentiated into actual osteoblasts. These tumors rarely go on to the point of actual bone trabeculae formation. It is known specifically as the *periosteal fibrosarcoma*, although coming from periosteal cells as it does, it should be included in the group of osteogenic sarcomata. In many textbooks this particular tumor is included among the fibrosarcomata because of its histologic appearance.

In this condensed discussion of the osteogenic sarcoma, we are forced to generalize to a considerable extent. From the practical standpoint, the usual tumor of bone tends to occur most frequently in the long bones and near one or the other end of the

PLATE LVII

TUMORS OF BONE

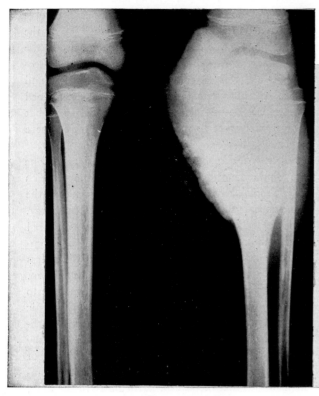

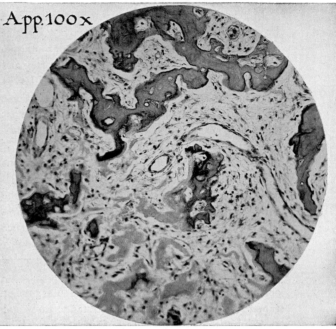

FIG. 235.—X-RAY—TIBIA: OSTEOGENIC SARCOMA.—
CASE 95.—Observe asymmetric enlargement of epiphyseal end of diaphysis with increased density, loss of normal landmarks and fuzziness of periphery resulting from radiating spicules of bone invading soft tissues.

FIG. 236.—CASE 95.—Low power photomicrograph showing sclerosing type of osteogenic sarcoma with atypical bone trabeculae, osteoid tissue, abnormal calcification and diffuse fibrosis. App. 100 x.

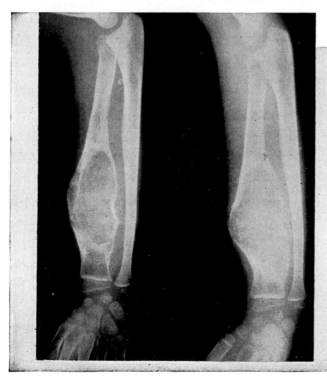

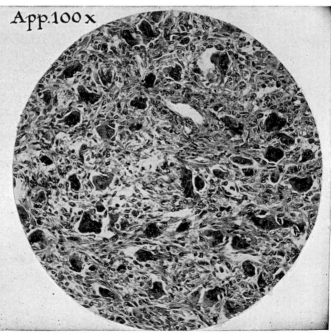

FIG. 237.—X-RAY—ARM: GIANT CELL TUMOR OF RADIUS.—
cf. CASE 96.—Typical fusiform enlargement of epiphyseal end of diaphysis with extensive demineralization and cystic degeneration of lesion centrally

FIG. 238.—CASE 96.—Low power histologic appearance. Irregularly arranged fibrous tissue stroma with presence of innumerable characteristic giant cells. App. 100 x. (See Fig. 83 and 217.)

diaphysis. No bones are exempt from such neoplastic degeneration, however. Thus, we find that another comparatively common site for osteogenic sarcomata is seen in the sacrum or the ilium in or near the sacro-iliac joint.

In general, osteogenic sarcomata are characterized by the production of abnormal bony trabeculae which, in the x-ray, appears as an irregular enlargement of the area involved, including both cortex and medulla. Typically, spicules of bone more or less at right angles to the cortical surface are seen. These spicules of bone tend to be somewhat broader at their base so that the lesion which tends to be fusiform becomes blurred at its periphery.

Microscopically, these tumors show all gradations of bone formation with varying degrees of vascularization. On the basis of the relative vascularity, bone formation and bone destruction, the tumors are classified in sub-varieties. This is of practical importance from the prognostic standpoint. Roughly speaking, these tumors with the more adult, sclerosing type of bone formation tend to have a somewhat more favorable prognosis whereas the extremely vascular type of tumor is much more prone to metastasize early and to exhibit the higher degree of malignancy. The terms applied to these variations in the histologic picture are as follows:

Telangiectatic Type.—These are the tumors which present extreme vascularity, the tumor cells frequently forming the walls of huge vascular sinusoids. As a result of this circulatory picture, areas of necrosis and hemorrhage are frequently seen.

Sclerosing Type.—(Fig. 235 and 236) These tumors are more often slowly growing and involve particularly the cortex, in contradistinction to the telangiectatic type, which is more apt to arise in the medullary portion of the bone. The degree of osteogenesis and cell differentiation is much greater and more calcium is laid down in the newly formed trabeculae. It is this variety which is somewhat slower in respect to metastasis, and in which there are a few five-year cures on record.

Osteolytic Type.—(Fig. 241) Occasionally, one may find among these osteogenic tumors one in which osteoclastic activity becomes so prominent that the bone appears to dissolve away as viewed by the x-ray. The osteoclastic activity may at times be confused with benign giant cell formation. There *is* accompanying osteogenesis, however, although this is less striking than the sclerosing form of the condition.

No attempt can be made in the space available to go into greater detail. In the treatment of osteogenic sarcoma we are dealing with one of the most hopeless forms of malignancy. Intensive irradiation may control cases at times. Amputation is the rule, but by the time diagnosis has been established it is common to find that metastasis, particularly to the lung, has already occurred. In large series of cases, with these radical methods of therapy employed early and in skilled hands, the mortality has been reduced from almost a hundred per cent to about eighty-five per cent. For the most part, these tumors are found in children and young adults, although no age group is entirely immune to their occurrence.

ILLUSTRATIVE CASE

CASE 95. (Ref. #S-230)
Diagnosis.—Bone—osteogenic sarcoma.
Patient was a white male of 16 years, who was admitted to the hospital with the following history: Four months before admission the patient received several slight injuries in the region of the right knee during basketball practice. He was not incapacitated at the time. Gradually he developed a limp because of an aching sensation on motion. There was a gradually increasing limitation of motion in the right knee. This produced no pain except with motion. For the four or five weeks preceding admission, swelling around the knee joint appeared and this increased steadily, even with two weeks' rest in bed and local applications of heat.
Past History.—The child was a full-term, normally delivered male infant who was artifically fed after the third month. At the age of two he developed blindness in the left eye as the result of a neoplasm. The eye was enucleated and a diagnosis of a retinoblastoma was

made, with an unusual amount of cellular proliferation. No recurrence of this tumor developed. He had a tonsillectomy at the age of nine years. He had had none of the usual childhood diseases and in all other respects had been entirely healthy. A review of his various systems was entirely negative. One year preceding the present condition, he complained of some stiffness of the right knee while playing basketball. This seemed to subside spontaneously, however, and he had given it no thought.
Physical Examination.—Physical examination presented a picture of a normal, healthy, well-developed, well-nourished young white male, who appeared his given age. His head was normal in contour. His right eye reacted normally to light and accommodation. He had an artificial left eye. Ears, nose and throat were negative. Chest was symmetrical. Heart and lungs were apparently normal. Abdomen: There were no masses or tenderness. Extremities were negative except for fusiform swelling of the right knee with limitation of mo-

PLATE LVIII
TUMORS OF THE BONE
Variants of the Osteogenic Sarcoma

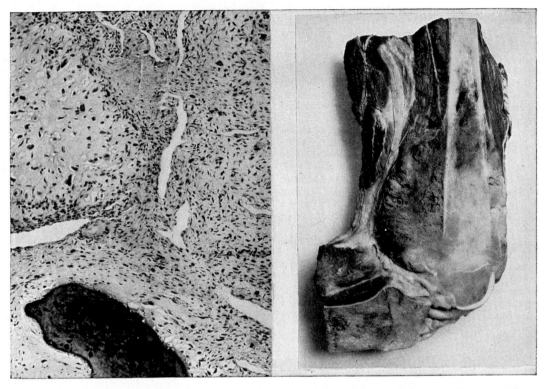

Fig. 239.—Osteochondrosarcoma.—Observe marked variation in appearance of tumor, with cells differentiating from embryonic connective tissue through abortive cartilage and osteoid tissue up to actual bone formation. App. 100 x.

Fig. 240.—Femur—Osteogenic Sarcoma.—Gross photograph of cross section of tumor showing its characteristic location at the epiphyseal end of the diaphysis and its extension to the soft tissues.

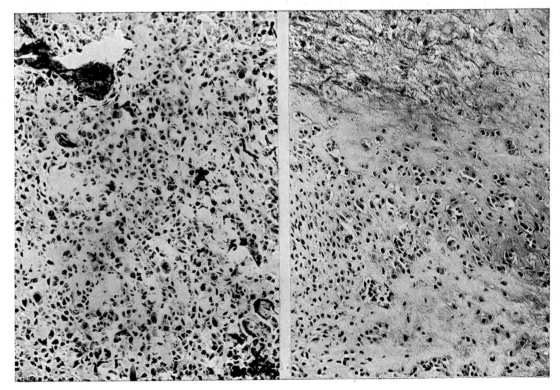

Fig. 241.—Osteogenic Sarcoma—Osteolytic Type.— Note necrotic bone (left upper) undergoing absorption, and proliferation of abortive osteoid tissue by pleomorphic, hyperchromic and anaplastic cells. App. 100 x.

Fig. 242.—Osteochondromyxosarcoma.—Another variant of the osteogenic sarcoma characterized by abnormal cartilage formation, marked myxomatous degeneration and absence of typical bone production. App. 100 x.

tion. This swelling was relatively uniform in appearance grossly. On palpation there was a large, firm mass attached to the bone. On pressure, this caused slight pain. The motion of the knee joint was limited at 170° extension and 100° flexion. The circumference of the leg was seventeen inches as compared to twelve and one-half inches on the opposite side.

Laboratory Findings.—Red blood cells, 5,020,000 with 99% (15.5 grams) hemoglobin. White blood cells 9,600 with 56% polynuclears, 33% lymphocytes and 11% monocytes. Urinalysis was negative, except for occasional very slight traces of albumin.

X-ray examination showed a neoplastic process involving the lower 18 cm. of the right femur. Both cortical and medullary portions showed both osteolysis and osteogenesis. The osteogenetic changes predominated. Spicules of new bone formation were seen extending outward into the soft tissues. Many of these were at right angles to the cortical surface. The tumor showed evidence of invasion of the epiphysis. No evidence of metastatic lesions in the chest or elsewhere were found. A diagnosis of osteogenic sarcoma was made radiologically.

On the basis of the history and radiologic findings, a confirmatory biopsy was done and the diagnosis of osteogenic sarcoma confirmed.

Operative History.—An amputation of the leg at the hip joint was performed, and the specimen was submitted for pathologic study.

Pathological Report.—Gross Description.—Gross examination showed a large, more or less fusiform tumor mass involving the lower half of the femur. This had invaded the soft tissues and was surrounded by a mass of edematous muscle and subcutaneous tissue. The specimen was split longitudinally and a diffuse neoplastic process found replacing the marrow cavity and involving the cortex extensively. It had invaded the epiphysis and extended into the joint cavity.

Microscopic Description of the Tumor.—(Fig. 235 and 236) Microscopic examination of the tissue shows the characteristic picture of osteogenic sarcoma. The tissue is extremely cellular. The cells are large, although they vary much in size and shape. They possess a light, basophilic cytoplasm, large nuclei made up of a deep staining nuclear membrane and a scant scattering of chromatin particles. Nucleoli are variable, but for the most part they are small, bluish bodies. Numerous multinucleated cells containing from four to eight or ten nuclei are encountered. Between the cells there is a hyaline ground substance which in some places has the contour of bony spicules of cancellous bone, but without the laminated markings or haversian canals. Spicules of disintegrated bone are encountered. Areas of hemorrhage and necrosis, as well as thin-walled blood sinuses are observed. In a few areas, the arrangement of the large cells described about the hyaline osteoid masses is typical of the osteoblastic pattern. Many bizarre mitotic figures are encountered.

BENIGN GIANT CELL TUMOR

The next most important type of tumor involving bone, from the standpoint of numbers, is seen in the so-called benign giant cell tumor of bone. This may be single, or it may occur in multiple form involving many of the long bones. This, likewise, tends to occur at the diaphyseal ends of the long bones. It arises usually in the medullary portion of the bone, although not necessarily symmetrically, and causes more or less fusiform local expansion of the cortex with thinning. The periphery of the tumor in these cases is usually smooth as compared with the periosteal reaction noted in the osteogenic type. There is a marked demineralization with the formation of lacunar areas of cystic degeneration, which become filled with soft fibrous tissue. These contain innumerable tumor giant cells with their nuclei characteristically centrally placed. This type of giant cell has been described (Fig. 83 and 217) in the chapter on chronic inflammation in contrast to the tumor giant cell seen, as for example in the fibrosarcoma (Fig. 84 and 218). As a matter of practical interest, the more nuclei that one finds in these cells the less the indication is of possible subsequent malignant degeneration.

The picture, radiologically, is very characteristic.

This shows loculated, demineralized cavitation and enlargement of the bone locally. It is seen particularly in association with parathyroid hyperplasia or neoplasm. Several cases have been cured by the surgical removal of tumors of the parathyroid. In general, the giant cell tumor is benign in nature and does not metastasize. However, spontaneous pathological fractures of the bone may occur as the result of thinning of the cortex. Rarely, they may undergo malignant degeneration. Such cases then run the course of other malignant tumors of the bone. These are apt to be confused with the osteolytic form.

The treatment of these cases is first, parathyroid control as indicated; and second, radiation. They should probably not be operated upon except, perhaps, for diagnostic biopsy, in doubtful instances, unless there is evidence of a sudden increase in the rate of growth. It is only the exceptional instance that requires any radical, surgical form of treatment. Many cases have been treated successfully, especially where fracture has occurred, by curetting out the contents of the neoplastic area and filling this cavity with bone chips and blood clot to act as foci of osteogenesis. Amputation should not be necessary but has been done in many instances with a mistaken

PLATE LIX

TUMORS OF THE BONE

MYELOMATA

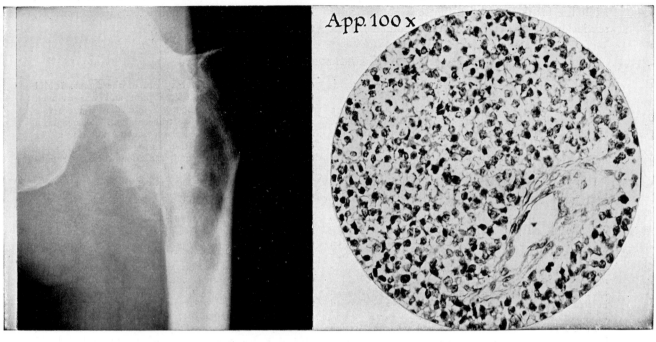

FIG. 243.—X-RAY—FEMUR: EWING'S ENDOTHELIAL MYELOMA.
—CASE 97.—Tumor arising in medullary canal of shaft of
bone and extending asymmetrically into soft tissues. Extensive irregular demineralization.

FIG. 244.—CASE 97.—Low power photomicrograph to illustrate
the monotonous uniformity in appearance of the cells and their
arrangement; sheets of cells having typical ovoid, vesicular
nuclei, indefinite cytoplasmic outlines and rare mitotic figures.
App. 100 x.

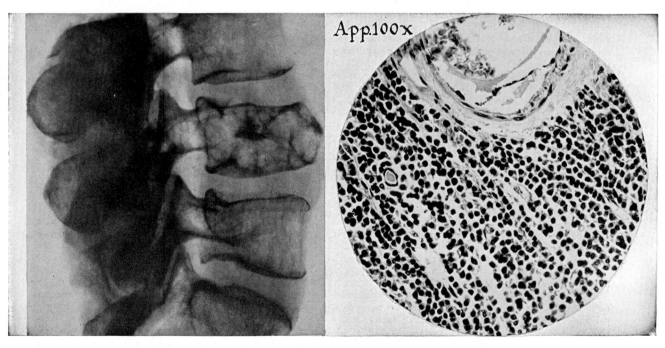

FIG. 245.—X-RAY—VERTEBRAE—PLASMA CELL MYELOMA.—
CASE 98.—Punched out areas of demineralization of body of
vertebra suggesting metastatic tumor invasion, and the resultant deformity from weight bearing.

FIG. 246.—CASE 98.—Low power photomicrograph.—Tumor
made up of strands or stalks of typical plasma cells, supported
by a delicate stroma of capillary vessels and connective tissue.
App. 100 x.

diagnosis or inadequate knowledge regarding the natural history of the disease.

The benign giant cell tumor is a tumor of young adult life for the most part. There is no particular sex incidence. The etiology of the condition is most obscure. Cases have followed trauma of varying degree and this is believed by many to be an important factor in the development of the tumor. In those instances where parathyroid activity is responsible, the treatment becomes obvious.

ILLUSTRATIVE CASE

CASE 96. (Ref. #S-123)

Diagnosis.—Bone—benign giant cell tumor.

Patient was a single, white female of 25 years, a hosiery worker by occupation. She was admitted to the hospital complaining of progressive swelling of the left knee region for ten months to a year accompanied by intermittent dull, aching pain and weakness of the leg on walking.

Present Illness.—The present illness dated back about two years before admission when the patient fell on an icy pavement and injured her left knee. She had no incapacity with this injury at the time, but about three months later she noticed increasing weakness of the leg when walking. In fact, when she put her full weight on the affected side, the knee would more or less give way under her. About one year before admission, approximately one year after her injury, she noticed swelling around the knee joint. This swelling had slowly increased in size during the interval and had been accompanied by intermittent, dull pain.

Past History.—As a child, she had whooping cough but none of the other contagious diseases. She was subject to frequent sore throats, but had no history of rheumatic fever. A review of her systems otherwise was irrelevant. Her cardiorespiratory system was negative. Gastro-intestinal system showed a moderate amount of constipation which was readily controlled with laxatives. Genito-urinary history was negative except for a rather definite polyuria with nocturia two to three times per night. Catamenic history was normal. Menses began at fourteen years of age and were regular every thirty days.

Physical Examination.—Patient was a fairly well-developed and well-nourished young white woman, who was lying comfortably in bed. Her skin and mucous membranes were somewhat pale. Head was grossly negative. Eyes, ears, nose and throat were negative. Neck showed slight enlargement of the cervical lymph nodes, particularly on the left. The thyroid was not palpable, and no abnormal pulsations were heard. Chest was of the phthisical type. Râles were heard throughout. Heart was negative. Abdomen was scaphoid. No masses were palpable. Extremities were negative except for the involvement of the left knee. There was a uniform swelling of the knee area. On palpation, a bulging mass about 8 x 10 cm. was felt involving the left internal condyle of the femur. The patella did not seem involved. The mass was not painful, nor was any fluctuation noted. There was marked limitation of motion, apparently of a mechanical nature.

Laboratory Findings.—Red blood cells, 3,400,000 with 60% hemoglobin. White blood cells 11,300 with 67% polynuclears and 29% lymphocytes. Urinalysis was negative.

X-ray examination of the left femur showed a large osteolytic area of demineralization with erosion of the cortex involving the distal 15 cm. of the femur. It did not, however, invade the knee joint and was confined to the diaphysis. Throughout the eroded area there was a great deal of coarse bone trabeculation. The neoplasm had extended into the soft tissues on the anterior aspect of the femur. A presumptive diagnosis of benign giant cell tumor was made and radiation therapy recommended.

Subsequent Course.—The patient was given an intensive course of x-ray treatment, and the lesion locally definitely improved with marked reduction in its size. However, osteogenesis was not satisfactory as should have been expected, and the patient subsequently developed another area of similar osteolysis in the left index finger involving the proximal phalanx and another area in the proximal end of the right humerus. On the basis of these multiple lesions and the failure of the patient to respond as satisfactorily to irridiation therapy as it was felt she should, it was decided to investigate this patient more thoroughly from the standpoint of parathyroid pathology. Laboratory studies showed a calcium of 12.7 mgm., a phosphorus of 3.2 mgm. and blood chlorides of 300 mgm. An exploratory operation was performed in an effort to remove one or more of the parathyroids in an attempt to reduce the parathyroid activity. A small cyst the size of a cherry was found on the posterior aspect of the lower pole of the left lobe of the thyroid, which was removed for pathological study, and a small plaque of yellowish tissue from the right side in the same relative position was also removed.

Pathological report of this tissue showed a diffuse hyperplasia of the parathyroid tissue. This could not be considered as a true adenoma, but as one of those diffuse processes containing many Wasserhelle cells. Accompanying this operative procedure, the phalanx was removed because of the extensive involvement of the bone with almost complete destruction of the cortex accompanied by a pathological fracture. Following this operative procedure, the patient showed steady improvement in the lesions involving the femur and the humerus. The treatment was combined with supplementary irradiation.

Pathological Report.—Gross Description.—The gross specimen consisted of the entire finger. This was split longitudinally and a diffuse neoplastic process was found involving the entire proximal phalanx. The medulla was replaced by a hemorrhagic and grayish colored mass of tumor tissue which had completely destroyed the cortex and had invaded the soft tissues surrounding the bone.

Microscopic Description of the Tumor.—(Fig. 237 and 238) There is a background of connective tissue showing a considerable amount of fibroblastic proliferation with a prominent collagen development forming closely woven interlacing bundles. Among these connective tissue cells are seen many large multinucleated giant cells measuring 40 to 60 micra in diameter. These are of the characteristic variety seen in such tumors with their nuclei centrally placed for the most part. The nuclei themselves are ovoid, with a fairly well defined nuclear membrane and scattered chromatin rods and granules. There is no particular tendency toward hyperchromatism.

In addition to these cells, a considerable mononuclear cellular infiltration of the stroma is observed. The tumor is relatively vascular with a good many small capillaries visible in the section, accompanied by hemorrhage into the tumor tissue.

MYELOMATA

Ewing's Tumor (endothelial myeloma).—This tumor, which was first separated by Ewing in 1920 from other tumors involving bone also tends to occur in children and young adults before the age of thirty. It usually arises within the medullary canal of one of the long bones, particularly the femur, tibia, humerus or fibula, but may involve the scapula or ilium initially. The exact histogenetic origin of this tumor is not completely agreed upon. Ewing's original thought was that it arose from the endothelium of the marrow spaces. Most people today believe it to be of reticuloendothelial origin and therefore not to be classed as a myeloma, but as a reticulum cell sarcoma.

The tumors tend to be expansive, producing rather fusiform enlargement of the bone and extending through the cortex gradually to involve the soft tissue. At times, this may stir up sufficient periosteal reaction to simulate osteogenic sarcoma. One particularly significant diagnostic feature of this type of tumor is that it tends to sooner or later involve multiple bones. Whether this is the result of actual metastasis or a multicentric stimulation of tumor production is not known. This is quite unlike true osteogenic sarcoma, which rarely, if ever, shows secondary bone lesions. It is a slowly growing tumor, which metastasizes late. Pathological fracture may occur and is sometimes the first symptom of the condition. Many cases respond fairly well to radiation, but the great majority of cases tend to become progressive regardless of any form of therapy.

As a result, the prognosis, in general, is very poor. Death results usually in a matter of two to three years, accompanied by pulmonary metastasis and multiple bone involvement. A few permanent cures are on record, however.

Histologically, the tumor is characterized by the presence of a more or less uniform proliferation of round, ovoid or polyhedral cells arranged in solid, monotonous sheets. Occasionally, some tendency toward perivascular proliferation is seen. The nuclei are relatively pale-staining, with a delicate cell nuclear membrane and chromatin granules. There is little or no cytoplasm demonstrable in the majority of these cells, which are in apposition to one another by what appear to be poorly formed fibrillar reticulum structures. The reticular nature of the tumor may be brought out by special silver stains. Mitoses vary in number, but in general are relatively few as compared with those occurring in the other malignant tumors of bone, and those which are seen are fairly typical in appearance.

ILLUSTRATIVE CASE

CASE 97. (Ref. #S-311)

Diagnosis.—Femur—Ewing's tumor (endothelial myeloma).

Patient was a white Hebrew male, aged 24, who was admitted to the hospital with the chief complaint of pain in the right hip radiating to the knee, of four months' duration.

Present Illness.—The present illness began eighteen months before his present hospitalization. At that time, he noted swelling of his hip with some limitation of motion. He went to a hospital and received a course of ten x-ray treatments, following a biopsy of an inguinal lymph node. He improved considerably following his discharge from the hospital and remained free from symptoms for a little over one year. At that time his hip again became swollen and he developed the radiating pain referred to as his chief complaint. He returned to the hospital and received another series of x-ray treatments two months before the present admission. The swelling decreased considerably in amount, but this time he did not get any great relief from his pain. About one month ago, his hip again became swollen and stiff, and prevented his being able to get around except with great difficulty. Over those four months, he had lost thirty pounds in weight and had noticed increasing weakness and fatiguability. He came to the hospital to see if anything further could be done for his relief.

Past History.—His past medical history was noncontributory. He had the usual childhood diseases. He had not had rheumatic fever. He had had no more than the average number of mild upper respiratory infections. His gastro-intestinal, cardiovascular and genito-urinary systems were normal. He denied venereal infection.

Physical Examination.—The patient was a well developed young white male adult, who showed marked weight loss. His physical examination was essentially negative except over the right hip region. His head was normal in contour. Eyes, ears, nose and throat were negative. His chest was clear throughout. Heart was not enlarged and showed no murmurs. His abdomen was flat. External genitalia appeared negative. The arms and left leg were negative. There was considerable post-radiation pigmentation of the skin over the right lower abdominal quadrant and over the right hip. The hip was painful on motion and there was a very marked limitation of motion present. No lymphadenopathy could be detected.

Laboratory Findings.—Blood count: Hemoglobin, 8.5 grams; red blood cells, 3,500,000. White blood cells, 8,750 with 88% polymorphonuclear leukocytes of which 19 were nonfilamented and 69 were filamented forms; lymphocytes 10%, monocytes 1% and basophiles 1%. Urinalysis: Yellow, acid, 1.014, very slight trace of albumin; no sugar; occasional hyaline casts. Wassermann negative.

X-ray suggested the probable diagnosis of Ewing's tumor of the femur with metastatic lesions in the lungs. Biopsy was recommended for pathological confirmation.

Subsequent Course.—The patient ran a progressively downhill course in spite of intensive radiation and died six weeks after admission. This represented a total time interval of somewhat under two years, although it is probable that the actual onset was somewhat earlier than the clinical history suggested.

Pathological Report.—Gross Description.—Tissue was obtained by biopsy from the right hip and from a subcutaneous nodule which was in the scalp. These consisted of soft, hemorrhagic, necrotic tumor tissue embedded in bone fragments in the femur.

Microscopic Description of a Section from the Hip Biopsy.—(Fig. 243 and 244) Sections from the bone show a degenerative process of the bone with considerable osteolysis. The marrow spaces are increased in size and show considerable edema and vascularity. Moderate osteoblastic activity can be demonstrated in certain areas. Many of the marrow spaces contain masses of tumor cells which are arranged around vascular spaces, some of which are lined by endothelium and others by tumor cells. These latter cells are irregular in outline, varying from ovoid to somewhat spindle shape. The nuclei are oval, lightly chromatic with scattered granules and rods of chromatin. There is a certain monotony to the structure of this neoplastic process which is entirely consistent with the diagnosis of Ewing's type of endothelial myeloma.

Plasma cell myeloma (multiple myelomata).—This tumor is one which is presumably of myeloid origin rather than of actual bone origin. The usual and characteristic cell type is the plasma cell, so that these tumors are ordinarily spoken of as plasma cell myelomata or *plasmacytomata*. They occur almost invariably in individuals past forty years of age and are characterized by the multiplicity of lesions. These tend to develop first in the marrow spaces of the flat bones, notably the skull, but later spread to the other bones, including the spine and the long bones. The process is apparently an invasion of the bone tissues with resulting osteoclasis and demineralization. This accounts for the multiple punched out lesions which can be demonstrated scattered through the membranous bone. In a small percentage of these cases Bence-Jones bodies can be found in the urine, as confirmatory diagnostic evidence.

Histologically, these tumors appear as cords of typical plasma cells arranged between delicate connective tissue and capillary stalks showing little or no stromal support. Mitoses are difficult to find in the majority of these cases, and many believe that these cells more frequently multiply by amitosis than by mitosis. The distribution, the age incidence and the appearance of the lesions, roentgenologically, render diagnosis usually easy. Prognosis is invariably fatal, the cases running an average duration of about two to three years after diagnosis is established. Occasionally, they may run a very much more rapid course, dying within a few months.

Diagnostically, all of the tumors of bone may, through replacement of marrow by tumor cells, gradually produce an anemia. This is particularly true, however, of the two latter tumors which are more likely to be multiple and involve much more of the active bone marrow. In the case of the usual osteogenic sarcoma or benign, giant-cell tumor of bone, the development of an anemia is less striking as these tumors are usually so well localized.

ILLUSTRATIVE CASE

CASE 98. (Ref. #S-172) (Courtesy of Drs. A. Ornsteen and S. Levine, of Jewish Hospital, Philadelphia, Pa.)

Diagnosis.—Bone—plasma cell myeloma.

Patient was a white male of 56 years, who was admitted to the hospital complaining of persistent headache.

Present Illness.—The onset of the present illness was about six months before admission when the patient first noticed the development of headaches, which became almost continuous. At first, they were right-sided but soon became bilateral. They seemed much worse at night. Dimness of vision developed in the right eye and he likewise had occasional periods of diplopia. There was no weakness or paralysis of any of his muscles. He had frequent nosebleeds.

Past History.—His past history was essentially negative. A review of his systems gave no information pertinent to his present illness.

Physical Examination.—Head was normal in shape. Pupils were regular and equal and reacted well to light and accommodation. There was no nystagmus. There was right internal deviation with strabismus. There was contraction of the right visual field on the temporal side.

Vision in the right eye was markedly diminished. There was no cyanosis or jaundice. The left eye was normal. Nose and throat were negative. Chest was symmetrical. There was impaired resonance of the apices and right middle lobe. Breath sounds were diminished at the right base. Over the fifth rib in the left axillary line, a small tender mass about the size of a walnut was palpated. Heart was not enlarged. There was a presystolic murmur heard at the apex. Blood pressure was normal. Abdomen was negative. The prostate was enlarged and somewhat tender. There was no generalized peripheral adenopathy.

Laboratory Findings.—Urine was negative for Bence-Jones protein. The reaction was acid; specific gravity, 1.012 to 1.016; albumin (cloudy); sugar, negative, few hyaline and granular casts. Mosenthal Test, specific gravity 1.006 to 1.010 over a period of ten hours. Blood count: hemoglobin, 33 to 52%; red blood cells, 1,850,000 to 2,950,000; white blood cells, 7,000 to 15,000 with 69% polymorphonuclears, 30% lymphocytes and 1% eosinophiles. Blood calcium 10.2 mgm. Blood phosphorus 5.0 mgm. Blood urea, 29 to 77 mgm. Blood sugar, 96 mgm. Blood culture sterile. Sputum examination was negative for tubercle bacilli.

X-ray examination revealed numerous areas of osteolysis throughout the skull. They were well circumscribed, sharply defined and varied in size. The floor of the pituitary fossa was eroded. The posterior clinoid process was partially destroyed. The floor of the fossa was destroyed with consequent invasion of the sphenoid bone. The pineal body was calcified. There was diffuse osteoporosis of the ribs on both sides with destruction of localized areas in the 7th rib in the axillary line. The shoulder girdles showed osteolysis in the head of the humerus, the upper third of the shaft of the humerus and in the body of the scapula and clavicle. Involvement of the spine was also noted (Fig. 245). Similar areas of osteolysis about the size of a nickel were seen in the bones of the ilium, ischia and pubes. Both femora likewise showed similar lesions. This distribution of osteolytic lesions to the skull, ribs, shoulder girdles, pelvis, etc. favored the diagnosis of multiple myelomata.

Subsequent History.—The patient went rapidly downhill and died shortly after his admission to the hospital, as a result of pneumonia.

Autopsy Findings.—Postmortem examination showed marked emaciation, confirmatory evidence of the bone lesions as involving the skull and ribs. No invasion of the brain was found. There was a diffuse lobar pneumonia involving the left lung and right lower lobe. There was an old calcified apical tuberculosis. Heart was negative except for senile arteriosclerosis of the coronaries. The bodies of the lumbar vertebrae were found involved in the neoplastic process. The liver, spleen, pancreas, gastro-intestinal tract and kidneys were negative.

Microscopic Examination of One of the Tumor Nodules.—(Fig. 245 and 246) In general, the morphology of this tumor is that of a diffuse overgrowth in the marrow cavity with extension to the cortex, and even to the soft tissues, of cells which appear to belong to the plasma cell variety. In the typical case, as here, the entire tumor is made up of these cells appearing characteristically as between delicate connective tissue and capillary supporting tissue. This presents almost the monotony of the histologic picture as seen in Ewing's type of endothelial myeloma, but the cells are more characteristic and definitive in outline. They are for the most part cells ranging from ten to twelve micra in diameter with a typical lymphoid nucleus with the usual peripheral distribution of the chromatin in coarse granules. The cytoplasm is uniformly homogeneous and stains dark purplish-red. Mitoses are rare but may occasionally be seen. It is by the rather characteristic arrangement of these cells in linear, cord-like fashion, as well as by areas where they occur in almost solid sheets that the microscopic diagnosis is readily established.

CHAPTER XXVI
TUMORS ARISING FROM MUSCLE AND PIGMENT CELLS
PART I
TUMORS OF MUSCLE

Tumors of muscle may arise either from smooth muscle cells, in which case they are called *leiomyomata,* or from striated muscle cells as *rhabdomyomata.* The great majority of the tumors of muscle are of the smooth muscle variety. They may occur at any age, although much more commonly they are seen before middle life. The great majority of the smooth muscle tumors are of a benign nature, whereas practically all tumors of striated muscle origin are malignant in character.

Smooth Muscle Tumors.—The smooth muscle tumors may develop in any tissue where smooth muscle cells are normally found. The most common site for such tumor development is in the uterus as the so-called *"fibroid."* This is frequently spoken of as *"fibromyoma"* on the basis of the unusually prominent connective tissue stroma. We believe with most pathologists that the type cell from which any tumor arises should be accepted as the cell of origin, and that regardless of the amount of desmoplastic reaction which occurs this merely represents a secondary proliferation of the stroma. On this basis, these tumors should be called *"leiomyomata."*

In the uterus, the leiomyomata may occur as subserous, intramural or submucous nodules. They may be single or multiple. They vary in size from a few millimeters to tumors weighing 15 to 20 pounds. There is a curious racial selectivity, it having been estimated that as high as 80 per cent of Negresses show tumors of this type. On the other hand, tumors of the uterus among Malay or brown race are extremely uncommon, and the Caucasian race seems to occupy an intermediate position in this respect. For a complete discussion of the leiomyomata of the uterus, the reader is referred to Cullen's classical monograph.

Less frequently, tumors of smooth muscle may arise in any tissue where smooth muscle exists. This includes the walls of blood vessels, the musculature of the intestinal tract, the gallbladder, the urinary bladder, and even the erector pili muscles in the skin. For the most part, these tumors are discrete, localized, slow-growing benign lesions, many of them showing a tendency to regression. Aside from pressure symptoms, they are of little clinical significance. Occasionally, however, such tumors may undergo malignant degeneration. These have been described particularly in relation to the uterus and the gut. Even when they become frankly malignant they tend to remain localized for a relatively long period of time. They extend chiefly by direct invasion of the tissues locally, rather than by distant metastasis. In the case of the uterus, however, such sarcomatous change is apt to be associated with an increase in the vascularity of the tumor and blood vessel invasion may take place. When this occurs, metastatic lesions may be found widely disseminated but most commonly, as would be expected, in the lung.

Histologically, these tumors are made up of irregular, interlacing, purposelessly arranged bands of smooth muscle fibers, usually showing complete adult differentiation and cause little difficulty in diagnosis. They are embedded in a connective tissue stroma which frequently undergoes extensive hyaline degeneration. The average leiomyoma has a very limited blood supply which accounts for the not infrequent hyaline and cystic degeneration which is seen as the tumors increase in size, and their nourishment is correspondingly cut down. The tumors tend to grow peripherally so that the degenerative changes are apt to be found centrally with the more active cell growth around the margin of the tumor. The tendency of these tumors is to grow slowly and to compress the surrounding normal structures. This results in the development of a true connective tissue capsule, and clinically these tumors may be shelled

PLATE LX
PIGMENTED TUMORS

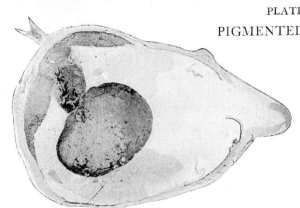

FIG. 247.—EYE: MALIGNANT MELANOMA.—Microtessar photograph of section through entire eye to show the pigmented nature of the lesion and its origin from the retina, growing out into the vitreous. App. 2 x.

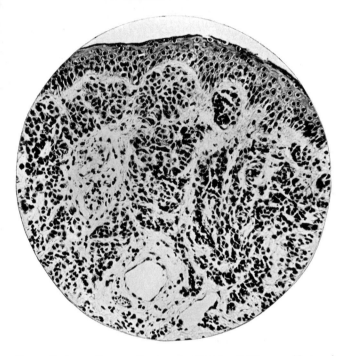

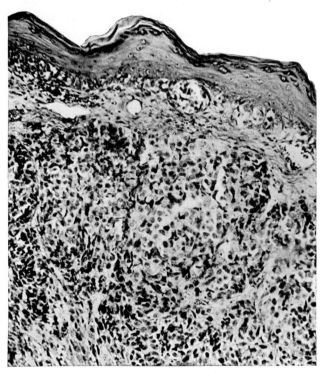

FIG. 248. SKIN: BENIGN PIGMENTED NEVUS.—CASE 102.—Nests of typical "nevus" cells (melanoblasts), which by their grouping suggests a relationship to the nerve ending. Overlying epithelium is thinned. App. 100 x.

FIG. 249.—SKIN: MALIGNANT MELANOMA.—By comparison with Fig. 248, note increased cellularity, presence of both pigmented and pale non-pigmented cells, complete disorder of architecture, with definite tissue invasion. App. 100 x.

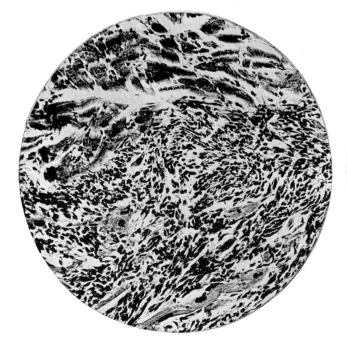

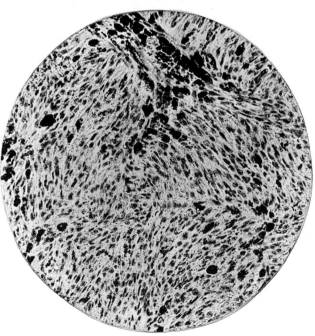

FIG. 250.—HEART: METASTATIC AMELANOTIC MALIGNANT MELANOMA.—CASE 103.—Spindling of cells, almost complete absence of pigment, and purposeless interlacing arrangement of cells suggest fibrosarcoma, but *some* pigment, history and involvement of *heart* establish diagnosis readily. App. 100 x.

FIG. 251.—From Fig. 247.—Again, observe close similarity in appearance of tumor to that of a fibrosarcoma. Scattered large, melanin-containing cells, however, reveal basic character of lesion. App. 100 x.

out of their capsule very readily and with little bleeding because of the comparatively few uterine vessels entering the tumor substance.

When such tumors become malignant, they may at times be distinguished with great difficulty from tumors of connective tissue origin. This is the result of the loss of their characteristic cell membranes and myoglia fibers. This is further complicated by the fact that not infrequently the connective tissue stroma tends to revert toward a more embryonic type of cell with a similar loss in the production of the typical collagen and fibroglia fibers. Indeed, in many cases it is hard to tell whether or not the stroma itself is not equally malignant. The cells develop anaplastic features with atypical and multiple mitoses, hyperchromatism and a tendency for the nuclei to become round or ovoid instead of spindle. Such

malignant myomata usually are extremely vascular, especially when seen in the uterus. With the development of these malignant features, a markedly increased blood supply usually develops. In the more malignant of these tumors, the muscle cells seem to actually form the walls of large vascular sinusoids much as occurs in the uterine wall, with the implantation of the ovum and the development of the placenta in pregnancy. Tumor giant cells, with extraordinarily pleomorphic nuclei are found in moderate numbers. Hyperchromatism of both the nuclei and cytoplasm is striking. Such tumors microscopically frequently appear more malignant histologically than they behave clinically. The reason for this has already been mentioned, the tendency toward local invasion rather than lymphatic or vascular extension, except in rare instances.

ILLUSTRATIVE CASES

CASE 99. (Ref. #S-130)

Diagnosis.—Uterus—leiomyoma showing hyaline degeneration.

Patient was a Negress of 36 years, admitted to the hospital because of menorrhagia and metrorrhagia.

Present Illness.—Her present illness began about six months before admission and was characterized by marked irregularity of her periods associated with prolonged and profuse menstruation, the intervals being only a few days apart. This was accompanied by marked dysmenorrhea. This latter symptom was of much longer duration. The patient had not been pregnant, according to her history, and had never had a miscarriage or abortion.

Past History.—Her past history was unsatisfactory and apparently irrelevant. She remembered nothing of her early life. She had been married about twelve years and had never had any children. A review of her systems was essentially negative, although no reliance could be placed on her statements.

Physical Examination.—Patient was a well-developed and well-nourished Negress. Her head was normal in contour. Eyes, ears, nose and throat were apparently normal. Chest was well developed and symmetrical. Heart was normal in size and there were no murmurs. Her lungs were clear throughout. Abdomen was moderately prominent. There were no definite masses or viscera which could be palpated. There was a feeling of discomfort rather than actual pain or tenderness on palpation over the lower portion of the abdomen. Rectal and vaginal examinations revealed a large, irregular, nodular uterus but no other masses or tenderness. There was a profuse mucoid, blood-stained discharge from the cervix. A diagnosis of multiple myomata of the uterus was made and operation advised.

Laboratory Findings.—Red blood cells, 3,100,000 with 62% hemoglobin. White blood cells, 9,600 with 71% polynuclears and 24% lymphocytes.

Subsequent History.—The patient was operated upon and a uterus, containing about one dozen spherical tumor

masses ranging in size from a pigeon egg to that of a large orange, was removed.

Pathological Report.—Gross Description.—Specimen consisted of a uterus which had been amputated above the cervix. This contained a number of typical leiomyomata. These were submucous, subserous and intramural in distribution causing distortion of the uterine canal. The smaller ones, on section, showed typical pearly white, tough, dense interlacing bundles of fibrous appearing tissue. The larger ones presented grayish, translucent areas of hyaline degeneration in addition.

Microscopic Description of a Section from One of the Myomata.—(Fig. 229 and 230) The tissue, histologically, is made up of interlacing bundles of spindle-shaped cells having no apparent purposeful arrangement. The characteristic nuclei and cell outline, as well as their deeper staining qualities and absence of intercellular fibers differentiate these as smooth muscle cells. These tumor cells are supported by a connective tissue stroma of varying density. In places it is difficult to distinguish between compressed fibroblasts and the smooth muscle cells (This differentiation may be readily established by the use of the special Van Gieson's picric acid-fuchsin stain, which colors smooth muscle yellow and connective tissue red). Where collagen is abundant, no such difficulty is encountered. It will be noted that there is a very inadequate blood supply to the tissue. As a result, extensive hyaline degeneration of the collagenous material has taken place.

Under high power, these degenerative changes with swelling and fusing of the collagen matrix can be better seen. As this process develops, actual cell death may occur with edema and cystic degeneration.

CASE 100. (Ref. #S-266)

Diagnosis.—Uterus—leiomyosarcoma.

Patient was a white unmarried woman of 55 years, who was admitted to the hospital with the chief complaint of progressive increase in size of the lower abdomen accompanied by a moderate amount of pain.

Present Illness.—The patient first noticed that her abdomen was increasing in size about six months before admission. At that time she had an attack of acute indigestion with nausea and vomiting, and on examination by a physician, an abdominal mass was found which was thought at that time probably to be a floating kidney. Her gastro-intestinal upset was apparently unrelated as no recurrence of those symptoms was noted. The patient noticed that this mass continued to increase in size, and at the time of admission was about the size of a full-term pregnancy. It was accompanied by low back pain radiating to the pelvis.

Past History.—The past history was irrelevant and inadequately given. A review of her systems showed no significant symptomatology. She had had occasional upper respiratory infections of a mild degree. There were no cardiorespiratory symptoms otherwise. Her gastro-intestinal system had been negative except for the one described upset, and for a rather persistent constipation. Her catamenia had always been normal up to her menopause six years ago.

Physical Examination.—The patient was a well developed middle-aged appearing woman who showed no acute symptomatology. Her head was negative. Eyes, ears, nose and throat were negative. She had an artificial denture for the upper jaw. Heart and lungs were negative. Abdomen was protuberant. There was a large mass in the lower abdomen, which was about the size of a nine months' gestation. This mass was very firm and extended up to a point three fingers' breadth below the costal margin. It was thought that a suggestion of a fluid wave could be obtained and a tentative diagnosis of ovarian cyst was made. The extremities were negative. In view of the obvious surgical problem, no gynecological examination was made.

Laboratory Findings.—Red blood cells, 4,000,000 with 78% hemoglobin. White blood cells, 11,400 with 72% polynuclears. Urinalysis was negative except for a slight trace of albumin.

Operative History.—An exploratory operation was done and the mass found to involve the uterus. A panhysterectomy was done with the removal of the tubes and ovaries as well. At the time of operation, there was a large tumor mass approximately 17 x 23 cm. growing from the fundus of the uterus and attached by a broad base. The tumor was so degenerated that fragments of it had broken off and were found free in the pelvis.

Pathological Report.—Gross Description.—Specimen consisted of an enormously enlarged uterus weighing 1700 grams. The uterine canal could barely be identified so completely had the tumor process involved the uterine wall. On section, innumerable myomatous nodules were found varying considerably in size and appearance. Some of the smaller of these were hard, whitish masses, discrete and encapsulated, which on section showed rather characteristic interlacing strands of tissue. Others of the tumor masses showed extensive hemorrhage and necrosis. One of the largest, which had an approximate diameter of 17 cm. was ill-defined and seemed to merge with the uterine wall.

The tubes and ovaries were essentially normal, but the broad ligament on the right side showed a similar intraligamentous, myomatous tumor with the same necrotic, friable consistency as the large tumor mass in the uterus.

Microscopic Description of a Section from the Large Necrotic Tumor of the Uterus.—(Fig. 233) Histologic examination of this tissue shows a great deal of necrosis and hyaline degeneration, which has resulted even in beginning calcific deposit. Many areas, however, are seen which are composed of an extremely cellular tissue made up of interlacing bundles of large spindle cells. The cytoplasmic boundaries are not readily distinguished, although the tissue does show considerable fibrillar structure. In this stroma are found many large pleomorphic, hyperchromatic, atypical nuclei varying in size and shape from round to spindle. Some of these cells show large nucleoli, but in most instances they are extremely small. Many atypical mitotic figures are observed as well as a considerable number of large, multinucleated tumor giant cells. Other sections show variation in this picture with histologic features ranging from questionable malignancy to frank wild, unrestrained tumor growth. Considerable hemorrhage is present, and there appears to be a marked increase in the blood supply to this tumor. Many large vascular spaces, apparently being outlined by tumor cells rather than by definitely defined endothelium may be seen.

Striated Muscle Tumors.—Tumors arising from the peripheral musculature are so rare as to almost be nonexistent. The most common site for striated muscle tumors or *rhabdomyomata* is found in the heart where they may occur as discrete tumor nodules in the myocardial wall. Such tumors might be considered in certain instances as theoretically benign as they rarely metastasize. More often, however, they present such marked histologic features of anaplasia of the cells that they must be considered as malignant. More frequently than the simple rhabdomyoma arising from already existent musculature must be cited that form of the tumor which is seen usually arising in the region of the kidney or bladder and usually occurring in children. This is believed to-day to represent the one-sided development of a complex teratoma, and as such should perhaps best be classified under that heading. However, certain such tumors consist, with the exception of their connective tissue and vascular stroma, exclusively of striated muscle cells and are more frequently designated by the term rhabdomyoma for this reason.

Characteristically, microscopically, the rhabdomyomata show cells of varying size and degree of differentiation. Their nuclei likewise vary greatly in size. In the heart particularly, one finds the so-called "spider cells," enormous cells 40 to 80 micra in diameter, with light-staining cytoplasm containing a few granules and in which small focal areas of longitudinal and cross striation may be identified. In other areas of such tumors, the cells are characteristically spindle in form and again show varying degrees of striation. In the more rapidly growing of the teratoid type of rhabdomyomata, many of the cells at first glance appear as simple spindle cells which might easily be confused with fibroblasts in their undifferentiated form. Such cells frequently lack any suggestion of cytoplasmic structure and may only show occasional fibers between the nuclei tending to outline the cell body in a vague sort of way.

These cells may be very difficult to differentiate from the stroma and the diagnosis in certain instances becomes dependent upon the finding of occasional cells with the characteristic muscle striae. This is particularly difficult when the cells tend to occur in bundles, as they not infrequently do and to be cut in cross section so that they appear merely as focal collections of nuclei with coarse cytoplasmic strands.

ILLUSTRATIVE CASE

CASE 101. (Ref. #S-237)
Diagnosis.—Kidney—rhabdomyosarcoma.

Patient was a white female child of 5 years, admitted to the hospital because of a large mass in the right side of the abdomen, which had been increasing in size.

Present Illness.—This mass first was noticed about three months before admission. It had been slowly increasing in size since that time until it reached about the size of a child's head. She had had considerable pain accompanying this, particularly in the lower back region.

Past History.—The child had not had any previous illness of any significance. She had been a normally delivered child and had been breast fed for the first year of her life. She had had no nutritional disturbances and had apparently been normal in all respects up to the onset of the present illness.

Physical Examination.—The patient was a well developed, but somewhat emaciated young, white child. Head was normal in contour. Eyes, ears, nose and throat were negative. Chest was symmetrical. Lungs were clear. Heart was not enlarged and showed no murmurs. Abdomen was asymmetrically enlarged with a mass on the right side. This was not tender and did not fluctuate on deep palpation. No fluid was apparently present in the abdomen. The extremities were negative. External genitalia appeared normal.

X-ray examination of the child showed a large tumor which was retroperitoneal as nearly as could be determined. This seemed fixed in position and was not related to the liver. It was felt that this represented a tumor of the kidney.

Subsequent Course.—She was given a course of irradiation with a temporary regression in the size of the tumor. The tumor, however, began to grow again more rapidly and the patient went progressively and rapidly downhill, dying two months after admission to the hospital.

Laboratory Findings.—On admission, she had a count of 4,100,000 red blood cells with 83% hemoglobin. White blood cells were 10,200 with 71% polynuclears.

As the disease progressed, and under the intense irradiation, the picture fluctuated considerably. Just before death there was a severe secondary anemia with a red blood count of only 2,300,000 with 58% hemoglobin. There was a moderate leukopenia with 6,400 white blood cells showing only 34% polynuclears.

Autopsy Findings.—The body showed marked emaciation but normal skeletal development. The examination was essentially negative except for a large tumor involving the entire right kidney. This weighed 1,200 grams and measured approximately 25 x 18 x 14 cm. The tumor evidently arose as a rather circumscribed lesion but had extended to diffusely infiltrate the entire renal substance. It suggested having sprung from the pelvic portion of the kidney. The mass was somewhat firm and nodular, but showed many areas of necrosis and hemorrhage. It was grayish-pink in color as a whole, with a definite white appearance to the well preserved cellular areas of the tumor. It lacked the yellow discoloration so commonly seen in hypernephromata.

Microscopic Description of Tissue from the Tumor.—(Fig. 234) Histologic examination of the tissue shows the tumor to be made up of interlacing bundles of fibers. This is not dissimilar in appearance to a fibrosarcoma at first glance. However, by more careful study the cells are seen to have actual cytoplasmic outlines for the most part, although the intercellular collagenous fibrils with the routine hematoxylin and eosin stain seem to merge with the tumor cells. By the use of phosphotungstic acid-hematein technique, the presence of definite longitudinal and cross striations is demonstrated and the independent nature of these cells in respect to the stroma. The cells, for the most part, are spindle in appearance, relatively uniform in size and show comparatively few mitotic figures. They do, however, show considerable variation from the normal appearance of striated muscle as they are nearly all much smaller in size and do not show the degree of differentiation nor the regularity of striation development which are seen in the normal striated muscle from myometrial origin.

PART II

PIGMENTED TUMORS

Pigmented tumors may arise wherever pigment producing cells exist. Thus, they are most commonly found in the skin and in the eye. Less frequently, they may arise in the central nervous system or even in the mucous membranes. Such pigmented tumors which arise from the retina are invariably malignant, although they may have a long interval between the appearance of the primary tumor and the development of the secondary metastatic lesions. On the other hand, those tumors arising in the skin may be either benign or malignant. The benign form is spoken of as a *nevus;* the malignant as a *malignant melanoma.*

There are few tumors which have occasioned so much confusion and discussion as this particular group, and in any presentation of them it is difficult to know where best to include them. With the recent work of Masson it has been shown conclusively that histogenetically these pigmented tumors arise in relation to the neuroepithelial derivatives of the end-organs. By special staining methods it can be demonstrated that nerve fibers are present in the characteristic nests of tumor cells. For this reason perhaps, it would be best to include this entire group of pigmented tumors with the tumors of the nervous system. Custom, however, has decreed that they should be taken up as a special variety of tumor because of the rather striking clinical features which differentiate them from all other tumors of the nervous system.

In former years, because of the fact that pigmented tumors may occur which present very striking differences in their histology, the tumors were divided into two major groups; one a tumor spoken of as a melanocarcinoma, in which large polyhedral cells predominated; the other called a melanosarcoma, because of the predominance of spindle cells. Today, it is recognized that both cell types may well exist side by side within the same tumor, and indeed within the same microscopic field. To avoid further confusion from the histogenetic standpoint, the terminology current today has been adopted, using malignant melanoma as a generic term to cover all such malignant pigmented tumors. The exact relationship of the melanoblast in the development

of these tumors is of extreme interest, but it is generally believed that these cells are basically the actual cell of origin.

To further complicate the problem, it is well known that many tumors which belong morphologically and histogenetically in this malignant melanotic classification show little or no evidence of any pigmentation whatsoever either grossly or microscopically. Various theories regarding this apparent paradox have been raised. Certain investigators believe that the failure of the melanoblasts in these tumors to produce pigment is dependent upon the rapidity of growth, with the cells dividing at such a rapid rate that they do not have time to differentiate to the point where they produce their characteristic pigment. On the other hand, many such melanotic tumors, when studied histologically, show no such evidence of rapid growth and yet fail to produce pigment except perhaps in minimal amounts. As has been discussed in Chapter IV on Pathological Pigmentation, Laidlaw and others have demonstrated the fact that for pigmentation to develop, it is necessary that the tissues contain an oxidase, dihydroxyphenylalanine, a substance closely related chemically to adrenalin. Thus, the activity of the melanoblast seems to be dependent upon both a nervous and a chemical or hormonal stimulation. These factors render the whole problem of melanotic tumors one which is far from settled. These few comments have been introduced merely to illustrate the confusion which exists regarding this type of tumor.

Benign Nevi.—From the practical standpoint, these tumors are comparatively easy to recognize. In the benign nevus we have a considerable range in the appearance of the lesion, both grossly and microscopically. The familiar term, "mole," is a synonym for this variety of tumor and it is only a question of degree in deciding whether an individual localized area of increased pigmentation should be clinically called a *freckle* or a *mole.*

Histologically, there is little difference save in degree. In either case, there is an accumulation of the so-called "nevus cell," a small polyhedral or ovoid cell which tends to occur in clumps. With silver stains, it is found that these cells usually surround the fibers of the nerve ending. Such aggregations of cells are usually sharply demarcated from the deeper tissues by a rather definite, thickened corium. However, no attempt at capsule formation exists. In the more marked cases of mole formation, we find that there may be a large, elevated plaque, which even contains hair follicles. These larger nevi are usually heavily pigmented by contrast to the nonelevated variety. The great majority of nevi remain benign throughout their existence, and not infrequently after middle age tend to show regressive changes, at times completely disappearing. Occasionally, however, such lesions, frequently as the result of chronic irritation, will undergo malignant change. This is particularly true of the large, pigmented, hairy nevi which frequently show papillary hyperplasia of the overlying epithelium. Histologically, such tumors should be differentiated from epithelial papillomata with pigmentation, in which the pigment is typically in the basal epithelial cells, although the two lesions tend to merge at times.

*

ILLUSTRATIVE CASE

CASE 102. (Ref. #S-107)

Diagnosis.—Pigmented nevus, benign.

Patient was a white woman of 52 years, who was admitted to the hospital because of marked debility following an attack of influenza.

Present Illness.—Present illness began about three weeks before admission when she had a fairly typical story with fever, chills, generalized malaise and pain in all her bones and muscles accompanied by weakness. She showed some temporary improvement and then suffered a relapse of her condition and was referred to the hospital.

Past History.—Past history was irrelevant. A review of her systems was unimportant except for the fact that she had known she had had heart disease for two or three years. She had always been of a nervous temperament, but in other respects had been normal.

Physical Examination.—Physical examination showed a well-developed, moderately well-nourished middle-aged woman, who did not appear acutely ill. Head was negative. Eyes, ears, nose and throat were normal. Skin was negative except for a somewhat elevated, large pigmented nevus on the abdominal wall. This measured 3 cm. in its greatest diameter. The chest was symmetrical. Heart was slightly enlarged. Blood pressure was elevated registering 180/110. The lungs showed a few crepitant râles throughout. There was no definite dullness, however. Abdomen showed poor muscle tone, and was somewhat protuberant.

Subsequent Course.—The patient asked to have this nevus removed because she had heard that a certain number of them became cancerous. Because of her nervous temperament it was deemed advisable to accede to her request in this respect as well as because of the fact that the nevus was of the elevated, deeply pigmented type which might undergo such change. Otherwise, the patient made an eventful recovery from her upper respiratory infection and was discharged improved.

Pathological Report.—**Gross Description.**—Specimen consisted of a soft, sessile, deeply pigmented, nevus-like tumor measuring 3 cm. in length by 1.5 cm. in breadth, and being elevated nearly 1 cm. above the skin level.

Microscopic Description of the Nevus.—(Fig. 248) Histologic examination of the tissue showed the superficial epithelial layer to be thinned and the rete pegs for the most part absent. Here and there some attempt on the part of the epithelium to undergo hyperplasia with superficial keratinization is noted. Beneath the superficial epithelium are found nests of typical small ovoid or polyhedral nevus cells. By special silver staining technique these can be demonstrated to occur around terminal nerve filaments. Many show intense pigmentation. In others, the cytoplasm shows no pigment. There is some deposition of pigment in the interstitial tissues. This is accompanied by moderate fibrosis and chronic inflammatory mononuclear cellular infiltration. The lesion is sharply demarcated from the underlying corium by rather dense, hyalinized collagen.

Malignant Melanomata.—The malignant melanoma is one of the most "malignant" tumors found in human beings. This malignancy is due to its extraordinary tendency to invade the blood stream early and thus metastasize widely to every tissue of the body. It is, from the practical standpoint, the only tumor which almost regularly invades the heart muscle, the peripheral striated muscle of the body, the brain, the thyroid, the pancreas, and all those other structures which usually escape metastatic involvement, even although the tumor cells are blood-borne. As a result, clinical cases showing metastatic melanomata usually run a rapidly fatal course, seldom living more than a year, and often dying within a few weeks after the metastatic process has been recognized.

The great majority of such malignant melanomata result from the malignant transformation of benign nevi. Exceptionally, however, malignant melanomata may apparently arise spontaneously and be malignant from the outset. One group of cases is worthy of comment in this connection. Those tumors arising from the retina as melanomata rarely metastasize until late, and then not infrequently only to the liver, and as a single large mass. Cases are on record in which such delayed metastatic involvement of the liver has not appeared for as long as thirty years after the enucleation of the eye containing the primary tumor.

Histologically, these tumors are so variable in appearance as to make their diagnosis difficult, ranging from a rather characteristic spindle-cell type which contains variable amounts of pigment and was formerly considered as a *melanosarcoma,* up to tumors made up of large polyhedral cells which were felt to be epithelial in origin and which for many years were called *melanocarcinomata.* Many of these tumors show the cells in combination, however. There is a tendency toward alveolar arrangement with a delicate compartment-like connective tissue stroma. Another feature to recall in attempting to diagnose

a melanoma is the frequency with which such tumors may show but little pigment production. Under these circumstances one is guided much by the rather characteristic alveolar architecture of the tumor and the presence of occasional intracellular granules of dark brown pigment. It is only the exceptional instance in which some pigment may not be found. In the more pigmented tumors, much of this pigment will be found intracellularly, but a considerable amount of it will be deposited in the interstitial tissue spaces. It is usually deeper in color than any of the pigments of hematogenous origin, but if uncertainty exists, hemosiderin may be ruled out by appropriate staining methods, with the Prussian blue reaction, the melanin remaining unchanged in color.

ILLUSTRATIVE CASE

CASE 103. (Ref. #S-186)

Diagnosis.—Heart—malignant melanoma.

Patient was a Negress of 43 years, admitted to the hospital complaining of cough and blood streaked sputum following hemoptysis two weeks previously.

Present Illness.—Her present illness began subjectively two weeks before admission with this hemoptysis and cough. This was accompanied by fever, but the patient had no definite chills. She complained of a severe pain in the right side of her chest.

Past History.—She remembered very little regarding her childhood. A review of her systems was essentially negative. She had never had any particular upper respiratory tract symptomatology except for a pain in her chest about a year before the present illness, which subsided spontaneously. She had never been heart conscious. She had never had any gastro-intestinal symptoms other than chronic constipation. Her genito-urinary history had been negative and her catamenic history had been normal. A year before admission, she had had a nodule appear on her toe, which had required amputation at another hospital, but no further details regarding this could be obtained.

Physical Examination.—Physical examination showed a fairly well-developed and well-nourished middle-aged Negress, who did not appear acutely ill, although she showed rapid respiration and had a somewhat anxious appearance. There was a suggestion of icterus to her sclerae. Head was normal in shape. Eyes, ears, nose and throat were otherwise negative. Heart was normal in size. There were no murmurs heard. Blood pressure was 140/94. Lungs showed a decrease in tactile fremitus at both bases with definite dullness over the left base and an inconstant friction rub in the left axilla. The abdomen was moderately distended. Extremities: The great toe of the left foot was absent. The entire left leg was somewhat smaller than the right.

Laboratory Examination.—Urinalysis was negative. Red blood cells, 2,600,000 with 58% hemoglobin. White blood cells, 38,400 with 84% polynuclears. Schilling count suggested an acute suppurative infection with a marked shift. Blood chemistry was negative. Sputum examination

showed a hemolytic streptococcus predominating. No pneumococci were found. No tubercle bacilli were found. Influenza bacilli were present in considerable numbers.

Subsequent Course.—The patient developed an extension of her pneumonic process in the left base with a generalized involvement of both lungs. Her temperature rose to 103° and remained elevated until her death one week after admission.

Autopsy Findings.—External examination of the body was essentially negative except for the absent toe. The peritoneal cavity was negative. The pericardial cavity showed a serous effusion. Heart was moderately enlarged. On section, it showed several polypoid, soft, grayish white tumor masses springing from the upper wall of the left ventricle, from the apex and from the posterior surface. The valves were negative. The right ventricle likewise showed a few sharply circumscribed metastatic tumor nodules. The pleural cavities each contained a considerable amount of dark, bloody fluid with many adhesions. Both lungs showed many necrotic tumor nodules one of them in the left lower lobe being as large as a lemon. Accompanying this was a secondary pneumonia. Actual invasion of the blood vessels could be demonstrated grossly in the lung by the tumor tissue. The liver, curiously, showed no tumor nodules. The spleen and kidneys showed several tumor masses.

Microscopic Description of Section of Tumor Nodule from Heart.—(Fig. 250) The heart muscle is seen microscopically to be infiltrated by a rapidly growing spindle cell type of sarcoma. This is difficult to identify under low power at first because of the relative absence of pigment. Most of the cells are spindle in outline with elongated, irregular nuclei and a considerable amount of interstitial connective tissue stroma. The nuclei furthermore show considerable hyperchromatism and some pleomorphism. There are a moderate number of mitotic figures, most of which are typical in appearance, although some atypical ones are found. The tumor as a whole is practically nonpigmented. Only by careful search here and there a few tumor cells are found which contain pigment. With the presence of this small amount of pigment and without the preceding history of a tumor of the toe which required amputation less than one year before the patient's death, it might be difficult to differentiate this particular case from a simple fibrosarcoma. Indeed, it becomes necessary to stain this pigment differentially by the use of Perl's reaction to be sure that this small amount of pigment is not hemosiderin, although

Note: See Fig. 42 and 249 for additional examples of malignant melanotic tumors.

Fig. 249 comes from a case in which a nevus underwent malignant change with the transition of the tumor from a simple nevus to a frankly malignant infiltrating malignant melanoma. This can be seen in the illustration where the tumor is diffusely infiltrating the tissue. A considerable amount of pigment may be seen in this tumor mostly within the cells. The cells, it will be noted, are polyhedral in type in this instance corresponding to the older terminology of melanocarcinoma.

its distribution within the tumor cells rather than within the phagocytic mononuclear cells is convincing. Its invasive character is well brought out by microscopic examination of the periphery of the tumor nodule where it is seen extending between the muscle bundles for a considerable distance from the main tumor mass.

Fig. 247 and 251 represent a primary melanotic tumor arising in the retina of the eye and metastasizing to the liver. Here, the similar spindle appearance of the cells as observed in Case 103 is apparent. It represents an intermediate lesion in respect to pigment production. In areas, large masses of pigment may be noted. In other areas, the cells are completely free from pigment production. Note the rather typical septate arrangement of the cells. This case occurred in a patient whose eye was removed three years before the secondary hepatic involvement caused the patient's death.

CHAPTER XXVII
TUMORS OF ENDOTHELIAL ORIGIN

In the group of tumors which are usually considered under this heading, only those of blood vessel or lymphatic origin may unquestionably be traced histogenetically to true endothelium. One difficulty which presents is one's inability to define an endothelioblast. Thus, tumors of mesothelial origin, including the serosal cells lining the pleura, pericardium, peritoneum, joint cavities and bursae, as well as certain tumors arising from the dura; and indeed, tumors of the reticulo-endothelial tissues are not infrequently included under this term, *"endotheliomata."* For convenience, we shall include those tumors of mesothelial and dural origin at this time, realizing thoroughly that there is a great deal of difference of opinion as to their exact histogenesis and classification. We shall consider, in the following chapter, the tumors of reticulo-endothelial origin along with those tumors arising from lymphoid structures, although this may well be considered a wholly arbitrary treatment of the problem.

ANGIOMATA

Hemangiomata.—The hemangioma is a tumor arising from vascular endothelium. In its commonest form, it is seen as the so-called "birthmark." It is made up of numerous capillary blood vessels lined by a single layer of endothelium. This may assume one of two forms or may occur in combination.

THE CAPILLARY HEMANGIOMA.—This type of blood vessel tumor is composed of innumerable small masses of endothelial cells which may occur as columns or sheets, but which gradually develop lumina and tend to present a coiled appearance in the subcutaneous tissue, histologically. The size of the lesion likewise shows a wide difference in extent. Some of the smallest are no larger than the ordinary freckle, two to three millimeters in diameter, and on the other hand, large lesions occupying almost half of the face may be present. Owing to the marked vascularity of these lesions, the overlying skin appears discolored. The degree of dilatation of these vessels varies greatly in the individual cases. They are usually found immediately beneath the true skin rather than in the deeper subcutaneous tissues. They are ordinarily entirely benign lesions remaining stationary in size. They may, however, show evidence of progression in diameter. Rarely these tumors may undergo neoplastic hyperplasia and become true angiosarcomata. When this occurs, the endothelium proliferates and may be seen growing from the wall of these new formed vessels with almost papillary projections into the vessel itself as well as into the surrounding tissue. The tendency for these malignant angiomata is to start in a peripheral vessel and to extend along the course of the vessel usually on the venous side of the circulation toward the trunk. In the most marked cases the process becomes almost generalized and the patient may die as the result of invasion of vital areas or as the result of hemorrhage from traumatic rupture of the tumor. The benign tumors ordinarily tend to be circumscribed and sharply demarcated from the surrounding tissue by a zone of connective tissue condensation serving as a pseudocapsule.

CAVERNOUS HEMANGIOMA.—In this group of cases the question has often been raised as to whether the lesion is a true neoplasm or whether it merely represents a developmental defect. The microscopic appearance of such a lesion is one of large vascular sinusoids rather than a proliferation of new-formed capillary channels. One example of this type of lesion is seen in the liver where single or multiple dark reddish purple areas are noted, usually on the surface of the liver, but when multiple frequently within its substance. This particular lesion is spoken of as a *cavernoma,* and is rather generally considered as a

PLATE LXI
TUMORS OF ENDOTHELIAL ORIGIN

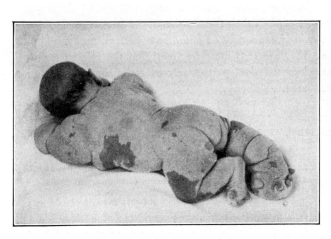

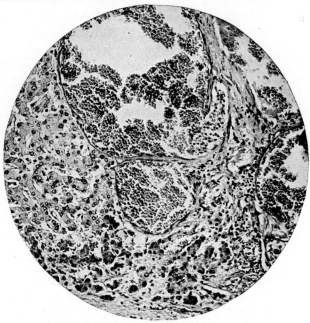

FIG. 252.—MULTIPLE LYMPHANGIO-HEMANGIO-ENDOTHELIOMATA.—CASE 104.—Gross photograph of infant showing multiple congenital lesions, with associated lymph stasis and elephantiasis.

FIG. 253.—LIVER: CAVERNOMA (CAVERNOUS HEMANGIOMA).—CASE 105.—Enormous dilated vascular spaces filled with red cells separated by connective tissue septa and embedded in normal liver parenchyma. App. 100 x.

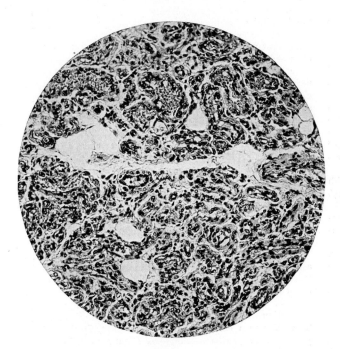

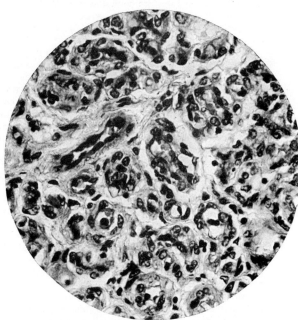

FIG. 254.—SKIN AND SUBCUTANEOUS TISSUES: CAPILLARY HEMANGIOMA.—CASE 104.—Multiple coil-like masses of capillary endothelium, some showing lumen formation and distended with blood. App. 100 x.

FIG. 255.—High power detail of Fig. 254 better revealing arrangement of endothelial cell nests with beginning lumen formation and the delicate connective tissue stroma of the lesion. App. 200 x.

pseudotumor and developmental anomaly. In its essential histology, however, it cannot be differentiated from a similar cavernous subcutaneous hemangioma. The larger hemangiomatous birthmarks are apt to be of this cavernous type. They usually appear relatively cyanotic because of the stasis of blood within these dilated channels. Occasionally, as in the case of the capillary angiomata, such cavernous lesions may, on occasion, undergo malignant degeneration.

One sound reason for believing that these vascular lesions are not true tumors, except as they undergo malignant change, is found in the fact that they almost invariably occur as congenital lesions. Attempts to explain their distribution are rather unsatisfactory. Angiomata may be found anywhere on the body, but they are seen most frequently on the face as a unilateral lesion, particularly over the cheek and nasal area.

ILLUSTRATIVE CASES

CASE 104. (Ref. #S-145)
Diagnosis.—Skin—capillary hemangioma.

Patient was a female child of 8 months, brought to the hospital acutely ill with what the parents thought was a severe cold. (Fig. 252)

Present Illness.—The present illness began three days before admission as a mild cold with a discharge from the nose and some coughing. The baby felt feverish the second day of her illness and as she did not seem to improve, the parents brought her to the hospital.

Past History.—The baby was born with a number of large, reddish birthmarks. The most extensive of these were found over the back and thigh regions, although several smaller ones were present on other parts of the body. In addition, there appeared to be some involvement of the lymphatic system with the gradual development of an elephantiasis of the right leg. In other respects the infant appeared to be symptomless, except for the apparent upper respiratory infection. These lesions did not seem to interfere with the normal development and growth of the baby otherwise. The patient was brought to the hospital to find out if anything could be done to alleviate this condition.

Physical Examination.—The outstanding physical findings were those relating to the congenital angiomatous lesions which apparently involved both the blood vessels and the lymphatics. In addition, there was a diffuse bronchopneumonia present involving the entire right side of the chest. This was evidenced by alterations in breath sounds and fremitus and by the presence of numerous crackling râles. Physical examination otherwise was negative.

Laboratory Findings.—Red blood cells, 3,600,000 with 72% hemoglobin. White blood cells, 26,800 with 92% polynuclears.

Subsequent Course.—The patient went rapidly downhill and died three days after admission of her pneumonia.

Autopsy Findings.—At autopsy an almost confluent, diffuse bronchopneumonia involving the entire right lobe with some beginning pneumonic consolidation in the left lower lobe was found. In addition, moderate secondary toxic degenerative changes with congestion of the spleen as a prominent feature were seen. The essential angiomatous lesions were unusually marked and sections were taken for microscopic study. Tissue was taken from a small angioma from the skin of the baby. Grossly it appeared as a small, elevated, pinkish red, rather firm lesion which was sharply demarcated from the underlying structures.

Microscopic Description of the Lesion.—(Fig. 254 and 255) The overlying epithelium is normal in appearance save for perhaps some slight thinning and underdevelopment of the rete pegs. Beneath this, embedded in the corium, is found an irregular mass of endothelial cells most of which show the presence of lumina. These are distended in part by red cells. The cells appear relatively large and less mature than the ordinary endothelial cells lining blood vessels and there is some suggestion that this may be an actual proliferative lesion as occasional mitotic figures may be encountered. There is no evidence of invasion of the deeper tissue and to all intents and purposes this remains as a simple benign superficial type of hemangioma.

CASE 105. (Ref. #S-103)
Diagnosis.—Liver—cavernous hemangioma.

Patient was a Negro, seventy years old, admitted to the hospital with marked arteriosclerosis, in a state of coma as the result of a cerebral accident.

Present Illness.—The present illness began about five days before admission with what was clinically diagnosed as a "stroke." Since that time, the patient had shown marked incontinence. He had developed a progressive disorientation, aphasia, amnesia and a gradual loss of speech, sinking slowly into coma.

Past History.—The past history was not obtained due to the condition of the patient.

Physical Examination.—The patient was a senile colored male. His pupils reacted sluggishly to light. There was a bilateral arcus senilis. Chest was emphysematous. Lungs showed râles at both bases. Heart was moderately enlarged. Blood pressure was 215/125. Abdomen was essentially negative. Central nervous system: The patient showed a left-sided paralysis. He went steadily downhill and died forty-eight hours after admission.

Autopsy Findings.—At autopsy, the patient showed a marked generalized arteriosclerosis with right cerebral thrombosis and early softening. There was marked toxic hypertrophy with myosclerosis as the result of coronary disease. There was marked emphysema with hypostatic congestion and terminal pneumonia on the right side. The liver was enlarged due to congestion. It showed a prominent *congenital hemangioma* about 2.5 cm. in diameter. This was roughly wedge-shaped and measured about 2.5 cm. in diameter, lying immediately beneath the capsule of the liver in the right lobe. In addition, he showed chronic passive congestion of the lungs, spleen

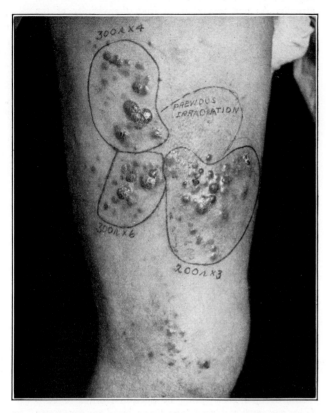

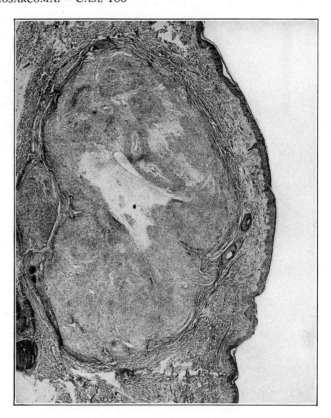

FIG. 256.—GROSS PHOTOGRAPH OF RIGHT THIGH.—Illustrates the hemorrhagic, elevated, irregularly nodular appearance of the lesions. Area marked "previous irradiation" indicates transient radio-sensitivity of tumor.

FIG. 257.—MICROTESSAR PHOTOGRAPH OF TYPICAL SINGLE SUBCUTANEOUS NODULE, showing pseudo-encapsulation, thinning of overlying epithelium and central area of myxomatous degeneration. App. 10 x.

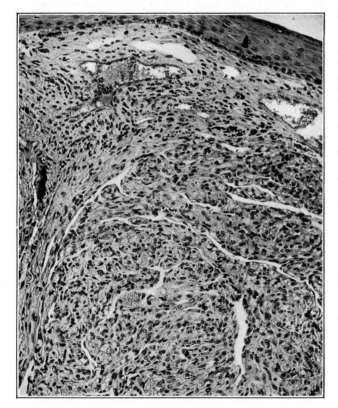

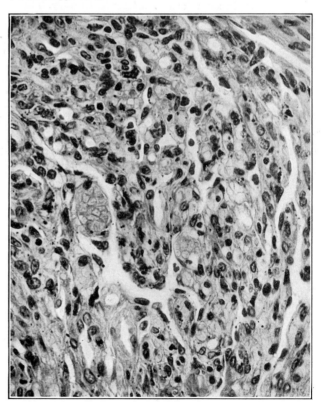

FIG. 258.—HIGH POWER VIEW OF AN AREA FROM A SIMILAR NODULE.—Ill-defined nests and cords of endothelial cells, showing considerable nuclear hyperchromatism, occasional mitoses and merging with surrounding corium. App. 100 x.

FIG. 259.—HIGH POWER DETAIL FROM FIG. 258.—Observe abortive attempts at vessel formation, some strikingly elongated, pleomorphism and hyperchromatism of cells, and generally wild histologic disorder of architecture. App. 200 x.

and kidneys, and a chronic prostatitis with marked hypertrophy.

Microscopic Description of a Section of the Liver Cavernoma.—(Fig. 253) Microscopic study of the tissue shows a number of large endothelial lined sinusoids filled with red cells. No evidence of any activity on the part of these endothelial cells can be observed. They are supported by a delicate connective tissue stroma and appear to be entirely normal. The liver cells immediately adjacent to the lesion show some slight compression atrophy. As one moves away from the vicinity of the lesion, the liver cells become normal in appearance. There is nothing which suggests a true neoplasm in this picture. It would appear to represent a congenital anomaly of the blood vessels in this area. One is forced by exclusion to the diagnosis of a simple cavernous hemangioma or cavernoma.

KAPOSI'S MULTIPLE HEMORRHAGIC SARCOMA. —An extremely unusual and interesting type of tumor was first described by Kaposi in 1872. Its exact classification has been a matter of considerable uncertainty. It occurs chiefly in adults in the southeastern part of Europe and around the Mediterranean, Black and Caspian Seas. It is usually associated with local vascular lesions and is frequently preceded by trauma. It is slow in its development. The lesions appear as rather elevated vascular nodules which become pigmented. Many of them may heal spontaneously with considerable fibrous scarring. They usually arise in one or another extremity, but sooner or later they involve the gastro-intestinal tract or other structures, and end fatally. Whether they should be considered as of infectious origin or whether they represent true tumors is difficult to decide. In the last analysis, they behave more like malignant neoplasms, and in their histology, they suggest a tumor arising from vascular endothelium and presenting features of low grade malignant change. From the practical standpoint, it seems better to include this as a form of angiosarcoma rather than as one of the infectious granulomata, in which category it is usually placed, as the lesions seem to grow along the vessels progressively.

ILLUSTRATIVE CASE

CASE 106. (Ref. #S-315)

Diagnosis.—Kaposi's multiple hemorrhagic sarcoma.

Patient was a white male of 35, (Fig. 256) born in Austria. Several months before admission, he developed some bluish nodules in the skin and subcutaneous tissue about the size of a dime. These were more or less painful in nature and tended to bleed readily. These tumors increased in numbers and appeared in groups, the earliest, involving the right foot; subsequent crops around the knee and thigh of the same side, the lesions thus seeming to follow the course of the blood vessels. Under intensive irradiation of individual lesions, they regressed to a considerable extent with the accompaniment of scar tissue formation. One of these masses was removed for histologic examination. The man's history in all other respects was entirely negative.

Pathological Report.—*Gross Description.*—Specimen consisted of a small nodule approximately 1.5 cm. in diameter, which was reddish brown in color and embedded in the subcutaneous tissue. The specimen included a small, elliptical portion of the skin overlying the tumor nodule and a wide margin of subcutaneous fat.

Microscopic Description of Section from Lesion.— (Fig. 257, 258 and 259) The tissue histologically shows localized angiomatous proliferation. It is sharply circumscribed from the surrounding epithelium and corium by a condensation zone of connective tissue as a pseudocapsule. Within this area, a diffuse proliferative reaction of endothelium is seen. In places, sheets of these cells are noted. In other places, a tendency toward lumen formation is found. Some of the lumina are filled with red cells. Others seem to contain only a coagulated serum. Between the endothelial cells and capillary buds, actual hemorrhage has occurred with secondary cellular infiltration, particularly by large mononuclear phagocytes, with the production of hemosiderin. Mitotic figures can be observed here and there. The cells as a whole appear to be regular in morphology and to show no striking pleomorphism or anaplasia. This lesion might well be considered as a low grade malignant angiosarcoma, as a malignant capillary hemangioma or as has been suggested by the English school, a hemangio-endothelioma.

Lymphangiomata.—Just as we may find the hemangioma as a subcutaneous type of lesion, so we may find a similar endothelial counterpart arising from the endothelium of the lymph vessels. Likewise, we may find both capillary and cavernous types of such lymphatic endothelial tumors. The more common variety is of the capillary type. This whole group of angiomata are at times difficult to differentiate from inflammatory obstruction of the vessels with telangiectatic or lymphangiectatic dilatation and tortuosity. The lymphangiomatous group also raises the question as to whether the lesion represents a true tumor or is a developmental congenital anomaly. One particular form of the lymphangioma is seen as the so-called *"hygroma colli,"* a cavernous type of lymphangioma seen in the neck region in newborn or very young babies. More rarely even than in the case of the hemangiomata, these lym-

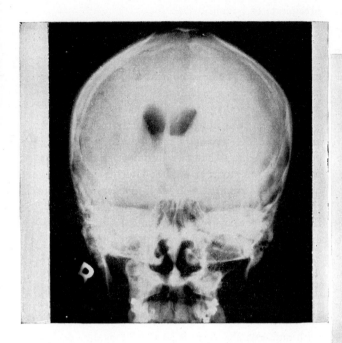

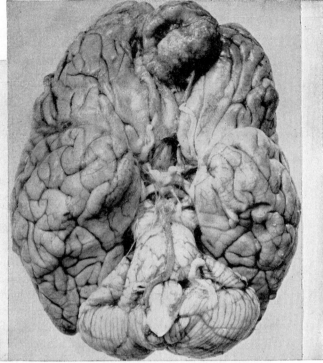

FIG. 260.—SKULL: MENINGIOMA. ROENTGENOGRAM.—Shows distortion of right lateral ventricle as a result of localized pressure from the tumor.

FIG. 261.—BRAIN: MENINGIOMA.—Gross photograph of base of brain with irregularly spherical, grayish, walnut-sized, encapsulated tumor mass causing distortion of frontal lobes.

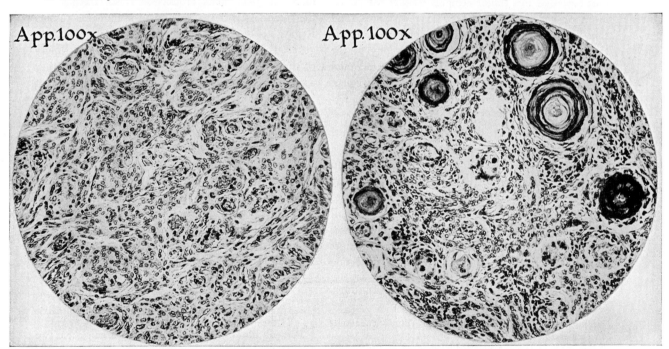

FIG. 262.—Photomicrograph from an area presenting the characteristic whorl-like arrangement of the tumor cells embedded in a septate connective tissue stroma.

FIG. 263.—Photomicrograph from an area illustrating the typical laminated, calcified psammoma bodies arising in such isolated whorls of tumor tissue.

phangiomata may undergo malignant change and become sarcomatous. Indeed, at times the two may be seen in combination as a hemangio-lymphangioma.

Histologically, one cannot differentiate between them at times, except by the contents of the capil-laries or sinuses. In the hemangiomata, the endo-thelial lined spaces are filled with red cells; in the lymphangiomata, with a pale pink granular staining precipitate of lymph.

MENINGIOMATA (DURAL ENDOTHELIOMATA)

Among those tumors which tradition has grouped with the endotheliomata is the meningioma. The source of this tumor is definitely from the meninges, but whether it comes from the mesothelial lining cells of the dura, from the vascular endothelium of the pia arachnoid sinuses, or from the connective tissue stroma of the dura is still a debatable question. An argument in favor of its endothelial or meso-thelial origin is seen in the fact that it is ordinarily an extremely slow-growing tumor which remains al-most invariably clinically benign except for pressure symptoms. It is hard to conceive of a fibrous tissue tumor so regularly remaining as a benign lesion. Likewise, the architectural details of the meningio-mata rarely conform to any other simple connective tissue tumor pattern. In any event, however, the tumor grows slowly but steadily and ultimately is liable to cause death as the result of sufficient increase in size to produce marked intracranial pressure, par-ticularly pressure upon vital centers. It is remarkable that although this tumor remains outside the actual brain or cord, except in very rare instances, and thus is not a true replacement type of tumor, never-theless, the growth is so slow that atrophy of the central nervous tissues takes place and intracranial pressure is slow in developing. In the cord region, such tumors may easily produce paralysis from pres-sure on the cord itself. The tumor usually appears as a more or less ovoid mass with a well defined compression capsule. It varies in size from a lesion a few millimeters in diameter to tumors as large as an orange. When in contact with the skull, particularly in relation to the suture lines, there is very apt to be extension of the tumor into and through the skull with the development of subcutaneous tumor masses in the scalp. Such tumors frequently produce changes in the skull by which the localization of the lesion may be accomplished. Rare forms of this tumor occur as plaques covering wide areas of brain surface or even extending along the cord as a sheath.

Clinically, these tumors are usually seen in adult and middle life. Actually many of them probably begin in childhood but only attain a size sufficient to produce symptoms at a much later date. There is no particular difference in their incidence between the two sexes, and it is one tumor which clinically, if recognized early enough, should result with op-erative measures, in a permanent cure.

Histologically, these tumors are made up of whorls of a more or less spindle type of cell. Many of these appear to be arranged around small blood vessels. Gradually with the growth of these numer-ous individual whorls, the blood supply is interfered with and centrally there is an area of hyaline degen-eration. This subsequently may become calcified with the production of laminated calcific bodies spoken of as *psammoma bodies*. Indeed, in certain of these tu-mors this psammoma production is so striking that the tumor itself is spoken of as a psammoma tumor. Regardless of their origin, they are likely to have a generous connective tissue stroma. The blood supply of these tumors is usually relatively slight, and they appear grossly as pearly gray or white tumors. Not infrequently they may show areas of degeneration and necrosis as a result of this inadequate blood sup-ply. Certain of these tumors tend to become ad-herent to the skull bones over the point of origin. As they progress they tend to produce pressure upon the skull with resultant atrophy of the inner plate and a tendency toward stimulation of the periosteum of the outer plate. Tumor cells may be seen invading the bone itself, and an identical histologic picture may be found in the subcutaneous tissues when the tumor extends through the skull.

ILLUSTRATIVE CASE

CASE 107. (Ref. #S-214)

Diagnosis.—Meninges—meningioma (dural endotheli-oma).

Patient was a white married woman of 54 years, who was admitted to the hospital complaining of sudden, sharp pains in the left side of her face and an ataxic gait to the left.

Present Illness.—Her present illness began about two and one-half years ago with pain in the lower and upper jaws radiating toward the tragus. These were followed

PLATE LXIV
TUMORS OF ENDOTHELIAL ORIGIN

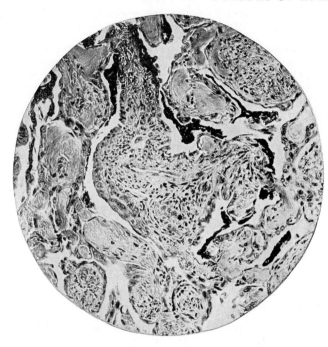

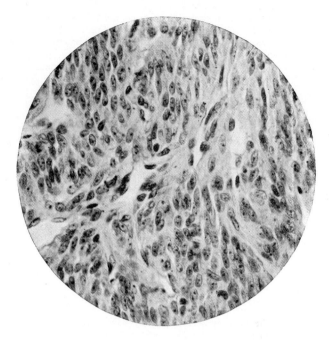

Fig. 264.—Foot: Synovioma.—Case 108.—Photomicrograph illustrating the tendency for the cells to attempt to reproduce serosal lined spaces, as well as to occur in undifferentiated fashion. App. 100 x.

Fig. 265.—Synovioma.—Case 108.—Higher power photomicrograph of a less differentiated area which shows the typical ovoid, vesicular nuclei of the tumor cells. App. 400 x.

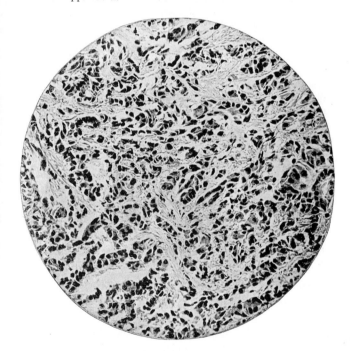

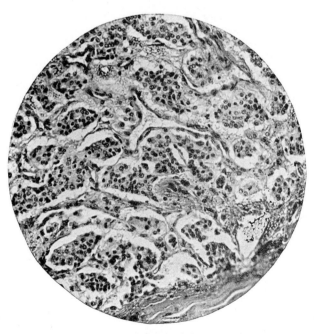

Fig. 266.—Lung: Pleural Endothelioma.—Case 109.—Photomicrograph showing attempted differentiation of tumor cells toward atypic pleural serosa. Note pleomorphism, hyperchromatism, density of stroma and carcinomatous appearance of tumor. App. 200 x.

Fig. 267.—Carotid Body Tumor: "Perithelioma."—Case 110. Photomicrograph to illustrate the characteristic nests of undifferentiated cells in relation to the vascular stroma. App. 200 x.

by a burning sensation, and could be brought on by touching the left side of the nose. All of her teeth were removed on that side with no relief of symptoms. These pains increased in intensity during the course of the year. There was very little headache and no nausea or vomiting. There was no vertigo and no diplopia but about one year ago the patient began to stagger somewhat in her gait, tending to fall toward the left. One year before admission the patient felt her left leg becoming a little stiff. There were no sensory changes.

Past History.—Past history was essentially negative. A review of her systems showed nothing of significance. There was never any history of a severe illness except a nervous breakdown three years before her present admission. Her cardiorespiratory system was apparently negative. Gastro-intestinal history showed no significant features. Genito-urinary and catamenic histories were negative. Menopause was five years earlier.

Physical Examination.—The patient was a somewhat emaciated woman with a dry, loose skin. Her head was normal in shape. Pupils were moderately dilated and reacted well. There were some nystagmoid movements and a definite bilateral corneal hypalgesia. Fundi were negative. Visual fields were negative. The other cranial nerves showed no involvement. Deep tendon reflexes were hyperactive. The abdominal reflexes were possibly absent, but difficult to evaluate because of flabbiness of the musculature. Cerebellar tests showed some tendency to past-pointing and awkwardness in pronation and supination. The patient could stand only on a wide base, and showed a definite tendency to fall towards the left or backwards. On the basis of the history and physical findings, it was felt that the patient probably had an intracranial mass lesion, very probably a tumor in the left cerebellar or cerebellar-pontine area.

Laboratory Findings.—Blood count showed 4,400,000 red blood cells with 88% hemoglobin (14 grams). White blood cells, 11,700 with 32% polymorphonuclear leukocytes and 65% lymphocytes. Urinalysis was essentially negative on several occasions, except for a very slight trace of albumin. Serology was negative.

X-ray examination of the skull suggested an angle tumor on the left side. This was based on the fact that there was a sharply circumscribed, oval-shaped opacity projecting into the shadow of the foramen magnum on the left side of the anteroposterior projection.

Operative History.—A bone flap was removed over the left cerebellar hemisphere. The dura was exposed over the posterior fossa. There was a large, soft, vascular tumor in this area extending toward the cerebellar-pontine angle, as well as through the incisura of the tentorium. The 7th nerve was freed from the tumor; the 8th nerve was involved and was removed by electrocautery. The sensory root was sectioned to eliminate further pain. In addition, a walnut sized, calcified tumor was found extending toward the pontine area. This was separated from the nerve roots and removed.

Pathological Report.—*Gross Description.*—Specimen consisted of about ten fragments of tumor tissue as well as a walnut-sized, rather solid, almost spherical tumor mass. These varied in consistency on section, some of them being very soft and hemorrhagic; the larger being very firm and grayish-white in color.

Microscopic Description of the Tumor.—(Fig. 260, 261, 262 and 263) Examination of the tissue histologically shows the tumor as a whole to be made up of interlacing bundles of spindle cells. Scattered through these cells are found concentrically arranged cells likewise showing some tendency toward spindle-shaped nuclei and cytoplasm. Some of these seem to be arranged around minute capillaries. Many of them show diffuse hyaline degeneration, and the development of psammoma-like bodies. Some are definitely calcified. One unusual feature of this particular tumor is seen in the fact that some of the longitudinal bundles of fibers likewise show this same degenerative change. These areas, if viewed in cross section, would create the picture of spherical psammoma bodies, but viewed longitudinally show changes which are particularly striking. The picture varies considerably from the interlacing bundle-like masses of tissue which resemble a fibrous tissue tumor in places, to these areas where concentric whorl-like arrangement of the cells has occurred with the development of the characteristic psammoma bodies.

SYNOVIOMATA

The synovioma is a specific tumor arising from the serosal cells lining the joint cavities and the bursae. From the histogenetic standpoint, they might better be classified as mesotheliomata than endotheliomata, but as in the case of the meningiomata, it has been found that a topographical anatomical nomenclature has served a very useful purpose in separating this particular group of tumors from the vast confusion of the other endotheliomata. In these cases, the tumor attempts to reproduce the tissue of origin. This is modified by a marked stromal proliferation which distorts the picture in many instances. There is a tendency toward papillary proliferation in this group of tumors at times so that there is a suggestion of resemblance to epithelium. In the literature, some of these cases have been classified as carcinomata. From the histologic standpoint, no generalities can be made regarding their appearance, for each tumor is a law unto itself and no two tumors appear identical histologically.

In general, they may be differentiated from carcinomata by their relatively large, ovoid nuclei and the absence of the typical epithelial nucleoli. Even this criterion is not absolute as nucleoli may be present at times in some of the cells. Mitoses are variable in number and in character. Cells tend to be fairly well differentiated with less anaplasia than is seen in many of the tumors. There is a generous connective tissue stroma which frequently shows hyaline degeneration and necrosis. There is a striking tendency for perivascular proliferation of the cells in pseudo-whorl fashion, which in itself serves to group these tumors among the endotheliomata. As a rule the tumors are relatively slow-growing and remain localized for long periods of time. Excision has been accomplished successfully in a limited number of cases. More often, particularly in those tumors arising from the joints where complete excision of the membrane of origin is technically next to impossible, recurrence has been prone to take place. Ultimately these tumors undergo malignant change and pulmonary metastasis is liable to be the end stage in the clinical picture. With radical surgery, a high percentage of recovery should result. With irradiation, little or nothing may be expected other than a very transitory regression in the size of the tumor.

ILLUSTRATIVE CASE

CASE 108. (Ref. #S-291)

Diagnosis.—Os calcis—synovioma.

Patient was a white Jewish male, aged 29, who was admitted to the hospital complaining of pain in the right foot near the heel.

Present Illness.—Five years before admission, the patient injured his right heel on a pavement which he struck in falling. This was followed by transitory pain for some days. Since that time the patient had had sporadic episodes of similar pain in the right heel. This had never been severe enough to interfere with walking. The present attack, however, was much more intense in nature and began one week before admission. This became steadily worse until he required crutches to get around. He was referred to the hospital for study and surgical treatment.

Past History.—His past history was irrelevant. He had had the usual childhood diseases. A review of his systems was noncontributory. He had had no more than the usual quota of upper respiratory infections. He had no gastro-intestinal symptoms and no weight loss. Genito-urinary history was negative. He denied venereal infection.

Physical Examination.—Physical examination revealed a well-developed, well-nourished young adult male. His head was negative. Eyes, ears, nose and throat were negative. Chest was symmetrical. Heart was not enlarged; there were no murmurs. Lungs were clear. Abdomen was normal. Genitalia were negative. Extremities were negative except for moderate swelling around the heel of the right foot.

Laboratory Findings.—Red blood cells, 5,180,000; hemoglobin, 14 grams. White blood cells 9,600 with 82% polynuclears of which 24% were nonfilamented and 58% were filamented forms. Urinalysis was negative. Wassermann was negative. Blood chemistry showed a serum calcium of 11.4 mgm., and a phosphorus of 3.9 mgm. Phosphatase was 3.4 Bodansky units. X-ray examination of the foot showed some slight loss of bone detail in the os calcis. The cortex itself did not appear unduly thin. No definite diagnosis was made by x-ray, but the question of possible osteomyelitis or tumor was suggested.

Operative History.—The os calcis was exposed and found to be filled with soft, grayish-pink tumor tissue continuous with a sausage-shaped tumor apparently arising from the tendon sheath beneath the longitudinal arch of the foot. Amputation was advised as a result of these findings, and the leg was amputated at its middle.

Pathological Report.—*Gross Description.*—Specimen consisted of a foot amputated in the mid-leg region. There was a large sausage-like tumor apparently arising from the tendon sheaths beneath the arch of the foot. This was continuous with a tumor mass which invaded the os calcis and left only a thin, bony shell of cortex.

Microscopic Description.—(Fig. 264 and 265) Sections microscopically present a picture of a moderately rapidly growing neoplasm of sarcomatous appearance. The cells are atypical in appearance. They tend for the most part to be round or ovoid with large nuclei having rather prominent nucleoli, a dense nuclear membrane but a vesicular appearance of the nucleus itself. The cells are regular in size but in many places are spindled with their nuclei becoming correspondingly elongated. There is marked tendency for the cells to grow around thin-walled spaces which are hard to identify as to whether they are lymphatic or angiomatous. Many of the spaces apear to be definitely lined by the tumor cells. In other areas there is a nest-like arrangement of cells in a septate connective tissue stroma. The differential diagnosis in this case comes down to the elimination of an endothelial myeloma of bone origin, a periosteal fibrosarcoma or a synovioma, presumably of tendon sheath synovial mesothelial origin. By differential stains and considering the gross appearance and apparent origin of the tumor, the first two of these diagnoses seem to be comparatively easily eliminated and a final diagnosis of synovioma or endothelioma is made.

MISCELLANEOUS ENDOTHELIOMATA

A. The primary tumors which arise from the serosal cells of the pleura, pericardium and peritoneum are further examples of this confused group of so-called endotheliomata or mesotheliomata. They are comparatively rare tumors, in general, although those arising from the pleura are more common than the others. In the case of the pleural endotheliomata, two varieties are encountered. In the first place, there is a tumor in which the serosal cells tend to multiply in markedly papillary form. The cells retain their cuboidal appearance, although they are apt to increase in size and to show atypical mitoses.

Because of the cuboidal appearance of the cells and the papillary architectural picture, these tumors are frequently included among the carcinomata. They have, as a rule, a very delicate connective tissue and vascular stroma, and tend to spread over the entire surface of the pleural cavity from their point of origin. Gradually as the tumor becomes more and more bulky, the lung becomes compressed and atelectatic and is ultimately replaced by tumor tissue.

B. The other type of pleural endothelioma is a more solid type of tumor in which there is a very dense connective tissue stromal response. The cells in this instance are more apt to occur in sheets and nests. The tumor is relatively avascular and large areas of necrosis are often seen. It presents very little of a characteristic diagnostic nature and the diagnosis is usually arrived at by exclusion rather than because of its specific appearance. The cells, however, are liable to show a slight tendency to spindle. Their nuclei are ovoid and have a well-defined nuclear membrane with coarse, scattered chromatin and without any striking nucleolar development. At times it is difficult to differentiate this lesion from a reticulo-endothelial sarcoma, and indeed, these tumors may well have a more or less common origin.

ILLUSTRATIVE CASE

CASE 109. (Ref. #S-118) (Courtesy of Dr. Robert Schless, Jewish Hospital, Philadelphia, Pa.).

Diagnosis.—Lung—primary endothelioma.

Patient was a girl of 9 years, admitted to the hospital because of weakness and shortness of breath.

Present Illness.—For a rather indefinite period of months, the child had had a poor appetite for which she had been given tonics. A few days before her admission, she was sent home from school because of weakness and shortness of breath. She was put to bed. She started to cough; a fever set in, and she began to vomit everything taken by mouth. She then complained of a sore throat and pain on the right side. Her cough was dry and non-productive. There was cyanosis of the lips.

Past History.—In infancy, she had whooping cough and measles. At the age of five years, she had a tonsillectomy and adenoidectomy. Otherwise, her development had been normal. There was no history of familial disease, and a review of her systems was negative, except for a long persisting vaginal discharge.

Physical Examination.—Patient was a thin, white, acutely ill appearing girl, breathing rapidly and shallowly. There was no cyanosis or peripheral edema. The left pupil was smaller than the right. Ears, nose and pharynx were negative. Neck showed a moderate cervical adenopathy. Heart was of fair tone. There were no murmurs. Rhythm was regular. The heart was displaced to the right. Chest showed diminished expansion on the left side. There was fullness of the interspace on the left side. Tactile fremitus was decreased. Percussion note was flat over the entire left chest. Grocco's sign was present on the right posterior chest. Breath sounds were distant over the left apex and absent below. There were no râles in either side of the chest. Temperature was 104.4°; pulse 124 and respirations 36.

Laboratory Findings.—Red blood cells, 3,800,000 with 62% hemoglobin. White blood cells, 16,500 with 55% polymorphonuclear leukocytes, 43% lymphocytes and 2% monocytes. Urinalysis: acid reaction; specific gravity 1.025; trace of albumin; occasional hyaline casts; no red blood cells; 3 to 5 white blood cells per high power field. Blood Wassermann was negative. Blood platelets 155,000. Bleeding time was 2½ minutes. Coagulation time was six minutes. Tuberculin test: 1:1,000, negative; 1:100, negative.

Subsequent Course.—Repeated thoracenteses showed the presence of serosanguineous fluid, which had about a normal differential blood cell count, with the addition of many unidentified large polyhedral cells, principally pleural in origin. During this time, she received radiation and improved temporarily in condition. Eight months after the onset, subsequent x-ray examination showed the mass in the chest was again increasing in size. She developed a recurrence of temperature, and a severe progressive anemia. An aspiration biopsy was done and a tentative diagnosis of endothelioma of the pleura was made. The patient went progressively downhill and died approximately nine months after the definite onset of symptoms.

Autopsy Findings.—At autopsy, the entire left lung was found involved in what appeared to be a primary malignancy with metastasis by contiguity to the second and fifth ribs on the left. There was atelectasis of the remaining portion of the left lower lobe. The right lung showed compensatory emphysema. The other viscera showed only evidence of toxic degenerative changes.

Microscopic Description of Section from the Lung.—(Fig. 266) Histologic examination of the tissue shows numerous clusters of polyhedral cells possessing small hyperchromatic nuclei. Many of the nuclei contain nucleoli. There is considerable pleomorphism with a good deal of variation in the size and shape of the cells. Many mitoses are present. Some of these are atypical. The stroma is very dense in consistency and shows extensive hyaline degeneration. The tumor cells show marked invasive properties. There is a great deal of necrosis and hemorrhage throughout the tumor tissue, which involves the stroma as well. In places, the cells are arranged in solid cords. Numerous islands of abnormal tumor cells are seen. Here and there, remnants of lung tissue can be identified with clumps of alveolar cells. The tumor presents many features which render it extremely difficult of diagnosis histologically. It illustrates the importance of knowing the clinical history and course of the disease as well as the microscopy in order to arrive at a correct diagnosis.

C. *Ewing's Endothelial Myeloma.*—For the sake of completeness, it is well to recall that the endothelial myeloma or Ewing's tumor represents again a tumor of presumptive endothelial cell origin. Whether to include it in this group of tumors or to put it in the reticulo-endothelial class, which will be discussed in the next chapter, is one of those decisions which is largely a matter of personal opinion.

D. *Carotid Gland Tumor (Perithelioma or Endothelioma of the Carotid Gland; "Potato Tumor").*—Occasional instances of a tumor arising from the carotid gland have been reported. These are likely to grow to a considerable size, from which the name "potato tumor" has developed clinically. These tumors usually occur in young adults. They arise behind the bifurcation of the carotid artery, which often becomes completely surrounded by the tumor tissue and in some instances even invaded. They rarely metastasize distantly but tend to extend locally in all directions. It is a slow-growing tumor as a rule with cases on record of as long as thirty years' duration. The tumors can usually be successfully removed surgically, although because of their close association to the carotid sheath, accidental hemorrhage or nerve injury are occasional complications of the operation.

Microscopically, these tumors are perhaps best classed as a variety of endothelioma, more often spoken of as a *perithelioma*. The cells are rather large and polyhedral. They have a rather characteristically granular cytoplasm and contain chromatin so that on gross section the tumor frequently has a yellow color. The cells are grouped in alveolar fashion but without lumen. They are embedded in a hyperplastic vascular stroma. Not infrequently, secondary degeneration with cystic development in the nests of tumor cells takes place. They appear to be a definitely specific tumor; but because of their general structure and difficulty of classification from a histogenetic basis, they are usually included in the group of endotheliomata. Some of them may show a very striking perithelial arrangement of their cells, which has given rise to this terminology in describing them.

ILLUSTRATIVE CASE

CASE 110. (Ref. #S-316)
Diagnosis—Carotid gland—peritheliomata.

Patient was a white female of 65 years, who was admitted to the hospital because of a mass on the right side of her neck, the size of an orange, which had been slowly increasing in size.

Medical History.—The patient was admitted to the hospital with a long history of numerous complaints, the most marked of which was this mass on the right side of the neck, which pulsated and caused her considerable discomfort. She had had arthritis for a number of years, with considerable disability as a result. For the eight years preceding her admission, she had suffered from varicose veins, which required the use of supportive bandages. Six years earlier, she had had a nervous breakdown and had been hospitalized for two months. For several years, she had known she had high blood pressure and had had dyspnea on exertion associated with palpitation and numbness of the extremities. The mass had appeared about three years ago and had slowly been increasing in size. It had not been at all tender but had caused her considerable annoyance on moving her head laterally.

She could not remember any of her childhood medical history other than to be sure that she had not had any serious illness. She was rarely bothered by colds or sore throats. Her gastro-intestinal system had been essentially negative except for constipation. For the few days immediately preceding her admission, however, she had had considerable nausea and had vomited on several occasions. She had never noted any blood in her stools. Her menstrual history was negative. This began at the age of fifteen, and she had her menopause at the age of forty-two. She had had a hysterectomy three years later as the result of the development of an ovarian cyst.

Physical Examination.—The patient was a fairly well-developed and somewhat-undernourished elderly white female. Head was normal in shape. There was a moderate amount of gray hair. Her eyes reacted sluggishly to light and accommodation. Conjunctivae were pale. Nose and throat were negative. She had two artificial dentures. Tongue protruded in mid-line. Examination of the neck showed a bulging mass which extended to the midline. This caused some difficulty in swallowing. The mass, on palpation, seemed rather soft and elastic and there was a definite pulsation felt. A bruit could be heard readily on auscultation. Marked prominence of the superficial veins in the neck was noted. Chest was symmetrical. Lungs were essentially negative. Heart was not enlarged, but there was a harsh systolic murmur heard at the apex, which was not transmitted. Blood pressure was 206/76. The abdomen was almost scaphoid. The liver was greatly enlarged nearly a hand's breadth below the costal margin and was somewhat tender on palpation. The extremities: the peripheral vessels were very tortuous and sclerotic. The fingers and toes showed considerable deformity as the result of her arthritis. Marked varicosities were noted on the lower extremities.

Laboratory Findings.—White blood cells, 6,200 with 58% polynuclears and 35% lymphocytes. Urinalysis was negative. Chemistry was within normal limits. Wassermann was negative.

X-ray examination: Fluoroscopy and films showed a mass in the neck at the level of the angle of the jaw, which encroached upon the hypopharynx to a considerable extent. A few irregular calcific opacities were noted within the mass. The X-ray examination was not conclusive in respect to definite diagnosis. The possibility of aneurysm or some neoplastic process was raised.

Operative History.—On the basis of these findings, the patient was advised to have an exploratory operation. This arose apparently at the bifurcation of the carotid found between the jugular and carotid. In addition, a solid tumor with a dark, hemorrhagic surface was found. This arose apparently in the bifurcation of the carotid and completely surrounded the vessel at that point.

Pathological Report.—*Gross Description.*—Specimen consisted of two masses of tumor tissue measuring approximately 5 x 4 x 3 cm. each. Passing through the substance of this tumor tissue could be seen a large arterial vessel. The tumor on section was yellowish-pink in color, moderately firm in consistency and seemed well encapsulated from the surrounding soft tissues.

Microscopic Description of a Section from the Tumor.—(Fig. 267) Histologic study of the tissue shows a tumor made up of nests of rather large cells, which vary considerably in their morphology. Some of these are polyhedral in outline. Others tend to be spindle. They seem to surround rather characteristically, capillary vessels and are found in rather concentric fashion in these areas. Supporting these nests of tumor cells is a fairly generous connective tissue septate stroma. This is well vascularized. The nuclei of the tumor cells are fairly uniform in size and shape and have a stippled appearance. There is some hyperchromatism, but only rare mitotic figures are found. This arrangement of the cells in discrete nests with a suggestion of peritheliomatous distribution establishes the diagnosis as a tumor of carotid gland origin. Its classification is of some uncertainty in respect to histogenesis. It seems best to consider these tumors as a rather highly specialized variety of endotheliomata, perhaps more accurately a peritheliomata.

CHAPTER XXVIII

TUMORS AND TUMOR-LIKE LESIONS OF THE LYMPHATIC, HEMATOPOIETIC AND RETICULAR TISSUES

The tumors arising in the lymphoid and reticulo-endothelial systems have long been a source of confusion and controversy to clinicians and pathologists alike. Most of these pathological processes present fairly well defined clinical pictures, and in many instances the pathological diagnosis is equally well defined. The etiology, however, of this group of cases is completely obscure, and whether some of these conditions should be considered as true neoplasms or whether they represent inflammatory hyperplasia with a possible infectious etiology is still the subject of dispute. All gradations from a well defined localized lymphosarcoma arising in a regional group of lymph nodes through the various diffuse lesions with invasion of the tissues distantly as is seen in some of the leukemoid and leukemic conditions serve only to confuse the issue.

For practical purposes, it seems best to consider this entire group of cases as true neoplasms. The great majority of these lesions sooner or later, if left untreated, with the single exception of the theoretically possible benign lymphoma, will run a typical malignant course and end fatally. Their response to irradiation is only further confirmatory evidence of their inherently neoplastic nature. They make up a very large and important group of cases from the standpoint of numbers and mortality, and the differentiation of inflammatory lesions which simulate such neoplastic pictures in the lymphoid tissues is of particular importance to the pathologist, the surgeon and the patient alike. Upon the pathologist's ability to differentiate these lesions depends the entire subsequent course of treatment and an estimation of the probable prognosis.

A classification of these lesions as suggested by Callendar from the Lymphatic Tumor Registry in the American Journal of Pathology represents the most satisfactorily workable plan. This, it will be noted, includes certain as yet unestablished varieties of lesions based on wholly theoretical assumptions that such lesions may develop from each and every cell type. This is as rational a thought as is the development of theoretical synthetic chemical substances by a knowledge of their structure. A consideration of these various types of lesions individually follows.

CLASSIFICATION OF TUMORS AND TUMOR-LIKE CONDITIONS OF THE LYMPHATIC, HEMOPOIETIC AND RETICULAR TISSUES †

Adult cell type	Lymphocyte	Myelogenous		Reticulum cell	
		Granular leukocytes	Red blood corpuscles	Reticulocyte monocyte	Hodgkin's disease
Reactions	* "Lymphoma" Lymphocytosis	Leukocytosis	Symptomatic polycythemia	* Gaucher's disease Niemann-Pick disease	Localized (sclerosing)
Proliferations of neoplastic type	Leukemic lymphocytoma 1. Chronic 2. Acute	Leukemic myelocytoma 1. Chronic 2. Acute	1. Polycythemia vera (Syn. Erythemia) 2. Leukemic erythrocytoma	Leukemic reticulocytoma (Syn. Monocytic leukemia)	←———
	Aleukemic lymphocytoma 1. Diffuse 2. Nodular	Aleukemic myelocytoma 1. Single 2. Multiple (Syn. Multiple myeloma)	* Aleukemic erythrocytoma	Aleukemic reticulocytoma	Generalized (cellular)
Malignant Tumors	Lymphosarcoma 1. Aleukemic 2. Leukemic (Syn. Lymphatic leukosarcoma	Myelosarcoma * 1. Aleukemic 2. Leukemic (Syn. Myelocytic leukosarcoma) Chloroma	Erythrosarcoma * 1. Aleukemic 2. Leukemic	Reticulum cell sarcoma	Sarcomatous

* Type not observed in Registry.   † Callendar, G. R., Am. Jour. Pathology, Vol. 10, p. 443, July 1934.

PLATE LXV
TUMORS OF LYMPHOID TISSUES
HODGKIN'S DISEASE.—CASE 114

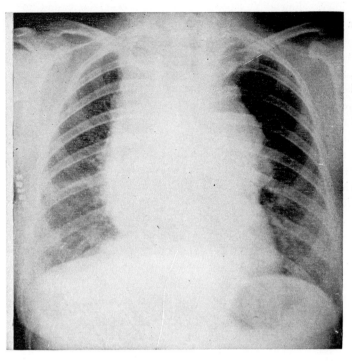

FIG. 268.—ROENTGENOGRAM—CHEST.—There is marked enlargement of the mediastinal shadow due to involvement of the lymph nodes in the process.

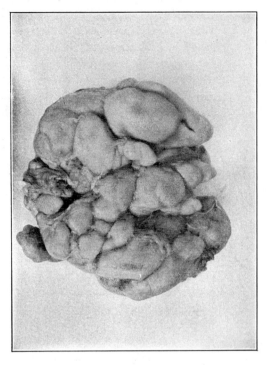

FIG. 269.—LYMPH NODES.—Gross photograph showing a mass of greatly enlarged, discrete nodes, the cut surface of which presents grossly the characteristic translucent, homogeneous "fish flesh" appearance.

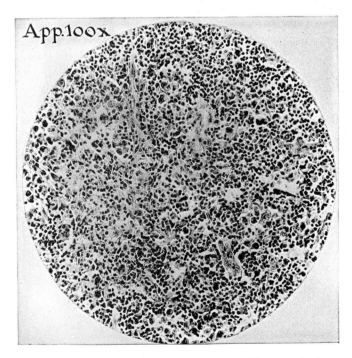

FIG. 270.—LYMPH NODE.—Photomicrograph to illustrate the loss of normal lymphoid architecture, the reticulo-endothelial proliferation and the presence of large numbers of characteristic Reed-Sternberg giant cells. App. 100 x.

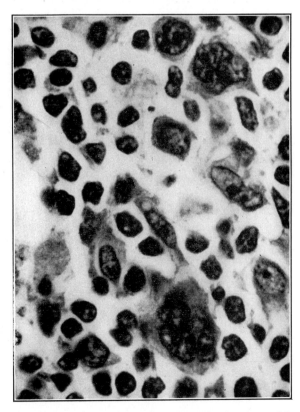

FIG. 271.—LYMPH NODE.—High magnification in which the characteristics of the multinucleated Reed-Sternberg cells are better shown. App. 1000 x.

LESIONS ARISING FROM THE LYMPHOCYTE

Benign Lymphoma.—With the term "benign lymphoma," we are treading on uncertain territory. Whether such a lesion actually exists as a true neoplasm in contradistinction to a simple inflammatory hyperplasia is debatable. Many pathologists will not concede this possibility. On the other hand, many pathologists have described cases which seem best to fit into such a category. Owing to the extremely labile nature of lymphoid tissue in relation to inflammatory processes generally, it obviously is difficult at times to tell whether a lesion is inflammatory in nature or is neoplastic. Ewing and others, however, report local lesions with marked increase in size of the lymphnodes which remain relatively stationary in their appearance over long periods of time. Removal of such tissue histologically shows the presence of simple lymphoid hyperplasia. The outstanding feature histologically of this condition is the persistence of the normal lymphoid architecture which, however, is usually exaggerated. Lymph follicles are larger than normal with extremely prominent germinal centers and wide collars of small lymphocytes. There is a diffuse increase of the lymphoid cells in the remainder of the node, and such crowding of the tissue by lymphocytes frequently results in a moderate reticulo-endothelial hyperplasia. Mitotic figures are rarely noted, although they may occur occasionally. One of the most significant features histologically is the fact that all the cells are normal in appearance. It is doubtful whether such a diagnosis may ever be made accurately on histologic grounds alone; but where there is a clinical history of a persistent localized involvement of lymphoid structures, with a microscopic picture of this nature it seems reasonable to consider such a lesion as a true benign neoplasm (see Fig. 272).

LYMPHOCYTOSIS.—As commented upon in the outline, lymphoid tissue may easily be stimulated to activity by a wide variety of conditions. In the simplest type of lymphoid stimulation we see a resultant outpouring of lymphocytes into the blood stream with a rise in both the relative and absolute numbers of such cells. This is particularly seen in childhood and in association with some of the more common children's diseases. Pertussis is perhaps the most outstanding of these, and indeed it is not uncommon to find the lymphoid cells which normally number approximately 2,500 to 3,000 per cubic millimeter (25 per cent to 30 per cent) increasing up to as high as 100,000 or more. This, in itself, may, on occasion, cause difficulty in diagnosis, raising as it obviously does the question of leukemia as will be discussed in subsequent paragraphs.

INFECTIOUS MONONUCLEOSIS.—Another lesion which falls in the same category as lymphocytosis as a result of infection is seen in the condition known as *"infectious mononucleosis."* In this condition, which likewise is apt to be seen in children or young adults principally, we have enlargement of the lymph nodes regionally, and particularly involving the cervical nodes. The picture is further complicated by an increase in the white blood cells ranging as high as 20,000 to 25,000, with large lymphocytes predominating. For this reason, the condition may, at times, be confused with a leukemic picture or some other condition associated with a lymphocytosis.

Clinically, it is usually accompanied by a low-grade fever, a feeling of lassitude and malaise, and may become complicated by a mild degree of secondary anemia. The disturbing and confusing element in this condition is seen in the long duration of the clinical history, which again causes confusion in diagnosis. The establishment of such diagnosis is of tremendous importance because the mortality of infectious mononucleosis is nil, whereas the mortality of leukemia is ultimately invariably fatal. A positive heterophile antigen develops in the course of this condition in a considerable proportion of the cases. This is of value, when it is present, in excluding leukemia. Biopsy examination of the tissue of lymphnodes removed from such cases is not always comforting to the uninitiated. There is a diffuse lymphoid hyperplasia chiefly of the medium and larger type cells. This results in considerable distortion of the normal architecture with a tendency toward loss of follicles or their apparent merging with the stroma of the node. Mitoses are not rare by any means, and hyperchromatism is also sometimes seen. Due to the chronicity of the lesion, fibrosis and reticular hyperplasia are apt to be present. Not infrequently eosinophilic infiltration also occurs. For this reason, the condition may at times be confused with Hodgkin's disease. Because of the ultimate fatal outcome of this latter condition, the responsibility of the pathologist is obvious.

PLATE LXVI

TUMORS OF LYMPHOID TISSUES

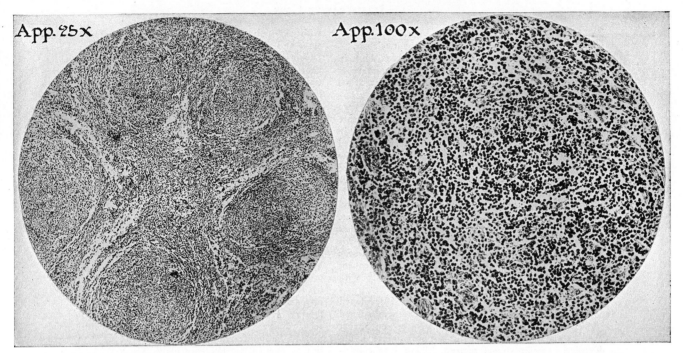

FIG. 272.—LYMPH NODE: BENIGN LYMPHOMA.—The outstanding diagnostic features—the increase in size of the lymph follicles, especially of their germinal centers, and the preservation of the normal architecture of the node—are well demonstrated. App. 25 x.

FIG. 273.—LYMPH NODE: INFECTIOUS MONONUCLEOSIS.—CASE 111.—Diffuse lymphoid hyperplasia and infiltration modifying the normal architecture of the node, readily confused with more serious lesions, lymphosarcoma, leukemia and even Hodgkin's disease. App. 100 x.

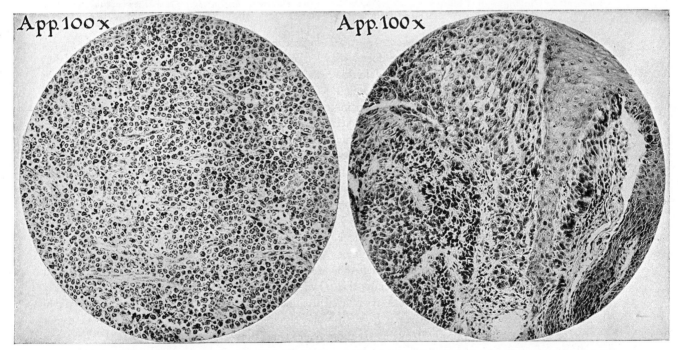

FIG. 274.—LYMPH NODE: LYMPHOSARCOMA.—CASE 112.—Highly malignant, invasive neoplasm showing a monotonous histologic pattern completely destroying the normal architecture of the node, and composed of atypical large lymphocytes showing many mitotic figures. App. 100 x.

FIG. 275.—TONSIL: LYMPHO-EPITHELIOMA.—CASE 113.—Note the composite nature of the tumor, with both nests of atypical lymphoid cells (at left), and malignant epidermal tissue (centrally), invading the adjacent mucosa. App. 100 x.

ILLUSTRATIVE CASE

CASE III. (Ref. #S-317)

Diagnosis.—Lymph node—infectious mononucleosis.

Patient was a white male student of 25 years, born in the south. He was submitted to the hospital complaining of sore throat, headache, malaise, weakness and marked bilateral cervical adenopathy.

Present Illness.—The present illness began about two weeks before admission when he developed a slight sore throat. This continued without any marked increase in symptoms for several days and then became complicated by diffuse muscle and joint pains, particularly in the lumbar back region. There was a marked feeling of lassitude and weakness. The lymph nodes in his neck began to swell and became slightly tender.

Past History.—The patient had the usual childhood diseases, including measles, whooping cough and mumps. He also had had typhoid fever at the age of twelve and had had a mild tertian malarial infection. During his school years in the north, he had developed a chronic sinusitis with several attacks of bronchitis and frequent colds. These had always subsided spontaneously with only minimal symptomatic treatment.

Physical Examination.—Patient was a well-developed and well-nourished young, adult male. Head was normal in appearance. Eyes were negative. Nose and throat showed rather marked injection of the soft palate, uvula and entire retropharyngeal mucosa. There was considerable postnasal, greenish-gray purulent material seen on direct examination. The cervical nodes were moderately enlarged and slightly tender. Chest was symmetrical. Heart and lungs appeared negative. Abdomen was negative. Genitalia and extremities were negative.

Laboratory Findings.—Red blood cells, 5,070,000 with 14 grams (82.6%) hemoglobin. White blood cells, 10,950 with 36% polynuclears and 46% lymphocytes; 11% monocytes and 1% eosinophiles. Of these cells, occasional lymphoblast forms and Türck irritation cells were seen. Repeated examinations showed essentially the same differential count, but the white cells rose to 20,150, about 10% being immature lymphocytes. Repeated examinations for malarial parasites were negative. Agglutination for *B. typhosus, Para A and Para B, and B. abortus* were negative. Heterophile antibody reaction was positive.

Subsequent Course.—With the coöperation of the patient, a biopsy specimen of one of the cervical glands was removed.

Pathological Report.—*Gross Description.*—The gross appearance of the node showed moderate hyperplasia. The node was grayish-pink in color and succulent in appearance. There were no gross diagnostic features.

Microscopic Description of the Node.—(Fig. 273) Histologic examination presents a picture of diffuse lymphoid hyperplasia. The lymph follicles are enlarged, but more striking than the enlargement of the germinal centers is the diffuse infiltration of the entire gland by large lymphocytes. Many of these are immature in appearance and suggest blast forms. Rare mitotic figures are encountered. Occasional eosinophiles are seen. There is a moderate reticulo-endothelial hyperplasia. The differential diagnosis is not easy to establish on microscopic evidence alone. Many of the features of this node could be duplicated in Hodgkin's disease.

Progress Notes.—Over a period of about six months, the blood count gradually returned to normal. During this interval the patient remained essentially symptom-free after the subsidence of his acute upper respiratory tract infection except for persistence of the enlarged nodes.

Lymphosarcoma (Malignant Lymphoma).—Under this heading will be considered those forms of lymphocytic malignancy which arise *locally* in the lymph nodes or in lymphoid tissue such as is found in the gastro-intestinal tract with or without an increase of lymphoid cells in the peripheral blood stream. This is in contradistinction to the leukemic process in which there is *generalized* lymphoid activity, again with or without apparent increase of these cells in the peripheral blood stream. The leukemic picture will be taken up separately in a consideration of leukemia as a whole.

Theoretically, at least, lymphosarcoma may occur in two forms, depending upon whether the tumor arises from the small adult lymphocyte or from the young, less-well-defined larger type. Practically, this differentiation is not maintained, and both types of cell may be found in the same tumor. In general, as a tumor becomes malignant, the tendency is for the cells to be of the more immature, large form. The diagnosis of lymphosarcoma is largely a histologic one and depends upon the microscopic examination of biopsy material. There are certain, fairly well defined criteria for the establishment of the diagnosis. In the first place, there is usually a marked loss of architecture. Of course, if the lesion is early enough, this loss of architecture may not be so prominent a feature as is usually true. In the second place, there is diffuse infiltration of the peripheral lymph sinuses and capsule of the lymphnode. This infiltration furthermore is not confined to the capsule, but extends through the capsule as perivascular invasion of the surrounding structures. In the third place, the type of cell is so characteristic as to make the diagnosis usually fairly simple. The cells are fairly uniformly large in size. They tend to show marked hyperchromatism, and mitotic figures are unusually prominent as a rule. Atypic mitoses are less frequently seen perhaps in tumors of lymphoid origin than in most other forms of malignancy. There is a monotony to the architecture of such a tumor as it causes little or no stromal proliferation and likewise stimulates very little vascular development, although there is usually an adequate blood supply. Grossly, such lymphnodes are almost milky white in color, uniform in appearance on cut section and extremely friable in consistency due to the lack of stroma.

Such tumors are extremely radio-sensitive and may even be permanently cured by intensive irradiation therapy, in a small percentage of cases. The difficulty in histologic diagnosis lies in the fact that the leukemic node may present an almost identical his-

tology at times, and because the localized lymphosarcoma may subsequently become a generalized process involving lymphoid structures throughout the body with the ultimate development of a leukemia. Thus, the whole problem of lymphoid stimulation becomes an extremely complex one with these numerous variants of the picture merging so closely with one another as to render their exact diagnosis among the most difficult histologically, as well as clinically.

ILLUSTRATIVE CASE

CASE 112. (Ref. #S-193)
Diagnosis.—Lymphosarcoma.

Patient was a white female married housewife, 29 years old. She was admitted to the hospital with the chief complaint of enlargement of the glands of the neck accompanied by a general feeling of malaise and frontal headaches.

Present Illness.—The patient stated that she had been in her usual good health until about two months before admission. At that time she noticed a feeling of discomfort in her throat as if something were caught there. This required a constant clearing of her throat. She developed a rather persistent nervous sort of cough. At that time she noticed a slight swelling at the base of the neck on the right side. About three or four weeks ago following exposure to cold and wet, she developed a severe cold. The glands on both sides of her neck began to swell and became prominent. They had not been particularly painful, however, and she had not noticed any reddening of the overlying tissues. She had had a feeling of easy fatigability for the past several weeks, particularly since the onset of her cold. There was a recurrence of this upper respiratory infection as a grippe-like infection for the past few days and she complained of a persistent slight hacking cough.

Past Medical History.—As a child she had the usual infections, including mumps and diphtheria. At the age of three she had a double mastoidectomy and she had been subject to a mild upper respiratory infection throughout her entire history. At the age of eleven, she was said to have had gastritis and from that time until five years ago, she had intermittent attacks of vague gastro-intestinal disturbances, associated with excessive belching after meals. Five years preceding admission she was operated upon for a chronic appendicitis and her condition had improved since that time. A review of her various systems showed nothing of significance. She had worn glasses for about fifteen years. There had been a few sore spots over the sternal area during the past few weeks. She had noticed occasional slight shortness of breath upon exertion. Her menstrual history had been entirely normal with the last period being one week before admission.

Physical Examination.—The patient was a young white woman who did not appear acutely ill and complained of nothing except "lumps in the neck." Head was essentially negative. Pupils reacted normally to light and distance. Hearing was normal. Teeth were well taken care of. Tonsils had been removed. Nose and throat, in general, were negative. The thyroid was not enlarged.

The anterior and posterior cervical lymphnodes were diffusely enlarged. The supraclavicular nodes, especially on the right side showed definite increase in size. Heart and lungs appeared within normal limits. Blood pressure 124/80. Abdomen was negative except for the right lower quadrant scar. In addition to the cervical lymphnode enlargement there was generalized enlargement of the peripheral nodes including the axillary and inguinal.

Laboratory Findings.—Red blood cells, 2,870,000 with 41.6% (6.5 grams) of hemoglobin; and a color index of 0.74. White blood cells, 7,000 with 25% polynuclears of which 19% were nonfilamented and 6%, filamented forms; 61% lymphocytes, 10% monocytes, 1 promyelocyte and 3 myelocytes as well as 5 nucleated red cells, seen in making the differential count. Urinalysis was essentially negative. Kolmer, Kahn and Kline tests were all negative.

X-ray examination: Fluroscopy and films of the thorax revealed a soft tissue mass in the anterior mediastinum which merged with the left border of the heart shadow causing slight posterior displacement of the trachea.

Operative Record.—The patient was advised to have a lymphnode removed for biopsy study, which was done, and a gland 2.5 cm. in diameter was excised from just above the clavicle posterior to the belly of the sternocleidomastoid muscle.

Pathological Report.—*Gross Description of Surgical Specimen.*—Specimen consisted of three lymphnodes, two of them measuring only approximately 0.5 cm. in diameter while the other measured 1.2 x 0.5 cm. They were firm, grayish-white in color, well encapsulated and on section had a uniform appearance with an absence of necrosis.

Microscopic Description of Section Through the Lymphnodes.—(Fig. 274) Histologic study reveals an almost complete loss of normal architecture. The nodes are made up of almost solid masses of lymphoid cells which, for the most part, are medium-sized. There are numerous mitotic figures showing all stages of mitosis. The capsule is definitely thickened and richly infiltrated by lymphocytes. These cells also infiltrate the pericapsular fat. With the loss of lymph follicles, the loss of peripheral sinuses, the infiltration of the stroma, capsule and perinodal tissue and the presence of innumerable mitotic figures, the diagnosis of lymphosarcoma cannot be avoided.

Subsequent History.—The patient was given intensive irradiation therapy, but in spite of this went rapidly downhill, dying two months following the establishment of the diagnosis. Unfortunately autopsy permission was not obtained to study the extent of the process.

Lympho-epithelioma.—A tumor which is difficult to classify, fits best perhaps into this group of lymphoid lesions. This is the so-called lympho-epithelioma, a tumor which arises almost regularly in the tonsil or the posterior nasal pharynx in relation to the ring of adenoid and lymphoid tissues. It is a difficult tumor to classify because both the epithelium and the underlying lymphoid tissues seem to take part in the malignant process. By some it is classified among the so-called "mixed tumors." We are inclined to believe that it represents basically a tumor of lymphoid tissue with the stimulation of the overlying epithelium to undergo malignant change. This epithelium, as a rule, is not the adult, well-defined squamous type but represents the incompletely differentiated type of epithelium sometimes spoken of inaccurately as "transitional cell epithelium," which is found at the base of the tonsillar crypts, for example. For this reason these tumors are sometimes designated as "transitional cell carcinomata." Earlier in the history of the recognition of this group of tumors, the term "primary endothelioma" of the tonsil was made, which corresponds to this same tumor, the nature of which has been so clearly established by Ewing.

Basically, the diagnosis of this type of tumor is made by finding a diffuse neoplastic hyperplasia of the undifferentiated transitional cell epithelium and the underlying lymphoid tissue. Whether these cells should not more accurately be considered as reticulum cells than true lymphocytes, or whether both are involved in the process is still somewhat debatable, but the similarity in appearance of neoplasms of the reticulum cell type and the typical lymphosarcoma is so well recognized as to require no further comment. These tumors are apt to be extremely small in their primary site, and often pass unnoticed and unrecognized. A metastatic lesion with enlargement of the regional lymphnodes, or even distant metastasis in the lung, may be the first evidence of the condition. The tumors are commonly seen in the young adult group, and it is rare to encounter them in individuals past the age of forty. Fortunately, the tumor is extremely radio-sensitive, and a number of cases are on record of permanent recovery following extensive irradiation. On the other hand, late recurrence is by no means unusual, and not an inconsiderable number of these cases go on to die ultimately of their disease in spite of combined surgical and x-ray therapy.

ILLUSTRATIVE CASE

CASE 113. (Ref. #S-314)
Diagnosis.—Lympho-epithelioma.
Patient was a single white male, a weaver by occupation, who was admitted to the hospital because of difficulty in swallowing solid food for the past year preceding admission. During the preceding six weeks, even liquids had occasioned him trouble as a sensation of a lump in the throat on the right side, accompanied by sharp shooting pains on the right side of his neck radiating to the back of the ear.

Present Illness.—About one year before admission, after eating an orange, he felt a lump in the right side of his throat. The patient thought nothing of it at the time, but the lump had persisted to the present time. Shortly after this, he noticed that solid food seemed to lodge in this region, but after repeated swallowing efforts, food finally went down. During the six weeks preceding admission he had had a great deal of difficulty in getting even soft solids down because his ability to swallow was so impaired. He had no cough, but cleared mucus from his throat occasionally. He had no history of dyspnea. There was a loss of weight of about ten pounds during the past five weeks.

Past History.—The past history was irrelevant. His mother and father died of old age. He had had typhoid fever at the age of seventeen, in addition to the usual childhood diseases; but since then had had no difficulty until the onset of the present illness.

Physical Examination.—The patient was small and poorly nourished. He showed an obvious loss of weight

but was not cachectic. He was not hoarse, but there was a curious change in the voice sounds. Eyes and nose were negative. There was compensated edentia of the upper jaw. Two teeth remained in the lower jaw. Hypertrophied and infected tonsils were present. There was a mass of adherent tissue extending from the edge of the epiglottis on the right to the base of the tongue, so that the interior of the larynx was not visualized. The right pyriform sinus was involved also by what appeared to be tumor. There was enlargement of the lymph nodes in the right anterior cervical chain. Chest was of the phthisical type. Sternum was depressed. Some wheezing sounds and a few râles were heard in both upper lobes. Voice sounds were modified but this was probably not intrapulmonary in origin but transmitted from the larynx. Heart was negative. Abdomen was negative. Extremities were essentially negative. A working diagnosis of probably malignancy of the larynx was made.

Laboratory Findings.—White blood cells, 10,150 of which 63% were polynuclears and 27% lymphocytes. Urinalysis was negative.

Direct Laryngoscopy.—The entire epiglottis showed a granular, proliferating mass which also involved the base of the tongue. The intrinsic part of the larynx seemed to be normal. A presumptive diagnosis of carcinoma of the epiglottis and base of the tongue was made.

X-ray Examination.—Soft tissue masses at the base of the tongue had displaced the epiglottis distally and posteriorly. Apparently these tumor masses had in some way interfered with the passage of food so that the food was diverted into the vallecula on the left side instead of passing through the pharynx in its usual manner.

Nothing remarkable was seen in the chest. Lung fields appeared clear. There were old, pleural, diaphragmatic adhesions most marked on the right side.

Operative Record.—A biopsy specimen was taken to confirm the diagnosis.

Pathological Report.—*Gross Description of Biopsy.*—Specimen consisted of several small fragments of grayish-pink tissue.

Microscopic Description.—(Fig. 275) Histologically, the tissue is partially covered by a poorly differentiated pseudostratified layer of epithelium. Where present, these cells seem to fuse as irregular, deep projecting spurs with a hyperplastic round cell tissue suggesting lymphoid cells. In the subepithelial areas these are packed together in large masses as nests with here and there a suggestion of follicle formation. In places, these masses of lymphoid-like cells project toward the surface. They all show marked hyperchromatism with round or oval vesicular nuclei. Atypical mitotic figures are fairly prominent. Deeper in the structure, these clusters of cells seem to elongate and anastomose as clumps fusing with the superficial epithelial-like spurs.

Subsequent Course.—He ultimately developed metastatic lesions in the hip, scalp and lungs and died four years after the onset of his illness, although responding amazingly well for a time to irradiation.

LESIONS OF THE RETICULUM CELL

Under this heading will be found a considerable number of pathological processes which relate to the reticulo-endothelial system generally. Many of these are in the nature of a metabolic disturbance affecting the metabolism of lipoids in particular. Among these may be mentioned Gaucher's disease, Niemann-Pick's disease, Hand-Christian-Schuller syndrome and Hurler's disease (gargoylism). These are obviously non-neoplastic in nature and need not be considered further at this time.

Hodgkin's Disease.—In the group of lesions involving the reticulo-endothelial system, Hodgkin's stands out as one of the important and confusing diseases. Whether this should be classified as of infectious etiology or as a neoplasm varies with the individual opinion of the authors. It is considered by many as one of the infectious granulomata; by others wholly on a neoplastic basis. It presents certain features suggesting its possible infectious nature. Among these may be cited the fact that there is often definite fever. This is apt to be of an intermittent nature and is seen particularly in the so-called "Pel-Ebstein" variety, in which splenic involvement is particularly striking. A wide variety of organisms have been recovered from the lesions, but the reproduction of the disease in experimental animals has met with little success. L'Esperance has shown that there is a very striking similarity in the clinical and histologic picture in certain cases of Hodgkin's disease to the avian form of tuberculosis, and has reproduced a picture not unlike the original lesion in chickens inoculated with material from human cases of the disease. Her feeling in this respect seems to be that Hodgkin's disease represents a clinical syndrome which may be caused by a wide variety of etiologic agents of which the avian tubercle bacillus may well be one.

Clinically, the disease usually starts as a painless enlargement of a group of superficial lymphnodes, most commonly in the cervical region. Primary involvement of the mediastinal or retroperitoneal or other peripheral nodes is by no means uncommon, however. As the disease progresses, there is gradual involvement of all of the reticulo-endothelial organs including the spleen. The progress of the disease is further evidenced by the development of a severe anemia due to bone marrow involvement. The skin is involved in the same type of tissue reaction with marked cellular infiltration. Clinically, this is accompanied by intense itching. Gradually, the patient becomes emaciated and weak, presenting the typical cachectic appearance of malignancy, and is very apt to die of intercurrent upper respiratory infection. So far as is known, the disease is uniformly fatal, or at least it has proven to be fatal in all cases in which the diagnosis has definitely been established by pathologic examination. Whether or not milder forms of the disease exist in which recovery may result spontaneously, or as the result of irradiation therapy is not known. It is certain, however, that the course of the disease may be materially modified by radiation therapy and many cases are on record whose lives have been prolonged three, five and even ten years as the result of such treatment. Left alone, the cases progress steadily to a fatal exodus, usually within two to three years at the most. Surgical treatment is merely palliative and to-day has largely been replaced by radiation, except as an accessory means of relieving symptoms.

The pathology of the disease is best seen in the lymphnodes. Usually a group of nodes is involved. They are markedly enlarged but remain discrete in contradistinction to the matting together of such nodes in tuberculosis and other inflammatory lesions.

On section, however, a rather characteristic yellow-ish-pink homogeneous appearance usually described as resembling the flesh of fish is noted.

Microscopic examination of the lesion shows a tendency toward obliteration of the normal architecture of the lymphnode by a diffuse reticulo-endothelial hyperplasia, by lymphoid hyperplasia and by fibrous tissue proliferation. Scattered through this picture, which resembles in many respects inflammatory hyperplasia may be found typically the characteristic cells of Hodgkin's disease, the so-called Dorothy Reed, or Sternberg cells. These are large cells with pale staining cytoplasm and elongated vesicular nuclei. Many of them are multinucleated with two to four or more lobulated nuclei. Their nuclear membrane stains intensely and the nucleus itself likewise contains a considerable number of deep-staining, scattered granules of chromatin. These cells are more numerous in the earlier stages of the disease and as the process continues, the hyperplastic picture is replaced by a diffuse fibrosis, which frequently shows extensive hyaline degeneration and necrosis. Embedded in this connective tissue stroma

not infrequently aggregations of lymphocytes are found which may even reproduce actual follicles. As a more irregular accompaniment of the histologic findings should be cited a rather characteristic eosinophilic infiltration.

A certain number of cases may present a frankly sarcomatous histology. In these instances, there is extensive infiltration of the capsule with invasion of the surrounding structures. The stromal cells seem to play a part in this malignant form of the disease, and a picture not unlike a diffuse fibrosarcoma may be observed. Necrosis of a rather caseous type is prone to occur and the cellular reaction around such lesions at times is very suggestive of an atypical tuberculosis. It is in this type, particularly, that the possible relationship to the avian form of the tubercle bacillus has been suggested.

Rare cases of Hodgkin's disease have been reported arising in almost every organ where reticulo-endothelial cells exist. Included among these should be mentioned the gastro-intestinal tract, the thymus and even the thyroid, as well as the bone marrow.

ILLUSTRATIVE CASE

CASE 114. (Ref. #S-75)
Diagnosis.—Lymphnode—Hodgkin's disease.
Patient was a white male, thirty-six years of age, admitted to the hospital because of swelling of the knee joints accompanied by marked itching of the skin.
Present Illness.—About one year ago, the patient noticed a feeling of vague discomfort in the arms and legs. This was followed by transitory attacks of swelling and redness, which responded well to salicylates. The picture since then had been characterized by a loss of strength. He had periods of normal temperature which alternated irregularly and at intervals of several weeks with fever of seven to ten days' duration. The fever might start with a chill. Adenopathy of the cervical and inguinal nodes had developed. In the beginning, a diagnosis of endocarditis was considered, but repeated blood cultures and continued observation led to the abandonment of this diagnosis. There had been no weight loss and no evidence of cardiac failure. There had been no cough at any time.
Past History.—The past history was not particularly significant. Measles was the only childhood disease. He had been in good health up to the onset of his present condition. He had had his tonsils out at the age of twenty-two following an attack of severe sore throat. He had no recurrence of upper respiratory infection since that time. His family history was negative. His social history was likewise negative. He was married and had one child, aged eight, who was living and well. His occupation was that of a metal worker in a shipyard where he had been employed for twelve years.
Physical Examination.—Patient was a well-developed

white adult male about one hundred thirty-five pounds in weight, lying fairly comfortably in bed. Head was normal in size and shape. Eyes and ears were negative except for a slight inflammation of both upper and lower lids. Nose was negative. Tongue was coated. All molars had been extracted on the lower jaw. Neck: There was a generalized bilateral enlargement of all of the cervical lymphnodes to a moderate degree with one large gland along the right anterior cervical chain. Heart and lungs were negative. Blood pressure was 110/60. Abdomen was symmetrical and negative on examination. Spleen was not palpable. Extremities were negative.
Laboratory Examination.—Red blood cells, 3,550,000; hemoglobin 72%. White blood cells 11,100 with 85% polynuclears, 12% lymphocytes, 2% large monocytes and 1% eosinophiles. Smears showed no abnormalities of the white blood cells. Urinalysis was negative. Wassermann was negative.
X-ray Examination.—(Fig. 268) There was slight enlargement of the hilar shadow on each side. There was a soft tissue shadow which presented smooth outlines and homogeneous density. It was probable that these represented enlarged nodes. With the associated history of fever, itching, adenopathy, weakness and secondary anemia, a diagnosis of Hodgkin's seemed most probable.
Subsequent Course.—On the strength of the indefinite history and the generalized cervical adenopathy, it was recommended that one of the lymphnodes be removed for diagnosis.
Pathological Report.—*Gross Description.*—Specimen consisted of a smooth, firm, well encapsulated lymphnode measuring 4 x 2.6 x 1.3 cm. On section the cut

surface was pale gray, homogeneous, translucent and had a fish flesh appearance suggestive of Hodgkin's disease.

Microscopic Description of Lymphnode.—(Fig. 269, 270 and 271) Microscopic study of the cervical node reveals some portions to be quite dense and cellular, while in other areas the stroma is much less dense and the cells likewise less numerous. The cells tend to show marked pleomorphism. Many large mononuclears are present in conjunction with a diffuse reticulo-endothelial hyperplasia. Many typical multinucleated Dorothy Reed

cells are present. As a whole, there is an increase of fibrous stroma throughout the gland. The lymph follicles are distorted and largely destroyed as also are the peripheral lymph sinuses. There seems to be some increased vascularity. Frequent mitotic figures are observed. Occasional eosinophiles are encountered. Some definite areas of necrosis are present. In these areas the cells show pyknosis and karyorrhexis. The picture as a whole presents the characteristic features of a relatively acute type of Hodgkin's disease. It illustrates particularly well the Reed-Sternberg giant cell feature of the histology.

Reticulo-endothelial Sarcoma (Retethelioma).—As a definite neoplasm of the reticulo-endothelial system should be mentioned a tumor which, as demonstrated by the use of special reticulum stains, is derived from the reticular cells. As has been already mentioned, this tumor is extremely difficult at times to differentiate from tumors arising strictly from the lymphocytic series, and such differentiation should perhaps best be made on the basis of such special stains. It is a tumor which, like the frank lymphosarcoma, is radiosensitive and almost melts away under adequate therapy. A considerable proportion of

permanent arrests or cures may be expected with such tumors. One of the commonest sites for this particular variety of tumor is seen in the form of a large, bulky, retroperitoneal tumor which reaches enormous proportions, often measuring as much as fifteen to twenty centimeters in diameter and weighing several kilos. Surgically, such tumors are apt to be inoperable because of their extent and location and thus irradiation is offered as the most promising form of therapy, although by no means always resulting permanently in a cure, but almost certainly causing regression of the lesion for a variable time.

ILLUSTRATIVE CASE

CASE 115. (Ref. #S-105)

Diagnosis.—Lymphnode—reticulum-cell sarcoma.

Patient was a white male of 78 years, who was admitted to the hospital complaining of pain in the region of the left hip.

Present Illness.—The patient stated that he was in good health until six weeks preceding his admission when he noticed severe pain in the left hip region accompanied by swelling and difficulty in walking. The pain was more or less constant, but worse on motion of the extremity. The pain seemed much worse at night. It was not affected by a change of position particularly, and was relieved only by sedatives. The patient did not think that the swelling had increased much since he first noticed it, but the pain had become much more intense.

Past History.—Patient had been a normal, healthy child who had had the usual childhood diseases. He had never had any serious illness previously. He had occasional sore throat and colds. His weight had fluctuated a good deal, but he had not noted any progressive loss of weight during the past several years. His family and social histories were irrelevant. There was no history of cancer in his family.

Physical Examination.—Physical examination showed a well-preserved, elderly, white male resting on his side to relieve the pain in his hip. There was moderate generalized arteriosclerosis noted of the peripheral vessels. Head was of normal contour, partially bald. Eyes, ears, nose and throat were negative except for a slight icteric tinge to the sclerae and skin. The chest was symmetrical and resonant throughout. Heart showed slight enlargement, but the sounds were of good quality and regular. The abdomen was moderately tense as the result of a voluntary spasm to prevent pain on motion of his extremity. The liver seemed somewhat enlarged, about two

fingers' breadth below the costal margin in the anterior axillary line. The spleen was enlarged and palpable three fingers' breadth below the costal border. There was an irregular, firm mass felt in the upper right quadrant. This felt about the size of a plum. There was tenderness in both flanks with a questionable fluid wave. There was no particular pain or tenderness on deep palpation. There was asymmetry of the pelvis posteriorly with prominence of the left buttock. This was the result of a firm mass apparently growing from or attached to the left ilium. The mass was fairly uniform in consistency and smooth in outline. Rectal examination showed rather prominent external and internal hemorrhoids. The prostate was negative.

Laboratory Findings.—Urinalysis was negative. Red blood cells, 4,400,000 with 10.5 gm. of hemoglobin (78%). White blood cells, 4,800 with 65% neutrophiles. Wassermann negative. Gruskin skin test for malignancy was faintly positive.

X-ray Examination revealed bone absorption and destruction of a portion of the left ilium. This extended to involve the sacro-iliac joint and suggested extension of the soft tumor into the bone rather than a true metastatic lesion.

Subsequent Course.—A biopsy of an inguinal lymph node was performed for diagnosis.

Pathological Report.—*Gross Description.*—Specimen consisted of two pieces of pink tissue which presented no gross features of diagnostic significance.

Microscopic Description of Tissue from the Tumor.—Histologic examination of the tumor shows it to be composed of masses of large cells with vesicular nuclei and having but little and barely discernible cytoplasm. These cells are found infiltrating the striated muscle tissue with extensive secondary degeneration of the muscle cells. These show hyaline change and loss of nuclei. The cells of the tumor have large, prominent nucleoli sometimes as many as five or six within a nucleus. Numerous multilobulated nuclei are seen. Marked pleomorphism and anaplasia are present. Both normal and atypical mitoses are seen in large numbers. The stroma of the tumor appears to be almost negligible and to be made up only of a few delicate connective tissue strands

Ewing's Tumor of Bone.—In this connection, again, should be mentioned Ewing's tumor of bone, which from the standpoint of classification offers so much difficulty. As has been already emphasized by many investigators, this tumor is believed to be de-

supporting a rather generous capillary vascular supply. Some areas of hemorrhage and necrosis may be observed. With special silver stains, the cytoplasm of these cells is found to trail off into typical reticulum, which fuses to create a supporting stroma of its own for the tumor cells. On the basis of this differential staining procedure, the tumor is diagnosed as a reticulum cell sarcoma or so-called retethelioma.

rived from the reticulo-endothelial system of the bone marrow and on that basis should be included in any discussion of the tumors of the reticulum cell. See Chapter XXV for a consideration of the actual pathology and an illustrative case.

TUMORS OF THE MYELOID CELL

Myelosarcoma.—Just as tumors may arise from the lymphocyte and from the reticulum cell, so may tumors arise on occasion from the myeloid cells. This condition may be differentiated from leukemia only in that there are focal tumor masses rather than diffuse myeloid infiltration of the tissues. Such a distinction may seem artificial to a very large extent but occasional cases are encountered which fit into such a concept. Usually, such tumors are associated with a leukemic blood picture at some stage or other in the development of the process, but this does not necessarily have to occur. One such case which we have seen occurring in a child presented all the usually accepted criteria for such a diagnosis. Over a period of nearly seven years the tumor has remained localized, although continually recurring, and at no time has there been apparent involvement of the peripheral blood stream in a leukemic infiltration. Such a tumor may well be called a localized myelosarcoma corresponding to the localized lymphosarcoma with which we are so much more familiar.

Chloroma.—As a variant of this lesion is the condition known as chloroma, in which tumor-like nodules occurring in the bone marrow and of definite grayish green color when exposed to the air may be seen. Such cases usually are associated with the presence of Bence-Jones protein in the urine. This lesion is more likely to be seen in the younger age group, particularly in young adult males, and invariably terminates fatally, often in less than six months. When it occurs in older individuals, its course may be considerably prolonged.

Unlike the other forms of myeloma, extension of the process to the lymphnodes as well as distant nodular metastasis is the rule rather than the exception. Histologic diagnosis is made by finding cells of the myeloid series, eosinophilic myelocytes, or their precursors, tending to predominate. A relative increase in the maturation forms of the myeloid cells in the peripheral blood is frequently encountered, accompanied by a low grade anemia. This is of the myelophthisic variety, the red cells being crowded out.

LESIONS ARISING FROM THE RED CELL DERIVATIVES

Symptomatic Polycythemia.—Just as we may have a proliferation of the lymphocytes or the leukocytes in the peripheral blood, so may we have an increase in the number of red cells under varying physiological conditions. By symptomatic polycythemia is meant an increase in the number of adult red blood corpuscles which results from alterations in altitude, for example, or as the result of hemoconcentration as seen in shock. No neoplastic consideration enters into this picture.

Of the theoretical malignant lesions arising from the red cell should be mentioned cases of *polycythemia vera* and instances in which local metastatic lesions occur showing active hematopoiesis. As reported in the Tumor Registry series, one such case of erythrosarcoma has been observed, characterized by the presence of polycythemia, multiple metastatic lesions, and terminating fatally. This rare condition is mentioned merely for the sake of completeness in discussing the classification as presented.

CHAPTER XXIX

THE LEUKEMIAS

By leukemia is meant a condition which affects the blood-forming organs and is usually manifested, as the term implies, by an increase in the number of the white cells in the peripheral blood. Its etiology is still unknown. By many it is believed to be an infectious disease, by others a neoplastic disease. In this respect it is similar to Hodgkin's disease and may be compared furthermore to this condition in that it invariably ends fatally. The problem is further complicated by the fact that many cases of leukemia go through a phase in which there is no demonstrable increase in the number of white cells seen in the peripheral blood (aleukemic leukemia), and indeed, certain cases of frank leukemia at autopsy may never have shown any such peripheral blood picture.

The leukemias are divided into three major types, depending upon the cell of origin, as follows: 1. *Lymphoid leukemia* (lymphatic leukemia, lymphadenosis or leukemic lymphocytoma); 2. *myeloid leukemia* (myelosis or leukemic myeloma); and 3. *monocytic leukemia* (leukemic reticulocytoma, or reticulo-endotheliosis). These lesions may furthermore be divided into acute and chronic forms, and as has already been commented upon, likewise into aleukemic forms which may be localized or generalized. These various forms have been indicated in the classification presented in the preceding chapter.

Leukemia, in general, may perhaps best be considered as a neoplasm arising from the various blood-forming cell elements just as other tumors of fixed tissues do. The inherent difference between leukemia and any other malignant tumor is merely that we are dealing with a circulating tissue confined normally within the blood vessels, but a mobile tissue designed to transport the cells to the various portions of the body as needed physiologically, or as part of the defense mechanism against infection. Obviously such a tumor cannot be surgically removed, so that here is one group of cases which can be attacked only by radiation. The x-ray treatment of leukemia offers definite benefit, often with the regression of the leukemic state, relief from symptoms for varying intervals and invariably prolongation of life often for several years. In the last analysis, however, even radiation merely delays the outcome. This is, perhaps, not surprising when one realizes the diffuse invasion of all the tissues of the body by these malignant cells, and it is perhaps amazing that such striking benefit results from the rather diffuse type of treatment which has to be employed over the more active bone marrow, blood-producing areas. A consideration of the various types of leukemia follows.

LYMPHOID LEUKEMIA

Acute Lymphoid Leukemia.—Lymphoid leukemia occurs in two varieties, the acute and chronic. The acute variety is commonly seen following some acute upper respiratory infection and for that reason the relationship to a possible infectious etiology has been emphasized. It is characterized by the generalized enlargement of lymph nodes, usually of the spleen; by the development of a rapidly progressive anemia and by the presence of abnormal cells of the lymphoid series in the peripheral blood stream. The total white cell count may rise rapidly to as high as one hundred or two hundred thousand, although more frequently counts of forty, fifty or sixty thousand are seen. The overwhelming numbers of abnormal and early lymphoid cells, particularly lymphoblasts and large lymphocytes, render the diagnosis usually easy.

Clinically, it must be differentiated from acute *infectious mononucleosis,* in which an increase in the number of large lymphocytes likewise occurs. In this latter condition, however, very few atypical cells or lymphoblasts are found in the peripheral blood. In acute leukemia, there is usually fever, and the patient runs a rapidly progressive downhill course, dying not infrequently within a matter of three to six months after its onset.

Chronic Lymphoid Leukemia.—In the chronic form of the disease, which it is said may follow an acute stage, but is more commonly seen as such from the outset, we find a similar generalized enlargement of the peripheral lymph nodes, enlargement of the spleen and often of the abdominal and retroperitoneal nodes as well. Fever and any suggestion of infection are much less common. The white cell count is apt to be somewhere between fifty and one hundred thousand, although at times it may exceed this considerably. The cells predominantly are of the small lymphocytic variety. Many atypical lymphocytes are seen and include a moderate number of the early blast forms. The patient responds fairly well to radiation and the disease may be controlled for a comparatively long period of time. The condition is more prone to be seen in young adults, although it may occur at any age from infancy to old age. There is a gradually developing myelophthisic replacement type of anemia and the patient is very apt to die of intercurrent upper respiratory infection. At autopsy, besides the generalized enlargement of the lymphoid tissues including the spleen, and lymphoid activity of the bone marrow, there is found striking infiltration of the viscera, particularly the liver and kidneys. In many instances, this occurs in almost nodular focal areas; in the liver, particularly in the portal areas; and in the kidney in the midportion between the tubules.

Microscopic examination of the tissues shows the blood vessels to be filled with the lymphoid cells and extensive perivascular lymphoid infiltration to have taken place. Careful study will reveal many early, immature cells.

ILLUSTRATIVE CASE

CASE 116. (Ref. #S-171)
Diagnosis.—Acute lymphatic leukemia. (Acute lymphadenosis) (lymphoid leukemia).

Patient was a white male child of 4 years, admitted to the hospital with the chief complaint of swollen glands in the neck.

Present Illness.—The patient was perfectly well until a month before admission when his mother noted that he had a cold accompanied by swelling of the cervical lymph nodes. This enlargement was not very prominent and caused the child no discomfort at the time. He was seen by a physician, who treated his upper respiratory infection, and the child improved considerably, but the lymph nodes instead of decreasing in size continued slowly but steadily to increase. Since that time there had been an intermittent low grade temperature rarely exceeding 100° until the three or four days preceding admission when it rose to 102°. Associated with this rise in temperature was marked anorexia, abdominal pain and severe constipation requiring an enema. The child had not complained at any time of pain in the neck. He had rather marked itching of the skin generally, however. He had no chills. There was no bleeding of the gums and no blood in the stool. He had had several severe nosebleeds during the week before admission.

Past History.—The child had been rather susceptible to upper respiratory infections almost since birth. He had had otitis media at the age of six months; pneumonia at one year of age and frequent colds and sore throats for the next two years, at the end of which time a tonsillectomy was done. Since that time he had seemed to improve until the onset of his present illness.

Physical Examination.—The patient was a well-developed but pale-appearing young boy about four years of age in appearance. His head was normal in contour. Neck was markedly swollen and his nodes could be palpated as discrete in character. Eyes, ears, nose and throat appeared to be essentially negative except for rather marked pallor of the mucous membranes. The chest was symmetrical. Lungs were clear. Heart was not enlarged. There was a soft systolic murmur at the apex. Abdomen was enlarged on the left side on inspection, and a mass was felt which moved with respiration and was in the position of the spleen. It had a distinct notch and was not tender on palpation. The liver was also enlarged three fingers' breadth below the costal margin. Examination of the rest of the peripheral lymph nodes showed generalized enlargement of the axillary nodes and possibly some slight enlargement of the anterior and posterior cervical, the supraclavicular, and inguinal nodes.

Laboratory Findings.—Blood count on admission showed a red count of 3,500,000 with 45% hemoglobin. The white cell count was 319,200 cells with 4% polynuclears, 71% lymphocytes and 25% abnormal immature lymphoid cells. Blood platelets 46,700. Other laboratory findings were negative.

Examination of the Blood Film.—(Fig. 276, 277, 278 and 290) The majority of the cells as seen in the blood film are fairly well differentiated, large sized lymphocytes as evidenced by the loss of nucleoli and the massing of the chromatin into coarse clumps. A few cells may be observed which represent the smaller, adult type, which differ only from the larger forms in their size. The remainder of the cells, however, are composed of atypical or early blast forms in which nucleoli are prominent. Many of the cells are indistinguishable from early myeloid cells. They are recognized chiefly by the coarser arrangement of the chromatin, the well defined nuclear membrane and the tendency to preserve a perinuclear halo. Azure granules in the later intermediate forms may occur in small numbers. More striking, however, are the abnormal cells in which lobulated nuclei, even with actual segmentation and vacuolization of the cytoplasm are seen. In such cells, the presence of azure granules in large numbers is commonly found. Among these atypical cells may well be included the so-called Türck irritation cell which is generally considered to be of lymphoid origin.

On the basis of these findings a diagnosis of acute

PLATE LXVII

FIG. 276.—NORMAL LYMPHOCYTES— MATURATION FORMS.

Upper Row.—Cells 1-4 represent the large lymphoid cells.

Middle Row.—Cells 5-8 represent intermediate sized cells.

Lower Row.—Cells 9-12 represent the usual small type cell.

Left Column.—Cells 1, 5 and 9.—Early lymphoblasts.

Second Column.—Cells 2, 6 and 10.—Immature lymphocytes.

Third Column.—Cells 3, 7 and 11.—Mature lymphocytes.

Right Column.—Cells 4, 8 and 12.—Old large, intermediate size and small lymphocytes, the two former with typical azure granules in the cytoplasm.

FIG. 277.—ACUTE LYMPHOID LEUKEMIA (LEUKEMIC LYMPHADENOSIS).

Cells 1, 2, 3, 4 and 5.—Atypical large lymphocytes.

Cells 6 and 7.—Badly degenerated "smudge" lymphoid cells.

Cell 8.—"Basket" cell.

Cell 9.—Polymorphonuclear leukocyte for comparison as to size.

Cell 10.—Polychromatophilic red cell.

FIG. 278.—DEGENERATIVE FORMS OF LYMPHOCYTES.

Upper Row.—Cells 13, 14, 15 and 16 show degenerative changes, characterized by vacuolization of cytoplasm and irregularity in arrangement of chromatin of nucleus. Turck's "irritation" forms.

Lower Row.—Cell 17.—Plasma cell.

Cell 18.—Rieder cell—nuclear division, evidence of pathologic maturation.

Cell 19.—"Smudge" cell.

Cell 20.—"Basket" cell with loss of all cell detail.

FIG. 279—CHRONIC LYMPHOID LEUKEMIA (LEUKEMIC LYMPHADENOSIS).

Cell 1.—Atypical large lymphocyte.

Cells 2 and 3.—Intermediate lymphocytes.

Cells 5-10.—Small lymphocytes.

Cells 11 and 12.—"Smudge" cells.

Cell 13.—"Basket" cell.

Cell 14.—Polymorphonuclear leukocyte (oxidase stain).

Cells 15 and 16.—Red cells—macrocytosis; polychromatophilia.

Cell 17.—Small lymphocyte.

[*Courtesy of Dr. Walter J. Crocker, Philadelphia General Hospital Atlas of Hematology (in preparation).*]

PLATE LXVII

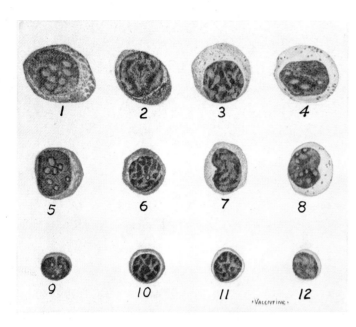

Fig. 276

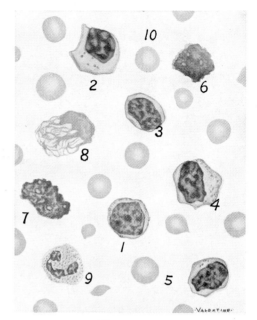

Fig. 277

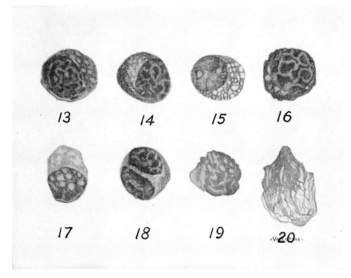

Fig. 278

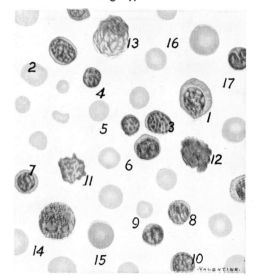

Fig. 279

lymphatic leukemia was made and the child was recommended to have x-ray therapy.

Subsequent Course.—X-ray treatment gradually over a period of three weeks brought his white blood count down to 30,000 with 13% polynuclear leukocytes and 79% adult lymphocytes. There were 8% immature abnormal lymphoid cells. In the meantime, the red blood count dropped to 1,900,000 with 5.5 grams (35%) hemoglobin. He did not tolerate his irradiation well, and he went rapidly downhill in spite of therapy, dying approximately three weeks after his admission, a total time interval of less than two months since the onset of his symptoms.

Autopsy Findings.—The body showed very marked anemia with generalized lymphadenopathy particularly involving the cervical glands. Lungs showed diffuse congestion with hemorrhage at both bases and a terminal pleural effusion on the right. The liver, spleen and kidneys were all greatly enlarged and grossly showed leukemic infiltration.

Note: In the chronic form of this disease, essentially the same histopathology is met in the viscera, except that the cells are for the most part small adult lymphocytes instead of being the large, atypical, immature young forms seen in the acute picture.

Examination of Blood Film of Chronic Lymphatic Leukemia.—(Fig. 278 and 279.) In the chronic form, the blood smear differs from that of the acute form, principally, in the fact that the cells are chiefly of the small variety even as seen in the peripheral blood. Degenerating forms of lympho-

Microscopic Description.—(Fig. 281, 282 and 283) Microscopic examination of the bone marrow, liver and other viscera shows essentially the same microscopic picture. The lymphoid tissues are replaced by a diffuse proliferation of large and medium sized lymphocytes. This produces an almost uniform histopathology, with obliteration of the peripheral sinuses and even invasion of the capsule and pericapsular tissues. Replacement of the normal bone marrow structures takes place and almost no evidence of active red cell production can be seen in these sections. The liver, kidneys and lungs particularly show diffuse infiltration of the tissue spaces by lymphocytes. This is particularly found in the portal areas although due to the increase in cell count generally, the sinusoids and vessels are likewise distended with the neoplastic lymphoid cells. The picture is one of diffuse infiltration rather than localized metastasis. Many atypical cells may be identified with mitotic figures suggesting the malignant nature of the process.

cytes, particularly so-called *smudge* cells are apt to be numerous. Among the cells are usually found some atypical forms, particularly those in which the nuclei show beginning segmentation or differentiation, the so-called *Rieder* cells. The nuclear chromatin is characteristic, as in all lymphoid cells, but it is particularly striking how little cytoplasm exists in these leukemic small lymphocytes. The examination of the red cells usually shows a moderate hypochromic anemia and a tendency for a relatively low platelet count.

MYELOID LEUKEMIA

Myeloid leukemia is, in many respects, similar to the lymphoid type, except that it involves the myeloid series of cells. In this case, lymph node involvement is much less frequently encountered except as a late manifestation of the disease with secondary infiltration of the tissues. On the other hand, the spleen is involved early and is enormously increased in size. Indeed, in myeloid leukemia, the spleen attains the greatest actual and relative increase in size which it does in any disease. The liver, likewise, is greatly enlarged and the patient develops a severe anemia by the same mechanism as in the lymphoid type. Both the acute and chronic forms occur, but the chronic variety is by far the more common. Myeloid leukemia is apt to be seen in the older age group, and chronic myeloid leukemia is commonly seen in individuals in their forties and fifties as compared with the lymphoid incidence in the second and third decades of life.

The diagnosis is usually established by the finding of atypical and early myeloid cells in the peripheral

blood, notably the presence of myelocytes and myeloblasts. The cell count in myeloid leukemia is prone to be considerably higher than in the lymphoid type and counts ranging as high as one million and two million white cells per cubic millimeter of blood are by no means uncommon. It must have been from such myeloid leukemic cases that the original name was suggested, for the blood in these cases with high white counts is definitely of a grayish color (Fig. 284).

At autopsy, these cases of myeloid leukemia show similar but more extensive general visceral involvement. Recognition of the condition is made by the identification of the cells and for this purpose special staining methods may be necessary, such as the various trichrome stains including May Grünwald, Giemsa and the like.

In the aleukemic form of these leukemias in which no increase in the cells in the peripheral blood exists, or in which only an occasional atypical or early type cell is observed, bone marrow puncture with smear preparation from the sternal marrow is a method of great value in establishing the diagnosis. By this method cell counts may be made showing the relative maturation of the cells. If an abnormal index is obtained, then evidence that the lesion is of a leukemic nature is readily confirmed.

ILLUSTRATIVE CASE

CASE 117. (Ref. #S-258)

Diagnosis.—Myeloid leukemia, chronic.

Patient was a white male of 46 years, who was admitted to the hospital because of pallor and weakness.

Present Illness.—The present illness began approximately eight months before admission following a severe attack of tonsillitis. Since that upper respiratory infection he had become steadily weaker and had shown increasing pallor and listlessness. During the preceding two months, the patient had noticed red hemorrhagic spots beneath the skin. Some of these were ecchymotic in appearance and persisted for a week or more. He also complained of frequent nosebleeds. There had been no hemoptysis or hematemesis. He had not noticed any abnormalities regarding his stool or urine, which had shown no gross blood.

Past History.—The patient had been entirely well up to his present illness. He did not recall any of the usual childhood infections. He had not been particularly susceptible to upper respiratory infections. He had not had otitis media nor chronic sinusitis. Cardiorespiratory history was negative. He had no significant gastro-intestinal disturbances. Genito-urinary history was normal. He denied venereal disease.

Physical Examination.—On admission, physical examination showed a pale, fairly well-developed and well-nourished, middle-aged white male. He appeared weak and listless, lying quietly in bed. His skin was dry. Musculature showed poor tone. There were numerous small petechial hemorrhages seen rather generally distributed over the chest and extremities. There was a large ecchymotic spot beneath the left clavicle and several smaller ecchymoses in the right axilla and right popliteal fossa. Head was normal in shape. Eyes reacted normally. Nose showed several hemorrhagic crusts. Pharynx was negative. There was generalized lymph adenopathy present which involved the cervical, axillary and inguinal nodes. Chest was symmetrical. Lungs were clear. Heart was not enlarged and showed no murmurs. The liver was palpable a hand's breadth below the costal margin. The spleen was immensely enlarged reaching the umbilicus mesially and the crest of the ilium inferiorly. It was not tender on palpation.

Laboratory Findings.—Blood count on admission showed 1,790,000 red cells with 6 grams of hemoglobin. White blood cells, 152,000 with 15% adult polymorphonuclear leukocytes, 12% lymphocytes, 8% monocytes, 6% adult eosinophiles, 34% myeloblasts, 13% promyelocytes and 12% myelocytes.

Examination of Blood Smear.—(Fig. 285, 286, 287, 288 and 289) Many types of myeloblasts, some of them of atypical appearance may be observed. The majority of them show a characteristic round or oval nucleus with a finely woven arrangement of the chromatin and three or four nucleoli showing no well-defined nuclear membrane. The characteristic perinuclear halo, as seen in the lymphoblast, is largely lacking. The atypical forms, however, show marked variation first of all in the size of the cells from the large macromyeloblast to the small micromyeloblast scarcely distinguishable from lymphoid cells. Occasional cells may contain the so-called Howell bodies. They may show vacuolization of the cytoplasm and atypical nuclear division as in the case of the lymphoblast. As the cells undergo maturation in the smear, numerous of the premyelocytes and adult myelocytes are also identified. The granules appear within the cytoplasm of the cell and show the differential staining characteristics toward eosinophilic, basophilic and neutrophilic reactions. These differences may be recognized as the cell develops from the large blast form to the more nearly adult differentiated myeloid cell. Indentation of the nucleus appears. The loss of nuclear detail and the beginning suggestion of lobulation of the nucleus all indicate the intermediate changes in the transition of the cell toward the final maturation form.

Subsequent History.—On the basis of the blood picture and the clinical picture a diagnosis of myeloid leukemia was made and the patient referred to the x-ray department for radiation therapy. The patient showed marked improvement temporarily under this therapy, with a sharp reduction in the number of cells and in the size of the spleen. This, however, was only transitory in nature and although the patient's life was undoubtedly prolonged for a period of nearly two years, he ultimately succumbed to his disease.

Autopsy Findings.—Autopsy examination revealed a marked enlargement of the liver and spleen, the liver at that time weighing 3600 gm. and the spleen, 2100 gm. Similar leukemic infiltration of the other viscera was noted.

Microscopic Description of the Bone Marrow and Viscera.—(Fig. 290, 291 and 292) Histologic examination of the bone marrow shows marked hyperplasia of the myeloid elements. Many myeloblasts and premyelocytes as well as more mature myelocytes are seen occurring almost in solid sheets and largely replacing the red cell elements of the marrow. Here and there a few small islands of active hematopoiesis may be observed. The lymph nodes show marked distortion of the normal architecture. Only rare follicles can be identified. There is a marked increase in the reticulum of the node and the entire node is infiltrated with myeloid cells in various stages of development and maturation. Eosinophilic myelocytes predominate rather strikingly in the visceral lesions. In the liver, this infiltration is marked. It occurs both in the portal areas and in scattered foci throughout the liver parenchyma. The sinusoids are particularly distended with myeloid cells. Similar histologic invasion of the tissues is seen in the sections of the lung and kidneys.

PLATE LXIX
THE DEVELOPMENT OF THE GRANULOCYTES

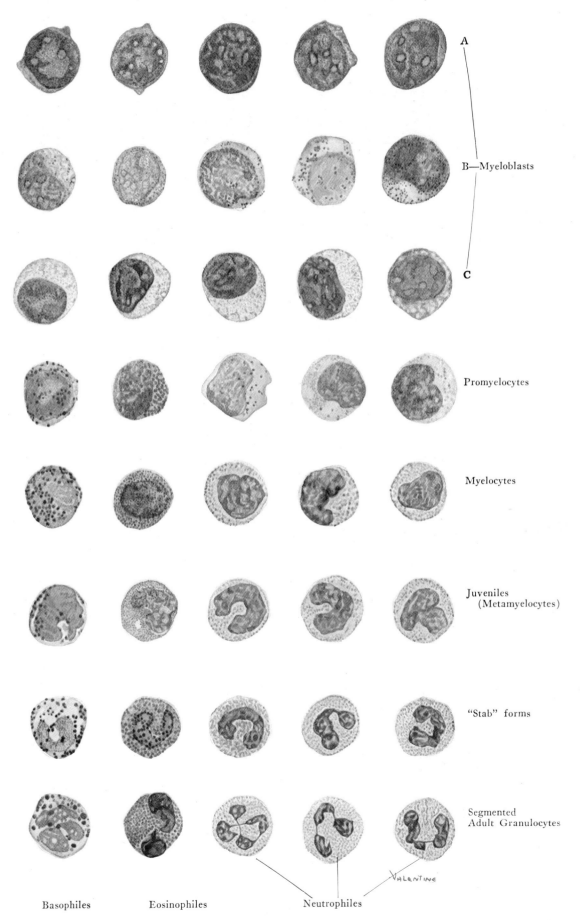

A

B—Myeloblasts

C

Promyelocytes

Myelocytes

Juveniles
(Metamyelocytes)

"Stab" forms

Segmented
Adult Granulocytes

VALENTINE

Basophiles   Eosinophiles   Neutrophiles

FIG. 284

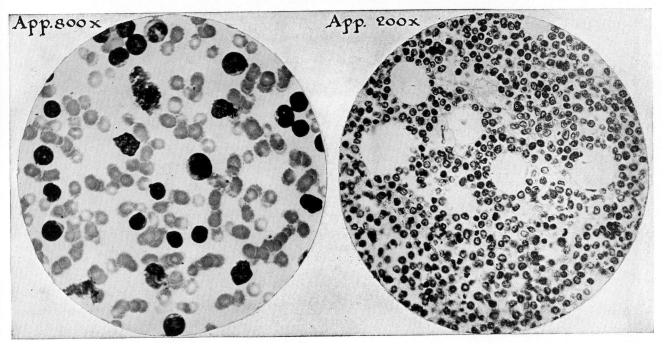

FIG. 280.—BLOOD FILM.—Note increase in lymphoid cells of blood with many atypical early blast forms and degenerated "smudge" cells. Red cells show moderate hypochromic anemia. App. 800 x. (See also Plate LXVII.)

FIG. 281.—BONE MARROW.—The normal hematopoietic tissue has been crowded out by diffuse infiltration of abnormal lymphoid cells. App. 200 x.

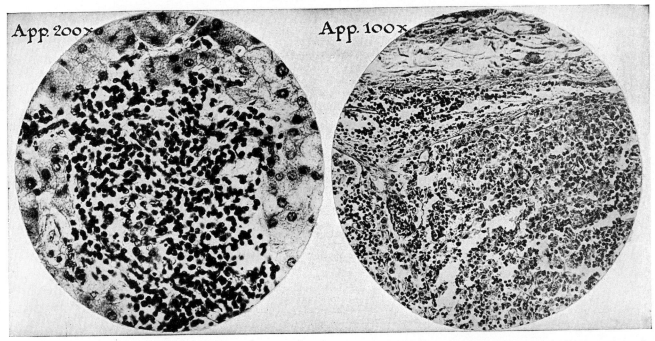

FIG. 282.—LIVER.—Extensive leukemic infiltration of the liver, most marked in portal areas, by lymphoid cells of varying stages of maturity is apparent. App. 200 x.

FIG. 283.—LYMPH NODE.—Photomicrograph to illustrate the typical crowding of the peripheral sinuses, the relative absence of capsular invasion and the distortion of the normal architecture by the leukemic cells. App. 100 x.

PLATE LXX

FIG. 285.—GRANULOCYTES—COMMON DEGENERATIVE FORMS.

Cell 1.—Toxic stab agranulocyte.—Nuclear hemogeneity; occasional Freyfeld's toxic granules.

Cell 2.—Stab cell.—With a few scattered Freyfeld's toxic granules.

Cell 3.—"Smudge" cell.—Swollen degenerated nucleus; no cytoplasm.

Cell 4.—Stab cell.—With many Freyfeld's toxic granules.

Cell 5.—Segmented leukocyte.—With beginning "basket" formation.

Cell 6.—Juvenile cell.—Doehle's inclusion bodies.

Cell 7.—Juvenile cell.—Typical "basket" cell degeneration.

Cell 8.—Segmented leukocyte.—Doehle's inclusions; vacuolated cytoplasm.

FIG. 286.—CHLOROMA.

Cells 1, 2, 3, 4 and 5.—Myeloblasts.—"A" coin, round type.

Cell 6.—Intermediate type lymphocyte.

Cell 7.—Stab form neutrophilic granulocyte.

Cells 8 and 9.—Myeloblasts "A" type.—Positive peroxidase reaction.

FIG. 287.—ACUTE MYELOID LEUKEMIA (ACUTE MYELOSIS).

Cells 1, 2, 3, 4, 6, 7 and 8.—Myeoblasts "A" type.

Cells 5 and 9.—Micromyeloblasts.

Cell 10.—Myeloblast "B" type with azure granules.

Cell 11.—Basophilic myeloblast.

Cell 12.—Early promyelocyte with persistent marginal basophilism, but cytoplasm chiefly neutrophilic yellow. Note the few persistent azurophile granules.

Cell 13.—Myeloblast (probably "A" type), showing mitosis.

Cell 14.—Eosinophilic myeloblast.

Cell 15.—Small lymphocyte.

Cells 16 and 17.—Myeloblasts.—Positive peroxidase reaction.

FIG. 288.—SUBACUTE OR CHRONIC MYELOID LEUKEMIA.

Cells 1 and 3.—Myeloblast.—"A" type.

Cell 2.—Myeloblast.—Intermediate between "A" and "B" types. Note beginning azure granulation, but deeply basic cytoplasm.

Cell 18.—Micromyeloblast.—"A" type.

Cell 6.—Myeloblast.—"B" type.

Cell 4.—Myeloblast.—"C" type.

Cell 5.—Promyelocyte.

Cell 17.—Micromyeloblast.—"B" type.

Cell 7.—Myelocyte.

Cell 16.—Micropromyelocyte.

Cell 9.—Micromyelocyte.

Cell 10.—Basophilic myelocyte.

Cell 19.—Eosinophilic myelocyte.

Cell 8.—Juvenile granulocyte.

Cell 11.—Microjuvenile granulocyte.

Cells 12 and 13.—Stab granulocyte.

Cells 14 and 15.—Segmented granulocyte.

Cell 20.—Normoblast.

Cells 21 and 22.—Red cells showing polychromatophilia.

[Courtesy of Dr. Walter J. Crocker, Philadelphia General Hospital, Atlas of Hematology (in preparation).]

PLATE LXX

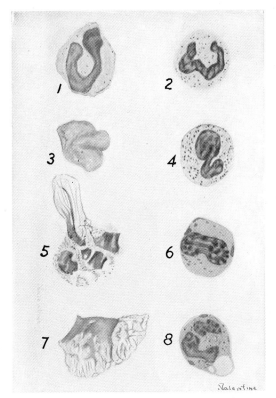

Fig. 285

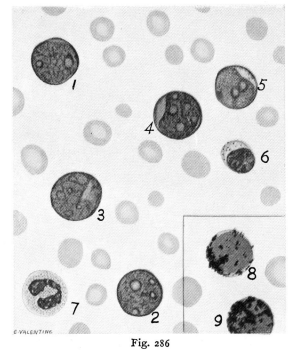

Fig. 286

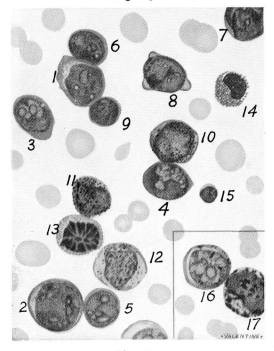

Fig. 287

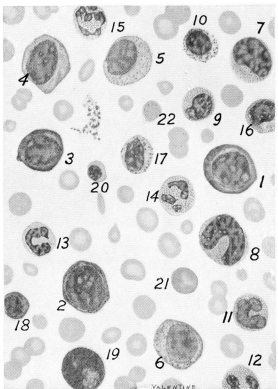

Fig. 288

MONOCYTIC LEUKEMIA

In recent years it has been recognized that the reticulocyte of the bone marrow and other reticulo-endothelial organs may equally well give rise to a leukemic picture. Most of these cases which to-day are recognized as reticulo-cell leukemia were formerly grouped in the lymphoid cases. The reader should, perhaps, be referred to laboratory manuals on hematology for the more minute criteria used in the establishment of this diagnosis.

From the clinical standpoint, the cases cannot be particularly well differentiated from the lymphoid variety. They are more often seen in the younger age groups and tend to show generalized lymph node involvement. The blood counts are likewise usually in the lower figures and the differential diagnosis becomes a matter of identification of the large cells, which are found in the peripheral blood and in bone marrow smears.

At autopsy, the same general features of anemia with lymphoid infiltration of the tissues generally is observed. With routine staining methods, using hematoxylin and eosin, it is doubtful whether an accurate differential diagnosis could be made. The final diagnosis as has been emphasized depends upon the identification of these cells, which usually requires special staining methods. The group as a whole is of about the same degree of radiosensitivity as is true of the lymphoid group. Ewing's tumor may well represent the localized aleukemic form of the disease just as multiple myelomata are grouped in the aleukemic myelocytoma group in the registry classification. For practical reasons, it serves our purpose merely to call attention to the fact that this form of leukemia does exist, and that among hematologists it is becoming of increasing importance in recent years.

ILLUSTRATIVE CASE

CASE 118. (Ref. #S-318)

Diagnosis.—Monocytic leukemia.

Patient was a white male of 28 years, who was admitted to the hospital complaining of swelling of the right jaw accompanied by weakness and a persistent cough.

Present Illness.—The patient was perfectly well until five weeks before admission when he noticed that there was marked swelling of his right jaw. He attributed this to an infected tooth and had a second molar extracted. This gave no relief to the patient, and his jaw increased steadily in size. His dentist sent him to the hospital for more thorough medical study. Accompanying this swelling of his jaw, he had had localized intermittent attacks of dull pain. He had noticed considerable anorexia and a loss of ten pounds in weight during approximately one month's period, which he attributed to his lack of appetite, and his inability to eat because of his jaw. He had grown progressively weaker on exertion and had noticed marked constipation during the preceding two weeks. He had no other specific symptoms or complaints.

Past History.—His family history was negative. His occupation was that of a sheet metal worker, which seemed to have no relation to his present illness except that, because of its heavy nature, his fatigability was increased. He had had the usual childhood diseases, including scarlet fever and diphtheria. He had always been more or less subject to recurrent attacks of tonsillitis, but had never had his tonsils removed. He had always been strong and healthy up to the onset of his present condition. A review of his systems was non-informative.

Physical Examination.—Physical examination showed a well-developed, well-nourished young, white male. His head was normal in shape except for the swelling of his jaw. Pupils reacted normally. Nose was negative. Ears showed a moderate deafness, particularly on the left.

Examination of the mouth showed a necrotic, sloughing ulcer of the lower jaw around the site of the extracted molar. His teeth, in general, were in very poor condition showing marked caries. The mucous membranes were pale. There was a large, fluctuating mass approximately three inches in diameter, anterior to the parotid gland and overlying the mandibular and malar bones. The regional lymph nodes were not appreciably enlarged. The cervical nodes, likewise, were palpable but not significantly enlarged. The chest was symmetrical. Heart and lungs appeared negative. Abdomen showed a moderate obesity. There were no palpable masses or tenderness. Neurologic examination was negative.

Laboratory Findings.—On admission, the patient showed a red blood count of 2,510,000 cells with 38% hemoglobin (6 grams) and a white blood count of 7,650 cells of which 15% were polynuclears, 27% lymphocytes and 58% monocytes. Of the monocytes, 6% were immature abnormal forms.

X-ray examination for evidence of a neoplasm of the jaw bone was negative. The entire swelling seemed to be limited to the soft tissues.

Examination of the Blood Smear.—(Fig. 512 and 513) Examination of the blood film shows a preponderance of the large monocytic cells. These are particularly identified by the curious infolding of the nuclear membrane in the younger forms. The morphology of these cells varies so extremely that their recognition is dependent to a large extent upon the elimination of the more characteristic features of the myeloid and lymphoid cells. The nuclei are rather similar in appearance to those of the myeloblast in the early forms in respect to the reticular nature of the chromatin, but rarely contain more than one or two nucleoli, which is more characteristic of the early lymphoid cell. In this respect they are intermediate in position. As the cell matures, however, characteristic indentation and folding of the nucleus upon itself, with the development of cytoplasmic vacuoles and oxidase granules renders its recognition from cells of the myeloid or lymphoid series comparatively definite. In the later typical forms, the tendency for the development of a horseshoe nucleus with its pale blue cytoplasm containing azure and oxidase granules is perhaps as nearly typical as any one criterion which may be advanced. However, in the pathological forms, the atypical appearance of the nuclei with simple indentation is a feature which makes their identification more difficult. Indeed, in the reported cases in the literature, a large percentage of so-called monoblastic leukemias has subsequently shown definite development into the myeloid form of the disease. Under such circumstances it is easy to believe that failure to recognize these atypic forms of the monocytic cells is responsible for the mistake in diagnosis. Practically, monocytic leukemia is a rare disease which is not even accepted as a clinical entity by all pathologists.

Subsequent Course.—The patient was in the hospital for a total period of only two weeks during which his white count slowly rose from the aleukemic phase which existed at the time of his admission to a count of 52,400

cells, of which 90% were of the monocytic series. Irradiation therapy in this case was of no avail and the patient went downhill rapidly and died.

Autopsy Findings.—At autopsy, the chief findings were those of a diffuse infiltration of the viscera by the characteristic leukemic cells. This was not as prominent a feature as was found in either the preceding lymphoid or myeloid forms of the disease. Indeed, the spleen was scarcely larger than normal, weighing but 180 gm. The liver, likewise, weighed only 1480 gm. The lungs showed marked congestion with a terminal pneumonic consolidation of the right base.

Microscopic Description.—The local tumor mass in the jaw region was found on histologic examination to represent a localized infiltration of the tissues, which might tend to classify this case on the basis of our outline in the reticulum cell sarcoma position associated with a leukemic phase. For practical purposes, it seems best to consider this as a leukemic reticulo-endotheliosis or monocytic leukemia with infiltration of the tissues of the jaw as the result of the infected tooth, which probably aided in this initial localization of the leukemic cells.

POLYCYTHEMIA VERA

(Syn: Leukemic Erythrocytosis or Leukemic Erythrocytoma)

Much uncertainty exists as to where to place a lesion familiar clinically, known as polycythemia vera or Vaquez's disease. As suggested in the Lymphatic Tumor Registry, this condition seems to represent the counterpart of the malignant leukemia lesions of the other bone marrow cells as seen in the peripheral blood. The characteristic finding is a progressive increase in the number of red cells. In the earlier stages, these red cells all appear of adult and fully maturated forms. As time goes on, however, more and more young forms appear and with the increase of these young nucleated forms, a definite leukemic picture not infrequently is seen

from the gross standpoint. Cell counts ranging up as high as twelve and fourteen million red cells may occur; death finally ensues. The patient's life may be prolonged by repeated bleeding in an attempt to keep the viscosity of the blood to functional levels, and by the repeated administration of intravenous diluents for the same purpose. The disease is one of middle life, much more prevalent in males than females, and runs a slowly progressive course over a period of months or years. Like the other forms of leukemia its etiology is obscure. It is perhaps best considered in this group of tumor-like lesions of the hematopoietic system.

PLATE LXXI

TUMORS OF HEMATOPOIETIC TISSUES

MYELOGENOUS (MYELOID) LEUKEMIA (CF. CASE 117)

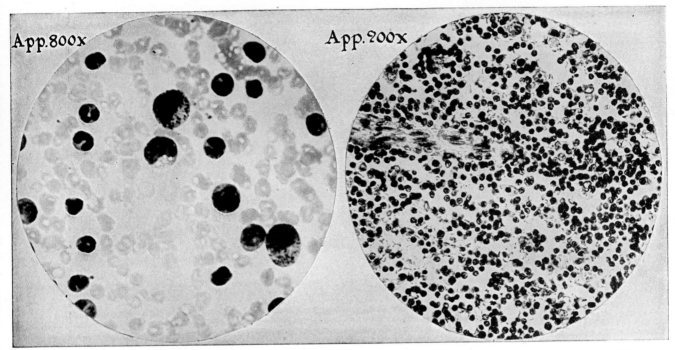

FIG. 289.—BLOOD FILM.—Note marked increase in total number of white cells, most of which are abnormal immature forms belonging to the granulocytic series. Hypochromism of red cells is marked. (See also plates LXIX and LXX.) App. 800 x.

FIG. 290.—BONE MARROW.—The extensive infiltration of the marrow cavity by the leukemic cells has replaced the normal hematopoietic tissue. App. 200 x.

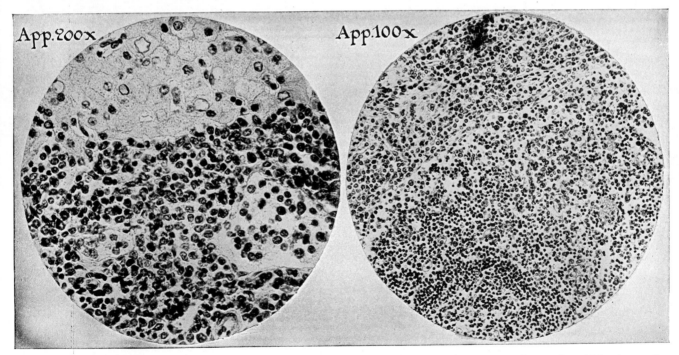

FIG. 291.—LIVER.—Widespread, diffuse and focal infiltration of the liver by the immature leukemic myeloid cells. App. 200 x.

FIG. 292.—LYMPH NODE.—Photomicrograph which shows the gradual encroachment upon a persistent lymph follicle by the infiltrating myeloid leukemic cells. App. 100 x.

CHAPTER XXX

TUMORS OF THE NERVOUS SYSTEM

Tumors which arise from the various component cells of the nervous system seem to confuse the average pathologist, as well as the medical student, more than those arising from any other tissue. Actually, their identification should be no more difficult than that of any other group of tumors, and much simpler than the recognition of the various endothelial, lymphoid and reticular cell tumors discussed in the preceding chapters. From the practical standpoint, the tumors of the nervous system fall into only a comparatively few types, each with fairly definite clinical and pathological features. These are based on the embryological development of the several cells. This will be reviewed very briefly here. The schematic presentation of Bailey probably offers the clearest concept of the maturation of these cells. It should be remembered that tumors can arise from any of these cells at any point in their differentiation. Like tumors from other tissues, the degree of malignancy roughly parallels the degree of cell differentiation. Neoplasms developing from adult cell types such as the astrocyte or oligodendroglia correspond in a general sort of way to the simple benign fibromata, leiomyomata, or adenomata. On the other hand, tumors arising from undifferentiated cells such as the medulloblast or primitive spongioblast present the same malignant features as are seen in fibrosarcomata, leiomyosarcomata or frank adenocarcinomata. Another point to remember in connection with the development of the various tumors of the central nervous system, notably those of glial cell origin, is that they occur with equal frequency in the spinal cord as in the brain itself.

Among the very earliest structures to appear embryologically are the medullary plates on the dorsal surface of the embryo. These develop by invagination of the dorsal ectoderm to form a groove. The folds of this groove fuse dorsally to make the neural tube. In the fully developed individual this tube is represented by the ventricular system of the brain and the central canal of the spinal cord.

The walls of the neural tube consist at first of columnar epithelial cells—the medullary epithelium—precursor of all the adult cell types. This may differentiate in several directions and the transition be readily followed in all its stages—into choroidal epithelium, pineal cells and into neuroblasts and spongioblasts either directly or through an intermediate form, the medulloblast.

On the neuro-epithelial side certain of the medullary epithelial cells show enlargement of their nuclei which assume a spherical form and a vesicular structure. The cytoplasm develops an affinity for silver. At this stage, the cell has no protoplasmic processes and is spoken of as an *apolar neuroblast*. Gradually it goes through bipolar, unipolar and multipolar phases, until the fully differentiated *neuron* or nerve cell emerges.

On the neuroglial side, on the other hand, other of the medullary epithelial cells, especially those of the ventricular aspect of the neural tube elongate, develop cilia and become *primitive spongioblasts*. Certain of these cells split off from the straight line of maturation, lose their cilia and eventually become the lining cells of the ventricular system or *ependyma*. Because of the essentially epithelial nature of these cells they are considered by some to belong to the neuro-epithelial derivatives rather than to the neuroglial tissue. The great majority of the primitive spongioblasts go through the more usual maturation phases of bipolar and unipolar development to become converted ultimately, after passing through a stage in which they are known as *astroblasts,* to adult *astrocytes.* Just as the primitive myeloid cell may differentiate into acidophilic, basophilic or neutrophilic adult forms, so may the astroblast give rise to two types of adult cells, the (a) *fibrillary* and the (b) *protoplasmic astrocytes.*

These astrocytes represent one of the three major supportive glial cells of the central nervous system. These are sometimes spoken of as the *macroglial* cells, and from these cells may be derived one of the more benign forms of brain neoplasms, the *astrocytoma.*

PLATE LXXII
TUMORS OF THE CENTRAL NERVOUS SYSTEM
GLIOMATA

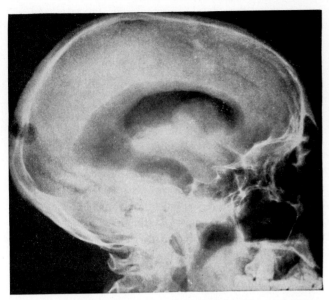

FIG. 293.—ENCEPHALOGRAM: BRAIN TUMOR.—CASE 120.—Showing a large tumor mass protruding into lateral ventricle.

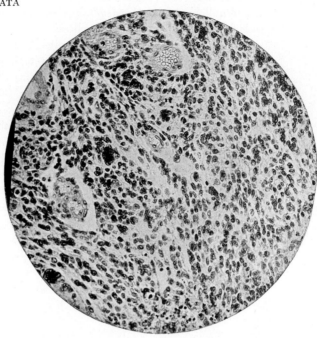

FIG. 294.—BRAIN: SPONGIOBLASTOMA.—CASE 120.—Tumor composed of numerous unipolar and bipolar glial cells with characteristic oval nuclei containing abundant chromatin, and showing rare mitoses. App. 100 x.

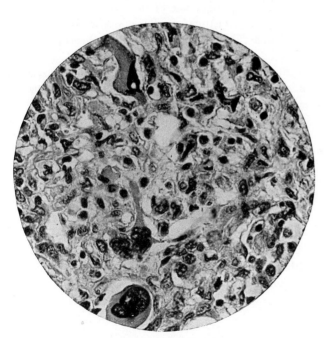

FIG. 295.—BRAIN: GLIOBLASTOMA (SPONGIOBLASTOMA) MULTIFORME.—CASE 121.—Tumor made up of variously appearing primitive glial cells with a striking tendency toward the formation of large multinucleated tumor giant cells and presence of numerous mitoses. App. 400 x.

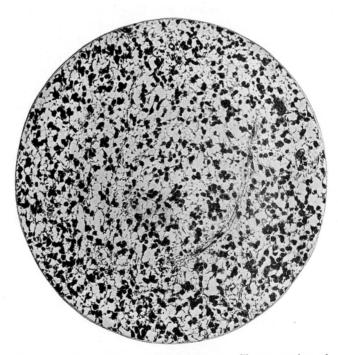

FIG. 296.—BRAIN: ASTROCYTOMA.—CASE 119.—Tumor consists of a feltwork of fibrils between which the characteristic astrocytes may be identified by their dendritic processes (Cajal's technique). The cells have small hyperchromic nuclei and scant, star-shaped cytoplasm. App. 100 x.

As a totally independent derivative directly from the medulloblast, the *oligodendroglia* develops as a second of the supportive glial cells of the central nervous system. These cells are smaller than the macroglia and usually have several protoplasmic processes. They may be identified with certainty only by some one of the many silver stains. Their function is both supportive, and in inflammatory or degenerative lesion, phagocytic. In this respect, they behave much as the microglia does. These cells may give rise to tumors, but only very occasionally. They are tumors of very slow expansile growth, entirely benign in nature, usually cerebral in location occurring clinically symptomatically as a rule in older individuals ordinarily past forty years. They are characterized particularly by calcification, which helps render the preoperative diagnosis possible.

The third variety of glial cells is known as the *microglia* or *Hortega cell*. These are small, bipolar or occasionally multipolar cells, which are believed to be derived from the mesenchyme and not from ectoderm. They migrate through central nervous tissues where they develop protoplasmic processes and become supportive elements. Equally important, however, is their phagocytic function in the inflammatory and degenerative diseases of the brain. Gradually, under such environmental circumstances they lose their protoplasmic processes, become ovoid or rounded and take up broken-down myelin and cellular debris. This has been commented upon in the section on poliomyelitis.

In tissue culture, these cells grow readily and cannot be differentiated morphologically or functionally from tissue histiocytes grown in the same manner. Dunning's recent studies in this field are most convincing. Furthermore, no tumors derived from this type of cell are known to exist. This may be considered added evidence of their origin outside the nervous system, for all other varieties of glial tumors are recognized.

TUMORS OF GLIAL ORIGIN

Macrogliomata.—From these introductory comments, it appears that of the so-called "glioma" group of tumors, actually all but a very few neoplasms are derived from the primitive spongioblast or glioblast in the course of its development. In recent years, there has been a tendency for neuropathologists to attempt to subdivide these tumors into a vast number of subvarieties with the object of evaluating prognosis through such histologic criteria. Much of value has been learned by this procedure, but for practical purposes it has been found that they may be reassembled into three major types:

ASTROCYTOMA.—An essentially benign tumor arising from completely differentiated macroglial cells or astrocytes.

SPONGIOBLASTOMA.—A tumor of intermediate malignancy arising from one or another of the developmental phases of the spongioblast with unipolar cells or bipolar cells at times predominating, but usually presenting a mixed picture.

GLIOBLASTOMA MULTIFORME (spongioblastoma multiforme or gliosarcoma).—A tumor of high malignancy, rapidly growing, invasive, and invariably fatal, arising from the undifferentiated primitive spongioblast or glioblast.

Standing on either side of this main stem line of gliomata, as illustrated in Bailey's schematic presentation, are the oligodendrogliomata and ependymomata.

Oligodendrogliomata.—As has been emphasized in the preceding discussion, the oligodendroglioma represents a benign form of glioma, which probably has its onset in childhood or early adult life, but due to the slow rate of growth rarely produces symptoms until middle age. It is an extremely rare tumor, the diagnosis of which is quite apt to be made before operation because of the characteristic calcification which occurs as the result of the slow growth, the inadequate blood supply and the resultant breakdown of the tissue with subsequent calcific deposit. Its location as a cerebral lesion eccentrically placed rather than as a mid-line tumor likewise aids in this differential diagnosis. The use of encephalography in recent years has been of added diagnostic value.

PLATE LXXIII
TUMORS OF THE CENTRAL NERVOUS SYSTEM

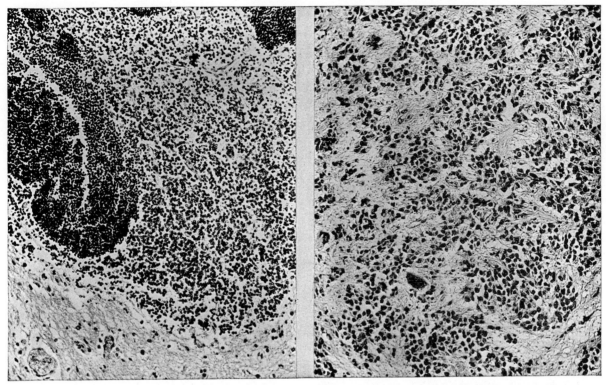

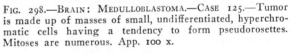

Fig. 297.—Brain: Pinealoma.—Case 126.—Photomicrograph of a pinealoma invading the brain substance and composed of its characteristic central hyperchromic small glial-like cells (left) surrounded by a zone of larger, paler-staining cells with vesicular nuclei. App. 100 x.

Fig. 298.—Brain: Medulloblastoma.—Case 125.—Tumor is made up of masses of small, undifferentiated, hyperchromatic cells having a tendency to form pseudorosettes. Mitoses are numerous. App. 100 x.

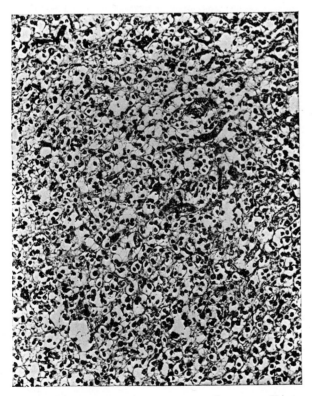

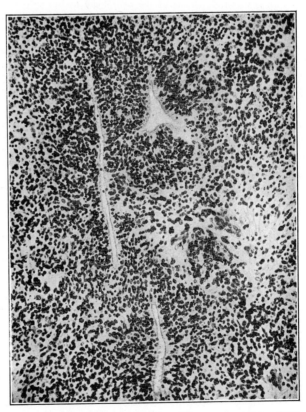

Fig. 299.—Brain: Oligodendroglioma.—Case 122.—Tumor is composed of closely packed, ovoid or rounded cells, with small, hyperchromatic nuclei surrounded by clear cytoplasm and sharply defined cell membrane, thus giving a halo effect. App. 100 x.

Fig. 300.—Eye: Retinoblastoma (Neuroblastoma).—Case 124.—A very cellular, malignant tumor composed of small, extremely hyperchromatic cells in places showing fibrillar processes which have a tendency to converge about a clear space producing pseudorosettes. App. 100 x.

ILLUSTRATIVE CASES

CASE 119. (Ref. #S-326)

Diagnosis.—Astrocytoma with cystic degeneration.

Patient was a white male of 27 years, who was admitted to the hospital in a deep stupor.

Present Illness.—The history of his present illness was obtained from his wife. So far as she could recall, the onset was six years before the present admission when the patient had a convulsive seizure. This subsided spontaneously and nothing further happened until two years later when he had another similar convulsion. Since that time he had had two other similar attacks which had been been controlled by large doses of phenobarbital. Five weeks before admission he developed aphasia. This was not complete but was very definite. He developed weakness in the right arm while working. His occupation was that of an accountant. Three weeks before admission, he developed headaches, which became more and more severe. One week preceding admission he became semi-stuporous, which became more and more profound until he was finally seen by a physician and sent to the hospital.

Past Medical History.—His past history was entirely irrelevant. He had had the usual childhood diseases. No family history of cancer, tuberculosis or mental disease was obtained. He had been married for five years. He had one child living and well. A review of his systems was noninformatory. He denied venereal disease.

Physical Examination.—The patient was a prematurely bald white male, who was lying in profound stupor and appeared severely dehydrated. Eyes were difficult to examine because of his condition. Nose and throat seemed normal. Chest was symmetrical. Heart and lungs showed nothing abnormal. Abdomen was negative. Extremities were negative outside of the neurologic findings. Neurologic examination: The pupils reacted sluggishly to light. Eyegrounds showed bilateral choking of one to two diopters. Percussion of the head revealed a suggestion of dullness over the left temporal area. Supra-orbital pressure showed marked weakness of the right facial muscles. The right upper extremity was paretic and the right lower extremity was not as strong as the left. Incontinence of urine was present.

Laboratory Findings.—Red blood cells, 7,250,000 with 102% hemoglobin. This was the result of hemoconcentration from dehydration. White blood cells, 10,700 with 72% polynuclears and 24% lymphocytes. Wassermann was negative. Blood chemistry: urea nitrogen 40 mgm. and Plasma CO_2 was 44 volumes per cent.

X-ray examination suggested a lesion of the left temporo-parietal area, presumably a neoplasm.

Subsequent Course.—Exploratory operation was urged, and a craniotomy was performed. Just above the angular gyrus and behind the ascending parietal convolution, a firm tumor mass about 4 cm. in diameter was exposed. This was removed without undue surgical difficulty and sent to the laboratory for diagnosis.

Pathological Report.—*Gross Description of Surgical Specimen.*—Specimen consisted of an almost spherical tumor mass about 5 cm. in diameter. This was grayish-pink in color and rather spongy in consistency with a large area of cystic degeneration filled with clear fluid. There was increased density of the white matter around the tumor tissue.

Microscopic Description of Section Through the Tumor.—(Fig. 296) Histologic examination of the tissue shows a mass of large, somewhat pleomorphic cells embedded in what appears to be gliomatous stroma. A few small areas of hemorrhage into the tissue are seen. Several areas of cystic degeneration are noted. In the routine hematoxylin and eosin-stained preparations, it is impossible to identify the tumor with any degree of certainty. Accordingly, special stained preparations with the gold method of Cajal are utilized to demonstrate the basic cell of origin. This is found to be the astrocyte, which is readily recognized by this staining procedure with its characteristic dendritic processes.

CASE 120. (Ref. #S-331)

Diagnosis.—Spongioblastoma.

Patient was a Hebrew female child of 9 years, admitted to the hospital because of attacks of excruciating pain of a migratory nature.

Present Illness.—Her present illness began about six months before admission when she first noticed intermittent attacks of headache with vague pains which seemed to shoot down the back of her neck and involve her shoulders and arms and later her legs. These pains subsided after several weeks, two of which she spent in bed; but about two months before admission they recurred with increasing severity and had been almost continuous since that time. Associated with these pains had been numerous attacks of vertigo and a continuation of the headache. For the past three months she had had attacks of double vision. She had no interference with smelling or hearing.

Past History.—As a child she had always been nervous and frail, and had been accused of being temperamental with her playmates. She had had otitis media at the age of one and one-half years with a running ear for nearly one year. She had had measles and chicken-pox in addition. She had a tonsillectomy at the age of six. There had been no other serious illness. A review of her systems revealed little of importance. During the attacks of pain, she had had some dyspnea. She had no other respiratory or cardiac symptoms. She had had many attacks of nausea and occasionally vomiting. These had been of several years' duration. She seemed to have a relatively "weak stomach" and had a great deal of belching following the taking of food.

Physical Examination.—Physical examination showed a thin, underweight, nervous child who did not appear acutely ill but cried intermittently and complained of dizziness. Her skin was dry but showed normal turgor. Her skeletal make-up was of the small bone variety with a normal trunk and extremity ratio. Head was normal in shape. Her pupils reacted sluggishly to light. There was a slight right-sided mesial nystagmus. Ears, nose and throat were negative. Chest was symmetrical. Heart and lungs appeared normal. Abdomen was negative. Extremities appeared negative. Reflexes were normal except for a slightly decreased left knee-jerk.

Laboratory Findings.—Red blood count on admission, 4,600,000 with 13 grams of hemoglobin. White blood cells 8,150 with 55% polymorphonuclear leukocytes. Urinalysis was negative. Spinal fluid was essentially negative with only a slight increase in globulin.

X-ray examination by ventriculogram showed a markedly widened coronal suture and the presence of a tremendous tumor which apparently arose in the 3rd ventricle and pushed upward into the greatly dilated right lateral ventricle. This had shut off the left ventricle so that it could not be visualized. (Fig. 293)

Operative History.—On the basis of these findings, an exploratory operation was done, and one of several tumors found was removed for histologic examination.

Pathological Report.—*Gross Description.*—Specimen consisted of a mass having the consistency of brain tissue and measuring 10 x 4 x 3 cm. It was pale grayish-pink in color and appeared to be covered on one side by a fine membrane in which numerous dilated capillaries could be made out. On section, several small hemorrhagic foci of necrosis were noted.

Microscopic Description of Tissue from the Tumor.—(Fig. 294) Examination of hematoxylin-eosin-stained sections reveals a neoplasm in which there are interlacing bundles of cells possessing long fibrils. Some are unipolar and some are bipolar cells. Fibrils are formed by the terminal processes. They occur in great numbers between individual cells. Most of the cells are spindle in outline; some are irregular. There are numerous blood vessels within the tissue, and it is from the connective tissue surrounding these vessels that the neoplastic cells seem to radiate.

Under high magnification, the cytoplasm of these various cell elements is eosinophilic and is finely granular. The nucleus varies considerably in shape; many are round, some are spindle. There is a definite nuclear membrane, a few coarse, poorly-defined chromatin granules and one or two deep-staining nucleoli. Many of the nucleoli appear vacuolated. Mitotic figures are not encountered.

CASE 121. (Ref. #S-332)
Diagnosis.—Glioblastoma multiforme (spongioblastoma multiforme or gliosarcoma).

Patient was a forty-five year old white male, who was admitted with the chief complaint of headache, vomiting, and dizziness of three weeks' duration.

Present Illness.—Patient was in his usual good health until about three weeks before admission when he began to develop severe headaches, which were chiefly localized to the vertex. He had marked projectile vomiting without nausea, and a sensation which he best described as dizziness, but which was not typical. These symptoms subsided after two or three days and he attributed them to some digestive upset. They recurred, however, ten days later with greater severity and since that time, they had been almost continuous. For the past several days, his family noted that he had been incoherent, disoriented and markedly apathetic. This even approached lethargy at times.

Past History.—Past history was irrelevant for the most part. His family physician stated that the patient had always been of an emotionally unstable type with alternate periods of depression and exaltation. Other than this, to his knowledge, the family history had no bearing on the present condition. He had not noted any particular character or behavior changes. He is believed to have had all the usual childhood diseases, but had never had any serious illness otherwise. He had had occasional qualitative attacks of indigestion and occasional mild upper respiratory infections. He worried a

great deal about himself at these times and had been more or less under medical supervision for many years on this account. Genito-urinary history was negative and he denied venereal disease. He had been married for a number of years but had not had any children.

Physical Examination.—The patient was a well-developed, fairly well-nourished, middle-aged white male. He appeared almost lethargic and could be aroused with difficulty. Even when aroused, he showed only momentary attentiveness, was incoherent and rather disoriented, and had marked lapses of memory of recent events. Head showed no gross deformities. Hearing was apparently slightly diminished bilaterally. Pupils were small but reacted normally. There was no nystagmus. Vision was apparently normal. Ophthalmologic examination showed three diopters of choking of the disks. Numerous retinal hemorrhages with beginning scarring were also noted. Nose and throat appeared negative. Chest was symmetrical. Heart and lungs showed no abnormalities. Abdomen was normal. Extremities were negative. Neurologic examination showed a positive Romberg and slightly hyperactive reflexes generally. A positive Babinski was present on the left and a right facial weakness.

Laboratory Findings.—Red blood cells, 4,570,000 with 86% hemoglobin. White blood cells, 15,000 with 64% polynuclears. Urinalysis was negative. Wassermann was negative.

X-ray examination showed the pineal to be displaced dorsad about 5 mm. There was no evidence of erosion of the skull. These findings suggested a mass lesion, probably neoplastic in nature, and in conjunction with the history and physical findings suggested a left frontotemporal localization.

Subsequent Course.—Exploratory craniotomy was performed and a large cystic tumor filled with yellow xanthrochromic-like fluid was found in the right frontotemporal region. On opening the cyst, large masses of tumor tissue were found as bosselated lesions protruding from the lining. Owing to the extent of the tumor, it could not be removed completely. As much tumor tissue as possible was taken out, however, and with the collapse of the cyst and the decompression, it was hoped that the patient's life might be prolonged for many years. Because of the cystic nature of the tumor, it was thought at the time of operation that it was most likely a glioma of the astrocytic type.

Pathological Report.—*Gross Description of Surgical Specimen.*—Specimen consisted of several fragments of tumor tissue, the largest being a rather discrete nodule 3 cm. in diameter. Its external surface was somewhat nodular and was pinkish gray in color.

Microscopic Description of a Section Through the Tumor Nodule.—(Fig. 295) There are areas where elongated spindle cells occur in bundles with a suggestion of bipolar spongioblastic development. On the other hand, there are areas, especially between these bundles, of more or less completely undifferentiated large, pleomorphic tumor giant cells. These are scattered through the tumor and vary greatly in size. Some contain two or three or more nuclei. The nuclei are stained deeply. The chromatin is dense. Nucleoli are present and vary considerably in size. In some areas, marked necrosis and hemorrhage are present. Everywhere the tumor shows a generous vascular supply. The picture is that of a rapidly growing malignant glioma arising apparently from the undifferentiated primitive glioblast or spongioblast.

ILLUSTRATIVE CASE

CASE 122. (#S-325)
Diagnosis.—Oligodendroglioma.

Patient was a white male, of 49 years, admitted to the hospital with the chief complaint of headache.

Present Illness.—The patient was in his usual good health until about six weeks before admission when he developed severe and progressive attacks of headache. He would wake up in the morning with it present, and it remained more or less constant throughout the day, becoming usually more severe toward evening. The pain was of an aching, pressure type and was generalized over the occiput and vertex, less marked over the frontal area. The pain had been so severe at times that it even awakened the patient. About one month before admission he noticed beginning numbness of his left hand. About a week before admission, he began to have attacks of nausea and vomiting, usually most severe before breakfast. He went to an oculist thinking that perhaps his eyes were responsible and had glasses prescribed for himself, which had not helped in relieving his symptoms.

Past History.—The patient had the usual childhood diseases. He had had an incipient tuberculosis and had been in a tuberculosis sanatarium for about a year when he was eighteen years of age. He had had a submucous resection of his turbinate on the left side in his early twenties and had also had his appendix removed several years earlier. A review of his systems otherwise showed nothing relevant.

Physical Examination.—The patient was a well developed and nourished middle-aged white male. Facies showed slight ptosis of the left eyelid. Pupils were irregular but reacted normally to light and accommodation. The nose showed some deviation of the septum. Throat was negative. Chest was normal. Heart and lungs showed nothing of significance. Abdomen was negative. Extremities were negative. Reflexes were normal except for the presence of a suggestive Romberg sign.

Laboratory Findings.—Red blood cells, 5,200,000 with 16 grams (95%) hemoglobin. White blood cells, 11,900 with 74% polynuclears. Urinalysis was negative. Serology: blood Kolmer-Wassermann was negative. Spinal

fluid examination showed a clear, colorless fluid with only four cells. The colloidal gold curve, Kolmer-Wassermann reaction and chemistry were essentially negative.

X-ray examination showed a calcified tumor lying between the base of the skull and the arch of the atlas. The apical or mesial portions of the petrous pyramids were eroded as a result of increased intracranial pressure. On the basis of the location and the calcification of the lesion, the possibility of its being an oligodendroglioma was suggested.

Operative History.—The atlas and axis were both decompressed by removal of their laminae, and a large decompression of the foramen magnum was made. The dura was incised and a large tumor exposed. The tumor apparently arose from within the fourth ventricle, growing out through the foramen of Magendie down the posterior lateral surface of the cord and up over the cerebellum. There was an attachment to the vermis and to the right cerebellar hemisphere. The floor of the fourth ventricle was visualized after the tumor was removed.

Pathological Report.—*Gross Description of Surgical Specimen.*—The specimen consisted of two masses of tumor tissue each approximately 5 cm. in diameter. They were pinkish in color, and soft and friable in consistency except for numerous areas of calcification. They were nodular in appearance and made up of homogeneous, semi-translucent tissue.

Microscopic Description of a Section Through the Tumor.—(Fig. 299) Histologic examination of the section reveals a loose fibrillar tissue supporting many nuclei. The nuclei are for the most part round. There is a nuclear membrane and a scattering of extremely fine chromatin particles within the nucleus. There are no nucleoli. It is noteworthy that in the region of blood vessels there is an attempt at palisading of nuclear elements. In some areas, the cells with real vascular feet are encountered. Areas of calcification are also observed. A number of thick-walled blood vessels may be seen, some of which are fibrosed and the lumen obliterated.

Ependymomata.—The ependymoma belongs less obviously to the group of glial tumors arising as it does from the lining cells of the ventricular system. Like the oligodendroglioma, it is essentially benign in itself, except for its location. The ependymoma is usually a mid-line tumor arising most frequently in the roof or the floor of the third or fourth ventricle; less frequently, eccentrically, from the lateral ventricular ependyma. Typically, the tumor consists of rather large cells with elongated protoplasmic processes. One of the most striking features of these tumors is their tendency to attempt to reproduce cavities simulating the ventricular system, with a resultant alveolar or rosette appearance.

ILLUSTRATIVE CASE

CASE 123. (Ref. #S-327)
Diagnosis.—Spinal cord—ependymoma.

Patient was a white male of 41 years, admitted to the hospital complaining of low back pain of six months' duration.

Present Illness.—The present illness began rather suddenly with an attack of sharp pain in the lower lumbar region on coughing. Similar attacks of pain recurred at increasing intervals and the patient noticed that they

could be brought on by very slight lateral motion of the body or even of the head. For the two months preceding admission, the pain had been almost continuous with radiation down the left leg on almost the slightest motion. About six weeks before admission, he complained of some numbness in both feet, but more marked in the left. He also noted that he was unable to detect the temperature of his bath water, which almost resulted in a serious burn. For approximately two weeks he had noticed some weakness of his extremities on walking upstairs.

Past History.—The early history was irrelevant. He had had the usual childhood infections. A point which seemed of possible significance was that the patient had always been subject to upper respiratory infections, and that about two months before the onset of his present symptoms he had had a severe tonsillitis, which had required bed rest for ten days. As a result, following this infection he had his tonsils removed, eight months before admission, but this had been followed a month later by another severe upper respiratory infection. The patient recalled that about a year prior to the onset of his present illness he had fallen, landing rather hard on his sacrum. This had resulted in some transitory disability in walking for a week or ten days.

Physical Examination.—Physical examination revealed a well-developed and well-nourished, middle-aged white male. His head was normal in contour. There was a small subcutaneous sebaceous cyst noted in the left temporoparietal region. Eyes reacted normally and his pupils were regular. Ocular movements were normal. Smell and hearing were normal. Examination of his other cranial nerves was negative. Examination of his neck was negative. Chest was symmetrical. Heart and lungs seemed to be within normal limits. Examination of his upper extremities was negative. The left lower extremity was negative. There was some slight difference in size of the right and left calves, the right measuring 1 cm. less in circumference. The epicritic sense was absent over the entire right lower extremity. Pain, temperature and vibratory senses were markedly impaired on the same side and up to the second lumbar level. Spine: There was marked tenderness on pressure over the lower lumbar spine and severely radiating pain could be elicited in that region by the slightest lateral motion.

Laboratory Findings.—Urinalysis was negative. Blood count was normal with 4,990,000 red blood cells and 90% hemoglobin. White blood cells, 6,750 with 54% polynuclears and 38% lymphocytes. Blood Wassermann was negative. Spinal fluid examination showed a moderate increase of globulin and total proteins with a slight re-

duction in chlorides. The fluid was colorless and contained 7 cells per c. mm. The colloidal gold and Kolmer-Wassermann reactions were normal.

Operative Record.—On the basis of these findings a laminectomy was done with the exposure of what appeared to be a hemorrhagic tumor mass involving the intramedullary portion of the cord. This was removed so far as possible, but because of its extremely friable and hemorrhagic nature it was felt that probably some tumor might well have been left behind.

Pathological Report.—*Gross Description of Surgical Specimen.*—Specimen consisted of several fragments of hemorrhagic, necrotic, grayish-pink tissue embedded in a mass of blood clot.

Microscopic Description of a Section of the Tumor.—Histologic examination of the tissue shows nests of cells with a tendency to cohere so that the cytoplasmic outlines are indistinct in these areas. The nuclear markings are not so coarse as is commonly seen in neoplastic cells. The nucleus is ovoid or spindled in form having a definite nuclear membrane and a large nucleolus. In a few areas, these cells are seen arranged more or less radially about the blood vessels. Where this occurs, they are more definitely spindled in form and the nuclei seem a little richer in chromatin. There is a very striking tendency for the cells to produce rosettes with the nuclei at the base of the cell away from the pseudolumen, and for the cytoplasmic processes of the cell to point toward the lumen. Stained with phosphotungstic-acid hematein and by the silver method these cells are easily identified as ependymal in origin. Some of them suggest rather primitive ependymal spongioblasts while others show rather more complete differentiation toward the adult type. The entire picture is complicated by hemorrhage and secondary degenerative changes with considerable cellular infiltration. Much of the hemoglobin has broken down and has been taken up by large mononuclear phagocytic cells. Some of these with small, round, eccentrically placed nuclei suggest typical Gitter cells. The lesion, as a whole, may best be considered as a somewhat atypical ependymoma.

TUMORS OF NEURO-EPITHELIAL ORIGIN

Neuroblastoma.—Tumors arising from the various neuro-epithelial derivatives are much less frequently encountered in the central nervous system. Just as in the case of the gliomata, it is theoretically possible to find such tumors developing at any stage in the differentiation of the nerve cell from the primitive medulloblast to the adult neurone. Practically, tumors of both the neuroblastic and adult neurone type are found more commonly in the peripheral nervous system than in the brain and spinal cord. One exception to this statement is true, the comparatively frequently encountered tumor of the eye, which arises from the retina. It is a highly malignant tumor of childhood, which remains for a considerable period of time as an intra-ocular tumor, but sooner or later invades the tissues locally and metastasizes

both by the lymphatic and blood streams. This tumor is frequently termed a "glioma," but incorrectly, as no glial fibers can be demonstrated in its composition by use of any of the more specific stains. The neoplasm is made up of small round cells with the typical nucleus containing, as a rule, a definite nucleolus. There is a tendency on the part of the cells to elongate to form potential rods and cones. In the course of this differentiation, they are frequently found arranged in pseudo-rosette fashion, but lacking the typical lumen seen in the true rosette of the ependymal type of tumor. The neoplasm has an extremely high mortality, very few cases being operated upon during the stage in which they are still intra-ocular. Unfortunately, the lesion is very commonly bilateral and may even be present at birth.

ILLUSTRATIVE CASE

CASE 124. (Ref. #S-190)

Diagnosis.—Neuroblastoma (retinoblastoma).

The patient was a white female infant of 15 months, referred to the hospital because of an intra-ocular tumor of the right eye.

Present Illness.—The child bumped her left eye about two weeks before admission and was taken to a physician, who told the parents that the left eye was perfectly normal but that the right eye had a tumor in it. The parents had noticed since that time that the color of the pupil was becoming a milky gray.

Past History.—No familial predisposition was known. The baby was a perfectly normal, full-term infant, who was breast fed for the first eight months of her life and had had an uneventful nutritional history since that time.

Physical Examination.—The patient was a normal-appearing infant. Head was normal in shape. The fontanels were closed. The right eye presented a whitish-brown reflex. The left eye appeared normal. Ophthalmoscopic examination of the eyeground showed a neoplasm, which because of its grayish color and absence of pigmentation suggested a glioma. Nose, ears and throat were negative. Chest was symmetrical. Lungs were clear. Heart was negative. Abdomen was negative. Extremities were normal.

Laboratory Findings.—Red blood cells, 5,790,000 with 72% hemoglobin. White blood cells, 9,650 with 17% polynuclears, 76% lymphocytes, 3% monocytes and 4% eosinophiles. Urinalysis was negative.

Subsequent Course.—The patient's family were advised to have an enucleation of the right eye. This was done and a gold ball inserted in place of the eye. No recurrence was observed at the end of a year.

Pathological Report.—*Gross Description of Surgical Specimen.*—Specimen consisted of an encapsulated right eyeball. The optic nerve had been cut at the margin of the globe. Externally, the eye appeared normal. This was fixed *in situ* and then split in half subsequently, and a tumor mass partially filling the posterior chamber, attached to the retina was noted. This was grayish-white in color and occupied about half the vitreous.

Microscopic Description of Section Through the Tumor.—(Fig. 300) Histologic examination of the tissue shows a portion of the eyeball with its several structures. Continuous with the retina is found a neoplastic overgrowth of retinal cells. These are for the most part small, round cells with scanty cytoplasm. Some of the nuclei are strikingly hyperchromatic and occasional mitotic figures are seen. Many of the cells show a fibrillar structure and in places definite "rosettes" are seen with the fibril pointing toward a pseudolumen with the nuclei placed peripherally. No pigment is found to suggest a melanotic tumor. The arrangement of the cells with the rather characteristic rosette picture and the presence of the typical fibrils which are best brought out by such stains as phosphotungstic acid-hematein clinch the diagnosis as a tumor of nerve cell origin. These are variously termed as neuro-epitheliomata of the neuroblast type or quite frequently erroneously, as gliomata. Because of their location in the eye arising from the retinal layer, it is customary to speak of this particular type of tumor topographically as a retinoblastoma.

MISCELLANEOUS TUMORS OF THE CENTRAL NERVOUS SYSTEM

Medulloblastoma.—Among the most malignant of the brain tumors is the medulloblastoma, a rapidly growing neoplasm which is found for the most part in children, as a midline lesion. Cases are on record in which the tumor has not appeared until as late as the sixth decade, but by far the majority of these tumors run their uniformly fatal course before the end of the second decade. The tumor is an infiltrating, soft, hemorrhagic-appearing tissue which has a tendency to appear as an intraventricular lesion. This is likely to be followed by symptoms of obstruction to the circulation of the cerebrospinal fluid with a result-ant hydrocephalus of the more familiar internal type.

Microscopically, the tumor is made up of small undifferentiated cells which may or may not suggest their origin from the primitive medullary epithelium. In view of the histogenesis of the medulloblast, it is difficult to decide whether this tumor should be classed with the neuro-epithelial tumors or whether it should be considered as a glial tumor. The same tendency toward pseudorosette formation which is evidenced in the neuroblastoma is a common finding. Like the neuroblastomata, however, they lack the true rosette formation of the ependymomata.

ILLUSTRATIVE CASE

CASE 125. (Ref. #S-328)

Diagnosis.—Medulloblastoma.

Patient was a white woman of 34 years, admitted to the hospital complaining of headaches, ringing in the right ear, weakness and vomiting.

Present Illness.—The onset of the present illness began indefinitely about seven years before admission. At that time she had some headache. She had occasional attacks of vomiting associated with the headache. This was most marked usually in the morning, and occurred almost daily during the attacks. About three years ago she noticed tinnitus of the right ear in conjunction with these same attacks of headache and vomiting, which had increased in frequency and severity. For the preceding three years, she had complete amenorrhea following a pregnancy. During pregnancy she felt improved and was free of headache. For about one year she had become progressively weaker until at the time of admission, she was unable to walk without support. Six months before admission, she had been to another hospital where a diagnosis of pituitary tumor was made and she received thirty-two x-ray treatments without benefit.

Past Medical History.—She had never had any serious illness until the onset of her present condition, except for an attack of influenza in the 1918 epidemic. A review of her systems was negative up to the present illness. She had been married fourteen years and had four living children. She had had no miscarriages.

Physical Examination.—Her physical examination was essentially negative except for the neurologic findings. Head was normal in contour. Eyes showed delayed bilateral corneal reflexes and lateral nystagmus. There was partial deafness of the right ear. Reflexes in general were not exaggerated and were equal on both sides. There was very slight intimation of cerebral incoordination. There was a general wasting of the musculature, but the skin showed a normal turgor. Heart and lungs were negative. Abdomen was normal. No masses or tenderness were noted.

Laboratory Findings.—Urinalysis was negative. Red blood cells, 3,400,000 with 70% hemoglobin. White blood cells, 4,150 with 68% polynuclears. Wassermann was negative. Basal metabolism was minus 32%. Glucose tolerance was negative. Blood chemistry was negative. Spinal fluid showed an increased protein and sugar content. Cell count was normal. Wassermann and colloidal gold tests were negative.

X-ray examination showed marked dilatation of the third and lateral ventricles. In addition, there was complete erosion of the posterior clinoid processes and displacement of the pineal gland, dorsad, caudad and toward the right. On the basis of these findings it was recommended that craniotomy be done, but the patient died suddenly before any operative procedure could be attempted.

Autopsy Findings.—The autopsy was restricted to an examination of the brain. The brain was removed in the usual fashion and the sella turcica found flattened out and shallow, with complete erosion of the clinoid processes. The pituitary likewise was compressed into a button-like structure in the fossa. The convex surface of the brain showed marked flattening of the convolutions. The interpeduncular space was widened and distended. There was a large, hemorrhagic-appearing mass, which protruded from between the dorsal aspect of the medulla and cerebellar tonsil. Sections through the midline of the brain showed moderate dilatation of the lateral ventricles and the third ventricle. The fourth ventricle was apparently obliterated by a huge tumor mass measuring 6 x 2 cm. The tumor appeared to extend laterally for a distance of about 2 cm. into the cerebellum proper in a markedly invasive fashion.

Microscopic Description of the Tumor.—(Fig. 298) Histologic examination of the tumor presents a rather characteristic picture of a medulloblastoma. There is a coarse stroma with the cells arranged both in nests and separately, with interlacing fibrillar structures. In some areas the cells seem to be arranged about thick-walled blood vessels. The nuclei are ovoid or rounded with coarse chromatic granules. Occasional mitotic figures are seen. Some larger hyperchromatic nuclei are found. A suggestion of beginning polar dendritic processes is noted here and there. By the use of silver stains, other forms of more thoroughly developed glial tumors are ruled out and the diagnosis of medulloblastoma is made. This is in keeping with its cerebellar midline origin. It is somewhat unusual in its spread to obliterate the fourth ventricle and to extend as widely as it did.

Choroidal Papilloma.—Rarely, a tumor may arise from the choroid plexuses. It is derived from the choroidal epithelium covering the vascular capillary bed and grows as a slow-growing papilloma does elsewhere. Unfortunately, owing to its location, it may be followed by a fatal outcome, although ordinarily benign histologically. It is an extremely rare lesion, and probably some of the reported cases may well represent metastatic adenocarcinomata from other foci, as these lesions are readily to be confused with such metastatic tumors.

Pinealoma.—Another of the rare tumors of the central nervous system is a tumor which arises from the pineal body. This has best been described in a monograph by Globus. Theoretically, at least, two forms of the tumor may occur as we find that the cells in differentiating from the primitive medullary epithelium produce a glial supportive element and the small round cell of the parenchyma. Practically, such tumors always arise from both types of cell. However, some of them may theoretically and histologically be benign, while others derived from the earlier stages of the development of these cells may be frankly malignant from the outset. From the practical standpoint, they are both invariably fatal. They are likely to grow slowly and sooner or later to invade the corpora quadrigemina and break through into the ventricular system, producing a secondary hydrocephalus and defects in hearing.

The diagnosis is based upon the finding of typical large polyhedral pineal parenchymatous cells and the supportive glial-like cells. These tumors usually occur between the ages of five and fifteen and for some reason are much more frequently seen in males. It is rare to see such tumors beyond the second decade of life, although a few instances have been reported.

Illustrative Case

CASE 126. (Ref. #S-287)

Diagnosis.—Pinealoma.

Patient was a white male child of 2½ years, admitted to the hospital because of a multiplicity of progressive neurologic symptoms.

Present Illness.—There was no definite date of onset as the lesion was probably congenital in nature. The first symptoms which were noted occurred at about the age of one year when the child seemed to be a little slow in learning to creep. The whole mental development went on fairly normally. However, it was noted that there was a suggestion of a hydrocephalus at the age of about fifteen or sixteen months. This was very slow in developing and did not become appreciable until two or three months before the child's admission. An internal strabismus was noted and a certain clumsiness in the use of his extremities followed by a tendency to toe in. None of these symptoms were of a sufficiently severe nature to arouse much anxiety on the part of the parents or the family physician until quite suddenly, the child went into a profound stupor.

Past History.—Aside from these neurologic symptoms, the past history was negative. The child had been artificially fed after the third month of his life, but had never had any gastro-intestinal disturbances. He never had had any upper respiratory or other infection.

Physical Examination.—Patient was a well-developed, somewhat undernourished male child about two years of age in appearance. Head showed a slight suggestion of hydrocephalic prominence of the frontal and parietal areas. There was a rather marked internal strabismus. Nose and throat were negative. Chest was symmetrical. Heart and lungs appeared within normal limits. Abdomen was somewhat distended. No masses or tenderness could be elicited. Extremities showed a moderate tendency toward inversion.

Laboratory Findings.—Red blood cells, 4,200,000 with 78% hemoglobin. White blood cells, 12,800 with 18% polynuclears, 81% lymphocytes and 1% eosinophiles. Urinalysis was negative. Spinal puncture was done to relieve the pressure and the fluid was found to be under considerably increased pressure and to be slightly opalescent. The cell count was 18, all lymphocytes, so far as could be determined. No changes in the protein composition of the fluid were noted. Wassermann was negative.

Subsequent Course.—The patient went progressively downhill and died with the clinical diagnosis of possible brain tumor and definite obstructive hydrocephalus.

Autopsy Findings.—Autopsy findings were entirely negative except for the presence of a large, hemorrhagic tumor mass approximately 10 cm. in diameter which arose from the region of the pineal body, infiltrated the corpora quadrigemina, and broke through the brain tissue into the left lateral ventricle, which was entirely filled with tumor tissue.

Microscopic Description of a Section Through the Tumor.—(Fig. 297) Histologic examination of the tissue presents the typical arrangement of the cells as seen in the pineal gland. There is a central core of small round glial-like cells made up of small nuclei, which are intensely hyperchromatic in their staining reaction. Many of them contain a definite nucleolus, but this cannot be demonstrated in others. Surrounding these cores of glial tissue are seen the characteristic large polyhedral pineal cells with their more vesicular rounded or oval nuclei and coarse granular arrangement of their chromatin. The cytoplasm is well defined by a cell membrane and stains intensely with the eosin dye.

CHAPTER XXXI

TUMORS OF THE PERIPHERAL NERVOUS SYSTEM

In a consideration of tumors arising from the peripheral nervous system, we have to consider the lesions which arise, not only in the main nerve trunks in relation to the central nervous system, but in the tumors of the sympathetic nervous system as well. The tumors arising from the nerve trunks may show marked variation. In the preceding chapter, we have discussed those tumors arising in the central nervous system, particularly those which are found involving the brain and spinal cord. In this part of the discussion, we shall consider those tumors which are derived from the nerve fibers and their associated coverings. Logically, to be completely inclusive, one should incorporate not only the tumors of the peripheral nervous system, but likewise those derived from the autonomic sympathetic structures.

From the practical side, it is comparatively easy to enumerate those tumors which are of common occurrence and of importance, and we shall restrict our discussion to these more familiar varieties. As has been emphasized in some of the earlier chapters referring to a rather wide range of neoplasms, the relationship to such lesions as the pigmented melanomata, and to the so-called "carcinoid" of the appendix with its characteristic argentophil cells, brings up problems of theoretical and hypothetical interest but of little practical importance. The tumors of the peripheral nerves may be considered in the simplest fashion as arising from the nerve fibers alone as neuromata, from the sheath fibers alone as Schwannomata or perineural or endoneural fibromata or in combination, as in the case of the neurofibromata of Von Recklinghausen's disease. At times, such tumors may go on and undergo malignant transformation when they become spoken of as neurogenic sarcomata. In addition to these relatively obvious varieties, we occasionally encounter a tumor which is made up of both ganglion cells and nerve fibers, which we speak of as a ganglioneuroma.

From the sympathetic nervous system, we find that tumors may arise from the small round cell primitive neuroblasts as malignant neoplasms usually found in the medulla of the adrenal, or as benign tumors arising from ganglion cells or as chromaffinoma (paraganglioma or pheochromocytoma), representing the adult differentiation forms of the primitive sympathetic neuroblast. These last two tumors are ordinarily benign in nature in contradistinction to the extremely malignant neuroblastoma, which metastasizes widely, occurs usually in children under the age of five and runs an invariably rapidly fatal course.

ACOUSTIC NEUROMA

In connection with these tumors of the peripheral nerves must be included the acoustic neuroma or cerebellar pontine angle tumor. This is identical in structure with the perineural tumors of the peripheral nerve as far as its histology is concerned. It is believed by many observers, as the result of Masson's brilliant work, to be derived from the sheath of Schwann. Opinions vary regarding this, however, and others contend that it is derived from the perineural fibrous tissue (Penfield, Bailey et al). At all events, the tumor is ordinarily a relatively small, encapsulated lesion which is important chiefly because of its pressure relationships with displacement of the normal structures of the brain and brainstem. It rises in relation ordinarily to the acoustic nerve, as its more familiar name implies. With these comments in mind, it is easy to understand why the tumor is frequently spoken of as a Schwannoma, as a neurinoma, or as a neurilemmoma.

The microscopic diagnosis is easily established, the tumor being composed of long, delicate fibers with elongated nuclei. These present a rather characteristic palisading, which is in itself almost diagnostic. In places where this palisading is not so prominent, the lesion might be almost mistaken for a meningioma, as the cells become somewhat larger and tend

PLATE LXXIV

TUMORS OF THE NERVOUS SYSTEM

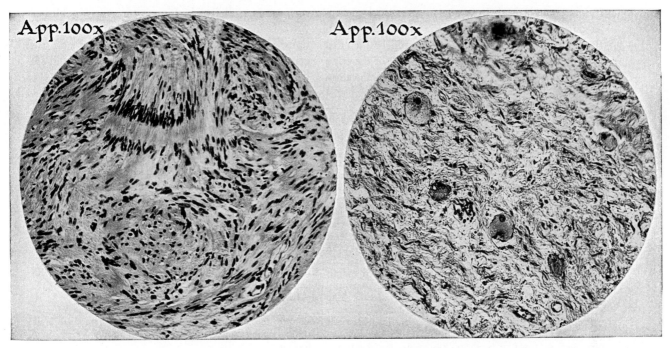

FIG. 301.—EIGHTH CRANIAL NERVE: ACOUSTIC NEUROMA (NEU-RINOMA, SCHWANNOMA, ETC.).—CASE 127.—Tumor is composed of typical interlacing fibers in which "palisading" is the out-standing feature. App. 100 x.

FIG. 302.—MEDIASTINUM: GANGLIONEUROMA.—CASE 130.—Tumor consists basically of relatively mature, purposelessly arranged nerve fibrils, scattered throughout which may be seen typical large ganglion cells. App. 100 x.

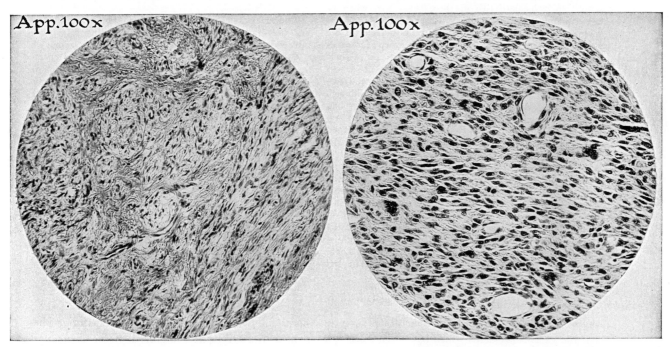

FIG. 303.—PERIPHERAL NERVE: NEUROFIBROMA.—Interlacing fasci-culi of well differentiated connective tissue together with others of neurogenic origin. (Identifiable by special staining.) App. 100 x.

FIG. 304.—THIGH: PERIPHERAL NERVE.—NEUROGENIC SARCOMA.—CASE 129.—Tumor cells are chiefly spindle-shaped, with taper-ing, hyperchromic nuclei, and ill-defined cytoplasmic processes. Multinucleated tumor giant cells and numerous mitoses are strong evidence of its highly malignant and invasive character. App. 100 x.

to occur in more or less whorl-like fashion. Special staining methods bring out the essential neurofibromatous nature of the lesion. In this connection the concept that the meningioma should be included in this group, as a tumor of nerve sheath or covering cells cannot be entirely overlooked. Indeed the term leptomeningioma is often applied diagnostically to such tumors. Bailey in his most recently published work is inclined strongly to the view of the essentially similar identity of the meningioma and the neurinoma. This has been discussed in detail in Chapter XXVII relating to the endotheliomata.

ILLUSTRATIVE CASE

CASE 127. (Ref. #S-173)

Diagnosis.—Right acoustic neuroma.

Patient was a white male of 48 years, who was admitted to the hospital complaining of progressive neurologic symptoms relating particularly to loss of vision.

Present Illness.—Present illness apparently began two years before admission with attacks of frontal and occipital headache. Accompanying these headaches there was slow but progressive loss of hearing in the right ear. As this deafness developed, he also noticed a progressive anesthesia of the right side of his face and during the past year had had progressive loss of vision in the right eye. He complained of occasional attacks of dizziness. More recently, he noted some ataxia and vertigo. The vertigo was usually ushered in by a premonitory aura. On occasions he had noticed some pain on the right side of the face. This was usually of a dull, aching nature, but at times was sharp and radiating from the lower border of the ear to the angle of the jaw.

Past History.—The patient had had the usual diseases of childhood, including mumps, measles, chickenpox, whooping cough and scarlet fever. He was particularly subject to colds until two or three years ago when he began taking vaccine treatments. A review of his systems was noncontributory. He had had to wear glasses for the past twelve years, but did not use them except for reading. He never had any earache or abscess in his ear, nor any history of mastoiditis. He had had several attacks of frontal sinusitis, but these subsided under local treatment. He had had a slight speech defect since childhood. His gastro-intestinal history was negative. He never had any genito-urinary symptoms.

Physical Examination. Patient was well developed and well nourished. He did not appear acutely ill. His memory and orientation were good. Head was normal in shape. Nose and throat were negative. Chest was symmetrical. Lungs were clear. Heart was not enlarged and there were no murmurs. Abdomen was somewhat obese with poor muscle tone. No masses were palpable. Genitals were negative. Extremities were negative. Neurologic examination showed a slight ataxia, but no spasticity. Investigation of his cranial nerves showed nothing significant in connection with the olfactory nerve. There was a temporal hemianopsia of the right eye. The left eye was normal. Pupils reacted normally to light and accommodation, and the eyeballs were freely movable in all directions. There was no nystagmus. There was an area of anesthesia over the mandibular division of the 5th nerve, reaching the angle of the mouth on both upper and lower lips. Pain sensation was present. Corneal reflex was diminished on the right. The 7th nerve showed no involvement. The 8th nerve showed deafness of the right ear. The 9th, 10th, 11th and 12th nerves showed nothing significant. Reflexes were slightly exaggerated but otherwise normal.

Laboratory Findings.—Red blood cells, 4,250,000 with 80% hemoglobin. White blood cells, 6,850 with 63% polynuclears. Urinalysis negative.

X-ray examination: There was a small area of erosion in the petrous portion of the right temporal bone near its mesial cephalic end as seen in the vertex projection.

Subsequent History.—On the basis of the x-ray findings which were somewhat inconclusive, the clinical history and the neurologic examination, a tentative diagnosis of right cerebellar pontine angle tumor was made and operation advised.

Operative History.—The patient was operated upon and the diagnosis confirmed with the finding of a definite right angle tumor, which was successfully removed.

Pathological Report.—*Gross Description.*—The specimen consisted of several pieces of grayish-white tumor tissue removed from the right cerebellar pontine angle.

Microscopic Description of the Tumor.—(Fig. 301) Histologic study of the tissue shows interlacing bundles of fibers within which are many spindle-shaped nuclei. Where these bundles are seen in cross-section, there is considerable vacuolization, giving the characteristic structure of nerve fibers. The nuclei vary considerably; some are deep-stained, tend to be only slightly oval or almost round; others are elongated and stain more lightly and have a distinctly basket network of chromatin. These apparently represent fibroblasts. There are other cells lying among these just described that show a considerable degree of pleomorphism; others a light staining, but definite nuclear membrane and a fine scattering of chromatin particles, which appear to be the nuclei of nerve cells.

AMPUTATION NEUROMA

The actual tumors of the peripheral nerves present the various problems which have been discussed. It is theoretically possible, at least for a tumor composed solely of axis cylinders to develop. Practically this is not seen except as a proliferation of the nerve fibers following an amputation as a reparative phenomenon. As is well recognized, nerve fibers will continue to grow as long as the nerve cell is not destroyed. This is one of the first principles in the surgical repair of traumatic injuries of nerves, to

PLATE LXXV

TUMORS OF THE NERVOUS SYSTEM

Von Recklinghausen's Disease (Neurofibromatosis)

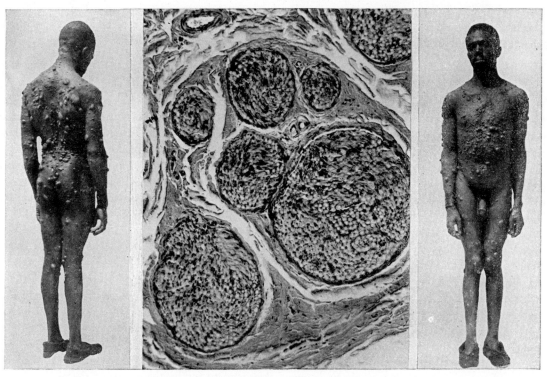

FIG. 305.—NEUROFIBROMA-
TOSIS.—POSTERIOR VIEW.

FIG. 306.—SCIATIC NERVE: DIFFUSE NEUROFIBROMA-
TOSIS.—CASE 128.—Photomicrograph illustrating diffuse
perineural fibrosis producing marked thickening of
nerve trunk. App. 100 x.

FIG. 307.—NEUROFIBROMA-
TOSIS.—ANTERIOR VIEW.

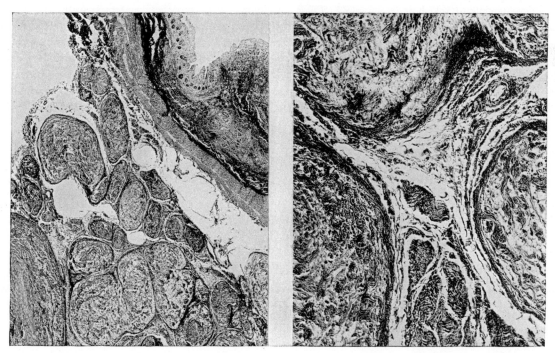

FIG. 308.—MESENTERIC SYMPATHETIC NERVE PLEXUS:
NEUROFIBROMATOSIS.—CASE 128.—Note proliferation of
all elements of nerve, but especially of the nerve
sheath. App. 10 x.

FIG. 309.—High power magnification of Fig. 308 to
better demonstrate the neuronal as well as the sheath
cell hyperplasia. App. 100 x.

Fig. 306, 308 and 309 are by courtesy of the *Am. Jour. Cancer,* Volume 31, "A Case of Diffuse Neurofibromatosis," Aegerter,
E. E. and Smith, L. W.

unite the two ends of the severed nerves so that the nerve fiber may grow along its original tract and ultimately reëstablish function. When this union is not possible as the result of an amputation, then these nerve fibers still proliferate and develop as a nodular, fibrillar growth in the amputation stump. They are likely to be associated with marked pain but cannot be considered as true tumors, although they are commonly spoken of as amputation neuromata.

NEUROFIBROMA

Simple Neurofibroma (PERINEURAL FIBROMA, ENDONEURAL FIBROMA, NEURINOMA, NEURILEMOMA, SCHWANNOMA).—(Fig. 303) By the very multiplicity of synonymous terms applied to this neoplasm, may be recognized the uncertainty regarding its histogenesis. In the tumors of the peripheral nerve trunks, invariably some portion of the sheath likewise takes part in the neoplastic process. Two major schools of thought have gradually developed, represented in this country by Masson who considers that the tumors are essentially of Schwann cell origin, and by Penfield and Bailey who believe that the tumors are derived from the highly specialized fibrous tissue sheath cells of the endo or perineurium. It would appear from the practical standpoint that these tumors are most simply considered as neoplasms arising from any or all of the component parts of the peripheral nerve. It seems reasonable to assume that the activator of the neoplastic process might well influence all the structures of the nerve, rather than show any selective stimulation of one or another of the various cells of which it is composed. These tumors may be either single or multiple. Usually, they are entirely benign, but at times, like other tumors, they may undergo malignant transformation and become definitely invasive tumors with metastatic capacities. As such, they are known as neurogenic sarcomata.

Von Recklinghausen's Disease or Diffuse Neurofibromatosis.—(Figs. 305 and 307) As has just been indicated, the neurofibromata are frequently encountered as multiple lesions. In many instances, there seems to be a definite familial history associated with the production of enormous numbers of such tumors. They vary from the so-called "neurofibromata occulta," which are represented usually by curious coffee colored, oval pigmented areas in the skin to large, pedunculated tumor masses sometimes as large as 10 to 15 cm. in diameter. They arise as neurofibromata involving both the nerve fibers and the nerve sheaths of the peripheral nerves, particularly the terminal filaments. With their overgrowth they become not infrequently oedematous and pedunculated and present an extraordinary picture occurring as they do over the entire body and tissue. Less often is the face found involved in this process. In general, they tend to follow the course of the nerves, but in the more marked cases, this is difficult to observe. In some instances the lesion may not be restricted to the peripheral nerves but may likewise be found to involve the sympathetic system as well. By the use of special staining methods to demonstrate the presence of nerve fibers, these tumors always show their presence embedded in the mass of perineural tissue. In this way it may be considered as a composite, or true "mixed" tumor involving as it does the highly specialized connective tissue of the nerve sheath and the actual nerve fiber itself.

ILLUSTRATIVE CASE

CASE 128. (Ref. #S-330)

Diagnosis.—Diffuse neurofibromatosis.

Patient was a white female child of 2 years, admitted to the hospital because of progressive weakness of her legs resulting in inability to walk.

Present Illness.—The present illness began about three weeks before admission with an attack of diarrhea. This was followed by anorexia and generalized progressive weakness. The day before admission, she had a convulsion lasting fifteen minutes and followed by profound sleep. Following the convulsion, the child complained of pain in the back of her head and appeared irritable. The mother thought that there had been a progressive drowsiness since the onset.

Past History.—The past history was essentially negative. The family history was irrelevant. The child had had none of the usual childhood diseases. She had been normally delivered and had been breast fed for the first ten months of her life. She was perfectly normal otherwise.

Physical Examination.—The child was emaciated, with a prominent, lax abdomen. The head measured 51 cm. in circumference. There were numerous pigmented and relatively hirsute oval lesions present on the trunk and lower extremities representing sites of neurofibromatosis occulta. Eyes showed moderate internal strabismus. The right pupil was wider than the left. The pupils reacted very sluggishly. Examination of the ears was un-

PLATE LXXVI
TUMORS OF QUESTIONABLE NERVOUS SYSTEM ORIGIN

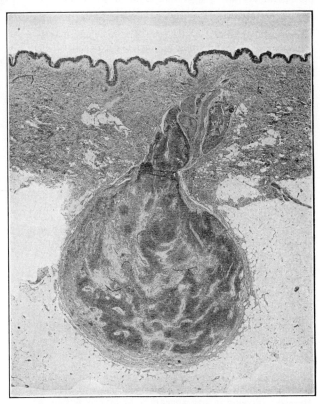

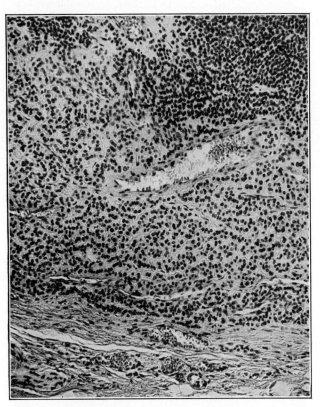

Fig. 310.—Skin: Glomus Tumor.—Case 131.—Microtessar photograph showing a cross section of the entire tumor with its relationship to the surrounding tissues and its general composition histologically. App. 5 x.

Fig. 311.—Glomus Tumor.—Case 131.—Photomicrograph of tumor including a portion of its capsule. Note the myoneural, vascular constituents of the neoplasm. App. 200 x.

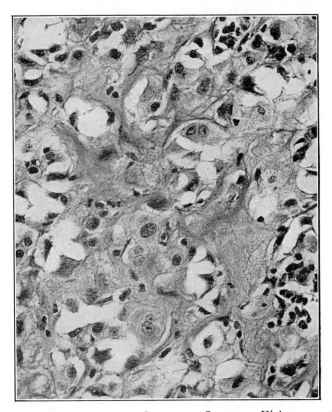

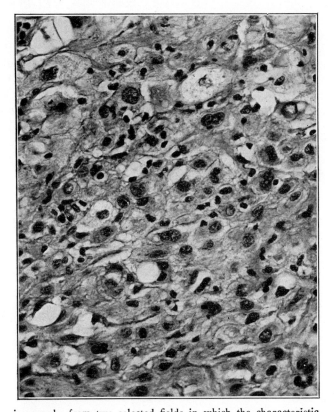

Fig. 312 & 313.—Skull: Chordoma.—Case 132.—High power photomicrographs from two selected fields in which the characteristic tumor cells may be observed. Cells are large with indistinct cytoplasmic borders, tending to be vacuolated (Fig. 313). In other areas the cells tend to line spaces filled with mucinous material. App. 600 x.

satisfactory, but the child apparently did not hear much. Abdomen: There was moderate nuchal rigidity with pain on motion. The child lay in a flexed position on the side. Reflexes were variable.

Laboratory Findings.—Red blood cells, 5,140,000 with 13 gm. of hemoglobin. White blood cells, 9,900 with 82% polynuclears, 16% lymphocytes and 2% basophiles. Spinal fluid showed increased pressure of 36 mm. Mantoux test was negative.

Ophthalmological Examination showed primary optic atrophy.

Neurologic Consultation suggested Tay-Sachs or Schilder's disease, or a posterior fossa neoplasm in association with hydrocephalus.

X-ray Examination, including encephalography, showed marked hydrocephalus and a dome-shaped opacity between the lateral ventricles, suggesting a Rathke's pouch tumor.

Subsequent Course.—The patient went progressively downhill and ultimately died four months after the onset of her symptoms.

Autopsy Findings.—Emaciation was very marked. There was definite hydrocephalus with unequal pupils. Irregular, macular, pigmented, chestnut colored hirsute lesions of the skin were noted. On opening the abdomen, a diffuse hyperplasia of what appeared to be plaque-like masses of nerve tissue could be seen in the mesentery and mesocolon as well as in the hilar notch of the spleen. No visceral pathology of any importance was found except that the adrenals were hypoplastic. There was a neoplastic, fusiform, bulbous enlargement of the optic nerve and chiasm on opening the head and exposing the brain, and marked enlargement of all the cranial nerves. On sectioning the brain, there was a large tumor involving the thalami and in direct continuity with the neoplastic processes of the optic chiasm. The entire peripheral nervous system was found to be involved in diffuse enlargement of the nerve trunks.

Microscopic Description of Sections from the Nerves.—(Fig. 306, 308 and 309) The histology may be summarized as representing an amazing generalized diffuse hyperplasia of the central, peripheral and sympathetic nervous systems. In the peripheral system all three components of the nerve structure are involved. As evidence of an increase over normal of the axone tissue, the fibrillar plaques in the mesentery are cited. These are in reality poorly defined nerve tumors. With differential stains the plaques are seen to consist of masses of interwoven peripheral nerve axones with proportionately normal Schwann sheaths and a massive increase in supportive connective tissue. Their relation to the enlargement of the mesenteric lymph nodes and the distended lymph vessels is problematic.

The remarkable increase in the size of the peripheral system as demonstrated by the brachial and sciatic nerves appears to be due to the proliferation of fibrous connective tissues. The actual number of axones is apparently within normal limits. The perineural sheaths show extreme thickening with some increase in the endoneurium.

The ganglia and trunks of the sympathetic plexuses show an increase in the ganglion cells and fibrils. The most striking characteristic of these sections, however, is the hyperplasia of the Schwann sheath. This hyperplasia appears to be responsible for the major part of the enlargement seen grossly.

Sections from other parts of the body show a diffuse hyperplasia of the terminal nerve fibrils. This is especially notable in the pericardium and corium of the skin. Here the increase in size appears to be largely due to the increase in the fibrous connective tissue of the sheath rather than to axonal proliferation.

NEUROGENIC SARCOMA

Not infrequently a tumor is encountered, usually in an extremity, and more frequently in a relatively young adult which raises considerable difficulty in diagnosis until histologic examination of the tissue is made. The tumor is apt to arise deep in the musculature and at times appears definitely to be related to the periosteum. This always brings up the possibility of the tumor being a periosteal fibrosarcoma or an osteogenic tumor. As a rule, they are slow growing and of a relatively low grade malignancy. Usually, they arise from the outset as malignant tumors although because of the low grade of malignancy, it is not infrequent for this to be overlooked even histologically. Less often the benign neurofibromata (neurinomata or perineurofibromata) may undergo malignant change and develop invasive characteristics. It is usually extremely difficult to establish relationship to any of the larger nerve trunks. The diagnosis is established on the basis of beginning pleomorphism, hyperchromatism, the presence of occasional anaplastic cells, mitotic figures and tumor giant cells in a tumor which in other respects resembles closely the simple neurofibroma. There is apt to be a tendency even toward palisading at times. The cells are spindled and occur as individual fibers usually, although interlacing bundles and whorls are not infrequently encountered. Here particularly the use of differential staining methods is helpful.

ILLUSTRATIVE CASE

CASE 129. (Ref. #S-241)

Diagnosis.—Neurogenic sarcoma.

Patient was a white female of 59 years, admitted to the hospital because of a mass in her left thigh.

Present Illness.—The present illness began about eight months before admission when the patient first noticed a tiny lump on the inner aspect of her left thigh. The patient paid no attention to this lesion and sought no medical advice at the time, largely because of the psychological fear of the necessity for surgery. The lump grew steadily until at the time of admission it was about 15 cm. in diameter.

Past History.—The patient was always well as a child and remembered no serious illness. Six years before admission, the patient developed a lipoma on her back which was removed. While she was in the hospital recovering from that operation, it was noticed that she had a small mass in her right breast. This proved to be a carcinoma and was likewise removed by radical mastectomy. There had been no recurrence during these six years. A review of her systems otherwise was negative. Her menstrual history had been normal and her menopause had occurred twelve years before admission. She had had no bleeding since that time.

Physical Examination.—Physical examination showed a well developed, well nourished elderly white female. Head was normal in contour. Pupils were regular and equal and reacted normally. Nose and throat were negative. Chest was negative except for a linear scar where the right breast had been removed. There were no nodules palpable along the line of scar or in the axilla. The left breast was normal. Lungs were clear. Heart was not enlarged and there were no murmurs. Abdomen was negative. Extremities: The upper right arm showed some slight lymph edema as the result of the radical mastectomy. The left arm was negative. The right leg was negative. The left leg showed a large, somewhat ovoid mass on the inner aspect of the thigh. This mass was firm, movable laterally, but fixed in the long axis of the leg. It was somewhat bosselated externally and extended deep into the adductor group of muscles.

Laboratory Findings.—Red blood cells, 5,060,000 with 85% hemoglobin. White blood cells, 13,350 with 87% polynuclears, 10% lymphocytes and 3% monocytes. Urinalysis was negative.

Subsequent History.—The patient was advised to have the tumor removed, to which she agreed. A large, bosselated tumor about 12 x 15 cm., originating in and involving the adductor muscles and extending from the tuberosity of the ischium down the thigh was excised. There was no apparent involvement of the bone nor attachment to the femoral vessels or sciatic nerve. The tumor was extremely firm and on cut section was almost cartilaginous in consistency. It appeared well demarcated from the tissue but not definitely encapsulated.

Pathological Report.—*Gross Description of Surgical Specimen.*—The specimen consisted of a lobulated mass measuring 14 x 19 cm. Externally, it was ragged and numerous knobs from 2 to 7 cm. in diameter projected from its surface. In one area there was a patch of adipose tissue. In another there were strips of voluntary muscle. In portions of muscle there was invading fibrosis as well as a white, pearly tissue from the mass itself. Sections through the mass revealed nodules from 1 to 6 cm. in diameter embedded in an edematous connective tissue. Cut surface of the nodules was yellowish-white, somewhat translucent and revealed interlacing fibers. Some showed an edematous, soft, brownish center. While the edges of the nodule were sharply defined, they were not smooth, but crenated. The nodules tended to bulge from the incised surface.

Microscopic Description of Section Through the Tumor.—(Fig. 304) Histologic examination of the tissue shows a picture of interlacing bundles of fibers that possess deeply-stained, spindle-shaped nuclei. There is considerable pleomorphism of the nuclei. Some of them are many times the size of the more frequently-occurring type. Where the nuclei are more mature, the fibers tend to be wavy; where they are larger and less mature, polarity is lost and fibers are indistinct. There are areas where this cellular lesion is definitely infiltrating both fat and muscle. Multinucleated tumor giant cells are common in the more cellular areas. Considerable anaplasia and hyperchromatism of the cells is observed. Mitotic figures, both typic and atypic, are numerous. Differential stains, including phosphotungstic acid-hematein, Masson's trichrome and Mallory's connective tissue blue reveal the neurogenic nature of the tumor.

GANGLIONEUROMA

The ganglioneuroma represents a tumor which is composed of adult nerve cells and delicate nerve fibers. It may be found occasionally within the central nervous system, but it is much more frequently encountered arising from groups of ganglion cells in some of the peripheral ganglia. Not infrequently such tumors are encountered in the retroperitoneal tissues. A considerable series has accumulated arising in the mediastinum. Closely related to this same type of tumor is the ganglioneuroma of sympathetic neuroblastic origin found chiefly, primarily in the medulla of the adrenal or anywhere that sympathetic nerve tissue exists. The tumor, being composed as it is of well-differentiated, adult cells, is ordinarily a slow-growing, benign lesion which should be amenable to surgery when it is located in a position where surgery is possible, but unfortunately often escapes recognition clinically until too late for such therapy.

ILLUSTRATIVE CASE

CASE 130. (Ref. #S-135)

Diagnosis.—Ganglioneuroma.

Patient was a white, married female of 26 years, admitted to the hospital because of a productive cough of about seven months' duration.

Present Illness.—The present illness began with a rather severe cold which "went down on her chest" and resulted in a persistent cough which continued long after the upper respiratory infection seemed to have disappeared. The cough increased in severity as time went on. At the time of admission she raised on the average of about a pint of thick, yellow mucoid sputum daily, which was occasionally blood streaked. She noticed marked dyspnea on the slightest exertion but had no dysphagia. She had not had chills or night sweats, or pain in her chest; but she complained of feeling extremely weak and having lost about twenty-five pounds in the two months preceding admission.

Past Medical History.—The past medical history seemed to be irrelevant. She had had all the usual childhood diseases including scarlatina. She had pneumonia as a child, but had not been particularly susceptible to upper respiratory infection since. A review of her systems otherwise was essentially negative. She had had occasional attacks of qualitative dyspepsia and had been moderately constipated. She had been married for six years and had had one child who was living and well.

Physical Examination.—At the time of admission the patient was a fairly well developed cachectic and anemic-appearing young white woman who was extremely weak and toxic. Head was of normal contour. Pupils were moderately dilated. The nose and throat appeared negative. Chest was symmetrical but the patient had marked difficulty with breathing using all her accessory muscles. There was definite lagging of both lungs. There were crackling and crepitant râles all over the right lower lobe. There was dullness on both sides but more marked on the lower left. Heart sounds were distant and feeble. No murmurs were made out. Blood pressure was 108/56. There was marked clubbing of the fingers. The abdomen was scaphoid. No masses or tenderness could be made out. Extremities: There was no edema of the lower extremities.

Laboratory Findings.—Red blood cells, 2,500,000 with 54% hemoglobin. White blood cells, 18,900 with 79% neutrophiles, 17% lymphocytes and 4% monocytes. Urinalysis showed a slight trace of albumin but was otherwise negative. Sputum examination: There were no tubercle bacilli, spirochetes or mycoses found. Numerous gram-positive cocci in chains and clumps were present. Blood Wassermann was negative.

X-ray Examination.—There was an abnormal fuzzy density present in the caudal portion of both lung fields. This presented a peculiar moth-eaten appearance. The character and distribution of the density suggested chronic pulmonary suppuration.

Subsequent Course.—The patient went steadily downhill in spite of everything that could be done for her, including several transfusions and postural drainage of her lungs.

Autopsy Findings.—A diffuse bilateral suppurative pneumonitis with multiple lung abscesses was found. In addition a bilateral, secondary purulent pleuritis and empyema was also found. This diffuse suppurative process had obscured the presence of a large tumor mass measuring 19 x 12 cm. which arose from the vertebral column just below the root of the lung. This had displaced the left lung upward and outward and had caused a marked atelectasis particularly of the lower lobe at the hilus. The tumor was sharply circumscribed and covered by parietal pleura. On the cut surface, it was grayish-white in color. It was firm in consistency but not hard. Bands of what appeared to be fibrous tissue ran through it as interlacing bundles. No pathology was found in the abdominal viscera.

Microscopic Description of Section Through the Tumor.—(Fig. 302) Histologic examination of the tissue shows the tumor to be made up of interlacing bundles of delicate fibrillar structures. Scattered through this tissue are seen the nuclei. These appear to be of two varieties, one definitely of the modified connective tissue type, elongated and spindle in outline with characteristic rounded ends; the other, a more ovoid or almost round nucleus with a rather prominent nucleolus and scattered chromatin granules. Embedded in this mass of interlacing fibrillar background are found occasional enormous cells which present the picture of typical adult ganglion cells. Some of these show actual axone and dendritic processes. Others appear somewhat degenerated and as large, ovoid cells with enormous round nucleoli which have a sharp nuclear membrane and one or more prominent acidophilic staining nucleoli. It is not hard to visualize the presence of Nissl granules in the cytoplasm of these cells in some areas. Special staining methods by modified Masson technique, by phosphotungstic acid and by silver stains demonstrate conclusively the nature of this tumor.

SYMPATHETIC NERVE TUMORS

Tumors arising from the sympathetic nervous system are found chiefly in the adrenal and will be discussed at greater length in the chapter devoted to that organ. Briefly, we find the tumor varies somewhat in its behavior. For some poorly-understood reason tumors arising from the right adrenal tend to metastasize early to the liver, whereas tumors arising from the left adrenal are much more likely to metastasize to the skull and orbit. These two varieties have been named after the observers who first recorded these peculiarities, as the Pepper type and the Hutchinson type. Both of them represent tumors of the neuroblastic variety composed of small round cells with little or no cytoplasm and tending to develop rosette formation. They occur in nests and clumps embedded in a rather loose and necrotic poorly vascularized connective tissue stroma.

The *chromaffinoma* is such a rare tumor as to merit only passing comment. It is usually seen in the older age group as a small, well encapsulated, benign lesion and is found, as a rule, accidentally at autopsy. It is easily identified by its usual rather bright yellow chromaffin pigment. Several cases have been suspected before death because of an associated paroxysmal hypertension as the result apparently of a functional activity on the part of the tumor cells to produce an excess of adrenalin. The tumor is likewise of interest because in many of the reported cases, there has been an associated generalized neurofibromatosis of the Von Recklinghausen type, implying some possible common etiologic factor in many of these various neurogenic neoplastic processes.

There are certain other miscellaneous tumors which are somewhat difficult to classify, but which are perhaps best considered at this point in relation to the nervous system. Among these must particularly be cited first, the so-called "glomus tumor" arising from the cutaneous end organs; and second, the chordoma, a tumor derived from persistent noto-chordal cells at either end of the vertebral column.

Glomus Tumor (Glomangioma).—The glomus tumor has in recent years occasioned considerable interest. Thanks are due to Masson, who was the first to recognize the inherent nature of these entirely benign cutaneous lesions. The tumor arises from the normal glomus body, which may be found anywhere in the skin. The most frequent site for these tumors, however, is immediately under the fingernails, where due to almost constant pressure, they are particularly painful. The tumor might be described as a mixed tumor because it is composed of a confusion of the various elements which go to make up the normal neuro-myo-arterial anastomosis. This consists of a network of small arterioles and venules or capillaries, which are embedded in masses of characteristic, large, polyhedral typical glomus cells and non-medullated fibers. That the majority of these vascular synapses are actually arterial or venous in nature is seen by the fact that many of them contain smooth muscle cells in their walls. It is believed that normally this glomus body is an important structure in regulating the superficial capillary circulation of the skin and thus maintaining the skin temperature.

When tumors arise from such a structure, they are composed of all of these cell elements including the vascular endothelium, the smooth muscle cells, the non-medullated nerve fibers and the typical glomus cells. In the tumors, the glomus cells seem to be the most important from the standpoint of numbers and for that reason it seems more logical to include this tumor among the neurogenic group than among the angiomatous neoplasms. From the clinical standpoint, these tumors are extremely painful, particularly on the slightest pressure; and occurring as they do for the most part on the extremities, they are peculiarly subject to pressure or to injury. Excision of the tumor mass results in a permanent cure and in instantaneous relief from the pain. So far as is known, the tumor is always benign in nature and neither infiltrates locally, nor metastasizes distantly. Its typical subungual localization has not been very satisfactorily explained.

ILLUSTRATIVE CASE

CASE 131. (Ref. #S-384)
Diagnosis.—Skin—glomus tumor.
Patient was a white female of 60 years admitted to the medical clinic because of a "chronic bronchitis" of about six years' duration.
Present Illness.—Recently she had noted that her cough was becoming worse and that she had considerable dyspnea on exertion. She also noticed swelling of her feet and ankles towards evening, almost regularly, and at times this would persist throughout the day. She had had a small lump on the side of her right buttock for a period of fourteen years. This had always been extremely painful on the slightest pressure but had not increased in size. She was worried about it for fear that it was "cancer."
Past Medical History.—The patient had had an uneventful childhood history from the standpoint of any serious illness. She had had her appendix removed and had had a complete pan-hysterectomy for fibroids. A review of her systems was essentially negative except for a chronic sinusitis of many years' standing. Her gastro-intestinal history was negative. Genito-urinary history had been negative until the development of moderate nocturia during the past few years. Three years before her present admission, she had had a "nervous break-down" and had been sent to a sanitarium for three months.
Physical Examination.—The patient was a well-developed and nourished elderly white woman who did not appear acutely ill. Her head was negative. Eyes reacted normally. Nose and throat showed a marked deviation of the septum and a prominent post-nasal drip. There was no tenderness, however, over any of the sinus areas. The tonsillar tissue appeared atrophied. Chest was symmetrical. Lungs showed a few râles at both bases. Heart was somewhat enlarged to the left with a loud systolic apical murmur. Blood pressure was 190/100. Abdomen was negative except for a mid-line scar. There was an exquisitely tender nodule about 1cm. in diameter, which was somewhat bluish-red in color on the lateral aspect of the right buttock. Palpation of this nodule was followed by radiating pain through the pelvis to the anterior abdominal wall. Extremities were negative.
Laboratory Findings.—Laboratory findings were essentially negative. Red blood cells, 4,900,000 with 12.5 gm. of hemoglobin. White blood cells, 8,850 with 62% polymorphonuclear leukocytes. Urinalysis was negative except for a slight trace of albumin and a moderate number of leukocytes. Blood chemistry was negative. Wassermann was negative.
Subsequent Course.—The patient was advised to have the tumor nodule excised for the relief of pain. This was done. The remainder of her story appeared to be one of chronic hypertensive cardiovascular disease and she was followed in the medical out-patient department for this condition with marked improvement in her symptomatology.
Pathological Report.—*Gross Description.*—The specimen consisted of a somewhat elliptical piece of skin 1.5 cm. in length. Centrally placed in this tissue was found a small, pea-sized, reddish-brown, elevated nodule which extended for a short distance into the deeper

subcutaneous fat. It was sharply circumscribed on section and suggested the possibility of a glomus tumor.

Microscopic Description of a Section Through the Tumor Nodule.—(Fig. 310 & 311) Histologic examination of the specimen shows the lesion to be composed of a variety of tissues. In general, the underlying architecture suggests a tangled network of intercommunicating capillary vessels. However, on high power it is seen that these vascular spaces are surrounded in many instances by collections of rather large, polyhedral cells with small round nuclei and a rather pale granular cytoplasm. Smooth muscle cells can be identified between many of the angiomatous channels. The entire lesion histologically is sharply demarcated by rather dense connective tissue stroma. The picture is a classical example of a glomus tumor arising from the neuro-myo-arterial junction. The various cells playing a part in this tumor are readily identified as endothelium, smooth muscle and the typical glomus cells embedded in a plexus of non-medullated nerve fibers.

Chordoma.—The chordoma, as was shown in the outline of the classification of tumors in Chapter XXII, might perhaps most accurately be considered as of hypoblastic origin, and as such occupies a position midway between the true tumors of the central nervous system and the tumors of mesothelial origin. In the development of the embryo, the notochord becomes obliterated in the formation of the vertebral column, but occasionally cells may persist at either pole in the vicinity of the pituitary fossa and the coccyx where they may give rise to a characteristic tumor. Such tumors are invariably midline in origin but due to pressure in one direction or another from surrounding structures, this midline origin may be difficult to determine clinically. The tumor may occur at all ages, but is perhaps most often seen in the young adult age group. The tumors are slowly, but persistently growing in character and may attain a considerable size. In the head region, they not infrequently involve the sphenoid and ethmoid sinuses and may be associated with marked obstruction to breathing. In the sacrococcygeal region, they not uncommonly may go unrecognized for long periods of time, particularly when they grow into the pelvis. Not until they cause pressure symptoms does their diagnosis become suspected.

Grossly, the tumors are likely to be of a curious elastic consistency, whitish in color, often with translucent areas where the tumor cells are massed in sheets. Not infrequently, hemorrhage may occur. The tumor rarely metastasizes but recurs with discouraging regularity in those cases where surgery has been attempted. So few of them have been treated that very little knowledge concerning their reaction to irradiation is available, but all evidence points to a high degree of radioresistance.

From the histologic standpoint, the diagnosis is often difficult to make. In the typical case, the tumor is found to consist of large, irregularly shaped cells which occur in sheets and have a tendency toward lumen or pseudolumen formation. The cells, for the most part, are filled with a gelatinous appearing substance which sometimes is confusing in diagnosis. In general, the cells are diffusely vacuolated and were it not for their distorted forms might readily be mistaken for the foam cells of a hypernephroma. The cytoplasm is variable in amount but there is a fairly generous amount of connective tissue as a rule. This may show extensive hyaline or mucinous degeneration. At times, as the result of pressure and the slow rate of growth, the cells may become even more distorted than usual and have a spindle form, which is confusing, so that they may resemble a fibrous tissue tumor or a liposarcoma.

ILLUSTRATIVE CASE

CASE 132 (Ref. #S-385)

Diagnosis.—Skull—chordoma.

Patient was a forty-two year old white female housewife who was admitted to the hospital with the chief complaints of blindness, dizziness, headaches, and bladder incontinence.

Present Illness.—The onset of the present illness was somewhat indefinite, but the patient dated her symptoms to about one year before admission when she began having almost constant severe headaches accompanied by beginning failure of vision in the left eye. This blindness was progressive and by the end of six months, she was totally blind in the left eye and her sight was already markedly impaired on the right side. This had gradually increased until a few days before admission she had completely lost the sight in both eyes. The headaches had likewise continued almost constantly. They were rather diffuse, but the point of maximum intensity was usually over the vertex. They seemed to start at the base of the skull and to radiate to the vertex where the pain became localized. For a month or more, the patient had also noted incontinence of urine at frequent intervals. This likewise had been more marked recently. Accompanying these symptoms she had had a good deal of dizziness so that she did not dare to walk alone, even around the house. She stumbled frequently and had very little sense of direction. About six months before admission, she had a spell of vomiting which lasted for several days, but this had not recurred since that time. She had no definite convulsions. She had not had any menstrual period for eleven months. Her sister stated that the patient had been mentally "queer" in recent months, that she had seemed to have a marked polydipsia and a ravenous appetite.

Past Medical History.—In reviewing her history it appeared that the onset of her headaches might more properly date back nearly twenty years. At that time, they were sudden in onset and were localized over the vertex occurring perhaps once or twice a day. These were always more severe just prior to her menstrual periods. A review of her systems otherwise was essentially non-informatory. She had had the usual childhood diseases but did not think she had ever had scarlet fever or rheumatic fever. Her gastro-intestinal history had been negative previously. She had never been subject to upper respiratory infection nor had she been heart conscious. Her genito-urinary history was negative. Menstrual history began at the age of twelve and had been regular. The flow had been scanty and rarely lasted over two days. This had not been accompanied by dysmenorrhea.

Physical Examination.—The patient was a very large, obese, middle-aged white woman. The skin of her face was heavy and coarse, especially around the forehead. There was moderate ptosis of both eyes. Pupils were unequal, the right being larger than the left. The corneal reflexes were acute. The palpebral fissure on the right was larger than on the left and there was a nystagmus on moving the eyes to the right. Upward rotation of the eyes was not possible. There was complete loss of vision. There was a definite right facial weakness of the peripheral type. There was deviation of the tongue to the left, but it showed no atrophy or tremor. Hearing seemed impaired. Voice was somewhat masculine in type. Hands were slightly large, but her sister stated that large hands and feet were common to the entire family. Chest was symmetrical. Heart was negative. Lungs were clear. Abdomen was obese but otherwise negative. Extremities showed diminution in the patellar reflexes and a suggestive Babinski on the right. Sensation appeared normal.

Laboratory Findings.—Blood count on admission showed 4,320,000 red blood cells and 13 gm. of hemoglobin. White blood cells, 6,000 with 69% neutrophiles. Urinalysis was essentially negative. Serologic tests were negative.

X-ray examination of the skull showed the sella turcica to be practically destroyed. The anterior clinoids were approximately twice as far apart as normal. The sphenoid bone and the entire basilar process of the occipital bone had been destroyed, and the foramen magnum had lost its ventral rim. A few flakes of calcification were seen in what might be described as the suprasellar region. The impression gained from a study of the skull film was that there was a tumor present which might have arisen in the basilar process of the occipital bone, although a pituitary tumor or Rathke's pouch tumor could not be wholly excluded.

Subsequent Course.—The patient agreed to an exploratory operation, and an attempt was made to remove a large tumor mass which was found beneath the pons. Due to the condition of the patient and the location of the lesion, however, this was impossible and only a small portion was removed for diagnostic purposes.

Pathological Report.—*Gross Description.*—Specimen consisted of several fragments of rather gelatinous tumor tissue. This presented no gross features of diagnostic value.

Microscopic Description of a Section Through the Tumor Tissue.—(Fig. 312 & 313) There is a very heavy, dense, fibrous stroma which in some places shows extensive hyaline degeneration. In many areas, it likewise shows diffuse mononuclear cellular infiltration. This connective tissue tends to form trabeculae surrounding clumps and sheets of cells, many of which attempt to outline irregular lumina. These are filled with a homogeneous mucinous-appearing material, some of which has been taken up by large mononuclear phagocytic cells. The cells making up this tumor tissue are large and irregularly outlined. Their cytoplasmic borders are indistinct. The cytoplasm has a pale eosinophilic staining reaction. The nuclei vary greatly in size and shape, but for the most part they are relatively round. Some appear to have crenated nuclear membranes. There is a liberal scattering of fine chromatin particles with small, rather light staining nucleoli in most of the cells. The cytoplasm appears both finely and coarsely vacuolated and in some areas, the same mucinous appearing material is recognized as seen in the clear spaces outlined by these cells. Many of the cells are closely packed together so that they appear almost as a syncytium. The picture is almost classical in its appearance as representing a relatively slow-growing neoplasm of notochordal cell origin.

CHAPTER XXXII

BENIGN TUMORS OF EPITHELIAL ORIGIN

The classification of the tumors of epithelial origin in its simplest form is much less complex than the nomenclature applied to the various mesoblastic tumors already studied, but tumors of epithelial origin far outnumber the mesoblastic type and practically each organ gives rise to specific tumors having a rather characteristic life history and course. This complicates the study of the epithelial tumors far beyond the simple problem of nomenclature.

In general, we have two types of epithelial tumors; those arising from superficial covering epithelium such as the skin and certain of the mucous membranes; the other from the various glandular organs. Their histology varies tremendously and the interpretation of these varying histologic pictures becomes of extreme importance from a prognostic standpoint. Of the benign tumors arising from the epithelial cells, there are, as just indicated, two major types: first, papillomata arising from surface epithelium, and second adenomata, tumors arising from glands of tubular, acinar or other type. In both of these one of the outstanding histologic features is the relatively normal relationship which is maintained between the epithelial and the connective tissue stromal elements. This, as has been emphasized, is of significance in relation to malignancy.

THE PAPILLOMATA

The papillomata are tumors composed of branching, lobulated, cauliflower-like epithelial overgrowth with a stroma consisting of a core of connective tissue, each containing a blood vessel. These tumors may arise from any portion of the superficial covering type of epithelium. They are most frequently seen on the skin, particularly about the face and around the anal and genital folds. They are not to be confused in these latter sites with the inflammatory condylomata either of the broad syphilitic type, condyloma latum; or the pointed acute infectious type, condyloma acuminatum.

They occur in several forms, the most characteristic of which is as a hyperplasia of the surface epithelium which is thrown up into papillary folds. The degree of keratinization varies a great deal. Some of these tumors show this to an extreme, and are spoken of as horns (cornua), especially when they occur as they frequently do on the forehead or scalp area. Many of these tumors are pigmented. A well recognized group of so-called pigmented papillary nevi is found which has as its basis a true nevus with a superimposed papillary proliferation of the epithelium. Lesions which appear similar in many respects are the warts (verrucae), which represent an inflammatory hyperplasia associated with infection. True warts are transmissible and are produced apparently by a filtrable virus, as filtrates will cause their production when inoculated into the skin.

Within the buccal cavity, especially in the antrum of Highmore, in the posterior pharynx and even in the larynx, we may find pedunculated papillomata having a narrow pedicle which expands into a typical papilloma. These are quite distinct from the true polyps previously described as representing basically an allergic inflammatory reaction of the mucosa resulting in mechanical edema. In the gastro-intestinal tract, at times, true papillomata may develop, but as a rule papillary tumors occurring in these areas belong to the adenomatous group of lesions and are more frequently spoken of as polyps, although incorrectly on the basis of our previous interpretation of polyp formation (Fig. 315). Loosely the term polyp is applied to pedunculated lesions of mucous membranes.

ILLUSTRATIVE CASE

CASE 133. (Ref. #S-106)
Diagnosis.—Pigmented papilloma with hyperkeratinization.

Patient was a white woman of 50 years, who was admitted to the hospital with a high fever, weakness and dyspnea.

338

PLATE LXXVII
BENIGN TUMORS OF EPITHELIAL ORIGIN

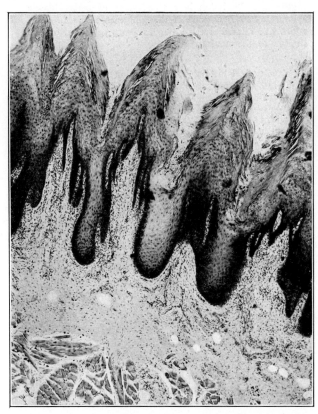

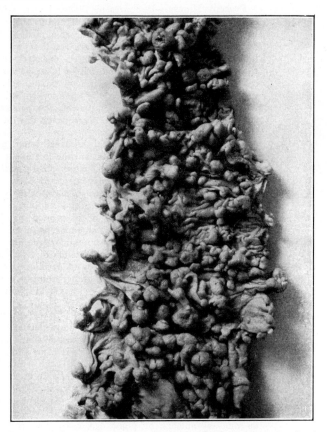

FIG. 314.—SKIN: PAPILLOMA.—CASE 133.—Excessive overgrowth of the epithelium both superficially as keratinizing papillae, and downward as exaggeration of the rete pegs. Basement membrane intact—uniform, orderly cell growth. No evidence of malignancy. App. 100 x.

FIG. 315.—COLON: POLYPOSIS.—CASE 87.—Entire mucosa involved in a diffuse polypoid hyperplasia, some of the lesions verrucous-like in appearance, others definitely pedunculated.

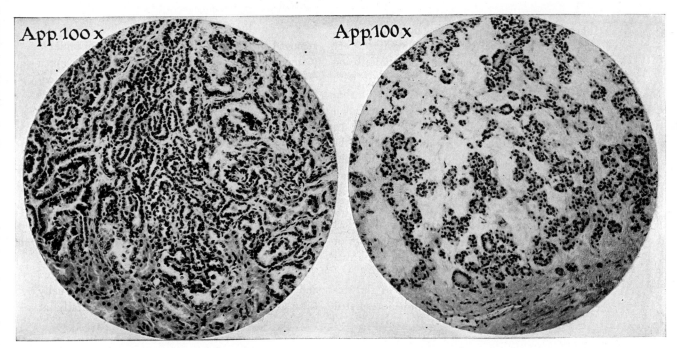

FIG. 316.—KIDNEY: FETAL ADENOMA.—CASE 134.—A sharply demarcated but indefinitely encapsulated mass of proliferating small, hyperchromatic cells with a tendency towards tubule formation. App. 100 x.

FIG. 317.—THYROID: FETAL ADENOMA.—CASE 135.—Encapsulated nodule showing epithelial hyperplasia as small cuboidal cell lined follicles, a few of which contain colloid. Stroma is characteristically gelatinous in appearance. App. 100 x.

Present Illness.—Her present illness began with a sudden onset characterized by a chill and a sharp rise in temperature to 103°. This was accompanied by difficulty in respiration. Inability to care for the patient at home led to her being brought to the hospital on the third day of the disease. A diagnosis of lobar pneumonia caused by Type 3 Pneumococcus was made, this organism being recovered from the sputum. In spite of all that could be done for the patient, she progressed steadily downhill and died on the seventh day of her illness.

Autopsy Findings.—A typical bilateral lobar pneumonia involving both lower lobes and the left upper lobe was found, in the stage of gray hepatization. In addition, evidence of toxic myocardial degeneration, toxic myocarditis, toxic hepatosis and nephrosis along with typical toxic splenitis was observed. Incidental findings at autopsy were those of a series of pigmented papillary lesions of the skin which occurred almost in girdle distribution around the waist. These numbered perhaps 100 and varied in size from a few millimeters to a lesion 1.5 cm. in size. They consisted of elevated papillary projections of the skin surface with a rather sharply demarcated base and presented varying degrees of pigmentation.

Microscopic Description of One of These Lesions.—(Fig. 314) Histologic examination shows the transition of the epithelium from normal to the characteristic papillary proliferation noted grossly. There is a marked overgrowth of the surface epithelium which is thrown up into papillary folds. It is associated with excessive keratinization. The rete pegs are broad and flattened. The underlying tissues contain clumps of cells, some of them suggesting nevus cells. The basal layer of the skin contains an unusual number of pigmented cells. The epithelial cells are all regular in appearance and show normal maturation and differentiation. Well defined spines can be identified in the deeper layers of the skin. There is no

evidence of invasion of the tissues. There is nothing to suggst that the lesion is a true tumor of melanoblastic origin. It represents one of those pigmented papillomata which are related to the group of neuro-epithelial tumors similar to the nevi in origin.

For a typical history and description of benign polypi of the intestinal mucosa, the reader is referred to CASE 87, (Ref. #S-217), Chapter XXIII. The polypoid lesions are well illustrated in Fig. 315.

Diagnosis.—Intestine—polyposis.

They occur as pedunculated or sessile lesions arising in the mucosa of the colon, particularly of the sigmoid portion of the large intestine. A zone of transition microscopically may be observed from the normal mucous glands to the neoplastic tissue. This is characterized by an increase in the size of the cells, usually with a definite tendency for increased activity on the part of the cells to produce an excess amount of mucus, with many of these cells appearing as dilated goblet cells. They are arranged in single or multiple layers upon a fibrous stalk usually containing a central nutritional vessel. The basement membrane remains intact and no evidence of invasion of the stroma is found. This is the most significant and important of all the microscopic criteria available in differentiating the benign from the malignant adenomatoid polypi of the gastro-intestinal tract. So frequently does some degree of anaplasia and even hyperchromatism exist in these lesions that to the beginning student of pathology, they offer a difficult problem of diagnosis. In general, however, it may be observed that the cells as a whole tend to be fairly uniform in size and well differentiated even although they may appear hypertrophic.

For a history and histologic description of a case of malignant papilloma of the bladder, refer to CASE 134 in this section and to Fig. 566 and 568 in Chapter LVII.

THE ADENOMATA

The adenomata are legion. They occur in varying forms, sometimes as very solid tumors with a very dense connective tissue stroma; at other times being made up of almost solid glandular elements with very little stroma. They may occur in any epithelial glandular organ. Perhaps the three most common sites are the breast, the ovary and the thyroid. In addition, frequent sites of election which may be mentioned are the gastro-intestinal tract and the endometrium of the uterus. Less frequently adenomata are seen in other organs such as the liver, pancreas, parathyroid, etc.

The gastro-intestinal adenomata, for the most part, as mentioned above, appear as papillary or polypoid tumors in direct continuity with the normal lining mucosa. They tend to be pedunculated and to show varying degrees of hyperplasia of the epithelium. Many of these tumors are to be interpreted

as a pre-malignant lesion which, unless completely removed surgically, is likely to recur and to undergo malignant degeneration. Similar polypoid adenomata are encountered in the uterus arising from the endometrial glands.

More discrete adenomata are those found, for example, in the kidney (Fig. 316) and in the thyroid (Fig. 317). In the kidney we find small isolated nodules varying in size from a few millimeters to a few centimeters in diameter. These are made up of twisted glandular or tubular epithelial structures attempting to reproduce tubules. It is thought these are, according to Cohnheim's theory, misplaced renal cells which were intended to form kidney tissue, but becoming displaced, resulted in these benign lesions. These tumors have little or no appreciable stroma and their vascular supply is slight. They are usually encapsulated and are found only incidentally at autopsy. The thyroid adenomata represent another problem which will be considered in greater detail in regard to thyroid pathology in general. Let it be said at this time that considerable uncertainty exists as to the development of these lesions. Many observers hold that they represent irregular evolutional and involutional changes of the gland and are not true tumors. Others believe that at least certain of these are true neoplasms. In either event they occur as solitary or multiple nodules, well encapsulated for the most part, and made up of cords and trabeculae of undifferentiated epithelium in their simplest embryonal form, or of minute follicles without colloid in their most common form. Again they show little or no appreciable stroma and tend to undergo cystic degeneration as a result of inadequate blood supply.

In the breast we find the development of lesions which are spoken of as adenofibromata because of the relative increase in amount of connective tissue stroma. McFarland believes that all represent variants of the so-called periductile adenofibroma. The term adenofibroma or fibro-adenoma has been applied to this group because of the disproportionate amount of stroma. In the more glandular appearing of these tumors the stroma tends to show myxomatous degeneration. These appear to represent the more undifferentiated or embryonal type of tumor comparable to the embryonal adenoma of the thyroid just described. The more adult type is seen in the lesion commonly called intracanalicular adenofibroma in which the connective tissue proliferates, forming papillary ingrowths distorting the lumen of the tumor glands and ducts so that at times the tumor appears as a fibroma in which branching epithelial structures may be seen simulating compressed ducts. Again, as in the case of the thyroid, many of these lesions may represent involutional changes in the breast and not be true tumors at all.

In the ovary we see a combination of lesions resulting essentially in the development of adenomata which undergo extensive cystic degeneration as the result of secondary activity on the part of the cells lining these gland-like structures. Such tumors arise from the ingrowth of the serosal cells covering the ovary and not as originally thought from follicular epithelium. They may be serous or pseudomucinous in their content; they may be unilateral or bilateral. They may range in size from a lesion not more than 1 cm. or less in diameter up to enormous tumor-like masses weighing as much as eighty pounds.

Histologically, they are usually multilocular cysts lined by columnar epithelial cells which tend to show extensive papillary proliferation (Fig. 323). These cells are either goblet or serous in nature secreting their corresponding fluids which gives rise to the character of the cyst contents. In general, they are considered under the heading of benign cystadenomata of the ovary. Certain of them, however, may undergo malignant degeneration as will be shown subsequently in a consideration of the malignant epithelial tumors in the chapter devoted to a consideration of the pathology of the female genital organs.

ILLUSTRATIVE CASES

CASE 134. (Ref. #S-10, S-50 and S-109)
Diagnosis.—Kidney—congenital fetal adenoma.

Patient was a white male of 57 years, admitted to the hospital because of pain in the lumbar region, recent persistent vomiting and marked loss of weight.

Present Illness.—The present illness began about one year before admission when he complained of vague, general malaise with attacks of indigestion. About four months before admission, these symptoms became much more marked with almost constant nausea and frequent attacks of vomiting. These were accompanied by low back pain, which had incapacitated him for about three weeks. This had forced him to remain home from work and to spend most of his time in bed. It was accompanied by marked weakness, and the loss of a considerable amount of weight. Associated with these gastro-intestinal symptoms, he had noticed that he had passed considerable bright blood by rectum. His stools, however, had been constipated and he had considerable difficulty, on defecation, on account of hemorrhoids, he thought. It was subsequently discovered, from a son, that the patient had had marked frequency of several years' duration, associated with burning and pain on urination. This had been accompanied on several occasions by hematuria and the passage of gravel.

Past History.—What past history the patient could provide was irrelevant. He had no recollection of any childhood diseases and did not recall that he had ever been seriously ill previously.

Physical Examination.—Physical examination revealed an emaciated, elderly white male, who appeared moribund. His head was normal in contour. Eyes, ears, nose and throat were negative. Lungs were essentially negative. Heart sounds were of poor quality. Respirations were shallow. Blood pressure was 98/64. Abdomen: An irregular, firm, nodular, lemon-sized mass was felt in the right lower quadrant. It seemed fixed to the deep tissues. The prostate was enlarged and boggy. There was some edema of the lower extremities. Neurologic examination was essentially negative.

Laboratory Findings.—Urinalysis: Specific gravity 1.012; albumin 2 plus, red blood cells 2 plus. Blood urea nitrogen 250 mgm. on admission, which rose to 420 mgm. before death.

Subsequent Course.—The patient went rapidly downhill, into coma, and died in apparent uremia.

Autopsy Findings.—The body was that of an emaciated, elderly-appearing white male. In the right lower quadrant of the abdomen, apparently attached to the muscles and entirely retroperitoneal was a large, soft tumor mass measuring 8 cm. in diameter which surrounded the right iliac artery and ureter. The ureter above this mass was markedly dilated; the left ureter likewise was dilated throughout its course. The bladder was about the size of a man's fist, and relatively hard. The mass, on section, was seen to represent a metastatic retroperitoneal lymph node from a soft, yellowish necrotic tumor filling the entire bladder cavity when it was opened and inspected. On the anterior wall of the bladder, a craterform, ulcerated mass was seen representing the point of origin of the tumor. There was no apparent extension to the prostate or rectum. The kidneys were both somewhat enlarged. Their capsules stripped with difficulty because of several small whitish nodular lesions in the cortex to which they were adherent. The largest of these measured 1.5 cm. in diameter. On section, these suggested metastatic tumor tissue.

Microscopic Description of a Section from the Kidney.—(Fig. 316) (Ref. #S-10 and S-109) Histologically, the section shows a portion of the persistent kidney tissue which presents evidence of moderate arteriosclerosis of the medium sized vessels particularly. It is accompanied by some fibrosis of the glomeruli. Rather well demarcated from the kidney structure is seen a definite tumor. This is made up of small cords of hyperchromatic cells somewhat smaller than the usual tubular epithelial cells. There is some tendency toward the development of lumina, as if to form tubules. There is likewise a tendency toward papillary proliferation of these cells in many places. There is a very delicate connective tissue stroma with a corresponding capillary type of blood supply. There is no evidence of invasion of the kidney substance. The cells are uniform in size and regular in arrangement. This lesion represents a congenital, benign adenoma found incidentally and is not a metastatic tumor mass from the bladder cancer.

Diagnosis.—Bladder—malignant papilloma.

Microscopic Description of a Section from the Bladder Tumor.—(Fig. 568) (Ref. #S-50) Histologic examination of the tissue reveals a point where transition from the relatively normal mucosa to a typical undifferentiated rapidly growing papillary adenocarcinoma of the bladder is seen. In this tumor the cells still retain a considerable degree of differentiation so that they resemble for the most part the cells of origin. There is, however, some anaplasia with hyperchromatism of nuclei and cytoplasm. In addition, many mitotic figures may be observed. There is a relatively small amount of connective tissue stroma which develops as a core in each of the papillary masses. This tumor shows an inadequate blood supply and many areas of necrosis may be observed. The picture suggests origin from a benign papilloma, which over a period of time has gradually undergone the characteristic malignant change with invasion of the musculature and surrounding tissues so characteristic of this type of tumor.

Diagnosis.—Thyroid—fetal adenoma.

Patient was a white female, forty-three years of age, admitted to the hospital with the chief complaints of extreme nervousness, recent loss of weight, insomnia and excessive vaginal bleeding at her periods.

Present Illness.—Her present illness began about six years before admission. At that time, the patient was treated for hyperthyroidism by irradiation. She improved markedly for a time, but had had recurrent attacks of nervousness accompanied by palpitation at intervals. During the two years preceding admission, these symptoms were more marked. Her nervousness had been heightened by an "eczema" over the right ankle associated with severe itching of the skin. She stated that she had lost some thirty-five pounds during the past two months. She felt weak and was very easily upset emotionally. She had required sedatives almost daily to sleep. Her catamenia had always been irregular, but her flow had been more profuse during the preceding two years with the periods becoming increasingly close together.

Past History.—Her past history was irrelevant.

Physical Examination.—The patient appeared well developed and nourished. She was mentally clear, but seemed rather apprehensive and nervous. Her eyes were staring in appearance, associated with some slight exophthalmos. There was definite lid lag. There was a visible fullness in the thyroid region of the neck that extended down to the manubrium. This was symmetrical, firm in consistency without palpable nodules. No bruit was heard. Heart was slightly enlarged and its rate, rapid, ranging from 100 to 120. Lungs were negative. Extremities: There were numerous superficial varicosities of both lower legs. There was a macerated exfoliating lesion with several small ulcerated areas over the right lateral malleolus. The patient had had a basal metabolic rate of plus 23 previously and was put on Lugol's solution for ten days preoperatively.

Operative History.—A partial thyroidectomy was done.

Subsequent Course.—The patient improved steadily with the pulse rate falling to normal and her subjective symptoms likewise improving.

Pathological Report.—*Gross Description.*—Specimen consisted of three pieces of thyroid tissue, the largest measuring 6 x 4 x 2.5 cm. Two of these presented the rather typical appearance of a hyperplastic thyroid. They were beefy red in color, moderately firm in consistency and on section showed a diminution in colloid. The third fragment contained a tumor nodule occupying practically the entire mass. This showed a dense fibrous capsule which sharply demarcated it from the remaining thyroid tissue.

Microscopic Description.—(Fig. 317) Section histologically shows a tumor made up of irregular cords and interlacing trabeculae of rather hyperchromatic cuboidal epithelial cells somewhat reminiscent of adult thyroid epithelium. However, there is beginning acinar formation. No colloid is demonstrable. There is a moderate sinusoidal and capillary intertrabecular blood supply with a delicate connective tissue stroma. The capsule is composed of dense connective tissue which sharply demarcates the tumor from the surrounding structures. No mitotic figures are observed. The outlying thyroid tissue shows compression atrophy.

Case 136. (Ref. #S-232 and S-319)

Diagnosis.—Adrenal—benign, subclinical, cortical adenoma.

Patient was an Italian male of 39 years, who was admitted to the hospital because of an increase of central nervous symptoms resulting from a previous accident.

Present Illness.—His present illness began approximately one and one-half years before admission when he had fallen to the floor and hit his head. He was knocked unconscious and remained so for several hours. Subsequently he had persistent headache. Shortly thereafter, he developed paralysis of the left side. A diagnosis of subdural hemorrhage was made at that time, and a right subtemporal decompression was performed which gave him marked relief. A small draining sinus in the operative scar persisted, however, in spite of repeated operative procedures designed to close it. A few days before admission, he developed a complete left homonymous hemianopsia and marked diminution of visual acuity on the left.

Physical Examination.—The patient was a well-developed and fairly well-nourished middle-aged Italian male lying quietly in bed. His head was essentially normal in shape. There was a large scar area over the operative site, and in the middle of this was noted a small draining sinus, which was slightly moist with a thin, serous exudate. Eyes: There was marked sluggishness of the left pupil. The ears were negative. Nose and throat were negative. Chest was symmetrical. Heart and lungs appeared normal. There were no abnormalities of the breath sounds or of the heart sounds. Abdomen was negative. Extremities showed marked weakness of the left side, particularly of the leg.

Laboratory Findings.—Red blood cells, 4,200,000 with 81% hemoglobin. White blood cells, 14,800 with 87% polynuclears. Urinalysis was negative except for a slight trace of albumin. Spinal tap yielded a clear fluid with twelve cells, all lymphocytes. A diagnosis of probable brain abscess was made and a craniotomy done to drain the abscess area.

Subsequent Course.—The patient did well postoperatively for several days and then developed secondary meningitis and died one week later.

Autopsy Findings.—The general visceral pathology in this case was negative as far as significant pathology is concerned. The heart showed a terminal toxic myocarditis of mild grade but playing a part in his death. Liver, spleen, pancreas and kidney were negative. The adrenals were of practically normal size except for the presence of a small cortical adenoma on the right. This appeared as a large pea-sized nodule on the surface of the adrenal cortex. The cause of death was found to be a diffuse streptococcic meningitis arising by extension from the draining abscess cavity in the brain.

Microscopic Description of Section from the Adrenal Gland.—Section histologically through the adrenal gland shows for the most part a normal relationship of cortex and medulla. The various zones of the cortex can be well differentiated. In addition, however, there is a small, almost spherical nodular area in the cortex which is composed of cords of pale, vacuolated cells resembling essentially the normal adrenal cortex epithelium. These have a characteristic sinusoidal blood supply. No mitotic figures are noted. The cells appear somewhat larger than normal cells but in other respects show no evidence of any abnormality. Whether this degree of incidental cortical hyperplasia as an adenoma may have had any clinical significance is extremely doubtful.

Diagnosis.—Brain—abscess; *Streptococcus hemolyticus.*
Microscopic Description of Brain Abscess (Ref. #S-319.)—Cf. Fig. 649) Examination of the tissue histologically from the brain abscess shows a very striking suppurative liquefaction necrotic process with a cavity filled with broken-down leukocytes and cellular debris. By the Gram staining method, the presence of bacteria in short chains can be made out in the exudate. There is no very sharp line of demarcation between the abscess cavity and the brain substance where the leukocytic infiltration merges with the actual liquefaction necrosis. An attempt at glial proliferation is observed in some areas. In addition to the localized abscess may be observed a very acute encephalitis in those portions of brain at some little distance from the abscess cavity. Here, petechial hemorrhages are seen around blood vessels. Many vessels show thrombosis. There is considerable perivascular mantling of the vessels with the Virchow-Robin's spaces filled with inflammatory cells of all sorts. Degeneration of nerve cells is observed with swelling of the cytoplasm and a loss of nuclear detail, loss of Nissl granules and changes in the appearance of the dendritic processes and axones.

Diagnosis.—Breast—adenofibroma, intracanalicular and pericanalicular.

The history and microscopic description of a case of adenofibroma of the breast are given in Case 8. (Ref. #S-108) (Fig. 21), Chapter II.

A supplementary description of this benign adenomatous lesion at this point is perhaps indicated. It is believed that the tumor should be considered as one of glandular origin in spite of the enormous amount of connective tissue stroma which develops. The tumor arises from the glandular epithelium of the breast probably as an embryonic displacement of normal acinar epithelium, which failed to unite with its respective excretory duct. As a result it tends to proliferate independent of the gland as a whole and, as was observed in the original description, may show the same changes which take place in the normal breast with each menstrual cycle. With the inability to dispose of any secretory material, these glands act almost as a foreign body in producing connective tissue stimulation in the effort to wall them off and isolate them from the rest of the breast. This results either in a simple productive fibrosis around each acinus, the so-called pericanalicular type of adenofibroma; or as a diffuse fibrosis of the stroma as a whole with compression of the acini into tubular-like structures, the so-called intracanalicular type of fibro-adenoma of the breast.

CHAPTER XXXIII

TUMORS OF SURFACE EPITHELIAL ORIGIN

The tumors which arise from the surface epithelium of the skin or mucous membrane are generally spoken of as the *epitheliomata*. More particularly, this term has become applied to those malignant tumors specifically arising from the squamous epithelium of the skin. It is in this group of tumors that the most significant work in the gradation of malignancy has been accomplished.

BASAL CELL CARCINOMATA

The basal cell carcinomata represent a group of tumors which arise from the skin or the skin appendages, including the sweat glands, sebaceous glands and hair follicles. They represent a totally distinctive group of cases which run an entirely characteristic course. They arise from the basal cell layer of the skin epithelium and for that reason would appear to represent a particularly undifferentiated type of cell which by analogy to our mesoblastic tumors should be among the most malignant of our epithelial neoplasms. Practically, however, it is easy to demonstrate that these tumors instead of rating among the highly malignant are among the least malignant tumors of the entire carcinomatous group.

Rodent Ulcer.—The commonest variety of this type of tumor is the so-called "rodent ulcer," which appears most frequently on the face, especially around the nose and orbit. These tumors may occur anywhere on the body but are most frequently seen, aside from the face, on exposed areas such as the back of the hand, the foot, etc. The tumor grossly consists of a slightly elevated, localized lesion in the skin at the outset. If one looks at this microscopically it will be found that there is a marked proliferation of the basal layers downward which, however, all stop abruptly at a single level and which remain sharply demarcated from the deeper structures (see Fig. 318). The cells are small and compact, tending to be hyperchromatic, with little cytoplasm. Mitoses are only rarely encountered. There is no evidence of pigmentation in these tumors to confuse them with the nevi, which they somewhat resemble at the beginning of their course. They characteristically remain localized, extending from the central area very slowly, but have a tendency to invade locally after a long period of time. It is from this gnawing character of these tumors that the term "rodent ulcer" was derived. They are likely to ulcerate early and to become secondarily infected so that the infection is often a more serious matter than the original neoplasm. They rarely metastasize and when in the exceptional instances they do, it is usually by the lymphatic route to the regional lymph nodes. They are extremely radiosensitive and are likewise amenable to surgical removal, if in an accessible area. They show little or no tendency to recur. In the very aged, it is not uncommon to find dozens of these early basal cell types of lesions developing all over the skin of the face and neck region. These tumors may be disregarded from the mortality standpoint, as long as they are identified early and properly treated. If neglected, however, they may be extremely destructive locally and even become malignant.

Illustrative Case

CASE 137. (Ref. #S-112)

Diagnosis.—Basal cell carcinoma (rodent ulcer).

Patient was a white male of 63 years, who was admitted to the hospital because of an ulcerated lesion on his face, just lateral to the right orbit.

Present Illness.—This mass first appeared about two years before his admission, and had been slowly increasing in size. At the outset, it had simply seemed to be a somewhat pigmented, thickened layer of skin. This tended to desquamate slightly, and the patient had thought it was only some type of skin irritation. He had applied salves locally without any particular relief or improvement. It had never bothered him particularly from the symptomatic standpoint. About one year before admission, it had first shown evidence of breaking down with a central area of ulceration. The ulcerated nature of this

346

PLATE LXXVIII
TUMORS OF EPITHELIAL ORIGIN

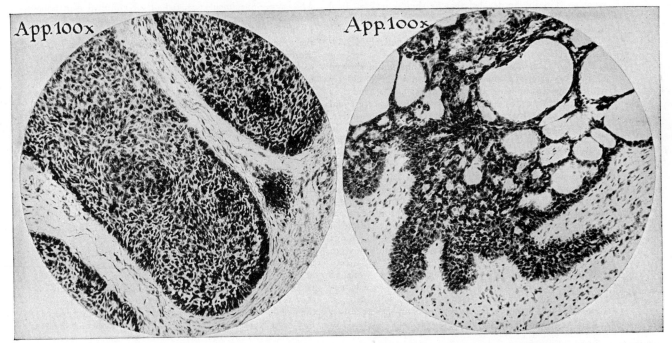

FIG. 318.—SKIN: BASAL CELL EPITHELIOMA (RODENT ULCER).—CASE 137.—Tumor composed of cells arising from basal layer of epithelium with their characteristic almost columnar appearance. Lesion is well defined with no evidence of invasion of the corium. App. 100 x.

FIG. 319.—SKIN: BASAL CELL EPITHELIOMA (ADENOID CYSTIC TYPE).—CASE 138.—Basal cell type of tumor, but with striking tendency toward pseudolumina formation. Cells uniform in size, hyperchromatic, well differentiated. Lesion is demarcated from corium by a pseudocapsule. App. 100 x.

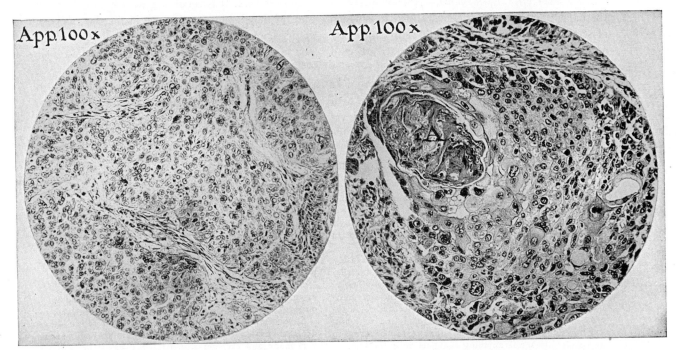

FIG. 320.—CERVIX UTERI: SQUAMOUS CELL (EPIDERMOID) CARCINOMA.—GRADE IV.—CASE 142.—Tumor composed of highly undifferentiated epithelial cells showing moderate pleomorphism, many mitoses, and invading uterine wall extensively. App. 100 x.

FIG. 321.—ESOPHAGUS: SQUAMOUS CELL (EPIDERMOID CARCINOMA.—GRADE III.—CASE 141.—Tumor shows marked malignancy. Cells are hyperchromatic, extremely pleomorphic with countless atypic mitoses and tumor giant cell formation. App. 100 x.

process had become more and more apparent as time went on. Finally, he decided that he should seek medical advice regarding the process because of its failure to heal under his own care.

Past History.—His past history was entirely irrelevant in relation to the present illness.

Physical Examination.—Physical examination showed a well developed, somewhat undernourished, elderly white male who did not appear acutely ill. His head was normal in contour. Eyes were negative. Pupils were equal and reacted normally. Nose and throat were negative. There was an ulcerated lesion approximately 2 cm. in diameter lateral to the orbit on the right side. This showed a central area of ulceration filled with a scablike mass of necrotic tissue and blood clot. The edges of the lesion were sharply demarcated and rather firm in consistency. The whole lesion was slightly elevated above the skin surface. The picture grossly presented the typical appearance of a basal cell carcinoma of the "rodent ulcer" type. The remainder of the physical examination was essentially negative and irrelevant. Heart and lungs were normal. Abdomen was negative. Extremities were normal.

Laboratory Findings.—Laboratory findings were of no significance. Red blood cells, 4,500,000 with 80% hemoglobin. White blood cells, 6,700 with 71% polynuclears. Urinalysis was negative. Blood Wassermann was negative.

Subsequent History.—The patient was advised to have the lesion excised because of its proximity to the orbit, rather than to have it treated by radiation therapy. This was done and an elliptical incision made with the removal of the lesion and the underlying subcutaneous tissue.

Adenoid Cystic Epithelioma.—A sub-variety of the basal cell type of carcinoma is seen in a lesion most commonly found in the eyelid, but which may occur generally in the skin. This is ordinarily a small tumor about the size of a large pea, which remains discrete for a long period of time (Fig. 319). It possesses the usual characteristic manner of growth of this group of tumors, however, with slow invasion of the tissues. Various theories regarding its

Pathological Report.—*Gross Description of Surgical Specimen.*—Specimen consisted of an elliptical skin fragment 3.5 cm. in length by 2.5 cm. in diameter. In the middle of this was a typical ulcerated epithelioma of the "rodent ulcer" type, which measured nearly 2 cm. in diameter. It was sharply demarcated from the underlying subcutaneous fat by a densely hyalinized-appearing layer of the corium.

Microscopic Description of Section Through the Ulcer.—(Fig. 318) Histologic examination of the tissue presents a large cellular nodule in the derma. The overlying epiderm is almost completely destroyed; just a few strands of flattened, hyalinized epithelium mark its site. Here, too, there are a number of mononuclear and polymorphonuclear leukocytes. Toward either side of the nodule the epiderm gradually takes on a more normal appearance and its component layers are easily recognizable. Its epithelial pegs are long and narrow. At one point they seem to fuse directly with one of the cellular masses, forming the tumor. The tumor itself is more or less circumscribed and almost completely globular; condensation of the surrounding connective tissue has formed a capsule; it is about 3 mm. in depth. It consists of irregularly-shaped accumulations of cells, the most peripheral of which are columnar elements arranged as they are in the rete layer or generative layer of the skin, the whole arrangement being that in which the generative cells were first evenly placed in position and the remaining cells of the mass later irregularly scattered within the space thus formed. All these cells possess reticular nuclei that stain very lightly. The nuclear membrane is thin. The nucleoli are small. Mitotic figures are rare. These cell masses are supported by a loose stroma.

origin are held. It is believed generally to arise from some of the glandular structures in the skin, and the cystic character of the tumor is the result of occlusion of small acinar structures formed by the tumor cells in their attempts to reproduce the structure of origin. No more serious significance need be given these tumors clinically than any of the other forms of basal cell tumors.

ILLUSTRATIVE CASE

CASE 138. (Ref. #S-229)

Diagnosis.—Skin—basal cell carcinoma (adenoid cystic type).

Patient was a sixty-one year old white male admitted to the hospital because of a small nodule about 2 cm. in diameter at the lateral end of the left eyebrow.

Present Illness.—The patient stated that this lesion began about two years ago and had been slowly increasing in size. It was slightly elevated, firm in consistency and showed no evidence of ulceration. It was not painful, but it had grown to such an extent that it interfered somewhat with his vision. A friend had told him that this might be cancer and for that reason he came to the hospital to see if anything could be done for him.

Past History.—The past history was entirely irrelevant.

Physical Examination.—Physical examination showed

a well-developed, well-nourished white male, apparently about sixty years of age. His head was normal in contour and entirely negative except for the small tumor in the left eyebrow, already described. Eyes, ears, nose and throat were entirely negative. He had two false dentures. Chest was symmetrical. Heart and lungs were apparently negative. Abdomen and extremities were negative.

Laboratory Findings.—Laboratory findings were unessential. Red blood count was normal. White blood cells, 9,200 with 67% polynuclears. Urinalysis was negative.

Subsequent Course.—A tentative pre-operative diagnosis of basal cell carcinoma of the cystic adenoid variety was made and excision advised. This was done, and six months post-operatively, nothing but a linear scar at the site of the operation could be demonstrated. There had been no evidence of a recurrence.

PLATE LXXIX
MALIGNANT TUMORS OF SURFACE EPITHELIUM
SQUAMOUS CELL (EPIDERMOID) CARCINOMATA OF VARYING GRADES OF MALIGNANCY

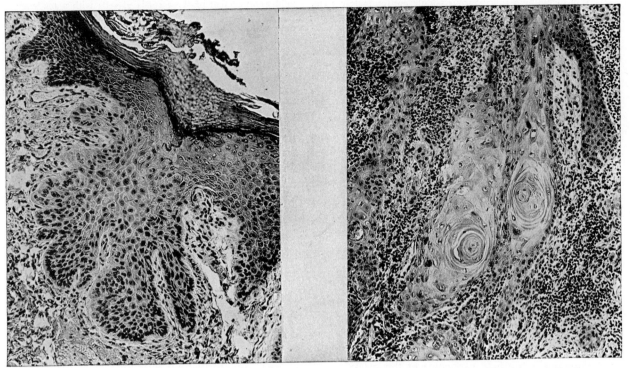

FIG. 322.—LIP: GRADE I.—CASE 139.—Hyperplasia of squamous cells, with exaggeration of rete pegs, nuclear hyperchromatism, beginning pleomorphism, occasional mitoses, probable beginning invasion of corium, but cells still largely differentiated with intercellular bridges. App. 100 x.

FIG. 323.—ANUS: GRADE II.—CASE 140.—Cells show more marked evidence of malignancy than in Fig. 322. Tongue-like masses of epithelium invading corium. Cells show striking effort at differentiation with prominent keratinization as "pearls." Moderate hyperchromatism of nuclei. App. 100 x.

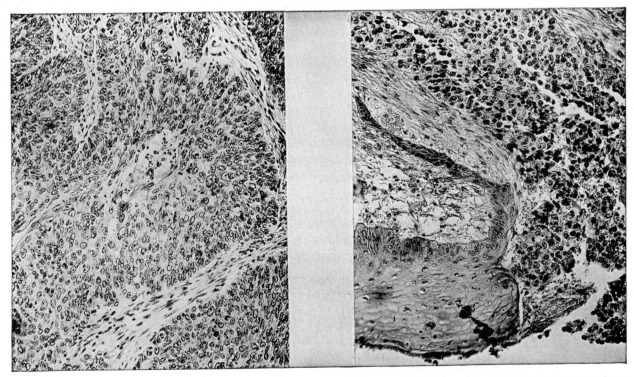

FIG. 324.—CERVIX UTERI: GRADE IV.—CASE 142 (cf. Fig. 320).—Solid nests and sheets of totally undifferentiated cells with atypical nuclei, prominent nucleoli, marked desmoplastic stromal reaction, and secondary inflammatory cellular infiltration. App. 100 x.

FIG. 325.—SKIN: ABDOMEN.—X-RAY CARCINOMA.—GRADE III.—CASE 143.—Section shows margin of tumor where relatively normal but thickened epithelium merges with poorly differentiated tumor tissue. Cells are large, hyperchromatic, with many mitoses. Picture complicated by ulceration. App. 100 x.

Pathological Report.—*Gross Description of Surgical Specimen.*—Specimen consisted of an elliptical section of skin including a subcutaneous nodule approximately 2 cm. in diameter. This was firmly united to the surface epithelium, but was sharply demarcated from the deeper subcutaneous tissues grossly.

Microscopic Description of Section Through Tumor. (Fig. 319) The tumor is found to be composed of cells arising from the basal layers of the epithelium. Cords of these cells are found extending well into the corium, but they remain sharply demarcated from the deeper tissues by a pseudocapsule of dense connective tissue. A feature of this particular lesion is the apparent cystic adenoid arrangement of these cords of cells with a tendency to form pseudolumina which become filled with a pale, pink-staining, almost homogeneous material representing serum. The cells are uniform in size, hyperchromatic in appearance, and show only rare mitotic figures which are normal in appearance. There is nothing noted microscopically to suggest actual malignant change, and the clinical history in this case bears out the diagnosis of a basal cell carcinoma of the cystic adenoid variety.

Sweat Gland Adenomata.—A third variety of tumor having its essential origin similarly from the basal layer cells is seen in the occasional sweat gland adenoma. These tumors are usually deeper in their location arising as they do from actual sweat gland epithelial cells, probably by displacement of such cells in the development of the gland. They are localized subcutaneous tumors usually adherent to the superficial skin, but freely movable in the deeper layers. On section, they are found to be made up of small round acini or arborescent glands having the characteristic double layer arrangement of the cells, with a well defined basal membrane. Rarely, such tumors may undergo frank malignant change and become true adenocarcinomata. More often, they remain as localized lesions with the usual characteristics of the basal cell group, except for the extraordinary faithfulness of glandula reproduction.

SQUAMOUS CELL (EPIDERMOID) CARCINOMATA

The most important group of surface epithelial tumors is that vast group of tumors generically classified as epidermoid or squamous carcinomata. These arise in many locations, the most important of which numerically are first, carcinoma of the cervix uteri; second, carcinoma of the lip and tongue in the male; and third, a miscellaneous group of cases involving the skin anywhere and the mucous membranes lining the larynx and esophagus most frequently.

In addition, there is another group of tumors found occurring in the bladder and the pelvis of the kidney, which arises from the lining mucous membranes as a transitional type of epithelium and is frequently spoken of as *transitional cell epitheliomata*. They may well be classified with the general group of squamous cell tumors.

In the group of epidermoid carcinomata, we find all gradations of differentiation from tumors showing marked keratinization and so-called epithelial "pearl" formation down to tumors made up of small undifferentiated cells in which the pavement epithelial origin is often almost indeterminate. The most benign form of this group of squamous cell carcinomata is the so-called *"acanthoma"* in which the actual intercellular bridges of the prickle cells of the skin can readily be made out. From this essentially benign lesion we pass through varying gradations of malignancy up to tumors in which extreme anaplasia, hyperchromatism and undifferentiation exist. In these more malignant forms, mitotic figures abound both as normal nuclear figures and with the development of abnormal multilobulated tumor giant cells (Fig. 320, 321, 322, 323, 324 and 325).

The outstanding characteristic histology of this entire group of tumors is their invasion of the underlying structures. Instead of the neat, orderly arrangement of the epithelial cells as noted in the basal cell type, we find irregular sized and shaped cords or sheets of cells extending down into the deep tissue, often actually invading muscle. Likewise, the tendency toward lymphatic extension both by direct growth along the lymphatics and by embolic involvement of the regional lymph nodes is the usual course of these tumors. In rare instances, even blood stream invasion may occur with a resultant generalized carcinomatosis and multiple visceral metastases.

No amount of description can cover the vast variation in the microscopic picture which one finds in these tumors. Another prominent feature of the usual histology of these tumors is seen in the appearance of the stroma. It has no definite morphologic neoplastic characteristics itself, but is apt to be diffusely infiltrated by inflammatory cells of all varieties. In certain locations, notably the cervix, this cellular infiltration is particularly prone to be eosinophilic to a high degree. The theory regarding the differences in tissue tension in respect to the development of the stroma and the invasion of the surrounding structures is of interest in this respect. Many pathologists feel that the desmoplastic reaction of the connective tissue stroma represents an equally important diagnostic phenomenon and feel that these connective tissue cells, in spite of their innocent appearance, possess biologic characteristics of malignancy.

Many of these tumors are of importance, not only because of their ultimately fatal neoplastic nature, but because of more immediate obstructive mechanical phenomena. This is obviously particularly true of those tumors involving the hollow viscera such as the larynx, esophagus, gastro-intestinal tract and bladder. Many patients die as the result of such obstruction or as the result of secondary infection following emergency surgical procedures.

From the standpoint of therapy, two courses are open to the physician. In many instances, surgery with the local excision of the lesion is adequate and gives permanent relief. In general, the earlier the diagnosis is established, the more likely surgical intervention will prove successful. The other method of treatment available is some form of irradiation. This is often the only method available because of the location of the particular tumor or the extent of the lesion. Roughly speaking, these tumors vary inversely in proportion to the differentiation of their

cells in their response to radiation. Paradoxically from the clinical standpoint, a tumor of Grade IV malignancy made up almost entirely of highly undifferentiated rapidly growing cells is perhaps more likely to respond successfully to intensive irradiation than is a tumor of much less marked malignant characteristics morphologically. The importance of pathological diagnosis and gradation of the degree of malignancy by histologic methods from a biopsy specimen of the tumor becomes apparent in relation to the above statement. It should be the responsibility of the pathologist, on the basis of his diagnosis, to make recommendation as to the preferable form of therapy and, in a general way, if irradiation is recommended, to indicate the approved method and dosage.

The entire group of epidermoid carcinomata, regardless of gradation, has a tendency to develop more and more marked malignant characteristics as time goes on. In no group of tumors is it more important for early diagnosis to be established and therapy to be instituted if we are to continue to reduce the mortality from this most serious and numerically most common type of cancer.

ILLUSTRATIVE CASES

CASE 139. (Ref. #S-320)

Diagnosis.—Squamous cell carcinoma (epidermoid carcinoma), Grade I.

Patient was a white male of 39 years, who was admitted to the hospital because of a small lump on his lower lip for about one year.

Present Illness.—The present illness began about one year preceding admission, when he noticed a small, pimple-like nodule on the left side of his lower lip. He went to a physician who removed it surgically. Three months later it had recurred and was somewhat larger. He returned to his physician who again removed the lesion locally. About one month before admission it began to recur again and he decided to come to the hospital for treatment.

Past History.—The patient had scarlet fever as a child, but none of the other childhood diseases so far as he was aware. He never had any serious illness. A review of his systems was essentially negative. He was married and had two children. The only etiological factor which he could think of in conjunction with the development of this lesion was the fact that he was an almost constant pipe smoker for many years. He had given it up, however, since the first appearance of the lesion.

Physical Examination.—The patient was a well developed, well nourished adult male who showed no abnormal physical findings. Head was negative. Eyes, ears, nose and throat were normal. Tonsils were present but showed no gross evidence of significant pathology. Teeth were in fair condition. The left lower lip showed a small

lesion approximately 1 cm. in diameter. There was a very slight suggestion of umbilication centrally with a small crust suggesting possible beginning ulceration. The mass was freely movable and not adherent to the deeper structures. No enlargement of the regional lymph nodes was noted. Heart and lungs were normal. Abdomen was negative. Extremities were negative.

Laboratory Findings.—Blood count and urinalysis were both of negative significance.

Subsequent Course.—He was advised to have the lesion removed and a follow-up course of radiation applied. A wedge-shaped mass was removed from the left lower lip measuring about 2 x 3 cm.

Microscopic Description of Surgical Specimen.— (Fig. 322) The stratified squamous epithelium is hyperplastic, with thickening and elongation of the interpapillary pegs. The basement membrane is intact. The cells of the germinal layer show nuclear irregularities with increase in the size and number of nucleoli and a few mitotic figures, all of which appear to be regular. The corium contains sweat-glands, salivary gland tissue and hair follicles. The corium is infiltrated with round cells most of which are plasma cells. At least one area is definitely neoplastic. On close scrutiny, intercellular bridges and even an attempt at pearl formation are revealed.

CASE 140. (Ref. #S-321)

Diagnosis.—Squamous cell carcinoma (epidermoid carcinoma), Grade II.

Patient was a white female of 58 years, admitted to the

hospital because of a large mass around the anal orifice.

Present Illness.—About three years before admission, the patient noticed an irritation around the anal orifice on defecation. She had paid no particular attention to this at the outset, believing it to be a hemorrhoid. However, she found that slowly there was a thickened plaque-like mass which developed at the site of the irritation. The lesion had bled on numerous occasion. She had had no treatment for it other than local application of ointments on the recommendation of her druggist. Recently, she had noted that the mass had increased considerably in size and was much more painful than it had been previously. It had been bothering her considerably, even on walking.

Past History.—She believed she had all the ordinary diseases of childhood, and influenza in the 1918 epidemic. Otherwise, she had had no serious illness. She had been married, but her husband died of cardiac disease. Two children were living and well. A review of her systems was essentially negative. She had no more than the usual number of mild upper respiratory infections. Her cardiovascular system was negative. She had occasional attacks of qualitative dyspepsia and for the past twenty years had suffered from marked constipation, which she believed was responsible for the development of the anal lesion.

Physical Examination.—Physical examination showed a well-developed, well-nourished, elderly white female lying comfortably in bed. Head was normal in shape. Eyes, ears, nose and throat were negative. She had a slight enlargement of the thyroid bilaterally. Lungs were clear throughout. Heart was not enlarged and there were no murmurs. Abdomen showed no tenderness and no palpable masses. Extremities were negative. In the anal region, there was a plaque about 3 cm. in diameter along the right aspect of the sphincter. It was not particularly tender or painful on palpation. It was elevated approximately 1.5 cm. above the remainder of the skin surface. The edges of this mass were of almost cartilaginous hardness. Centrally, some umbilication and a small area of erosion were noted.

Laboratory Findings.—Blood count and urinalysis were of no significance.

Subsequent Course.—The patient was advised to have the lesion excised locally and this to be followed by a course of radiation postoperatively. This was done. The mass was removed by a large wedge-shaped excision and sent to the laboratory for diagnosis.

Pathological Report.—*Gross Description of Surgical Specimen.*—Specimen consisted of an irregularly wedge-shaped piece of tissue measuring 3.5 cm. on the surface and about 1 cm. at the base. There was a thickened plaque of tissue approximately 1 cm. in thickness, which faded out into the deeper tissues as infiltrating bands of grayish-white. There was some superficial ulceration with a crust adherent to the surface.

Microscopic Description of Section Through the Tumor.—(Fig. 323) Histologic examination of the tissue presents the typical picture of a squamous carcinoma of low grade malignancy. The tumor is found to be made up of cells which show a very striking tendency toward keratinization, the entire superficial layer being made up of keratinized cells. Toward the base of the lesion, the tumor tissue may be seen infiltrating the subcutaneous fat as tongue-like masses of cells. Even deep in the tissue there is a striking tendency for keratinization with

typical pearl formation. The pearls are made up of concentrically arranged epithelial cells which centrally show this keratinizing feature. In addition, many definite prickle cells with their intercellular bridges may be recognized. There is a moderate amount of pleomorphism with occasional atypical mitotic figures. The basal layer of these malignant cells is fairly well maintained, although in places it has definitely broken through. The entire process is accompanied by a very extensive secondary inflammatory lesion with polynuclear and mononuclear cellular infiltration. There is, likewise, secondary productive fibrosis as a result of the combined neoplastic and inflammatory irritation.

CASE 141. (Ref. #S-111)

Diagnosis.—Esophagus—squamous cell carcinoma, Grade III, with extension to trachea.

Patient was a colored male of 59 years, admitted to the hospital because of difficulty in swallowing.

Present Illness.—The patient's present condition began at least five years before his present admission at which time he first noticed some difficulty in swallowing. He was seen by his family physician, who referred him to a hospital for x-ray studies and treatment. No particular improvement followed a series of x-ray treatments, and his symptoms persisted tending to increase in severity. He gradually developed inability to swallow solid foods and was only able to take liquids. This he felt accounted very largely for the fact that he had lost over fifty pounds of weight.

Past History.—His past history was irrelevant and unreliable.

Physical Examination.—The patient was a fairly well developed, emaciated, elderly colored male. Head was normal in contour. Pupils reacted normally. Ears were normal. Nose was negative. Buccal cavity was negative but there was considerable congestion of his posterior pharynx. There was marked swelling of the neck, chiefly in the midline but extending somewhat more to the right. On palpation a mass could be felt more or less fusiform in outline but not definitely encapsulated, and integral with the tissues of the neck. The skin over this area showed moderate pigmentation, the result of x-ray therapy. Chest was symmetrical. Lungs showed a few crepitant râles but no dullness. Heart sounds were normal. Abdomen was scaphoid. There were no palpable masses. Genitalia and extremities were normal.

Laboratory Findings.—Red blood cells, 3,400,000 with 68% hemoglobin. White blood cells, 12,600 with 74% polynuclears. Urinalysis was negative.

Subsequent Course.—The patient was given another course of x-ray treatments, and it was planned to do a gastrotomy when he suddenly developed a diffuse bronchopneumonia and died after three days of illness.

Autopsy Findings.—Autopsy revealed a tumor which apparently took its origin from the first portion of the trachea. This extended to completely surround the esophagus and had produced an ulcerative fistulous tract between the esophagus and trachea. The lungs showed a diffuse, patchy bronchopneumonia with beginning abscess formation. The regional lymph nodes all showed metastatic tumor tissue. The remainder of the viscera showed nothing of significance.

Microscopic Description of a Section of Tumor from the Esophagus.—(Fig. 321) The major portion of the section is composed of masses of tumor cells with a definite and fairly abundant stroma made up of loosely arranged fibrous tissue, some of which is undergoing myxomatous degeneration. There is a small amount of involuntary muscle observed near one surface. Along this same surface may be seen normal stratified epithelium. This merges with the definite neoplastic process in which the tumor cells show rather striking pleomorphism and occasional mitotic figures. There is considerable variation in the size of the cells. There is a tendency in certain areas for the cells to be arranged in somewhat laminated fashion and to show definite keratinization. Such epithelial pearl formation is rather striking for a tumor apparently arising from the tracheal mucosa and establishes fairly definitely an oesophageal origin for the lesion. No basement membrane can be found. There is definite evidence of infiltration of the tumor cells into the musculature and connective tissue of the esophagus.

CASE 142. (Ref. #S-322)

Diagnosis.—Squamous cell carcinoma of the cervix (Grade IV).

Patient was a white married female of 42 years, who was admitted to the hospital because of severe bleeding from the vagina associated with pain.

Present Illness.—The present illness dated back nearly two years. At that time she noticed that her menses, which previously had been regular, became prolonged and the intermenstrual period markedly irregular. She went to a physician who ascribed these symptoms to the beginning of her menopause, and on physical examination found evidence of fibroids, which were treated by radium implantation and irradiation with marked improvement. Approximately one year went by when she again developed vaginal bleeding and a recurrence of right lower quadrant pain. This tended to radiate to the lumbar region. Examination at this time revealed the presence of a fungating growth from the cervical canal.

Past History.—She had had the usual childhood diseases, including diphtheria and scarlet fever at the age of seven. She never had any other serious illness. She had been married for twenty years and had had seven children all of whom were living and well. She had never had any previous operative history. A review of her systems was essentially negative. Her menstrual history began at the age of thirteen and was always regular up to the onset of the present illness.

Physical Examination.—The patient was a well-developed, obese, middle-aged white female. Head was negative. Eyes, ears, nose and throat were normal except for very poorly kept teeth. Chest was symmetrical. Lungs were clear. Heart was not enlarged and showed no murmurs. Abdomen was pendulous. There was no tenderness. No masses could be felt. Extremities were negative.

Laboratory Findings.—There was a moderate anemia present. Red blood cells, 3,320,000 with 69% hemoglobin. White blood cells, 6,850 with 67% polynuclears. Urinalysis was negative. Blood Wassermann was negative.

Gynecologic examination was done in conjunction with a curettage and an ulcerated, fungating, cauliflower-like growth was found growing from the anterior wall of the cervical canal. Tissue was taken for pathological diagnosis.

Subsequent History.—The uterine cavity was curetted and 100 mgm. of radium were inserted in two capsules

of 50 mgm. each; one in the fundus and the other in the cervical canal for twenty-four hours. One week later, fifty additional milligrams of radium were inserted into the cervical canal and six radium needles implanted in the cervix itself, surrounding the tumor mass.

The patient went on for five months developing a rectovaginal fistula with a gangrenous cystitis. A metastatic tumor was found by x-ray in the right lung. The patient went steadily downhill, finally dying as a result of complications and metastasis associated with carcinomatosis.

Autopsy Findings.—There was carcinoma of the cervix with extension to the body of the uterus; a rectovaginal fistula; stenosis of the ureters with resultant bilateral hydronephrosis, and an abscess of the right lobe of the liver. There was a metastatic tumor in the right lower lobe of the lung and along the retroperitoneal, perivertebral and pelvic lymph nodes.

Microscopic Description of Original Biopsy Specimen from Cervix.—(Fig. 320 and 324) Histologic examination of the tissue presents evidence of a typical surface epithelial type of carcinoma which should be classified as of Grade IV malignancy. The cells are arranged in nests and sheets with little suggestion of differentiation. There is no keratinization and no pearls are noted. The tumor is found extensively in the musculature. There is marked superficial ulceration with a very intense cellular infiltration of the surrounding tissue. There is a thrombosis of several of the medium-sized vessels.

CASE 143. (Ref. #S-323)

Diagnosis.—Skin—squamous cell carcinoma, Grade III.

Patient was a white married housewife fifty-eight years of age, admitted to the hospital complaining of an ulcerated area of her abdominal wall following x-ray therapy.

Present Illness.—Patient had a history of six pregnancies, with all but first child weighing from twelve to seventeen pounds at birth. Following last pregnancy patient bled excessively every two or three weeks. Her physician said the uterus had not involuted properly and advised x-ray therapy which was given at weekly intervals for five years, without controlling hemorrhage until the end of the five year period. Shortly after starting x-ray treatments "red spots" appeared on the abdomen. Three years before admission, when bathing, skin rubbed off one of these areas. This exfoliation increased in extent and would not respond to local application of various types. Eight months before admission a large mass appeared in the ulcerated area which had spread continuously in size.

Past History.—Excellent health until age of twenty-one. In 1923 had influenza. At that time also had indefinite pain in right lower quadrant. Saw a physician who discovered a mild diabetes and she was put on a diabetic diet with considerable fluctuation of weight. Urine examined every six months since and diabetes thought to be under control. No other information given in history.

Laboratory Findings.—Urine: sp.g., 1.028; albumin, slight trace. Sugar present. Blood: red blood cells, 2,760,000. Hemoglobin, 6 gm. White blood cells, 7,546. Blood chemistry: 250 mgm. sugar.

Subsequent Course.—Patient was prepared for operation by controlling her diabetes with insulin. Excision of the abdominal wall mass was done under spinal anesthesia and a plastic closure performed.

Pathological Report.—*Gross Description of Surgical Specimen.*—Specimen consisted of three pieces of tissue representing the several margins of the ulcerated lesion.

Microscopic Description of a Representative Skin Area Through the Ulcerated Lesion.—(Fig. 325) At one side of the section, the floor of an ulcerated lesion is observed covered by necrotic cellular detritus and fibrin. Beneath this inflammatory exudate, however, definite granulation tissue is observed. Along the margins of this granulation are seen typical neoplastic cells which merge with a definite squamous cell type of carcinoma, which occupies the surface area on the edge of the ulcer. Near the periphery somewhat thickened but fairly normal stratified epithelium may be seen. For the most part, the tumor tissue is formed by masses of immature epithelial cells. They are round or oval in form and show little cohesion. There is no preservation of the intercellular spines. Huge disproportionately sized nuclei with rather delicate nuclear membranes and a liberal scattering of fine chromatin particles are found. Most of the cells show large metachromatic nuclei. Areas of attempted keratinization and pearl formation are seen. Mitotic figures, both typical and atypical are noted. The stroma is relatively avascular and hyalinized, the result of the irradiation.

CHAPTER XXXIV

TUMORS OF GLANDULAR ORIGIN OR ADENOCARCINOMATA

(Illustrated by a Series of Malignant Tumors of the Breast)

In the preceding chapters, we have considered the benign tumors of epithelial origin and the malignant tumors arising from various types of surface epithelium. In this chapter, a consideration of the malignant tumors arising from glandular epithelium will be presented. A series of cases taken from the various forms of cancer of the breast is presented to illustrate the several types of such tumors which may arise and whose counterparts may be seen in most of the other glandular organs. Certain of the other viscera, however, give rise to rather special types of carcinomata which will be discussed in the following chapters.

Tumors of the breast may be divided first of all into those arising from the duct epithelium and those arising from the acinar epithelium itself. This is likewise true of other glandular organs having a duct system such as the liver and the pancreas. In the breast, the tumors which arise from the duct epithelium far outnumber those derived from the acinar cells. This ratio is not as striking in some of the other viscera as we shall see in the section devoted to a consideration of the special pathology of these organs individually.

The histologic picture which carcinoma of the breast presents is almost infinite in its variation. This renders a classification of these neoplasms extremely difficult at times and makes it almost impossible to estimate with any exactness the degree of gradation of malignancy unlike the case in respect to the sur-

face epithelial tumors. Attempts at grading the breast carcinomata have been notoriously unsuccessful except in a very broad way, indicating a relatively low grade or a definitely high grade of malignancy. Even by this method of gradation many discrepancies will occur in the clinical results at the end of any five-year period, which is the established time unit for the determination of a so-called "cure."

From a practical standpoint, it is comparatively simple to classify the malignant tumors of the breast into the following major groups:

1. CARCINOMA SIMPLEX
   (a) SCIRRHOUS
   (b) MEDULLARY
2. ADENOCARCINOMA
3. COLLOID OR MUCOUS CARCINOMA
4. PAGET'S DISEASE

These all actually being derived from acinar or duct epithelium must be considered in the broad sense as variants of the adenocarcinomata. It is furthermore possible to subdivide the second group of so-called "adenocarcinomata" into a considerable number of subvarieties such as comedocarcinoma, inflammatory carcinoma and so forth. No good purpose is served in this discussion to elaborate on the basic nature of the malignant process. The student is referred to the more complete discussions of these tumors as they may be found in Cheatle and Cutler's monograph.

CHRONIC CYSTIC MASTITIS

In any consideration of the tumors of the breast, the problem of chronic cystic mastitis must be taken into account. As a precursor of many cases of cancer of the breast, we have a history of the development of a chronic inflammatory lesion, which is seen much more frequently in women who have borne children. It is thought to be the result largely of inflammatory

occlusion of ducts with milk stasis, resulting in the accumulation of secretion within the duct or acinus or to cyclic changes. This is followed usually by a hyperplasia of the lining epithelium which assumes a cuboidal form and stains intensely, as a rule, with eosin. In many instances, compensatory attempts at function are seen in the proliferation of these cells

PLATE LXXX
TUMORS OF GLANDULAR EPITHELIAL ORIGIN

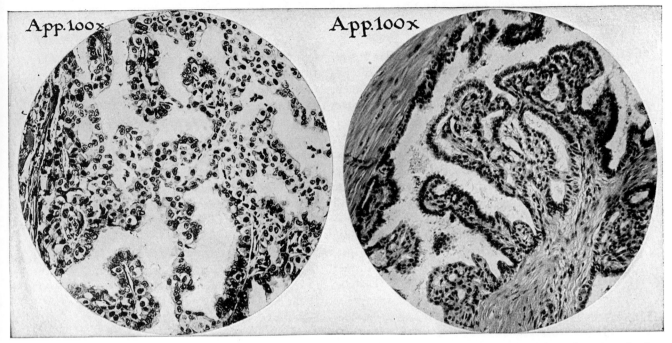

FIG. 326.—BREAST: INTRADUCTILE PAPILLOCARCINOMA.—CASE 147. —Tumor composed of proliferating duct epithelium thrown up into plicated folds and showing secondary acinar formation. Cells atypic in appearance with prominent nucleoli, moderate pleomorphism and occasional mitotic figures. Early invasion of duct wall is present. App. 100 x.

FIG. 327.—OVARY: PAPILLARY CYSTADENOMA.—CASE 247.—Section from wall of ovarian cyst showing papillary proliferation of lining epithelial cells with secondary pseudoacinar production. Cells are uniform in size; mitoses are absent; no evidence of invasion is seen. App. 100 x.

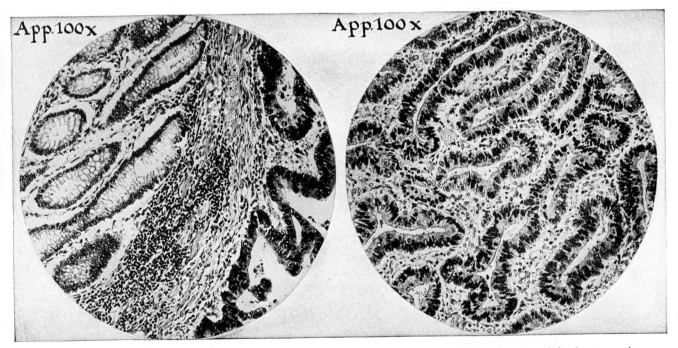

FIG. 328 and 329.—SIGMOID: ADENOCARCINOMA.—GRADE II.—In Fig. 328 the normal mucosa is seen at the left, the tumor tissue at the right. In Fig. 329 the character of the tumor is better observed. The acinar arrangement is well preserved, but the cells are large, with hyperchromatic nuclei and prominent nucleoli. Stroma is moderate in amount and infiltrated secondarily by inflammatory cells. App. 100 x.

even to form papillae. Frequently such spaces will be lined by these cells four and five deep instead of the usual single layer. This suggests a work hypertrophy with a functional exhaustion of the cell. Similar changes may be noted in other glandular organs, particularly in the thyroid in involuted glands following hyperthyroidism. The basement membrane in these cases of chronic cystic mastitis remains intact and there is no evidence of invasion of the surrounding interstitial normal breast stroma. This, however, may show considerable chronic mononuclear cellular inflammatory infiltration. For the novice this represents one of the most difficult lesions to differentiate from true tumor and, indeed, for the experienced pathologist it frequently offers difficulty in interpretation as to where benignancy ends and malignancy begins.

Many cases of chronic cystic mastitis are further confused by the fact that this hyperplastic glandular epithelium is prone to follow the cyclic changes of the breast associated with the menstrual cycle. This fact is frequently overlooked by the clinician and pathologist alike. Many breasts have been removed following biopsy examination of small nodules palpated in the breast and diagnosed as early carcinoma by the pathologist unfamiliar with this picture. On the other hand, it is true that in a certain number of cases of chronic cystic mastitis there is a stage which we may term *"precancerous."* This represents a clinical stage between the transitional period of simple inflammatory hyperplasia and the malignant change of these epithelial cells. Fortunately, only a very small percentage of such cases of chronic cystic mastitis actually undergo such malignant change. Opinions vary as to the percentage, but chronic cystic mastitis is one of the commonest lesions found in the female breast, whereas cancer is seen in only a relatively small percentage of individuals. Certainly not every case of cancer is preceded by this picture of chronic cystic degeneration as will be emphasized in the following paragraphs which represent rather typical clinical histories.

ILLUSTRATIVE CASE

CASE 144. (Ref. #S-113)

Diagnosis.—Breast—chronic cystic mastitis (Schimmelbusch disease).

Patient was a white woman of 42 years, admitted to the hospital because of a mass in her left breast.

Present Illness.—The patient stated that there had been a mass in her left breast for nearly three years. At first it had been stationary in size, but more recently it had seemed to be slowly increasing. A similar, but smaller, mass had been noted in the right breast and this also seemed to have increased somewhat. Neither lesion had been associated with any pain.

Past History.—The patient believed she had had all the usual childhood diseases. She had had no serious illness previously to require hospitalization. A review of her systems was essentially negative. She had had occasional mild upper respiratory infections. Gastro-intestinal history was the usual one of chronic constipation. Her genito-urinary history was negative. Menses had begun at the age of twelve and had been regular up to the present time, except during her several pregnancies. She had had six children, all living and well.

Physical Examination.—Physical examination showed a well developed and nourished middle-aged woman, who presented no evidence of disease other than the local breast pathology. Head was normal in contour. Eyes, ears, nose and throat were negative. Chest was symmetrical. Lungs were clear. Heart was not enlarged and showed no murmurs. Abdomen was moderately obese. No masses could be felt. Extremities were negative. Gynecologic examination revealed no pathology of the uterus or adnexae, other than a laceration of the cervix on the left. Both breasts were moderately enlarged, fatty and dependent. The left showed a generalized diffuse nodular enlargement of the glandular elements. This seemed to involve the entire breast. Several distinctly lobulated masses could be felt in the right breast. Some of these gave a sensation of fluctuation. Some were of such extreme density that they raised the question of possible malignancy. A tentative diagnosis of chronic cystic mastitis (Schimmelbusch disease) was made and left mastectomy advised.

Subsequent Course.—A simple left mastectomy was done. No enlargement of the axillary lymph nodes was noted at the time of operation.

Pathological Report.—*Gross Description of Surgical Specimen.*—Specimen consisted of a large breast measuring 15 x 12 x 10 cm. with overlying skin which appeared normal and showed no attachment to the deeper structures. The nipple and areola were normal. On section of the breast tissue there was noted a diffuse cystic degeneration of the glandular structures. These cysts varied in size from one to two millimeters up to cysts measuring 2.5 cm. Some of these were filled with clear fluid; others with a serosanguineous appearing material while others were gelatinoid in consistency. The stroma of this breast tissue appeared markedly increased in density.

Microscopic Description of Section Through the Breast.—(Fig. 332 and 333) Histologic examination of the breast tissue shows glandular structures of varying sizes. There is a marked hyperplasia of the lining epithelium which in many places is heaped up to several layers. Secondary acini formation is noted in these hyperplastic areas. The basal membrane appears intact everywhere in all the sections taken from this breast, and there is no definite evidence of malignant change. The cells, however, are hyperchromatic, relatively undifferentiated and suggest a potential precancerous state. Nothing can be found microscopically to suggest actual

PLATE LXXXI

TUMORS AND PSEUDOTUMORS OF THE BREAST

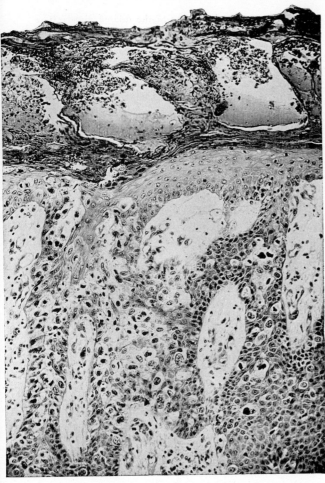

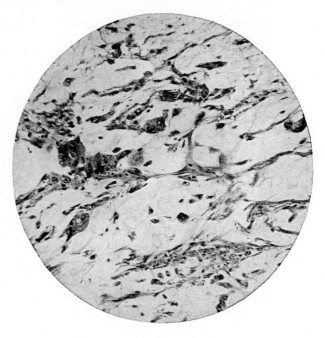

FIG. 330.—PAGET'S DISEASE.—CASE 149.—Crusted, eczematous surface exudate overlying the skin. At upper right, relatively normal epithelium is seen merging with typical tumor tissue below. Numerous large, pale, vacuolated Paget cells with atypical, hyperchromic nuclei abound. App. 100 x.

FIG. 331.—"COLLOID" CARCINOMA.—CASE 148.—Tumor cells seen in small groups within masses of mucinous material embedded in a connective tissue stroma. Nuclei are relatively small with prominent nucleoli. Cytoplasm is indefinite as a result of the excessive mucin production. App. 100 x.

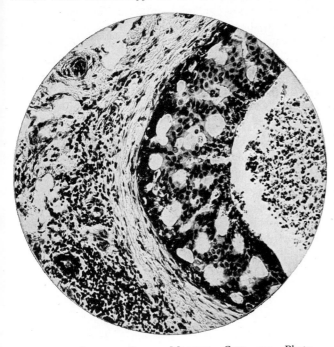

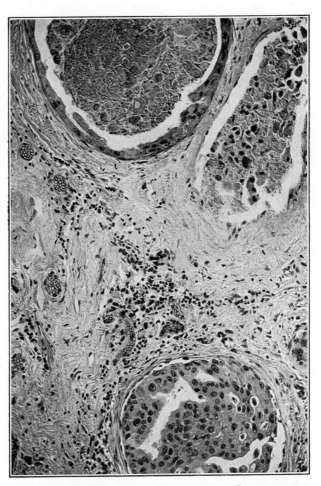

FIG. 332.—CHRONIC CYSTIC MASTITIS.—CASE 144.—Photomicrograph showing edge of a small cyst. Note intraductile proliferation of epithelium with secondary pseudo-acinar formation, and detritus in lumen. Wall of cyst shows marked lymphocytic cellular infiltration. App. 100 x.

FIG. 333.—CHRONIC CYSTIC MASTITIS WITH CARCINOMATOUS DEVELOPMENT.—Cf. CASE 144.—Area illustrated emphasizes the intraductile hyperplasia characteristic of cystic disease of the breast. Cells are large, atypical and in this instance have invaded the stroma. Note desmoplasia and chronic inflammatory cellular infiltration. App. 100 x.

invasion of the breast substance. There is a diffuse fibrosis of the stroma associated with considerable chronic mononuclear cellular infiltration around the acini. Many monocytes are found in some of the dilated glands. The picture is one of simple chronic cystic mastitis, but presenting many of the features of a precancerous state.

CARCINOMA SIMPLEX

The term "carcinoma simplex" is one which we would do well to eliminate from the literature as it is misleading. By this term we mean the development of a carcinoma arising from the cuboidal epithelium of solid glands. The commonest site for such tumors is seen in the breast. Actually, we are dealing with a form of adenocarcinoma because the tumors are derived from glandular or tubular epithelium. The outstanding characteristic of such tumors is their failure when malignant to develop the characteristic acinar arrangement of a more definitive adenocarcinoma. It is of clinical convenience to pathologically differentiate these more solid tumors of the breast from the true glandular carcinomata rather than insist on an exact terminology.

Scirrhous Carcinoma.—This is the commonest tumor of the breast and occupies the first place numerically in carcinoma occurring in women. It usually occurs in the upper outer quadrant of the breast where it forms a small dense nodule. The great majority of these tumors are painless at the outset and frequently escape observation for long periods of time, often being found accidentally. As the tumor increases in size, it tends to become fixed to the deep fascia and later to the skin, and frequently to the nipple itself. This results in a curious "orange rind" or "pigskin" appearance of the skin overlying the tumor, and of retraction of the nipple. The tumor usually occurs in the age group past the menopause with the most common age incidence being between 45 and 60. Cases have been reported in adolescents and occasionally are seen in young women during the child-bearing age. Such tumors are usually more likely to be of the medullary and rapidly-growing rather than the scirrhous slow-growing type.

It was from the characteristic gross appearance of such scirrhous tumors that the term, "carcinoma" (crab-like), was derived (Fig. 334). On section of such a tumor grossly, one finds a dense nodule varying in size from perhaps a few millimeters to larger lesions a few centimeters in diameter. These are irregular in outline and show ramifications which may extend along the lymphatics and fascial planes for long distances into the substance of the breast,

invading the fat and connective tissue stroma extensively. This is quite different from the benign circumscribed adenofibroma, the only point of similarity of these two tumors being at times their density. On section one can make out the dense scirrhous trabeculated stroma of the tumor. Indeed, it resembles a fibrous tissue tumor more than it does a true carcinoma. Grossly between the trabeculae, however, one may find small yellowish areas representing the hyperplastic epithelial elements and these may be associated with actual foci of necrosis.

Histologically, such tumors show a dense hyalinized connective tissue stroma between the strands of which nests of pyknotic small epithelial cells may be identified. At times these occur in cords (Fig. 337). In other areas, only two or three cells may be visible. No acinar arrangement is noted. Mitoses are difficult to find and are frequently absent. The characteristic invasiveness of the tumor into the surrounding breast tissue is perhaps as characteristic as anything histologically in relation to this type of tumor. At first glance and without experience one might underestimate the significance of this comparatively insignificant lesion and even fail to recognize its malignant qualities. It is, however, a most persistent tumor and simple excision is rarely if ever adequate. Because of its extreme density and great amount of connective tissue stroma, this particular type of carcinoma of the breast is also radioresistant, requiring massive doses to produce any effect.

The malignancy of these tumors may be said to be inversely proportional to the age with many exceptions to the rule. The later in life, however, that one of these tumors appears, the less malignant its course, as evidenced by the history in Case 145 (Ref. #S-251) of an elderly woman who was known to have had her tumor for over fifteen years before operation. The danger of this type of scirrhous carcinoma is not in the local lesion, but through its characteristic habit of metastasizing by direct lymphatic extension or embolic extension to the regional axillary lymph nodes. This may even proceed through the lymphatic plexuses and lead to intra-abdominal metastasis. In addition, we find direct extension to the pectoral muscles and even

PLATE LXXXII
MALIGNANT TUMORS OF GLANDULAR EPITHELIAL ORIGIN
Carcinoma (Simplex) of the Breast

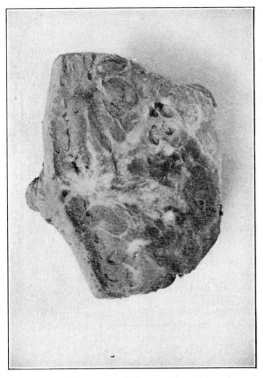

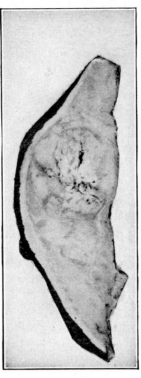

Fig. 334.—Scirrhous Carcinoma.—Case 145.—Gross photograph of cross section through breast showing dense tumor mass arising in ducts beneath nipple and extending in typical "crab-like" fashion through breast substance.

Fig. 335 and 336.—Medullary (Encephaloid) Carcinoma.—Case 146.—Gross photograph of large, soft, grayish-pink tumor, as seen in cross section, involving almost the entire breast, but seemingly rather sharply demarcated from the surrounding tissues.

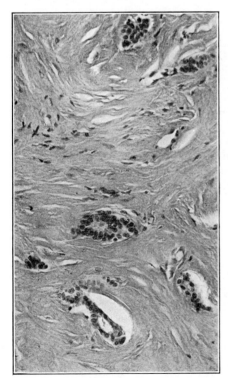

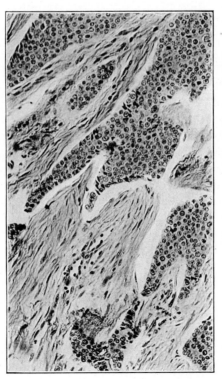

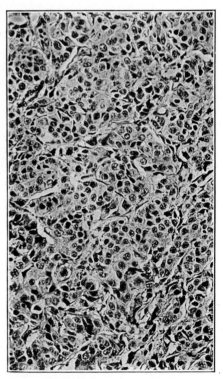

Fig. 337.—Scirrhous Carcinoma.—Case 145.—Photomicrograph of Fig. 334 showing characteristic dense, hyalinized connective tissue stroma with rare clumps of compressed, small, hyperchromatic epithelial cells. Mitoses are rare. A suggestion of acinar arrangement is present. App. 100 x.

Fig. 338.—Carcinoma Simplex.—Photomicrograph illustrating the difficulty in differentiation of the scirrhous and medullary forms of carcinoma of the breast. Both scirrhous and medullary features may be observed in this field. App. 100 x.

Fig. 339.—Medullary Carcinoma.—Case 146.—Photomicrograph of Fig. 335 and 336 showing a rapidly growing, highly undifferentiated cell tumor growing wildly in cords and trabeculae. Cells hyperchromatic, anaplastic, pleomorphic and showing atypic mitoses. App. 100 x.

invasion of the chest wall. In advanced cases in which the degree of malignancy seems to become heightened terminally, we find at times a generalized carcinomatosis with invasion of the blood stream and metastases everywhere but particularly in the lungs and bones.

ILLUSTRATIVE CASE

CASE 145. (Ref. #S-251)

Diagnosis.—Breast—scirrhous carcinoma.

Patient was a white woman of 62 years, admitted to the hospital because of a lump in her left breast, which had been recently increasing slowly in size.

Present Illness.—The patient first noticed this lump more than fifteen years ago. It had remained approximately the same size without causing her any symptoms until a few months before admission. It was never painful and had never occasioned her any worry. Occasionally, she had had a slight aching sensation in the breast associated with the lump when she felt particularly tired.

Past History.—Her past history was apparently irrelevant as far as any details which could be obtained. The patient had had an uneventful medical history except for a panhysterectomy for myomata of the uterus at the age of forty-seven, the year following her menopause. A review of her systems otherwise was essentially negative.

Physical Examination.—The patient was a fairly well-developed but poorly-nourished, white female who appeared her given age. Head was normal in contour and covered with sparse gray hair. Eyes showed a beginning arcus senilis on the left. Pupils were regular and reacted normally. Ears, nose and throat were negative. There was no peripheral adenopathy. Chest itself was symmetrical, but the breasts were different in size. Lungs were clear throughout. Heart was not enlarged and showed no murmurs. Abdomen was flat. No masses or viscera could be palpated. Extremities were negative. The left breast was considerably larger than the right. There was an extremely dense, irregular mass approximately 4 cm. in diameter, which was chiefly in the upper outer quadrant, but extended to underlie the nipple. This mass was firmly adherent to the overlying skin and nipple causing considerable retraction and the characteristic

"pigskin" appearance of the overlying skin. The tumor was also fixed to the deeper structures, and apparently to the chest wall.

Laboratory Findings.—Red blood cells, 3,200,000 with 73% hemoglobin. White blood cells, 8,600 with 67% polynuclears. Urinalysis was negative.

Subsequent Course.—The patient was advised to have a radical mastectomy. This was done and the entire breast with the underlying muscles and axillary nodes removed. The patient's immediate postoperative recovery was uneventful, and a year later she had shown no recurrence.

Pathological Report.—*Gross Description of Surgical Specimen.*—Specimen consisted of a breast approximately 10 x 8 cm. in diameter. This contained a dense tumor nodule approximately 3 cm. in diameter, which on section presented the characteristic appearance of scirrhous carcinoma. There was a very dense fibrous trabeculated stroma in which could be seen yellowish islands of tumor tissue. It was adherent to the underlying skin. No enlargement of the axillary lymph nodes was noted, and on section no evidence of metastatic tumor tissue could be found grossly. There was definite invasion of the muscle tissue, however, on the undersurface of the tumor mass.

Microscopic Description of Section Through the Tumor.—(Fig. 334 and 337) The tumor represents the typical scirrhous type of carcinoma simplex, consisting for the most part of an extremely dense hyalinized connective tissue stroma in which scattered islands and nests of compressed atrophic tumor cells may be seen. They are hyperchromatic and scarcely can be identified as epithelial in nature. In other areas some slight suggestion of pseudo-acinar arrangement can be made out, although this particular tumor represents one of the most pure examples of an uncomplicated scirrhous carcinoma which one can encounter.

Medullary Carcinoma.—The medullary or encephaloid type of adenocarcinoma is fortunately much less frequent. The term, "encephaloid," was derived again from the gross appearance of the tumor which is usually of a soft, grayish-pink color and consistency not unlike the appearance of brain tissue. It is similar in nature to the scirrhous type but very much more rapidly growing so that little or no connective tissue stroma by comparison with the scirrhous type has an opportunity to develop. Even these tumors may appear relatively orderly in their arrangement, consisting of nests of cells separated by a few connective tissue strands. The cells may be comparatively uniform in size, not unduly pyknotic, but showing invariably numerous mitotic figures. In the more rapidly growing of this type of medullary tumor we may find marked anaplasia and distortion

of the cells even to the point of tumor giant cell formation with multiple atypical mitoses (Fig. 336).

Histologically, the increased size of the nucleolus in relation to the size of the nucleus is striking in the typical carcinoma of the breast. This has been described as resembling an owl eye, and such cells are described as "owl cells" (Fig. 339). Even the recognition of a single such cell in an aspiration needle biopsy from such a tumor is sufficient in the minds of some pathologists to establish the diagnosis of carcinoma. In the rapidly growing medullary type of carcinoma simplex, the lymphatic metastasis is not prominent. Blood stream invasion occurs much more frequently and as a result pulmonary and bony metastases are comparatively common. The medullary type of tumor is likely to be seen in the younger age group, particularly in association with pregnancy, or to occur following pregnancy during the early lactation period. Such cases are apt to exhibit a hypermalignancy with the entire course of the disease symptoms lasting only a matter of a few months.

As has been previously noted in the general discussion of tumors, it is in this group, particularly when occurring in the lactation period following pregnancy, that striking benefit is obtained at times by sterilization of the patient, either surgically or by x-ray. This is of interest in raising the question of whether excess ovarian secretion may not well have been the important factor in the production of the tumor and with its cessation, the resulting regression in tumor growth. Unfortunately this result is obtained only in a very small percentage of such medullary tumors.

The chief difficulty in differential diagnosis histologically between the scirrhous and medullary types of carcinoma is seen by examining numerous areas from the same tumor. Almost invariably one may find areas of scirrhous tumor and areas of frank medullary or encephaloid activity (Fig. 335 and 338). It is this which makes gradation so impossible

from a satisfactory standpoint. It is in this group of tumors that we see how variable the rate of growth in different parts of the same tumor may be and that while a tumor may start as a slow-growing scirrhous type, it may subsequently undergo frankly increased malignancy with the development of the medullary type of picture. This is particularly true as seen in the metastatic nodules. From the therapy standpoint, breast cancer still is in a comparatively unsatisfactory state. The most approved methods today usually combine irradiation with surgery. Once diagnosis has been established irradiation is used to cause tumor regression to the point where surgery may be hoped to be effective. Then radical mastectomy with the removal of the regional lymph nodes is the method of choice. This may or may not be subsequently followed by another course of irradiation depending upon the opinion of the particular group treating such cases. If taken early, cancer of the breast should be curable in perhaps 80 per cent of cases. If left alone, it will be invariably a fatal disease so that the aim of all of us interested in the cancer problem is the establishment of early diagnosis and treatment.

ILLUSTRATIVE CASE

CASE 146. (Ref. #S-114)

Diagnosis.—Lymph node—metastatic medullary breast carcinoma.

Patient was a young white married woman, thirty-eight years of age, who was admitted to the hospital because of a mass in her right breast which was increasing rapidly in size.

Present Illness.—The patient had been delivered of a normal child, her third, three months before admission to the hospital. The pregnancy had apparently been entirely uneventful and she had not noted any difficulty with her breasts during this period. However, shortly after lactation developed she noted a small, somewhat tender mass in her right breast in the upper outer quadrant. This had increased rapidly in size so that by the time she came to the hospital it involved almost the entire breast.

Past History.—Her past history was largely irrelevant. She had had a normal childhood with the usual diseases. She had never had any serious illness. A review of her systems was essentially negative. She had occasional upper respiratory infections and a mild qualitative dyspepsia at times. Her genito-urinary history was negative. Catamenia began at thirteen and had been regular. She was married at twenty-five and had had two children previously. There was no history of cancer in any of her immediate family.

Physical Examination.—The patient was a well-developed, well-nourished adult white woman who showed nothing abnormal except for the local pathological process involving her breast. Head was normal in

contour. Eyes, ears, nose and throat were negative. Lungs were clear throughout. Heart was not enlarged and there were no murmurs. Abdomen was negative. Extremities were negative. Gynecologic examination showed a moderate laceration of the cervix. Examination of the breasts showed the right to be nearly twice the size of the left. The right was the seat of a large tumor mass approximately 10 to 12 cm. in diameter. This was resilient in consistency rather than dense, as would be expected in the typical scirrhous type of tumor. It was well defined marginally and seemed to involve the nipple with a beginning retraction. The mass was adherent to the deeper structures. Several markedly enlarged axillary lymph nodes were palpated, the largest being the size of a walnut. Both breasts showed active lactation, but the secretion was slightly blood tinged from the right breast.

Laboratory Findings.—Red blood cells, 3,100,000 with 68% hemoglobin. White blood cells, 14,200 with 78% polynuclears and 21% lymphocytes. Urinalysis was negative.

Subsequent History.—A tentative diagnosis of probable medullary carcinoma of the breast was made and radical mastectomy advised. This course was followed and the breast, with the underlying muscles and axillary nodes removed surgically. Unfortunately, pulmonary metastasis had already occurred, although not demonstrable by x-ray at the time. The patient ran a rapid downhill course, dying six months after the onset of the disease with diffuse metastases.

Pathological Report.—*Gross Description of Surgical Specimen.*—Specimen consisted of a large, asymmetrically formed, somewhat fatty breast with the nipple slightly retracted. Embedded in the breast substance was an irregularly outlined, rounded tumor mass approximately 12 cm. in diameter. This was relatively soft in consistency. Section through this showed no demarcation of the tumor tissue from the surrounding glandular structures. Indeed, invasion of the musculature could be made out grossly. The axillary lymph nodes were greatly enlarged, several of them the size of walnuts. These were soft in consistency on section, grayish-pink in color and showed numerous foci of necrosis and hemorrhage representing break-down of metastatic tumor tissue.

Microscopic Description of Section Through One of the Axillary Lymph Node Metastases.—(Fig. 339) Sections microscopically through this lymph node show large masses of hyperplastic epithelial cells practically replacing the lymph node. Here and there nests of lymphoid cells can still be identified and the peripheral sinuses and capsule are still discernible in places. Most of the section, however, is made up of nests of rapidly growing hyperchromatic small ovoid or round tumor cells with large nucleoli and many mitotic figures. These nests of cells are separated by a very delicate connective tissue stroma.

ADENOCARCINOMA

In this group of cases many observers include only those cases arising from the actual acinar epithelium. This makes up a relatively small group. The tumors of this type tend to be bulky and in their early stages almost encapsulated. They tend to break through the capsule and to fungate through the skin. They likewise are late in developing regional metastasis. The majority of these tumors probably arise from the epithelial lining of the cysts in chronic cystic mastitis.

Practically, we should include the various forms of carcinoma of the breast which show definite adenomatoid structures in this general heading of adenocarcinoma. There are several more or less characteristic types. The first is the typical adenoma malignum which occurs as solitary, moderately anaplastic, rather orderly papillary adenocarcinoma. These tumors are particularly seen in the large ducts just beneath the nipple. Many of these cases are given the name of intraductile papilloma in the more benign forms and intraductile papillocarcinoma in the more malignant forms. The cells are cuboidal or cylindrical, granular, vacuolated, or opaque, often atypical, and variously termed accordingly.

ILLUSTRATIVE CASE

CASE 147. (Ref. #S-234)

Diagnosis.—Breast—intraductile papillocarcinoma.

Patient was a white female of 70 years, admitted to the hospital with a history of a lump in her left breast of approximately a year's duration.

Present Illness.—So far as the patient could recall, she first noticed this small mass in the breast about one year before admission. This had recently begun to increase in size. Previously, it seemed to be stationary and to cause her no pain. In the three months preceding admission, however, it had been accompanied by a marked stinging pain. It was not tender on palpation. Expression of the breast showed a small amount of serosanguineous discharge from the nipple. The patient thought the lesion was an inflammatory process probably, and so resorted to localized massage by a doctor. It was following this treatment that the lesion began to increase relatively rapidly in size and to be accompanied by considerable black and bluish discoloration of the overlying skin.

Past History.—Her past history was apparently totally irrelevant. The patient had very little recollection of her earlier history. So far as she could recall, in reviewing her various systems, she had had nothing of an unusual nature. Her catamenic history was normal. Menses had begun at the age of twelve and her menopause occurred at the age of fifty-two, nearly twenty years before her present illness.

Physical Examination.—The patient was a well-developed, well-nourished, elderly white female who showed, however, some recent weight loss. Head was normal in contour. There was a moderate amount of almost white hair. Eyes were negative. Nose and throat were negative. She had two false dentures. Chest itself was symmetrical. Lungs were somewhat emphysematous on auscultation. Heart was not enlarged and showed no murmurs. Abdomen was negative. Extremities were negative. Examination of the breasts showed two nodular masses in the left breast, one measuring about 10 cm. in diameter; the other approximately 5 cm. These seemed to merge with one another. They were tense and hard on palpation except near the surface beneath the nipple where there was a suggestion of fluctuation. There was marked reddish-blue, hemorrhagic discoloration of the skin overlaying these masses, and the skin was adherent to them. The nipple was markedly retracted. Pressure on the nipple produced a small amount of serosanguineous discharge. No nodes could be palpated in the axilla.

Laboratory Findings.—Urinalysis was negative. Red blood cells, 3,100,000 with 73% hemoglobin. White blood cells, 6,400 with 69% polymorphonuclear leukocytes.

Subsequent Course.—The patient was advised to have a radical mastectomy. This was done with a simple removal of the breast and axillary nodes, but without the removal of the underlying pectoral muscle.

Pathological Report.—*Gross Description of Surgical Specimen.*—Specimen consisted of a moderately fatty breast 18 x 9 cm. in size. There were several cysts found on section, the largest representing the tumor mass noted clinically. The walls of these cysts were smooth for the most part except that of the largest one. Here the cyst was filled with tumor tissue, the result of papillary pro-liferation of the lining epithelium. The largest of these papillary masses measured 5 cm. in diameter. They were soft, friable and reddish-gray in color. The cysts con-tained some serosanguineous fluid.

Microscopic Description of Section Through the Tumor.—(Fig. 326) Section histologically shows marked papillary proliferation of the epithelium. These cells are irregular in size and shape and arrangement. They vary in depth from one or two cells up to eight or ten cells.

A second more malignant form involves whole segments of ducts or their associated glands in any part of the breast producing multilobulated tumors. Such tumors are also apt to be cystic and papillary, but the papillae are smaller in size with the develop-ment of secondary alveoli.

A third form, a malignant type of adenocarcinoma is seen which is of a very similar nature with but little evidence of adenomatoid structure persisting. Traces of papillary proliferation may persist, but the papillae tend to fuse into solid masses. Anaplasia is very marked. These tumors merge with the previ-ously described medullary type of carcinoma simplex and should best be considered under that heading. Several other terms will be found in the literature in respect to certain types of these tumors.

Comedo Carcinoma.—This represents a rather

There is considerable anaplasia, hyperchromatism and loss of polarity. The stromal connective tissue consists of delicate stalks containing small blood vessels. Definite invasion of the wall of the cyst and of the surrounding breast tissue is made out. However, this represents a relatively early stage of malignant degeneration of a lesion which undoubtedly had existed for many years as an intraductile papillary adenocystoma, but has devel-oped through trauma and chronic irritation into a typical intraductile papillocarcinoma.

characteristic group in which the entire breast is transformed into a dense fibrous mass involving the nipple and skin, and on section it is marked by prominent yellow streaks or focal areas which rep-resent ducts filled with necrotic detritus and tumor cells. This material may be expressed much as the comedones of the skin and from this gross appearance the name has been developed. It tends to occur most commonly in small atrophic breasts in which there is little fat tissue.

Inflammatory Carcinoma.—In certain cases we find a diffuse, usually medullary type of carcinoma associated with marked generalized inflammation of the entire breast which appears reddened, is painful on palpation and appears to be the site of a diffuse acute inflammatory process. It is one of the most rapidly developing carcinomas of the entire group.

COLLOID OR MUCOUS CARCINOMA

This type of tumor very definitely belongs in the group of adenocarcinoma, but is usually considered separately because of its distinctive clinical and path-ological features. The tumor is slow in developing, but if left alone will reach the largest dimensions of any type of cancer of the breast. It remains en-capsulated until late and likewise is slow to metasta-size. It owes its slow course to degenerative mucoid

changes which interfere seriously with the nutrition of the tumor cells. It is characterized by many areas of necrosis and hemorrhage, often going on even to cystic degeneration. Its therapy is wholly surgical, and unfortunately recurrence is quite prone to fol-low. Due to its relatively low cellular content and the presence of so much inert mucin, it will not respond to radiation to any extent.

ILLUSTRATIVE CASE

CASE 148. (Ref. #S-324)
Diagnosis.—Breast—mucous colloid carcinoma.

Patient was a white female of 56 years, who was ad-mitted to the hospital because of a large mass in her left breast.

Present Illness.—The onset of the present condition was approximately ten years before admission. At that time, the patient first noticed a small lump in the left breast while dressing one morning. She went to her local physician who recommended that she be kept under observation for a few weeks to see whether there was any suggestion of increase in the size of this lesion to indicate cancer. She had not noticed any appreciable change in the size of the mass and it gave her no dis-comfort so that she disregarded her physician's advice

and did nothing further about the lesion. It remained practically the same size for a matter of three or four years and then started to slowly grow. Because of the absence of pain or discomfort and the fear that she would be told she had cancer, she failed to do anything about the condition until her present admission. During the interval it had increased tremendously in size until the breast was nearly twice as large as the other. More recently it had bothered her because of the feeling of weight associated with the mass, but she still had no definite feeling of pain other than a dragging sensation. She had not noted any bleeding or discharge of any sort from the nipple.

Past Medical History.—The patient's past history was essentially irrelevant. She had had the usual childhood diseases. She had been married at twenty and had had five children, all of whom were living and well. A review of her systems revealed nothing of significance in relation to her present illness. Her menopause had occurred eight years ago.

Physical Examination.—The patient was a well-developed, somewhat obese, middle-aged, white woman. Head was normal in contour. Hair was iron-gray in color. Pupils were regular and equal. Nose and throat were negative. The thoracic cage was symmetrical. Lungs were clear. Heart was not enlarged. Abdomen was obese. There were no masses or tenderness which could be made out. Extremities were negative. The left breast was nearly twice the size of the right. This was the result of a large mass which occupied apparently all of the glandular portion of the breast substance. There was some slight retraction of the nipple and a suggestion of adherence to the skin evidenced by a "pigskin" appearance. The mass was soft and elastic in consistency. It was fairly well demarcated and did not appear to be fixed to the chest wall.

Laboratory Findings.—Red blood cells, 3,600,000 with 75% hemoglobin. White blood cells, 8,700 with 71% polynuclears. Urinalysis was negative. Blood Wassermann was negative.

Subsequent History.—The patient was advised to have a radical mastectomy. This was done with a complete dissection of the axillary lymph nodes, none of which could be demonstrated on physical examination nor at the time of operation to be involved in the pathological process.

Pathological Report.—*Gross Description of Surgical Specimen.*—Specimen consisted of a large, fatty breast containing a huge mass, practically replacing the entire breast substance. The specimen in its entirety measured 30 x 18 x 12 cm. Section through this showed the tumor to be of a gelatinous consistency with numerous areas of what almost suggested cystic degeneration and necrosis. It presented grossly the typical appearance of the so-called "gelatinous" or "colloid" carcinoma of the breast.

Microscopic Description of a Section Through the Tumor Mass.—(Fig. 331) Histologic examination of the tumor tissue shows it to be made up of nests of mucinous material embedded in a connective tissue stroma of varying density. This connective tissue background consists of trabeculae of collagen with a few small capillary vessels. The vascular supply seems extremely small and several areas of necrosis and degeneration are seen. The tumor cells occur for the most part in small clumps more or less centrally situated in masses of mucoid material. Here and there some persistence of the cell detail can be made out. For the most part only rather compactly compressed cells with round or ovoid nuclei can be identified. These nuclei show rather prominent nucleoli and scattered chromatin with a dense nuclear membrane. The cytoplasm of the cells is difficult to identify but apparently the cells have shown an extraordinary degree of mucous production to the point where the cell membranes have ruptured and remaining cytoplasm becomes compressed. The mucoid material in the tissue spaces stains rather intensely with the basophilic dyes, as is characteristic of mucin.

PAGET'S DISEASE

Paget's disease represents a special form of cancer of the breast which is associated with a primary involvement of the nipple. This clinically precedes the development of a deeper tumor arising from the ducts, and which probably always coexists, though some disagreement regarding this feature of the condition is encountered in the literature.

The onset, clinically, is characterized by an eczematous thickening of the epithelium of, and around the nipple, associated with a bloody discharge or actual ulceration. This is persistent over a long period of time and is invariably followed by a definite carcinomatous picture in the deeper structures. Extension of this eczematous lesion over the entire breast even to the axilla and much of the thorax may

occur. The underlying carcinoma apparently arises concomitantly in the large ducts and develops as a definite adenocarcinoma.

Histologically, these cases are characterized by a hyperkeratinization of the surface epithelium, marked proliferation of the duct epithelium and very characteristic hydropic degeneration of the tumor cells particularly in the squamous epithelium of the nipple. These cells have hyperchromatic, pyknotic nuclei which stand out prominently against vacuolated cytoplasm; mitoses are frequent. These atypical cells are spoken of as Paget cells. The course of the disease is rapid and by the time the breast tumor is recognized clinically the outcome is almost invariably fatal.

ILLUSTRATIVE CASE

CASE 149. (Ref. #S-231)

Diagnosis.—Breast—Paget's disease of the nipple.

Patient was an Italian woman of 54 years, admitted to the hospital with a history of having a lump in the right breast for a period of a little more than a year.

Present Illness.—So far as the patient knew, this mass in her right breast first appeared a little over a year before admission. She had noted it while bathing. It had

been slowly increasing in size since that time. She had been to another hospital and had received a series of nine x-ray treatments, but these had not seemed to be effective in halting the growth of the mass. In addition to the actual presence of the lump in her breast, it was somewhat painful on occasions. She had had a crusting lesion which had involved the nipple and had been associated with some bleeding at times. This eczematous picture of the nipple had existed for a considerably longer period than the lump itself according to the patient. She had treated it at intervals with local applications of various ointments. These had effected temporary improvement, but the process had recurred in spite of treatment.

Past History.—The patient's history was relatively unimportant. She had had the usual childhood diseases. She had never had any serious illness before. A review of her systems showed that she had never been particularly susceptible to upper respiratory infections nor to gastro-intestinal disturbances. Menses began at the age of eleven and had been fairly regular throughout her life. She had been married and had had eleven children. Menopause had occurred two years before admission, at about the time the eczematous condition affecting the nipple had developed.

Physical Examination.—The patient was a well-developed, obese, middle-aged, Italian female. Head was negative. Eyes, ears, nose and throat were negative. The chest itself was symmetrical. Heart and lungs were within normal limits. Abdomen was so obese that it was difficult to tell whether any of the viscera were palpable. Extremities were negative. The breasts were large, fatty and pendulous, the right being somewhat larger than the left. There was an area of deep pigmentation over the skin of the breast on the right side in relation to the nipple. This was assumed to be the result of x-ray therapy. On palpation of the breast, a mass approximately 6 cm. in diameter in the right lateral lower quadrant was noted. This was firmly attached to the deep tissues. It was relatively dense in consistency. There was a crusted lesion over the nipple area and areola, which extended beyond the areola over about 3 cm. of the skin. On pressure, a small amount of sero-sanguineous discharge was obtained from the nipple. There were no definitely palpable lymph nodes in the axilla.

Laboratory Findings.—Red blood cells, 3,300,000 with 74% hemoglobin. White blood cells, 5,800 with 72% polynuclears. Blood Wassermann was negative.

Subsequent Course.—The patient was advised to have a radical mastectomy. This was done. The breast and underlying muscles were removed along with the axillary lymph nodes.

Pathological Report.—*Gross Description of Surgical Specimen.*—Specimen consisted of a large, fatty breast approximately 30 x 20 cm. in diameter. The nipple showed some retraction and was covered with a sanguineous, crusted, scab-like exudate. This extended over the entire areola and involved part of the surrounding skin. On section, a tumor mass about 8 cm. in diameter was found somewhat lateral to the nipple line, but definitely in relation to the ducts. This was ill-defined and merged with the surrounding structures where it infiltrated. Definite infiltration of the musculature was noted. On section, the tumor was grayish-pink in color and relatively soft in consistency, although many areas of connective tissue trabeculation could be made out. Toward the nipple, areas of hemorrhage and necrosis could be seen.

Microscopic Description of Section from the Tumor Including the Nipple.—(Fig. 330) Histologic examination of the tissue presents the typical picture of Paget's disease. There is a crusted mass of exudate on the surface of the epithelium over the nipple area made up of necrotic cells and fibrin. Beneath this, varying degrees of differentiation of these cells are observed with some keratinization. The most striking feature is the presence of a large number of pale, vacuolated, distended, swollen cells which show hydropic degeneration. The nuclei here are pyknotic and show atypical mitoses. The epithelium invades the deeper tissue in irregular fashion but does not show characteristic epidermoid carcinomatous degeneration. On tracing the duct epithelium from the nipple area, it will be observed that there is definite adenocarcinomatous degeneration present. The cells are hyperplastic, being four, five or six layers deep instead of the usual single layer. They are anaplastic, and poorly differentiated. Most of them have lost their polarity and are hyperchromatic. There are many mitotic figures, rupture of the basement membrane and invasion of the stroma. There is concomitant desmoplastic proliferation of the stroma and secondary chronic inflammatory cellular infiltration.

CHAPTER XXXV
SPECIAL TYPES OF EPITHELIAL TUMORS

In this chapter will be considered a group of tumors which perhaps might well be left to be discussed under the respective organs in which they arise. They present such striking features clinically and pathologically, however, as to make it seem advisable to include them at this time as a group of somewhat unusual neoplasms. It is this group of tumors particularly which has become classified on the basis of their anatomical origin quite as much as on the basis of their histogenesis. There are four of these which should be considered from this standpoint: first, those tumors arising from the liver, known as either *hepatomata* when they appear to be derived from liver cells, or as *cholangiomata* when they arise from bile duct epithelium; second, the *hypernephromata* which is a term loosely used to include tumors arising specifically from the adrenal cortex or from misplaced adrenal cortical cells in the kidney, and also frequently including tumors actually of renal tubular origin; third, the *adamantinoma,* a variety of tumor arising for the most part in the jaw bone in relation to misplaced cells of the tooth bud; and finally, fourth, the so-called *"Krukenberg tumor,"* which is typically found as bilateral metastases in the ovaries in association with a primary tumor of the gastro-intestinal tract.

CARCINOMA OF THE LIVER

Hepatoma.—Tumors of the liver may arise either from the liver cells or from the bile duct epithelium and accordingly present two distinct pictures. The liver-cell type of tumor is by far the more common, although in this country neither type of tumor occurs with any great frequency. The usual history of hepatoma (liver-cell type) is one of neoplastic development on the basis of chronic irritation in association with a preëxisting biliary cirrhosis. For this reason, these tumors are in general more frequently encountered in the Far East and in tropical countries where bacterial diseases and parasitic infestations of the gastro-intestinal tract abound. (See Case 82 (S-309), Chapter XXI, page 215.) The great majority of these cases occur as multicentric tumors arising in a dozen or more places in the liver simultaneously. Occasionally one may find a single larger tumor nodule which suggests a unicentric origin with extension to the other parts of the liver. Most of these tumors may be considered essentially as benign adenomata at the outset, but a considerable proportion of them subsequently undergo malignant degeneration. They usually grow by expansion and become confluent as a result of fusion of several tumor nodules. They tend to remain localized to the liver and to extend very slowly to the regional lymph nodes. In only extremely rare instances has distant metastasis occurred.

ILLUSTRATIVE CASE

CASE 150. (Ref. #S-192 and S-117)
Diagnosis.—Liver—malignant hepatoma.
Patient was a young white male, twenty-five years of age, admitted to the hospital because of enlargement of the abdomen associated with marked loss of weight.
Present Illness.—According to the patient, his symptoms began approximately six months before admission. The onset was indefinite in its nature. He developed a feeling of malaise and easy fatigability. He noted that his abdomen felt a little full, and that this was accompanied by vague qualitative gastro-intestinal symptoms. He had a little anorexia. Following a meal, he had more or less gaseous eructation. Bowel movements were irregular in character. A local physician thought his condition was one of some gastro-intestinal disturbance and very possibly related to ulcer development, and put him on a restricted, modified, Sippy diet. The symptoms progressed, however, but his chief complaint was enlargement of his abdomen, which gave him a very heavy, uncomfortable feeling and a sense of fullness. This even seemed at times to interfere with breathing, producing moderate dyspnea. In spite of the increase in the size of his abdomen, he had noted a persistent loss of weight which worried him considerably.
Past History.—The patient had had an uneventful medical history as a child other than the milder con-

PLATE LXXXIII

MISCELLANEOUS TUMORS OF EPITHELIAL ORIGIN

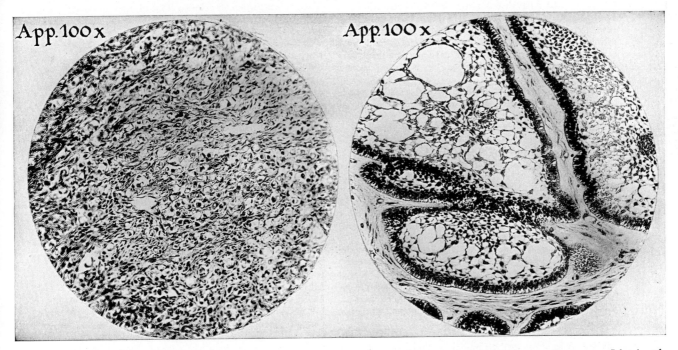

FIG. 340.—STOMACH: KRUKENBERG CARCINOMA.—CASE 154.—
Tumor is composed of small ovoid cells with eccentrically placed
hyperchromatic nuclei and vacuolated cytoplasm ("signet-ring"
cells) lying scattered throughout a diffuse cellular connective
tissue stroma. App. 100 x.

FIG. 341.—MANDIBLE: ADAMANTINOMA.—CASE 153.—Islands of
tumor tissue composed of a central core of imperfectly differentiated stellate pulp cells limited by a layer of primitive
enameloblasts. Note cystic degeneration and dense stroma.
App. 100 x.

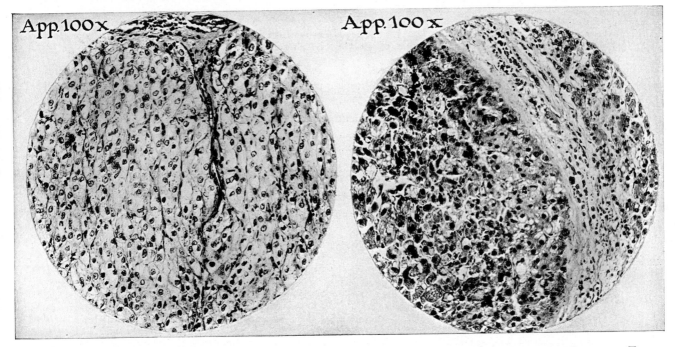

FIG. 342.—KIDNEY: HYPERNEPHROMA.—CASE 152.—Tumor composed of cords of large, pale cells with small nuclei, and a
delicate stroma similar in appearance and arrangement to the
adrenal cortex. App. 100 x.

FIG. 343.—LIVER: MALIGNANT HEPATOMA.—CASE 150.—Tumor
composed of very large polyhedral cells resembling liver cells
in their morphology and staining. Compare normal liver at
right. Marked pleomorphism, many mitoses and occasional
tumor giant cells (cf. Fig. 208). App. 100 x.

tagious diseases. There was no history of rheumatic fever. He had no previous gastro-intestinal disturbances. He had not had his appendix removed. A review of his systems in general was non-informatory. He had had the usual quota of mild upper respiratory colds and sore throat. He had no pulmonary or cardiac symptoms. His genito-urinary history was negative and he denied venereal infection.

Physical Examination.—Patient was a fairly well-developed but emaciated, young, white adult male. Head was normal in appearance. He presented a markedly anxious facies. Eyes were normal. Nose and throat were negative. Chest was symmetrical. Heart was not enlarged and there were no murmurs. Lungs were clear. Respiratory rate was slightly increased to about 28 per minute. Abdomen was markedly distended, which made a detailed examination difficult. There was, however, an irregular mass outlined in the epigastric region. The tissues were generally markedly anemic and there was a suggestion of an icteric tinge to the sclerae. Genitalia were negative. Extremities were negative.

Laboratory Findings.—Red blood cells, 2,300,000 with a hemoglobin of 5.5 grams (41%). White blood cells, 12,600 with 78% polymorphonuclear leukocytes. Urinalysis, negative. Blood Wassermann, negative. Blood chemistry was essentially negative, although there was a slightly increased icterus index. Liver function tests, including bromsulphthalein, were negative.

Subsequent History.—Exploratory laparotomy was advised to establish the diagnosis. At the time of operation, what appeared to be a generalized carcinomatosis of the abdomen with masses filling the mesentery and omentum as well as retroperitoneal nodes were found. In addition, an enormous tumor mass was seen in the liver. The condition was recognized as inoperable and tissue was merely taken for a histologic diagnosis. The patient went progressively downhill, dying approximately six weeks after his admission.

Autopsy Findings.—The body was that of an ex-

tremely emaciated white male with marked pallor and a slight suggestion of icterus. The peritoneal cavity contained about 500 c.c. of thin, sanguineous fluid. Throughout the entire peritoneal cavity generalized carcinomatosis was noted, the nodules completely studding the mesentery, mesocolon, omentum, peritoneum and the surface of the viscera. The liver was greatly enlarged weighing 3,250 grams. On the pleural surface there were many tumor masses which were restricted to an area about 13 cm. in diameter. These showed umbilicated surfaces and were pinkish white in color, and rather firm in consistency, although tending to show foci of necrosis. When the liver was sectioned, there was found a large spherical mass 10 cm. in diameter in the upper portion of the right lobe. This was similar in appearance to the other nodules noted.

Microscopic Description of a Section Through the Liver.—(Fig. 343) Histologic examination of the liver tissue shows a somewhat unusual picture as compared to the usual malignant hepatoma. This has occurred in the first place in an unusually young individual which may account for the extreme degree of malignancy noted. The tumor tissue is made up of irregular cords and trabeculae of cells, many of them occurring in sheets. Little or no tendency toward true lobule formation is made out. There is very marked anaplasia of the cells, but many of them still retain their characteristic polarity. One of the outstanding diagnostic features is the large size and roundness of the nuclei and the enormous nucleoli which so definitely suggest liver cells. Marked hyperchromatism and many atypical mitoses are seen. Occasionally the cells suggest true tumor giant cells. The picture is one of frank carcinoma of the liver. This apparently started as a unicentric lesion with subsequent metastatic spread and is unusual in its implantation and subserosal lymphatic permeation in its metastatic course, as most tumors of the liver remain relatively localized to the liver itself, or in the immediate adjacent regional lymph nodes.

Cholangioma (Bile-duct type).—This lesion is even less frequently observed than the liver-cell type of neoplasm. This is more likely to occur as a unicentric tumor with extension along the lymphatics to other portions of the liver. This is identical in appearance to tumors arising in the gallbladder or bile ducts distal to the liver in respect to the biliary tract.

It consists of overgrowth of bile duct epithelial cells, usually as an adenocarcinoma. At times one may find metaplasia to the squamous type of cell occurring in such tumors and confusion with primary liver-cell tumors may even arise in atypical cases. The mode of extension is lymphatic and metastasis is much more often encountered than in the liver cell variety.

ILLUSTRATIVE CASE

CASE 151. (Ref. #S-238)
Diagnosis.—Liver—cholangioma malignum.
Patient was a fifty-four year old white male admitted to the hospital complaining of swelling of his abdomen with soreness on the right side.

Present Illness.—The patient dated the onset of his present illness to an automobile accident three weeks before admission. Since that time he had had vague abdominal complaints chiefly of a qualitative dyspeptic nature. He had a marked anorexia with a great deal of gas in his stomach following the taking of food. He had a persistent constipation, which was entirely foreign to his usual colonic habits. He also had noted since that time that his abdomen had gradually increased in size.

Associated with the constipation, he had observed that there was a progressive loss of pigmentation until at the time of admission, his stools were practically clay-colored, dry, and crumbly in consistence, although he had no definite jaundice.

Past History.—His past history was essentially negative. He had had the usual childhood infections. He had had occasional gastro-intestinal upsets. He had an attack of acute appendicitis for which he had been operated upon. A review of his systems otherwise was non-informatory. His cardiorespiratory system was essentially negative. Genito-urinary history was normal. He was married and had had two children. A review of his family history showed that his father died of chronic nephritis, and his mother of some form of intra-abdominal cancer.

Physical Examination.—Patient was a pasty complexioned, fairly well nourished and developed middle-aged white man. Head was negative. Eyes, ears, nose and throat were normal. Chest was symmetrical. Heart was essentially negative. Lungs: There was some change in the breath sounds and percussion note in the right lower chest. There was no rise in temperature, however, and the pulse was normal. Abdomen was rotund. There was some dullness in the flanks and a fluid wave was elicited. The presence of this fluid made it difficult to be sure whether the liver was or was not definitely palpable. Genitalia negative. Extremities were negative.

Laboratory Findings.—There was a moderate secondary anemia. Red blood cells, 3,600,000 with 74% hemoglobin. White blood cells, 13,900 with 84% polymorphonuclear neutrophiles. Wassermann was negative. Urinalysis was negative.

Subsequent Course.—Abdominal paracentesis was done, and 2,700 c.c. of cloudy yellow fluid removed from the abdomen. He progressed steadily downhill, receiving several paracenteses, with a total of 12,000 c.c. of fluid being removed. He gradually became stuporous. His pulse became imperceptible and he died.

Autopsy Findings.—On opening the abdomen, about 700 c.c. of turbid, amber fluid were found. The liver was enlarged and somewhat hobnail with sharply circumscribed grayish-white areas, apparently neoplastic in nature. These nodules ranged in size from two to ten centimeters, some of the larger ones showing central umbilication. The heart and lungs were negative except for an old adhesive pleuritis. Kidneys were essentially negative. Gallbladder, common duct and the hepatic ducts as far as the liver substance showed no evidence of malignancy.

Microscopic Description of a Section Through a Tumor Nodule in the Liver.—(Fig. 495) The tissue histologically shows marked compression atrophy of the liver cords around the tumor nodule. The tumor apparently arises in the duct epithelium of the portal area and is quite unlike the characteristic liver cell type of primary tumor of the liver. The cells are smaller and tend to retain to some extent their columnar or cuboidal form, and there is a marked tendency toward lumen formation suggesting attempted duct development. Mitotic figures will be noted scattered throughout the tumor tissue. There is a moderate amount of anaplasia with some loss of polarity, definite hyperchromatism and occasional large tumor giant cells. The picture is one of a typical bile duct epithelial type of malignancy of the liver.

HYPERNEPHROMA

This tumor is perhaps best known as the Grawitz tumor. There is a sharp distinction to be drawn between tumors arising definitely in the adrenal gland and tumors arising in the kidney substance. In the first instance we are dealing with true hypernephroma; in the second instance, we may be dealing with adrenal rest tumors and thus with true hypernephroma, but more commonly we are dealing with similar appearing tumors of the kidney itself, which arise from tubular epithelium. This distinction is perhaps of only academic interest because the two tumors behave very similarly clinically and are generally considered under the single term of hypernephroma by the urologists. The tumor starts as an adenomatoid lesion in the cortex of the kidney substance usually. It tends to have a capsule or to develop one as it grows by lateral expansion. It is more frequently seen in the upper pole than elsewhere. Gradually it extends through its capsule, producing painless hematuria, and invades very characteristically the venous circulation. There it frequently grows as a solid cord of tumor tissue to completely fill the renal vein on the affected side. It may even grow into the vena cava and extend up to the auricle of the heart. Typically this venous involvement gives rise to metastatic nodules in the lung where discrete circumscribed semi-encapsulated metastases arise which, by radiologists, are termed "cannon-ball" metastases because of their large size and almost spherical appearance. This is a late manifestation of these tumors. Early recognition and removal surgically of the involved kidney gives rise to a very high percentage of cures. The tumors are only moderately radio-sensitive.

ILLUSTRATIVE CASE

CASE 152. (Ref. #S-262)
Diagnosis.—Kidney—hypernephroma.
Patient was a white woman of 62 years, who was admitted to the hospital because of severe lower back pain radiating down the leg posteriorly. This had been associated with incontinence of urine and marked constipation.

Present Illness.—The present illness began about three weeks before admission with a sudden sharp pain which radiated down both legs. Lying on her left side brought some relief. She had had three similar attacks previously, one, two and four years apart. These attacks lasted only a few days and were relieved by rest. She had had some numbness of her feet during the two or three weeks immediately preceding her admission.

Past History.—The patient's previous history was irrelevant. She had been married for forty years and had seven living children. She had her menopause ten years preceding admission. A review of her systems showed nothing of significance in respect to the present illness.

Physical Examination.—Physical examination showed a rather elderly woman with no particular objective evidence of disease other than a moderate arteriosclerosis, except for the local picture involving the abdomen. Head was normal in contour. Eyes, ears, nose and throat were negative. Chest was symmetrical. Heart and lungs were negative. Abdomen: There was a large, firm, freely movable mass in the left upper quadrant extending to the midline at the level of the umbilicus and about three fingers' breadth below it in the left lower quadrant. A tentative diagnosis of kidney tumor was made and operation recommended.

Subsequent History.—A left nephrectomy was done and the kidney was removed through the usual left loin incision. A large tumor mass the size of an adult head and producing almost complete destruction of the kidney substance was removed. The patient made an uneventful recovery.

Pathological Report.—*Gross Description of Surgical Specimen.*—Specimen consisted of a kidney with a large tumor mass measuring 18 x 15 x 12 cm. On section, this had a soft, grayish-pink color with numerous areas of hemorrhage. In addition, many yellowish areas suggesting necrosis could be seen. The tumor was so soft and friable that in handling it, it was difficult to prevent its falling in pieces.

Microscopic Description of a Section Through the Tumor.—(Fig. 342) Histologic examination of the tissue presents the typical picture of true adrenal type of tumor or hypernephroma. This consists of masses of tumor cells arranged in sheets, cords, and in places simulating the adrenal fascicular layer. There is no suggestion of lumen formation. The cells are uniform in size, pale in staining quality and suggest the usual vacuolization of typical adrenal cortex. In places, the picture almost reproduces that of normal adrenal cortex. No mitoses are noted and no definite evidence of malignant transformation can be made out. The subsequent course in this case depends upon whether renal invasion has taken place with the potential metastatic lesions in the lungs, which have thus far not shown evidence of development. Prognosis should be guarded, but may well be good.

ADAMANTINOMA

There is a group of tumors arising for the most part in the maxilla in relation to the teeth. They may generically be spoken of as *odontomata*, or teeth tumors. The most common variety is the so-called "adamantinoma," which arises from misplaced cells of the enamel organ, the enameloblasts. It is made up of these cells arranged around pulp spaces such as one sees in the usual tooth structure. Within this mass of cells may be found a core of so-called *"star cells,"* which are vacuolated. These produce a curious interlacing architecture, which is the result of the highly specialized cytoplasmic ridge-like arrangement of these epithelial cells. Tumors of the odontomatous group may be found occurring as simple or dentigerous cysts. In other instances, they are seen as solid tumors of imperfectly formed or fused teeth and are spoken of as composite odontomata. The dentigerous cyst is a cystic odontoma arising from the tooth follicle and is benign in character. Similar tumors may be found in other locations notably in tumors of the craniopharyngeal region arising from the rudimentary inclusions of the hypophyseal duct. Here they may behave like basal cell carcinomata eroding the sphenoid bone and sella turcica, ultimately producing pressure symptoms leading to death. For more detailed discussion see Chap. LXVIII.

ILLUSTRATIVE CASE

CASE 153. (Ref. #S-139 and S-165)
Diagnosis.—Jaw—cystic adamantinoma.

Patient was a white female of 15 years, admitted to the hospital because of a swelling of the left mandible.

Present Illness.—The onset of the present illness was about four weeks before admission. At that time she had noted a swelling of the jaw beneath the bicuspid tooth. This had slowly progressed in size, but had not been associated with any particular discomfort or pain.

Past History.—The child had had a normal, uneventful history. She had had the usual minor childhood diseases. She had not been particularly subject to upper respiratory infection. She had had no difficulty with the eruption of her teeth. Gastro-intestinal history was negative. Menses began at the age of fifteen and were regular.

Physical Examination.—Physical examination showed a normal, well-developed, well-nourished adolescent young white female. Head was normal in shape. Eyes were regular and reacted normally. Ears and nose were negative. There was a hard tumor mass about 3 cm. in diameter, which involved the middle portion of the left mandible. The tumor was not tender on palpation and appeared well localized. Some devitalized gum tissue was seen around the margin of this tumor with no apparent cervical lymph node enlargement. Heart and lungs were negative. Chest was symmetrical. Abdomen was negative. Extremities were normal.

Laboratory Findings.—Red blood cells, 4,800,000 with 88% hemoglobin. White blood cells, 8,200 with 64% polynuclears. Urinalysis was negative.

Subsequent Course.—A tentative diagnosis of adamantinoma was made and operation advised. This was done and the tumor removed, including the point of origin from the jaw itself. Recovery was uneventful, and there had been no recurrence at the end of two years.

Pathological Report.—*Gross Description of Surgical Specimen.*—Specimen consisted of a nearly spherical piece of tissue of almost bony hardness measuring 3 cm. in diameter. A small piece of easily recognizable bone was attached to one side. This represented the point of origin of the lesion. On section, the cut surface showed numerous spicules of bone forming a shell. Internally, there appeared to be a cystic network of stroma. This was pale in color and soft in consistency.

Microscopic Description of Section Through the Tumor.—(Fig. 341) Sections histologically show a tumor made up of what appear to be edematous structures with lumina filled with clear or granular pink-staining material. Around each of these areas of cystic degeneration will be found a layer of small hyperchromatic cells more or less resembling basal cells, but actually representing enameloblasts. Inside this layer of cells is found a loose, rather myxomatous-looking tissue which represents the pulp of the tooth organ. It is most distinctive histologically and unlikely to be confused with other tumors. Essentially this represents a type of tumor which usually remains benign, but at times may undergo malignant transformation like any other epithelial tumors. In this instance, no evidence of malignancy is found.

KRUKENBERG TUMOR

In 1896, Krukenberg first described a tumor of the ovary under the name of *"fibrosarcoma muco-cellulare carcinomatoides."* This was invariably bilateral in distribution and involved both ovaries diffusely, but with only moderate enlargement of the organs. Characteristically, the tumor was found to be composed of groups of small round or ovoid cells with an eccentrically placed nucleus and cytoplasm which was filled with a large vacuole often producing a signet-ring appearance of the cell through crowding of the nucleus to one side. Furthermore it was noted that very commonly other lesions of a similar histopathology could be found in the gastro-intestinal tract. These were believed to be metastatic. With our present concept of the condition, we are inclined to believe that the primary lesion is in the gastro-intestinal mucosa arising from the small mucous cells deep in the glands, and that the ovarian lesions are the metastatic ones. This belief is founded on the fact that similar signet-ring carcinomata may be found in males with almost as high an incidence as in females. The belief today held by most pathologists is simply one of unexplained tissue selectivity in respect to these metastases as in the case of other specific tissue affinities. Because of the nature of the process there is a high mortality associated with the disease as a whole, although individual cases are still alive long after the accepted five-year-period of cure. Whether this type of lesion represents the precursor of the more extensive large, bulky, gelatinoid tumors of the stomach and colon is problematical, as no comparable ovarian involvement is found in this latter group.

ILLUSTRATIVE CASE

CASE 154. (Ref. #S-162)

Diagnosis.—Stomach—Krukenberg carcinoma.

Patient was a white male of 57 years, admitted to the hospital with the chief complaint of a gnawing pain in the stomach after meals.

Present Illness.—Patient stated that the onset of his present illness was about three months before admission. This pain was first noticed following the taking of food and had become progressively worse. It was of a gnawing or boring character and seemed to radiate to the interscapular region, lasting for about one hour. It had been accompanied by some nausea, but no vomiting. He had had considerable gaseous eructation, which had not been relieved by alkalies. He had had marked obstipation. His appetite had remained good, but he had eaten little in the few weeks before admission because of the pain induced by food. He had noticed that he fatigued more easily during the preceding three months. He had a history of excessive use of alcohol for about fifteen years. He had lost eighteen pounds in the past three months. There had been no jaundice.

Past History.—His past history was apparently irrelevant. He had had no previous symptoms pointing to any gastro-intestinal disturbance. A review of his cardio-respiratory and genito-urinary systems was likewise negative.

Physical Examination.—Physical examination showed a well-developed, fairly well-nourished, middle-aged man with a slightly sallow complexion. The superficial veins around the umbilicus were suggestive of a caput medusae. Head was negative. Eyes, ears, nose and throat were negative. Chest was symmetrical. It was of a somewhat emphysematous type. The heart and lungs were essentially negative. The abdomen was distended. There was some tenderness just below the umbilicus in the midline. The liver margin could not be felt. There was no apparent ascites. The extremities were negative.

Laboratory Findings.—Red blood cells, 3,800,000 with 78% hemoglobin. White blood cells, 7,600 with 64% polynuclears. Urinalysis was negative. Serology was negative.

X-ray Examination: There was an area of narrowing seen in the pyloric antrum, and there was a marked gastric residue of about 90% at the end of six hours. There was a large organic lesion in the distal end of the stomach which was producing a high degree of obstruction, and in view of the short history, the diagnosis of carcinoma was considered the most probable.

Subsequent Course.—The patient was advised to have an operation for the relief of the obstruction. A subtotal gastrectomy was performed. His progress following this radical operative procedure was unsatisfactory. He developed a postoperative, diffuse peritonitis as the result of sloughing of the wound edges around the gastrojejunostomy from autolytic digestion of the tissues, and he died a week later.

Pathological Report.—*Gross Examination of Surgical Specimen.*—Specimen consisted of the distal 15 cm. of a stomach and 4 cm. of duodenum. The pylorus measured 8 cm. in circumference when opened. There was an annular thickened area involving about one-half of the specimen. The mucosa overlying this thickened area seemed to be intact, but there was diffuse infiltration of the submucosa and muscular wall.

Microscopic Description of a Section Through the Stomach Wall.—(Fig. 340) Histologic examination of the tissue shows at one side of the section a portion of the stomach mucosa, which presents evidence of inflammatory hyperplasia. The remainder of the mucosal surface shows superficial ulceration with fibrinopurulent exudate firmly adherent to it. Beneath this surface layer is seen a diffuse infiltration of the submucosa and entire wall of the stomach by small round or oval cells, many of which contain mucous droplets which have pushed the nuclei to one side, producing so-called "signet-ring cells." These show little or no tendency toward acinar arrangement and occur in sheets and cords or as individual cells. There is no architectural pattern to be noted. The cells apparently arise from the small epithelial cells at the base of the glands. There are numerous mitotic figures, although none of the cells appear particularly anaplastic. There is considerable hyperchromatism, and the degree of infiltration is indicative of the malignant nature of the process.

CHAPTER XXXVI

MIXED AND TERATOID TUMORS

Teratoid tumors represent complex tumors arising from cells ranging all the way from primitive undifferentiated totipotential cells up to cells forming one or more germinal layers during the course of their differentiation. They are not true tumors in the strict sense of the word, but rather abortive attempts at forming a fetus. Such tumors are particularly found at the poles of the body, springing from the roof of the mouth or from the coccygeal region and are nearly always midline in origin except in relation to the gonads. They should perhaps be discussed better under the heading, teratology.

MIXED TUMORS

The term, "mixed tumors," is used in two distinct ways. In its simplest implication, the term is applied to lesions in which two adult tissues seem to both play a part in the neoplastic process. Numerous examples of this have been encountered in the preceding chapters, the lympho-epithelioma, the fibro-adenoma, etc. The more exact use of the term is restricted from the practical standpoint to two tumors. These are the so-called "mixed tumors" of the parotid gland and of the kidney. In these tumors, it is generally conceded that there are at least two germ layers represented, which have arisen from partially differentiated somatic blastomeres. Such tumors are slow-growing as a rule, and while they not infrequently undergo malignant change sooner or later,

yet if they are recognized early enough it is possible to completely extirpate them with a permanent clinical cure. More often, complete extirpation is unsuccessful and recurrence is the rule. This is particularly true of the parotid or other salivary gland tumors of a similar nature.

The "mixed tumors" of the kidney are more often considered to-day as representing a one-sided development of a complex teratoid tumor than as a simple "mixed tumor." This is the tumor which we have already discussed briefly as the Wilm's tumor, giving rise not infrequently to the rhabdomyosarcomatous picture, although at other times retaining a definite alveolar structure embedded in a sarcomatous stromal background.

ILLUSTRATIVE CASES

CASE 9. (Ref. #S-220)
Refer to Chapter II, Page 17 and Fig. 19. The patient was a young thirty-year-old white male, who had had a swelling under the jaw for several months. This was operatively removed and found to represent a typical so-called "mixed tumor" of the parotid gland.

In CASE 101 (Ref. #S-237), Chapter XXVI, Page 268 and Fig. 234, it will be recalled that this patient was a five-year-old child who developed a rapidly growing tumor of the kidney which was found at autopsy to be an embryoma of the kidney with a one-sided development as a rhabdomyosarcoma.

DERMOID CYST

In addition to the above mentioned varieties of so-called "mixed tumors," we see tumors which are most frequently found involving the ovary or testis. The commonest type of this group is the one which we see in the ovary developing as the so-called "dermoid cyst" (Fig. 359), a tumor made up usually of cells derived from two germinal layers. The usual picture is a cystic tumor of variable size ranging

from 1 cm. or smaller up to large tumors 20 or 30 cm. in diameter. These tumors usually show a papilla-like structure at one point in the wall, and in this papillary projection may be found a wide variety of tissues histologically. All types of surface epithelium may be found ranging from simple stratified mucosa through the more complex skin derivatives including hair follicles, sebaceous and sweat

PLATE LXXXIV

MIXED AND TERATOID TUMORS

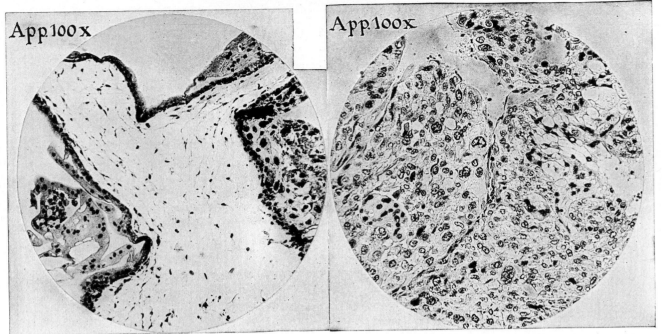

FIG. 344.—UTERUS: HYDATIDIFORM MOLE.—CASE 157.—Photomicrograph of a chorionic villus showing edema and myxomatous degeneration of its core. The overlying Langhans' layer is intact, while the syncytial cells are undergoing adenomatous proliferation (left). App. 100 x.

FIG. 346.—UTERUS: CHORIOCARCINOMA (CHORIOEPITHELIOMA).—CASE 158.—Sheets of anaplastic Langhans' cells, showing pleomorphism, hyperchromic nuclei, numerous mitotic figures both typic and atypic, and inconspicuous groups of syncytial cells. App. 100 x.

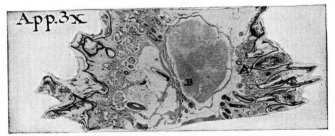

FIG. 345.—OVARY: TERATOMA.—CASE 115.—Microtessar photograph in which the varying tissue constituents are apparent. App. 3 x.

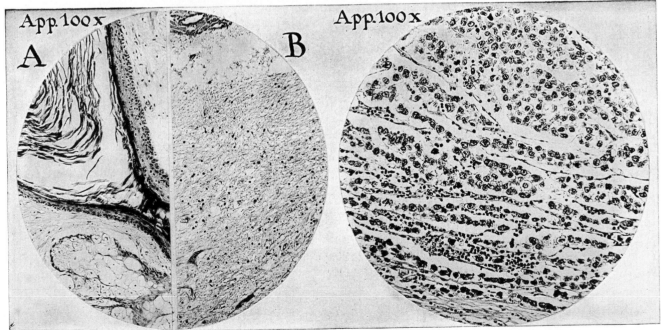

FIG. 347.—OVARY: TERATOMA.—CASE 155 (See Fig. 345).—Area "A": Photomicrograph showing stratified squamous epithelium with sebaceous glandular and hair follicle formation, as well as keratinization. Area "B": Tissue shows an abortive attempt at reproduction of the central nervous structures, with glia, nerve cells and even membrane formation. App. 100 x.

FIG. 348.—TESTIS.—EMBRYONAL CARCINOMA (SEMINOMA).—CASE 156.—Tumor is composed of cords of large cells resembling undifferentiated spermatogenic cells, with large, pale-staining nuclei having a rather characteristic arrangement of the chromatin. A few mitoses are present. App. 100 x.

glands up to such complex structure as abortive tooth development. The mesoblastic element is represented by various imperfect attempts at cartilaginous and bone development as well as connective tissue and fat formation. These tumors likewise are perhaps best considered as an intermediate developmental form of the potentially complex teratomata. Not infrequently tooth structure can be identified.

TERATOMATA

In the more complex of the teratoid tumors, we find in addition to the mesothelial and ectodermal derivatives a third germ layer representing the endoderm. This is evidenced by the presence of attempted organoid formation. Unrelated bits of abortive gastro-intestinal mucosa, thyroid gland, pancreas and even central nervous system tissues will be found side by side. These latter complex teratomata are more likely to be solid tumors with perhaps here and there small areas of cystic degeneration in contrast to the dermoid cyst, with its single large cavity. Such tumors usually are found in the ovary or testis, but may occur anywhere in the midline, especially at the sacral end of the vertebral column. Intrathoracic teratoid tumors occurring in the mediastinum are likewise by no means rare. They offer an extremely difficult problem both from the standpoint of diagnosis and therapy, which must be surgical.

ILLUSTRATIVE CASE

CASE 155. (Ref. #S-256)

Diagnosis.—Ovary—dermoid cyst (teratoma).

Patient was a white woman of 32 years admitted to the hospital because of left lower abdominal pain.

Present Illness.—The onset of the patient's symptoms began approximately six weeks before admission when she complained of a dragging sensation in the pelvis associated with sharp, severe pain in the left lower quadrant which radiated down the thigh and to the lumbar back region. These symptoms followed the delivery of a normal child six weeks earlier.

Past History.—Her past history did not appear particularly pertinent except that about one year earlier she had been told by a physician that she had "inflammation of her ovaries." She was treated by her physician with marked improvement. Other than this, her past medical history was negative. She had had the usual childhood diseases. She had not had any history of rheumatic fever. Her cardiorespiratory system was negative. Her gastrointestinal history was negative. Menstrual history began at the age of twelve and had been regular. She was married at the age of twenty-three and had two previous children.

Physical Examination.—The patient was a well-developed, well-nourished, young white woman who did not appear acutely sick. Her head was negative. Eyes, ears, nose and throat were normal. Chest was symmetrical. Breasts were large and lactating. Heart and lungs were negative. Abdomen was distended particularly in the lower portion. There was obvious tenderness and pain in the pelvic region. Vaginal examination: A large, well-rounded mass could be palpated in the cul-de-sac, which was extremely tender. The uterus seemed to be in good position.

Subsequent Course.—A tentative diagnosis of an ovarian tumor with a twisted pedicle was made and exploratory operation advised. This was done and the left ovary was located in the cul-de-sac. It was deep purplish in color and suggested beginning gangrene. This was easily removed by severing the pedicle. The patient had an uneventful recovery.

Pathological Report.—*Gross Description of Surgical Specimen.*—Specimen consisted of a gangrenous-appearing ovary measuring 6 x 5 x 4 cm. The ovary itself showed extensive cystic degeneration, the major portion being made up of a large cystic cavity filled with sebaceous material and a hair ball. The lining of this cyst was smooth except for an area 2 cm. in diameter from which the hair was seen growing. In addition, there was a large corpus luteum seen in the wall of the cyst.

Microscopic Description of Section Through the Wall of the Cyst.—(Fig. 345, 347, and 359) Histologic examination of the tissue presents a variable picture. As is characteristic of this type of tumor one may find all varieties of epithelial lined cysts. Some of these are lined by squamous epithelium showing marked keratinization; others appear to be of a simple mucous membrane type of pavement epithelium without keratinization. Innumerable glandular structures can be identified including sebaceous and sweat glands. Embedded in the stroma will be found other types of tissue. Especially noteworthy is the area containing an abortive attempt at brain formation with characteristic supportive glia and occasional, atypical nerve cells. The hair follicles noted grossly likewise may be observed and depending upon the particular section studied, areas of other attempted organoid structures may be identified, including several islands of cartilage.

EMBRYONAL CARCINOMATA

In addition to these solid teratoid tumors, or embryomata as they are frequently termed, we may find a much more primitive type of tumor arising from undifferentiated germinal epithelial totipotential cells. These cells, instead of differentiating as they must have done in the development of the complex teratomata, simply have retained the power to multiply and reproduce themselves in a manner similar to other carcinomata. They are made up of enormous round or polyhedral cells with large spherical nuclei containing scattered chromatin granules and usually rather prominent nucleoli. The cells occur in long strands supported only by a thin, delicate capillary and connective tissue supportive stroma or in nests where, because of an inadequate blood supply, they frequently show large areas of necrosis. Such tumors are prone to invade the blood stream and develop distant metastases, especially in the lung.

At any time, any of these complex teratoid tumors may show neoplastic changes of any of their incompletely differentiated tissues so that carcinoma or sarcoma may occur either independently or in combination within the same tumor. Such carcinomatous, or sarcomatous lesions may show their distinctive adult metastatic distribution. In general, it is true that the teratoid tumors, other than this group of embryonal carcinomata or dysgerminomata, remain as benign neoplasms, and if removed surgically rarely, if ever, recur. Even in this latter group permanent cures are obtained in many instances.

ILLUSTRATIVE CASE

CASE 156. (Ref. #S-263)

Diagnosis.—Embryonal carcinoma (malignant embryoma, seminoma) from the testis.

Patient was a male Negro of 29 years, who was admitted to the hospital with the chief complaint of marked swelling of his abdomen.

Present Illness.—About one year before admission, he first noticed a swelling in his left groin. He stated that there had always been a lump in this region, that he had never had a testis in the left scrotal sac and had been told that this lump was an undescended testis. This grew rapidly in size and was very painful. He went to a physician who sent him to the hospital for treatment. The tumor was excised locally, and he was given a course of intensive x-ray therapy. This was six months before the present admission. He felt much better for a period of two or three months and then noticed that his abdomen was beginning to increase in size. For the past three months this had increased progressively. It had given rise to considerable discomfort locally and apparently to pressure on his diaphragm, as he had complained of increasing dyspnea. There was no edema of his lower extremities. He returned to the hospital to see if further x-ray treatment would relieve him of these two symptoms which bothered him.

Past History.—His past history was irrelevant and unreliable.

Physical Examination.—The patient was a well-developed and well-nourished, young adult male Negro. Head was normal in contour. Pupils were regular and equal and reacted sluggishly. Mouth showed marked dental caries. Nose and throat were otherwise negative. Chest showed moderate dullness over the lower half of the lungs with suppression of the breath sounds. Heart was pushed upward and did not appear to be definitely enlarged. There was a rough, systolic, apical murmur. Blood pressure, 135/90. Abdomen was so markedly distended that it was impossible to palpate any of the viscera or to be sure whether any definite masses were present. There was a marked fluid wave demonstrated. The scrotum was small and firm. The right testis appeared normal. The left testis was absent. Extremities:

The left thigh and leg were somewhat swollen. The right appeared normal. Reflexes were normal.

Laboratory Findings.—Urinalysis was negative. Wassermann was negative. Blood count was within normal limits.

Subsequent Course.—The patient had repeated paracentesis and thoracentesis with the removal of a total of some 18,000 c.c. of bloody fluid from the peritoneal and pleural cavities. He went progressively downhill, dying three weeks after admission.

Autopsy Findings.—Autopsy examination showed a left orchectomy scar. There was a large retroperitoneal tumor representing a metastatic extension of the left testicular tumor. This extended further to involve the omentum, the mesenteric, retroperitoneal, paravertebral and pelvic lymph nodes. It had also gone through the diaphragm and involved the mediastinal nodes, and was present as blood borne metastases throughout both lungs. Similar metastatic tumor tissue was found in the adrenals and in the brain.

Microscopic Description of a Section Through One of the Metastatic Tumor Nodules.—(Fig. 348) Histologic examination of the tumor tissue shows a typical embryonal type of carcinoma of testicular origin. The tumor is made up of solid sheets and cords of large round or polyhedral cells, with enormous nuclei. The nuclei have a sharp nuclear membrane and scattered chromatin granules. There are large nucleoli present. The tumor varies a great deal in its blood supply, but in general shows a rather generous capillary vascular stroma. It is this vascular background which tends to produce the rather characteristic architectural arrangement of the tumor tissue. Many areas of necrosis and hemorrhage are found where the cells cannot be identified and where secondary leukocytic infiltration has occurred. The cells, in general, resemble closely those of the undifferentiated early cells of the reproductive tubules, but in their neoplastic overgrowth fail to show any striking tendency toward tubule formation. The cells have apparently lost their power of differentiation and are capable solely of reproduction. Mitotic figures are innumerable with many large atypic mitoses.

TUMORS OF THE FETAL MEMBRANES

In the development of the fetus during pregnancy, occasionally degenerative lesions may be found which affect the placenta and its membranes. The simplest of these conditions results in the development and ultimate delivery of the so-called "hydatidiform mole." In this condition we find a hydropic degeneration of the chorionic villi with an obliteration of the central arteriole of the villus and the accumulation of fluid within the interstitial tissues until the villus hangs like a grape from its central point of attachment. This mole development usually occurs in the second half of pregnancy and many patients go on to what they believe nearly full-term with gradual increase in the size of the uterus due to the slow growth of this mole. Were the end of the story in such cases simply one of uncomplicated miscarriage and delivery of the mole, this would not be a particularly disquieting condition. Unfortunately, however, a rather high percentage of cases of hydatidiform mole show definite malignant change involving the fetal ectodermal membranes with the development of a choriocarcinoma.

This is characterized by neoplastic overgrowth of both the Langhans' and syncytial ectodermal cells; marked changes in the nuclei are observed with the development of atypic mitotic figures, tumor giant cells, extreme hyperchromatism, pyknosis and all the usual histologic criteria of malignancy. More impressive than the cytologic changes themselves, however, are the evidences of invasion and early metastasis by way of the blood stream to the lung, where multiple large spherical metastatic nodules develop ending with the death of the patient. Unfortunately, invasion occurs so early in this condition that one is not justified in any great delay in advising radical surgical measures, with the removal of the uterus. Obstetricians and gynecologists vary somewhat in their opinions as to the factor of safety in these cases. It has always seemed to us, personally, that each case was a problem in itself dependent upon the age of the woman and the importance of any subsequent pregnancy to her. If histologic evidence was not convincing of the malignancy, then it seems justified to observe such a patient for a period of two or three months, with a subsequent examination of her uterine scrapings to determine whether there is any evidence of tumor development. If the process is frankly malignant at the time the mole is delivered, then hysterectomy is the only possible solution; but unfortunately, it is already too late in many instances.

As a complication, in certain tumors arising in the testis which are potentially so far undifferentiated as to give rise to fetal structures, a choriocarcinoma (chorio-epithelioma) may arise as an apparent primary tumor of the testis and run a similar malignant course if not interfered with. Here, fortunately, the lesion may be detected comparatively early in its development and by the surgical removal of the involved testis, recovery may at times be effected permanently.

ILLUSTRATIVE CASES

CASE 157. (Ref. #S-119)

Diagnosis.—Hydatidiform mole.

Patient was a white woman of 27 years, admitted to the hospital because of a threatened miscarriage.

Present Illness.—The present illness began suddenly with profuse vaginal bleeding on arising in the morning during the seventh month of her pregnancy. Previous to this, apparently her pregnancy had been proceeding normally and she had been able to do her regular housework.

Past History.—Her past medical history was entirely irrelevant in relation to the present illness. She had had a normal childhood with the usual diseases. She had never had any serious illness. She had been married three years. This was her first pregnancy. She was one of four normal children and so far as she was aware there had been no history of miscarriage, of cancer or other familial disease in either her own or her husband's background.

Physical Examination.—The patient was a well-developed, well nourished, young white woman who showed no external evidence of illness. Head was normal in contour. Eyes, ears, nose and throat were negative. Chest was symmetrical. Breasts showed considerable enlargement and a small amount of excretion could be expressed from the nipples. The heart and lungs appeared normal. The abdomen was prominent and resembled in size approximately a full-term pregnancy. The extremities were negative. Gynecologic examination was not done with the thought in mind that subsequent surgical intervention might be necessary.

Laboratory Findings.—Laboratory findings were essentially negative. The blood count showed a slight secondary anemia with 3,800,000 red blood cells and 74% hemoglobin. White blood cells were slightly elevated—12,600 with 81% polynuclears. Urinalysis was negative, except for many red cells as the result of the hemorrhage.

Subsequent Course.—The bleeding subsided temporarily on bed treatment, but was followed six hours later by the spontaneous expulsion of a large mass from the uterus. This presented the characteristic appearance of an hydatidiform mole. It resembled a mass of polypoid, grape-like structures supported by a delicate stroma. In addition, a dead and badly macerated small fetus could be identified.

Microscopic Description of a Section Through the Mole.—(Fig. 344) Histologic examination of the tissue presents the characteristic picture of a simple hydatidiform mole. The chorionic villi may be identified as the nucleus of the individual cyst-like structures noted grossly. These consist of an edematous, delicate fibrillar connective tissue stroma in which the central arteriole or capillary has been obliterated. Covering these edematous villi will be identified the characteristic Langhans' and syncytial cells. In addition, considerable hyalinized necrotic tissue may also be identified representing the decidual elements of this degenerated placenta.

CASE 158. (Ref. #S-170)
Diagnosis.—Choriocarcinoma.
Patient was a white female of 30 years, admitted to the hospital because of hemoptysis and vaginal bleeding.

Present Illness.—The patient had a history of having passed an hydatidiform mole six months earlier. At that time the uterus had been completely curetted and histologic examination of the mole at another hospital had shown no evidence histologically of malignancy. She had been told to return to the hospital at the end of three months for a check-up examination and curettage. In the absence of symptoms, she had neglected this and did not seek medical attention until the sudden onset of rather severe hemorrhage.

Past History.—The patient had had a normal and uneventful childhood medically. She had been married at the age of twenty-eight, and her first pregnancy had resulted in the aforementioned hydatidiform mole. A review of her systems was essentially irrelevant.

Physical Examination.—The patient was a young white woman about thirty years of age. Head was normal in contour. Dry blood was present in both nares, Eyes were negative. Pupils were regular and equal. Nose and throat otherwise were negative. Chest was symmetrical. Numerous râles could be heard over both sides of the chest scattered rather uniformly throughout the lobes. On percussion, several doubtful areas of diminished resonance were detected, but these were so uncertain in extent that it was impossible to say whether actual dullness was present or not. The heart appeared normal in size and no murmurs were present. The abdomen was moderately prominent. The liver edge was felt just below the costal margin. The uterus was sufficiently enlarged to be palpable by abdominal examination just above the brim of the pelvis. It felt rounded and smooth in outline. Extremities were negative. Gynecologic examination showed a bloody discharge from the cervix with moderate dilatation of the canal.

Laboratory Findings.—Red blood cells, 2,800,000 with 62% hemoglobin. White blood cells, 14,200 with 78% polynuclears, 19% lymphocytes and 3% monocytes. Urinalysis, by catheter specimen, was essentially negative. Blood Wassermann was negative.

X-ray examination showed the lungs to be studded with dozens of small, spherical, metastatic tumor nodules 2 to 3 cm. in diameter.

Subsequent Course.—The patient remained in the hospital for approximately 3 weeks and died of profuse hemorrhage from rupture of one of the metastatic lung nodules into a bronchus.

Autopsy Findings.—At autopsy, very little additional was found other than a diffuse infiltrating tumor filling the uterine canal and invading the musculature. In addition, the rather sharply circumscribed metastases in the lungs were noted numbering perhaps fifty or more. These nodules were bright red in color and showed diffuse hemorrhage. One of them in the right upper lobe was the source of hemorrhage into the right secondary bronchus. There was a terminal bronchopneumonia which was a contributory cause of death.

Microscopic Description of a Section from the Primary Uterine Tumor.—(Fig. 346) Histologic examination of the tissue presents the characteristic features of the so-called choriocarcinoma or chorionic epithelioma. This represents a tumor derived from the fetal membranes of the placenta and thus differs from any other tumor. The characteristic Langhans' and syncytial cells may readily be identified. The great majority of these cells appear essentially normal and do not present very strikingly the usual evidence of malignant anaplasia. Here and there hyperchromatism of the nuclei and the presence of atypical anaplastic cells may be noted. Mitoses, both typical and atypical are present in moderate numbers. The most outstanding histological feature by which diagnosis can be made, however, is the evidence of direct invasion of the uterine musculature with degenerative changes affecting muscle cells and stroma.

CHAPTER XXXVII

TERATOLOGY (*Abnormal and Defective Embryologic Development*)

MULTIPLE BIRTHS

The largest number of multiple births in humans is unknown. Authentic records up to six exist. Twins occur about once in 88 births, triplets once in 8,000, quadruplets once in 400,000 and quintuplets about once in 10,000,000 births. As interference in growth in simultaneously developing embryos is in itself very rare, and the results are essentially similar to those occurring in twins, such defective development will be considered entirely from the standpoint of twins in this brief outline.

Gemini (Twins)

Gemini Aequales

Heterologous Twins.—May be of the same or different sexes—develop from entirely separate ova (hetero-öphal), each with its own placenta and membranes (dichorial). No double monster has ever been seen in twins of different sex.

Homologous (identical) Twins.—Must be of same sex, developing as they do from a single ovum (mono-öphal); and are identical in every particular, anatomically, physiologically, mentally, etc. The theories regarding their development are:

FIRST. The separation of the primary blastomeres —in this case each embryo has its own chorion and amnion and so do not interfere with each other in development.

SECOND. By the development of two primitive streaks and the division of the germinal area into two equal parts. They may have separate or fused amnions, a common placenta (monochorial), and their umbilical cords may be separate in their insertion into the placenta.

THIRD. The theory of determination: in which chemical or hormonal activators distributed through the ovary play a part. This is one of those wholly hypothetical and as yet unconfirmed hypotheses.

Gemini inaequales

Inequality of twins usually results from disease or accident to one during the latter part of intra-uterine existence, and thus is not a developmental defect. If one dies it may become a flattened mass of tissue called *fetus papyraceus.*

Developmental defects are most commonly the result of asymmetry of blood supply to the two embryos, the more favorably placed in respect to the placental circulation, appropriating an ever increasing proportion, until the circulation of the weaker becomes dominated by the stronger even to the exclusion of the development of its heart. Such a creature, without a heart, is spoken of as an *acardiac monster,* or an *omphalosite* (deriving its blood supply through the umbilical vessels). Various forms of such acardiac monsters occur:

1. *Hemiacardius* (acardius anceps)—general body configuration is recognizable.
2. *Holoacardius acephalus*—a headless acardiac.
3. *Holoacardius acormus*—a monster with a head but no body.
4. *Holoacardius amorphous* (fetus amorphous) —shapeless mass of tissue.

If interference in development of twins occurs early enough, the tissues of one may become confused with those of the other to form *Diaxial (double) Monsters.* Because of identical polarity the developing embryos always have their heads pointing in the same direction, so such conjoined monsters are always conjoined head to head; or tail to tail—never head to tail. Likewise, because in development they

386

PLATE LXXXV

TERATA

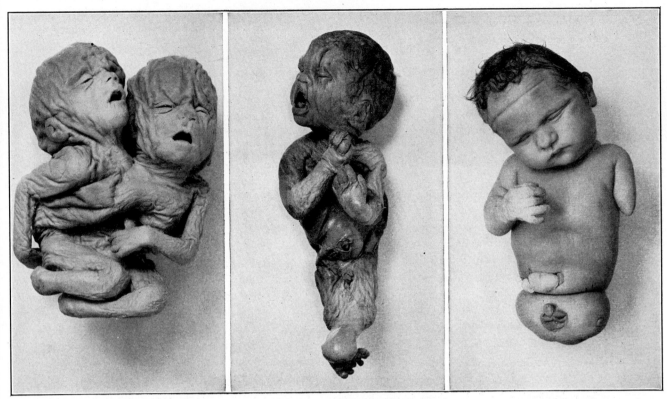

FIG. 349.—DOUBLE MONSTER (DICEPHALUS). FIG. 350.—SIREN TYPE OF MONSTER (URO-MELUS). FIG. 351.—ECTROMELUS (PHOCOMELUS).

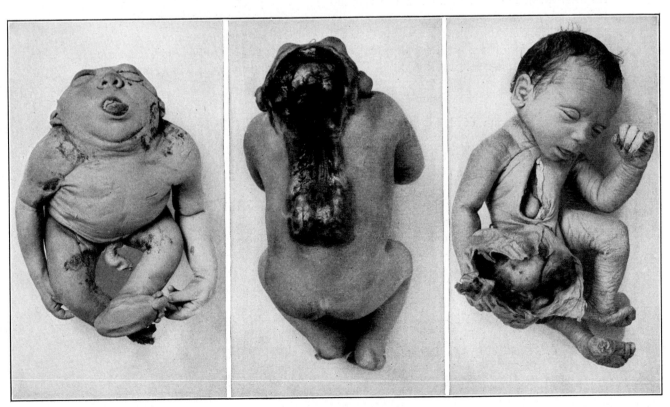

FIG. 352.—ANENCEPHALY. FIG. 353.—CRANIORACHISCHISIS. FIG. 354.—CELOSOMA (THORACO-ABDOMINAL).

naturally face one another, the union is usually anterior.

Double monsters may arise either by (1) secondary partial coalescence following original complete primary separation (diaxial) or (2) by dichotomy of one or both ends of a single axis (monoaxial). The following major types may be identified:

DIAXIAL (DOUBLE) MONSTERS

I. *Duplicitas symmetros*—in which conjoined twins are equal.
  1. *Craniopagus*—in which the fusion is at head end.
  2. *Thoracopagus*—in which the fusion is ventral.
  3. *Pygopagus*—in which fusion is at hip region.

II. *Duplicitas asymmetros*—in which one twin develops imperfectly as an acardiac *parasite*—the healthy normal twin being called the *autosite*.
  1. *Craniopagus parasiticus*—parasite attached to head.
    a. *Epignathus*—parasite attached to upper jaw (commonest type); other varieties depending on point of attachment are called *hygonathus, paragnathus, augnathus*, etc.
  2. *Thoracopagus parasiticus*—parasite attached to torso.
    a. *Epigastrius*—parasite consists of a head only.
    b. *Heterodymus*—parasite consists of a head and shoulders.
    c. *Heterotypus*—parasite consists of a head, body and limbs.
    d. *Heteropagus*—parasite consists of limbs only.
  3. *Pygopagus* (or *Ischiopagus*) *parasiticus*—attached to pelvis.
  4. *Inclusio fetus in fetu*—parasite within body of autosite.

MONOAXIAL DOUBLE MONSTERS

In reduplication by fission there is merely some splitting of a single embryo. Always some part of the median axis remains intact. In case of both anterior and posterior dichotomy (anacatadidymus) there may be a close resemblance to conjoined diaxial symmetrical twins. More often fission is unipolar, and typical monsters result, as follows:

I. *Anadidymi*—cephalic dichotomy.
  1. *Dicephalus*—two-headed monster (Fig. 349).
II. *Catadidymi*—caudal dichotomy.
  1. *Dipygus*—anomalous reduplicative development of genitals and lower extremities, with three or four legs at times.

MONSTERS RESULTING FROM ARRESTED DEVELOPMENT

I. Defective closure of dorsal groove forming neural canal.
  1. Conditions affecting the skull and brain.
    a. *Triocephalia*—no head; merely a knot of tissue.
    b. *Cranioschisis*—no closure of cranial sutures, with escape or failure of brain substance to develop.
      a'. *Anencephaly*—commonest type; absence of brain from collapsed cranium (occipitally) with typical "frog" face (Fig. 352).
    c. *Craniorachischisis*—defect of skull and vertebrae (Fig. 353).
    d. *Microcephaly*—inadequate development of brain and premature development and closure of cranium (Fig. 637).
II. Arrested development at the superior embryonal pole in the region of the face.
  1. *Trigonocephaly*—narrowness of skull with approximation of orbits.
  2. *Cyclocephaly*—more or less absence of olfactory organs with development of rudimentary fused visual organs in midline.
    a. *Cyclopia*—complete or incomplete; single orbit with fused eye.
  3. *Arhinencephaly*—rudimentary or complete absence of nose.
    a. *Ethmocephaly*—rudimentary proboscis of soft tissues.

PLATE LXXXVI
CYSTS

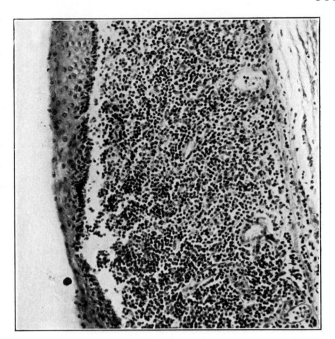

FIG. 355.—NECK: BRANCHOGENIC CYST.—CASE 159.—Photomicrograph which shows an infected, ulcerated, squamous epithelial lined cyst wall and a subepithelial layer of lymphoid tissue, both of which are infiltrated by inflammatory cellular exudate. App. 100 x.

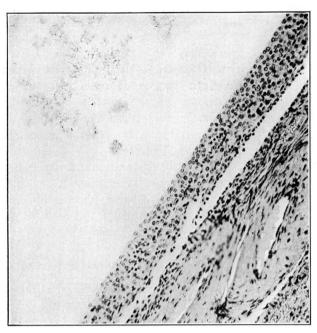

FIG. 356.—OVARY: FOLLICULAR CYST.—Section through a portion of the wall of one of the cysts seen in Fig. 358. It is lined by normal follicular epithelium several layers deep. Lumen contains a pale, serous coagulum. App. 100 x.

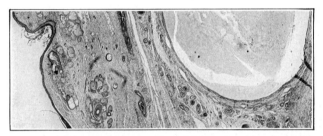

FIG. 357.—OVARY: DERMOID CYST.—Low power photomicrograph showing a small follicular cyst at bottom and the wall of a large dermoid cyst at top. Note skinlike epithelium with its usual appendages. App. 10 x.

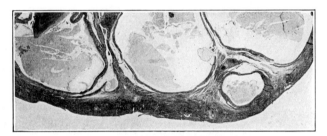

FIG. 358.—OVARY: FOLLICULAR CYSTS (see Fig. 356).—Multiple simple cysts developing in persistent ovarian follicles. App. 10 x.

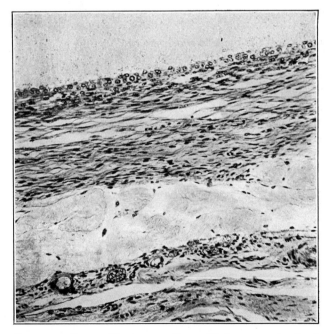

FIG. 359.—OVARY: FOLLICULAR CYST.—High power detail of wall of cyst from Fig. 357. This is apparently lined by flattened connective tissue and filled with a serous, albuminous material. App. 100 x.

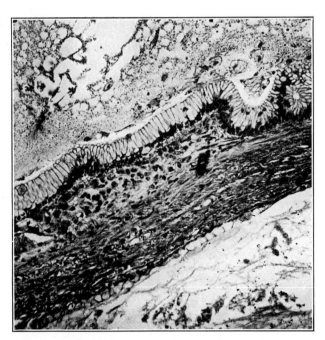

FIG. 360.—OVARY.—PSEUDOMUCINOUS CYSTADENOMA.—CASE 252.—Photomicrograph of cyst wall lined by tall, pale, columnar epithelial cells with hyperchromic, basally placed small nuclei. Lumen filled with granular pseudomucinous material derived from the lining epithelium. App. 100 x.

4. *Rhinocephaly*—a tuberous proboscis located above fused eyes.
5. *Otocephaly*—union or approximation of ears because of rudimentary or absent lower jaw or mouth.
   a. *Synotia*—fusion of ears.
6. Several other less common anomalies exist —not listed here.

III. Arrested development at inferior embryonal pole:
   1. *Ectromelus*—having abortive limbs.
      a. *Amelus* (legless).
      b. *Micromelus* (stunted legs).

c. *Phocomelus* (rudimentary limbs attached to trunk.) (Fig. 351.)

2. *Symmelus*—having imperfect pelvis and fused legs.
   a. *Uromelus*—fused legs with a single foot.
   b. *Sirenomelus*—fused legs with no feet (Fig. 350).

IV. Arrested Development in the Midline:
   1. *Celosomus*—body cleft with eventration; including exstrophy of heart, bladder, etc., in marked cases (Fig. 354).

ANOMALIES RESULTING FROM ARRESTED DEVELOPMENT

I. Anomalies affecting cephalic region: most of these will be found in relation to the embryonal fissures of the face.
   1. Sequestration dermoid cysts (Fig. 346).
   2. Basal cell carcinomata (Fig. 318 and 319).
   3. Branchial cysts (Fig. 355).
   4. Mixed tumors of salivary glands (Fig. 19).
   5. Harelip and cleft palate.
      a. single.
      b. double—resulting from failure of lateral buds to fuse with nasal process. May extend to involve uvula and hard palate as well.

II. Anomalies affecting caudal region—confusion in development of cloaca, allantois, omphalus, etc.
   1. Meckel's diverticulum.
   2. Exstrophy of bladder.
   3. Hypo- and epispadias, etc.

Theories.—(1) (Fournier) Monstrous development may be traced to the existence of syphilis in the antecedents of the child, as expressed by an exhaustion of the developmental force. This theory while in the ascendancy for many years has been completely discarded. (2) The theory of maternal impressions also has been thoroughly discarded because such changes would have to occur within the first two weeks of fetal development and the usual incident cited as causing the stigma rarely occurred until the latter part of pregnancy. (3) Present theory is based much more practically on our more thorough knowledge of embryology, and is dependent chiefly on mechanical factors. The great wonder is not that monsters occur, but that they occur so seldom. Even an hereditary factor must be considered in certain cases, although this is a difficult thing to wholly explain.

CYSTS

A problem which always presents itself is where to include a consideration of the various types of cysts, which are found pathologically. It seems perhaps more logical to consider them at this time in relation to the developmental defects as a large proportion of them fall under this classification. However, there are other cystic lesions which are less well-defined and offer more difficulty of classification. In the broad sense of the term, "tumor," in the older literature, the cysts were included as one division, while the true neoplasms made up the other major group of lesions. Certain of the cysts should be included as true tumors; others as defects in development, while still others represent mechanical inflammatory and degenerative lesions which are better termed "pseudocysts." A brief attempt at classification of the various forms of cystic diseases which are encountered pathologically is appended for convenience and consideration. It is fully appreciated that this is by no means complete.

CYSTIC ADENOMATA

True Cystomata.—In this group of lesions must be included those true tumors which develop usually as proliferative neoplasms from the various glandular organs. Among the most important of these should be mentioned the tumors of the ovary and of the thyroid. Less frequently, similar cystadenomata are found involving the pituitary, and even the kidney. These will be considered under the respective organs in which they occur (Fig. 356, 358, 359 and 360).

CYSTS ARISING FROM DEVELOPMENTAL DEFECTS EMBRYOLOGICALLY

In this group belong the various lesions which have already been commented upon previously in the preceding section. The dermoid sequestration cyst results from infolding of the ectoderm along the normal lines of closure of the embryonic clefts as has been indicated. In this group may even be included a possible explanation for the distribution of a great majority of the basal cell carcinomata, as McFarland has brought out in his consideration of these tumors. The entire group of midline defects such as spina bifida, the meningoceles and encephaloceles, should be included also.

Likewise, in this group should be included those cysts which result from the persistence of fetal structures which normally disappear. Most important in this group should be considered the branchial cleft cysts (Fig. 355), those of the thyroglossal duct, Rathke's pouch cysts, Meckel's diverticulum and the like. Other examples of cysts of this variety are those seen which arise from persistent remnants of the urachus of the wolffian ducts, of the mullerian ducts and even of the mesonephritic ducts. In this group, the parovarian cysts at times become of clinical and pathological importance. Of this group, the branchial cleft cysts are probably of the greatest significance as they not infrequently undergo neoplastic development, becoming true tumors, which may indeed undergo malignant transformation and give rise to squamous carcinomata similar in character to those arising from the surface epithelium elsewhere.

As a lesion which is difficult to classify must be considered the so-called *"polycystic kidney"* or congenital cystic disease of the kidney. This is generally believed to be due to failure of the tubules of the developing kidney to succeed in fusing with the corresponding glomerular unit. This results in multiple cystic lesions in the kidney. They are always bilateral in distribution and are of grave significance to the life of the individual, although many individuals unfortunately afflicted with this condition may survive until middle age. Unexplainable on this same basis is the fact that associated with this condition not infrequently one finds cystic lesions affecting the liver and pancreas, and even the lung so that the term "polycystic disease" is sometimes applied to this combined congenital picture.

PARASITIC CYSTS

The cysts which result from parasitic diseases have already been discussed in the chapter relating to those infestations. Suffice it to say at this point that the hydatid cyst resulting from Taenia echinococcic infestation is the most impressive of this group in man. Cysticercus disease resulting from Taenia solium infestation and the small cysts resulting from Trichina infestations are examples of this group.

RETENTION CYSTS

Of the other varieties of cysts should be mentioned the so-called retention cysts which result from the occlusion of some duct. Thus, obstruction of the parotid or submaxillary ducts may result in cystic dilatation. Similarly, in the biliary tract or in the pancreatic duct, obstruction from calculus, infection or outside pressure may result in similar cystic changes in those structures. Another comparable lesion is seen in the sebaceous cyst, already described as a pseudotumor (Chapter XXIII, Case 87, page 236, Fig. 222). These should not be considered as true cysts but merely as mechanical lesions which result from obstruction in some form. Included in the usual classification of cystic lesions, likewise,

must be mentioned those accumulations of fluid occurring in closed cavities, particularly in relation to
the serous lined spaces of the bursae, joints and tendon sheaths. The degenerative changes in the tendon
sheath with resultant pouch-like dilatation, known as

the ganglion, falls in this category. Likewise, those
inflammatory changes seen at times as a sterile type
of arthritis or an inflammatory bursitis are considered by some as cystic lesions. These might well be
listed as pseudocysts.

Pseudocysts

Finally, there is the group of so-called "false
cysts" or pseudocysts which result from mucoid degeneration or from hemorrhage with subsequent
liquefaction. Such lesions may be seen in old infarcts
or in tissues, the site of extensive hemorrhage. It is

best perhaps to disregard this group in any consideration of the various forms of cystic disease and to
consider them only as degenerative lesions affecting
the organ or tissue in which they occur, although
they were always included, in the older texts.

Illustrative Case

Case 159. (#S-333)
Diagnosis.—Branchial cyst (infected).
Patient was a white, married male of 47 years, admitted to the hospital because of a lump in the left side
of his neck, which had been bothering him for several
weeks.
Present Illness.—Following a cold six months before
admission, the patient developed a small lump in the
left side of his neck, which had gradually increased in
size, until at the time of admission it was about the size
of a lime. It was not particularly tender or painful.
There was no appreciable swelling around the mass and
the skin was not reddened. It disturbed the patient
chiefly as a psychologic and cosmetic problem rather than
as anything more acutely serious.
Past History.—He had the usual childhood diseases
including scarlet fever. He had had no previous operations. Had never been sick enough to require hospitalization. Patient had a history of marked frequency of
colds over many years. More recently he had been better
in this respect following the use of cold vaccine. In association with these subsequent upper respiratory infections, he had had some difficulty with his hearing on occasions. He had shown a slight loss of weight during the
past few weeks but had had no disturbance of his appetite or digestive tract. Had no history of cough or expectoration.
Physical Examination.—Patient was a well-nourished,
middle-aged, white male in no acute pain or distress.
Head was essentially negative. Eyes, ears, nose and
throat were normal. Tonsils showed moderate enlargement and suggested a mild, chronic inflammatory process. Neck: On the left side there was what appeared to
be an enlarged cervical lymph node about the size of a
lime. This was tense but had a suggestion of fluctua-

tion. It was not matted down. It appeared isolated.
There was no redness of the overlying tissues and there
was no notable tenderness or pain on pressure. Heart
was not enlarged and appeared to be normal in all
respects. Lungs were clear and resonant throughout.
There were no râles. Abdomen was negative. Extremities were negative.
Laboratory Findings.—Red blood cells, 5,220,000 with
86% hemoglobin (14.5 grams). White blood cells, 12,500
with 78% polynuclears of which 10% were nonfilamented.
The patient was advised to have the mass in his neck
excised locally.
Operative Record.—The nodule in the neck was exposed and excised intact. It appeared fluctuant and on
section there appeared to be merely a shell of tissue filled
with thick, pea-green, purulent material which was
thought to probably be tuberculous in nature.
Pathological Report.—*Gross Description of Surgical
Specimen.*—Specimen consisted of the wall of a cyst,
which measured in its collapsed state about 4 x 2.5 cm.
The inner surface was rough and trabeculated.
Microscopic Description of Section Through the
Cyst.—(Fig. 355) Histologic examination of the cyst-
wall shows the tissue to be made up of a fairly dense
fibrous connective structure and lined by a definite layer
of stratified squamous epithelium. Lying between these
two structures is a fairly abundant amount of lymphoid
tissue. This varies somewhat in amount in different
parts of the section. Some areas of the lining epithelium
are ulcerated away, leaving an infected granulation-like
structure richly infiltrated with small round cells and
polymorphonuclear leukocytes. This leukocytic infiltration extends in some places rather deep into the wall of
the cyst. There is no histological evidence of tuberculosis
present.

CHAPTER XXXVIII
DISEASES OF THE HEART

ENDOCARDITIS

In a consideration of the diseases which primarily affect the heart, three conditions stand out preeminently as most important numerically. These are represented first, by the group of conditions which affect primarily the endocardium and are considered clinically under the general heading of endocarditis; second, coronary artery disease, which is one of the most important causes of death statistically; and finally, the large group of degenerative lesions affecting the myocardium, which may result from a very wide range of etiologic factors. In addition, there is a group of cases which arises as the result of developmental defects resulting in the various clinical forms of congenital heart disease. There are occasional rare cases of neoplasm. For convenience, the lesions of the heart may also be approached from the standpoint of the three anatomical structures; the endocardium, the myocardium, and the pericardium. This is a rather arbitrary division based wholly on anatomical grounds and from the practical standpoint clinically is of comparatively little significance as the great majority of pathological processes which affect the organ are likely to involve all three elements. However, it is true that occasional instances are encountered both clinically and pathologically in which the pathology seems to be restricted to one or another of these three structures and where this occurs the consideration of the pathological findings logically follows the more usual anatomical approach. This is particularly true of pericardial lesions many of which represent extensions of lesions elsewhere in the chest; as for example the development of an acute pericarditis from contiguity in a case of infection of the pleura. Thus, it is seen that in this important organ the usual arrangement of the material in the clinical order of malformations, circulatory disturbances, toxic lesions including the various degenerative and infiltrative processes, infectious diseases and neoplasms becomes a difficult problem. With this explanation in mind, let us turn to a consideration of those conditions which affect primarily the endocardium from the clinical standpoint. In this group of lesions must be included first of all rheumatic fever; second, subacute bacterial endocarditis and third, acute ulcerative bacterial endocarditis. It will be noted as the discussion progresses that the actual involvement of the endocardium is more often restricted to that portion covering the valves and particularly involving the mitral valve. For this reason, it might be more accurate to speak of these diseases as "valvulitis" rather than "endocarditis." However, many cases are found in which the inflammatory process extends beyond the valves involving especially the endocardium of the auricle and for this reason the time-honored nomenclature will be followed.

RHEUMATIC FEVER

Rheumatic fever is an acute infectious disease affecting the fibrous tissue of the body, characterized by the formation of tiny miliary lesions which are best seen in the myocardium and are known as Aschoff bodies. Grossly, the most spectacular lesions are seen in the heart and joints.

Valvular Lesions (Fig. 361).—The valvular endocardium shows typical small verrucous or wart-like vegetations along the line of contact, arranged much like a chain of beads, measuring 2 or 3 mm. in diameter, firmly attached and not easily dislodged, most commonly found in the mitral valve but may be present on the aortic, and less commonly on the other valves.

Histologically, the affected valve shows edema and the presence of a productive exudate consisting of fibroblasts, large phagocytic mononuclears, plasma cells, lymphocytes, and an occasional polymorphonu-

PLATE LXXXVII

HEART—RHEUMATIC CARDITIS

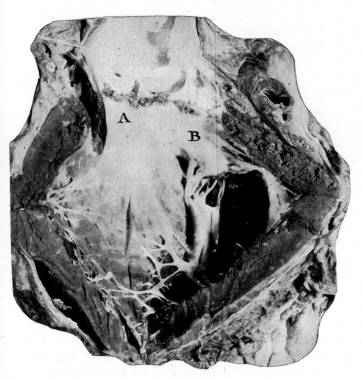

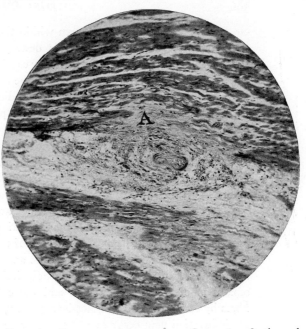

FIG. 362.—RHEUMATIC MYOCARDITIS.—CASE 160.—Section of myocardium showing typical fibrillary Aschoff body (A) with degenerative changes in the adjacent muscle fibres. App. 75 X.

FIG. 361.—HEART: RHEUMATIC ENDOCARDITIS.—CASE 160.—Verrucose vegetations along the line of contact of aortic cusps (A), an older mitral lesion (B) with thickening and shortening of chordae tendineae. Adhesive pericarditis.

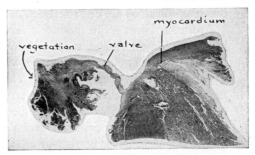

FIG. 363.—VALVE LESION.—CASE 160. App. 3 X.

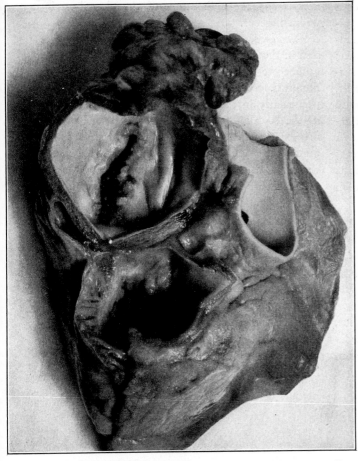

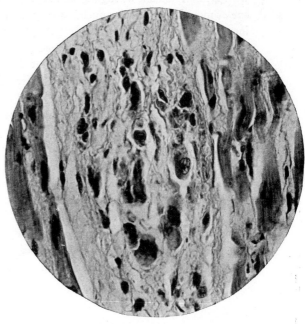

FIG. 365.—RHEUMATIC MYOCARDITIS.—CASE 160.—Aschoff body showing swollen, interlacing collagen and typical large Aschoff cells. Some contain two nuclei ("owl" cells). Others tend to have basophilic staining cytoplasmic streamers. App. 200 X.

FIG. 364.—HEART: RHEUMATIC ENDOCARDITIS; MITRAL STENOSIS.—CASE 161.—Thickened and calcified mitral valve seen from the base of the heart. The function is impaired, the valve incapable of opening beyond the slit illustrated (buttonhole mitral).

clear. Young capillaries may be seen within the leaflet. The endothelium (Fig. 363) is destroyed beneath the vegetation. The vegetation consists of platelets and some fibrin. Examination of the chordae tendineae shows the presence of Aschoff bodies, the healing of which results in shortening. If the patient survives the acute stage of the disease, the valve will be healed by fibrous tissue, the contraction of which leads to stiffening and shortening of the cusps. Calcification and adhesions also frequently occur in the older lesions still further impairing the function.

Myocardial Lesions.—The changes which are seen in the myocardium are of both the exudative and proliferative nature. The exudative phase of the picture is characterized by a rather variable amount of interstitial edema, characterized histologically by separation of the muscle bundles and the collagen fibers by serum. In addition, not infrequently, cellular infiltration may occur in the more severe cases. This is chiefly of the mononuclear variety with large mononuclear cells, lymphocytes, and plasma cells predominating. The proliferative reaction is seen in the development of the characteristic Aschoff bodies.

ASCHOFF BODY.—The proliferative reaction is best studied in the Aschoff body of the myocardium. It consists of small pinpoint lesions not visible to the naked eye, oval in shape, located to one side of a small vessel in the connective tissue stroma. Typically, there are four zones which may be fairly readily identified: (1) A center of necrotic collagen; (2) a variable number of Aschoff cells which surround this area. These are large, round or oval cells, with a small amount of slightly basic cytoplasm and one or more large vesicular nuclei usually with prominent nucleoli; (3) A zone of lymphocytes, plasma cells and rarely an occasional polymorphonuclear; (4) Around the edge, proliferation of fibroblasts which show varying degrees of adult differentiation in an attempt to wall off the lesion.

Several of these miliary lesions may coalesce and actually become visible to the naked eye as tiny pale elongated areas which have the morphology of a millet seed, in the myocardium (Fig. 362 and 365). In addition to the Aschoff body in the myocardium the heart muscle fibers show degenerative changes (marked myocardosis) and the interstitial tissue, inflammatory edema. This is spoken of as myocardosis and consists of fatty and hydropic degeneration of the cytoplasm of the cells. In the more severe

cases, this may go on to actual myocarditis and the accumulation of phagocytic leukocytes.

Pericardial Lesions.—Not only do these inflammatory changes occur in the endocardium and myocardium, but they may be found extending to involve the pericardium as well. The reaction when seen in the pericardium is characterized by the presence of an acute inflammatory reaction with variable amounts of fibrin laid down on the serosal surface. This is accompanied by a marked dilatation of the blood vessels and a very considerable cellular infiltration of the epicardium. Not infrequently, actual Aschoff bodies may be identified in this zone of inflammatory changes which present the same microscopic features as those seen in the myocardium. As the lesion progresses, the fibrinous exudate tends to undergo organization from both the parietal and visceral surfaces. This will form adhesions and, if the patient survives the acute stage of the disease, the end result may be the obliteration of all or a considerable part of the pericardial cavity. This produces a gradually increased strain upon the heart with a very marked work hypertrophy. The inflammatory pericarditis may extend beyond the pericardium itself to involve the pleura or even the mediastinal tissues and result in similar inflammatory fibrosis and the obliteration of the pleural cavity with adhesions.

Extracardiac Lesions.—The proliferative changes seen in the development of the Aschoff body are not confined to the heart by any means but occur in the fibrous tissues of the body more or less generally, but particularly in the subcutaneous tissues of the skin as the so-called rheumatic nodule. Likewise, they may be seen histologically in the connective tissues around the joint cavities and around the blood vessels of the viscera. In every instance of the development of an Aschoff body, there seems to be a predilection for its localization just outside the smaller vessels but unlike the usual inflammatory reaction, it tends to be asymmetrical in position rather than uniformly perivascular in distribution. Furthermore it is a specific lesion which is found *only* in rheumatic fever.

Theoretically, it is of interest to note that the lesion in the course of its development goes through a number of rather characteristic phases. The work of Gross in this regard may be considered as almost classical in its thoroughness and clearness. The lesion

PLATE LXXXVIII
SUBACUTE BACTERIAL ENDOCARDITIS.—CASE 162

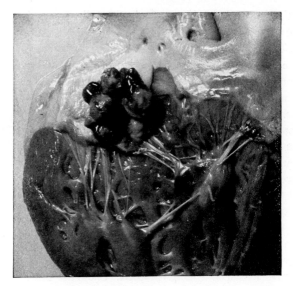

FIG. 366.—HEART: VALVE LESION.—Mitral valve showing large, polypoid vegetation.

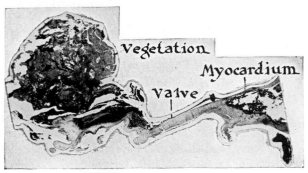

FIG. 369.—MITRAL VALVE VEGETATION. App. 5 x.

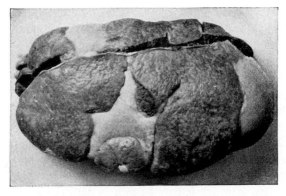

FIG. 367.—SPLEEN: INFARCTION.—Gross spleen showing three pale, slightly depressed areas of infarction, the result of embolism.

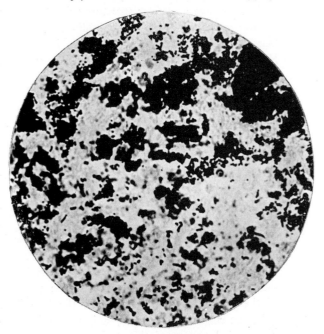

FIG. 370.—High power photomicrograph showing masses of S. viridans in vegetation. App. 900 x.

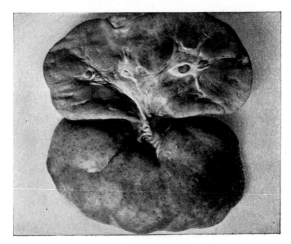

FIG. 368.—KIDNEY: FOCAL EMBOLIC GLOMERULAR NEPHRITIS AND INFARCTION.—Tiny characteristic reddish dots seen scattered over the surface give rise to the term "flea bitten kidney."

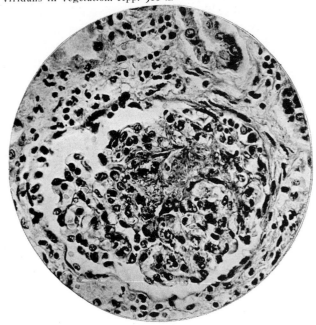

FIG. 371.—KIDNEY—FOCAL EMBOLIC GLOMERULAR NEPHRITIS.—Glomerulus with hyalinized thrombus obstructing a capillary loop of the tuft. App. 200 x.

starts as a rather indefinite accumulation of mononuclear cells which in many instances are rather difficult to identify histogenetically. They fall into a rather jumbled pattern which Gross speaks of as the mosaic form. Gradually the identity of these (Fig. 365) cells makes itself apparent with the appearance of typical "owl-eye" cells, consisting of large nuclei with extremely prominent nucleoli and appearing in pairs. These "owl-eye" cells are specific from the histological standpoint for recognition of the developing rheumatic lesion. A stage further in the development of the Aschoff body is seen when the cells begin to assume a fibrillar structure with the fibers tending to be laid down in longitudinal bundles so that an ovoid appearance of the lesion is assumed. Following the appearance of this fibrillar stage of the lesion, frank fibrosis develops with what might almost be described as a pseudo-capsule of fibroblasts with the typical Aschoff cells still present centrally in the lesion. This represents the fully developed stage of the lesion. From that point on the changes are those associated with the gradual disappearance of the lesion as a result of a fibrous scar tissue replacement.

The presence of histologic Aschoff bodies is diagnostic of rheumatic fever, but their absence by no means excludes the existence of the disease, for it has been shown by Gross and others that in many of the milder cases it requires almost serial section of the heart to be able to demonstrate the presence of the typical diagnostic lesion. In the healed or quiescent stage of the disease, it is extremely common to find no recognizable Aschoff bodies on careful microscopic study of the heart. To Gross also should go the credit for the recognition and realization of the rather selective distribution of the Aschoff lesions in the heart. He has demonstrated time and time again, if such lesions are present, they will always be found in sections taken from the wedge of muscle tissue at the base of the several valves, and his recommendation that uniform sections should always be taken from hearts for study from these selected areas, has added tremendously to our evaluation of the rheumatic lesion.

Etiology.—The etiology of rheumatic fever is one of the moot problems of medicine. The pendulum has swung through a wide arc in the course of the past quarter century. Numerous investigators have come forward with claims for one or another agent as the cause of the disease. It is generally accepted that rheumatic fever must be classed among the infectious diseases, and that there appears to be some close relationship in the development of the disease to one of the streptococci. Whether this is a specific organism or not is still entirely a matter of conjecture. There are those advocates of the hemolytic streptococci theory, and there are those who believe that the organism belongs to the non-hemolytic group of streptococci. There are those who are convinced that the disease is primarily a virus infection and that if the streptococcus plays any part, it is as a secondary invader. There are those who believe that the entire clinical picture of rheumatic fever and even the pathological lesions are the result of tissue allergy from sensitization to some one or another of these various strains of streptococci. There are those who believe that avitaminosis is an essential part of the picture before the disease may develop. The possibility of focal infection such as chronic tonsillitis remains one of the favorite conceptions in respect to etiology. From the above statements, it seems apparent that the exact nature of the etiologic agent is still most assuredly in doubt. On the other hand, there seems to be but little question that a streptococcus is responsible to a very large extent for many of the manifestations of the disease, probably not as a specific infecting agent but through the action of its toxins either directly or through some previous tissue sensitization.

Clinically, rheumatic fever is very largely a disease of childhood, appearing most frequently in its acute manifestations between the ages of five and ten years, although it may be seen in early infancy and may not occur until adult life. It is characterized frequently and particularly in the childhood form by a history of previous streptococcus infection of the tonsils and throat. In a very considerable percentage of cases, this acute upper respiratory infection is followed by chorea or St. Vitus' dance, as it is commonly called. In other instances no such definite history of throat infection can be elicited. The symptoms are those of an acute or subacute inflammatory process involving a succession of joints, accompanied by swelling, redness and pain. This is combined usually with fever and malaise. Many mild cases subside spontaneously and show no evidence of cardiac involvement clinically either at that time or later. Others, however, may go on to develop pro-

PLATE LXXXIX
DISEASES OF THE HEART

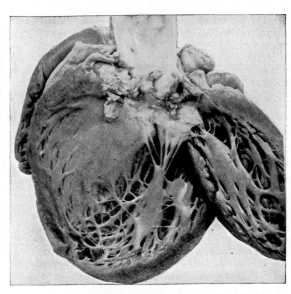

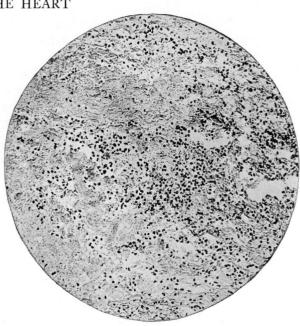

FIG. 372.—ACUTE BACTERIAL (ULCERATIVE) ENDOCARDITIS.
—Cf. CASE 163.—Large friable reddish-gray vegetations involving both the valvular and mural endocardium of the mitral valve with ulceration and perforation of the cusps.

FIG. 373.—VEGETATION—ACUTE BACTERIAL ENDOCARDITIS.—CASE 163.—Photomicrograph of vegetation in which the fibrin and platelets are undergoing liquefaction necrosis. App. 10 x.

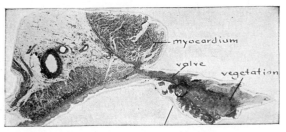

FIG. 374.—VALVE LESION—ACUTE BACTERIAL ENDOCARDITIS.—CASE 163. App. 3 x.

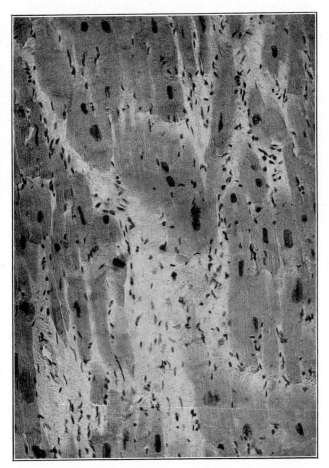

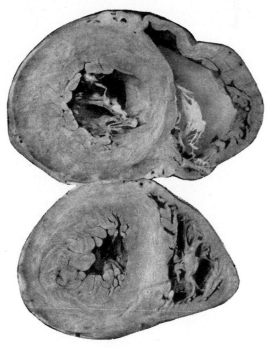

FIG. 375.—HEART—MYOSCLEROSIS.—CASE 164.—Section of the hypertrophied myocardium showing rather diffuse interstitial replacement fibrosis. App. 400 x.

FIG. 376.—HEART—HYPERTROPHY (CONCENTRIC).—CASE 164.—Tangential section: the left ventricle has undergone marked concentric hypertrophy associated with malignant nephrosclerosis.

gressive involvement of the heart manifested by the presence of valvular murmurs, most frequently involving the mitral area. In some instances the disease progresses steadily to a fatal exodus within a comparatively short period of time. More often, however, the disease subsides after a few weeks in its acute form. The fever disappears, the joint symptoms vanish as if by magic, leaving no residual pain or disability and it is only several months later that evidence of cardiac damage gradually manifests itself, with dyspnea, cyanosis, anorexia and a wide variety of other symptoms. The child, on examination, is found to have a heart which is considerably enlarged, particularly on the right side. There is commonly a soft, blowing, systolic murmur heard over the mitral area. Less frequently involvement of the aortic, tricuspid and pulmonic valves is found in the order named. As time goes on the cardiac symptoms become more pronounced, the liver becomes greatly enlarged and may extend as much as a hand's breadth below the costal margin. The patient's appetite remains poor; the nutrition as a result is impaired; not infrequently a cough is developed with the raising of "rusty" sputum, until finally the patient dies of intercurrent infection, usually a pneumonia, or of cardiac decompensation.

At autopsy, in the typical case of advanced rheumatic heart disease, as may be expected from the clinical symptomology, the heart is found to be enlarged. Upon the duration of the disease and the severity of the valvular lesions will depend the extent and distribution of the hypertrophy. There may be extensive calcification of the mitral valve to such a degree that it will not even admit the tip of the finger. This is the characteristic end lesion of a severe mitral valvulitis resulting in mitral stenosis and insufficiency. The great majority of cases show only the mitral valve involved.

Another large group shows combined mitral and aortic valve involvement. Less frequently the other valves show similar changes. Rarely the aortic may be involved alone but these are merely variants of the basic pathology. The secondary manifestations resulting from those disturbances in circulation is seen in a very striking passive congestion of the viscera, particularly of the lungs and liver. These changes are all considered from the pathological standpoint in the series of case histories which follow.

Rheumatic Pneumonitis.—In recent years, particular attention has been called to the fact that the rheumatic picture not infrequently may be seen as a true interstitial pneumonitis. For many years it was held that the changes which were found in the lung were entirely the result of the chronic passive congestion with resultant thickening of the alveolar walls and some secondary incidental cellular infiltration. The work of Gross and others has shown, however, that this cellular reaction is a true inflammatory response, which is seen almost exclusively during the active acute exacerbations of the disease clinically. Indeed, around the smaller bronchioles in conjunction with a peribronchial interstitial fibrosis, it is at times possible to find lesions which are indistinguishable from Aschoff bodies.

ILLUSTRATIVE CASES

CASE 160. (Ref. #S-181 and S-183)

Diagnosis.—Acute rheumatic pancarditis.

Patient was a white female age 13, who was admitted to the hospital complaining of pain in the chest and of dyspnea.

Present Illness.—The present illness began about one year before her present admission. At that time she had a severe attack of tonsillitis, which kept her in bed for about ten days. Following this infection, within a month, she developed multiple joint symptoms. These consisted of painful swelling of the fingers, wrists, ankles, elbows and shoulders. This was accompanied by a moderate fever. The joint pains subsided on bed rest and the administration of salicylates. Following this acute attack of typical rheumatic fever, she seemed to be entirely well and was able to attend school and to carry on her usual normal physical activities for several months. About six months before admission, however, she first noticed some slight dyspnea on exertion and on examination by a physician at that time, a diagnosis of heart disease was

made and the child restricted in her physical activities. She had no joint symptoms at that time and her physician felt that the cardiac picture was a residual lesion and that the rheumatic process was quiescent. She went along uneventfully until about one month before admission when she began to complain of pain in her chest and dyspnea with the very slightest exertion. This had been accompanied by a recurrent flare-up of her joint lesions and the patient had been in bed during this preadmission period.

Past History.—The patient had had no previous history of any serious illness. She had been a normally delivered, healthy infant and had had an entirely uneventful nutritional history. She had not been unduly susceptible to upper respiratory infections. A review of her systems up to the onset of her present illness was noninformatory.

Physical Examination.—Physical examination showed a well developed, well nourished adolescent girl who appeared somewhat older than her given age. Head was normal in contour. Eyes were negative. Ears were negative. Nose and throat were negative. Tonsils had been removed. The chest was symmetrical. The heart was greatly enlarged to the left reaching the midaxillary line. There was a loud systolic blowing murmur best heard over the apex and transmitted to the left axilla and to the scapular region. Her lungs showed a few crepitant râles at the bases. Temperature was 103° on admission and her pulse ranged from 100 to 130. Blood pressure was 108/58. Her abdomen was slightly prominent and the liver edge was felt three fingers' breadth below the costal margin. The spleen was questionably enlarged. The extremities showed some slight reddening and swelling over the ankles and wrists. There was no apparent involvement of the other joints. No nodules could be felt in the skin.

Laboratory Findings.—Red blood cells, 4,300,000 with 83% hemoglobin. White blood cells numbered 13,200 with 76% polynuclears. Blood sedimentation rate was twice the normal. Blood cultures taken at repeated intervals were uniformly negative. Urinalysis showed occasional traces of albumin and a few red cells at times.

Subsequent Course.—The patient became progressively worse, developed definite cardiac decompensation and died with clinical evidence of terminal bronchopneumonia.

Autopsy Findings.—Pleura: There was a bilateral hydrothorax. Lungs showed edema and terminal bronchopneumonia. Heart weighed 550 gm. and showed marked hypertrophy and dilatation of the right side. The myocardium was soft, flabby and pale reddish gray in color (Fig. 361). The mitral, aortic and tricuspid valves showed a number of small verrucous vegetations arranged along the line of contact, together with thickening of the cusps. The pericardium (cf. Fig. 103, 104, 105 and 106, Chapter XIII) was the site of fibrinous pericarditis. There was marked chronic passive congestion of the liver, spleen and kidneys.

Microscopic Description of a Section Through the Myocardium.—(Fig. 362, 363 and 365) Histologic examination of the myocardium reveals the muscle fibers pale and irregularly stained. There is marked interstitial edema. The most conspicuous feature, however, is the presence of many Aschoff bodies usually occurring near an arteriole. These lesions are ovoid in shape, and consist of an area of central necrotic collagen, around which appear numerous irregularly shaped, oval or rounded Aschoff cells. Some of these contain more than one nucleus. Mononuclear cellular infiltration including particularly plasma cells and lymphocytes is prominent. At the periphery of the lesion there is considerable proliferation of young fibroblasts. In some instances, the wall of the arteriole itself may appear to be incorporated in the development of the Aschoff body. Accompanying the process, marked granular, fatty and hydropic degenerative changes affecting the adjacent muscle fibers have occurred.

Under high magnification, the Aschoff cells are found to have a definite cell membrane with a slightly basic staining cytoplasm and a vesicular nucleus with prominent chromatic masses. The cell outlines, however, are frequently indefinite. Some of the cells have more than one nucleus producing the typical "owl cell," pathognomonic of rheumatic disease.

A similar case illustrating the pericardial lesion has already been referred to in Chapter XIII, Case 47 (Ref. # S-2), page 118, and Fig. 103, 104, 105 and 106.

CASE 161. (Ref. #S-55)

Diagnosis.—Heart—rheumatic fever; mitral stenosis and regurgitation.

Patient was a girl, age 13 years, admitted to the hospital with the picture of cardiac decompensation.

Present Illness.—The onset of the patient's present illness dated back five years to her first attack of rheumatic fever at the age of eight years. This was preceded by tonsillitis and a severe attack of chorea. She had been followed carefully in the heart clinic since that time. She had had at least three recurrences of the acute picture which required bed rest for periods of several months at a time. For the six months preceding her present admission she had had repeated periods of marked cyanosis accompanied by dyspnea on the slightest exertion. She likewise complained of pain over the precordium at intervals, which radiated at times to the left scapular region. She was admitted to the hospital in a moribund condition in acute cardiac collapse.

Two months before her death, physical examination of her chest showed a heart which was greatly enlarged causing a marked precordial thrust with each beat. A loud, rumbling systolic murmur was heard throughout the precordium loudest over the mitral area. On resolution, this was thought to be a double mitral murmur. The liver was greatly enlarged, nearly three fingers' breadth below the costal margin. The spleen was not palpable, but there was tenderness in the splenic area.

Laboratory Findings.—Laboratory findings were not significant except for a rather constant leukocytosis averaging about 15,000 cells with 80% polymorphonuclears, over the last six months of her life. Blood sedimentation index was likewise consistently high. She died shortly after her admission.

Autopsy Findings.—At autopsy, the heart (Fig. 364) was greatly enlarged, more particularly on the right side. The mitral valve showed a marked sclerosis and stenosis with a fish mouth, slit-like lumen. There was considerable scarring of the endocardium of the auricle. The lungs both showed marked chronic passive congestion and what appeared grossly to suggest a rheumatic interstitial pneumonitis. The spleen and kidneys were likewise the seat of a marked chronic passive congestion. The liver presented the typical nutmeg appearance of chronic passive congestion.

This case illustrates the significant features of the late manifestations of the rheumatic lesions. These are dependent upon the scarring of the involved valves and result in productive fibrosis of the tissues. Secondary degenerative changes follow and calcification develops as an almost regular sequence. This results in a rigid valve, which presents varying degrees of obstruction to the blood flow as a stenosis. Due to the contraction of the scar tissue, there is usually a defect in the valve, even after complete healing has occurred. This produces the clinical picture of regurgitation and may be recognized by the characteristic timing of the murmur in respect to the cardiac cycle. As the result of such obstructive and incompetent valves, marked circulatory changes follow. In a simple mitral case uncomplicated by other valvular involvement a right ventricular hypertrophy may be expected. Where other valves are involved, modification of this picture obviously results. The cause of death in the usual case of rheumatic fever is the result of marked chronic passive congestion and cardiac dilatation resulting ultimately in failure. As accessory findings pathologically, as secondary manifestations of this pathology, must be cited the marked chronic passive congestion of the lungs, liver, spleen, kidneys and entire gastro-intestinal mucosa which result in clinical signs and symptoms of those respective organ systems. We have seen some of the results of such pathology with the production of rusty sputum, hemosiderosis of the spleen and shall have occasion to see these other lesions in the consideration of the special pathology of the various organs individually.

Microscopic Description of Tissues from This Case. —Histologic examination of the tissues from this case confirms the gross findings in their entirety. The outstanding changes are seen as a diffuse interstitial myosclerosis resulting from chronic passive congestion.

SUBACUTE BACTERIAL ENDOCARDITIS

Subacute bacterial endocarditis represents the next most important form of valvular disease of the heart. It likewise represents one of the most discouraging diseases from the standpoint of therapy with which we have to deal, having an almost uniformly ultimately fatal outcome with the duration of the disease varying from a matter of a few months to as long as three to four years. It is characterized clinically by running a subacute febrile course, which may simulate a wide variety of clinical conditions and thus offer great difficulty in diagnosis. The lesions are restricted very largely at the outset to the endocardium of the valves with later involvement of the myocardium and extension of the process occasionally to the mural endothelium of the auricles. The great majority of the symptoms are the result of embolic lesions in other organs.

The etiology of subacute bacterial endocarditis is a nonhemolytic streptococcus, in over 95 per cent of cases. The diagnosis is made by the demonstration of the organism in blood culture. This may require repeated attempts as the organisms may be present in only small numbers at times. It is believed by many pathologists that subacute bacterial endocarditis is almost always engrafted upon a rheumatic valvulitis. There are many cases, however, in which such a relationship is extremely difficult to demonstrate.

Valvular Lesions.—The valvular lesions in the case of subacute bacterial endocarditis are quite different from the small verrucous-like beading of the valve seen in rheumatic fever. In this disease, the vegetations are large and polypoid in appearance (Fig. 366). They are usually soft and friable, and reddish in color. They frequently measure as much as 1 to 1.5 cm. in diameter. They are located usually along the line of closure of the valve just as in the case of rheumatic endocarditis and frequently the characteristic thickened, fibrous, bead-like lesions of rheumatic fever may be seen involving the remainder of the valve. As the vegetation grows in size, it frequently spreads to the base of the valve and even over the mural endocardium, particularly of the auricle.

Histologically, the vegetation is found to be made up for the most part of platelets and fibrin in the meshes of which countless red cells are seen. With appropriate staining methods, masses of bacteria may also be observed (Fig. 369 and 370) growing in almost colony fashion. Under oil immersion, these clumps of bacteria may be resolved into typical cocci, many of them occurring in chains. The diseased leaflet usually shows evidence of a previous valvulitis with thickening and vascularization. There is usually a productive exudate present, which further suggests rheumatic fever. It is made up of many large mononuclear phagocytes, plasma cells and lymphocytes along with a fibroblastic proliferation. In some instances, actual Aschoff bodies may be demonstrated.

Myocardial Lesions.—Careful examination of the myocardium histologically usually shows small areas of necrosis containing many polynuclear leukocytes. These are essentially minute metastatic embolic abscesses and are known as Bracht-Wächter bodies. Accompanying these focal areas of myocarditis may also be observed varying degrees of degeneration of the muscle fibers. These are much less conspicuous as a rule, however, than those seen in rheumatic fever. Inasmuch as these lesions are of an embolic nature and occur at irregular intervals rather than at a single time, it is not uncommon to find patchy areas of fibroblastic proliferation and even minute fibrinous scars, representing the healing process of these Bracht-Wächter bodies.

Embolic Phenomena.—It is a common finding in subacute bacterial endocarditis for multiple embolic lesions in the viscera to develop as the result of fragments of the vegetations being swept off into the circulation, as is true of embolism in general. It depends upon the localization of these fragments as to the nature of the subsequent embolic phenomena. Typically, in organs with terminal arterioles, infarction results. This is particularly common to find in the spleen (Fig. 367) and kidney (Fig. 368 and 371). Owing to the difference in size of the emboli, many other different types of lesions may result: painful cutaneous nodules, focal embolic glomerular nephritis, petechial hemorrhages of the skin and mucous membranes, infarcts of the brain and cord, and not infrequently retinal hemorrhages as well as the more striking large infarcts already commented upon. Due to the fact that this embolic material is largely composed of bacteria, the resultant lesions frequently show the secondary manifestations of infection with abscess formation. More often, however, owing to the low grade of virulence of the organism, a subacute inflammatory response rather than actual abscess formation is found.

ILLUSTRATIVE CASE

CASE 162. (Ref. #S-54, S-182, and S-267)

Diagnosis.—Heart—subacute bacterial endocarditis.

Patient was a twenty year old white female admitted to the hospital because of fever and listlessness.

Present Illness.—Six weeks before admission she noticed that she became easily fatigued and generally lost interest in everything. She became markedly apathetic and noted intermittent attacks of being feverish, while at other times she alternated with a feeling of chilliness almost approaching a true chill. She had lost about ten pounds in weight during the two months preceding admission. Two weeks before she became hospitalized she first noticed a number of small red spots scattered pretty generally over her body. They appeared in crops and would be painful for a day or so, then become purplish and fade away. She noted several of these painful lesions under the finger nails. She complained of pain in the left groin and also noted at this time that her urine was dark red.

Past History.—She had a normal childhood. She had had measles at the age of seven. She had several attacks of tonsillitis and for that reason had her tonsils removed at the age of ten. Six years before her present illness she was rejected for insurance because of a leaky heart. At that time, however, she was not incapacitated and led a normal life including participation in school athletics. She did not give any definite history of rheumatic fever, chorea or scarlet fever and had had no other serious illness. She had been worried about her heart because of the fact that she had been rejected for insurance on a second attempt about a year before her present admission, but she had never been actually heart conscious. On account of her history it was thought that she might have a focus of infection in relation to her teeth. X-ray examination revealed several apical abscesses and the teeth of the upper jaw were removed. No improvement in her condition followed.

Physical Examination.—The patient was a well developed and nourished young adult white female. Head was normal in contour. Eyes: There were several pinpoint hemorrhagic spots noted in the conjunctivae. Pupils reacted normally to light and distance. The upper teeth were missing. The lower teeth appeared in good condition. No enlargement of the peripheral lymph nodes was noted. No subcutaneous nodules were demonstrable. The chest was symmetrical. Lungs were clear throughout. Heart was moderately enlarged to the left. There were both a presystolic and a systolic mitral murmur and a faint diastolic murmur heard over the aortic region. The fingers showed some slight clubbing and cyanosis of the nail beds. A small "splinter" hemorrhage under the right index finger nail was seen. Scattered clumps of minute petechiae were seen over the trunk and lower extremities. The abdomen was negative in other respects. The extremities were normal. No abnormal reflexes were noted.

Laboratory Findings.—Urinalysis: Specific gravity, 1.027; 1 plus albumin; occasional red blood cells; granular and hyaline casts. Blood count: Red blood cells, 4,200,000 with 78% hemoglobin. White blood cells, 20,000 with 86% polymorphonuclear neutrophiles. Blood culture was positive for Streptococcus viridans on three occasions. Electrocardiogram showed slight exaggeration of the PR interval.

Subsequent Course.—Three days after admission, the patient developed several petechiae of the right palm. Temperature ranged between 97° and 104°, septic type. The patient became progressively worse. Two months after admission she developed weakness of the right arm and leg, evidence of a cerebral embolus; and slurring of the speech was noted. Patient continued to grow weaker and died about three months after the onset of the first symptoms.

Autopsy Findings.—The heart was slightly enlarged. The myocardium was pale in color and softer than normal. Examination of the aortic valve revealed several cauliflower vegetations (Fig. 366), the largest 11 mm. in diameter, quite friable, reddish-gray in color, and situated along the line of contact, which interfered with complete closure of the valve. The most striking lesion, however, was seen in the mitral valve where a large lobulated vegetation was located, occupying the major portion of one leaflet and measuring over 3 cm. in diameter. It was pinkish gray in color and was covered with postmortem dark reddish clot. Both the aortic and mitral valves were slightly thickened. The papillary muscles were hypertrophied and the chordae tendineae were thickened and slightly shortened. The left ventricle was hypertrophied. Several large infarcts, both recent and healed in character, were found in the spleen (Fig. 367). The kidneys showed multiple infarcts and a typical focal embolic glomerular nephritis characterized by minute punctate hemorrhagic spots giving the appearance of the so-called "flea-bitten" kidney (Fig. 368 and 371).

Microscopic Description of Section Through the Mitral Valve and Vegetation.—(Fig. 369 and 370) The vegetation is composed of platelets and some fibrin with a cap of recent blood clot. In the underlying valve the endothelial lining is entirely destroyed and the valve is considerably thickened due to proliferation of fibroblasts. The fibroblasts can be seen growing into the actual vegetation in an attempt to organize this material. At the base of the valve an inflammatory cellular infiltration of the tissue is seen, consisting chiefly of many large mononuclear cells and occasional polymorphonuclears. It is difficult to completely evaluate the obvious double lesion, the older lesion suggesting a rheumatic picture with its cellular infiltration and the increase of old fibrous scar tissue; the newer, subacute process being represented by the recent connective tissue reaction. Further evidence of the relatively acute nature of the process is seen in a few minute areas of liquefaction necrosis of the valve itself. This is associated with marked polynuclear infiltration. Sections stained by the Gram-Weigert method reveal the presence of large numbers of organisms throughout the vegetative process (Fig. 370).

Additional sections through the myocardium show the characteristic Bracht-Wächter bodies with minute focal areas of necrosis and connective tissue proliferation. Accompanying this focal lesion is seen a rather diffuse parenchymatous myocardial degeneration. There is a definite loss of cross striations of muscle fibers in places, and of the continuity of the muscle fibers. As in rheumatic fever, there is considerable interstitial edema. The picture in general is one of a moderate myocardosis with the complicating additional factor of the minute embolic lesions. The description of the focal embolic glomerular lesions will be found in the chapter devoted to a consideration of glomerular nephritis, page 650. A description of the resultant lesion following such embolic infarction of the spleen and kidney has already been described in Chapter I, Case 2, although this case was not bacterial in origin.

ACUTE BACTERIAL ENDOCARDITIS (ULCERATIVE)

A third form of endocarditis which bears no necessary relationship to rheumatic fever or subacute bacterial endocarditis is seen as a complication in many other serious infections elsewhere in the body. Almost all the pathogenic bacteria have at one time or another been associated with the development of such lesions. The diagnosis clinically is established on the finding of the specific organism in the blood stream coupled with the physical signs pointing to cardiac involvement in association with some infectious condition. The following organisms are those most frequently found as the causative agents: *Streptococcus hemolyticus* and *Staphylococcus aureus*. In addition, any of the other pathogenic organisms, including the *pneumococcus* and the *gonococcus, Bacillus influenzae* and *Bacillus typhosus*. Even the colon bacillus may less frequently gain access to the blood stream and localize on one of the heart valves. The disease runs a rapidly fatal course, the patient rarely surviving more than six or eight weeks. The symptoms are those of an acute infection with high fever, marked prostration, bacterial evidence of a septicemia, the development of cardiac symptoms and death, usually as the result of embolic lesions coupled with profound toxemia.

Valvular lesions.—The endocardial vegetations in acute ulcerative bacterial endocarditis vary considerably with the nature of the infectious agent. In general, they are apt to be large, cauliflower-like or polypoid lesions which are extremely soft and friable.

The valves become ulcerated and are often actually perforated or show deep lacerations along their margins. The vegetations tend to spread much more rapidly and extensively to the base of the valves and over both auricular and ventricular mural endocardium because of the ulcerative nature of the process which permits extension through the valve to the undersurface. Not infrequently the endocardium covering the chordae tendineae is involved. These likewise frequently ulcerate and break off with resultant more marked functional valvular disturbances (Fig. 372).

Microscopically, these lesions show a very much more acute inflammatory process. The valve cusp is swollen and ulcerated (Fig. 374) with extensive polymorphonuclear leukocytic infiltration of the deeper portions of the base. Marked liquefaction necrosis is present (Fig. 373). The vegetation is very similar histologically in appearance to that seen in subacute endocarditis except that there are many more leukocytes found in the fibrinous meshes.

Specific Embolic Phenomena.—Just as in the case of subacute bacterial endocarditis, portions of the vegetations may break off and gain access to the blood stream. These produce emboli characteristically in whatever location they occur. Owing to the higher degree of virulence of the infecting agent, however, the great majority of such emboli produce actual abscess formation. Death results from septicemia or embolism of some vital area, such as the respiratory centre of the brain stem.

CASE 163. (Ref. #S-57)

Diagnosis.—Acute ulcerative bacterial endocarditis. Pneumococcus, Type 2.

Patient was a seventeen-year-old Negress who was admitted to the Obstetrical Service for delivery.

Present Illness.—The patient was a primipara, who had had an entirely normal prenatal history and had been under constant observation during her pregnancy. The delivery was apparently normal, requiring sixteen hours. On the third day after delivery, she developed a pain in the lower abdomen accompanied by generalized rigidity and tenderness, particularly in the right lower quadrant. Temperature became elevated and was followed by a typical septic swing ranging from 96° to 105°, and accompanied by chills and sweats. Lochia had increased slightly in amount and had an offensive odor.

Past Medical History.—Her past history was irrelevant.

Physical Examination.—At this time, six days after delivery, physical examination showed a well-developed, well-nourished, acutely sick-appearing young Negress. Head was normal in contour. Pupils reacted normally. There was no enlargement of the cervical nodes. Chest was symmetrical. Heart was moderately enlarged diffusely. There was a loud systolic murmur heard best over the mitral area. Numerous crackling râles were heard at the bases of both lungs. Abdomen was rigid. Extremities were negative.

Laboratory Findings.—Red blood cells, 3,100,000 with 73% hemoglobin. White blood cells, 28,400 with 92% polynuclears. Urinalysis showed a moderate amount of albumin, occasional red cells but no casts. Blood Wassermann was negative. Blood culture revealed the presence of a Pneumococcus, Type 2.

Subsequent Course.—The septic temperature persisted. The patient became progressively worse. Three weeks after the onset of the first symptoms there developed evidence of central nervous involvement with projectile vomiting, stiffness of the neck and severe headache. At that time, spinal puncture yielded a cloudy fluid under 35 mm. of pressure and a cell count of 18,800 with 95% polymorphonuclear leukocytes. During the next few days, examination of the patient's chest showed further evidence of cardiac involvement, with localization of the murmur over the tricuspid area. The patient failed to respond to treatment and died forty-eight hours after the onset of the meningeal symptoms.

Autopsy Findings.—Brain and cord: There was acute purulent meningitis with several metastatic, cerebral abscesses. Lungs showed bilateral terminal bronchopneumonia. Heart: Acute ulcerative bacterial endocarditis was present involving chiefly the tricuspid valve. Along the line of contact and spreading to the base of the right cusp of the tricuspid were several large friable, reddish-gray vegetations which, as a group measured 3.25 x 2 cm. No actual perforation of the valve could be found, although the vegetation near the base of the valve had spread to the under-surface and had involved the chordae tendineae. The heart itself was moderately enlarged and the muscle tone was poor. There were definite focal abscesses found in the kidneys. The remainder of the viscera showed marked congestion.

Microscopic Description of Section from the Base of the Tricuspid Valve.—(Fig. 373 and 374) Histologic examination of the myocardium shows evidence of an acute inflammatory reaction characterized by diffuse leukocytic infiltration of the tissues. There is capillary dilatation and perivascular invasion of the stroma. Marked edema is present. Actual liquefaction necrosis is present to a considerable extent. The myocardium shows very marked degeneration with loss of striation and fatty vacuolization of the cytoplasm of the cells. Already some attempt at fibrous tissue repair is in evidence. The fibroblasts are all young in appearance and have as yet produced but little collagen. The valve itself is damaged almost beyond recognition. By gram stain, the presence of the characteristic organisms can be made out.

MISCELLANEOUS FORMS OF INFECTIOUS ENDOCARDITIS

STAPHYLOCOCCIC ENDOCARDITIS.—In the case of staphylococcic endocarditis, we find an acute ulcerative variety. The Staphylococcus, being such a highly lytic agent, is likely to produce particularly prominent multiple abscess formation when it gains access to the blood stream and develops metastatic embolic foci. It has an extremely high mortality when it involves the blood stream, which is still further heightened when valvulitis develops.

GONOCOCCIC ENDOCARDITIS.—As one of the more serious complications of gonorrheal infection must be mentioned the severe ulcerative endocarditis which is seen in a small percentage of cases. The mortality from this complication is cited in the literature as being approximately 95 per cent. Until recent years, no cases of recovery from proven gonococcic endocarditis could be found in the literature. More recently, an occasional case seems to have been cured by the use of artificial fever therapy.

SYPHILITIC ENDOCARDITIS.—Curiously, syphilitic endocarditis, with the single exception of extension from the aorta to the aortic valve, is only rarely encountered. It has already been considered in the chapter on syphilis and will be referred to again at greater length in the following chapter devoted to a consideration of the diseases of the blood vessels.

CHRONIC ENDOCARDITIS

By the term "chronic endocarditis" is meant ordinarily the quiescent or healed stage of rheumatic fever. From the above observations, it is apparent that with the single exception of syphilis, the various other types of bacterial valvulitis and endocarditis are almost invariably fatal conditions so that no chronic changes are likely to occur. The interest in chronic endocarditis lies not only upon the cardiac pathology *per se,* but in the effects upon the circulation in general. The local lesion is characterized by a marked deformity of the valve cusps. This is characterized by extensive fibrous thickening; by adhesions between the cusps; by thickening of the chordae tendineae with resultant inability of the valve cusp to completely close. There is often degeneration of these thickened valves largely as the result of local tissue ischemia. With this degeneration a secondary calcification occurs. Thus, we have as a final picture, valves which are both incompetent through contracted scars leaving a patency through which blood may flow in either direction and a stenosis as the result of this same scarring and secondary calcification, which in turn results in obstructive phenomena in relation to the flow of blood through the valve.

Although a great majority of chronic thickening with calcification of the valves is of rheumatic origin, occasionally, in older individuals, fibrous thickening with calcification is encountered in the aortic ring frequently accompanied by nodular calcification at the base of the aortic and sometimes the mitral cusps. The free portion of the valves are not affected and the function of the valve seems not to be impaired. It accompanies advanced atheromatosis of the aorta and arteriosclerosis in general. Likewise, at times, with or without thickening of the aortic and mitral rings, yellowish-gray opacities of the mitral cusps, particularly the anterior cusp, are seen. Sometimes these plaques may extend to involve the mural endocardium, particularly in the region of the undefended space. The lesions may be accompanied by moderate nodular calcification. In both of these cases atheromatosis of the aorta and mesial arteriosclerosis of the peripheral vessels is marked.

Effects of Valvular Disease.—Whether the lesion be obstructive or one resulting in insufficiency, the work of the heart is permanently increased, and in general, *hypertrophy,* with or without dilatation, may result. If the valvular lesions are progressive and lead to an exaggeration of the regurgitation or stenosis, the myocardial hypertrophy will progress until the coronary circulation becomes inadequate and is no longer capable of supporting the increased volume of musculature. When a physiological limit of hypertrophy is thus reached, a gradual dilatation of failure will be initiated and symptoms of congestive heart failure will begin to appear.

With a gradual rise in the venous pressure, as the result of the damming back of the circulation, especially in association with mitral stenosis, the viscera will generally show chronic passive congestion. The liver will be enlarged and painful, and as a result of possible pressure and certainly anoxemia, atrophy of the liver cords around the central portion of the lobule will follow. This was spoken of in the older texts as *"red atrophy."* Subsequently, fatty degenerative changes of the liver cells, even to the point of necrosis, becomes a common and striking finding. (Fig. 477, 478, 479 and 480.) In the kidney this chronic congestion produces a striking cyanosis of the organ and may even go on to impairment of glomerular function. This may result in renal failure, with a rise of the blood urea and nonprotein nitrogen and creatinine. In the gastro-intestinal tract chronic passive congestion is manifested by a dusky, cyanotic congestion and edema of the mucosa. This is often followed by disturbances of digestion.

Varicosities of the hemorrhoidal veins with subsequent thrombosis and the production of hemorrhoids is not an infrequent occurrence. The characteristic pulmonary changes resulting from congestion have been discussed in an earlier chapter. The typical picture of "brown induration" with dilated capillaries, thickening of the walls of the alveoli and the presence of a few red cells and large mononuclear phagocytes laden with hemosiderin is a familiar picture. In mitral stenosis, hemoptysis may be an important symptom and is due to capillary hemorrhages resulting from such congestion. Pulmonary edema of varying degree is always seen terminally. Finally, edema of the tissues generally, *anasarca,* results. This appears first in the lower extremities and dependent parts of the body as a result of gravitation, and tends to disappear with rest in bed. Gradually all the tissues become water-logged, together with accumulations of transudate in the serous cavities. The effects of valvular disease upon the heart have thus far been discussed in general. The specific results of the more important valve lesions follow:

MITRAL STENOSIS.—Mitral stenosis is the most common valvular lesion of the heart and is almost exclusively the result of the healing of acute rheumatic lesions. The stenosis or narrowing results from fibrous thickening and calcification of the mitral valve, sometimes accompanied by adhesions between the cusps and shortening of the chordae tendineae. The severity and frequency is much greater in women than in men. The obstruction to the passage of blood into the left ventricle results in: (1) hypertrophy and dilatation of the left auricle; (2) marked chronic congestion of the lung with pigmentation and fibrosis (brown induration), frequently accompanied by hemoptysis and recurrent attacks of pulmonary edema; and (3) marked hypertrophy of the right ventricle. Increased pulmonary pressure frequently results in atheroma formation in the pulmonary artery. The left ventricle is normal in size.

During the state of compensation no evidence of general venous congestion is seen, but when the limit of hypertrophy of the myocardium is reached the right ventricle dilates with subsequent relative insufficiency of the tricuspid and thus initiates the train of events terminating in congestive heart failure. During the course of the disease, thrombi may arise in the auricular appendage due to partial stasis in the auricle. Such thrombi may give rise to cerebral emboli, or, more rarely, "ball thrombi." In many cases auricular fibrillation still further embarrasses the heart resulting principally from the involvement of the left auricle in the rheumatic process with subsequent fibrosis. Extreme dilatation of the auricle may likewise play a part. Partial or complete heart block may follow extensive lesions in the neighborhood of the undefended space, thus disturbing the auriculoventricular conduction bundle.

Clinically, mitral stenosis gives rise to a presystolic thrill and murmur heard best at the apex and transmitted to the axilla. Its intensity is greater during the period of compensation, and gradually decreases as right heart failure progresses.

MITRAL REGURGITATION.—This is very frequently seen as a *functional* stretching of the mitral ring rather than as an organic lesion of the valve. The regurgitant murmurs heard very early in rheumatic fever are probably of this origin and are due to the myocardial weakness accompanying the disease. At times, the regurgitation is due to organic lesions such as laceration or perforation of the cusps or ulceration of the chordae tendineae as seen in acute bacterial endocarditis.

Mitral insufficiency is rarely seen in the pure form but almost invariably accompanies stenosis. It may be seen in rheumatic fever, acute and subacute bacterial endocarditis due to the presence of vegetations preventing the complete closure of the valves, and it may likewise complicate stenosis due to shortening of the chordae tendineae or scarring and contraction of the cusps. The results of mitral regurgitation are: (1) dilatation and hypertrophy of the left ventricle; (2) moderate dilatation of the left auricle; (3) chronic passive congestion of the lung and (4) hypertrophy of the right ventricle.

Clinically, a systolic murmur is heard best at the apex with accentuation of the pulmonary second sound. Evidence of systemic venous congestion becomes apparent with right ventricular incompetence.

AORTIC STENOSIS.—Aortic stenosis is uncommon in a pure form. It is most commonly observed as a result of the fibrosis and calcification of rheumatic lesions. Occasionally, the stenosis may be produced by nodular calcifications and fibrosis of the aortic ring in association with simple senile atherosclerosis. The result of aortic stenosis is a concentric hypertrophy of the left ventricle without dilatation. During the stage of compensation the rest of the heart is unaffected. Clinically, a rough rasping systolic murmur with thrill is present. The rate of the heart is slow; the pulse tracing shows a slow rise and fall. With the onset of left ventricular failure a diastolic murmur is also heard due to relative insufficiency of the mitral valve.

AORTIC REGURGITATION.—Aortic regurgitation in pure form is seen almost exclusively in syphilis of the aorta and aortic valves. It results from destruction of the elastica with subsequent stretching of the ring. The condition may occasionally accompany rheumatic valvulitis or subacute and acute endocarditis due to inability of the cusps to close on account of the vegetations interfering with the closure of the cusps. Similarly, aortic insufficiency may occur as a result of healed rheumatic lesions in combination with stenosis.

Aortic insufficiency during the stage of compensation results principally in a marked hypertrophy and dilatation of the left ventricle. Dilatation is necessary to accommodate the normal quantity of blood flowing through the mitral valve from the auricle and also that regurgitating from the aorta. As long as the left ventricle is capable of thus compensating for the leakage no evidence of general congestion will be seen. This type of dilatation is known as the "dilatation of compensation." As the disease progresses, dilatation of the mitral ring takes place with insufficiency of that valve and subsequent right-sided hypertrophy. In this condition, the heart may be tremendously enlarged as the so-called *"cor bovinum."* Clinically, a diastolic murmur is heard and the area of precordial dullness is increased both to the right and left. The pulse pressure is high with the diastolic reading approaching zero. Capillary pulsation, the so-called Corrigan pulse, is evident in the nail beds, etc.

TRICUSPID AND PULMONARY REGURGITATION AND STENOSIS.—Infrequently the tricuspid valve may be the site of chronic lesions usually due to rheumatic disease. They result in hypertrophy of the right ventricle, principally, followed later by its dilatation. Pulmonary stenosis is occasionally encountered likewise, usually as result of rheumatic disease. The rheumatic involvement is prone to occur in the presence of congenital defects in the interventricular septum and as a rule the aortic and mitral valves are likewise involved. The effect of the lesion is hypertrophy of the right ventricle. In congenital stenosis the hypertrophy of the right side may be extreme.

HYPERTROPHY AND DILATATION.—Hypertrophy of the heart is an increase in functional power accompanied by an increase in size and weight of the organ. Two types are usually described; concentric hypertrophy, in which the ventricular wall is thickened without increase in the size of the cavity; and the hypertrophy of compensation, which is an increase in the size of the cavity plus a normal or increased thickness of ventricular wall. Pure examamples of hypertrophy without dilatation are seen during compensation in the left ventricle in hypertension and in pure aortic stenosis. Compensatory hypertrophy and dilatation are seen to advantage in the left ventricle in aortic regurgitation in which the ventricular capacity is considerably increased with the ventricular wall normal, or increased in thickness.

DILATATION.—Dilatation is usually referred to as either compensatory dilatation (hypertrophy with dilatation) or the dilatation of failure. In compensatory dilatation the increase in capacity of the ventricle or auricle results from incompetency of the valve, the increased capacity thus compensating for leakage, and so making it possible for the heart to maintain its normal output. In the dilatation of failure, the increased capacity of the auricle or ventricle is the result of failure of the ventricle to empty itself completely, and it is a feature accompanying cardiac decompensation in valvular disease, and is an important immediate cause of death in many cases.

ILLUSTRATIVE CASE

CASE 164. (Ref. #S-374)
Diagnosis.—Heart—concentric hypertrophy; myosclerosis.

Patient was an Italian male, age 36, admitted to the hospital with the chief complaint of severe pain in his right side accompanied by attacks of vomiting.

Present Illness.—The patient stated that he was perfectly well until four months ago when he developed acute ivy poisoning. This persisted for some weeks and was very severe in character. It was accompanied by swelling of his legs. He subsequently developed a hernia for which he was operated upon at another hospital. He was discharged two months before his present admission, with a warning that he was suffering from kidney disease. Three weeks before admission, he developed severe pain in his right side and had several attacks of vomiting. He was treated by a physician with the diagnosis of acute appendicitis. He refused operation. The pain in his abdomen persisted, and he continued to have attacks of nausea, although his vomiting

ceased, until two days before his present admission. During this three week period he suffered from attacks of vertigo. For the week or ten days before admission, he had developed a moderately severe diarrhea. These complaints of pain, nausea, vomiting, diarrhea and marked frequency brought him to the hospital for thorough study.

Past Medical History.—The patient had never been seriously ill previously. He had had all the usual childhood infections but did not recall ever having suffered from rheumatic fever. A review of his systems was not particularly informatory. He had always had a fair appetite and had never had any serious gastro-intestinal symptoms previously. He had never been heart conscious. He never had any symptoms referable to his respiratory tract. He first noticed his frequency about one year before his present illness. This was about equally marked during the night as during the day. He had suffered for several years from occasional attacks of headache and complaining of a feeling of stiffness in his neck at times. He never had any edema of the ankles, except during his attack of ivy poisoning.

Physical Examination.—Patient was a fairly well developed and nourished white male, thirty-six years of age. His skin had a somewhat sallow appearance, but was otherwise negative. Eyes, ears, nose and throat were negative. Chest was symmetrical. Lungs were clear and resonant throughout. Heart was definitely enlarged to percussion. The heart sounds were of good quality. Both the aortic and pulmonary second sounds were accentuated. No murmurs were heard. The rhythm was regular and the rate rapid. Blood pressure was 260/140. Abdomen showed moderate tenderness over the gallbladder region. There was no tenderness in the renal area. Reflexes were negative. Several acute hemorrhages were noted in his retinae by ophthalmoscopic examination.

Laboratory Findings.—Blood count on admission showed 3,560,000 red cells with a hemoglobin of 8 gm., and a white count of 13,850 cells with 87% polynuclears. This white blood count dropped during the course of his stay in the hospital to an average of 7,500 with about 70% polynuclears. Urinalyses: Specific gravity 1.008 to 1.012; albumin variable in amount, but always present; no casts were seen; occult blood was present at times. Blood chemistry: Urea nitrogen was 127 mgm. on admission, which rose to 178 mgm. before death. Similarly the creatinine rose from 16.5 to 20.6 mgm. Plasma carbon dioxide on admission showed 32 volumes percent, which subsequently dropped to 18 volumes percent. Wassermann and Kline tests were negative.

Subsequent Course.—Two days after admission, the patient developed a sudden pain in his chest which radiated to the right shoulder. He developed a gallop rhythm and a friction rub all over the precordium. Electrocardiographic studies revealed a marked left axis deviation. Temperature, pulse and respiratory rate were not remarkable except that his pulse tended to range between 70 and 100. Blood pressure on admission was 260/140, but fell to 140/100 just before his death. His fluid intake was always considerably in excess of his output, although he did not develop any appreciable edema. He died in a typical uremic state.

Autopsy Findings.—Heart weighed 630 gm. There was marked concentric hypertrophy of the left ventricular wall, which measured 3.3 cm. in thickness while that of the right ventricle measured only 0.7 cm. (Fig. 376). The chamber of the right ventricle was semilunar in shape due to pressure from thickening of the interventricular septum. There were no valvular lesions noted. The lungs showed terminal congestion and edema. The liver was considerably enlarged and showed rather marked congestion. The kidneys presented the typical picture of a rather marked malignant nephrosclerosis. They were somewhat smaller than normal. The capsule stripped with difficulty. The surface of the kidney was granular. On section, the cortex was diminished in amount. The pelvic fat was increased.

Microscopic Description of a Section Through the Left Ventricular Wall.—(Fig. 375) Histologic study of the tissue presents evidence of marked hypertrophy of the muscle cells. The nuclei appear considerably increased in size. They tend to be hyperchromatic. The cytoplasm of the cells is likewise increased in amount and the striations appear very coarse. Varying amounts of degenerative changes are seen of a fatty and hydropic nature affecting the muscle fibers. In places, there is a considerable increased amount of connective tissue between the muscle fibers. Some of this fibrosis appears to be patchy in distribution and suggests a replacement type of fibrous tissue overgrowth, undoubtedly the result of some localized areas of myocardial degeneration. No evidence of rheumatic fever is seen. The coronary vessels show no very striking changes of an atheromatous nature.

CHAPTER XXXIX

DISEASES OF THE HEART (*Continued*)

PERICARDIUM, MYOCARDIUM AND CORONARY ARTERY DISEASE

PERICARDIUM

INFLAMMATORY LESIONS

From the pathological standpoint, the only lesions of importance relating to the pericardium are those of an inflammatory nature.

Pericarditis.—Chief among these is the pericarditis which is part of the picture of rheumatic pancarditis (Fig. 103). This has already been described in the discussion of rheumatic fever in the preceding chapter. Other infections which are liable to produce symptoms of a similar nature in affecting the pericardium are particularly the *Pneumococcus* and less often the *Streptococcus*. In addition, the *tubercle bacillus* occasionally may be the causative organism in the development of a pericarditis. From the clinical standpoint, the outstanding feature of pericardial involvement is seen as precordial pain which, however, is often absent. On physical examination, one may hear the roughened surfaces of the parietal and visceral pericardium rubbing against each other with each contraction of the heart or with respiration. As fluid accumulates from the acute exudate, this friction rub, as it is termed, disappears with the separation of the two layers of the pericardium. As the fluid absorbs, the friction rub frequently recurs. In many instances the serosal cells lining the pericardium are destroyed and organization of the fibrinous exudate from the parietal and visceral sub-pericardial tissue takes place. This may proceed to obliteration of the cavity completely as the so-called *chronic adhesive pericarditis*. Such obliteration of the pericardial cavity enforces upon the heart a marked strain which is compensated for by a work hypertrophy which is usually symmetrical in nature.

In the tuberculous form, the exudate within the pericardial sac is likely to be very profuse. This is in contradistinction to the picture in rheumatic fever in which a rather delicate fibrinous exudate is found on the pericardial surface. It is not infrequently associated with hemorrhage and even in some instances by calcification. The diagnosis of the tuberculous variety is readily made by the histologic demonstration of characteristic tubercles in the deeper layers of the epicardium. At times such tuberculous lesions may extend from the epicardium deep along the interstitial septum into the myocardium.

Pick's Disease.—There is a group of conditions which seem rather closely related, but which often present somewhat different features in respect to distribution of the lesion. These are generally considered under the term of *polyserositis*. The most common form of this inflammatory reaction of the serosae is usually known as Pick's disease, while Concato's name is also found applied to a similar related process. The lesion is characterized by marked thickening of the serosa, especially of the parietal pericardium. It likewise is seen involving the pleura and the peritoneum with a thickening of the peritoneal surface of the liver and spleen in the more advanced instances. In its initial phases, there is usually an increase of fluid in the serosal body cavities, but as the process continues the fluid appears to absorb and the serosal membranes develop their characteristic hyaline thickening. In the case of the pericardium, this is comparable, from the mechanical standpoint, to the adhesive pericarditis already described, forming as it does a constricting membrane, which interferes with cardiac action.

The other lesions of the pericardium are negligible for the most part. As part of the generalized picture of cardiac or renal failure, we may find the accumulation of fluid within the pericardial sac as a simple transudate without evidence of inflammation. Such a condition is spoken of as *hydropericardium*. Simi-

PLATE XC

DISEASES OF THE MYOCARDIUM

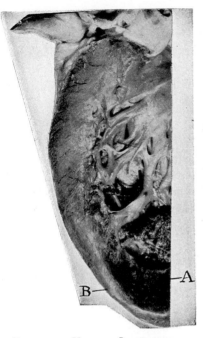

FIG. 377.—HEART: INFARCTION.—
CASE 165.—Cross section of heart
showing a recent infarct of the posterior wall, left ventricle, with in-
tracardiac thrombosis (A). The
scarring and fibrosis (B) of the
outer wall is the result of a former
coronary accident.

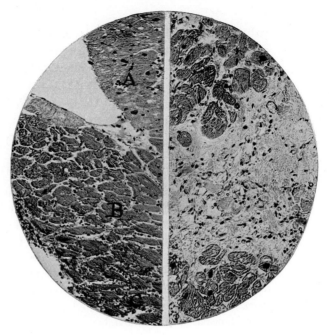

FIG. 378.—HEART: INFARCT.—CASE 165.—Photomicrograph (left
half) showing area of recent infarction (Fig. 377) with coagulation
and beginning liquefaction necrosis (b). Photomicrograph (right
half) from healed area of infarction with characteristic fibrosis.
App. 100 x.

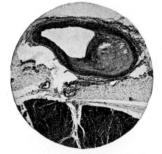

FIG. 379.—CORONARY ARTERY:
ATHEROSCLEROSIS.—Cf. CASE
165.—App. 5 x.

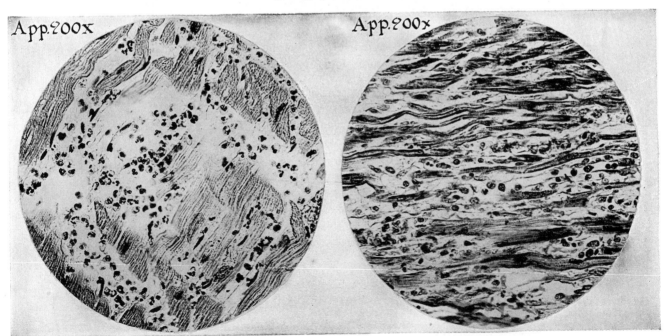

FIG. 380.—HEART: ACUTE DIFFUSE SUPPURATIVE INTERSTITIAL
MYOCARDITIS.—CASE 71.—Marked interstitial edema and polynuclear cellular infiltration. App. 200 x.

FIG. 381.—HEART: ACUTE DIFFUSE NON-SUPPURATIVE INTERSTITIAL
MYOCARDITIS.—CASE 72.—Advanced degeneration and necrosis of
myocardium with intercellular inflammatory edema and mononuclear cellular exudation App 200 x.

larly, as a result of stab wounds, traumatic injury, or of rupture of the heart, or of an aneurysm into the pericardial sac, the pericardium may become filled with blood clot to the point where it causes constrictive failure of the heart. In its various degrees, this condition is known as *hemopericardium*. A number of very brilliant surgical results have been obtained by operative measures in some of these traumatic cases of rupture of the heart wall, with complete recovery of the patients.

MYOCARDIUM

Congenital Anomalies

An entire volume could easily be devoted to a discussion of the congenital anomalies of the heart in the course of its development from a primitive single tube to the complicated adult, four-chambered mammalian pump. These have been described in detail by Abbott, to whose recent monograph the reader is referred for a more detailed discussion of this extremely interesting and important problem. From the more immediate practical standpoint, the congenital lesions can be considered briefly in respect to those lesions which we see comparatively commonly as congenital anomalies, but which are not incompatible with life. More striking anomalies are seen in the actual failure of the development of the heart at all, and in various degrees of ectopia which might better be considered in the problems of teratology.

In the development of the heart, as has been intimated, there is normally a rotation of the primitive vascular tube in the form of an "S." This is followed by fusion of these loops with subsequent development of the interauricular and interventricular septa and the formation of the valves. The great majority of the congenital defects result in some abnormality in the septal relationship. The four most common lesions which are found clinically and at autopsy are: (a) inter-atrial septal defect (patent foramen ovale); (b) interventricular septal defect; (c) patent ductus arteriosus and (d) pulmonic stenosis. In addition, coarctation of the aorta is a frequent accompaniment of some of these defects.

The *interauricular septal defect* is rarely of any great significance. It may be associated with cyanosis. If the defect is marked there may develop murmurs. In general, the development of symptoms from this relatively common lesion is seen as a result of other cardiac lesions with asymmetry of the right or left hearts, which result in the blood being shunted in excess to one side or the other of the circulation. As a matter of fact it has been estimated that as high as thirty to forty per cent of individuals show some defect in the foramen ovale, even into adult life. This is usually minimal, but is very prone to persist.

In the *interventricular septal defect,* we are very likely to find an associated pulmonic stenosis of varying degree. The two lesions are more or less compensatory, permitting as they do the blood to pass from the right to the left side of the heart. Abbott has shown that the usual etiology of this type of septal defect is basically dependent upon a deviation of the aortic bulb septum to the right, which results in the shutting off of the pulmonary artery from the aorta. If such a defect occurs alone, it is compatible with life but is usually accompanied by marked cyanosis and with the development of secondary circulatory disturbances, notably clubbing of the fingers.

Patent Ductus Arteriosus.—Normally in fetal life, the ductus arteriosus functions to pass the blood directly from the right side of the heart into the aorta inasmuch as there is no necessity for any pulmonary circulation in utero. At the time of birth, with the beginning function of the lungs, this vessel ordinarily undergoes atrophy and disappears by the end of the first month of life. It may, however, persist. In itself it produces no symptoms, as the balance of the circulation is maintained. In conjunction with pulmonic stenosis and interventricular septal defects, it becomes of importance as a means of maintaining life, as it offers the only opportunity for the blood from the right side of the heart to get into the lung for oxygenation. With this complicated compensatory mechanism, life is possible to be maintained; but such patients rarely survive into adult life, dying during childhood of some relatively mild intercurrent upper respiratory infection. Clinically such cases show cyanosis and clubbing of the fingers which should suggest the probability of such anatomical lesions.

Pulmonary Stenosis.—Pulmonary stenosis, in itself is incompatible with life, but in combination with the usual accompanying compensatory defects, as has been emphasized, it is possible for a patient to live, but at an almost vegetative level as a chronic cardiac invalid. The mechanism of this lesion has been discussed in relation to the previous forms of congenital heart disease.

Coarctation of the Aorta.—Coarctation of the aorta has been mentioned as another comparatively frequently encountered lesion which may occur. Transposition of the great vessels, the development of dextrocardia, and almost any conceivable combination of these many lesions have been reported. As long as a respiratory circulation can be maintained to any appreciable degree, so long may these cardiac cases live. When the anomalies interfere too much with the pulmonary circulation and concomitant oxygenation of the blood, then the patient must succumb of asphyxia as interpreted in its broadest sense, tissue anoxemia.

CIRCULATORY DISTURBANCES OF MYOCARDIUM

(Coronary Artery Disease)

The circulatory disturbances which affect the heart make up one of the most important chapters in medicine. They relate essentially to the various disturbances of the coronary circulation, which range all the way from the relatively mild spastic picture of simple angina pectoris to the advanced arteriosclerotic lesions of the coronaries with associated thrombosis, occlusion and myocardial infarction. To-day, coronary vessel disease represents one of the largest and most important groups of cases from the mortality standpoint.

The cause of coronary disease is still a matter of speculation. Its relationship to hypertension is discussed in the chapter on renal disease. Curiously enough, the lesions which are seen as the significant ones in coronary artery disease are those of the central type of arteriosclerosis; namely, atherosclerosis, rather than the diffuse hyperplastic sclerosis of other peripheral end-arteries, such as those seen in the kidney. Yet we find an antecedent history of angina in a great many cases of terminal coronary artery occlusion in which the mechanism must have some relationship to that which produces essential hypertension. This factor is thought to be in the nature of a nervous stimulus with resultant vasospasm and a transitory ischemia of the heart muscle. Just what this stimulating substance might be is wholly in the realm of hypothesis.

It is indisputable that the incidence of coronary disease is many times greater in those individuals who are subject to mental strain and responsibility than in those of a more phlegmatic disposition, who earn their living largely by physical effort. The disease rarely occurs under the age of fifty years. Clinically, it is ushered in with acute agonizing precordial pain, accompanied by dyspnea and evidence of cardiac collapse. If actual infarction has taken place a friction rub is frequently heard a few hours after the onset. The blood shows a moderate leukocytosis, which fact assists in differentiating this condition from pure anginal paroxysms in which coronary infarction has not occurred. In coronary artery disease, which often becomes a very important problem from the medicolegal standpoint, careful search of the coronary arteries at autopsy may fail to reveal any significant changes adequate to explain the sudden death which so commonly occurs even with the first attack of coronary symptoms. More often, however, a variable degree of atherosclerosis of the vessel walls may be recognized. The picture under these circumstances is one of atherosclerosis with plaques of varying size and thickness, at times almost shutting off the lumen of the vessel. In the typical case, this underlying atherosclerotic process is accompanied by the production of a thrombus which may or may not occlude completely the coronary artery involved.

The point of occlusion is usually found in the anterior descending branch of the left artery, but may occur anywhere in either vessel. Less often the occlusion may result from other causes such as bacterial emboli from an endocarditis. Syphilitic involvement of the aorta may extend to involve the ostia of the coronaries with resultant complete shutting off of the blood supply in extreme instances. The presence of a patent interventricular septum has been found to account at times for the presence of certain transposed embolic phenomena. However, by far the most important and most frequently encountered cause of coronary occlusion is the simple arteriosclerotic process either alone or complicated by secondary thrombosis.

The effect on the myocardium deriving its blood supply from the diseased vessel, varies from gradual degenerative changes in the mild case to frank coagulation necrosis as seen in the typical infarct in severe cases and spoken of as *myomalacia cordis*. In the mild case obstruction to the coronary circulation results in a localized anemia of the heart muscle and is accompanied by all the degenerative changes associated with such anoxemia. Fatty degeneration is perhaps the most outstanding of these phenomena, but in many instances it is difficult to detect either grossly or microscopically with the usual hematoxylin and eosin stained preparation. For its demonstration, either osmic acid impregnation of the tissues or frozen section technique with the use of one of the fat solvent dyes, such as Sudan III or Scharlach R is to be recommended. Under these circumstances the fat droplets which are usually extremely small in size can be readily recognized. There is a rather universal tendency for this to follow a somewhat symmetrical pattern with alternating areas of relatively uninvolved muscle fibers. When the process is marked enough, this results in the characteristic gross tigroid mottling which has already been described.

Accompanying this fatty degeneration, not infrequently, hydropic changes and granular changes of the cytoplasm are also demonstrable. One of the most striking lesions from this standpoint as seen in the heart muscle is the so-called fragmentation of the muscle fibers. This represents a fracture of the muscle fibers at the intercalary disks. This is seen much more strikingly in fixed preparations than in fresh tissues, and it is probable that at least some of this fragmentation is in the nature of an artifact.

In the severe case, when the occlusion becomes complete through the combined atherosclerotic and thrombotic processes, then infarction follows. Due to the rather extensive anastomosing circulation of the coronary system, such infarcts usually require the occlusion to be relatively near the proximal end of the vessel. Likewise the area of infarction which follows is extremely irregular in outline as contrasted to the almost geometrical pattern seen in other organs supplied by end-arteries, such as the spleen and kidneys. If this process is very extensive involving any of the major branches of the coronary and the patient survives for a long enough period for the complete degenerative changes to occur, a picture of softening follows which is spoken of as *myomalacia cordis* (Fig. 378B). This may perhaps best be described as the point at which the maximum

tissue changes occur. At this point the muscle shows coagulation necrosis. The cytoplasm loses its striations and tends to stain homogeneously and rather more intensely with eosin. The nuclei may not be seen or show marked degenerative pyknotic and karyorrhectic changes. In other areas, particularly near the edge, degenerative processes are paramount. The cells are enormously swollen and show fatty, granular and hydropic changes. Interstitial edema of the supportive stroma is seen and a variable amount of cellular infiltration follows. Accompanying this extensive degenerative softening of the wall of the heart, there follows obviously intimal damage with the development of a mural thrombus at the site of the involved area. This is in the nature of a protective mechanism and may at times aid in the reparative phenomena through its organization and with a resultant thickening of the endocardium. Unfortunately, however, at times fragments of such a thrombus may break off and be carried in the peripheral circulation to serve as a source of fatal embolus.

Gradually the musculature undergoes lysis and the phenomena of repair set in. The end result in such a case is replacement fibrosis which ultimately contracts down to typical scar tissue. Involving as it does most frequently the left descending branch, the apex of the left ventricle is the most frequent site of such extensive infarction. In healing, there is not infrequently left merely a thin, fibrous wall instead of the usual thick musculature. This at times may bulge to form an aneurysm. Occasional instances of rupture of such scarred areas have been reported.

The clinical course of the disease varies. Patients with coronary disease often die suddenly of cardiac failure within a matter almost of minutes after the onset of the attack. In these instances, it is fair to assume that a major branch of the myocardial circulation has been shut off. In other instances, the patient may survive for a period of a few days, but as the degenerative changes go on, a point is reached at which cardiac insufficiency develops. Less often, the patient survives for a long enough period for repair to follow.

In the milder forms of such circulatory disturbances, a moderate degree of anemia to the part follows. This may result in the actual destruction of a certain number of muscle fibers which are replaced by fibrous tissues. This is a typical example of the replacement type of fibrosis. This diffuse interstitial fibrosis may likewise result from various forms of toxic damage to the heart muscle, or even in the repair of focal areas of necrosis resulting from actual infectious lesions. Perhaps the most striking examples of such diffuse interstitial fibrotic scarring is seen in relation to some of the more severe infectious diseases such as diphtheria, scarlet fever and other streptococcic infections. This replacement fibrosis is frequently spoken of as chronic interstitial fibrous myocarditis (cf. Fig. 375). This is obviously a misnomer inasmuch as the lesions represent the healed stage of a degenerative process as a rule, which may or may not have been accompanied by inflammation during the course of its development. It seems more appropriate to use the simpler terminology of interstitial fibrosis, fibrous scarring of the myocardium or better still—*myosclerosis.*

The pain in coronary disease is one of the most striking features of the picture, and a great deal of experimental work has been done in an attempt to explain its mechanism. As was intimated in the early part of this discussion, no very adequate conception of the etiology of coronary artery disease exists, and the relationship of mental activity as a factor in stimulating the onset of the picture is a difficult one to explain. Some of the recent experimental evidence would point to the fact that vasospasm may be the result of a direct chemical stimulation of the nerve endings through the production of acetylcholine. This work still requires confirmation, but opens up an interesting experimental field in respect to the neurogenic relationship of many diseases relating to the circulatory system.

Lewis also considers the pain in coronary disease as chemical in origin, resulting from muscular activity in the absence of adequate blood supply. Lambert,

Boyd and others suggest that the pain originates from over-distention of the vessels, thus stimulating sympathetic nerve endings.

Although the mechanism of pain-production is uncertain and the exact point of origin is in doubt, its course is definite. Thus, due to stimulation arising in the heart, impulses are conveyed to the cardiac plexus with resultant precordial pain. By way of the sympathetics through the inferior cervical ganglion other impulses pass through the first and second dorsal and eighth cervical segments of the cord and are projected along the course of the nerves from these segments, giving rise to pain, particularly in the left arm.

Angina Pectoris.—The symptom-complex referred to as "angina pectoris" consists of recurrent attacks of precordial pain which are projected to the left arm, or at times to both arms. It most frequently follows cardiac strain, such as unusual physical effort or following a heavy meal. The paroxysms last for a short time, usually a matter of minutes, and then gradually disappear. The pain appears to be similar in character to that observed in coronary artery disease but less severe. Frequently individuals dying with coronary disease give a history of anginal seizures.

From the standpoint of pathology, little or no change may be found to account for the severe symptom-complex. The coronary arteries may or may not show a mild degree of atherosclerosis. As in coronary thrombosis, the exact mechanism which gives rise to the pain is in doubt. The pathology is most probably in the form of spasm of the arterioles with resultant ischemia of the heart muscle. If this be the case the pain in both disturbances is probably of common etiology.

ILLUSTRATIVE CASE

CASE 165. (Ref. #S-131)

Diagnosis.—Heart—coronary artery occlusion with subsequent infarction (myomalacia cordis); chronic interstitial fibrosis (myosclerosis).

Patient was a white male, 50 years old, admitted to the hospital with a fracture of the left fibula.

Present Illness.—The patient slipped while stepping off a curbstone and felt a sudden sharp pain in his left ankle. He was unable to walk and was brought to the hospital for treatment.

Past History.—The patient believed he had had the usual childhood infections. He had never had any serious illness until five years ago at which time he had a typical coronary thrombosis with subsequent infarc-

tion. This was corroborated by electrocardiographic studies at that time. Since that time he had been entirely free of any cardiac symptoms other than dyspnea on exertion and by leading a relatively quiet life, he felt perfectly well. A review of his systems was otherwise noninformatory. He never had any particular gastrointestinal disturbances. He was aware that he had a hypertension with a systolic blood pressure of 180, but this again had not occasioned him any symptomatic worry. His respiratory system was negative. Genitourinary system was negative.

Physical Examination.—Patient was a well-developed, well-nourished white male who did not appear his given age. Head showed no deformities. Eyes reacted normally. Nose and throat were negative. Chest was symmetrical. Lungs were clear. Heart was slightly enlarged to the left. No murmurs were heard. Blood pressure was 180/110. Abdomen was negative. Extremities showed localized swelling of the left ankle area.

Laboratory Findings.—Red blood cells, 5,200,000 with 86% hemoglobin. White blood cells, 9,700 with 71% polynuclears. Urinalysis negative. Wassermann negative.

Subsequent Course.—The patient's fracture was set and a plaster cast applied. X-ray examination showed perfect alignment of the two fragments.

During the third night of his hospitalization, he developed a typical precordial severe anginal pain which radiated down his left arm to the finger tips. This came on suddenly. It was extremely severe in character. He improved considerably over a period of several days and it was felt that he might recover from this particular coronary episode. However, on the seventh day after the attack, on attempting to sit up in bed, he was suddenly seized with a similar attack of precordial pain, which was excruciating in character. He collapsed and died in the course of one-half hour.

Autopsy Findings.—Heart: Acute infarction of the posterior wall of the left ventricle (Fig. 386). Bilateral coronary artery atherosclerosis. Left descending branch occlusion. Healed infarct at the left apex with thinning of the ventricular wall by fibrous scar. Mural thrombosis of the left ventricle. Right descending coronary artery thrombosis and obstruction. The heart showed moderate hypertrophy, chiefly left-sided. Lungs showed chronic passive congestion. The abdominal viscera likewise showed chronic passive congestion. There was a fracture of the left fibula showing early union.

Microscopic Description of Section Through the Heart Muscle.—(Fig. 377, 378, 379 and 386) Histologic study of the tissues includes a portion of the cardiac muscle with its overlying pericardium. This is the site of an organizing fibrinous pericarditis. The pericardium is markedly congested. The organizing fibrinous pericarditis is confined to a portion overlying an area of cardiac infarction. The underlying myocardium presents the typical picture of myomalacia cordis with extensive fatty and hydropic degeneration peripherally and actual beginning necrosis centrally. The degenerative muscle stains poorly. Some of the cells still show the persistence of the nuclei and vague suggestions of striation. The cells tend to be enormously swollen and to take the eosin dye more intensely. Many of the cells show complete loss of striation and either karyolytic or karyorrhectic changes of the nuclei. Such areas of degeneration and necrosis are seen frequently just adjacent to vessels which are apparently not involved by the process, indicating the relatively extensive collateral circulation which exists in the heart muscle and prevents the usual clear-cut area of infarction, which is usually observed in obstruction of terminal arteries. Where necrosis has gone on to a point of liquefaction, there is marked secondary polynuclear leukocytic infiltration. On the endocardial surface of the tissue an acute mural thrombus can be identified. The overlying endothelial cells have been destroyed and beginning organization of this thrombus by the subintimal connective tissue is observed. Examination of a section of myocardium from the left apex shows evidence of a diffuse interstitial fibrosis, which is best interpreted as a replacement fibrosis or scar formation in relation to a previous vascular accident of this same type.

INFLAMMATORY LESIONS OF THE MYOCARDIUM

The inflammatory lesions of the myocardium are divided into three groups under the following headings: (1) Myocarditis, characterized by an inflammatory exudate in the interstitial tissue usually accompanied by degenerative changes in the parenchyma; (2) Myocardosis. In this condition the interstitial exudate is insignificant, the major changes occur in the parenchyma, and are degenerative in character. This condition is also indicated by the term "acute parenchymatous myocarditis"; (3) Myosclerosis, characterized by local or diffuse fibrosis of the myocardium, replacement or productive in type, usually resulting following myocardosis or myocarditis, or some circulatory disturbance such as coronary artery disease. It is also spoken of as "chronic interstitial fibrous or fibroid myocarditis."

BACTERIAL MYOCARDITIS

Suppurative.—This process may be focal or of a diffuse interstitial variety. In the former, as part of a generalized bacterial septicemia focal lesions usually of an embolic nature may result in multiple abscess formation. This is particularly seen in the staphylococcic type of septicemia. In streptococcic lesions the picture is more likely to be of a diffuse nature. In subacute bacterial endocarditis occasionally focal lesions are met with which consist chiefly of accumulations of polymorphonuclear leukocytes and are spoken of as "Bracht-Wächter" bodies. The diffuse variety is particularly seen in the severe infections such as diphtheria (Fig. 380), where in addition to the usual degenerative changes a diffuse interstitial exudate is present, consisting chiefly of polymorphonuclear leukocytes. This condition has already been discussed in Chapter XIX and is illustrated by Case 71 (Ref. #S-153).

Diffuse Interstitial Nonsuppurative.—Occasionally a diffuse exudate of nonsuppurative toxic character is met with, particularly in association with streptococcal infections elsewhere in the body (Fig. 381). Here the majority of the cells are mononuclear in character. The condition has been discussed at some length under scarlatina, Chapter XIX, page 82, Case 72 (Ref. #S-150). If the patient recovers healing takes place with replacement or productive fibrosis.

RHEUMATIC MYOCARDITIS

The actual incidence of primary inflammatory lesions of the heart is comparatively slight. The most outstanding examples of actual myocarditis are seen in relation to rheumatic fever, but even here the exact etiologic agent is distinctly uncertain and whether the lesions which are seen in the heart muscle are the result of reaction to the specific infectious agent or are the result of some toxic manifestation from some distinct focus of infection in the nature of an allergic response are still problems requiring further investigation. For further detail the reader is referred to the preceding chapter where the subject has been discussed under rheumatic pancarditis (Fig. 362 and 365, Case 160).

SYPHILITIC MYOCARDITIS

It is uncertain whether the spirochaete of syphilis ever actually invades the myocardium to produce its characteristic reaction. With the single exception of Warthin, pathologists in general do not hold to the view that syphilitic myocarditis occurs as a diffuse infection. Occasionally, syphilitic gummata may be seen. They are prone to occur in the ventricular septum and are likely to produce heart block through involvement of the conduction bundle. At other times they may be found in the auricular wall.

MYOCARDOSIS (TOXIC MYOCARDITIS)

The term toxic myocarditis is one which is used very commonly to represent degenerative lesions of the myocardium, usually seen in association with acute infectious disease elsewhere in the body. The most striking examples of this perhaps are seen in such infections as diphtheria or typhoid. Under these circumstances, we find the usual fatty, hydropic and hyaline changes affecting the cytoplasm of the muscle fibers. Very frequently accompanying these degenerative cytoplasmic changes will be found an interstitial edema, often marked capillary dilatation and not infrequently mononuclear cellular infiltration. The changes are very similar in nature to those seen as the result of anoxemia through coronary circulatory obstruction and may even go on to the point of actual necrosis.

MYOSCLEROSIS (CHRONIC INTERSTITIAL FIBROID MYOCARDITIS)

In this condition of the myocardium, there is a local or diffuse increase in fibrous tissue throughout the affected portions of the heart (Fig. 375). Its etiology is varied. In the above conditions (myocardosis and myocarditis) a productive or replacement fibrosis follows the acute phases of the disease. Likewise, as a result of degenerative changes following anemia or ischemia due to coronary artery disease, a similar diffuse fibrosis may result. It will be seen, therefore, that fibrosis of the myocardium may follow many varied injuries to the heart muscle, but is especially related to circulatory disturbances.

HEART BLOCK

Disturbance in the impulse from the sino-auricular node through the conduction system may be caused by any lesion of the heart which may bring about pressure or destruction of these specialized conduction fibers. Some of the more important causes are severe acute myocarditis, severe degenerative lesions (myocardosis) as in diphtheria, typhoid fever, rheumatism, etc., fibrosis of the myocardium from coronary artery diseases or healing of acute inflammatory degenerative changes, syphilitic myocarditis, gumma, tuberculoma, tumors, calcareous infiltration about the aortic ring, etc.

TUMORS OF THE HEART

Primary tumors of the heart are extremely rare. The most common of these is the rhabdomyosarcoma. An example of such a tumor in the kidney has already been discussed in Chapter XXVI, and illustrated in Case 101 (Ref. #S-237), Fig. 234, page 268. It is in the heart that the characteristic "spider" cells representing the abortive development of attempts at the production of muscle are found. It will be recalled that these are enormous cells with large nuclei and characteristic areas in the cytoplasm showing both longitudinal and cross striations.

Likewise, as a rare tumor of the heart may be mentioned the fibroma, a case of which has been described in Chapter XXIV (Fig. 227).

Less frequently, other tumors arise from the various connective tissue derivatives such as chondromata, myxomata and even osteomata.

The heart is notoriously resistant to secondary metastatic tumor implantation. This is possibly very largely due to the arrangement of its circulation, the tumor cells having relatively little chance to get into the coronary vessels. The only tumor of importance in the group of metastatic lesions is represented by the melanosarcoma.

CHAPTER XL
DISEASES OF THE BLOOD VESSELS
PART I
ARTERIES

It long has been customary to base any discussion concerning the diseases of arteries upon the localization of the pathological process in respect to the various part of the vessel wall. Thus, the term "endarteritis" applies to disease beginning or essentially paramount in the intima; "mesarteritis," to conditions where the pathology is chiefly confined to the media; and "periarteritis," to those lesions in which the pathology is particularly restricted to the adventitia. Such a division is useful, but it must be recognized that many conditions involve the vessel as a whole.

For purposes of convenience, it also seems profitable to divide arteries into three groups in accordance with their size and structure; (1) the elastic type of vessel, represented by the large vessels such as the aorta and its immediate branches, where there is an abundance of elastic tissue in the media; (2) the medium size muscular type of vessel, represented by the radials, renals, mesenterics, etc., in which the media is made up chiefly of muscle; (3) a group consisting of the small arteries and arterioles, such as the arterioles of the splenic follicle, the interlobular arteries and afferent arterioles of the kidney. Each of the above have a somewhat different function to perform. In the aorta the vessel must rapidly expand to accommodate the large quantity of blood pumped at each beat of the heart and, distributed to its various branches, again to contract to its normal size. It is not particularly involved in the maintenance of a constant blood pressure, nor in the quantitative distribution of the blood to the various parts or organs. The intermediate sized vessel, with its muscular media, is capable of governing the quantity of blood distributed to any organ or section of the body by changes in its lumen, which may be maintained for long periods of time. The small arteriole again, plays an important rôle, not only in varying the amount of blood passing through to the part supplied, but also in maintaining and stabilizing the peripheral resistance, and thus having an important part in the maintenance of blood pressure.

An understanding of the structure and function of these important groups of arteries is of value in the proper interpretation of some of the pathological processes affecting them. Thus, in diseases, such as arteriosclerosis, it will be seen that the lesions, occurring in the various vessel groups, probably are the result of variation of the structure and function of the vessel, rather than any difference in the fundamental mechanism of the disease.

It is important also to remember that the nourishment of the blood vessels themselves is through arterioles entering from the adventitia and extending into the mid-portion of the media and sometimes almost to the intima. Apparently very little nutrition is received from the intimal surface. In the aorta the vasa vasorum take their origin from the intercostals near their beginning. In the medium size vessel the vasa vasorum arise some distance from the part of the vessel wall which they supply. These small nutrient vessels not only bring nourishment to the arterial wall but may likewise convey bacteria or other injurious agents.

Most diseases of the arteries fall into two important groups; first, infectious lesions in which the pathology is brought about by the presence of bacteria or their toxin; and secondly, degenerative lesions in which group the primary change is apparently degenerative in character.

PLATE XCI

Fig. 382.—Spleen, Hyaline Degeneration of Central Arteriole. Case 11. Cf. Fig. 25.

Fig. 384.—Kidney, Hyperplastic Arteriolar Nephrosclerosis. Case 233.

Fig. 386.—Heart, Infarction. Case 165. Cf. Fig. 377 and 378.

Fig. 383.—Adrenal, Acute Necrotizing Arteritis. Case 167. Cf. Fig. 393 to 397.

Fig. 385.—Kidney, Arterio-(athero)sclerosis. Case 169. Cf. Fig. 398 to 400.

Fig. 387.—Peripheral Artery, Monckeberg's Medial Medial Sclerosis. Case 169. Cf. Fig. 392.

PLATE XCI

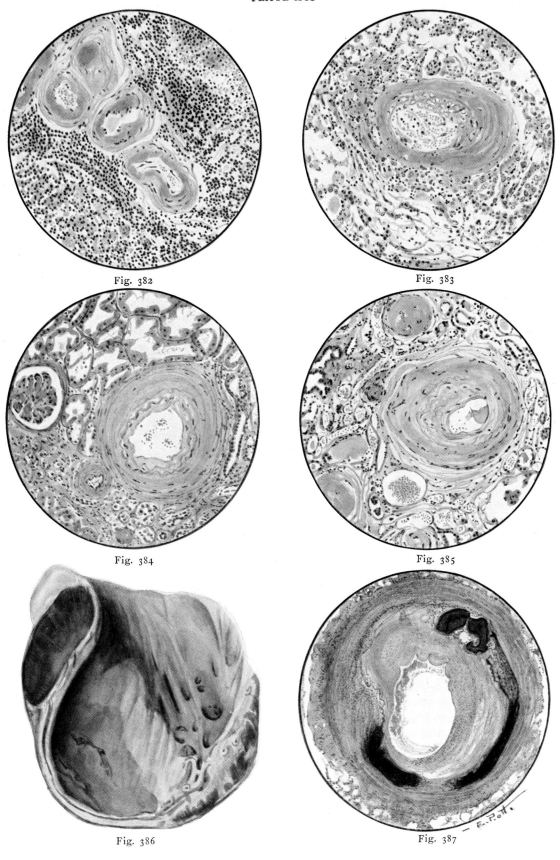

Fig. 382

Fig. 383

Fig. 384

Fig. 385

Fig. 386

Fig. 387

Inflammatory Lesions of the Arteries

Acute Arteritis (Infectious arteritis)

Acute arteritis is an inflammatory condition of the vessel wall brought about by the action of various bacteria and their toxins. It may be subdivided into two forms: (1) Acute periarteritis, in which the process begins in the adventitia or media, and (2) acute endarteritis, which results from the lodgment of an infected embolus or the formation of an infected thrombus within the lumen of the vessel with extension to the adjacent intima.

Acute Periarteritis.—Acute periarteritis is most commonly seen in vessels extending through an area of suppuration. The arterial wall is quite resistant to bacterial invasion, and it is not uncommon to find vessels traversing abscessed areas without marked involvement of the wall. Even when the vessel becomes infected from without the process extends slowly and is frequently halted by the external and internal elastic laminae. The organism may extend directly from the adventitia through to the media, but more commonly the bacteria are conveyed by the vasa vasorum into the media. If the process is rapid the wall softens and severe or fatal hemorrhage may result. If the process is slow a thrombus may form within the vessel, thus preventing at least temporarily, severe hemorrhage.

Secondary surgical hemorrhage is very commonly dependent upon such a periarteritis, the infecting organisms being present at times in the ligature. The wall of the cut vessel is particularly vulnerable since it has been traumatized. The suppurative process soon involves the wall extending to the thrombus which has formed within the vessel. Liquefaction necrosis soon leads to rupture of the vessel and hemorrhage.

Endarteritis.—Infectious endarteritis usually is the result of the lodgment of a septic embolus. This may arise in acute ulcerative endocarditis from a portion of vegetation breaking off and being carried to a small vessel. It also may be brought about by an embolus arising from an infectious thrombophlebitis, such emboli being carried through the heart to the lung where they produce an involvement of the vessel wall from within. A metastatic abscess may result by extension of the infectious process through the wall, or the weakening of the media may lead to production of a small mycotic aneurysm. In other cases, rupture of the vessel may occur with severe hemorrhage. Histologically, the involved portion of the artery is infiltrated with an exudate consisting mainly of polymorphonuclear leukocytes, with areas of liquefaction necrosis.

Acute Nonsuppurative Arteritis.—A form of nonsuppurative arteritis is seen occasionally in typhoid, scarlet fever, diphtheria and pneumonia, in which there is an involvement of the intima with subsequent thrombosis. The exudate is made up chiefly of mononuclears together with proliferation of the subintimal connective tissue. Sometimes the exudate may involve all coats, and there may be considerable accumulation of mononuclear exudate in and about the adventitia. The process is due, either to the organisms or their toxins, or both.

Tuberculous Arteritis.—In a tuberculous lesion arteries may be attacked from without by continuity of structure, the vessel being situated in an area of extensive caseation, or the organism may be conveyed to the media by way of the vasa vasorum. The resistance of arteries to even a tuberculous process is evidenced by their frequent persistence in acute ulcerative tuberculosis of the lung, extending across a portion of the cavity, the remaining tissue having undergone necrosis. At times, however, the involvement of the vessel leads to weakening of the wall and eventually rupture, with hemorrhage. In the average case of tuberculosis, however, severe hemorrhage is rare, since the arteries undergo thrombosis before extreme caseation and ulceration occur. This process is probably the result of an endarteritis brought about through the toxins of the organism with subsequent thrombosis, thus sealing the vessel before softening has occurred. Arteries may also be involved from the intimal surface by tuberculous emboli, particularly in hematogenous miliary tubercle.

Syphilis of Arteries.—The involvement of the arterial system in syphilis is rather diffuse. The most spectacular lesions, however, are seen in the aorta and in the smaller vessels, such as those of the meninges. The nature of the disease and the causative organism, the treponema pallidum, have been dealt with at some length in a previous chapter.

Syphilitic Aortitis.—The organisms are

brought to the aorta by way of the vasa vasorum and are found in the perivascular lymphatics. Thus, in the early stage of the disease, the exudate will be seen to follow the branches of the nutrient arteries in the adventitia and extending into the media.

Histologically, the lesions consist of accumulations of round cells, plasma cells and mononuclears in the perivascular lymphatics of the adventitia and media. At times the plasma cells may predominate; in other cases the lymphocytes. The chief damage to the vessel wall is degeneration and necrosis of the elastic tissue of the media. Numerous young vessels appear which are also associated with the perivascular exudate. After a time the areas undergo fibrous cicatrization, and the contraction of these lead to puckering of the wall which is such a prominent feature in the gross appearance of the lesions. The subintimal connective tissue proliferates, forming a plaque-like area. This proliferation was formerly considered to be due to the toxin of the organism. It is, however, probably a compensatory effort with the purpose of strengthening the wall at this point.

In most instances the organisms may be demonstrated in the involved areas, even after considerable healing has taken place. The damage to the elastic tissues of the vessel lead to weakening of the wall, frequently giving rise to local or general dilatation, with the formation of an aneurysm. In the early stages of the disease, in which histologically the changes are mainly degenerative and exudative, no gross changes in the appearance of the vessel can be noted. It is only after the intimal thickenings occur, together with the puckering resulting from varying degrees of healing, that the typical morbid anatomical appearance of the vessel becomes apparent. The lesions consist of smooth, pearly, slightly elevated plaques within the intima, from the edge of which linear wrinkles proceed, usually running in the longitudinal axis of the vessel. The process is most severe and appears earliest in the first 6 or 7 cm. of the aorta, probably due to the fact that the perivascular lymphatics are most abundant in this portion of the aorta.

The intimal thickenings may involve the opening of the coronary arteries, bringing about considerable narrowing of their orifices, and thus limiting the blood supply of the heart, although the process rarely extends to involve the coronary arteries to any marked degree. The damage to the elastic tissues

at this portion of the aorta, particularly the aortic ring, leads in many instances to relative dilatation with insufficiency of the aortic valve, even though the cusps apparently are normal.

In some instances the valves are affected with a cord-like thickening of the free edge and widening of the commissures between the valves. Such lesions tend to exaggerate the insufficiency which is already present due to the dilatation of the ring. These lesions are frequently spoken of as syphilitic endocarditis and are the most important cause of pure aortic regurgitation, leading to marked enlargement of the left ventricle of the heart. The extensive involvement of the first part of the aorta results in weakening of the wall with a tendency for saccular aneurysm to arise at this point (Fig. 125 and 126).

In the average case, the lesions become less numerous in the thoracic aorta and are usually absent in the abdominal portion. In atheroma the earliest and most severe lesions are apt to appear in the abdominal aorta and become less frequent in the thoracic portion and arch.

In many instances syphilitic aortitis is complicated by atheroma, so that both lesions are frequently found in the same aorta. The syphilitic plaques of the intima do not undergo softening nor do they calcify as is the rule in atheroma (Fig. 386). (Refer to cases 56 and 57 (Fig. 123 and 124, Chapter XV.)

SYPHILITIC ARTERITIS.—The effect of syphilis on the elastic type of vessel has just been described. In the muscular type or medium sized vessel, the changes produced lead to narrowing of the lumen. The first lesions are seen in the adventitia as perivascular accumulations which may extend to involve the media with degeneration of the elastic tissue and some atrophy of the muscle. At times the vessel is surrounded by a considerable collar of exudate made up of plasma cells and lymphocytes. The medial involvement, however, is less spectacular because of the relative abundance of muscle tissue in this coat which does not suffer to the same degree as elastic tissues. There is marked intimal thickening which is symmetrical, bringing about an obliterating endarteritis. The effects of such lesions are to decrease the nutrition of the part with probably eventual thrombosis. There is little tendency to weakening of the wall with subsequent aneurysmal dilatation or rupture. Such vessel changes are particularly seen in

PLATE XCII

DISEASES OF THE ARTERIES

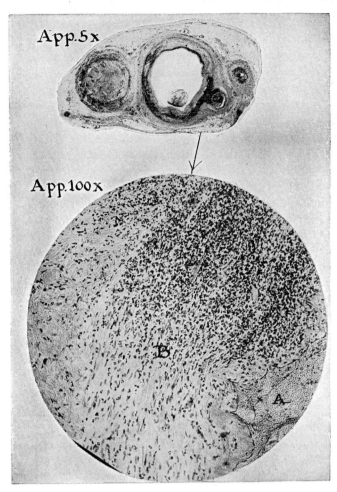

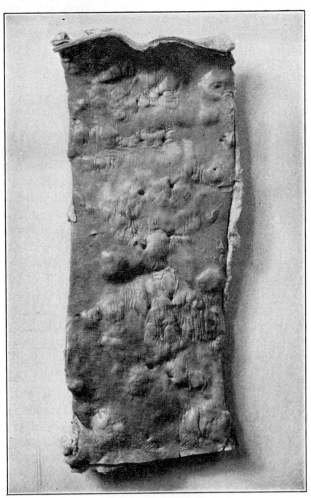

FIG. 388.—THROMBO-ANGIITIS OBLITERANS.—CASE 166.—Acute pan-arteritis with thrombosis involving the vein and artery, together with beginning perivascular fibrosis. App. 5 x.

FIG. 389.—THROMBO-ANGIITIS OBLITERANS.—CASE 166.—High magnification of the above (Fig. 388) showing extensive polynuclear infiltration of media and intima (B) and beginning thrombosis (A). App. 100 x.

FIG. 390.—AORTA: SYPHILITIC AORTITIS.—CASE 57.—Gross photograph of thoracic aorta which has been opened anteriorly. Numerous raised irregular grayish plaques showing linear striations are seen. (Cf. FIG. 124.)

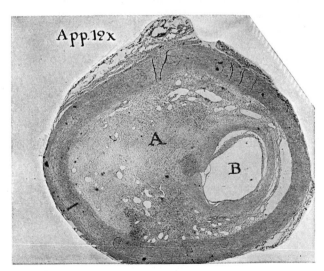

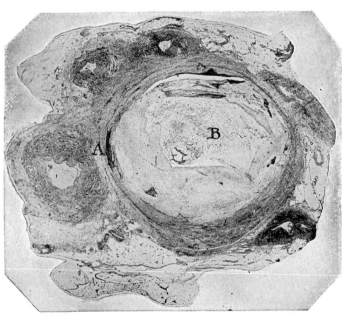

FIG. 391.—ARTERY: ENDARTERITIS OBLITERANS.—CASE 168.—Microtessar photograph to show marked reduction of lumen (B) as a result of endothelial and fibroblastic proliferation. App. 12 x.

FIG. 392.—ARTERY: MESARTERITIS WITH CALCIFICATION.—CASE 16.—The large central vessel shows extensive degeneration of the media with several areas of calcification (A). Atherosclerotic thickening of the intima and accompanying thrombosis with canalization is also present (B). App. 8 x.

the vessels of the central nervous system in association with meningitis, tabes, cerebrospinal syphilis and general paresis.

Rheumatic Arteritis.—In rheumatic fever the aorta and various arteries show definite changes. In the aorta the histologic appearance and distribution of the exudate much resembles that seen in syphilis, the exudate being found in the adventitia and to a lesser degree in the media around the nutrient vessels. The exudate, like that of syphilis, is made up of lymphocytes and plasma cells, but usually differs in having a few large mononuclear cells of the Aschoff type also present. At times, in the adventitia, rather typical Aschoff bodies may occur. The involvement of the media with degeneration of the elastic tissue is much less severe than in syphilis, and although the vessel wall would seem to be weakened by this process, aneurysms in association with rheumatic aortitis have not been recorded. The aorta shows little gross evidence of the disease, probably owing to the relatively small amount of damage and subsequent repair. The smaller arteries may show considerable necrosis and damage to the entire wall, thus somewhat resembling periarteritis nodosa. There is, however, no tendency to thrombosis of the vessel, healing of the wall proceeding without obliteration of the lumen.

Thrombo-angiitis Obliterans (Buerger's Disease).—This disease is characterized by an acute panarteritis and phlebitis probably of infectious origin, the exact cause of which, however, is unknown. It involves chiefly the deep vessels of the lower extremities, although cases have been reported in which the upper extremities have been affected. It is usually not recognized until the obliteration of the vessels leads to trophic ulcers or gangrene of the extremities. It is almost exclusively a disease of middle aged adult males, only a few cases having been reported in women. In the series of cases recorded by Buerger, the disease seems to have a particular predilection for Russian and Polish Jews. Subsequent reports, however, show that the disease is by no means confined to this group.

EARLY LESIONS.—The veins and arteries are invaded from without by an exudate consisting mainly of polymorphonuclear leukocytes. The process is patchy, involving various areas along the length of the deep vessels. The inflammatory process progresses by infiltration of the media and subsequently of the intima. Thrombosis results with obliteration of the lumen. The process is progressive, various vessels of the extremity being successively involved, thus gradually bringing about decrease in the nutrition of the part. Due to the collateral anastomosis little or no clinical evidence of the disease is manifest during this period, with the exception in about twenty per cent of the cases of painful red spots due to phlebitis of the superficial veins.

After a variable length of time the first clinical evidence of the disease may appear in the form of intermittent claudication, the patient complaining of pain and inability to walk after slight exercise, the claudication being due to inability of the superficial collateral circulation to longer maintain the muscles in a state of exercise.

There may be disturbances of the vasomotor control of the extremity with blanching of the leg when elevated, and painful redness in the dependent position. At this time any trivial injury may result in trophic ulcer of the foot. It is excruciatingly painful and tends not to heal. These changes are apparently due to involvement of the nerve trunk in the perivascular inflammatory and fibrotic process. Finally, gangrene of one of the toes may begin, gradually spreading to involve the greater part of the extremity, necessitating amputation. When the vessels are seen by the pathologist after the gangrenous extremity has been amputated, the acute manifestations have usually disappeared, the vessels showing obliteration by organized thrombi.

The process involves both the deep veins and arteries. The main vascular trunks are surrounded by a marked amount of scar tissue which also includes the nerve. The vessels are not uniformly involved throughout their length, the lesions being segmented in distribution frequently. Careful examination of the thrombosed vessel reveals no evidence of thickening of the intima or of asymmetric narrowing of the lumen previous to the formation of the thrombus, such as is observed in arteriosclerotic changes with secondary thrombus formation. There is an absence of calcification. Thus, the vessels of Buerger's disease are not visible in the roentgenogram as may be the case in arteriosclerotic gangrene.

PLATE XCIII
DISEASES OF THE BLOOD VESSELS

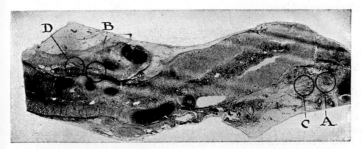

ARTERY-PERIARTERITIS
NODOSA.—CASE 167

FIG. 393.—ADRENAL.—Microtessar photograph illustrating several phases in the development of the lesion from the acute necrotic to the fibrous healed stage.

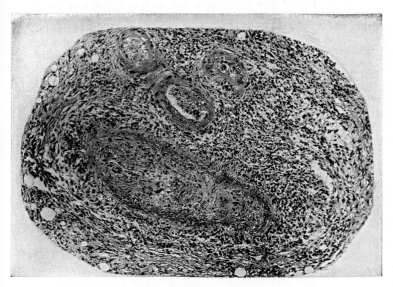

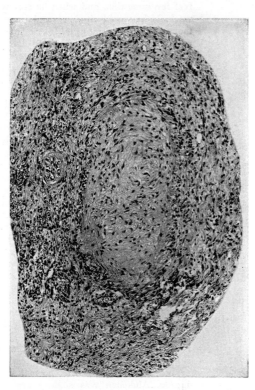

FIG. 394.—(VESSEL "A").—Acute necrotizing lesion with beginning repair. App. 100 x.

FIG. 395.—(VESSEL "B").—Late nearly healed lesion. App. 100 x.

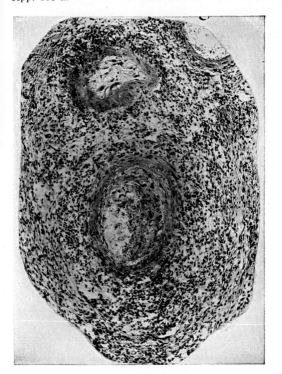

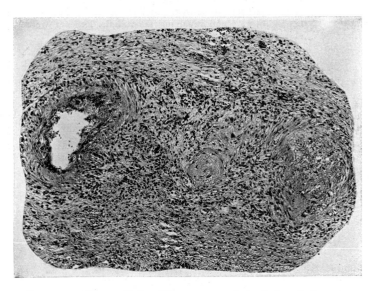

FIG. 396.—(VESSEL "C").—Acute hyaline necrotic phase. App. 100 x.

FIG. 397.—(VESSEL "D").—Three stages of the lesion. Left acute, middle healed, right thrombosis. App. 100 x.

CASE 166. (Ref. #S-358)

Diagnosis.—Thrombo-angiitis obliterans.

Patient was a Hebrew male of 48 years, admitted to the hospital complaining of an intermittent type of burning pain in his feet.

Present Illness.—The onset of the present complaint began approximately a year earlier. At that time, the pain was chiefly confined to the large toe of the left foot. He noticed it particularly when he had been on his feet for some time and when he was walking home from work. If he would sit down and rest for a short period, the pain would disappear. These intermittent attacks of pain had increased in frequency and severity until now at the time of admission they interfered seriously with his work. He noted that the skin over his feet would blanch with the onset of the pain and would appear reddened as the pain disappeared.

Past Medical History.—He had the usual childhood diseases as he recalled. He had had his tonsils removed at the age of ten. He was born in Austria but had lived in this country for the past twenty-five years. His diet had always contained a large amount of rye bread. He had always smoked a good deal averaging twenty to thirty cigarettes a day. He stated that he drank about a quart of whiskey a week. He was one of four brothers and sisters, all of whom were living and well. His father had died of apoplexy several years earlier, but his mother was alive and in good health. He was unmarried. A review of his systems was noninformatory. He had very few colds. Cardiorespiratory system was negative. He had had occasional qualitative attacks of dyspepsia. Bowels had been regular. Genito-urinary history was negative. He denied venereal infection.

Physical Examination.—Patient was a well developed, middle-aged white male who appeared nervous and restless. He complained of pain in both feet. Head was negative. Eyes, ears, nose and throat were negative. Chest was symmetrical. Lungs were clear. Heart was slightly enlarged to the left on percussion. There were no murmurs. Rhythm was normal. Blood pressure was 140/80. Abdomen was slightly protuberant. There was no tenderness. No viscera or masses could be felt. External genitalia were negative. Extremities: Skin over both feet showed a curious mottling suggesting the appearance of marble. No pulsation was felt in either dorsalis pedis or posterior tibials. These peripheral vessels were markedly sclerosed. Similar sclerosis, but less marked, was found involving the radials. Reflexes were negative.

Laboratory Findings.—Red blood cells, 5,250,000 with 11 gm. of hemoglobin (66%). White blood cells, 12,000 with 63% polynuclears. Urinalysis was negative.

Subsequent History.—The patient developed gangrene of the right large toe and a midthigh amputation was advised. This, the patient refused, but agreed to the amputation of his foot. This was done and the typical picture of diffuse thrombo-angiitis obliterans was found. The vessels above the point of amputation were definitely seen to be involved, and as was expected, the gangrenous process extended requiring subsequent midthigh amputation. A similar gangrenous process ensued in the other foot and a midthigh amputation was performed. The patient was discharged, and at last report was doing very satisfactorily with a pair of artificial legs.

Pathological Report: *Gross Description.*—The pathological specimen consisted of a serial accumulation of the right foot, the right leg and left leg with the attached foot, removed at different intervals. There was definite gangrene of the large and second toes on the right and beginning gangrene of the large toe on the left foot. The pathological interest in the specimen was centered in the vessels. These showed marked cord-like thickening and on cross section, at approximately the level of the ankle there was almost complete obliteration of the lumina not only of the arteries but of the venae comites. There appeared to be some collateral circulation which had been established as evidenced by a number of smaller vascular channels around the major vessels. In examining the vessels at the proximal end of the amputation, the lumina of the arteries was found widely patent although the walls seemed definitely thickened. The gross diagnosis was without much question that of thrombo-angiitis obliterans.

Microscopic Description of a Section Through a Group of Vessels from the Ankle Level.—(Fig. 388 and 389) Sections through the artery and venae comites at the ankle level show a diffuse organized thrombosis. The wall of the artery is somewhat thickened and shows considerable fibrosis. The lumen is practically obliterated by an organized thrombus which shows a small amount of canalization. A few mononuclear cells are seen in this organized connective tissue, some of which are laden with hemosiderin. Similar thrombotic lesions are seen involving both of the major venae comites. The process is late as seen in this histologic specimen and represents the end or healed stage of the condition with very little persistence of cellular exudation.

Periarteritis Nodosa.—This form of arteritis has an apparent predilection for the muscular type of medium and small sized arteries and arterioles, especially those of the gastro-intestinal tract, pancreas, spleen, liver, kidney, heart and vessels of the brain. The disease is usually ushered in with fever, prostration and a variety of severe symptoms referable to the organ showing the major vessel involvement. The process begins with acute periarteritis, but soon involves all coats of the vessels with necrosis of the media, thus weakening the wall and giving rise to small mycotic aneurisms. Thrombosis of many vessels also occurs. Rupture and hemorrhage are common. The exudate is made up chiefly of polymorphonuclear leukocytes with a few lymphocytes and mononuclears. The occurrence of these mycotic aneurisms and associated periarterial exudate along the course of the vessel wall leads to the nodular appearance of the vessel and thus the name. As a result of the occlusion of small arteries and arteri-

PLATE XCIV

DISEASES OF ARTERIES

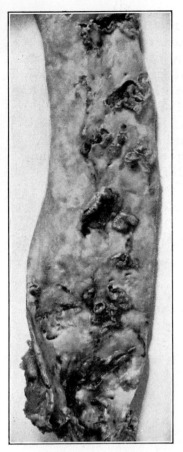

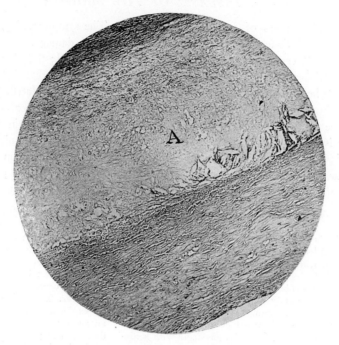

FIG. 399.—AORTA: ATHEROMA.—CASE 169.—Higher magnification from the area indicated in Fig. 400. Within the deeper layers of the intima is an area of lipoid degeneration containing rhomboid clefts originally occupied by cholesterin crystals. (A) A few fat-laden mononuclears may still be observed. App. 75 x.

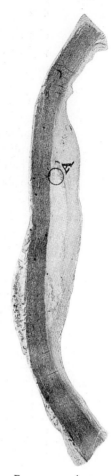

FIG. 398.—AORTA: ATHEROMA.—CASE 169.—Gross photograph showing advanced ulcerative atheromatous lesions.

FIG. 400. — AORTA: ATHEROMA. — CASE 169. — Microtessar photograph showing general characteristics of atheromatous plaques. App. 3 x.

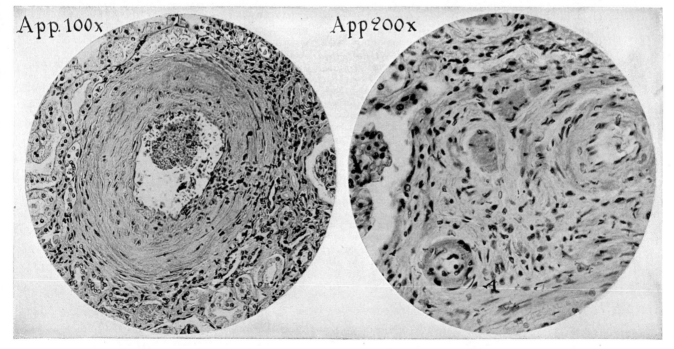

FIG. 401.—ARTERY: HYPERPLASTIC SCLEROSIS.—CASE 233.—Small artery within the kidney showing marked thickening of the wall as a result of subintimal fibrous hyperplasia. Reduplication of the elastic tissue may be revealed by special staining. 100 x.

FIG. 402.—ARTERIOLES: HYPERPLASTIC SCLEROSIS.—CASE 233.—Arterioles of the kidney with lumen much reduced by thickening of the wall as a result of endothelial and fibrous hyperplasia of the intima. App. 200 x.

oles small multiple areas of necrosis occur in the various organs and tissues affected. The disease is progressive so that vessels may be seen in all stages of involvement from the beginning of the periarterial exudate to the healed stage following the organization of the thrombus and the healing of the perivascular tissue with subsidence of the acute exudate. The disease is usually fatal within a few weeks.

The clinical diagnosis of the condition is rarely made due to the great variation in the symptoms.

The symptoms depend upon the organ showing the chief damage. Thus, coronary thrombosis may be simulated; the picture may be that of acute hemorrhagic pancreatitis, or at times mesenteric thrombosis may be simulated. The etiology is unknown. The theory that streptococci or their toxins may be the biologic factor in the presence of highly allergic tissues has been advanced and seems the most satisfactory explanation at present. Filterable virus may also be listed as a possible cause.

ILLUSTRATIVE CASE

CASE 167. (Ref. #S-175)

Diagnosis.—Adrenal—periarteritis nodosa.

Patient was a white male of 44 years, admitted to the hospital with the chief complaint of pain in the stomach.

Present Illness.—The onset of the patient's present illness was approximately one month before admission when he was seized with cramp-like pains in his legs. He had apparently been in his usual good health until that time. Two weeks later he consulted a physician with a history of similar cramp-like pains in his abdomen. Owing to the fact that he had worked with lead in a battery plant for over fifteen years, it was thought that he probably had an attack of lead poisoning. He was treated with this in mind by his physician, but without relief of his symptoms, and he was accordingly referred to the hospital for further study. At the time of admission, he complained not only of gastric cramp-like pains, but also of fleeting pains in his shoulders, arms, fingers and feet. He had also noticed occasional swelling of his feet and ankles, which persisted for several days at a time in spite of bed rest.

Past History.—As a child, he had had scarlet fever and typhoid fever and believed he probably had all the other minor childhood ailments. He had never had any serious illness except an attack of what was considered to be acute lead poisoning fourteen years before his present illness. This was supposed to be associated with an ulcer of his stomach. These were relieved by medical treatment and he had been completely free of symptoms during the interval, continuing his employment in a battery plant. A review of his systems was non-informatory. He had had no symptoms relating to his respiratory, cardiovascular or genito-urinary systems.

Physical Examination.—Physical examination revealed a well developed male, apparently quite ill and with severe pain in the upper abdomen. Head showed no abnormalities. Eyes, ears, nose and throat were negative. No lead line was present on the gums. The chest was symmetrical. Heart and lungs appeared normal. There was a blood pressure of 200/110. Abdomen was moderately distended and was diffusely tender. Liver was definitely enlarged and tender on palpation. There was visible peristalsis. No masses could be felt at the time of admission. Extremities were negative, in respect to reflexes and pain.

Laboratory Findings.—Red blood cells, 4,230,000 with 69% hemoglobin. White blood cells, 56,250 with 95% polynuclears. Kahn test was negative. Blood Chemistry: Plasma chlorides 537 mgm. Icterus Index 6%. Van den

Bergh indirect negative. Blood sugar 110 mgm. Urea 31 mgm. Urinalysis: Specific gravity 1.017 to 1.030; albumin 2 plus. Occasional granular casts.

Subsequent Course.—The pain in the patient's upper abdomen became practically continuous. It was boring in character. The patient was transferred to surgery and an exploratory operation revealed what appeared to be an acute pancreatitis. There was a serosanguineous exudate in the peritoneal cavity with evidence of necrosis of the head of the pancreas. The gallbladder was thickened, adherent and acutely inflamed. A cholecystostomy was performed, and drainage established. No stones were found in the gallbladder. The postoperative condition seemed good, but two days after operation, the patient became irrational and died a few hours later.

Autopsy Findings.—At autopsy the pancreas, liver, spleen and renal organs showed multiple areas of necrosis. At the head of the pancreas a larger area of necrosis showed evidence of hemorrhage into the parenchyma, and the adjacent fat showed fat necrosis. There was a fibrinous exudate of the adjacent organs and peritoneum together with a small amount of purulent exudate. A dissection of the pancreatic artery revealed the true nature of the disease in the form of bead-like nodules occurring along the course of the vessel and branches, some having undergone thrombosis. There were no stones in the gallbladder, although the walls were edematous and swollen.

Histologically, a periarteritis nodosa was seen in many of the vessels of the lung, spleen, kidney, liver, pancreas, adrenal, gallbladder and the brain, some showing recent thrombosis, others in various stages of healing. The adjacent portions of the organs showed necrosis.

Microscopic Description of a Section of the Adrenal. —(Plate XCII) Histologic examination of the adrenal as a whole under low power shows multiple foci of necrosis. These appear to be in relation to extensive degenerative lesions affecting the blood vessels. These are distributed irregularly throughout both cortex and medulla of the gland. (Fig. 393.)

Higher power study of the tissue shows the process to be largely confined to the smaller arteries and arterioles. The entire process of periarteritis nodosa may be observed by studying various of these vessels. In some areas the acute phase of the pathology is present. This consists of an acute periarteritis with extensive degeneration and hyaline necrosis of the arteriolar wall, accompanied by secondary thrombosis and proliferative changes in the subintima. The wall is infiltrated by leukocytes and there is a wide collar of inflammatory cells around the adventitia. The majority of these are polynuclears, but a few plasma cells, lymphocytes and mononuclears can be identified. (Fig. 383, 394 and 396.) In the more advanced lesions, the acute process seems to be subsiding to some extent and the inflammatory cellular exudate shows a gradual transition from the polynuclear to the mononuclear picture. There is marked reparative fibrosis found which in places suggests an attempt to wall off the development of a small mycotic aneurysm (Fig. 396). This diffuse reparative fibrosis is found not only in the adventitia but throughout the vessel wall, and in association with the organization of the almost regular thrombotic process which co-exists with the acute degenerative and inflammatory changes.

Endarteritis Obliterans.—Endarteritis obliterans is a condition in which the lumen of a vessel is narrowed or obliterated by thickening of the intima. The condition is seen normally in many physiological and pathological processes. The closure of the hypogastric vessels and ductus arteriosis are physiological examples. Endarteritis of syphilis and hyperplastic sclerosis of the small vessels in arteriosclerosis are also examples of pathologic varieties. In granulation tissue the vessels decrease in the resultant scar by a

In still other areas, almost complete replacement fibrosis may be found with complete obliteration of the vessel (Fig. 395), which appears as an irregular fibrous scar. These vessels have not proceeded to the ultimate point of a contracted cicatricial scar tissue, but still are in a stage where the connective tissue is relatively rich in loosely woven bundles of collagen. Accompanying this reparative fibrosis is seen a very extensive chronic inflammatory mononuclear cellular infiltration. The picture as a whole is entirely consistent with the thought that the inflammatory reaction is of an allergic nature in response to a severe streptococcic infection, but in the light of our present knowledge, this is still a theoretical hypothesis rather than a proven fact.

somewhat similar process. In Ayerza's disease the lesions in the pulmonary vessels are an endarteritis.

Histologically, the intima is thickened by proliferation of the endothelium or necrosis in the subendothelial connective tissue, or both. The condition is not a definite pathological entity, but is a term applied rather loosely to obliterating processes, in which the intimal thickening brings about limitation or occlusion of the lumen. It may have a physiologic, a toxic, a metabolic or a degenerative background.

ILLUSTRATIVE CASE

CASE 168. (Ref. #S-60)

Diagnosis.—Peripheral artery—obliterative endarteritis.

Patient was a colored male of 61 years, admitted to the hospital complaining of dyspnea and ankle edema.

Present Illness.—It is difficult to state with any degree of certainty when the present illness actually began. His immediate complaints dated back a period of about five months, during which time he had complained of intermittent attacks of diarrhea associated with severe colic-like pains in the abdomen. This had been accompanied by marked dyspnea on exertion and swelling of his ankles, particularly when he had been much on his feet. Most of his complaints otherwise were relatively indefinite and vague, but seemed largely to be dependent upon circulatory disturbances.

Past Medical History.—The patient had no idea of his childhood medical history. A review of his systems showed that he had been rather subject to colds for the past several years. He had never been heart conscious until the present admission when he occasionally noticed some palpitation in association with his dyspnea. His gastro-intestinal history was entirely negative, again except for the present illness. He had always had a good appetite and his bowels had always been regular. He had had no particularly significant genito-urinary symptoms other than occasional nocturia during the past year or so. He denied venereal disease.

Physical Examination.—The patient was an emaciated, fairly well developed, elderly male Negro. Head was not remarkable. Pupils reacted normally. Nose and throat were negative. Chest was symmetrical and was somewhat of the emphysematous, barrel type. There was a patchy consolidation noted on percussion in the left

upper lobe as evidenced by alteration in the percussion note. Here the breath sounds and voice sounds were likewise altered and there were a number of moist râles heard. Râles were likewise heard at both bases. The heart was definitely enlarged downward and to the left, with the apex impulse felt in the sixth interspace in the midaxillary line. There was a short, systolic, aortic murmur heard. The peripheral arteries were tortuous and sclerotic. There was a marked difference in the blood pressure on the right and left, that in the right being 176/70, while that in the left was 90/80. The abdomen was negative. The extremities showed moderate edema of the feet and ankles. At the time of admission, the temperature was 101° and fluctuated between 98° and 103° during the week he was in the hospital, the respirations ranging from 20 to 36.

Laboratory Findings.—Red blood cells on admission numbered 4,200,000 with 78% hemoglobin. White blood cells, 12,400 with 82% polynuclears. Urinalysis was essentially negative. Kahn test gave a three-plus reaction. Sputum examination revealed the presence of many streptococci, chiefly of the hemolytic type.

Subsequent Course.—The patient grew progressively weaker with evidence of increasing toxemia. He died quietly with no acute terminal episode.

Autopsy Findings.—The heart showed a chronic fibroid myosclerosis. There was marked atherosclerosis of the aorta with involvement of the aortic valve in a calcific process. The aortic ring showed diffuse fibrous thickening as well as the calcification at the base of all three cusps. The large and medium sized arteries all showed marked atherosclerosis. The left subclavian artery was almost obliterated at its source by what appeared to be an extensive atherosclerosis. Similar atherosclerotic endarteritic changes were noted in the vessels of the lower extremity. The lungs showed a patchy broncho-pneumonia in the left upper lobe and a terminal hypostatic type of pneumonia at both bases. The autopsy findings otherwise were negative. Nothing was seen to definitely suggest syphilis other than the possible fibrous thickening of the aortic valve.

Microscopic Description of a Section Through the Posterior Tibial Artery.—(Fig. 391) Histologic examination of the vessel shows marked thickening of the intima. This consists of a proliferative fibrous connective tissue reaction. In places, this shows myxomatous degeneration. There must have been a previous thrombosis as is shown by a rather marked organization of the tissue with the presence of many small blood channels. Much of the subintimal connective tissue has undergone hyaline degeneration. There are a few round cells scattered throughout this subintimal endarteritic fibrosis. Some of these are large mononuclear phagocytes filled with blood pigment. The media is involved in this arterial degenerative process with considerable hyalinization of the musculature. No typical Mönckeberg calcification of the media is seen and the elastic membrane can still be recognized. There is considerable mononuclear lymphocytic and plasma cell infiltration of the adventitia. The picture may best be interpreted as a simple obliterative type of peripheral endarteritis. Whether this could be considered as of syphilitic etiology is extremely debatable.

DEGENERATIVE DISEASES OF THE ARTERIAL SYSTEM

Arteriosclerosis

The term "arteriosclerosis" has for many years been applied to a group of lesions of the arterial vessels of the body, all of which are probably the result directly or indirectly of degenerative changes in the vessel. It is the most common form of vascular disease, and is almost universally present at autopsy in individuals dying past midlife. The lesions are quite varied in the different types of vessels, although they are probably the manifestation of the same process.

The etiology is still not definitely known, many theories having been propounded. The importance of the disease may be better appreciated when it is realized that the condition leads in most instances to decrease in the blood supply to the various important viscera, and is therefore directly or indirectly responsible for vital changes which eventually result in the death of the individual. The expression that "one is as old as his arteries" is essentially an expression of the degree of arteriosclerosis of his vessels.

The disease is characterized by three main types of lesions: (1) In the aorta and the large elastic type of vessel the lesion is an atheromatous one which may be better spoken of as *atherosclerosis;* (2) in the medium or muscular type of vessel the essential lesion is usually a degeneration of the media with subsequent calcification, an exaggerated form of which is known as *Mönckeberg's mesarteritis* (Fig. 387 and 392) and (3) in the small arteries and arterioles the lesions are mainly subintimal and are accompanied by proliferative changes. The process is usually known as *hyperplastic sclerosis.*

The degree of involvement of the vascular system is not uniform. In some cases atherosclerosis of the large vessels may predominate; in others the hyperplastic changes may predominate. In the usual senile variety of arteriosclerosis, the first two, atherosclerosis and medial calcification, are most frequently seen. In younger individuals the hyperplastic sclerosis may predominate. This is particularly true in cases in which hypertension is a symptom.

Atheroma, Atherosclerosis.—Atheroma is essentially a degenerative lesion of the intimal portion of the large vessels of the elastic type, such as the aorta and large size arteries. The lesions are seen in the majority of aortas in individuals past middle life, and vary considerably in severity. The abdominal aorta is usually more extensively involved than the arch or thoracic portions. Grossly, the lesions are patchy and at first appear as slightly grayish-yellow opacities of the intima. Later, they become raised due to the thickening of the subintimal connective tissue with necrosis of the deeper portions. This degenerative material is soft, yellowish and porridge-like, hence the name "atheroma" (athere, gruel and oma, swelling). In addition to scattered plaques there is a tendency for button-like atheromata to occur about the openings of the smaller branches of the aorta, particularly the intercostals. The lesions frequently show calcification (Fig. 398). They may ulcerate and subsequent thrombus formation may occur. At times, due to severe ulcerative changes, a dissecting aneurism may arise. The swelling of these atheromatous plaques has little effect upon the lumen of the aorta, but in the other arteries the plaque may considerably diminish the lumen. This is well seen in branches of the celiac axis, the coronaries, the renals and the cerebral vessels. (Fig. 379 and 385.)

Histologically, an atheroma of the aorta probably begins by the imbibition of blood plasma into the ground substance of the intima (Aschoff), probably as a result of an initial degenerative change in this part of the vessel wall. The etiology is due to factors not yet thoroughly understood. If the blood at the time has an abnormally high lipoid content, it is thought that the resorption of this fluid leads to its deposit in the subintima. Many large mononuclears soon accumulate which take up these lipoids. They become tremendously swollen and eventually die. There is proliferation of the subintimal connective tissue. Usually a few lymphocytes are seen at this stage. Later the portion of the plaque next to the media undergoes necrosis with accumulation of lipoids as globules and as needle-like crystals of cholesterol. In the superficial portions the thickened intima undergoes hyalinization. The innermost elastic layers of the media show fraying and fragmentation as they approach and enter the lesion. If the lesions are examined late, the fatty portions may be entirely calcified. The media and adventitia show little change (Fig. 399 and 400).

Many theories have been advanced to explain the initial changes which lead to the production of the atheromatous plaque. One of the first to be advanced was the increased strain brought about by arterial hypertension, considering that the increase in wear and tear upon the vessel wall was manifest by minor degenerative changes which eventually give rise to the typical lesion of atheroma. Some of the older writers have suggested that, in addition to the increased strain upon the vessel wall produced by hypertension, the nutrient vessels (vasa vasorum) are compressed in passing through the media, and thus the nourishment of the intima is diminished. Additional weight has been added to the hypertensive theory by the presence of atheroma in the pulmonary artery in severe cases of mitral stenosis where the blood pressure is increased. It must also be recognized, however, in this particular instance that, in addition to the increased pressure, the vessel itself may be injured by various products the result of chronic congestion. In conclusion, although hypertension may play a part in the production of atheroma, it must be recognized that, in a great majority of cases, clinical hypertension does not exist, and

that many individuals with marked elevation in blood pressure show no commensurate atheromatosis.

Many experiments have been performed on animals in which the blood pressure has been elevated for long periods of time, the results of which are conflicting. In most instances, there has been a failure in producing atheromatous lesions. Others consider the process as a reaction to the wear and tear on the vessels, the thickened atheromatous plaques representing compensatory strengthening of the wall which has been weakened by degenerative change.

Arteriosclerosis has been blamed on diets high in lipoid content in an attempt to explain the initial deposits in the earliest atheromatous lesions. Experimentally, Leary succeeded in developing lesions similar to those seen in man in the coronary artery of rabbits which had been fed with a diet containing large amounts of cholesterol. It is interesting to note in this connection that the extensive atherosclerotic lesions of diabetes with subsequent gangrenous changes have appreciably diminished with the discontinuance of the high fat diets which were formerly advocated in the treatment of the disease. An infinite number of toxic substances of endogenous or exogenous origin have been blamed as factors in the initiation of the lesions, but conclusive proof is absent. Some of the older writers refer to the absorption of metabolic waste products from the intestine in chronic constipation as important factors leading to ageing of the vessels. Bacterial toxins, various inorganic substances such as lead, etc., have been suggested. Experimental injections of nicotine have failed. Alcohol for a long time was considered as a possible irritant. It, therefore, becomes evident that as yet the exact etiology is unknown, but it seems to be the consensus of opinion that an irritant or group of toxic irritants initiate the process.

Medial Calcification and Sclerosis (Mönckeberg). —Degenerative changes in the media followed by varying degrees of calcification is observed in many cases of arteriosclerosis and is probably brought about by similar etiological factors as those discussed above. This calcification is not always confined to the muscular type of vessel but may occur following degenerative changes in the media of the aorta and the larger elastic type of vessel, thereby being associated with an atherosclerotic process. In old individuals at times, degenerative changes with extreme calcification of the large and medium sized muscular type of vessel are seen. These vessels are spoken of as "tracheate" or "pipe stem" arteries when occurring in vessels of the extremity. They are easily palpated in the radials and sometimes in the temporals. The vessels are tortuous and show patchy calcification partially surrounding the vessel, thus giving a "tracheate" appearance.

In diabetes, medial degeneration and calcification in many cases is extreme, affecting the muscular type of vessels. The process is associated with degenerative and atherosclerotic lesions of the intima. This intimal sclerosis tends to undergo calcification with narrowing of the vessel lumen and occasionally thrombus formation. The gangrenous lesions associated with the disease are due to such thrombosis. In the typical case of Mönckeberg's mesarteritis, on the other hand, such sclerotic degenerative changes in the small peripheral vessels are ordinarily lacking.

Histologically, there is marked degeneration of the media with calcareous infiltration occurring in patches (Fig. 387 and 392). When the condition is extreme, the lesions result in thickening of the wall, so that the intima is compressed and the lumen narrowed. Pressure atrophy may occur in the muscle of the infected media. The condition is usually associated with severe atheromatosis of the aorta with calcification. The condition has apparently no relation to hypertension.

ILLUSTRATIVE CASE

CASE 169. (Ref. #S-59 and S-359)

Diagnosis.—Aorta—atheroma, atherosclerosis.

Patient was a Negro of 78 years, admitted to the hospital in uremia.

Present Illness.—The history of the patient's illness was obtained from his daughter. He had been in his usual fairly good health until about two weeks before admission. At that time he complained of headache and nausea. He vomited two or three times that day and was confined to bed. He became progressively weaker and went into a semistupor about ten days after the onset of his symptoms. This was complicated by a very marked frequency at almost half hour intervals. He seemed to be becoming so definitely worse that it was felt he could be better cared for in the hospital, and was referred by his physician for that reason.

Past Medical History.—Very little information of significance was obtained from his daughter. She knew that her father was supposed to have a mild diabetes, which had been of many years' duration. He had never had any serious illness, most of his complaints being of a minimal nature. He had his right eye enucleated twenty-five years before following a traumatic injury, but other than these scattered bits of information, no really pertinent past history could be obtained.

Physical Examination.—Patient was a semicomatose, elderly Negro, fairly well developed but markedly emaciated. He could be fairly easily aroused, but his attention wandered rapidly. Head was normal in contour. Right eye was absent. There was marked sclerosis and tortuosity of the temporal vessels. His nose and throat were negative. There was a complete edentia. Chest was symmetrical. Lungs showed a few scattered fine moist râles, chiefly at the bases. Heart was not enlarged and no murmurs were heard. Abdomen was scaphoid. Extremities showed better muscle tone on the right than on the left. All the peripheral vessels of the arms and legs showed very extensive tracheate Mönckeberg's type of arteriosclerosis. No pulsation could be felt in the dorsalis pedis arteries.

Laboratory Findings.—Urinalysis was negative except for a slight trace of albumin. Blood examination showed a hemoconcentration with 7,700,000 red cells and hemoglobin of 14.9 gm., as a result of apparent dehydra-

tion. White blood cells similarly were increased in number to 14,200 with 81% polynuclears. Blood chemistry: Blood sugar 180 mgm.; blood urea 74 mgm.; CO_2 39 volumes per cent.

Subsequent Course.—The patient was given fluids intravenously and subcutaneously in an attempt to relieve his immediate dehydration picture, but he proceeded rapidly down hill and died twenty-four hours after admission.

Autopsy Findings.—The basic cause of death in this case was a very extensive generalized arteriosclerosis which affected not only the aorta and larger elastic type of vessels, but also involved the medium sized peripheral arteries in a very extensive Mönckeberg's medial type of arteriosclerosis. It even affected the smaller arteries and arterioles of the brain, kidney and heart. Such other findings as existed were relatively incidental to these disturbances of his circulatory system. The heart was not primarily at fault. It showed typical brown atrophy with thickening of the coronaries. Lungs likewise showed brown induration with some suggestion of slight terminal hypostatic congestion. The kidneys presented the typical picture of arteriosclerosis with deep, patchy, wedge-shaped fibrotic scarred areas (Fig. 385).

From the standpoint of the arteriosclerosis, the aorta presented the typical picture of simple senile atherosclerosis. This was most marked in the lower portion of the abdominal aorta and particularly involved the bifurcation. It was present throughout the length of the vessel but diminished in degree toward the arch. Many of these atheromatous plaques were calcified. Some of them were associated with secondary overlying thrombosis, and a few had actually undergone ulceration.

In the peripheral vessels, sections taken from the tibials as well as from the dorsalis pedis showed a textbook picture of medial sclerosis. The arteries were of the characteristic pipestem variety and were rigid tubes in appearance. Splitting such a vessel longitudinally, the tracheate arrangement of the calcium in more or less radial bands could be easily made out.

Microscopic Description of a Section Through One of the Aortic Atheromatous Plaques.—(Ref. #S-59) (Fig. 399 and 400) Histologic examination shows the intimal lining of the aorta elevated above the surface of the endothelium as a whole. Beneath this layer of somewhat thickened intima is found a grumous mass of degenerated material in which a few large mononuclear phagocytic cells can be seen. These are particularly prominent just beneath the intimal surface. Deeper in this patch of lipoid degeneration can be seen rhombic clefts representing actual cholesterol crystals, which have been dissolved out of the specimen. Growing in from the base and the sides may be observed a moderate amount of subintimal connective tissue proliferation. By the use of special elastic tissue staining technique on supplementary slides from the material, a fraying and splitting of the elastic fibers may be readily observed, and the internal elastic lamina, as such, is no longer identifiable. As a result of such diffuse atheromatous degeneration of the vessel wall, it is apparent that much of the normal elasticity of the vessel is lost and a tendency toward its becoming a relatively rigid tube as the result of the secondary cicatricial fibrosis occurs.

Diagnosis.—Tibial artery—peripheral, Mönckeberg's medial sclerosis.

Microscopic Description of a Section Through One of the Tibial Arteries.—(Ref. #S-359) (Fig. 387 and

Diffuse Hyperplastic Sclerosis.—This condition is seen to affect the small arteries and arterioles particularly of the viscera of the body. It is observed to advantage in the intralobular arteries and afferent arterioles to the glomeruli in the kidneys.

Hyperplastic sclerosis of the vessels in general was formerly considered to be definitely associated with hypertension, the degree of involvement somewhat paralleling the severity of the increase in arterial pressure. Recently, however, Moritz and Old have shown that this statement holds true only when applied to the vessels of the kidney. A comparison of the size and the degree of hyperplastic sclerosis of the smaller arteries of the body in hypertensive and non-hypertensive subjects reveals no diagnostic difference in the process in any of the organs with the exception of the kidney. In this organ in the non-hypertensive individual the arteries and arterioles show little or no involvement, whereas in hypertension the involvement is marked. Attempts to diagnose essential hypertension by muscle biopsy, therefore, would seem to have less import than was formerly conceded.

The general discussion of hypertension will not be considered at this point as it is taken up in Chapter LVI on nephrosclerosis. The condition may be suspected on gross inspection of the organ by the "wide mouth" appearance of the tiny vessels. The change is extreme in most cases of hypertension and by some

392) Histologic examination of one of these smaller muscular type of arterial vessels shows its typical arteriosclerotic degenerative features. Instead of the lesion being almost exclusively subintimal, the involvement of the media is immediately apparent. There is a swelling of the musculature with an interstitial hyalinization of the vessel wall. This undergoes further degeneration even to the point of necrosis and secondary calcification. For some poorly understood reason, this calcium tends to be deposited in relatively annular fashion as rings. Thus, in longitudinal section of the vessel, several such patchy areas of calcification may be observed at rather surprisingly regular intervals. In cross section, it is quite possible at times to have a complete band of such calcific deposit within a single section. Accompanying this medial involvement is a secondary subintimal fibrosis and thickening, which gradually results in a diminution in the caliber of the vessel lumen, in the more striking instances even to its complete obliteration. This represents the familiar peripheral type of arteriosclerosis which we believe is merely a variation in the general picture of arteriosclerosis as modified by the architectural structure of this particular type of vessel.

is thought to be a compensatory reaction to the increase in strain.

Histologically, there is thickening of the entire wall of the artery with a marked corresponding decrease in the size of the lumen. This is due to both hypertrophy of the muscular coat and hyperplastic thickening of the intima. In the tiny arteriole the change is mainly intimal (Fig. 384, 385, 401, 402). The thickening of the intima is accompanied by considerable increase in elastic tissue in the form of a number of concentrically-arranged elastic lamina spoken of as *reduplication*. For its demonstration the tissues must be stained by some modification of Weigert's technique for elastic tissue. The initial muscular hypertrophy of the media is replaced gradually by fibrous tissue sclerosis. The wall becomes less elastic and more or less rigid. In the afferent arteriole to the kidney the intimal hyperplasia is extreme, and the vessel lumen may be completely occluded. These vessels normally can be identified only with difficulty, whereas in hypertension they become quite prominent (Fig. 402).

Degenerative changes, such as hyalinization of the intima, are frequently seen as early manifestations, and are commonly found in the vessels of the spleen, pancreas, brain, etc., even in individuals without hypertension. In malignant hypertension hyalin necrosis may be a prominent feature and indeed is the *only* microscopic criterion for establishing the diagnosis.

Angiospasm (Neurogenic Vascular Disease)

That angiospasm may occur and be the chief factor in the production of pathology is probably conceded by all. The factors producing this spasm, however, are far more difficult to demonstrate. Most probably they are due to neurogenic disturbances in the vaso-motor control. In Raynaud's disease, characterized by symmetric gangrene, chiefly of the fingers or toes and occasionally occurring in other parts of the body, the superficial small arteries are involved in an angiospasm which is so prolonged as to result in these changes. Examination of the affected arteries fail to show definite organic basis intrinsic to the vessel. In angina pectoris the symptoms are apparently due to an ischemia(?) of the myocardium, brought about by spasms of the arteries. The abdominal crises of tabes seem best explained by angiospasm resulting from changes in the nervous system. Symptoms referable to the brain, which give rise to transient hemiplegia without evidence of organic disease, can possibly be explained by spasm of the arterioles. Angiospasm can be observed in the retina in conditions such as essential hypertension. It would seem that such angiospasm may bring about definite pathological changes in tissues or even organs without showing any demonstrable gross or microscopic lesions in the vessels affected.

Aneurysm

An aneurysm may be defined as a cyst-like mass containing blood and communicating with an artery. Two important varieties are recognized: (1) true aneurysms in which the sac is made up of one or more of the coats of the vessel wall; and (2) false aneurysms, in which the wall is made up by the surrounding tissues.

True Aneurysms.—These, in general, are usually due to some disease which results in weakening of the vessel wall, plus the strain associated with an increase in arterial pressure. The underlying etiology in probably ninety-nine per cent of aneurysms is vascular syphilis. True aneurysms are described as primary (spontaneous), dissecting and mycotic.

Primary (spontaneous) Aneurysm.—This type is by far the most common. It usually occurs in the elastic type of vessel, particularly in the aorta. It may be saccular, cylindric or fusiform in shape. The saccular variety is most often found involving the aorta and cerebral vessels, whereas the cylindric and fusiform varieties are more frequently encountered in the large arteries.

Dissecting Aneurysm.—This is a comparatively rare type, seen usually in the ascending portion of the arch of the aorta. It is characterized by a rupture of the intimal lining of the vessel, often in relation to an atheromatous plaque, with a resultant dissecting hemorrhagic process between the layers of the vessel wall. It may be relatively localized, or extend the entire length of the aorta.

Mycotic Aneurysm.—This is particularly a disease of the medium sized and small arteries. It is due to weakening of the wall as a result of some inflammatory process accompanied by necrosis. The necrosis may occur from within, following the lodgment of an infected embolus, as acute ulcerative endocarditis. Secondly, the process might be initiated from without. In periarteritis nodosa, for example, the necrotic process begins as a periarteritis but subsequently involves the entire wall. Or again, the lesion might result from the extension of a suppurative or tuberculous process in the surrounding tissues.

False Aneurysms.—These are usually the result of injury to the vessel wall through trauma, stab wounds, bullet wounds, fractures, etc. The hematoma thus formed is walled off by the surrounding tissues or organs, forming a sac which connects with the artery. Many so-called *arteriovenous aneurysms* are likewise of traumatic origin and result from injuries in which the artery and adjacent vein are lacerated with subsequent communication after healing. A few arteriovenous aneurysms are congenital in nature. They are the result of dilated arteriovenous channels which are formed without the usual interposition of capillary field. This type of lesion is spoken of as a *cirsoid aneurysm*.

ANEURYSM OF THE AORTA

Saccular Aneurysm.—The aorta is the most common site of aneurysm. It may be saccular, cylindric or dissecting in type. The saccular variety is the most common and is found almost regularly in the arch of the aorta particularly in the ascending portion. Etiologically, it is due to vascular syphilis which frequently brings about a patchy weakening of the media with subsequent ectasia. From the first portion of the aorta the aneurysm usually springs from the convex surface anteriorly and tends to extend forward pressing upon the sternum. Aneurysms arising from the transverse portion of the arch usually originate from the posterior wall and extend backward, pressing upon the trachea, esophagus, recurrent laryngeal nerve, upper dorsal vertebra, etc. Those arising from the descending arch also extend posteriorly, but they are not frequent. Occasionally, saccular aneurysms may arise from the thoracic aorta about the level of the diaphragm and also, but very rarely, from the abdominal portion. Aneurysmal dilatation with involvement of the sinus of Valsalva must also be mentioned, occurring in association with dilatation of the aortic ring and involvement of the aortic cusps in occasional cases of syphilitic aortitis.

Grossly, the aneurysm is roughly spheroid in shape with an opening into the aorta which is less than its greatest diameter (Fig. 126, Chapter XV). It is usually partially filled with a laminated thrombus which shows little or no attempt to organize. In rare instances such thrombi may undergo organization and endothelium may cover its surface. The wall of the aneurysm is made up chiefly of fibrous tissue, which may be of considerable thickness. The media is almost entirely lacking and apparently replaced by fibrous tissue. Early it may be seen as a degenerated and atrophied layer. The aneurysm progressively enlarges by stretching of the sac from a point near its origin in the aorta, where the wall is thinnest. This is where rupture usually occurs.

The symptoms of aneurysm are due to pressure of the tumor mass upon the adjacent viscera. Pain, which is the most constant symptom, may arise reflexly from stretching of the vessel wall and may be the result of direct pressure upon the nerves (intercostal or dorsal nerve groups). The pain also may originate from pressure and erosion of bone. The paroxysmal "brassy cough" in most instances is the result of pressure upon the trachea or bronchi; the hoarseness and weakness of the voice to pressure on the recurrent laryngeal nerve. Death results from rupture of the aneurysm into the pleura or pericardium in about one third of the cases, more rarely into the trachea or esophagus. Occasionally an aneurysm may erode through the sternum or ribs and rupture through the skin surface.

Cylindric or Fusiform Aneurysms.—Cylindric dilatation of the arch of the aorta is seen in a few cases of elderly males showing advanced atheromatous changes. The lesions may occasionally be of syphilitic origin with diffuse moderate involvement of the wall, although in most cases the atheromatous nature of the process is apparent.

Dissecting Aneurysm.—This interesting though relatively rare disease of the aorta results from a rupture or split of the intima with subsequent hemorrhage into the wall of the artery. The extension of this hemorrhage leads to separation of the arterial wall in the media. The most common site of origin of the aneurysm is in the ascending aorta. The aneurysm may extend to the aortic ring above or to the iliac vessels below. Commonly, the aneurysm ruptures into the aorta itself in the lower abdominal portion and circulation thus may be reëstablished with the aorta. Cases have been reported in which the aneurysm has been lined by endothelium and in which circulation took place within the aneurysm as well as within the aorta. Death may occur from rupture of the aneurysm into the pericardium, although occasionally it has followed its rupture into the pleural or peritoneal cavities.

PART II

THE VEINS

The veins, curiously enough, are not subject to the wide range of pathological changes which are seen affecting the arteries. Indeed, aside from the inflammatory process known as phlebitis which is inevitably accompanied by some degree of thrombosis, no lesions of particular clinical significance are encountered except the several varicosities, such as varicose veins of the legs, hemorrhoids, varicocele and oesophageal varices. The clinical importance of these lesions, however, cannot be overestimated.

PHLEBITIS

From the pathological standpoint phlebitis is always a potentially dangerous lesion, due to the fact that it is regularly complicated by thrombus formation. Accordingly, the term *thrombophlebitis* is perhaps more accurate as a designation for the process. The condition is of importance primarily from the mechanical standpoint, first, as being one of the most prolific sources of emboli, whether sterile or infected, and second, through its frequent local thrombotic obstruction to the circulation at the site of the inflammatory process.

Two forms of phlebitis are usually recognized— the infectious and the noninfectious. In the infectious type, there are several ways in which the inflammatory process may be initiated. (1) It may be traumatic in origin with the bacteria being carried directly to the vessel walls through cutaneous wounds, operative incisions, compound fractures, stab or bullet wounds. (2) The infection, on the other hand, may arise from mural implantation of bacteria in the course of some blood stream infection or simple bacteremia. (3) The infectious process may be of very low grade in respect to virulence, but may spread by direct continuity from some more distant focus. One of the best illustrations of this method of development is seen in the so-called *phlegmasia alba dolens* or "milk-leg" following childbirth. Here, there is usually some minimal, essentially saprophytic bacterial invasion of the uterine sinuses. This gradually spreads to involve the femoral vein in a typical thrombophlebitis, and results in swelling of the extremity due to interference of the venous, and often lymphatic return circulation. Finally, (4) extension of an infectious process through contiguity of structure may occur, such as is only too frequently seen in the resultant thrombosis of the lateral sinus from direct extension of an acute mastoiditis.

Non-infectious Phlebitis is seen most often as the result of traumatic injury. Bacteria are not introduced into the injured area, so that the inflammatory process remains sterile. Pressure from an intra-abdominal tumor or from pregnancy might be cited as possible causes for the development of such lesions. Post-operative thrombosis, especially following operations in the pelvis and around the gall-bladder area, is one of the complications which always makes intra-abdominal surgery a major risk even in the most skilled hands. Such thrombophlebitis is the chief source of that post-operative tragedy, pulmonary embolism. Certain of these lesions are accompanied by low grade, nonspecific bacterial infection as shown by post-mortem cultures, but bacteriologic investigation in the majority of such cases yields completely negative results.

In some of the pathologic processes which affect primarily the arterial side of the circulation it is by no means rare to encounter venous involvement as well. This is particularly true of that poorly understood disease, thrombo-angiitis obliterans. Indeed, when the pathologist has the opportunity to examine the vessels in these cases, i. e., at the time of amputation, the process is in a relatively quiescent, healed stage. One of the principal diagnostic points histologically is the regular involvement of the venous channels in an organized or organizing thrombophlebitis. We have likewise seen in various conditions, notably in hemolytic streptococcic infections of the body, that there not infrequently occurred an acute or subacute proliferative process involving the intimal endothelium of not only arterioles, but capillaries and venules as well, which seems to be wholly toxic in nature. In typhus, Rocky mountain spotted fever, meningococcemia and a host of other infections, minute bacterial emboli involving capillaries and tiny venules are seen, associated with petechial hemorrhage and a variable amount of inflammatory reaction of the vessel wall and surrounding tissues. No particular purpose seems to be gained by detailing the thousand and one diverse clinicopathological pictures which follow the involvement of the various veins individually.

ILLUSTRATIVE CASE

CASE 170. (Ref. #S-357)

Diagnosis.—Jugular vein—infected thrombophlebitis.

Patient was an eleven year old white male child admitted to the hospital because of pain over the right mastoid area following a measles infection complicated by otitis media.

Present Illness.—Twelve days before admission the patient came down with a typical measles having the characteristic rash and the prodromal upper respiratory aura. The rash began to subside the end of the fifth day and two days later the patient complained of a diffuse headache accompanied by pain in his right ear. The drum ruptured spontaneously with great relief to the patient. This was followed by involvement of the other ear and his physician opened the drum on this side, again with relief of the pain. Since that time, both ears had drained freely, but the patient had complained of intermittent intense pains all over the entire head. With the development of mastoid tenderness it was felt that he should be hospitalized with the thought of operation.

Past History.—The patient was a full-term, normally delivered infant who was breast fed for two months before being weaned. He had a normal nutritional history. He had had whooping cough at four years of age, tonsillitis at six years of age, following which the tonsils were removed. He had chickenpox at ten years of age. He had always been subject to frequent colds and had had frequent mild earaches previously, but never with abscess formation or rupture. His parents dated this tendency toward respiratory infection to a varioloid reaction following vaccination some four years earlier, which was accompanied by an attack of tonsillitis and earache. In all other respects the child had had an entirely normal history.

Physical Examination.—The patient was a well-developed, well-nourished, in fact somewhat overweight, male child who appeared almost to suggest the Frölich's syndrome. Skin was of fine texture and normal color. Head was somewhat larger than average measuring 53 cm., but there was no asymmetry. Hair was of unusually fine texture. Eyes were negative. Pupils reacted normally. Nose showed a mucopurulent discharge. There was a purulent discharge from both ears with considerable excoriation of the auricles. There was definite tenderness over the right mastoid process. Throat was negative. Chest was symmetrical. Lungs were clear. Heart was not enlarged and there were no murmurs. Abdomen was very obese but otherwise negative. Genitalia were poorly developed but both testes were descended. Extremities were negative. Neurologic examination was negative.

Laboratory Findings.—The blood picture on admission showed 3,280,000 red cells with 60% hemoglobin, and 16,560 white blood cells with 74% polynuclears. Urinalysis was negative.

X-ray examination of both mastoid areas showed an exudative mastoiditis, but without evidence of bone destruction at the time of admission.

Subsequent Course.—On the basis of the history, physical findings and x-ray report, bilateral simple mastoidectomy was done. The patient ran a prolonged course complicated by the development of a thrombosis of his lateral sinus on the right, which extended to involve the right internal jugular. This was removed surgically and for some time it was thought that the child was going to recover. He received eight transfusions during his stay in the hospital, but ultimately developed terminal meningitis from which he died.

Pathological Report.—*Gross Description.*—Specimen consisted of a portion of the lateral internal jugular vein, which showed complete thrombosis grossly.

Microscopic Description of a Section Through the Vein.—Histologic examination of the specimen shows an acute phlebitis. The wall of the vessel is diffusely infiltrated by inflammatory cells with polynuclear leukocytes predominating. Around the vessel, in the adventitial area, are likewise seen many inflammatory cells including plasma cells and lymphocytes as well as leukocytes. Hemorrhage has occurred to some extent into the perivascular interstitial tissue. There is likewise considerable edema and some fibrosis. The lumen of the vessel is completely filled with a laminated fibrinous thrombus in which leukocytes are seen in large numbers. Considerable hemolysis has occurred and some large mononuclear phagocytes containing hemosiderin pigment can be identified. Some of the fibrin of the thrombus appears to be undergoing proteolytic digestion and stains poorly. The lining endothelium has disappeared.

PHLEBOSCLEROSIS

A sclerotic thickening of the walls of the veins somewhat comparable to the sclerotic process as seen in the arteries may take place. It does not parallel the arterial process in any way, either in regard to age, incidence or extent. In fact it is seen almost invariably in young adults. It involves both the superficial and deep veins, especially of the lower extremities, but at times, of the upper extremities as well. Grossly the vessels appear thickened and cord-like. Microscopically the changes are similar to those seen in hyperplastic sclerosis of the smaller arteries and arterioles. Degenerative changes are ordinarily not found. The etiology is entirely obscure, but is believed to be toxic in nature.

Varicose Veins (Varices, Varicosities, Etc.)

By the term varix is meant a somewhat irregular, more or less tortuous dilatation of a vein, usually associated with some defect in the wall of the vessel or its valves, and brought about by some interference with venous return circulation. It is likely to result in impaired nutrition of the part with various secondary complications.

The three most common sites for the development of varices are seen (1) in the lower extremities and (2) as the result of chronic congestion, as internal or external hemorrhoids and (3) as the variocele of young adult males. Less frequently, especially in marked portal obstruction in relation to cirrhosis of the liver, the development of varicosities of the gastric and esophageal veins, and of the "caput medusae" around the umbilicus may be encountered, the esophageal type at times rupturing and causing fatal hemorrhage.

When the term *varicose veins* is used, it is ordinarily applied to the elongated, dilated, tortuous vessels of the lower extremity, seen in middle-aged or elderly individuals as a rule, and particularly in people whose occupation keeps them standing a great deal, such as motormen, and many factory workers. It rarely occurs in people who are active on their feet, maintaining their muscle tone as an aid to venous circulation.

It is generally held that some congenital factor exists in the form of some weakness of the muscular wall, or some defect in the development of the valves of the veins. In many instances, there likewise seems to be some deficiency in the support of the vessels by the surrounding adventitial structures. The obstructive phenomena which frequently initiate the process vary greatly, dependent upon the site involved. Pregnancy or tumors of the pelvis often precede the lesion in the leg, the scrotum and the vulva. Emphysema, fibroid lesions of the lung, and mitral stenosis may play a part in the development of varicosities of the systemic venous circulation, while cirrhosis of the liver correspondingly starts off the types associated with portal obstruction.

The *effect* of such varicosities varies again dependent upon location. In the lower extremities the circulation becomes sluggish, the tissues chronically congested, edematous and cyanotic in appearance. The nutrition of the tissues is impaired. Injuries to the overlying epithelium, ordinarily trivial in character, result in chronic, indolent, slow healing ulcers, on a brawny, indurated, chronic granulomatous appearing base. The reëstablishment of an adequate circulation to such an area is one of the most discouraging problems in therapy. Many schemes have been advanced, ranging from attempts at obliteration of the varicosities by the injection of irritants between two ligatures, to the actual removal of the vessel surgically. Considerable success appears to be attending the more recent obliterative thrombotic measures, not only in the extremities, but also in respect to hemorrhoidal varices.

This latter group, occurring both as internal and external lesions, is frequently accompanied by a very marked pruritis due to the inflammatory and congestive features. It likewise results in spontaneous thrombosis, usually the result of low grade infection, and is followed by subsequent fibrous scarring in a considerable proportion of the cases. Externally this appears as a series of ragged fibrous tabs around the anal orifice. It is found very commonly in association with chronic constipation.

Illustrative Case

Case 171. (Ref. #S-356)

Diagnosis.—Varicose veins—healed thrombophlebitis.
Patient was a white female of 42 years, admitted to the hospital with the chief complaint of varicose veins of the right lower leg with ulceration of the skin.

Present Illness.—The patient had had varicose veins for about twelve years following the delivery of a child, but these had never given her any trouble until comparatively recently. She dated the onset of her present illness to a period about six months previously when she noticed an abrasion of the skin on the medial aspect of her right lower leg. This was accompanied by a burning sensation. This rather painful burning sensation had become more severe and was practically constant. It kept her awake at night and had begun to affect her disposition. Recently, a second similar ulcerated area had begun to appear a little lower down on the same side of the leg.

Past History.—She had had the usual childhood diseases. A review of her systems was, generally speaking, of little significance except in respect to her last pregnancy. Her digestive system was negative. Urinary system was normal except for occasional nocturia. Menses began at fifteen and had always been regular. She had had two normal pregnancies. For the past several months she had had some irregularity of her periods and had noted hot flashes so that she believed she was approaching her menopause.

Physical Examination.—The patient was an obese, adult, middle-aged woman. Head was negative. Eyes, ears, nose and throat were negative. Chest was symmetrical. Heart and lungs were negative; but she showed a moderate hypertension with a blood pressure of 190/100. Abdomen was essentially negative. Examination of her right leg showed a typical varicose ulcer about 3 cm. in diameter on the mid-tibial medial aspect of the right leg. A similar scarred area was seen just above this present ulcer. Around these areas was marked discoloration of the skin with a few superficial, dilated, tortuous veins running laterally and cephalad. Due to the marked obesity, the underlying varicosities were barely visible.

Laboratory Findings.—Urinalysis was essentially negative. Red blood cells, 4,610,000 with 13 gm. (76.7%) hemoglobin. White blood cells, 11,500 with 64% polynuclears. Blood chemistry: Sugar 95 mgm. per 100 c.c.; urea nitrogen 14 mgm. per 100 c.c. Wassermann was negative.

Subsequent Course.—The patient was treated expectantly at first with rest in bed and local applications to the ulcerated area. The ulceration healed slowly but showed a marked tendency to break down as soon as the patient would be allowed on her feet for any length of time. As a result, it was felt advisable to excise the vessels showing the major amount of involvement. A phlebectomy was accordingly done and the patient showed marked improvement, being discharged two weeks later relieved of her symptoms.

Pathological Specimen.—*Gross Description.*—Specimen consisted of three sections of moderately thin-walled blood vessels. Two of them measured 10 cm. in length and the other measured 31 cm. in length. They averaged four to five millimeters in diameter. In one area there was a large aneurysmal dilatation which measured 1 cm. in diameter. The intimal surface of the vessels was somewhat irregular. The walls varied considerably in thickness.

Microscopic Description of Several of the Veins in Cross Section.—Histologic examination of the veins shows a marked dilatation of the vessels as a whole. The wall shows some hypertrophy of the musculature, but such thickening as is present is largely the result of increased fibrous tissue content. This is accompanied by a considerable intimal hyperplasia. There has evidently been thrombosis at some previous time in some areas with organization and subsequent hyaline degeneration, as the subintimal picture is asymmetrical in different areas. The picture might best be considered as a form of thrombophlebitis complicating the simple mechanical development of varicose veins.

PART III

THE LYMPHATICS

The lymphatics even less often than the veins are the site of any primary pathology. Inflammation in the form of *acute lymphangitis* is of significance in indicating the spread of an infection from a local area. This is seen most strikingly in streptococcic infections of the extremities as red painful streaks extending up the arm or leg to the axillary or inguinal lymph-nodes. It is usually accompanied by secondary acute lymphadenitis. The lesion itself, viewed under the microscope, is more accurately described as a peri-lymphangitis. The single-layered endothelial walled vessel shows dilatation—its lumen is distended with serum containing some leukocytes, but there are many more inflammatory cells found in the surrounding loose areolar structures as they have migrated through the wall.

Obstructive lesions to lymphatic circulation may result in lymphangiectasis, corresponding roughly to the varices of the venous circulation. More often the picture, however, is simply one of lymphedema with the accumulation of fluid in the tissues ordinarily drained by vessels or lymph nodes involved. Thus, the elephantiasis of the scrotum as seen in filariasis (Fig. 203) has already been mentioned in the chapter on parasitic diseases, which is the result of inguinal lymph node obstruction. The unilateral edema of an arm following a radical breast amputation with a complete lymphatic and lymph node dissection of the axilla for carcinoma again serves to emphasize the degree of pathologic change to which such obstructive or destructive lesions of lymphatic circulation may reach (Fig. 202).

CHAPTER XLI

DISEASES OF THE RESPIRATORY SYSTEM

UPPER RESPIRATORY TRACT

The pathological processes which affect the upper respiratory tract are among the most numerous in the entire field of medicine. They probably make up nearly half the cases seen by the average doctor in general practice. For this reason, it seems warranted to devote some time to a consideration of those conditions which are commonly encountered and which are rather lightly treated generally. From the practical standpoint, the diseases of the upper respiratory tract are relatively simple in respect to the pathology, the great majority of the cases falling under the heading of the more familiar infections. In addition, however, it must be remembered that there are a considerable number of neoplasms which give rise to very characteristic symptomatology and form the other major group of lesions affecting this part of the respiratory system.

To be entirely logical, any discussion of the various diseases of the upper respiratory tract should include those conditions which affect the bronchi as well as the nose, throat, larynx and trachea. However, it seems advisable to include certain of the diseases of the bronchi in conjunction with the diseases of the lung, inasmuch as they are so regularly associated with pulmonary pathological changes. Accordingly, the problems of bronchiectasis and bronchogenic tumors will be taken up later, in the discussion devoted to lung pathology.

PART I

NOSE

CONGENITAL ANOMALIES

The congenital anomalies of the nose belong perhaps more accurately in the discussion of developmental defects in the chapter on teratology. They result usually from defects in the development of the anterior maxillary process in relation to the two lateral bodies. Thus, such defects are commonly seen accompanying hare lip, particularly of the bilateral type. In this variety there is very commonly a defect in the development of the hard palate resulting in the so-called *"cleft palate,"* which communicates freely with the floor of the nares. From the standpoint of the rhinolaryngologist, deviation of the septum with various defects in the development of the turbinate bones are the most common anomalies encountered. Indeed, it is probably safe to say that better than ninety per cent of individuals show some degree of asymmetry in respect to the development of the septum. At times, this may result in actual deformity of the nose or may seriously interfere with the drainage of the accessory sinuses and require operative correction. More striking defects are occasionally seen as the result of absence of development of the nasal septum. Such lesions all are of comparatively little physiological significance but are particularly problems for the corrective efforts of the plastic surgeon.

CIRCULATORY DISTURBANCES

The most significant circulatory change which involves the mucosa of the nose is seen in relation to the various infectious diseases of the nasopharynx and will be considered in relation to them. However, there are many other etiologic factors, which may result in alterations in the circulatory mechanism. Irritations following the inhalation of irritating gaseous substances such as ammonia, formalin, chlorine and the like, result in a marked active hyperemia with a stimulation of the secretion of the mucous epithelial cells. Chronic passive congestion may occur as part of the generalized picture of circulatory changes associated with cardiac pathology or as the result of local lesions which interfere with the venous and lymphatic drainage. *Epistaxis* is a familiar condition which may be seen in association with many conditions. It may be the result of traumatic rupture of a vessel in association with a fracture of the nasal bone or from the rupture of a tortuous varicose vessel in association with acute, or chronic passive hyperemia. As a manifestation of Vitamin C deficiency or in association with various forms of purpura and particularly with leukemia of the myeloid type or as part of the picture of hemophilia, such epistaxis may assume significant proportions. Ulcerative lesions, particularly in association with some of the chronic granulomata, particularly syphilis and tuberculosis or rhinoscleroma may even result in fatal hemorrhage. Epistaxis is also an important diagnostic feature of so-called "vicarious menstruation."

Inflammatory Conditions of the Nose

Acute Inflammations.—Coryza (The Common Cold).—The acute inflammatory diseases of the nose may be fairly well summed up in a discussion of the common cold. In coryza, we are confronted with one of the major problems of medicine. Enormous advances have been made as a result of experimental work in many conditions, but up to the present time, very little has been accomplished in the control of this extremely important and common condition. It has been conclusively shown by Dochez and others during the past few years that the immediate causal agent in the development of acute coryza belongs in the group of filtrable viruses. Like all such substances, however, thus far it has been impossible to isolate it to identify its inherent nature. Whether the virus alone could be responsible for the production of the typical clinical picture or whether it requires the presence of other bacteria to initiate its attack is still somewhat problematical for the simple reason that it is impossible to completely sterilize the mucous membrane of the nasopharynx in respect to the normal bacterial flora. That the virus, however, is primarily at fault has been shown repeatedly by the development of an acute coryza both in experimental animals and in human volunteers by the instillation of filtrates from the nasal secretion of individuals in the acute stage of a coryza. The current view to-day which seems most satisfactory to explain the subsequent picture, both clinically and pathologically, implies that as a result of diminished resistance such as may be brought about, as Mudd has shown, by exposure to cold, with vasoconstriction of the vessels of the nasopharyngeal mucosa and resultant ischemia, this invasion of the tissues by the virus is followed by acute hyperemia and edema of the mucous membrane. This is seen clinically in the serous discharge which almost regularly initiates the typical cold. It is followed shortly after by the more characteristic thick, tenacious, glairy mucopurulent secretion which it is believed results from secondary bacterial invasion of the mucous membranes. The nature and course of the cold from that point on depends largely upon the nature of these secondary invaders. There is usually a mixed flora in which *Staphylococci, Streptococci* and *Micrococcus catarrhalis* predominate. Less frequently, the *Pneumococcus* and *Haemophilus influenzae* are recovered.

From the microscopic standpoint, the picture is one of acute inflammation. There is diffuse infiltration of the mucosa itself by leukocytes, which at times are seen actually invading the epithelium, but which are seen for the most part between the cells of the mucosa and deeper in the submucosa. Depending upon the severity of the process either degenerative changes of the mucous epithelial cells or actual necrosis occurs. This is accompanied by a considerable mononuclear cellular infiltration as well. The inflammatory process can be classified as all other acute inflammatory lesions, either as a simple catarrhal process or if the severity of the inflammation is sufficiently marked to produce an ulcerative and membranous type of inflammation, such a designation may be indicated. In diphtheria, for example, one may find a simple fibrinous type of exudate with the infection limited to the nares. This, of course, bears no relationship necessarily to an antecedent acute coryza, but occurring as it not infrequently does in extremely young infants, a similar mechanism as in other forms of acute coryza may be presumed. Similar acute inflammatory changes may be found at times in association with various allergic phenomena. Thus, the patient who is susceptible to the various manifestations of allergy, such as asthma, hay fever or certain types of rhinitis is likely to be particularly susceptible to such infection. A feature of particular interest in this respect is the extraordinary number of eosinophiles in the inflammatory exudate. These may even be identified in the nasal secretions.

Chronic Inflammations.—Both hypertrophic and atrophic forms of inflammation of a chronic nature may be encountered in the nasal mucosa. Not uncommonly, the chronic atrophic form of rhinitis may follow the hypertrophic picture, or it may occur independently from the outset. The character of the inflammatory reaction depends largely upon the activating agent. A number of the more important and common forms of such rhinitis will be discussed briefly.

Ozena (Chronic Fetid Atrophic Rhinitis). —This condition is one of the most difficult problems imaginable to handle from the clinical side. The picture, both from the clinical and pathological standpoints, is one of a chronic atrophic rhinitis associated with crusted, scab-like lesions on the mucosa and accompanied by a particularly fetid odor from which the disease derives its name. There is some suggestion that there may be a constitutional or mechanical explanation in part for this condition as it occurs almost entirely in the broad, flat-faced type of individual with rather prominent and somewhat vertically placed nares. The organism, which apparently belongs to the Proteus group, but which is believed by many to be a specific bacterium, the so-called Bacillus ozenae, can usually be recovered from the crusted lesions. At all events, the bacterium is of the putrefactive group and is responsible for the changes which take place in the tissues. Owing to the fact that the condition is not infrequently seen in congenital syphilis, it has been suggested that the basic underlying cause of the disease might well be of a luetic nature. This, however, has never been definitely established.

Syphilis.—Probably syphilis represents the most common of the chronic granulomatous lesions of the nose. It is seen both in congenital syphilis and as a later manifestation in the acquired form of the disease. As has already been emphasized, in the congenital syphilitic, there is a very frequent accompaniment of the process by secondary putrefactive bacterial invasion resulting in a similar ozena-like atrophic form of rhinitis. The process not infrequently extends to involve the septum in what might be considered as a gummatous type of lesion. This frequently breaks down with perforation and is followed by the picture of the so-called saddle-nose. In the acquired form of the disease, the lesions may be of two types. There may be involvement of the mucous membrane with the development of typical mucous patches. More commonly, however, the picture is one of gumma formation which involves the septum. This likewise, as in the congenital form, tends to break down and perforate, and gives rise to the typical depressed bridge of the nose, which is seen as one of the stigmata of syphilis.

Tuberculosis.—Tuberculosis of the nose is only found as a complication of tuberculosis elsewhere. It may be seen either as a tuberculide affecting the skin and subcutaneous tissues, or as a lesion of the mucous membrane resulting from extension of a tuberculosis of the larynx, pharynx, tongue, tonsil, or even of the lung. Clinically, it is rarely of any great significance. It is very likely to be unilateral and to appear upon the mucous membranes of one or more of the turbinates. As it develops, it tends to invade the cartilage of the septum and even the nasal bones. The diagnosis is established microscopically by the finding of the organism in scrapings from the local lesion or in actual histologic examination of biopsy material removed surgically.

Leprosy.—As has already been taken up in our consideration of leprosy as a disease entity, the early involvement of the nasal mucosa has been emphasized. Typically, this lesion appears as a small, tubercular nodule in the mucosa, especially on the septal side of the mucosa. Not infrequently, this may go on to ulceration with secondary infection, and as in the case of syphilis and tuberculosis, perforation of the septum may occur. From the diagnostic standpoint, the nasal mucosa is likely to be the first tissue infected and the last from which the infection disappears under treatment. Accordingly, diagnosis is usually made by examination of scrapings from the nasal mucosa and the progress of the therapeutic course of the disease may be roughly followed by such repeated examinations at intervals. Biopsy or autopsy material from such cases reveals the typical diffuse chronic granulomatous picture of leprosy. This is characterized by unusual vascularity and the presence of the typical lepra cells with the organisms within their cytoplasm.

RHINOSCLEROMA.—A disease which is rarely seen in this country and which appears to be found almost exclusively in individuals coming from central and eastern Europe is known as "rhinoscleroma." This is an extremely chronic granulomatous type of lesion which apparently starts ordinarily in the posterior part of the nose and extends both into the nose and into the pharyngeal tissues. It is characterized by an almost cartilaginous density of the submucous tissues. A small gram-negative bacillus, difficult morphologically to differentiate from *Bacillus pertussis* or *Hemophilis influenzae* may be recovered from scrapings or biopsy material from such cases.

Histologic examination of the tissues presents fairly characteristic features with the presence of large numbers of so-called Mikulicz cells. These are large cells several times the size of the other lymphoid and plasma cells seen in the tissues. They appear vacuolated and not infrequently are seen to contain small, fine, rod-like structures. Characteristically, so-called Russell hyaline eosin-staining bodies likewise have been described as occurring commonly in these cells in this condition.

GLANDERS.—Glanders is a disease which is most commonly seen involving the nasal mucosa and septum of horses, but may be transmitted to man and produce similar lesions. The process is again of the chronic granulomatous type with the development of nodular lesions, which tend to ulcerate and give rise to a profuse purulent secretion. The glanders bacillus may easily be recovered from the exudate. The diagnosis is largely established by such bacteriologic studies as the histologic features are not entirely specific.

TUMORS OF THE NOSE

Almost every variety of tumor has been described at one time or another as being found arising within the nose. However, they are usually relatively uncommon for some unexplained reason, as it is difficult to imagine any tissue more subjected to chronic inflammatory irritation than is the nasal mucosa. The most common neoplastic-like lesion which is found in the nose is the ordinary polyp. As has already been stated, this is not a true tumor but represents a curious mechanical process, the result of the accumulation of fluid in the submucosa, particularly in relation to some allergic inflammatory reaction. These polypi are most frequently seen arising from the lateral wall of the nose near the drainage canal of the antrum of Highmore. They soon become pedunculated with a narrow base and a pear-shaped, dependent mass, which may completely occlude the air spaces. Removal of these lesions by simple excision is frequently followed by their recurrence. So far as is known, they never undergo malignant metaplasia and should be considered in the nature of an inflammatory process rather than as a neoplasm.

The only tumor of any great importance in relation to the nose is probably that curious type of tumor variously called lympho-epithelioma, transitional cell carcinoma, or if located appropriately, the Schneiderian carcinoma. The local lesion may remain relatively small and apparently inoffensive, but may be manifested first clinically by metastatic involvement of the regional lymphoid structures. Occasional instances of squamous cell or adenocarcinoma are encountered, as are the even more rare instances of sarcomata.

PART II

PHARYNX, INCLUDING THE TONSILS

CONGENITAL DEFECTS

The congenital defects of the pharynx are comparatively uncommon. When they do occur, they are seen as the result of maldevelopment of the branchial clefts. The major lesions of the pharynx can best be considered under the general heading of inflammations.

INFLAMMATORY LESIONS

The great majority of the inflammatory processes of the pharynx are infectious in nature. In the preceding section, we have already described the changes which are seen in the nasopharyngeal mucosa in relation to the common cold of acute coryza. In addition to this rather widespread type of inflammation, we not infrequently encounter lesions which are primarily localized to the fauces and pharynx, itself, usually in relation to a primary infection of the tonsils. In considering the infectious diseases of the upper respiratory tract, it seems logical to utilize the tonsil as the major structure involved and recognize that many of these infections spread from the tonsils to the deeper structures of the neck giving rise to such conditions as retropharyngeal abscess, *Ludvig's angina* and a host of other similar severe lesions.

Acute Inflammations.—TONSILLITIS.—The tonsils must be thought of as part of the reticulo-endothelial system of the body. As such, they are generally believed to play a part in the development of immunity as well as to act in a somewhat comparable fashion to the lymph nodes and spleen in serving as an effective barrier against the extension of bacteria. The question as to the value of the tonsils is one about which there is no agreement among the rhinolaryngologists. In recent years, there seems to have been a definite tendency toward conservatism in respect to tonsillectomy, as the functions of the reticulo-endothelial and lymphoid tissues of the body have become more definitely established. Nevertheless, there are still many definite indications for the removal of the tonsils in the presence of definite pathology. Such indications may include a simple hypertrophy and hyperplasia of the organs if this increase in size reaches such proportions that it actually interferes with breathing or swallowing.

It is extremely difficult to evaluate the relative value of the tonsil in respect to infection. It has been shown very clearly that there is a definitely reduced incidence of many of the diseases of childhood in that group of children in whom the tonsils have been removed. Among these conditions should be cited particularly scarlet fever, diphtheria and rheumatic fever. Less definitely, poliomyelitis should be considered in this group. On this side of the argument of prophylaxis against infection many able clinicians have taken a definite position. It is our belief that it is not so much the presence or the absence of the tonsils which is the determining factor in these cases necessarily, as it is a more fundamental constitutional diathesis in which lymphoid hyperplasia generally as seen in the so-called lymphatic constitution is of apparent significance in respect to the relative frequency of infection. It is in this group of individuals that we find the great majority of acute bacterial infections occurring, in contradistinction to other constitutional types in whom metabolic disturbances, such as diabetes, are more likely to be seen.

Tonsillitis, or inflammation of the tonsil, may occur in a wide variety of forms. The most familiar is the typical so-called *"acute follicular tonsillitis."* In this condition there is an acute inflammatory reaction associated with superficial invasion of the tonsillar mucosa, including particularly that of the crypts, by leukocytes. There is an accompanying hyperplasia of the lymphoid elements and marked inflammatory changes affecting the germinal centers of the lymphoid follicles. The tonsils grossly are swollen and hyperemic. The exudate may be seen as pin-point, whitish spots protruding from the crypts. Often, this extends as a thin, membranous-like process over the surface of the tonsil itself. The usual etiologic agent in the production of this picture is a hemolytic Streptococcus. Similar acute inflammatory changes may be seen in the so-called epidemic sore throat, which is probably caused by a hemolytic Streptococcus, which some investigators believe to be specific.

SCARLET FEVER.—In scarlet fever, likewise, another disease of hemolytic streptococcic origin, a similar acute diffuse inflammation of the tonsil may be seen. In these two latter conditions, the characteristic follicular picture is often lacking and, indeed, the follicular type of infection is very apt to be associated with a mixed bacterial flora including the presence of a considerable number of staphylococci.

DIPHTHERIA.—The diphtheria bacillus has already been mentioned as another organism which most frequently initiates its infection in the tonsillar lesion, spreading from there to the naso-pharynx and down the respiratory tract. This is recognized by its characteristic dirty yellowish-gray pseudomembrane with its almost diagnostic odor. In diphtheria, the inflammatory appearance of the tonsils and pharynx is of a rather deep cyanotic red in contradistinction to the flaming redness of the streptococcic infections.

MEASLES.—In measles, again, the onset of the disease is usually characterized, as has been already mentioned, by an upper respiratory infection with a marked purplish congestion of the tonsils and pharynx and the development of a definite tracheitis with a mildly productive cough.

VINCENT'S ANGINA.—In Vincent's angina, the lesion is more necrotic and ulcerative in character and appearance. This is caused specifically by the combined spirochaete and fusiform bacillus of Vincent. It is less regularly found primarily involving the tonsil than any of the previously mentioned infections, but the tonsil usually becomes involved by extension even when the lesion starts elsewhere in the buccal mucosa.

AGRANULOCYTIC ANGINA (*Agranulocytosis; Malignant Neutropenia, Etc.*).—Agranulocytic angina is a clinical syndrome which has occasioned a great deal of investigation in respect to its etiology. It is a condition which is seen most frequently in middle-aged women and runs a rapidly fatal course in the severe cases, the patient seldom surviving a period of more than a week to ten days. It is characterized in the typical case by extensive superficial ulceration of the tonsils and surrounding tissues. The ulceration is only in the nature of an erosion at times, but there is apt to be a very extensive invasion of the deep tissue by the inflammatory process. This is characterized by marked edema as a result of serous outpouring into the interstitial tissue. From this serum precipitates out a network of fibrin. A few mononuclear inflammatory cells will be seen in the exudate. The outstanding feature of the pathology is the absence of leukocytes. On the ulcerated surface, a thin, membranous layer of fibrin may be deposited in which, again, only red cells and occasional mononuclears will be seen. As a result of injury to the vascular endothelium, hemorrhage is not infrequent in the exudate. Clinically, the patients show extreme prostration, usually having a high fever, and succumb rapidly to a profound toxemia.

Examination of their peripheral blood shows a complete repression of myeloid activity with the total white blood count dropping rapidly to less than a thousand. Indeed, in at least three instances which we have seen the count has fallen below four hundred white cells, all of which were lymphoid in character. The red cells are not appreciably affected and the picture appears to be one of some severe toxic depression of myeloid activity. Various bacteria have been incriminated, but no experimental work with which we are familiar has been presented in which the specificity of the infection has been demonstrated. Most frequently, a member of the hemolytic streptococci group of bacteria is found. Accompanying the streptococcic element, *Bacillus pyocyaneus* is also found in over half of the cases. It is our belief that the condition represents a curious individual constitutional reaction to infection rather than that it is a specific infectious disease.

Certain cases of agranulocytosis may be seen without any evidence of the associated mucosal pathology and a few instances of identical clinical pictures have been reported in which the ulcerative lesion was found in the vagina, rectum and even in the bladder. This further supports the hypothesis that the condition is not a specific infection, but a response on the part of the individual to overwhelming infection of any sort.

QUINSY SORE THROAT (PERITONSILLAR OR RETROTONSILLAR ABSCESS).—If the infection extends through the tonsillar tissue into the retrotonsillar or peritonsillar structures, and particularly if the infection is complicated by the presence of *Staphylococcus* with its tendency to produce localized abscess formation, not infrequently the patient will develop an acute suppurative process which, strictly speaking, is extratonsillar. This is characterized by enormous unilateral swelling of the throat with the tonsil protruding to a degree that interferes seriously with deglutition. Many such cases rupture spontaneously either laterally to the tonsil itself, or through one or more of the deep crypts. As long as the lesion remains localized, it is a matter more of discomfort than of danger, but at times such infection may spread through the tissues of the neck or invade the retropharyngeal tissues and form mechanical obstruction to breathing as well as give rise to toxic absorption from the infected area. Such abscesses may likewise be a source of blood stream infection with the familiar serious complications. Thus, retrotonsillar and retropharyngeal abscesses represent complications of the more superficial type of infections of the tonsil and pharyngeal mucosa, which do at times give rise to some of these more serious conditions.

Chronic Inflammations.—CHRONIC TONSILLITIS. —Chronic tonsillitis is again one of those conditions about which there is very little agreement among clinicians and pathologists. Almost any tonsil which shows enlargement is felt by the clinician to represent a chronic inflammatory hyperplasia or hypertrophy. Actually, as we have seen, many such cases are constitutional in origin. Like the appendix, however, the tonsil may be the seat of repeated acute infectious processes. Some of these may completely subside; others may linger on in a subacute or even chronic form. The crypts may become occluded by inspissated exudate and continue to fill up with additional cellular detritus until small cyst-like structures may be found, which can at times be evacuated by pressure. Such lesions may probably properly be considered as true chronic inflammatory processes. From the bacteriologic standpoint, there is usually a mixed flora, with, as a rule, saprophytic varieties of staphylococci, streptococci and the like being recovered. Such chronic inflammation may be manifested microscopically by marked enlargement of the lymph follicles, particularly of the germinal centers. Not infrequently the picture is accompanied by extensive fibrosis representing the healed scars of previous acute infections.

CHRONIC INFLAMMATION OF PHARYNX.—In the pharynx a chronic irritation of the throat is seen very commonly in people who smoke too much, and particularly in singers and public speakers, who use their voices extensively. This is accompanied very often by a thickening of the mucosa with the formation of small, granulation-like beads.

Microscopically, this usually is found to consist of a slight epithelial hyperplasia and accumulation of foci of lymphoid cells in the submucosa.

TUBERCULOSIS OF THE TONSIL.—Tuberculosis of the tonsil is a lesion which is seen not infrequently in childhood. In the routine examination of tonsils removed surgically, it is not uncommon to find as high as three to five per cent of such tonsils infected by the tubercle bacillus. Opinions vary greatly as to its significance in respect to being the portal of entry of the tubercle bacillus either in the usual picture of childhood tuberculosis or in the adult type of pulmonary infection. It seems fairly definite that a relatively high proportion of cases of cervical adenitis of a tuberculous nature occur in conjunction with tuberculosis of the tonsil. The infection is seen in several forms. Not infrequently in the child particularly, it may be recognized as an ulcerative lesion of the mucosa of the crypts. At other times, the lesions may appear as miliary tubercles within the tonsillar tissue itself. Depending upon the nature of the organism and the resistance of the individual, the lesion may progress either to caseation or more often to productive fibrosis. It is probable that the great majority of cases of tonsillar tuberculosis heal spontaneously.

SYPHILIS OF THE TONSIL.—Syphilis of the tonsil is seen particularly in the form of mucous patches. More rarely a primary infection of the tonsil may occur, and in conjunction with tertiary syphilis, occasionally actual gumma formation may be found.

TUMORS OF THE TONSIL AND PHARYNX

As has already been emphasized, the most important tumor of the tonsil is seen in the form of the so-called *"transitional cell carcinoma or lympho-epithelioma."* This has been discussed in Chapter XXVII relating to tumors of endothelial origin, and illustrated in Case 113 (Ref. #S-314), Fig. 275. Primary lymphosarcoma of the tonsil may also be found occasionally. Squamous cell carcinoma may rarely arise from the tonsillar mucosa, but more often is seen as an extension of such a lesion elsewhere in the mouth, especially arising on the lateral aspect of the tongue.

Benign tumors of mesothelial origin are occasionally seen, including particularly fibromata and chondromata. The comparatively rare tumor, the chordoma, may likewise first appear as a midline tumor of the pharynx arising from the sphenoid region; and rarely, an epignathus may be seen filling the pharyngeal cavity and protruding from the mouth of the monster.

PART III

LARYNX

Anatomically, there are comparatively few congenital lesions which are seen affecting the larynx which are compatible with life. Asymmetry in the development of the cartilages, or actual atresia may be encountered. From the practical viewpoint, the lesions of interest which are found in the larynx are represented particularly by the infections, either acute or chronic, and by certain tumors of the larynx which are almost specific in this region. The student is referred to the recent monograph of the Jacksons.

INFLAMMATORY LESIONS

Acute Inflammatory Lesions of the Larynx.— LARYNGITIS.—Laryngitis, or inflammation of the larynx, might be part of the general acute catarrhal inflammatory process seen in the common cold or coryza. It not infrequently may be seen secondary to such an acute infection of the nose and throat. It likewise is seen in a number of associated acute infectious diseases, notably in whooping cough, measles and scarlet fever. In diphtheria it is possible to have a localized infection of the larynx, but more often diphtheritic laryngitis is seen as an extension of the throat infection.

The pathology is similar to that of diphtheria elsewhere. It is characterized by the production of the typical "stag horn," fibrinous, pseudomembrane with little actual destruction of the underlying basement membrane except as such cases are complicated by secondary streptococcic or stapyhlococcic infection. In certain of the acute streptococcic infections, a true membrane in association with ulcerative, destructive lesions of the mucosa may simulate the picture of diphtheria.

Bacteriologic examination can resolve this problem in many instances, and the therapeutic use of diphtheria antitoxin in case of doubt is followed by loosening of the pseudomembrane promptly in diphtheria, whereas if the lesion is truly membranous and streptococcal in origin, such therapy has no effect upon the inflammatory process.

It should also be recalled that various toxic substances, particularly poisonous gases, which are inhaled may produce very severe acute inflammatory changes. In the more marked instances, such as occur in relation to mustard gas, actual ulcerative lesions with true membrane formation may result. This, in turn, may be followed by marked cicatricial stenosis as the process heals.

*Chronic Inflammations of the Larynx.—*The two outstanding chronic inflammatory processes which are seen in the larynx are tuberculosis and syphilis. In addition, however, certain forms of chronic catarrhal laryngitis are seen, again as in the case of chronic pharyngitis, particularly in heavy smokers and in people who use their voices a great deal, such as singers and public speakers. This is usually characterized by a hypertrophic picture in respect to the mucosa. Not infrequently an actual thickening of the mucous membrane is seen with the cells piled up several deep, and also, a chronic inflammatory infiltration of the submucosa by lymphoid cells even to the point of follicle formation accompanies the process.

TUBERCULOSIS.—Tuberculosis of the larynx is almost invariably secondary to pulmonary tuberculosis. The process is usually seen as multiple small serpiginous, superficial ulcers in the region of the arytenoids or vocal cords. This results in typical chronic granulomatous tuberculous tissue being formed in the sub-epithelial layers. It interferes with the mobility of the vocal cords and results in complete aphonia as the process extends, and in hoarseness in the earlier stages. From these areas, the ulcerative process tends to spread throughout the larynx, often in the deeper tissues, apparently by way of the lymphatics. In other instances, it spreads by direct continuity. The organisms may invade the deeper structures and produce an infection of the perichondrium with resultant caseation necrosis of the cartilaginous wall of the larynx. This may go on to a perforation into the esophagus, commonly followed by secondary inhalation pneumonia.

The histologic diagnosis of tuberculosis is readily established by biopsy, if it cannot be previously established by scrapings from the lesion with the demonstration of the bacteria. Like tuberculosis elsewhere, at times the lesions may simulate syphilis or neoplasm, and a diagnosis of any ulcerative lesion of the larynx should be established by definite biopsy procedure. In this way, many early cases of carcinoma may be picked up and many cases of chronic infectious granulomatous disease of the larynx may be recognized and differentiated from suspected malignancy. This is of great importance from the standpoint of therapy, as in the early malignancies, simple laryngofissure is an adequate procedure; whereas if the process is allowed to go on, complete laryngectomy becomes necessary.

SYPHILIS.—Syphilis of the larynx is of much less frequent occurrence, but is manifested by the same type of lesions seen elsewhere in mucous membranes, chiefly with the formation of mucous patches. As in the case of the nose, at times the spirochaete may invade the cartilage with the production of gumma and result in ultimate perforation between larynx and esophagus. The lesion is more prone to occur in the upper part of the larynx, in contradistinction to tuberculosis; but like tuberculosis may spread to involve the entire lining mucosa.

Other chronic granulomatous infections of the larynx do occur, but with comparative infrequency. Among these should be mentioned leprosy, glanders, and rhinoscleroma.

TUMORS OF THE LARYNX

Benign Tumors.—PAPILLOMA OF THE LARYNX. —The papilloma of the larynx is without question the commonest variety of neoplasm found in relation to this organ. It usually arises in or near the anterior commissure of the vocal cord. Jackson and Jackson, in their recent monograph on the Larynx and Its Diseases, report over six hundred cases seen in their clinic. They believe that inflammation plays an important part in their development, but recognize that some of them may be congenital. The tumor tends to be more or less pedunculated. It not infrequently occurs in multiple form. It may well be divided, for purposes of convenience, into two types; those seen in children, and those seen in later adult life. In children, there is a striking tendency for the process to be a self-limited one, although the tumors may recur almost as rapidly as they are removed for several years; but with the onset of adolescence, the process apparently stops. On the other hand, in the adult group, there is an even greater tendency for the lesions to recur after their removal, but in our experience, it is only rarely that a papilloma of the larynx ever undergoes malignant transformation, in spite of multiple recurrences. In the adult group, owing to the fact that a very large proportion of them seem to occur in people who use their voices a great deal, it is felt that mechanical strain may play a part in initiating the process, as a manifestation of chronic irritation.

Pathologically the tumors are typical fibro-epitheliomata composed of a dense stalk of connective tissue and covered by a proliferating, thickened, papillary type of epithelium. There is some suggestion of down-growth of the epithelial pegs into the stroma at times, but there is always a well-defined basement membrane and the cells are always well differentiated, tending to show intercellular bridges and to develop pearls at times.

Malignant Tumors of the Larynx.—The outstanding malignant tumors of the larynx are *squamous carcinomata*. These are seen particularly arising from the anterior third of the vocal cords in relation to the anterior commissure, in the same way that the benign papilloma does. Other locations for the primary development of such squamous cell carcinomata are seen as extrinsic lesions arising in the epiglottic, aryepiglottic folds and hypopharynx. These squamous cell tumors of the larynx show all the usual gradations in malignancy as based on histologic criteria, as do those of the cervix uteri or other organs. Many of them are of a relatively low grade malignancy showing striking cell differentiation with pearl formation. The nuclei in these cases show little anaplasia and only occasional mitotic figures. On the other hand, occasional instances of completely undifferentiated squamous cell tumors occur in which mitoses abound and in which extensive invasion of the deeper tissues is seen.

PART IV

TRACHEA AND BRONCHI

Lesions of the trachea and bronchi will be considered very largely in the following chapter relating to the inflammatory diseases of the lungs, as involvement of the respiratory tree under these circumstances is almost impossible to avoid. Like the rest of the upper respiratory tract, the most important lesions are those associated with the various inflammatory processes. In a certain number of such instances, the infection may be restricted to the trachea and bronchi without producing any definite pulmonary symptomatology. This condition is spoken of as *tracheobronchitis*. It may result from irritation by a wide variety of causes. As in the case of acute laryngitis, diphtheria, and streptococcic infections this may be accompanied by diffuse ulcerative lesions with actual membrane or pseudomembrane formation. As a rule, such lesions are followed by actual pulmonary infection as well.

In uncomplicated measles, it is highly probable that a simple acute catarrhal tracheo-bronchitis is the extent of the inflammatory process in the upper respiratory tract; but, as has been shown, very commonly there is an associated interstitial pneumonitis, and a secondary streptococcic pneumonia. In pertussis, the specific pathology of the disease may be said to be found only in the larynx and trachea. In this area, the pertussis bacilli may be found in myriads enmeshed in the cilia of the lining mucosa. This is accompanied by marked mucoid catarrhal inflammation, and one of the outstanding diagnostic features of the disease is seen in these almost gristle-like masses of tenacious, glairy mucus, in which the bacteria can be demonstrated. Moderate hyperemia of the sub-epithelial structures with extensive mononuclear cellular infiltration, almost exclusively lymphocytic in nature, is seen as part of this picture. Chemical irritation, particularly by steam and poisonous gases, result in a similar acute catarrhal or even ulcerative trachea bronchitis. The tracheo-bronchitis which follows ether anesthesia is familiar to all of us as another example of this type of lesion.

Chronic Bronchitis is characterized typically by a rather hyperplastic type of inflammation. The mucosa usually shows definite thickening, often with plication. There is marked hyperemia, but of a passive type, so that the tissues appear somewhat cyanotic. They are usually edematous. Chronic inflammatory cellular infiltration of a mononuclear, round cell type is found. This is often followed by reparative or productive fibrosis with cicatrization.

Etiologically, chronic bronchitis is somewhat difficult to explain in many instances. At times it may be the result of chronic infection as a result of chronic sinusitis. It is a common accompaniment of chronic valvular disease of the heart as part of the picture of chronic passive congestion, which in turn offers a particularly likely soil for recurrent infection.

Bronchial Asthma.—True bronchial asthma is believed to be a definite allergic condition. Anatomically, in true asthma the walls of the smaller bronchi and bronchioles are markedly thickened. This particularly involves the smooth muscle. The mucosa tends to show hypertrophic changes and there is usually a considerable amount of edema and congestion present. The glands are particularly active and show a great increase in their mucous production.

The submucosal tissues, particularly, but the walls of the bronchi as a whole, are diffusely infiltrated by chronic inflammatory cells in which eosinophiles are especially prominent as in many other allergic lesions.

Clinically, the condition is characterized by paroxysmal attacks of dyspnea with particular difficulty in expiration. This is explained on the basis of spasm of the bronchial musculature resulting in inability to empty the pulmonary alveoli. This results in rather marked emphysema of the lungs and is likewise frequently accompanied by areas of atelectasis where spasm or stenosis from secretion has blocked off certain of the smaller bronchi. In the sputum, it is often possible to demonstrate the typical Charcot-Leyden crystals and the Curschmann spirals as well as many eosinophilic cells.

The etiology is obscure, many cases apparently being sensitized in early childhood through food sensitization. In other instances, the sensitizing agent appears to be the result of previous infection. Even plant pollens, dust, and the dander of horses, dogs and other domestic animals may be causal agents in the initial sensitization.

Foreign Bodies.—Foreign bodies in the trachea and bronchi make up a very important part of the practice of the bronchoscopist. Almost every conceivable object small enough to pass through the larynx has been recovered at one time or another from the respiratory tree. The significance of such foreign bodies lies particularly in their location and in their composition. Some inert substance with smooth edges may produce very little in the way of a clinical problem. On the other hand, some substance such as a peanut which is definitely toxic in its local effect, may result in prompt necrotic changes of the tissue and secondary infection. In every case where a foreign body occludes a bronchus, this is followed by atelectasis. The atelectasis, in turn, may result in pneumonia, bronchiectasis, or a wide variety of other pathological conditions. These will be considered from the practical standpoint in the section devoted to suppurative lesions of the lung.

Tumors of the trachea and bronchi are discussed in Chapter XLV, in a consideration of the tumors of the respiratory system as a whole. The increase of cancer of the lung in recent years is noteworthy.

CHAPTER XLII

DISEASES OF THE RESPIRATORY SYSTEM (*Continued*)

THE LUNG

CIRCULATORY DISTURBANCES

Hyperemia (Active Congestion).—Hyperemia may be defined as an increased amount of arterial blood within the vessels of the lung. It occurs in the early stages of many inflammatory processes. In lobar pneumonia the stage of engorgement consists of a marked hyperemia of the affected portion of the lung. Histologically, the arterioles, capillaries and venules are distended with blood. The distention of the arteries, however, is rarely seen at autopsy or in histologic tissues since at death there is a tendency for the arteries to empty and the veins to become distended. Thus, the difficulty of differentiating the condition from passive congestion arises.

Passive Congestion.—Passive congestion of the lung is seen in two forms: (a) brown induration and (b) hypostatic congestion.

BROWN INDURATION.—This results from chronic congestion of the lung over a long period of time. It is usually due to left-sided heart disease, particularly mitral stenosis. The pulmonary blood pressure is raised and the capillaries are under chronic increased tension. The pulmonary artery frequently shows atheromatous plaques. As a result of the chronic congestion and increased pressure, occasionally diapedesis of red cells occurs into the alveolar wall, and at times into the air space itself. The red cells undergo hemolysis and the hemoglobin is converted into hemosiderin by large mononuclear phagocytic cells, the so-called "heart failure" cells, which are found in large numbers within the air spaces and even in the vesicular wall (Fig. 32 and 50). These phagocytic mononuclears are probably derived from the reticulo-endothelial tissues of the lung and are sometimes spoken of as "septile" cells. Previously, they were considered as desquamated lining cells of the lung alveoli. The pigment is likewise deposited within the lymph tissues of the lung, particularly in the peribronchial lymph nodes, to which it is apparently carried in the lymphatics directly by the phagocytic mononuclear cells.

Congestion likewise results in a certain degree of anoxemia with qualitative degenerative changes of the alveolar wall. This is followed by a varying amount of fibrosis. Grossly, the lung is firmer than normal and brownish in color. Hemoptysis is a frequent clinical finding in this condition due to capillary hemorrhage. Pulmonary edema may occur as a terminal condition or as a complication during the course of the disease (see illustrative case 22, Chapter IV, and Fig. 49).

HYPOSTATIC CONGESTION.—This is dependent upon several factors; the weakness of the cardiac action (right heart), deficiency in the respiratory effort, and the effect of gravity. It occurs during the agonal period and is most severe in bedridden, aged and debilitated individuals. The more prolonged the agonal period the more severe the congestion. Postmortem relaxation of the vessels with gravitation of the fluid to the dependent parts also contributes to the autopsy appearance of the picture, and must be evaluated carefully in the diagnosis.

It should be remembered that the pulmonary circulation is dependent primarily upon the action of the right heart but is augmented by the respiratory movements. Pulmonary hypostasis is, therefore, not always terminal but may also be of frequent occurrence in aged, debilitated individuals during the course of disease in which the patient is bedfast. The danger of confining aged individuals to bed in cases of fracture, etc., has long been recognized as predisposing to hypostatic congestion, since the three factors for its production are present. If the patient is allowed to lie in one position, there is a tendency for a slowing of the circulation in the dependent portions of the lungs, leading to relative anoxemia and increased permeability of the capillaries. Edema of this portion of the lung together with diapedesis of red cells into the alveolar walls and air spaces frequently follows. In such congested portions of the lung the vitality is markedly lowered and bacteria

PLATE XCV

DISEASES OF THE LUNG

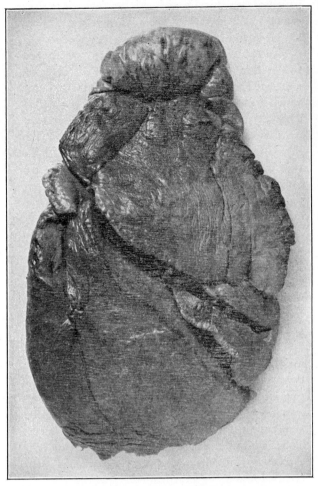

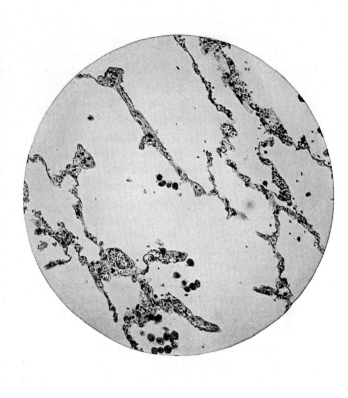

FIG. 403.—LUNG: BULLOUS EMPHYSEMA.—(cf. CASE 173).— Gross photograph of the right lung showing typical emphysematous bullae of considerable size at the apex and along the anterior margin.

FIG. 404.—LUNG: EMPHYSEMA.—CASE 173.—The air spaces are much enlarged, the alveolar walls thin. Terminal congestion has produced irregular bulging of the walls. App. 100 x.

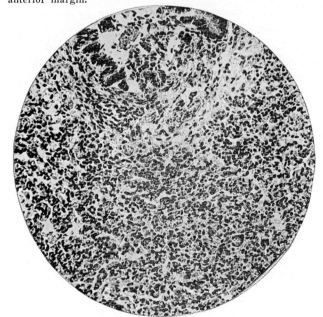

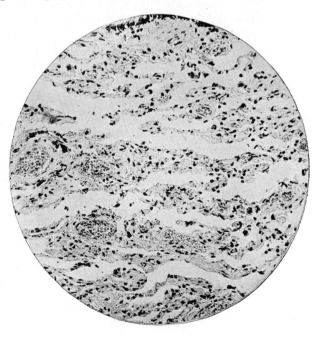

FIG. 405.—LUNG: ATELECTASIS (CONGENITAL).—CASE 174.—Typical fetal lung. A portion of the plicated mucosa of bronchus is seen above. The alveoli are airless and their walls in apposition. App. 100 x.

FIG. 406.—LUNG: ATELECTASIS (ACQUIRED).—CASE 175.—As a result of compression, by pleural effusion, the walls of the alveoli are approximated and the vesicles contain only a small amount of air. App. 100 x.

are readily able to gain a foothold with resultant terminal or hypostatic pneumonia.

Grossly, the condition is confined to the dependent parts of the lung, which are dark reddish or reddish-black in color. Normal crepitation is diminished. Large quantities of venous blood and serum can be expressed from the cut surface. Histologically, the vessels are markedly distended and red cells may be seen within the alveolar walls and within the air vesicles. A certain amount of edema practically always coexists. At times, the lung seems airless and is completely filled with a serous transudate, red cells and patchy areas of exudate made up chiefly of polymorphonuclear leukocytes and phagocytic mononuclear cells, representing the early stage of a hypostatic terminal pneumonia.

Pulmonary Edema.—Pulmonary edema may be local or general. It is a condition in which the serum is found within the vesicles of a portion of the lung. The local form is seen surrounding areas of inflammation, infarction, tuberculosis or neoplasm. The general variety may be acute or chronic, and may be seen in cases of chronic nephritis, arteriosclerosis with hypertension, chronic heart failure, following rapid paracentesis, during the course of severe septic processes, and in chronic congestion of the lung from whatever cause. It is frequently associated with hypostatic congestion as a terminal condition. Grossly, the lungs are heavy, voluminous, pit on pressure, crepitate to a diminished degree, and on section much frothy blood-tinged serum flows from the surface. Histologically, the capillaries are dilated, and most of the alveoli are filled with an almost homogeneous pink staining material. A few pigment laden large mononuclear cells may be present in the fluid. (See Fig. 49 and illustrative case No. 22.)

Infarction (Pulmonary Embolism).—This condition results from the occlusion of the pulmonary artery or its branches by the lodgment of an embolus or the formation of a thrombus. It is an all too frequent post-operative complication and is commonly due to an embolus arising from an area of thrombo-phlebitis near the site of the operation. Fat emboli may occasionally give rise to similar infarcts of the lung. These may arise as a result of trauma during operation, with globules of fat entering the venous circulation and being carried to the lung. They not infrequently are observed in accident cases following crushing injuries, especially fractures. They are probably overlooked in the routine exami-nation of hematoxylin and eosin sections, since their demonstration is only possible when frozen sections are made and stained for fat.

The results of embolism of the lung depend upon two factors, (1) the location and size of the vessel obstructed and (2) the nature of the embolus. If the vessel is small in size and the collateral circulation adequate, infarction does not develop. If collateral circulation is not established, a typical conical-shaped area of necrosis will result, the base of the cone being the pleural surface and the apex directed towards the hilus. A fibrinous exudate occurs over the affected pleural surface and gives rise to the symptoms of pain synchronous with the respiratory movement. This is a prominent symptom in this condition.

If the embolus is large enough to occlude the pulmonary artery at its bifurcation or in one of its major branches, death results in anywhere from a few minutes to a few hours, before evidence of actual infarction has time to develop.

The subsequent changes in the areas of infarction mainly depend upon the nature of the embolus or thrombus. If the embolus is infected by pyogenic organisms the area will soon be converted into a metastatic abscess. If the embolus consists of tumor cells a metastatic tumor nodule will result. If the embolus is bland the area of infarction will undergo characteristic degenerative and necrotic changes with eventual healing by cicatrization.

Infarction in general has been considered already in Chapter VI, so that only these essential features as relating to the lung are mentioned at this point. Typical pulmonary infarcts are seen as single or multiple sub-pleural dark-reddish black areas, 1 to 5 cm. in diameter, most frequently occurring in the lower lobe. On section, they are wedge-shaped, with their apices directed towards the hilus (see Fig. 52, 53, and 56, Cases 23 and 25).

Histologically, the area of infarction is surrounded by a zone of edema. Early, the infarcted area is packed with red cells. Hemolysis with varying amounts of pigment production follows (see Fig. 56). The affected alveolar walls undergo coagulation necrosis. Leukocytic infiltration is seen, aiding in the removal of necrotic material through its proteolytic and phagocytic action. Reparative fibrosis from the periphery completes the sequence, with the final development of a fibrous scar. The amount of such scar tissue is usually small and at autopsy the

PLATE XCVI

DISEASES OF THE LUNG (*Continued*)

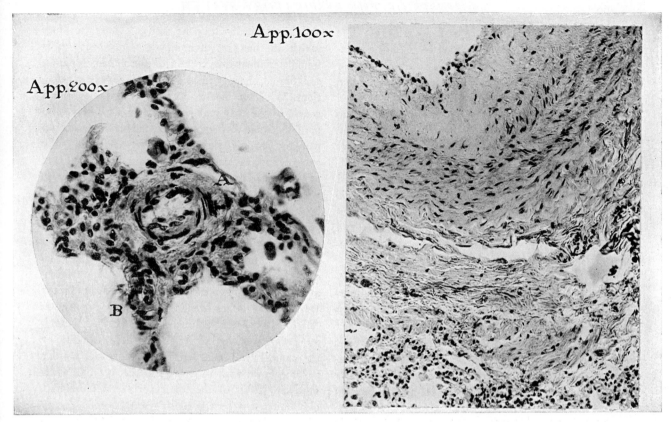

FIG. 407.—LUNG: AYERZA'S DISEASE.—CASE 172.—Pulmonary arterioles showing marked hyperplastic sclerosis with reduction in the size of their lumina (A and B). App. 200 x.

FIG. 408.—LUNG: AYERZA'S DISEASE.—CASE 172.—Photomicrograph of a portion of medium-sized pulmonary vessel in which marked thickening of the wall as a result of hyperplastic sclerosis, principally of the intima, has brought about considerable diminution in the size of the lumen. App. 100 x.

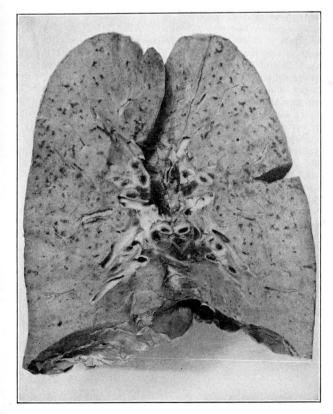

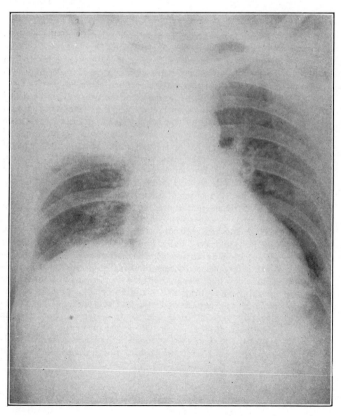

FIG. 409.—LUNG: LOBAR PNEUMONIA, GRAY HEPATIZATION.—CASE 177.—Gross photograph of right lung which shows a uniform consolidation throughout. This is grayish in color, airless and has the consistency of liver. Note the fibrinous exudate on the diaphragmatic pleura.

FIG. 410.—LUNG: LOBAR PNEUMONIA (cf. CASE 176).—Roentgenogram showing pneumonic consolidation confined chiefly to the upper right lobe.

small healed infarct may be easily overlooked. The pleural surface at first is covered by a fibrinous exudate which is confined to the area of infarction, and usually heals by organization without the production of adhesions (see illustrative case No. 25).

Ayerza's Disease.—The condition known as Ayerza's disease is one which has occasioned a great deal of confusion among clinicians and pathologists alike. As nearly as can be ascertained from the available literature, the condition which Ayerza described was characterized clinically by a polycythemia in which the red cells might even reach as many as ten million per cubic millimeter, intense cyanosis and marked dyspnea. It appeared to have some relationship to altitude. Pathologically, the findings were essentially those of an arteriosclerotic process affecting the pulmonary arterial system characterized particularly by hyperplastic sclerosis and endarteritis obliterans of the smaller arterioles. This was not infrequently accompanied by thrombosis. As a result of this marked interference with pulmonary ventilation, an increased load was thrown on the right side of the heart with resultant hypertrophy, dilatation and even right-sided failure.

The etiology of this condition as such is entirely obscure. A similar pathological picture both grossly and histologically may be seen at times in lungs which are the seat of a diffuse fibrosis such as is found accompanying certain of the pneumoconioses, and fibroid changes in relation to the chronic infections. We have seen at least three examples in the course of the past year in which an absolutely comparable histopathology could be demonstrated accompanying chronic rheumatic fever associated with extensive mitral valvulitis. It is our impression that at times rheumatic infection may be associated with very definite pneumonitis and may be accompanied by such hyperplastic sclerotic changes of the lesser pulmonary circulation. These changes to our minds are indistinguishable from those described as Ayerza's disease. To many physicians, the term "Ayerza's disease" is synonymous with syphilis of the pulmonary artery, but the demonstration of spirochetes in the vascular lesions has been conspicuous by its absence. All in all, we are inclined to believe that there is no specific pathological lesion which is diagnostic of the clinical syndrome described by Ayerza. By this statement, we wish to emphasize the fact that obliterative sclerosis of the lesser peripheral pulmonary circulation may be caused by a rather wide variety of etiologic agents, which still need further investigation.

ILLUSTRATIVE CASE

CASE 172. (Ref. #S-370)

Diagnosis.—Lung—hyperplastic sclerosis of the peripheral vascular bed (Ayerza's disease?).

Patient was a white female of 24 years, admitted to the hospital with a picture of acute cardiac decompensation associated with auricular fibrillation.

Present Illness.—The onset of the present illness dated back to a period about seven years earlier when a suspected diagnosis of congenital heart disease was made following the development of symptoms as a result of athletic competitive activities. Since that time the patient had had several periods of relative decompensation, which subsided upon bed rest and digitalization. The patient had been of a very striking cyanotic appearance ever since the onset of these symptoms. Her present attack of decompensation was apparently initiated by a mild upper respiratory infection.

Past Medical History.—The patient was a full-term, normally delivered baby. She never had any disturbances of nutrition as an infant. She had the usual mild childhood infections consisting of measles, pertussis and varicella. She had never had scarlet fever, diphtheria or anything suggesting rheumatic fever. She had been cyanotic in appearance at birth, and this had not been particularly noticed until the acute onset of her cardiac symptoms as previously noted, seven years before admission. Previous to that time she had never had any illness serious enough to require hospitalization. She had

had no operations. A review of her systems in general was negative. She was relatively subject to mild upper respiratory infections. Her gastro-intestinal history in general was negative, although she had a rather delicate appetite and was somewhat subject to constipation. Her genito-urinary history was negative. Menstrual history began at the age of twelve and had been regular, without any undue dysmenorrhea. She had been married two years earlier but had had no pregnancy, on the advice of her physician on account of her cardiac condition.

Physical Examination.—At the time of admission, the patient was extremely cyanotic and dyspneic, lying in bed in obvious distress. Head otherwise was not remarkable. Pupils reacted normally. Nose and throat were negative except for a dusky, cyanotic congestion of the mucosa. There was visible pulsation of the vessels in the neck with very prominent jugulars. The chest was symmetrical. It was slightly emphysematous in type with a definite increase in the antero-posterior diameter. The heart was greatly enlarged with the apex beat felt diffusely in the sixth interspace about the midaxillary line. The heart was in apparent fibrillation with a complete escape of the ventricles so that the ventricular rate was 60 while the auricular rate could not be definitely counted and was extremely irregular. What appeared to be a systolic murmur was noted over the apical area. The lungs were filled with moist râles which were most prominent at both bases. On percussion, some diminution in resonance was noted in the same basal areas. Abdomen was moderately prominent. The liver was greatly enlarged, being palpable a full three fingers' breadth below the costal margin. The spleen was believed to be palpable. The extremities were negative.

Laboratory Findings.—Blood count on admission showed 6,800,000 red cells with a hemoglobin of 108%, and a white blood count of 16,000 with 57% polynuclears. The sedimentation rate was increased. Blood chemistry was negative. Urinalysis was negative. Wassermann was negative.

Subsequent Course.—The patient continued steadily downhill, and died forty-eight hours after admission.

Autopsy Findings.—At autopsy, about 3,000 c.c. of fluid were found in the peritoneal cavity with about half as much in each of the pleural cavities, and approximately 300 c.c. of similar fluid in the pericardial cavity. There was generalized anasarca as well. The heart weighed 500 gm. and showed marked hypertrophy of all the chambers, but especially of the right auricle and both right and left ventricles. There was a marked pulmonary conus. The pulmonary artery measured 3.5 cm. in diameter just above the pulmonary valve and showed marked atherosclerotic deposits in the intima. There was an old calcified mitral valvulitis with almost complete stenosis, the valve being represented by a narrow, slit-like orifice 1.2 cm. in length by 0.3 cm. in diameter. The aortic valve, likewise, showed considerable thickening of its cusps along the free border. The tricuspid and pulmonic valves did not appear to be involved in the old rheumatic process. The lungs were unusually heavy and contained a large amount of fluid. The entire pulmonary arterial system stood out prominently on section of the lungs. Even the small, fine branches could be identified as being the seat of a diffuse sclerosis. The abdominal viscera showed very extensive chronic passive congestion, including the presence of markedly dilated esophageal varices.

Microscopic Description of a Section Through the Lung.—(Fig. 407 and 408) Sections through the periphery of the lung present a diffuse, chronic interstitial fibrosis. This is accompanied by marked mononuclear cellular infiltration. Toward the hilum, in some of the larger septa, these aggregations of cells almost simulate atypical Aschoff body formation. The impression is readily gained that this represents a true rheumatic pneumonitis. More striking than this aspect of the picture, which it is admittedly difficult to differentiate from the possible effects of simple chronic passive congestion, save that in the latter one would not expect to find the same degree of cellular reaction, are the outstanding changes in the blood vessels. The picture may best be described as a diffuse, hyperplastic, arterial and arteriolar sclerosis. This involves media and intima alike and is characterized by hyperplasia and hypertrophy of the musculature, which is accompanied by interstitial fibrosis. In addition, there is marked intimal proliferation with thickening of the subintima by connective tissue. Atheromatous degenerative changes may be seen in the major vessels. With elastic tissue stains, it is seen that the elastic laminae have been broken up and show marked reduplication and fraying. The picture is entirely consistent with the findings as described in the typical case of Ayerza's disease. Whether this can be considered as a true example of the clinical syndrome, or whether it should be considered as such only on the basis of the pathological findings, in the light of our present knowledge, seems irrelevant.

EMPHYSEMA

This condition is characterized by an excess of air within the lungs. It occurs in several forms as indicated in the following outline:

1. Interstitial

2. Vesicular (Alveolar)
   - Acute
     - Local or compensatory
     - Diffuse, acute visceral emphysema
   - Chronic
     - Large lung
       - hypertrophic
       - substantial
       - substantive
     - Small lung, senile or atrophic

Interstitial Emphysema.—In interstitial emphysema the air is found within the parenchymatous tissue itself of the lung and pleura. It is mechanical in origin, either the result of trauma, as, for example, a penetrating wound from a fractured rib, or from rupture of the air sac by excessive dilatation of the lung, as in violent coughing (whooping cough) or in strangulation. Grossly, blebs are usually seen on the pleural surface which can be pushed from place to place within the sub-pleural tissues or along the walls of the air spaces. Air may even be driven into the areolar tissues of the mediastinum and spread through the loose connective tissue of the neck. On palpation of such emphysematous tissues, a characteristic crackling sensation is imparted.

Vesicular Emphysema.—In the vesicular type, the vesicles are distended with an abnormal amount of air.

ACUTE LOCAL OR COMPENSATORY EMPHYSEMA.—Results from over-dilatation of those alveoli in the unaffected portions of the lungs, in association with an atelectasis or a pneumonic consolidation. For example, in lobar pneumonia, in bronchopneumonia, or in cases of atelectasis of a portion of the lung from whatever cause, the remainder of the lung undergoes compensatory dilatation. Grossly, the emphysematous areas stand out prominently against the darker compressed or consolidated tissues. These areas may be patchy and confined to individual lobules or the dilatation may be lobar in extent. Histologically, the vesicles are overdistended with air. Little change is seen in the alveolar wall since the process is usually of short duration.

ACUTE DIFFUSE VESICULAR EMPHYSEMA.—
This results from extreme effort to empty the lung
in cases of strangulation, and is usually associated
with interstitial emphysema. It may be encountered
at autopsy in hanged and drowned individuals.

CHRONIC HYPERTROPHIC; LARGE LUNG EM-
PHYSEMA.—This is the classical form. It is associated with the "barrel-shaped" chest in which the
antero-posterior diameter practically equals the transverse. The sternum is raised, the ribs are less oblique
and tend to become fixed in position. The chest is
hyperresonant and the area of cardiac dullness may
be obscured due to the tendency of the anterior edges
of the distended lungs to overlie the pericardium.
The respiratory movements are prolonged due to the
inelasticity of the lung and the tendency of the chest
to be fixed in the position of expansion. Grossly, the
lungs are pale and fail to collapse when the chest is
opened. Bullae 0.5 to 1 cm. in diameter are seen
along the anterior edge frequently. These represent
tremendously distended air spaces (see Fig. 403).
The lungs are large, inelastic, dry, pit on pressure,
and weigh less than normal. The air spaces are
easily seen, and are considerably larger than normal. Histologic examination of the tissues reveal
large alveoli with very thin stretched walls in which
the capillaries often appear distended but diminished in number. Many of these dilated air spaces
are found to represent a terminal bronchiole with
its vesicles, the walls of which have undergone
atrophy. As a result the tremendous diminution in
the aeration surface of the capillary field may be
readily appreciated (Fig. 404). This leads to an
increase of the work of the right heart since the
same volume of blood per minute must be aerated
and passed through the lung as in the normal organ.
It is accompanied by increased pressure of the pulmonary artery. Hypertrophy of the right ventricle is
at times marked, and after a variable time may be
followed by dilatation and evidence of general congestion. Polycythemia is usually present and is compensatory. Atheromata of the pulmonary artery are
likely to result.

The etiology of large lung emphysema is still obscure. Formerly, the disease was thought to be more
frequent among individuals whose occupation resulted in frequent increase of alveolar pressure, such
as glass blowers, or musicians who played the brass
or wood wind instruments. Reliable statistics, however, fail to show any apparent increased incidence
among such individuals. Emphysema tends to occur
in families, so apparently there is an hereditary factor. The theory has been suggested that in the emphysematous individual the lungs may be hypoplastic
but no convincing proof has been advanced. Another
theory which seems more tenable, is that a congenital
hypoplasia of the elastic tissues of the lung exists, so
that overdistention of the alveoli may lead to permanent dilatation. It would seem probable, therefore, that at least two factors play a part in the
development of emphysema: First, a congenital factor, probably in the form of decrease in the elastic
tissue of the lung, and secondly, some acute or
chronic condition resulting in overdistention of the
alveoli. This is particularly found in relation to some
obstructive type of lesion in which the vesicles are
forcibly distended, such as asthma, chronic bronchitis, bronchopneumonia, etc.

ILLUSTRATIVE CASE

CASE 173. (Ref. #S-13)
Diagnosis.—Lung—chronic hypertrophic emphysema.
Patient was a white male of 53 years, admitted to
the hospital complaining of edema of his feet and
dyspnea.
Present Illness.—The patient dated his present illness
back about one year when he first noticed dyspnea on
going upstairs and swelling of his feet towards evening.
This became so severe that he had to give up his work
as a porter shortly afterwards. He had had a succession
of colds and coughs throughout the preceding winter and
about three months before admission he consulted a physician because of his cough. He described it as of a
"wheezing" character. His physician told him that he
had cardiac asthma and recommended that he be hospitalized. This he refused at the time, but because of increasing weakness and the progressive nature of his

dyspnea and "wheeziness," he had become bedridden.
As a result he was sent to the hospital by his family.
Past Medical History.—His past medical history was
essentially irrelevant so far as could be ascertained from
the patient. He had had the usual childhood infections.
He did not ever recall having had anything in the nature
of hay fever or asthma, or any other allergic manifestations. He had not had rheumatic fever so far as he was
aware. He denied venereal disease. A review of his
systems showed that he had always been rather subject
to mild upper respiratory infections and had had a severe
case of influenza during the epidemic some fifteen years
previously. He had never had any gastro-intestinal
symptoms and up to a year earlier had never been heart
conscious. Genito-urinary history was negative.
Physical Examination.—The patient was a well developed, muscular white male about fifty years of age in

appearance. Head was negative. Eyes, ears, nose and throat were not remarkable. Chest was of the barrel-shaped type with the anteroposterior diameter only slightly less than the transverse. The obliquity of the ribs was greatly reduced and the chest was fixed in position. The lungs were full of wheezing râles and seemed generally hyperresonant, particularly in the upper part of both lungs. The heart was moderately enlarged on percussion, especially to the right. Sounds were distant. There were no murmurs. The abdomen was moderately prominent. There was some shifting dullness in the flanks, although no definite fluid wave could be obtained. External genitalia were negative. There was marked edema of the feet and ankles.

Laboratory Findings.—On admission, the patient had a red cell count of 5,200,000 with 14.5 gm. of hemoglobin, and a white blood count of 8,700 with 62% polynuclears. Urinalysis was negative except for a slight trace of albumin. Wassermann was negative. Blood chemistry was normal.

Subsequent Course.—The patient became progressively worse and died of apparent congestive heart failure about ten days after admission.

Autopsy Findings.—At autopsy there was a rather generalized anasarca with considerable ascites and a moderate amount of fluid in both pleural cavities and an increase of fluid in the pericardium. There was marked chronic passive congestion of the viscera, particularly the liver, spleen and the mucosa of the gastro-intestinal tract. The heart showed marked hypertrophy and right-sided dilatation. No valvular lesions were noted. Lungs presented the typical picture of so-called "large lung" or chronic vesicular emphysema. They were voluminous in appearance and failed to collapse when the chest was opened. Along the anterior edge, particularly at the apices, numerous enormous bullae, some measuring as much as 3 cm. in diameter were seen. There was a suggestion of atheromatosis of the pulmonary artery. No other changes of significance were found.

Microscopic Description of a Section Through the Lung Tissue.—(Fig. 404) Histologic examination of the tissue shows a somewhat thickened pleura at one side of the specimen. The alveoli of the lungs are much larger than normal. The alveolar walls appear stretched and are extremely thin in places, appearing only as a hair line. The capillaries seem reduced in number. Some of them appear markedly congested; others are almost completely collapsed. In places, there is a compensatory attempt at interstitial fibrosis. With elastic tissue stains, it is seen that the elastic fibers are diminished in number and show marked degenerative changes with fraying. Occasional large mononuclear cells are seen within the alveolar spaces. These tend to contain blood pigment. The picture is typically that of a simple chronic hypertrophic type of emphysema, but is somewhat obscured by an associated oedema.

CHRONIC ATROPHIC OR SENILE EMPHYSEMA (JENNER).—This is the type seen in old age and is scarcely comparable with the other forms of emphysema. The increase in the size of the air spaces is brought about as a result of senile atrophy of the lung parenchyma. The chest is smaller and flatter than normal and the obliquity of the ribs is increased. The lungs have lost their elasticity. There may even be small bullae present. Grossly, the air spaces present a similar dilatation to that seen in the hypertrophic variety. Histologically, the picture likewise resembles that of the large lung variety, but there is less evidence of thinning of the alveolar walls and there is usually an increase of fibrous tissue. There is apt to be an associated hemosiderin pigmentation.

ATELECTASIS (COLLAPSE, APNEUMATOSIS)

By definition, atelectasis is the reverse of emphysema, and as such is characterized by a diminished amount of air in the lung as the result of compression of the air vesicles. This condition may be congenital or acquired.

Congenital Atelectasis.—The congenital variety may be partial or complete, and results from a failure of the lung to expand at birth. This is usually due to one of four causes: (1) prematurity or too weak an infant, (2) plugging of a bronchus with blood or mucus, (3) malformations of the lung, including an imperforate bronchus and (4) congenital syphilis.

If the process be general, both lungs will be affected. A good example of bilateral complete congenital atelectasis is seen in stillborn infants. The lungs are reddish gray in color, they fail to crepitate, and sink in water. If the child breathes and only a part of the lung remains atelectatic the collapsed areas are darker in color, usually a purplish red, and tend to be slightly depressed. Likewise, they fail to crepitate. Histologically, the picture is that of fetal lung. The alveoli are small, airless and lined by cuboidal appearing cells (see Fig. 405; Illustrative Case No. 174).

ILLUSTRATIVE CASE

CASE 174. (Ref. #S-12)
Diagnosis.—Lung—congenital atelectasis.
Patient was a stillborn infant, who was born prematurely at about the end of the eighth month of pregnancy as the result of an acute appendicitis of the mother which required operative intervention. The mother was a normal appearing, well-developed, well-nourished young woman twenty-three years of age who had had a normal gestation up to the onset of her appendicitis. She had had two other children who were living and well.

Autopsy Findings.—The autopsy revealed an apparently normal seven or eight months' fetus. The head showed no abnormalities. Heart was normal in size and position. The foramen ovale was widely patent. The lungs showed complete atelectasis with no evidence of any expansion whatever. They failed to crepitate on palpation and sank in water. They were a deep, cyanotic, reddish color. There was no evidence of any congenital malformations or obstructions to the bronchial tree. The abdominal viscera all appeared normal.

Microscopic Description of a Section Through One of the Atelectatic Lungs.—(Fig. 405) Histologic study of the tissues shows a typical fetal type of lung with the pleural surface on one side of the section. The tissue may be identified by the presence of small bronchioles with rather characteristic high columnar epithelial cells, some of which show cilia. This mucous membrane shows considerable plication. There is some slight desquamation observed in the lumina of the bronchioles. The alveolar walls of the lung parenchyma are practically in apposition with each other. They are made up of delicate septa which show marked congestion of the capillaries. The lining cells appear almost cuboidal. There has been some slight escape of fluid into the potential alveoli as evidenced by pink-staining granular precipitate here and there.

Acquired Atelectasis.—In acquired atelectasis, an area which has been previously expanded becomes collapsed. Acquired atelectasis may be divided into two types according to cause: (a) *Compression atelectasis:* (Fig. 406) This variety results from fluids, gases or solids compressing the lung either from the pleural surface or from the mediastinum. Conditions such as pneumothorax, hydrothorax, empyema, tumors of the pleura, pushing up of the diaphragm from intra-abdominal lesions or pressure from an aneurysm may give rise to such compression atelectasis. Marked enlargement of the mediastinal lymph nodes such as occurs in Hodgkins' disease, pericardial fusion or even marked hypertrophy of the heart are other examples which may produce this picture; (b) *Obstructive atelectasis:* This type is due to bronchial obstruction either from within or from without. Tumor, exudates, or foreign bodies are among the important causes. Patchy areas of this form of atelectasis frequently accompany bronchopneumonia as a result of plugging of bronchioles by catarrhal exudate. The lobule affected undergoes atelectasis, while the uninvolved areas show compensatory emphysema.

ILLUSTRATIVE CASE

CASE 175. (Ref. #S-17)

Diagnosis.—Lung—acquired compression atelectasis.

Patient was a white female of 45 years, admitted to the hospital with the chief complaint of cough and shortness of breath.

Present Illness.—The patient's present illness dated back a matter of two or more years. Approximately two years before her present admission, the patient first noticed a lump in her right breast. This caused her no pain and she did nothing about it for several months. Subsequently, she consulted a physician who advised surgical intervention. A diagnosis of scirrhous carcinoma was made and radical mastectomy with excision of the axillary nodes was done. The patient made an uneventful recovery following the operation and had been free from symptoms since that time until about one month before her present admission.

Four or five weeks earlier, she noticed she began to have dyspnea on exertion. She thought very little of this as again it was not associated with any pain, but shortly after the onset of her dyspnea she developed a cough, which had persisted until after her present admission. Dyspnea increased so that it was present constantly as well as during periods of exertion. She believed that she had lost considerable weight in the preceding three or four months. She had become rather weak and was beginning to worry a good deal about her health.

Past Medical History.—Past medical history was entirely irrelevant. She had a normal childhood with the usual diseases. A review of her systems yielded little information of importance. She had the usual quota of mild upper respiratory infection. She never had had any gastro-intestinal symptoms other than rather chronic constipation. Genito-urinary history was negative. Menses began at the age of twelve and had been regular throughout her life. Her last period before admission had been two weeks earlier. She had had three healthy children who were all alive and well.

Physical Examination.—Patient was a fairly well-developed and well-nourished middle-aged white woman who showed some evidence of recent weight loss. Head was negative. Pupils reacted normally. Nose and throat were negative. The chest was somewhat asymmetrical in respect to the actual bony structure with relative prominence of the right side. There was a long linear scar representing the site of the amputation of the right breast along which several small dense nodules could be felt suggesting recurrent tumor tissue. The left breast was found to contain a large, hard mass which occupied almost the entire glandular portion of the breast. The skin was of the so-called "orange-rind" appearance. The lung findings on physical examination were very confusing. There was extensive dullness over both sides of the chest, which on the left was more marked, becoming completely flat on percussion. The breath sounds on the left were diminished and distant. On the right, in the apical area, they were almost bronchial in quality while at the base they likewise seemed diminished. It was difficult to make out the left border of the heart due to the flatness of the left side of the chest. The abdomen was moderately prominent. No masses or tenderness could be felt. The extremities were negative.

Laboratory Findings.—The patient had a blood count of 3,100,000 red cells with 63% hemoglobin and 11,200 white blood cells with 71% polynuclears. Urinalysis was negative. Wassermann was negative.

X-ray examination showed extensive bone involvement of the ribs on the right side. There was a huge mass filling practically the entire right side of the right lower half of the chest. There was a hydrothorax on the left side with a definite fluid level in the upright position. The lung could be demonstrated as showing marked compression atelectasis with displacement upward and outward. The heart was likewise displaced toward the chest wall.

Subsequent Course.—In view of the extensive nature of the process surgery was impossible, and x-ray treatment was given to the limit of tolerance. The patient, however, failed to improve and died two months later.

Autopsy Findings.—There was a diffuse adenocarcinoma of the left breast, in addition to the recurrent lesion on the right, with metastases to the thorax. This extended through the right chest wall involving the ribs, pleurae and right lung extensively. It likewise had extended to involve the diaphragm as well. The left pleural cavity contained about 1,200 c.c. of slightly turbid, amber colored fluid with a specific gravity of 1.020. The pleural surface was studded with numerous tumor nodules, which were grayish-white in color. The lung showed almost complete compression atelectasis as a result of the fluid.

Microscopic Description of a Section Through the Lung.—(Fig. 406) Histologic study of the tissue shows a thickened, subpleural connective tissue filled with metastatic adenocarcinomatous tissue. This can be seen spreading along the subpleural lymphatics as cords of tumor cells. In addition, the tumor has actually invaded the blood vessels in this area and beginning parenchymatous metastatic nodules are also seen. The lung parenchyma itself is almost completely collapsed with the alveolar walls in apposition in many paces. Even the bronchioles seem somewhat compressed and oval rather than round in shape. There is marked capillary congestion. Considerable diapedesis of red cells has occurred with their subsequent hemolysis and the development of hemosiderin. This is largely within the cytoplasm of phagocytic cells. There is very little evidence of inflammatory exudation in the lung substance.

Massive Collapse (Atelectasis) of the Lung.—Clinically, a post-operative form of acute massive atelectasis is described. It is characterized by a sudden onset accompanied by dyspnea and cyanosis. It is more prone to follow operations upon the upper abdomen and has been attributed to paralysis of the diaphragm on the affected side. Fluroscopic examination reveals no respiratory movement, with the diaphragm high and immobile.

Recently, Chevalier Jackson has shown that a similar massive atelectasis may follow the lodgement of a foreign body in a major bronchus. He feels that acute massive collapse of the lung may even result from the obstruction brought about by bronchial secretions which are not removed due to suppression of the cough reflex or the extreme weakness of the patient. The administration of a general anesthetic probably also contributes to its development, due to mucosal irritation, with resultant increased production of mucous secretion. The condition may readily be differentiated clinically since the collapse results in displacement of the heart towards the affected side, which is the reverse of that found in pneumonic consolidations. A somewhat similar picture is seen in the compression atelectasis of artificial pneumothorax.

Grossly, the lung in acquired atelectasis is apt to be pale in color, firm and practically airless. Histologically, the air vesicles are collapsed, the walls almost in opposition and the vessels congested. If the lung remains unexpanded for a considerable period of time diffuse fibrosis takes place with permanent destruction of the lung parenchyma. This end result is known by the older writers as the "cirrhosis of collapse" or *gray induration.*

CHAPTER XLIII

DISEASES OF THE RESPIRATORY SYSTEM (*Continued*)

THE PNEUMONIAS

From the standpoint of relative importance, the pneumonias occupy first place in respiratory pathology. By pneumonia or pneumonitis is meant an inflammation of the lung. This is usually infectious in nature, but may have some chemical irritation, such as one of the lipoids or poisonous gases as an etiologic factor. The pneumonias are divided on an anatomical basis into two major types: (1) *lobar pneumonia,* in which one or more entire lobes of the lung are involved uniformly, and (2) *lobular,* or more familiarly, *bronchopneumonia,* in which the inflammatory process is patchy in nature and develops in relation to the individual lobules. They are likewise classified very commonly on the basis of the etiologic agent insofar as such a method is applicable. Such a classification is not entirely satisfactory because it is quite true that at times the pneumococcus which is the usual cause of lobar pneumonia may, particularly in children and elderly individuals, result in a lobular type of the disease. Similarly, streptococcic infections, while usually producing a patchy type of bronchopneumonia, occasionally are found to be the cause of a very diffuse process with a lobar distribution. Thus, it will be seen that the strictly bacteriologic method of classification is open to criticism in respect to the anatomical type of pneumonia is produced.

Inasmuch as our efforts in this presentation are aimed at trying to simplify the picture as much as possible, we are inclined to follow the relatively common usage of making pneumococcus pneumonia synonymous with lobar pneumonia and to place all the other varieties of pneumonia in the bronchopneumonic group, and attempting so far as possible, to classify them on a bacterial etiologic basis. Even the use of some of the more common terms is confusing to the uninitiated and for that reason the following brief comments are made at this point. From the practical standpoint, although etymologically the words, pneumonia and pneumonitis, are synonymous, actually the term, pneumonitis, is ordinarily used in relation to an actual inflammation of the lung parenchyma itself, particularly as seen in interstitial pneumonitis. By contrast, the word, pneumonia, is usually applied to inflammations of the lung in which the inflammatory exudate is within the alveoli. This can be best considered as a surface exudate, the anatomical arrangement of the lung being designed simply to increase the surface area for gaseous exchange. With these reservations in mind, let us proceed to a discussion of the various types of pneumonia.

PART I

Lobar Pneumonia

(Pneumococcus Pneumonia; Pleural Pneumonia; Croupous or Fibrinous Pneumonia)

Classically, lobar pneumonia is an infection produced by one of the pneumococci which results in inflammatory consolidation of one or more lobes of the lung. Clinically, the typical case is ushered in abruptly with a chill, a rapid rise in temperature to 102 or 103 degrees, and is accompanied by severe dyspnea. There is a fastigium lasting anywhere from five to eight or more days during which the temperature remains elevated and the patient remains critically ill. If his resistance is low, and the virulence of the infecting organism high, it is during this period that the patient is likely to succumb to the infection. At the end of the fastigium, the temperature falls equally abruptly by crisis. The dyspnea

468

PLATE XCVII

DISEASES OF THE LUNG—Lobar Pneumonia

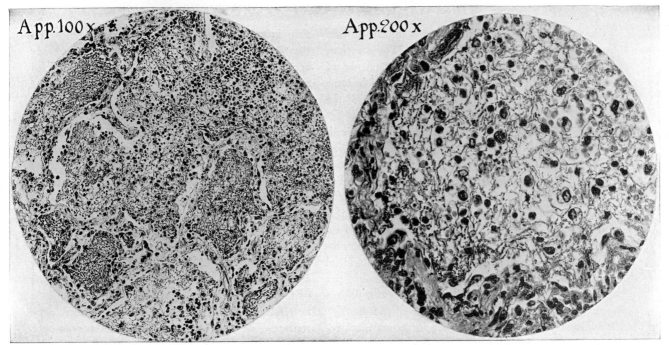

FIG. 411.—RED HEPATIZATION.—CASE 176.—All the vesicles of the lung are completely filled with acute fibrinous exudate. The alveolar walls are swollen and congested. App. 100 x.

FIG. 412.—RED HEPATIZATION.—CASE 176.—High power photomicrograph better showing the exudate composed of fibrillar fibrin, large mononuclear phagocytes and numerous red cells. Occasional polynuclears also may be observed. App. 200 x.

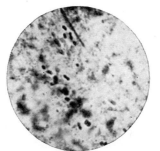

FIG. 413.—PNEUMOCOCCI FROM SPUTUM. App. 1000 x.

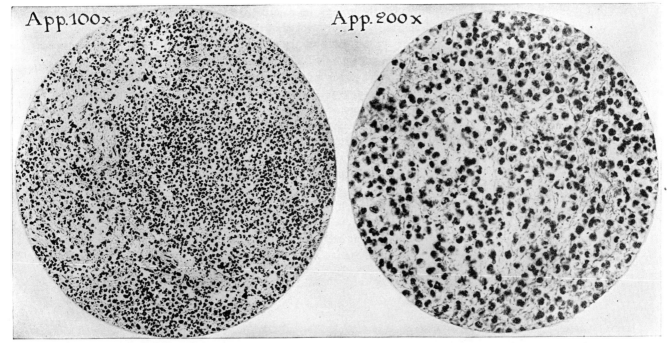

FIG. 414.—GRAY HEPATIZATION.—CASE 177.—The vesicles of the lung are shown completely filled with exudate in which most of the fibrin has disappeared. The alveolar walls are inconspicuous and the capillaries not congested. App. 100 x.

FIG. 415.—GRAY HEPATIZATION.—CASE 177.—High power photomicrograph of a vesicle showing exudate to consist chiefly of inflammatory cells in which polymorphonuclears predominate. Most of the fibrin has been removed by cytolytic autolysis. App. 200 x.

disappears and the patient recovers in the uncomplicated case by a slow convalescence. These various clinical stages correspond to a regular sequence of pathological changes which will be described in some detail in the section devoted to the pathology of the disease.

Etiology.—The etiology, as has been emphasized, is usually due to the *Pneumococcus*. The *Friedländer bacillus* was the first bacterium to be demonstrated from the lungs of patients showing the lobar distribution of the pneumonic process, but with our increased experience, bacteriologically, we now recognize that not more than one-half of one per cent of such lobar pneumonias are caused by this organism. Heffernon, in a review of thirty-three hundred and nineteen cases showed that over ninety-six per cent of cases were due to the pneumococcus, with a streptococcus as the principal other offender.

Great strides have been made in recent years regarding our knowledge of the pneumococci. Formerly, only four types were generally recognized, types 1, 2 and 3 being specific, and type 4 representing a heterogeneous group which did not show any of the specific characteristics of the other three groups. In the past few years, at least twenty-nine additional strains of pneumococci have been demonstrated by Cooper, Edwards and Rosenstein by the use of specific agglutination methods, as composing the principal members of the old type four. These additional twenty-nine types of pneumococci have been particularly studied by Bullowa and Wilcox in the metropolitan New York area in a recorded survey of over four thousand cases of infection. They have demonstrated that types 15 and 23 in adults and types 8, 28, 23 and 15 in children, in the order named, are associated with as high mortality figures as seen in respect to the more familiar types 2 and 3. In groups 1, 2, and 3, fortunately type 1 predominates both in metropolitan and rural areas throughout the world, as shown by Heffernon. Approximately thirty-three per cent of all pneumonic pneumonias are caused by type 1, which responds particularly well to the use of specific antiserum therapeutically.

Types 2 and 3 vary considerably in frequency from year to year, but again from Heffernon's figures covering nearly fifteen thousand cases, roughly twenty per cent are due to type 2 and eleven per cent to type 3. The remaining thirty-six per cent are divided among the other twenty-nine groups. Statistical information as to their relative incidence and the therapeutic value of their specific sera is slowly becoming available, but until more data has been accumulated, no very sweeping generalities can be made.

Mode of Transmission.—The mode of transmission of the organism is disputed. It is probable that it must be transmitted by individuals suffering with the disease, or as carriers by the aerogenous route through coughing, sneezing, etc. However, the organisms may be present in the nose and throat without producing symptoms until such time as resistance is broken down through fatigue and exposure to cold. This seems a more satisfactory explanation of the way in which the disease develops than the direct droplet infection theory because it is almost unheard of for secondary cases of pneumonia to develop in a hospital in spite of crowded conditions and close contact. The bacteriologic evidence to support such a theory is very slim, however, as only exceptionally does the normal mouth flora yield pneumococci to any extent.

The way in which the organism reaches the lung is likewise a matter of considerable difference of opinion. Three major routes have been suggested: (1) the older theory held that the organism was *inhaled directly* into the lung alveoli where it set up its characteristic reaction; (2) later the theory was advanced that the organism might reach the lung by the *hematogenous* route, in an attempt to explain the curious uniform lobar distribution. In this connection it must be observed that blood cultures are notoriously negative in pneumococcic pneumonia. That much abused term, "tissue specificity," in regard to the infection is likewise logically invoked at this point, but without contributing a great deal; and (3) more recently the work of Cecil, Blake and others points to a *lymphatic* method of distribution as the most likely since it is shown in experimental animals that the pneumococci can be demonstrated within the peribronchial lymphatics and the walls of the alveolus before they are present within the air spaces. That this is the probable method of spread is further borne out by the fact that the inflammation obviously spreads from the hilus to the periphery of the lobe and not infrequently extends in the hilar region to involve a small amount of lung tissue in the adjacent lobe. Apparently very little resistance is offered to the passage of the pneumococci by the lymphatics as they reach

PLATE XCVIII

DISEASES OF THE LUNG (*Continued*)

LOBAR PNEUMONIA (*Continued*)

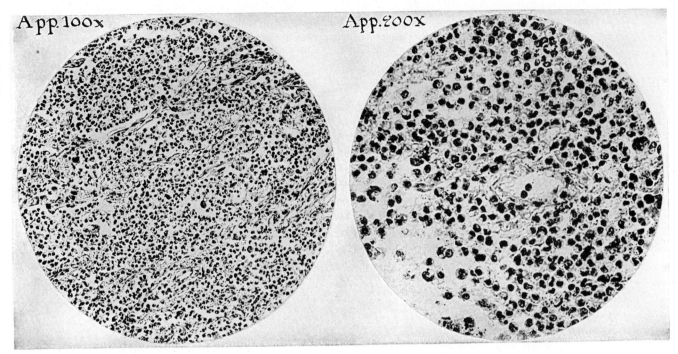

FIG. 416.—LATE GRAY HEPATIZATION; RESOLUTION.—The vesicles of the lung are seen filled with exudate in which the fibrin has completely disappeared. The alveolar walls are thin, almost transparent. App. 100 x.

FIG. 417.—LATE GRAY HEPATIZATION; RESOLUTION.—The exudate, as seen under the high power, is similar to that of gray hepatization except that the cells are poorly stained and show various retrograde nuclear and cytoplasmic changes. App. 200 x.

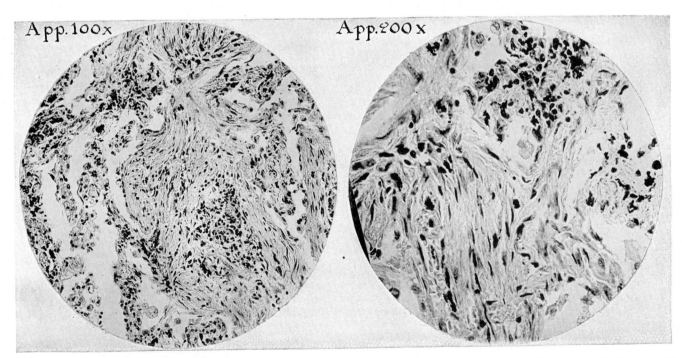

FIG. 418.—ORGANIZING PNEUMONIA.—CASE 178.—In the center of photomicrograph, a considerable mass of vascularized young fibrous tissue is seen within the vesicles. This apparently arises from the alveolar wall in the upper part of the section. App. 100 x.

FIG. 419.—ORGANIZING PNEUMONIA.—CASE 178.—A higher magnification of an area from Fig. 418. Proliferation of fairly well differentiated fibroblasts and new formed capillaries may be observed. App. 200 x.

the alveolar wall before any marked evidence of inflammatory reaction is seen. This is in contrast to certain cases of streptococcic pneumonia in which the organism apparently enters the lung in a similar fashion. In such cases the resistance to the extension of the infection is almost immediately manifested in the form of an acute inflammatory reaction, which impedes the spread of the organism uniformly throughout the lung and thus gives rise to patchy areas of bronchopneumonic consolidation.

Diagnosis.—The diagnosis of lobar pneumonia today is a combined clinical and laboratory procedure. The history itself is typical enough in the great majority of instances to establish the pneumonic nature of the infection. The physical findings further substantiate them, but it is upon the bacteriologic diagnosis of the type of Pneumococcus which is responsible for the particular case that modern therapy depends. Typing of pneumococci from sputum in former times was a long, tedious and somewhat uncertain procedure relying as we did wholly upon cultural methods and agglutination after the organism was obtained in pure culture. A great advance was made when it was discovered that the white mouse was susceptible to pneumococcus infection, and that the organism could be recovered in a matter of a few hours instead of a day or two. More recently, the time of diagnosis of the specific type of pneumococcus causing the specific infection in any given instance has been cut down to a matter of minutes through the use of Neufeld's technique in which sputum containing the organism is directly tested against specific immune sera (Fig. 413). A positive reaction consists in the visible swelling of the capsule of the organism. By this means, all thirty-two types can be rapidly tested. This ability to recognize the specific type promptly, it is anticipated, will result in the reduction in the mortality of the disease from the several other types in which specific anti-sera seem to be of actual therapeutic value, as in the case of Type 1 serum. In Type 1, the mortality has been reduced when serum is administered within the first twenty-four hours of the disease almost sixty per cent. It is still too early to know the relative value of the other sera, but Bullowa's figures certainly suggest that in at least several of these other types, equally promising results may be expected.

Pathology.—Typical lobar pneumonia affects one or more lobes of the lung simultaneously (Fig. 409),

the lower lobes being more commonly affected than the upper. However, at times the process may spread, so that at autopsy one lobe may be in a late stage of gray hepatization while the adjacent lobe may present a much earlier process. The consolidation can readily be demonstrated in x-ray (Fig. 410). The affected portions of the lung become completely airless as a result of the alveoli being filled with exudate. The unaffected portions of the lungs undergo compensatory emphysema. The consolidation also results in a decrease in the aeration surface of the lung with the result that the pulmonary arterial pressure is raised. This throws a considerable strain on the right heart. In fact, death results in a certain number of instances from right-sided heart failure brought about by a sudden increased demand from a seriously damaged lung.

The pathological changes can be divided conveniently into four stages which correspond very closely to the clinical course of the disease: (1) engorgement; (2) red hepatization; (3) gray hepatization and (4) resolution.

ENGORGEMENT.—*Grossly,* in the state of *engorgement* the lung presents a picture of active hyperemia or acute congestion. This stage of pneumonia is rarely seen at autopsy since death seldom occurs until later. Occasionally, due to extension of the nonpneumonic process to other lobes, during the course of the disease, it may be encountered. This acute phase may be difficult to differentiate from passive congestion which is likely to follow during the course of lobar pneumonia. The pleural surface at this time is usually smooth, glistening and fails to show any evidence of pleuritis. The lung crepitates throughout. On section, the cut surface is moist and congested.

Microscopically, in the state of *engorgement,* the organisms are found almost entirely in the peribronchial lymphatics and in the interstitial tissue of the alveoli. The alveolar capillaries are enormously engorged and some escape of fluid and red cells into the air spaces may be observed.

RED HEPATIZATION.—*Grossly,* in this stage which immediately follows that of engorgement, the pleural surface over the affected lobe is the seat of an acute fibrinous pleuritis. When the chest is opened the affected portions of the lung are found to be solidified, and form a complete cast of that portion of the thorax. The depressions produced by the ribs are plainly marked on the pleural surface. The con-

PLATE XCIX

DISEASES OF THE LUNG (*Continued*)

BRONCHOPNEUMONIA

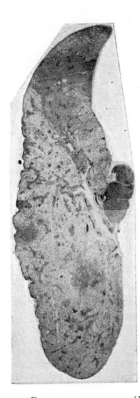

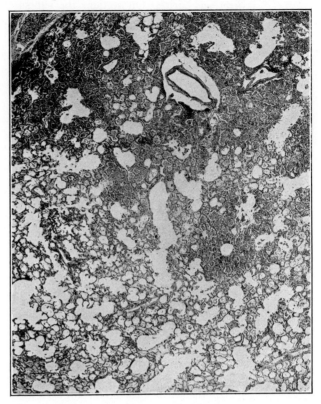

FIG. 420.—LUNG: BRONCHOPNEUMONIA (Interstitial).— CASE 180.—Histologic section of entire lung to show patchy distribution of lesions. Note the scattered areas of consolidation throughout becoming confluent in the upper lobe. Reduced ½.

FIG. 421.—BRONCHOPNEUMONIA (Lobular).—CASE 179.—The patchy involvement of groups of vesicles, theoretically lobules, interspersed with areas of emphysema and atelectasis is shown in this photomicrograph. App. 20 x.

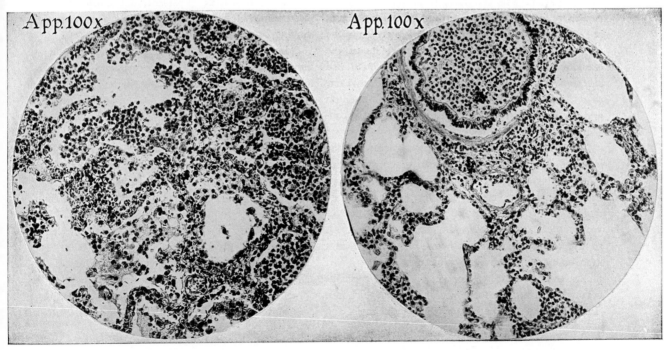

FIG. 422.—BRONCHOPNEUMONIA (Lobular).—CASE 179.—There are several vesicles which contain an exudate consisting almost entirely of degenerated polymorphonuclears. In others, large mononuclears predominate, while in still others fibrin is an important feature. App. 100 x.

FIG. 423.—BRONCHOPNEUMONIA (Interstitial).—CASE 180.—The striking feature in this case is the marked interstitial cellular infiltration with relatively little intra-alveolar exudate. Note secondary mucopurulent exudate within the bronchiole. App. 100 x.

solidation is lobar in distribution. The affected lobe is firm and airless. On section, the cut surface is reddish-gray, dry and slightly rough resembling ground glass in texture. This roughness is due to little plugs of fibrinous exudate sticking out of the vesicles. The lung is quite friable, thus somewhat resembling the liver, from which the term, "red hepatization," was derived.

Microscopically, red hepatization is initiated, in twenty-four to forty-eight hours after the onset, by the organisms entering the vesicles of the lung. They are accompanied by an outpouring of fluid exudate from which a meshwork of fibrin rapidly forms on the surface of the alveolus. This gradually fills the alveoli of the entire lobe involved (Fig. 411 and 412). The strands of fibrin pass through the interstitial pores of Cohn of the alveolar walls and the adjacent vesicles. The extent of the fibrinous exudate can be better appreciated if the sections be specially stained by Weigert's method in which the fibrinous exudate appears a dark blue, and the bacteria a blue black. The walls are still swollen, and the vessels distended with blood. Soon, a few polymorphonuclear leukocytes and large phagocytic mononuclears are added together with varying numbers of red cells. By the use of a bacterial stain such as Gram's, the enormous number of pneumococci within the alveoli and actually still in the alveolar walls may be appreciated. Large numbers of pneumococci can be demonstrated not only in the exudate, but also in the sputum. The cellular portion of the exudate is well preserved and the outlines of the leukocytes are distinct. Their numbers gradually increase as the disease progresses. The large mononuclears of the exudate were formerly thought to be desquamated alveolar lining cells. It has been shown, however, that they are derived from the reticulo-endothelium and are similar to histiocytes. They frequently contain phagocytosed debris.

GRAY HEPATIZATION.—The gross picture of the involved lung gradually changes so that by the fifth or sixth day the lung has a distinctly gray rather than red color on section. Death frequently occurs during this stage of the infection. *Grossly* the involved areas still are consolidated and fill the chest cavity, but the lung is less firm. The rib markings are usually not so definite by this time, however. The pleura over the affected portion of the lung is still covered by a fibrinous exudate of varying thickness. The cut surface of the lung is grayish and moist and

upon pressure, a purulent-appearing exudate can be expressed. The peribronchial lymph nodes are enlarged, grayish-pink in color and rather soft in consistency. They present the typical picture of an acute lymphadenitis.

Microscopically, as the lung passes from the stage of *red* to that of *gray hepatization,* the histologic characteristics likewise gradually change. The fibrin begins to contract, pulling away from the wall so that a clear space frequently exists between the exudate and the wall. The alveolar walls no longer appear swollen and the vessels no longer appear engorged. More and more polymorphonuclear leukocytes are added to the exudate. Many of these are in a poor state of preservation, with pyknosis of their nuclei and indefinite cytoplasmic outlines (Fig. 414 and 415). The red cells undergo hemolysis and disappear. The fibrin gradually undergoes lysis until only a small amount or none remains. Many of the phagocytic mononuclears are seen which contain hemosiderin; others are filled with cellular debris. In the favorable case the pneumococci have to a large degree disappeared. It is during this stage that most individuals die, usually between the fifth to eighth day.

RESOLUTION.—If the individual survives this period, the inflammatory process undergoes resolution. During this stage it will be noted that the lung, *grossly,* is fairly soft and has a peculiar translucent appearance. From the cut surface purulent exudate can still be expressed, but much of it has been removed by expectoration and absorption following extensive lysis.

Microscopically, with the appearance of the all important clinical feature, the crisis, no noteworthy change is seen in the appearance of the lung. During the next following days the exudate is gradually removed by absorption or expectoration in the stage known as *resolution.* Histologically, in this stage, only a few of the vesicles are filled with exudate. This consists of degenerated cells and debris, with large mononuclears predominating. The alveolar wall stains poorly at first. The alveolar wall capillaries are inconspicuous (Fig. 416 and 417). Ordinarily, the inflammatory process does not apparently result in any great amount of actual alveolar wall injury, and the lining cells regenerate. Fibrous thickening does not usually occur. Indeed, the lung is practically restored to normal so that subsequent examination grossly or histologically will fail to

PLATE C
DISEASES OF THE LUNG

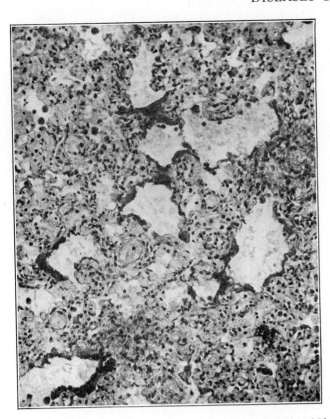

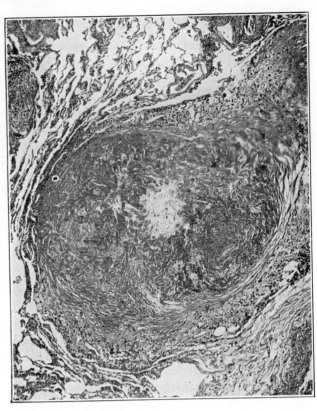

FIG. 424.—LUNG: BRONCHOPNEUMONIA (INTERSTITIAL).—(Cf. CASES 180 and 181).—The striking histologic feature is the presence of a hyalinized eosinophilic staining "asphyxial" membrane lining certain of the alveoli. Note likewise the abundant interstitial exudate. App. 100 x.

FIG. 425.—LUNG: SILICOSIS.—CASE 185.—A circumscribed avascular nodule composed of concentric hyalinized laminae of collagen, undergoing degeneration centrally, and with a peripheral pseudocapsular layer of productive inflammatory fibrosis. App. 50 x.

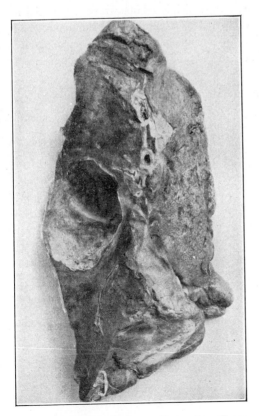

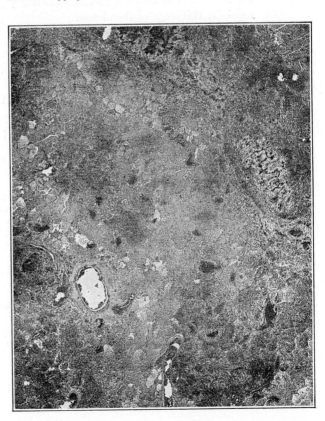

FIG. 426.—LUNG: ABSCESS.—CASE 183.—Gross photograph of large abscess cavity lined by a thickened pyogenic membrane, and which contained a quantity of thick, grayish-yellow pus.

FIG. 427.—LUNG: MULTIPLE BRONCHIECTATIC ABSCESSES WITH ASSOCIATED PULMONARY SUPPURATION (Cf. CASE 48—Fig. 110).—Note the abscessed areas arising as an extension of a suppurative bronchiectasis and the associated diffuse pneumonitis. App. 25 x.

show evidence of the previous inflammatory pneumonic process.

ORGANIZATION.—In certain cases, the patient, instead of having a classical drop in temperature by crisis over a period of a few hours, shows a gradual drop in his fever more like the picture seen in bronchopneumonia. This gradual return to normal is spoken of as lysis and is usually associated with a very different picture pathologically in the lung. Such cases represent instances of so-called "delayed resolution" and are usually complicated by a good deal of lung destruction, unlike the typical uncomplicated case of lobar pneumonia. Considerable difference of opinion exists regarding the nature of this process. Many observers hold that it is always associated with a simple pneumococcic type of lobar pneumonia which, due to specific individual differences in immunity response and to a presumed unusual virulence of the infecting organism results in a diffuse, destructive process. Others believe that this represents a complication of a pneumococcic lobar pneumonia by some secondary organism usually one of the streptococci, although the Friedländer bacillus and other organisms have been incriminated at times.

The pathology grossly is characterized by a lung which is extremely firm due to a widespread fibrosis. On pressure, little or no exudate can be forced from the alveoli as one would expect in an ordinary pneumonia at this stage of the disease.

Microscopically the picture consists of an organization of the fibrinous exudate by fibroblasts growing out from the alveolar walls (Fig. 418 and 419).

This is identical in its characteristics histologically as is the organization of fibrin in any other similar exudate. The fibrin, instead of being digested persists in the alveoli. This is due in part to the fact that for some unexplained reason the polynuclear leukocytes are not called out in adequte numbers. Thus, their proteolytic activity is absent in the inflammatory process. As a makeshift measure, the exudate accordingly undergoes this secondary type of repair by organization. This is manifested by a process comparable to granulation tissue with new capillary vessels and connective tissue growing into the alveolar spaces and in many instances completely obliterating them. Where lining alveolar cells have not been destroyed, they will proliferate to form abortive vesicles. Many of these are not connected with the bronchial tree and remain functionless.

BRONCHI IN LOBAR PNEUMONIA.—Nothing has been said up to the present time of the state of the bronchi. In the early stages, the mucous membrane is congested, reddish-gray in color, and the submucosa may be swollen. Inflammatory edema and considerable cellular exudate may be present. In red and later gray hepatization, the small bronchioles may contain first fibrin and later a pus-like exudate, some of which is expectorated. During gray hepatization and resolution the swelling disappears. There is some desquamation of the lining epithelium. There is apparently no damage to the elastic tissues or the muscular coat, which is an important differential feature as compared to streptococcic pneumonias. Thus, the classical pneumonococcic lobar pneumonia is not a factor in the production of bronchiectasis.

ILLUSTRATIVE CASE

CASE 176. (Ref. #S-21)

Diagnosis.—Lung—lobar pneumonia, stage of red hepatization.

Patient was a white male of 44 years, admitted to the hospital with marked pain in his chest, dyspnea and a high fever.

Present Illness.—Patient had a cold about two weeks before his present illness. He seemed to be recovering perfectly normally from this when suddenly, two days before admission, he developed a severe chill and a high fever. This was accompanied by marked dyspnea and a severe pain in the upper part of his right chest. This was made much worse by coughing. He noticed that he raised a small amount of sputum, which was "rusty" in color.

Past Medical History.—Past medical history was entirely irrelevant. The patient had had the usual childhood infections. He had never been particularly subject to upper respiratory infections. He had never been seri-

ously ill before and had never had any operations. A review of his systems was entirely negative.

Physical Examination.—Patient was an adult white male who appeared acutely ill. His breathing was rapid and shallow with marked dilatation of his alae nasi. He had a rather cyanotic appearance to his mucous membranes and nail beds. Head was not remarkable. Eyes, ears, and nose were negative. Throat showed a moderate dusky congestion of the pharynx. His chest was symmetrical but expansion was markedly restricted on the right side. There was marked dullness over the upper and lower lobes on the right with hyperresonance over the middle lobe area. Typical bronchial breathing was heard over the dull areas. The left lung was essentially normal on percussion and auscultation except for a few scattered crepitant râles, which disappeared on coughing. Heart rate was 132. Heart sounds were distant and seemed somewhat feeble. No murmurs were heard. Blood pressure was 120/80. Liver was somewhat enlarged, being palpa-

PLATE CI

DISEASES OF THE RESPIRATORY SYSTEM

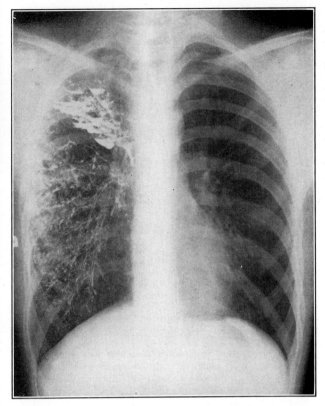

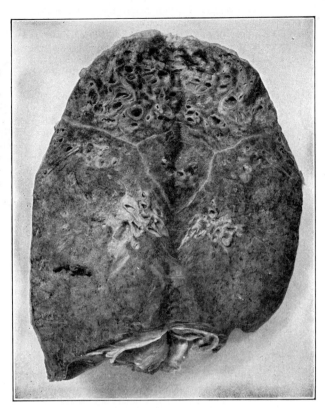

Fig. 428.—Roentgenogram: Chest—Bronchiectasis.—Case 184. —Extensive right upper lobe bronchiectasis revealed following lipiodol instillation.

Fig. 429.—Lung: Bronchiectasis.—Case 184.—Dilated, thick-walled upper lobe bronchi and bronchioles, with marked fibrosis of the surrounding lung parenchyma.

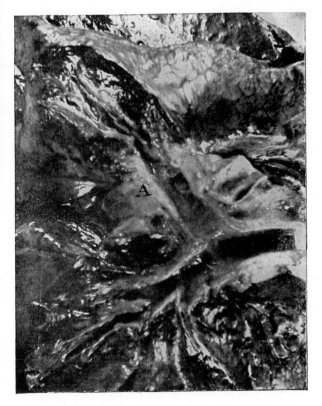

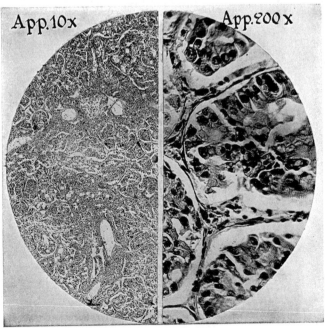

Fig. 430.—Lung: Bronchogenic Carcinoma.—Cf. Case 189.— Stenosis of right primary bronchus at (A) with distal atelectasis as a result of an endobronchial annual carcinoma.

Fig. 431.—Lung: Alveolar Carcinoma.—Case 190.—High and low power photomicrographs showing the alveoli of the lungs filled with tumor cells without infiltration of the walls and grossly resembling gray hepatization in lobar pneumonia.

ble two fingers' breadth below the costal margin. The extremities were negative.

Laboratory Findings.—On admission, the red cell count was 4,600,000 with 87% hemoglobin, and the white blood count was 17,000 with 80% polynuclears. Sputum was positive for Type 3 pneumococcus by the Neufeld technique. Urinalysis was negative.

X-ray examination showed complete consolidation of the right upper and lower lobes with an area of lung tissue containing air in the position of the middle lobe.

Subsequent Course.—Patient grew progressively worse. The white blood count, instead of rising as indicative of an adequate defense mechanism, fell to 7,000 with only 68% polynuclears. This was felt to be of extremely poor prognostic significance. The patient died on the fifth day following the onset of his disease.

Autopsy Findings.—Pericardium showed acute fibrinous pericarditis. Heart revealed marked myocardosis. Right pleura showed an acute fibrinous pleuritis. Right lung showed lobar pneumonia in the stage of late red hepatization. Left lung showed compensatory emphysema, congestion and pulmonary edema. There was parenchymatous degeneration of the liver; nephrosis of the kidneys, and toxic splenitis.

Lungs: The right lung filled the right chest completely. The upper and lower lobes were consolidated and airless throughout. Over their surface a thick fibrinous exudate was present. On section, the cut surface was dry, and pale reddish gray in color. The surface was slightly rough and granular. The middle lobe showed emphysema.

Microscopic Description of a Section Through the Lung.—(Fig. 411 and 412) Histologic examination shows the air vesicles to be filled with an acute fibrinous exudate. This is seen especially massed over the surface of the alveolar lining cells. In many places, strands of fibrin are seen passing between the cells of the alveolar wall. Many polynuclear leukocytes are seen in the section, some few of them in the interstitial tissue of the alveolar wall around the still dilated capillaries, but most of them have migrated into the air vesicles between the strands of fibrin. Here and there the fibrin shows contraction away from the alveolar wall leaving a clear space between the exudate and the wall. Many of the lining alveolar wall cells have become desquamated. In addition to the leucocytes and fibrin, there are large numbers of red cells in varying stages of hemolysis. Mononuclear phagocytes have converted much of the hemoglobin into hemosiderin which appears within their cytoplasm.

ILLUSTRATIVE CASE

CASE 177. (Ref. #S-197)

Diagnosis.—Lobar pneumonia, stage of gray hepatization.

Patient was a white male of 29 years, admitted to the hospital acutely ill.

Present Illness.—The patient's present illness began five days before admission at which time he developed a mild upper respiratory infection with a slight cough. This was followed the next day by a severe chill with a high temperature and a stabbing type of pain in his right chest. He likewise complained of extreme difficulty in breathing.

Past Medical History.—The patient's childhood history included all the usual minor contagious diseases with the addition of scarlet fever. At the age of fifteen, he had what was diagnosed as a mild attack of rheumatic fever characterized by fleeting joint pains and the development of a mitral valvular lesion, which, however, did not interfere with his normal activities except to limit his athletic ambitions. A review of his systems otherwise was negative. He had the usual number of mild upper respiratory infections, but had never had any serious illness. His gastro-intestinal history was negative. He denied venereal infection.

Physical Examination.—Patient was a young white male who appeared critically ill. Temperature was 104°, pulse 130 and respirations, 45 per minute. Head was normal in shape. Eyes reacted sluggishly. Nose was negative. Ears were negative. Throat was congested and contained a considerable amount of mucopurulent secretion. Chest showed marked limitation of expansion on the right side. There was dullness over the entire right lung with almost hyperresonance over the left lung. Heart was considerably enlarged to the left with the apex felt in the sixth interspace in the midaxillary line. A double mitral murmur was heard at the apex which was transmitted to the axilla. Moderate clubbing of his fingers was accompanied by marked cyanosis of the nail beds

and of the mucous membranes. Abdomen was somewhat distended. Liver was definitely enlarged two fingers' breadth below the costal margin. Extremities were negative.

Laboratory Findings.—On admission the red count was 4,600,000 with 87% hemoglobin, and the white blood count was 16,400 cells with 84% polymorphonuclear leukocytes. Sputum examination revealed a pneumococcus, which by the Neufeld technique was shown to be Type 15.

Subsequent Course.—The patient went progressively downhill, his cyanosis and dyspnea increasing. The blood count rose to 28,000 white cells with 92% polynuclears. Terminally, he showed acute cardiac decompensation and died three days after admission on the seventh day of his illness.

Autopsy Findings.—Heart showed acute bacterial endocarditis with fenestration of the mitral valve, old rheumatic valvulitis, hypertrophy and dilatation. The right lung showed lobar pneumonia in the stage of gray hepatization. The left lung showed compensatory emphysema. There was congestion of the spleen, liver, etc.

Lungs: The right lung was covered with acute fibrinous exudate. The entire lung was consolidated and airless. On section, the cut surface was grayish in color, moist and a pus-like exudate could be squeezed from the vesicles. Lymph nodes were enlarged and reddish-gray in color.

Microscopic Description of a Section Through the Lung.—(Fig. 414 and 415) Histologic study of the lung tissue shows a uniform pathological process with all the alveoli filled with a fibrinopurulent exudate. The fibrin shows a considerable amount of lytic degeneration and there is a great deal of granular debris. Many of the polymorphonuclear cells are necrotic in appearance with their nuclear chromatin broken-up. A considerable number of large mononuclear phagocytic cells are present in the exudate. These likewise show a considerable degree of degeneration. The tissue includes a portion of the pleura which is seen to be enormously thickened. This is the result of acute dilatation of the capillaries and diffuse seropurulent infiltration of the subpleural connective tissue. The serosal cells have largely been destroyed and there is an acute fibrinous exudate overlying the pleural surface. Sections stained by Gram's method show the presence of large numbers of organisms. Many of these are intracellular, the majority are found lying free in the alveolar exudate. The alveolar walls appear to be intact.

ILLUSTRATIVE CASE

CASE 178. (Ref. #S-22)

Diagnosis.—Lung—organizing lobar pneumonia.

Patient was a white male of 58 years, admitted to the hospital with the chief complaint of pain and swelling of the tongue.

Present Illness.—The patient's present illness began approximately a year earlier when he first noticed some thickening of the right side of his tongue. This became rather sore and an area of redness and swelling around this thickened mucosa was seen. His physician thought it to be a simple inflammatory process and treated it locally for several months. The inflammatory process more or less subsided, but the surface of the tongue seemed to become thicker and thicker. During this period, he paid very little attention to the lesion because it was not particularly painful. Recently, however, he noted a marked increase in his symptoms with swelling of the tongue, and extreme tenderness which interfered with his ability to swallow or to speak. During this interval he had lost about fifty pounds in weight.

Past Medical History.—His past medical history was entirely irrelevant in respect to his present illness. He had had the usual childhood infections. He had had no serious illness during his entire life. A review of his systems was essentially negative.

Physical Examination.—The patient was a fairly well-developed, emaciated, elderly white male. Head showed no gross deformity. Pupils reacted normally. Nose was negative. Tongue was markedly swollen, chiefly on the right side. It was fiery red in color. There was a whitish plaque of thickened epithelium which showed an irregular, serpiginous margin and an ulcerated central area. The anterior and posterior chains of cervical lymph nodes on the right were greatly swollen. The throat otherwise was negative. Chest was symmetrical. Lungs were clear. Heart was apparently negative. Abdomen was negative. Extremities were normal.

Laboratory Findings.—The laboratory findings, on admission showed a red blood count of 3,100,000 with 63% hemoglobin. White blood cells 12,100 with 79% polynuclears. Urinalysis was negative.

Subsequent Course.—A biopsy of the lesion revealed it to be a typical Grade II squamous cell carcinoma. It was treated intensely with radium implantation with marked regression of the primary growth. However, he had a very extensive reaction of his tissues with sloughing of the tumor. He developed what was believed to be an aspiration pneumonia, but on physical examination this was found to involve the entire right lower lobe. It came on suddenly with a chill and a temperature rising to 103°. Respirations averaged about 30 and his pulse 110. This process failed to clear up at the end of the usual ten days or two weeks, and a new area involving the other lower lobe developed. The patient succumbed to this second lobe infection. Sputum examination revealed the organism to be of a type 2 Pneumococcus.

Autopsy Findings.—At autopsy there were the remnants of the squamous carcinoma of the tongue, which showed extensive necrosis and ulceration with suppuration. There was a generalized metastatic tumor involvement of the cervical nodes on the right side. The lungs showed a massive terminal bronchopneumonia of the left lower lobe. The right lower lobe showed a typical unresolved pneumonia which seemed to have a large amount of connective tissue in it grossly, suggesting organization.

Microscopic Description of a Section Through the Lung.—(Fig. 418 and 419) Histologic examination of the lung tissue presents the typical picture of a diffuse organizing type of pneumonia. The alveolar walls show extensive destruction in many places. The entire lung architecture is distorted. The alveoli are filled with fibrinous exudate, which in many places shows complete replacement by connective tissue. This newly-formed fibrous tissue is seen growing out from the alveolar walls and carrying with it a new capillary blood supply. In places there is some remnant of the air sac seen as a somewhat crescentic space between the alveolar wall and a large mass of this potential scar tissue. In some places, persistent fibrin can be recognized. In many of the air spaces, large mononuclear cells are seen, many of them containing hemosiderin. A few persistent polymorphonuclears are likewise noted. The histologic picture is typical of a very extensive lobar type of pneumonia associated with destruction of the lung parenchyma and secondary fibrous tissue organization and repair.

PART II

BRONCHOPNEUMONIA

Bronchopneumonia in contrast to lobar pneumonia may be defined as a patchy type of consolidation scattered throughout both lungs, but usually more prominently in the lower lobes. It occurs particularly at the two extremes of age; in infancy and childhood, and in old age, although it may be seen at any time, particularly in relation to epidemic diseases of the respiratory tract, such as influenza.

Under the microscope, this patchy distribution of the pneumonic consolidation is found to occur in two major forms. On the one hand, we find a distribution which corresponds to the terminal alveoli of the anatomical bronchial lobule, which suggests a direct descending type of infection. On the other hand, we see a variety of bronchopneumonia, which is characterized primarily by a local peribronchial reaction which extends to those pulmonary alveoli adjacent to the bronchus or bronchiole. More will be said about these two varieties as the discussion proceeds. Strictly speaking, the old term, "lobular pneumonia," should be confined to the first of these two varieties.

Contributory Etiologic Factors in the Development of Bronchopneumonia.—Bronchopneumonia is a frequent complication of almost any of the infectious upper respiratory diseases, particularly measles, whooping cough, influenza, scarlet fever and diphtheria. It may be observed during the course of typhoid fever and glanders. A variety of bronchopneumonia is observed following the inhalation of irritating gases, such as chlorine, ammonia, bromine, nitrogen trioxide, mustard gas or phosgene. This is usually spoken of as *chemical pneumonia*. It is commonly observed as a terminal event and the immediate cause of death in elderly individuals or in bedridden patients suffering from wasting or debilitating diseases. This variety of bronchopneumonia is known as *hypostatic* or *terminal bronchopneumonia*. The insufflation of organic material such as blood, mucus, vomitus, fragments of adenoid or tonsillar tissue during operations upon the upper respiratory tract, leads to the development of a relatively localized variety of bronchopneumonia, which very commonly subsequently progresses to suppuration. This type is called *postoperative* or *inhalation pneumonia*. In children, particularly, the inhalation of various types of lipoid material, especially mineral oil as used in nasal sprays, and cod liver oil as employed for its vitamin value, may also result in the development of a type of bronchopneumonia spoken of as *lipoid pneumonia*.

Bacteriology.—Bronchopneumonia has no specific bacteriology as is the case in lobar pneumonia where the infection is almost regularly due to the pneumococcus. The streptococcus is the organism most frequently found in bronchopneumonia, but a host of other bacteria may be responsible for the secondary pneumonic consolidation of the lung.

It is highly probable that the development of many varieties of bronchopneumonia is preceded or accompanied by an underlying filtrable virus infection. Just as recent experimental work by Dochez in relation to the common cold or coryza and of Smith, Andrews and Laidlaw in respect to influenza has shown that these conditions are primarily caused by a filtrable virus with the secondary clinical picture depending upon the nature of the accompanying bacteria, so it seems highly probable that many of the various types of bronchopneumonia may be similarly initiated by a virus with the secondary symptoms caused by the subsequent bacterial invaders. The various forms of streptococci, but particularly the hemolytic variety are the most important of these secondary invaders, both from the standpoint of incidence and severity of the infection. The pneumococci are much less frequently seen, but particularly in infancy are prone to give rise to a bronchopneumonic rather than a lobar pneumonic picture when they invade the lung. The influenza bacillus, alone or in combination with other bacteria is also very frequently encountered. In the aspiration forms of pneumonia, the staphylococci are especially important. In the light of our present knowledge regarding the bacteriology of the upper respiratory tract, it is very difficult to evaluate the relative significance of the finding of any given type of organism in the sputum. The part played by the anaerobic bacteria is a field which is just beginning to be explored. It is quite conceivable that our whole concept regarding the problem of bacterial infection in the respiratory tract will undergo extensive modification within a comparatively brief period of time.

Clinical features of Bronchopneumonia.—In contrast to the sudden onset seen on lobar pneumonia, bronchopneumonia is ushered in by an insidious sequence of symptoms, usually starting as a mild upper respiratory infection and gradually extending clinically to involve the trachea and bronchi in an inflammatory process which may eventuate in the development of actual patchy consolidation of the lung. The course is usually prolonged. The physical findings and the symptoms vary from day to day. As one area seems to improve, a new area lights up and relapses are common. The spreading nature of the bronchopneumonic process has been compared to the smoldering of a brush fire, which as fast as it is beaten out in one place springs up again at some distant point. Clinically, the temperature rarely reaches as high a point as in lobar pneumonia. Unlike lobar pneumonia there is likely to be a rather wider diurnal range. The leukocyte count rarely rises as high, and the symptoms in general are less severe. Cyanosis is not as marked. Respiratory difficulty is not as prominent, but owing to the prolonged nature of the infection and the fact that the great majority of cases of bronchopneumonia occur in individuals whose resistance is low, there is a high mortality rate.

Mode of Transmission.—Rather more definitely than in the case of lobar pneumonia, bronchopneumonia appears to be a direct contact infection from one patient to another, although this is often not any more apparent than in many cases of the lobar type. The fact that the great majority of these infections start as mild upper respiratory lesions accounts for this more ready transmissibility. Blake and Cecil in their experimental work on streptococcic pneumonias in monkeys have shown that the organisms apparently enter the peribronchial lymphatics in much the same way as does the *Pneumococcus* in lobar pneumonia. They emphasize the fact that the marked inflammatory reaction which occurs in these peribronchial tissues is responsible to a large extent in preventing the spread of the infection throughout the lung as they feel that it leads to local inhalation and results in the patchy consolidation so familiar as bronchopneumonia. They further comment upon the fact that the entrance of the streptococcus into the lung tissue is greatly facilitated by previous inoculation of the animal by insufflation of influenza bacilli. This appeared to lower the animal's resistance. Such a mechanism offers the simplest explanation for the amazing variation in the clinical picture which is seen in the almost infinite forms of bronchopneumonia.

Pathology.—Grossly, the lung, which is the seat of a bronchopneumonic infection, shows many small, firm areas scattered through the parenchyma of both lungs (Fig. 420). This is not necessarily a symmetrical lesion, however, and the major pathological process may be found in one or more of the lobes. These consolidated areas often may be more satisfactorily palpated than seen. The pleural surface, as a rule, is smooth and glistening and free from any evidence of acute inflammation unless the area of consolidation is immediately beneath the pleura. Under such circumstances, a delicate fibrinous exudate may be found overlying the pneumonic area. The picture varies tremendously in different cases. At times the areas of consolidation are so numerous that

they become confluent and present a picture difficult to differentiate from a lobar pneumonia. This is particularly true of the more severe fatal cases of epidemic influenzal pneumonia.

Examination of the lung in bronchopneumonia either through the pleural surface or on cross section will show three distinct lesions: (1) the patchy areas of consolidation already described; (2) areas of atelectasis which result usually from obstruction of a bronchiole or bronchus in an area adjacent to the consolidated area (these are likewise congested in appearance and at times are difficult to differentiate from the actual area of consolidation); and (3) areas of compensatory emphysema. The emphysema is comparatively easily recognized as it tends to be lighter in color than the consolidated and atelectatic areas and to be somewhat elevated as compared to them on cut section. Not infrequently pressure upon the lung will result in the appearance of a small amount of pus-like exudate from the infected areas. This is likely to be particularly prominent about the terminal bronchioles.

The bronchi and trachea are usually of a reddish color which varies in its intensity depending upon the severity of the infectious agent. There is usually an associated catarrhal mucopurulent exudate which tends to cling to the congested surface. Not infrequently superficial erosion of the mucosa is present. It is this exudate which frequently plugs small bronchi and bronchioles and results in the atelectasis previously described. Such atelectasis likewise tends to be followed by extension of the infection to the atelectatic area and Coryllos has emphasized the importance of atelectasis as one of the factors in the spread of the bronchopneumonic process.

The ever changing physical signs are due in part to the fact that during paroxysms of coughing, the patient clears the exudate from some of these obstructed atelectatic areas so that dullness or changes in tactile or vocal fremitus occur with frequency. More important, however, in respect to these changing signs is the migratory nature of the infection from one lobule to another. Just as in lobar pneumonia, the various stages of consolidation and resolution follow so that as the lesion spreads from one area to another in the lung the picture will vary considerably, some places showing intense congestion; others being grayish in color as the result of leukocytic exudation, and still others becoming soft and undergoing liquefaction of the exudate.

Histologically, the picture of bronchopneumonia occurs, as has been intimated in two distinct forms; (1) *lobular* pneumonia (Fig. 422), a type in which exudate is chiefly confined to groups of alveoli which represent terminal lobules; and (2) an *interstitial* and peribronchial (Fig. 420 and 423) variety characterized by a very marked involvement of the respiratory tree with pneumonic consolidation of the alveoli immediately adjacent to the peribronchial tissues. This is easily recognized under the microscope by the collar-like arrangement of the exudate outlining the bronchial tree. The peribronchial inflammation is apt to extend out into the interstitial lung parenchyma for a variable distance and gives rise to a rather characteristic picture spoken of as *"interstitial pneumonitis."* In the milder forms of such inflammatory reaction, which are seen particularly in the early stages of such virus infections as measles and influenza, this interstitial pneumonitis is the only outstanding pathological feature. With the advent of secondary infection, however, the characteristic consolidation of the surrounding alveoli occurs and the picture becomes confused, being complicated not infrequently further by a typical lobular type of lesion as well. As has already been mentioned, in the more overwhelming type of infections, the inflammatory process involves so many contiguous lobules that the resultant picture is spoken of as a diffuse, confluent bronchopneumonia. It may involve the major part of one or more lobes of the lung and cause some confusion to the uninitiated in differentiating the process from that of lobar pneumonia.

In the interstitial peribronchial type of lesion, the inflammatory reaction of the respiratory tree is often extremely severe and is accompanied by extensive desquamation of the lining epithelium. This is followed by diffuse infiltration of the wall by exudative cells which, however, curiously enough, consist chiefly of mononuclears. This is advanced by many as further evidence of the presumptive virus nature of the underlying inflammatory reaction. In the larger bronchi, the process appears to be limited by the cartilaginous rings, but in the bronchioles where cartilage is absent, the involvement of the entire wall results frequently in weakening. This is followed in many cases by bronchiectasis. The inflammatory edema and inflammation extends out into the adjacent interalveolar septa as the process advances. This is followed by invasion of the vesicle by an exudate consisting of mixed cytology with a variable amount of fibrin. In certain types of bronchopneumonia, notably those due to streptococcic infections following measles, pertussis and influenza, there develops a membrane-like lining to the alveolus, frequently referred to as an *"asphyxial membrane"* (Fig. 424). This is similar in appearance to that seen in the pneumonia of the newborn following aspiration of amniotic fluid in labor. It is hyaline in appearance and takes the eosin stain intensely. In the more severe instances it is possible that this may act as an impermeable membrane and interfere seriously with pulmonary ventilation resulting in cyanosis of the patient. At times this membrane appears to represent a hyaline degeneration of the lining cells. At other times, it seems to consist of fused, hyalinized cellular debris and fibrin and at times it seems as if both factors were combined.

With these general comments regarding the nature of the bronchopneumonic process in contradistinction to that of lobar pneumonia, a brief discussion of some of the more important varieties seems to be of some value in gaining a clearer understanding of the subject.

BACTERIAL TYPES OF BRONCHOPNEUMONIA

Pneumococcic Bronchopneumonia.—As has already been emphasized, the *Pneumococcus* may at times give rise to a bronchopneumonia instead of the more usual lobar type. This is seen particularly in infants and young children and in the aged, where it is much more commonly encountered than the lobar picture. As a secondary invader in other upper respiratory infections, it likewise may result in a similar patchy pneumococcic consolidation of the lung, particularly in influenzal pneumonia. As the next most frequent secondary invader to the *Streptococcus,* the *Pneumococcus* is responsible for many of the very severe and confluent forms of such pneumonias. By many, the development of an "asphyxial membrane" in such infections is believed to be seen much more commonly in such secondary pneumococcic and streptococcic infections.

Streptococcic Pneumonia.—The lesion in the lung resulting from streptococcal invasion depends upon whether it is of the hemolytic or non-hemolytic type, and upon its virulence. In the average case, the resultant pneumonia is of the lobular variety, as described above. In the more severe cases, the areas become confluent and a consolidation of lobar extent may be produced. In every case there is considerable damage to the bronchioles causing weakening of the wall and ectasia. At times, due to marked tissue resistance, an interstitial pneumonitis results. This is prone to occur following the so-called "contagious"

diseases: measles, whooping cough, scarlet fever, diphtheria, and also influenza. Frequently in streptococcal pneumonias, rather striking vascular changes are seen. The wall and perivascular connective tissue may show inflammatory edema and cellular infiltration. This may be accompanied by varying degrees of degeneration and necrosis of the vessel wall itself, with the production of a true arteritis or phlebitis.

ILLUSTRATIVE CASE

CASE 179. (Ref. #S-20)

Diagnosis.—Lung—lobular bronchopneumonia.

Patient was a Negro of 66 years, admitted to the hospital complaining of a cough, feverishness and weakness.

Present Illness.—The onset of the present illness began about one month before admission at which time he developed a severe cold. This did not seem to clear up as it should and he noticed that he kept having mild chills at intervals accompanied by a definite fever. He had some increase in the rate of his respirations and was bothered by a productive cough, raising considerable thick, greenish-yellow, mucopurulent sputum. On two or three occasions he had noticed that this sputum was blood streaked. These symptoms had been accompanied by anorexia and several attacks of epistaxis.

Past Medical History.—The patient was known to have had scarlet fever in childhood. He believed he had all of the minor contagious diseases as well. He had never had any serious illness during his more active adult life. For the past several years he had suffered from headache and vertigo. He had been told that he had high blood pressure. He had also noticed at times a puffiness under his eyes in the morning, and for a year or more had had to get up at least three or four times a night to urinate. He had never had any operations and had never previously been hospitalized. A review of his systems otherwise was not particularly informatory. He denied venereal disease.

Physical Examination.—The patient was acutely ill and showed an almost stertorous type of breathing. At the time of admission, he was in a state of almost semi-stupor. Head was not remarkable. Pupils showed bilateral arcus senilis. Ears and nose were negative. Throat was moderately congested. Chest was symmetrical and somewhat emphysematous in appearance. His lung findings could better be described as diminished resonance over both bases than actual dullness. There were scattered râles throughout both sides of his chest, most marked at the lung bases. There was a questionable area of consolidation at the base of the right lower lobe. Heart was slightly enlarged. There were no murmurs. The blood pressure was 150/100. Abdomen was negative. Extremities were negative.

Laboratory Findings.—The blood count, on admission, showed 4,200,000 red cells with 78% hemoglobin, and a white count of 12,800 cells with 83% polymorphonuclear leukocytes, of which 15% were young forms. Urinalysis showed a strongly positive albumin test, and the sediment was found to contain many hyaline casts. Blood Chemistry: Urea was 90 mgm. on admission and

rose to 180 mgm. before his death. The creatinine correspondingly gave values of 6 and 14 respectively.

X-ray examination presented the typical fuzzy appearance of rather diffuse bronchial pneumonia.

Subsequent Course.—The patient went into profound stupor and died, with the clinical picture of a uremia complicated by a diffuse, patchy bronchopneumonia of nearly a month's duration.

Autopsy Findings.—Heart was moderately enlarged but showed no valvular lesions. The enlargement was of the concentric hypertrophic type, involving the left ventricle chiefly. The lungs showed a diffuse, patchy bronchopneumonia throughout all five lobes, but most marked in the right lower lobe where there was an area of consolidation about 5 cm. in diameter. The kidneys suggested a chronic glomerular nephritis. They were diminished in size, irregular in appearance on their cut surface and the capsule stripped with difficulty leaving many depressed scars.

Microscopic Description of Section Through the Lung.—(Fig. 422) Histologic examination of the lung tissue presents the typical picture of lobular pneumonia. The smaller bronchi and bronchioles show marked dilatation of the capillaries and lymphatics. This is accompanied by considerable perivascular cellular infiltration and edema of the tissues. Marked desquamation of the surface epithelium is seen. The lumen of the bronchi and bronchioles is filled with this desquamated cellular debris and mucus, as well as many inflammatory cells, chiefly broken down leukocytes. Scattered through the lung substance are found focal areas of inflammatory reaction. These seem to arise in relation to terminal bronchioles and their corresponding atria. The walls of the alveoli in these areas show marked congestion with dilatation of the capillaries and a variable amount of interstitial infiltration. More striking, however, is the inflammatory exudate within the alveolar spaces. This reaction varies in different parts of the lung. In some areas one can find a picture which corresponds closely to the stage of red hepatization in the lobar type of pneumonia. This is characterized by marked congestion and the presence of a fibrinous exudate with many red cells and beginning polymorphonuclear infiltration. In other areas a picture not unlike that of gray hepatization is seen where the fibrin is undergoing lysis and the exudate is composed almost entirely of polymorphonuclear cells, many of them showing marked degenerative changes. In still other areas, a picture corresponding to resolution is seen where little or no fibrin can be recognized in the exudate, but a great deal of broken down, purulent cellular debris is seen, and the cellular reaction is almost entirely mononuclear in character, with large mononuclear phagocytes predominating. The histology suggests a picture of a migratory, wandering type of infection, which involves first one branch of the bronchus and then another with one area showing early acute inflammatory changes, while others show the end stage of the infection, with the clearing up of the exudate.

ILLUSTRATIVE CASE

CASE 180. (Ref. #S-152)

Diagnosis.—Lung—acute interstitial pneumonitis with secondary peribronchial bronchopneumonia with pertussis.

Patient was a white female child of 2 years, admitted to the hospital on the twenty-first day of her illness with a clinical picture of pneumonia.

Present Illness.—The onset of the patient's illness dated back definitely to a period three weeks earlier when her parents first noted that she developed a cough. In going over the history more thoroughly, it was found that this represented an incubation period in respect to exposure to pertussis of ten days. The child developed the characteristic cough of pertussis and was acutely ill with the disease. She gagged almost constantly with her paroxysms and was unable to retain any appreciable amount of food. At the time of admission, she showed marked malnutrition. She had developed a temperature which seemed somewhat disproportionate to the usual picture of uncomplicated pertussis and showed a certain amount of difficulty with breathing, which worried her parents considerably. During the preceding twenty-four hours before admission the child had become almost stuporous. She was seen by a physician who immediately referred the case to the hospital for care.

Past Medical History.—The child had been a full-term normally delivered child and had had no previous illness. She had had no nutritional difficulties having been nursed for the first eight months of her existence and having been on a modified general diet since that time. She was exposed to whooping cough by a neighbor's child ten days before she developed any symptoms.

Physical Examination.—The patient was a fairly well developed but definitely dehydrated and emaciated two-year-old white female child. Head was essentially negative. Eyes showed an internal strabismus with considerable lateral nystagmus. There was no discharge from either ear. Throat was moderately congested. The cervical lymph nodes were definitely enlarged but not tender. Chest was symmetrical. Breath sounds were diminished over the entire chest and innumerable râles were heard over both lung fields. The heart did not appear to be enlarged and no murmurs could be heard. Abdomen was negative. Extremities showed hyperactive reflexes.

Laboratory Findings.—The red cell count was 3,200,-000 cells with 70% hemoglobin. White blood cells 86,000 with 98% small lymphocytes and 2% polynuclears. Urinalysis showed the presence of a considerable amount of albumin but no other abnormalities.

Subsequent Course.—The patient was in an almost moribund condition at the time of admission and went rapidly downhill dying twenty-four hours later. The diagnosis of bronchopneumonia complicating pertussis was made and the suspicion raised as to whether there might not be an actual encephalitis found at autopsy.

Autopsy Findings.—Pertussis from the history; diffuse interstitial pneumonitis and peribronchial bronchopneumonia; thymic atrophy; acute toxic encephalitis.

Microscopic Description of Section Through the Lung.—(Fig. 420 and 423) Histologic study of the lung tissue presents a typical picture of a descending type of infection relating to the bronchioles and peribronchial tissues. This is characterized by marked cellular infiltration of these structures with what appears to be an actual increase in the amount of peribronchial connective tissue. The inflammatory process extends out into the lung alveolar walls for a variable distance in relation to the peribronchial lesions. In this instance, the great majority of the cells are found to be small round cells of the lymphoid series, although many large mononuclear phagocytes and occasional plasma cells are also seen. Towards the lung tissue itself, more polynuclears begin to appear. Complicating this basic underlying picture of pertussis, pneumonitis and peribronchitis, is seen a secondary associated bronchopneumonia. This has obviously arisen through contiguity, the exudative picture being restricted to those groups of pulmonary alveoli surrounding the bronchi. They do not appear to bear any definite relationship to the terminal air vesicles of the individual bronchial lobule. This secondary pneumonia is characterized by the usual fibrinous and polymorphonuclear leukocytic outpouring into the air spaces. Here and there some suggestion of beginning asphyxial membrane formation is noted with hyalinization of the fibrin and the alveolar lining cells. Varying degrees of lysis of the fibrin and breaking down of the leukocytes are seen.

For another example of this same type of bronchopneumonia in a case of measles refer to Case 73 (Ref. #S-191), Chapter XIX.

Influenza, Influenzal Pneumonia.—Influenza in its mild form is characterized by inflammation of the upper respiratory tract in the form of a tracheobronchitis, frequently associated with infection of the accessory sinuses and accompanied by a low fever, marked prostration and leukopenia; in its severe form, by actual pneumonic consolidation accompanied by an unusual degree of dyspnea and cyanosis. The disease is ordinarily endemic and mild and the death rate low, but occasionally it is seen in pandemic form, rapidly spreading over the entire world and with a high mortality rate.

Etiologically, the disease is believed to be due to a filtrable virus, with the *influenza* bacillus, *streptococcus* and *pneumococcus* as secondary invaders. In the mild case, it is quite common to recover the influenza bacillus in almost pure culture from the throat. In the severe case, hemolytic streptococci usually predominate and often over-grow the influenza bacilli. Occasionally, the pneumococcus is recovered. Since the 1918 epidemic, an enormous amount of experimental work has accumulated in respect to the etiology of the disease. Either a virus alone, or a virus in combination with the influenza bacillus are the more generally held theories to-day. There are still those who maintain that the disease is due to the influenza bacillus alone. However, the experimental inoculation of pure cultures into the throats of volunteer workers and various animals has failed to substantiate this theory. The work of Shope on swine influenza, a disease which he proved was due to a virus in combination with the *Haemophilus influenzae suis* led to the belief that influenza was the result of a virus combination with the *Hemophilus influenzae*.

The recent work of Smith, Andrewes and Laidlaw has further established the virus origin of the disease. Using ferrets, they were able to produce infection by filtrates from the nose and throat of patients recovering from influenza. Pneumonic lesions were produced when the animals were anesthetized before injection of the virus. Serum obtained from animals recovering from the disease was found to neutralize the virus obtained from various parts of the world during the last epidemic. In view of this work, the virus etiology of influenza seems fairly well established although it is always dangerous to compare animal and human in experimental work.

It is possible that in mild cases which result in very slight lesions of the respiratory tract, the virus alone is responsible. In slightly more serious cases, with evidence of interstitial pneumonitis and peribronchial involvement, the influenza bacillus is probably in part responsible; whereas in the more exten-sive frank pneumonic consolidation seen in epidemic influenza and accompanied by a high mortality rate, organisms such as streptococci or pneumococci act with heightened virulence in the presence of this virus-influenza bacillus combination.

PATHOLOGY.—Pure virus lesions probably are represented only by a tracheo-bronchitis, with edema and mononuclear cellular infiltration of the trachea and bronchial walls, although a certain amount of interstitial pneumonitis and peribronchial exudate also may develop. With the addition of the influenza bacillus these features are accentuated. From the mucopurulent exudate within the bronchi and bronchioles, almost pure cultures of the organism may be obtained. Very few organisms are demonstrable within the alveolar wall or actually within the adjacent air spaces.

Extending from the terminal bronchioles into the adjacent alveoli, a hyaline membrane is frequently seen, which is apparently produced by hyalinization of the exudate and degenerated lining cells, as was particularly emphasized by Winternitz. It is quite similar to the "asphyxial membrane" seen in the stillborn infants (Fig. 424). Special staining technique reveals the presence of lipoid substances in the membranous material. Similar membrane formation is also seen in some of the more severe cases in which pneumococci (MacCallum) or streptococci are important secondary invaders.

In the more severe case in influenza with its high mortality, the lungs are edematous, rather heavy, and on section are moist. There are numerous hemorrhagic areas and the greater portion of the lung is filled with bloody fluid exudate. The pleura is frequently covered with a layer of fibrin. The consolidated areas are scattered throughout the lung and may be confluent in character. The bronchioles are prominent and filled with purulent exudate.

ILLUSTRATIVE CASE

CASE 181 (Ref. #S-380)

Diagnosis.—Lung—influenzal diffuse confluent bronchopneumonia.

Patient was a white male of 38 years, admitted to the hospital in acute respiratory distress.

Present Illness.—The patient was in his usual good health up to twenty-four hours before his admission. At that time he was working out-of-doors chopping wood. He noted that he did not feel quite as well as usual and had a rather chilly sensation. He thought that he developed a little temperature. He was unable to continue at his work after about an hour of these symptoms, which progressed in severity, and he went home to bed. He called his physician, who could not find anything definite on physical examination, and who suspected some upper respiratory infection. By midnight the patient started to break out into a cold sweat, which was accompanied by a mild chill and a rise in temperature to 101°. He became restless and somewhat dyspneic. In the morning, he attempted to eat a light breakfast, but the taste of food nauseated him and he vomited. At that time, he noticed his fingers and hands were of a deep purplish color. When his physician called in the morning, he made a tentative diagnosis of influenzal pneumonia and referred him to the hospital for confirmation of the daignosis.

Past Medical History.—The patient had been healthy all his life. He did not know whether or not he had had any of the usual childhood diseases. He had a somewhat similar upper respiratory attack about eight years earlier and had had a dry cough off and on for several years. This had not influenced his health in general. His appetite had been good and he had maintained himself in an excellent state of nutrition. He had had no genito-urinary symptoms and denied venereal infection.

Physical Examination.—The patient appeared completely prostrate lying apathetically in bed. He had a very definite cyanotic appearance. This was particularly prominent, in the mucous membranes and nailbeds. His head, otherwise, was not remarkable. Eyes, ears and nose were negative. Throat showed moderate congestion of the mucosa. Tongue was slightly coated. There was no cervical adenopathy. Chest was symmetrical. One could hear scattered, moist râles over both sides of the chest. There was surprisingly little change in the voice or breath sounds or to the percussion note in relation to the apparent severity of the patient's symptoms. The heart was not enlarged and no definite murmurs were heard. Abdomen was negative. Extremities were negative. The patient's temperature was only 97.3°. His pulse rate changed between 100 and 110, and his respirations were 36 per minute. His blood pressure was reduced to 100/68.

Laboratory Findings.—Red blood cells, 5,070,000 with 76% hemoglobin; white blood cells 4,800 with 67% polynuclears. Urinalysis showed a small amount of concentrated urine with a very slight trace of albumin and occasional red and white cells.

Subsequent Course.—The patient continued in the same prostrated condition during the brief thirty-six hours which he lived. During this time, the temperature never rose above 99°. The cyanosis increased. The dyspnea became more marked. He had a cough, which was of a dry, unproductive nature. There gradually developed definite dullness over the lower two-thirds of the left side of the chest posteriorly with bronchial breathing and increased tactile fremitus. The patient was given antipneumococcus serum and was kept in an oxygen tent,

without avail. He died with a striking picture of peripheral vascular circulatory failure, with cyanotic, cold, clammy skin.

Autopsy Findings.—At autopsy, there was marked right-sided dilatation of the heart. The lungs showed intense edema and congestion. They were apparently completely waterlogged. On section, a serosanguineous, frothy fluid literally poured from the cut surface and could be expressed from the lung much as water from a sponge. When this was done, it was found that there was a definite consolidation of the left lower lobe characterized by the presence of a fibrinous exudate, which appeared relatively gray, as compared to the surrounding cyanotic lung tissue. Moderate toxic degenerative changes of the heart muscle and of the abdominal viscera, particularly of the kidneys, were observed. No other specific pathology was found.

Microscopic Description of a Section Through the Lung.—(Fig. 424) Histologic study of the lung in this case reveals a diffuse congestion of the peripheral capillary pulmonary circulation. The alveolar walls are markedly thickened due chiefly to dilatation of the capillaries, but in part to edema and diapedesis of red cells into the interstitial tissue of the alveolar walls. Serum is present in enormous amounts, and red cells in large numbers in the alveoli. A considerable amount of fibrin can be seen, which has precipitated out of this extensive serous exudate. This gives a certain amount of rigidity to the tissues. Only rare polynuclear leukocytes can be demonstrated. Occasional large mononuclear cells are also seen. The picture microscopically might easily represent what one would expect the earliest stage of a lobar pneumonia after the initial engorgement might look like, except for the relative lack of white cells in the exudate.

From the gross standpoint, this serosanguineous picture is so typical of the early acute overwhelming type of influenza seen in epidemic years as to be utterly impossibly confused with any other condition. Even the beginning development of the asphyxial hyaline membrane can be demonstrated.

Cultures from this case yielded, both ante-mortem, and from the lung, at postmortem, pure growth of *Hemophilus influenzae*.

Staphylococcic Pneumonia.—This organism may be responsible for a patchy bronchopneumonia which frequently results in abscess of the lung. It occurs most commonly in the upper lobe and especially in the postoperative aspiration or inhalation type of pneumonia. This organism has also been found as a secondary invader in epidemic influenza. The mortality in conjunction with staphylococcic infection of the lung is extremely high.

Friedländer Bacillus Pneumonia (Bacillus mucosus capsulatis).—The *Friedländer bacillus* is a rare cause of lobar pneumonia, and occasionally is seen producing a more patchy form of consolidation. A striking feature of the exudate is its mucoid character. The mortality from this type of pneumonia is particularly high.

Terminal (Hypostatic) Pneumonia.— By this term is meant a form of bronchopneumonia which occurs as a terminal event, usually in debilitated or bedridden patients suffering from some chronic disease such as cancer, nephritis, malnutrition or in conjunction with a fracture, requiring prolonged immobilization, the patient being required to stay in one position. The pneumonia is only incidental in these cases, the patient really dying of his other disease, typically. The pneumonic process is usually preceded by hypostatic congestion and pulmonary edema. The hypostatic congestion may be extreme, leading to actual hemorrhage into the alveoli. With the lowered resistance of the tissues, and the presence of an almost ideal culture medium—blood serum—relatively virulent organisms may grow profusely but give rise to a relatively slight local inflammatory reaction characterized by an exudate consisting almost entirely of polymorphonuclears. There is usually no general reaction in the form of increased temperature or leukocytosis, etc. The consolidation occurs in the dependent parts of the lung where the circulatory stasis is greatest and is often difficult to recognize grossly at autopsy.

ILLUSTRATIVE CASE

CASE 182 (Ref. #S-121)

Diagnosis.—Lung—terminal diffuse confluent bronchopneumonia.

Patient was a female of 85 years, admitted to the hospital with a traumatic fracture of the neck of her right femur.

Present Illness.—The onset of the patient's present illness began by her slipping on a small scatter rug and falling to the floor on her right hip. She heard a crack and felt an excruciating pain in her hip region. She was unable to arise from the floor without help. A physician was called, who recommended her removal to the hospital for treatment.

Past Medical History.—Her past medical history was entirely irrelevant in relation to the present illness and terminal pathology. The patient had had apparently a totally uneventful medical history and had never been previously hospitalized.

Physical Examination.—Patient was a well-developed, elderly white female who appeared all of her given age of eighty-five. Head was negative. The patient's vision was very poor. There was a bilateral arcus senilis. Nose, ears and throat were negative. Chest was symmetrical. Lungs were clear. Heart was not enlarged. There were no murmurs. Abdomen was negative except for a certain amount of muscle spasm in the right lower quadrant in relation to the hip pathology. Extremities: The left leg was negative. The right leg showed an impacted fracture of the neck of the right femur with about one inch shortening of the leg. There was considerable swelling and hemorrhage of the soft parts around the bony fracture.

Laboratory Findings.—The laboratory findings were negative at the time of admission. The patient's red count showed 4,300,000 cells with 78% hemoglobin. White blood cells 8,600 with 74% polynuclears. Urinalysis was negative.

Subsequent Course.—The patient was of necessity confined to bed while the fracture was immobilized. About three weeks following admission, she developed a slight rise in temperature to 100.5°. This was accompanied by a non-productive cough. Physical examination at this time showed somewhat impaired breath sounds over the lower portion of both lungs together with many râles of crackling and crepitant nature. Heart sounds were distant, but no murmurs could be heard. The white blood count rose to 12,600 cells with 86% polymorphonuclears. This lung pathology increased in extent over the course of the next few days, and was diagnosed as a hypostatic pneumonia. The patient became progressively worse, gradually lapsed into unconsciousness, and died.

Autopsy Findings.—At autopsy, there was an impacted fracture of the right hip. Heart showed brown atrophy with terminal myocardosis and dilatation. Lungs showed very extensive hypostatic congestion in the bases and dependent portions. This was accompanied by pulmonary edema. There appeared to be actual consolidation of the bases on both right and left sides. Abdominal viscera showed moderate chronic passive congestion. The extremities, other than for the fracture, were negative.

Microscopic Description of a Section Through the Right Lower Lobe.—Histologic study of the lung tissue shows a diffuse confluent bronchopneumonic process. The great majority of the alveoli are filled with exudate, although here and there a few vesicles are seen which are not involved and contain no inflammatory material. The bronchi and bronchioles present evidence of a marked passive congestion of the mucosal vessels with considerable cellular infiltration of the soft tissues. This is both mononuclear and polynuclear in character. Many of the alveoli are filled with a serous exudate in which a few red cells and leukocytes are found. In others, the exudate is predominantly polymorphonuclear. In places, the picture almost suggests hemorrhage, the congestive features and diapedesis of the red cells into the alveolar spaces being so predominant. The picture, as has been suggested, varies considerably in different parts of the same slide as well as in different portions of the lung substance. In general, the reaction is one of polymorphonuclears with a variable number of large mononuclear phagocytes being found in different areas. Many of these are seen to contain hemosiderin. The picture is one of a diffuse confluent type of bronchopneumonia, which in this instance was definitely related to general weakness on the part of the patient, with circulatory failure. This resulted in hypostatic congestion of the lungs offering a perfect culture media for any bacteria which might be inspired and which, in the face of the reduced resistance of the patient, was able to give rise to this terminal pneumonic picture.

Aspiration (Inhalation or Insufflation) Pneumonia.—PNEUMONIA NEONATORUM.—This form of pneumonia is not uncommon in "stillborn" children. It apparently results from the insufflation of amniotic fluid in utero. No typical inflammatory cellular reaction is found. The walls of the alveoli are usually lined by an *"asphyxial"* membrane, which apparently results from hyaline changes taking place in the insufflated fluid which is rich in cells. The membrane stains an intense red with eosin and can be shown to contain lipoids and neutral fats by staining with Scharlach R or Sudan III. Very rarely, an area of consolidation results from bacterial invasion of the lung through transplacental infection from a mother with upper respiratory disease. The causative organism may be recovered usually from the blood stream under such circumstances. This represents a true intra-uterine fetal type of pneumonia and is seen in perhaps five per cent of stillborn infants or those dying shortly after birth.

POST-OPERATIVE PNEUMONIA.—The insufflation of infected material during the course of some operative procedure on the upper respiratory tract may result in patchy areas of bronchopneumonia which, due to the bacterial content of the material, usually progress to suppuration and gangrene. In pharyngeal diphtheria portions of the exudate may be insufflated, producing first atelectasis and later inflammation. During anesthesia or unconscious states, infected mucus or vomitus may likewise be inhaled. The lesions are likely to be definitely localized, most often occurring in the upper lobe, and to suggest an area of infarction in their earlier stages.

LIPOID PNEUMONIA.—The literature, in recent years, has been replete with accounts of various types of bronchopneumonia in which lipoid material has been found within the consolidated areas. The work of Pinkerton some years ago called our particular attention to the danger of the use of mineral oils in the form of nose drops in the treatment of upper respiratory infections, particularly in infants. Not infrequently, sufficient of this inert substance was inspired into the alveoli to set up a definite inflammatory reaction. The oil, being totally inert and almost incapable of being broken down, was usually associated with a large mononuclear, phagocytic type of cellular reaction. Not infrequently actual giant cell production was seen in an attempt to engulf this oily material. Often, this likewise would spread out as a film over the surface of the alveolar lining, and as in the case of the so-called "asphyxial" membrane,

seen in other forms of bronchopneumonia, is believed to play a definite part in producing cyanosis. Frozen section preparations from such lungs showed many fat droplets within the phagocytic cells in the exudate. Occasionally, such instances of lipoid pneumonia were followed, through impairment of lung function, with secondary bacterial invasion of the tissues, even to the point of producing a fatal bronchopneumonia.

The use of vegetable oils, particularly in the form of lipiodol, seems to have been attended with much less disaster. Lipiodol again appears to be a relatively inert substance, but in the course of time is apparently either completely eliminated from the lung through expectoration or is broken down and absorbed. At all events, it produces no reaction in the lung tissue and can be used with apparent impunity in outlining the bronchial tree. This has proven of infinite value in the recognition of obstructive lesions of the bronchi and in outlining areas of bronchiectasis or of atelectasis.

Just as in the case of mineral oils, so in the case of animal fats, used particularly to provide adequate Vitamin "A" and "D" intake in infants and young children, inhalation of the material may not infrequently take place. This animal oil, unlike either the mineral or vegetable oils used in medicine, is prone to set up a relatively acute inflammatory raction. This has been recently demonstrated most clearly by Graef. It results in a rather extensive bronchopneumonia with a mixed inflammatory cellular exudate, but one in which large mononuclear phagocytes tend to predominate in their efforts to remove the irritating substance, although at times the polynuclears are in excess.

PART III

SUPPURATIVE LESIONS OF THE LUNG, INCLUDING BRONCHIECTASIS

Suppuration of the lung results from the implantation of a wide variety of bacteria, particularly by those belonging to the pyogenic group. Not uncommonly, saprophytic organisms may be present either primarily or secondarily, and complicate the picture. The method whereby the infectious process is initiated varies, but there are at least four major groups of cases (1) those in which the infectious agent is brought to the lung by way of the bronchi; (2) those

in which the infection is brought from contiguous structures; (3) those of hematogenous origin; and (4) the postinflammatory group.

(1) The first group is by far the most important. It results from the insufflation of infected material usually admixed with blood, during the course of operations upon the upper respiratory tract, particularly when the patient is under a general anesthetic. It may occur after tonsillectomy or the removal of

adenoid tissue, or even following the abstraction of an infected tooth. Moore, in a survey of a large number of cases of tonsillectomy states that one in every twenty-five hundred or three thousand cases is followed by pulmonary suppuration. The possibility of the abscess in such cases being due to infected emboli must not be overlooked. Fetterolf and Fox maintain that many of the postoperative pulmonary abscesses are of this origin. The insufflation of infected material from suppurative processes in the upper respiratory tract, particularly during unconscious states, must also be included as a possible cause.

Aspiration pneumonias frequently progress to suppuration. The insufflation of foreign bodies is very commonly accompanied by subsequent ulceration and suppuration of the bronchi and adjacent lung tissue. Malignant tumors of the upper respiratory tract, particularly of the trachea and bronchi, may undergo necrosis with subsequent secondary infection. This material may likewise be insufflated and result in suppuration. Tumors of the esophagus may ulcerate into the trachea or bronchi, and result in similar aspiration and abscess formation.

(2) In the *hematogenous group,* the suppurative process develops following the lodgment of a septic embolus. It is most often seen in association with obstetrical and surgical operations on the abdomen complicated by an infectious thrombophlebitis. Such emboli usually produce an area of infarction first. This rapidly undergoes liquefaction necrosis and suppuration. The areas tend to be multiple and are often superficial in respect to the pleura. They not infrequently ultimately rupture into the pleural cavity producing an empyema. Occasionally, an abscess of the lung may follow some septic process which causes thrombosis of the lateral sinus and gives rise to infected emboli.

(3) Extension of the infectious process from adjacent structures is rare, but it may follow an empyema, an abscess of the liver with ulceration of the diaphragm, or a mediastinal abscess secondary to a perforating carcinoma of the esophagus. In many cases of bronchiectasis, suppuration of the adjacent lung sooner or later occurs. In traumatic wounds of the chest organisms may also be implanted in the lung.

(4) *Postpneumonic:* Postpneumonic suppuration occasionally occurs as a complication of lobar or bronchopneumonia. It is more frequent in the latter,

and is most likely to be seen in the streptococcic type. In this group of suppurative pneumonitis, the areas are apt to be multiple and evidence of the primary pneumonia may be seen in other parts of the lung.

Pathology.—In the inhalation group, the suppuration is in the form of a localized abscess most commonly found in the lower lobe of the right lung. This is explained on a mechanical basis dependent upon the more nearly straight position of the right main stem bronchus. The insufflated material, accordingly, is more apt to be carried into this portion of the lung. Many such abscess cavities communicate with a bronchus, so that their purulent contents are discharged as sputum. Such cavities may be demonstrated readily by x-ray, particularly, if lipiodol is used. Other abscesses become walled off, and in such closed abscesses, their x-ray demonstration may be difficult.

On section, grossly, the involved area is yellowish or yellowish-gray in color, the liquefaction necrosis is advanced, and fluid pus flows from the cavity. If the process has existed for any length of time, considerable fibrosis may be present around the area. This is particularly true in the abscesses following bronchiectasis. In most abscesses of the inhalation group, the pus has a putrid odor, and the tissues may show extensive necrosis. This is due to the action of numerous saprophytic, putrefactive organisms, many of which are anaerobes. If the suppurative process extends to involve any considerable part of the lung and is accompanied by extensive liquefaction necrosis with putrefaction and interference wtih the blood supply by thrombosis, the term "gangrene" of the lung is applied.

Abscesses from infected emboli are usually multiple, and most frequently occur in the lower lobe. Upon the lodgment of the embolus a cone-shaped area of hemorrhagic coagulation necrosis results. This is soon followed by liquefaction upon the advent of numerous polymorphonuclear leukocytes which are attracted to the site by the pathogenic organisms. As has been shown in our early consideration of the various types of inflammation, the presence of polynuclears alone does not constitute suppuration. It must be accompanied by liquefaction necrosis, and this side of the picture appears to be dependent very largely upon the character of the infecting organism.

In the typical acute abscess, three relatively distinct areas may be seen: (1) a central area of liquefaction necrosis consisting of large numbers of disintegrating polymorphonuclear leukocytes, much tissue debris, bacteria, fluid exudate (liquor puris), and occasionally degenerated tissue cells, particularly elastic tissue; (2) surrounding this, a zone of tissue showing coagulation necrosis. The air spaces in this part of the lesion are filled with a fibrinous exudate accompanied by varying numbers of red cells, and the entire area is infiltrated by numerous well-preserved polymorphonuclears. On the outer edge of this zone, marked congestion or hyperemia of the vessels of the alveolar walls may be seen; and (3) a peripheral zone of localized pulmonary edema merging with the normal lung parenchyma.

ILLUSTRATIVE CASE

CASE 183. (Ref. #S-408)

Diagnosis.—Lung—pulmonary abscess.

Patient was a white male of 48 years, admitted to the hospital because of asthma and a dry cough of several years' duration, and dyspnea.

Present Illness.—The patient stated that for nearly ten years he had had a very slight, dry cough with some shortness of breath. He never consulted a physician about this, however, until three months before admission, when his cough suddenly became worse, being loose and productive, with a considerable amount of blood streaked sputum, of about one week's duration. His dyspnea likewise became much more marked and the patient complained of severe pain in his chest.

Past Medical History.—The patient had had an uneventful medical history with the exception of an attack of influenza during the 1918 epidemic. He was married and had had seven children, all of whom were living and well. There had never been any history of cancer, tuberculosis, or lung trouble of any sort in his family. A review of his systems was entirely negative. He had no recollection regarding his childhood medical history.

Physical Examination.—The patient was a well-developed, well-nourished, middle-aged white male. Pupils were regular, equal and reacted normally. Ears, nose and throat were essentially negative. Teeth were in poor condition showing marked caries and pyorrhea. Tonsils were small, atrophic and buried. The posterior pharynx showed some chronic irritation. Chest was symmetrical and well-developed. It was somewhat barrel-shaped, with equal but somewhat limited expansion. Tactile fremitus was normal throughout. The percussion note was resonant except for a small area at the right base. The diaphragm had limited motion in this area. A few sonorous râles were heard at both apices. Heart was apparently negative. Blood pressure was normal. Abdomen was negative. Extremities: There was a possible beginning clubbing of his fingers and toes.

Laboratory Findings.—Blood count showed 3,800,000 red cells with 78% hemoglobin and a white blood count of 11,400 cells with 82% polynuclears, 13% lymphocytes, and 5% monocytes. Blood Wassermann was negative. Urinalysis was negative. Scrutum yielded only the usual mixed bacterial flora.

X-ray examination revealed a definite abscess cavity close to the mid-sagittal plane in the middle of the right lower lobe lung field. This had a definite fluid level and the cavity appeared to be about half full of fluid. Around this abscess area was found suppurative pneumonitis as visualized by abnormal density of the tissues.

Subsequent History.—The patient was treated by aspiration for several months with marked improvement. He was on his way to the hospital on one occasion when he was struck by an automobile and brought to the hospital in a moribund condition.

Autopsy Findings.—At autopsy, the patient showed multiple fractures of his skull with profuse subdural hemorrhage as the immediate cause of death. He likewise presented evidence of a chronic, suppurative pericarditis with many adhesions between the parietal and visceral layers. The lungs showed a huge right lower lobe abscess cavity (Fig. 426) with plugging of the right lower bronchus. This was complicated by a zone of suppurative pneumonitis, chiefly in the right middle lobe. The left lobe appeared entirely negative. The abdominal viscera were not remarkable.

Microscopic Description of a Section Through the Abscess Cavity Wall.— (Fig. 427) Sections histologically through the abscess wall of the lung present evidence of a typical chronic suppurative inflammatory process. There is a thick layer of fibrous tissue which makes up the wall. This is covered on its anterior aspect by a thin, fibrinopurulent exudate in which are found many broken down leukocytes and cellular debris. The connective tissue which serves almost as a capsule shows extensive hyaline degeneration. It likewise shows considerable chronic inflammatory cellular infiltration with lymphocytes and large mononuclear cells predominating. Surrounding the wall of the abscess, the lung parenchyma shows marked thickening of the alveolar process and a secondary suppurative pneumonitis with a purulent exudate filling many of the alveoli. This is not uniform in distribution. In some areas the exudate is frankly leukocytic; in others it is monocytic. Many of the alveoli are completely destroyed and replaced by dense fibrous scar tissue. In places, this almost resembles an organized pneumonia. The picture, in brief, is one of chronic suppuration with reparative fibrosis.

Gangrene of the Lung.—The line drawn between advanced suppuration and gangrene is indistinct. The etiological factors are similar in both processes, and in many instances gangrene is initiated by abscess formation. However, gangrene may be defined as a rapidly-spreading necrosis with involvement of the vascular supply, brought about by the action of various putrefactive bacteria, including saprophytes. The process is rapid and spreading in character. There is no tendency for fibrosis to develop, nor any attempt to wall off the process as is seen in the more localized suppurative lesion. On section, grossly, the gangrenous lung usually has a greenish cast, with a dark reddish-purple line of demarcation from the surrounding lung tissue. The gangrenous area is usually soft and mushy in consistency and may at times even be semi-fluid. It invariably has a very offensive putrid odor.

Bronchiectasis.—Bronchiectasis may be defined as abnormal dilatation of one or more of the bronchi. For purposes of description, it may be divided into congenital and acquired varieties. The acquired variety may be local or diffuse, dependent upon the contributory factors which cause the lesion.

CONGENITAL BRONCHIECTASIS.—In congenital bronchiectasis, due to failure of the normal development of the bronchi or lung tissue, bronchioles may terminate in saccular dilatations, which in the gross specimen give the lung a cystic appearance. The malformation is probably due to a failure of development of the alveoli from the primitive buds of the bronchial stalk, so that the bronchioles simply end as blind pouches which become enormously dilated as the lung is expanded. At times it is difficult or impossible to demonstrate the connection of these sacs with the bronchi, so that a diagnosis of polycystic disease of the lung has been made in a number of such cases. The spaces are lined with flattened epithelium, sometimes continuous with the bronchi. Clinically, the disease gives rise to recurrent sudden attacks of dyspnea and cyanosis in infancy. This is due to compression atelectasis brought about by rupture of one of the cysts into the pleural cavity, which causes collapse of the lung. Such congenital lesions are usually confined to a single lobe or at most to one lung only.

ACQUIRED BRONCHIECTASIS.—In acquired bronchiectasis the dilatation may be confined to a single bronchus or bronchiole, but more commonly involves the great majority of those of a lobe of the lung. The process may be unilateral or bilateral. It most frequently is seen in the lower lobes, but may occur anywhere in the lung. The condition is fairly common, from two to four per cent of adults coming to autopsy in a general hospital showing such lesions. The process often begins in childhood, particularly following infectious diseases such as measles, whooping cough, influenza and streptococcic bronchopneumonia. The diagnosis of most cases is made between the age of 20 and 40, although the process is almost always of gradual onset. Occasionally, cases are encountered, particularly in children, in which the course is more acute. These are prone to occur following streptococcal infections of the lung.

The bronchiectatic dilatation of the bronchus or bronchi may be cylindric, fusiform or saccular in form. The cylindrical type is more apt to be a diffuse process throughout a lobe involving the main bronchus and a number of its branches. The saccular form is frequently multiple and may occur in both the large and small size bronchi and bronchioles. The individual lesions vary greatly in size ranging from several millimeters to several centimeters in diameter. Usually, in the cylindrical form, if the dilatation occurs in both the large and small branches, the degree of dilatation is proportionate. The most common site of the lesion is in the lower lobe of the left lung, although not uncommonly, both lower lobes may be involved. This tendency of the process to remain localized to a single lobe is of great practical importance from the standpoint of therapy, for with modern surgical technique, lobectomy can be done in many cases.

Once bronchiectasis is established, the process is progressive with little or no tendency towards regression or spontaneous cure. Upon gross examination of the affected lobe early, the dilated bronchi or bronchioles are lined by mucous membrane frequently showing a moderate degree of hyperplasia. Considerable secretion may be seen within the lumen. The mucous membrane is congested and highly vascular so that only slight trauma such as coughing may give rise to small or large hemorrhages. This is an important clinical finding. If the lung is examined at a later stage, the mucous membrane has become atrophic, and the wall thickened by varying degrees of fibrosis. The submucosa, and at times even the muscle and elastic tissues, and even the cartilage may be replaced by such fibrous cicatrization. Ulceration of the lining epithelium is common. The lumen is usually filled with mucopurulent exudate. This may have a very offensive odor due to the presence of putrefactive changes of the exudate itself. Numerous spirochetes and spirilla, organisms of the Vincent variety, yeasts and particularly monilia and saprophytic organisms of other types have been isolated at times in symbiosis with the usual pyogenic bacteria.

The bacteriology of bronchiectasis of the lung is complicated and varied. A recent review of the fifty-nine cases from a metropolitan general hospital by E. H. Spaulding shows the flora to be predominantly anaerobic. Thirteen of the cases showed growth *only* on anaerobic culture. Suppuration of the lung may result in such cases by extension of the process through the wall of the bronchus. In the saccular variety, the tendency for secretions to accumulate and for putrefaction to take place is much greater than in the cylindric form. In such cases, change of position frequently brings about a paroxysm of coughing with expectoration of a considerable quantity of foul secretion. In addition to the clinical findings, the diagnosis is readily made in the average case of bronchiestasis by x-ray, particularly with the use of lipiodol.

The etiology of bronchiectasis varies greatly in the individual case. In general, however, several factors usually combine to bring about its production: (1) conditions weakening the bronchial wall; (2) traction on the bronchus from without; and (3) increase in intrabronchial pressure. The bronchial wall is frequently weakened in streptococcal pneumonias, particularly in those complicating the acute infectious diseases, measles, whooping cough, and influenza. The destruction of the elastic tissue and at times even the musculature of the bronchioles is well recognized in these conditions, with predisposition to subsequent dilatation. Traction on the bronchi or bronchioles from without is brought about particularly by the contraction of adhesions in chronic tuberculosis or other chronic fibroid lesions of the lung. Atelectasis also causes an increase in negative pressure with resultant traction on the unaffected bronchi and bronchioles, thus exerting traction from without. Increase in pressure within the bronchi is seen in connection with their obstruction, particularly in relation to expiration. This may be brought about by tumors, foreign bodies or tenacious exudates within the bronchi, or by compression from without by aneurysms or by enlarged peribronchial and mediastinal lymph nodes. The chronic cough seen in bronchitis probably has little bearing as an etiological factor, but true bronchial asthma is an important etiological factor in some cases.

ILLUSTRATIVE CASE

CASE 184. (Ref. #S-141)

Diagnosis.—Lung—chronic bronchiectasis.

Patient was a Negro of 44 years, admitted to the hospital with the chief complaint of a chronic productive cough of about two years' duration.

Present Illness.—The onset of the present illness was somewhat indefinite, but was dated back in the patient's mind to a severe cold and attack of pneumonia, which he had had a little over two years previously. Since that time he had had a cough which had varied considerably in severity. At times it had been nonproductive. Much of the time, however, he had raised a considerable amount of thick, tenacious, mucopurulent sputum. The amount of sputum had definitely increased during the previous few months. He had complained of marked weakness, lassitude and easy fatigability. At times he had noted some pain in the right chest with these coughing attacks. He had never noticed any night sweats or that he had had any definite fever. His chief concern was his increasing weakness and a recent loss of weight, although his outstanding symptom was his cough.

Past Medical History.—The patient's past medical history seemed to be comparatively irrelevant. He had had the usual childhood infections, including measles, pertussis, varicella and scarlatina. A review of his systems showed that he had always been rather subject to upper respiratory infections with an average of five or six colds every winter. Up to the onset of his present illness, however, he had had no serious symptoms relating to his respiratory system and had never been hospitalized. He had never been cardiac conscious. His gastro-intestinal history was entirely negative until his present illness when he had noted marked anorexia. His genito-urinary history was apparently nonpertinent. He had had gonorrhea as a young man, but denied syphilis.

Physical Examination.—Patient was a fairly well developed, but definitely undernourished, middle-aged Negro. His head was negative. Eyes, ears, nose and throat were negative. There was no postnasal discharge. Neck showed moderate bilateral cervical adenopathy. Chest examination showed definite asymmetry more pronounced on the left side. The right side definitely lagged and expansion was limited, particularly in the upper portion. Auscultation of the lungs revealed marked dullness and many coarse râles over the right upper lobe area. A few moist, crackling râles were heard in the base. The left lung appeared negative. Heart was not enlarged and showed no murmurs. Abdomen was negative. Extremities were normal except for beginning clubbing of the fingers.

Laboratory Findings.—The red cell count on admission showed 3,200,000 cells with 58% hemoglobin. The white blood cells numbered 11,300 with 78% neutrophiles. Urinalysis was negative on several occasions. Sputum examination was negative for tubercle bacilli, fungi and spirochetes. It was copious in amount and was of a tenacious, mucopurulent character. On one occasion it showed some blood streaking. A mixed bacterial flora was obtained in which streptococci of the viridans type predominated. Blood Wassermann was negative.

X-ray examination of the chest with lipiodol introduced in the Trendelenburg position revealed very extensive bronchiectasis of the right upper lobe (Fig. 428).

Subsequent Course.—Bronchoscopy was done on several occasions in an attempt to drain the bronchiectatic areas. The patient, however, developed a diffuse confluent bronchopneumonia of the left lung and died approximately ten days after admission to the hospital.

Autopsy Findings.—At autopsy there was moderate hypertrophy and dilatation of the heart noted. The lungs: (Fig. 429) the right upper lobe showed a diffuse chronic bronchiectasis with multiple bronchiectatic abscesses. Surrounding these areas, a diffuse fibroid type of pneumonia was found. The left lower lobe showed a very diffuse, confluent bronchopneumonia and was filled with a serosanguineous exudate. The other organs showed moderate toxic degenerative changes.

Microscopic Description of a Section Through the Lung.—Histologic examination of the lung tissue shows evidence of a chronic inflammatory process involving the bronchi. The walls of the bronchi have been practically destroyed and replaced by a thick, hyalinized layer of connective tissue. The diameter of these pathological bronchi is greatly increased. The walls of these bronchi are lined by a layer of chronic granulation tissue, which is diffusely infiltrated by chronic inflammatory cells. The lumina are filled with a purulent exudate consisting for the most part of broken down, necrotic-appearing polymorphonuclear leukocytes.

CHAPTER XLIV

DISEASES OF THE RESPIRATORY SYSTEM (*Continued*)

THE LUNG (Continued)

PART I

Chronic Granulomata of the Lung

In the preceding chapter the problems of the relatively acute infectious diseases of the lung have been considered. In this part of the discussion, a review of the more important chronic inflammatory conditions which affect the lung, including especially the infectious granulomata and the pneumoconioses, will be taken up. The particular interest in this group of diseases, as far as the clinician is concerned, is in how to differentiate them from tuberculosis. This is the all important point, and as we shall find, presents many difficulties to clinician, roentgenologist and pathologist alike. It is with this thought in mind that we proceed to a discussion of a few of the more outstanding of these conditions.

Tuberculosis of the Lung.—Tuberculosis is the most common and most important of the so-called infectious granulomatous diseases affecting the lung. It is caused by the tubercle bacillus and produces lesions characterized by the formation of histological tubercles. The process is often diffuse. The lesions are prone to undergo caseation necrosis and ulceration, and to heal by fibrosis and calcification. The disease is of great importance throughout the world, being responsible for about 8 per cent of all deaths. The incidence of the disease is very much greater, and in most communities almost one hundred per cent of adults will show evidence of healed, quiescent or active tuberculosis. Based upon the von Pirquet test, twenty per cent positives are obtained under 2 years of age, fifty-five per cent under 5 years, and ninety to ninety-seven per cent under 14 years of age. Opie, approaching the subject by the postmortem x-ray examination of lungs after removal from the body in a series of cases, was able to demonstrate presumptive evidence of tuberculosis in forty-three per cent of children from 2 to 5 years

of age, eighty to ninety per cent after the age of 12, and one hundred per cent after the age of 30. Ghon, in reporting his observations in 184 autopsies upon children, revealed the presence of primary tuberculous lesions in ninety-two per cent of cases. The truth of Bunyan's statement that tuberculosis is "the captain of the men of death" is thus substantiated.

INCIDENCE.—Although the incidence of the infection or the morbidity rate rapidly rises throughout childhood, the mortality curve sharply declines. Thus, the highest mortality is seen during the first year of life, when, it has been estimated, approximately seventy per cent of infants infected die. There is then a sharp drop in the figures, with an almost negligible death rate until the adolescent period. At that time a second peak in the mortality figures again is found between the ages of 20 to 30. This occurs earlier in the female who is subject to greater physiologic strain, especially with pregnancy and lactation, but it is equaled in the male figures a few years later. Following this young adult high-water mark, there is a gradual decline in the mortality rate. Statistical information presents evidence of the interesting fact that the death rate from tuberculosis is on the decline. Thus, since 1900 it has dropped from over 200 to less than 70 deaths per 100,000 at the present time.

ETIOLOGY.—The human type of tubercle bacillus is most frequently found as the cause of active tuberculosis in man, the bovine variety only being responsible for a relatively small number of cases. In this country it is due largely to the rigid control of tuberculosis among cattle used in the production of milk, and to the almost universal pasteurization or certification of milk sold. Where these regulations are not enforced bovine tuberculosis is much more

496

prevalent. In general probably less than two per cent of tuberculosis of the lung is due to the bovine type. In nonpulmonary tuberculosis, in a survey of cases by Griffiths, some years ago, as high as thirty-five per cent of cases of non-pulmonary tuberculosis were of bovine origin.

In tuberculosis, the lungs, with few exceptions, are always involved, either primarily or secondarily. It is true, however, that there are a few cases in which the tonsils, the cervical lymph nodes or the bones may be involved without definite lesions in the lung, although even in these cases it is frequently possible to demonstrate a healed or active lesion within the lung.

MODES OF INFECTION.—(1) inhalation, (2) ingestion, (3) cutaneous inoculation, (4) congenital. The modes of infection, together with discussion of tuberculosis in general have been considered under Chapter XVI.

Inhalation.—Infection in tuberculosis is one of immediate contact in the great majority of cases, whether as the primary infection of childhood, or the later secondary manifestations in adult life. Likewise, inhalation of tubercle bacilli directly from an infected case by the droplet method can be accredited with being the most common way of spreading the disease. From an open, ulcerative case of active tuberculosis, literally billions of organisms are sprayed into the atmosphere through coughing, sneezing or even in talking. These provide the usual source of infection for the subsequent case. It is quite true, as has been shown experimentally many times, that both street dust and house dust may contain tubercle bacilli. The latter, however, is the most dangerous, since the organisms tend to persist, due to their waxy covering, for several months. In out-of-door dust, however, the actinic rays of the sun soon destroy the organism. This infection of floor dust may be very significant in spreading infection among infants as they first learn to creep.

Ingestion.—Unquestionably, in some instances the tubercle bacilli may be ingested, particularly the bovine type, when the organism is present in milk, butter, cheese, etc. It may pass through the stomach successfully and subsequently penetrate the wall of the intestine, especially of the terminal ileum. Likewise, the routine study of tonsillar tissue following tonsillectomy shows the presence of unsuspected tuberculous infection in three to five per cent of cases.

This may well be the portal of entry in certain cases of cervical gland tuberculosis.

Cutaneous Inoculation.—Infection by the tubercle bacillus through the skin is occasionally seen in the "butcher's tubercle" and "pathologist's tubercle." These lesions, however, are probably of little importance as source of primary invasion of the organism.

Congenital.—Congenital infections are said to occur in rare instances. They likewise are not of great importance as a cause of primary tuberculosis.

We see, therefore, that the possibilities for the entrance of the organism are many, but it would seem that the bulk of evidence is still in favor of the direct inhalation of the organism into the lung by way of the respiratory tract.

The reactions of the tissues of the body to the presence and subsequent growth of the tubercle bacillus are complex and varied. They depend upon several factors: the degree of immunity and allergy on the one hand; the size and frequency of the dose of the organism and its virulence on the other. These have been considered in some detail in Chapter XVI where the problem of tuberculosis as a whole was reviewed in some detail.

PRIMARY OR SO-CALLED CHILDHOOD TUBERCULOSIS OF THE LUNG.—In the great majority of cases, the primary infection follows the inhalation of the organism into the depths of the lung. On reaching the alveoli the tubercle bacilli are taken up by the phagocytic mononuclear cells and conveyed to the lymphoid tissue of the alveolar septa. Very little other immediate reaction to their presence takes place, and the organisms tend to multiply. Soon, many or most of them are carried along the lymphatics to the regional peribronchial lymph nodes (Fig. 142, Case 60, Chapter XVI). After a variable interval of days, or even weeks; the tissues become allergic to the presence of the organism, and caseation follows. This primary caseous lesion is commonly seen in children, and is more and more frequently encountered in adults who have lived in districts free from tuberculosis and have thus escaped any previous primary infection.

If the lung be examined at this stage, an area of caseation is found, usually near the periphery, frequently less than 1 cm. in diameter, rather definitely set off from the surrounding tissues, grayish or yellowish in color and often surrounded by fibrous tissue forming a capsule. The peribronchial lymph nodes draining the area are considerably enlarged and show extensive caseation. The line of extension along the lymphatics from the primary lesion to the node can frequently be traced by tiny bead-like areas of caseation. Thus, primary tuberculosis is characterized by a caseous lesion in any part of the lung and by similar caseous lesions of the regional peribronchial lymph node. In the great majority of cases, except in early infancy, the resistance of the individual or his natural immunity leads to spontaneous healing by fibrosis and calcification. Similar changes take place in the affected peribronchial lymph nodes. Such healed lesions are commonly spoken of as "Ghon tubercles" (Fig. 142). In infants, as has been emphasized, death is apt to result from a rapidly spreading confluent tuberculous bronchopneumonia. This is brought about sometimes by extension of the caseous process from the lymph nodes into the bronchial wall with the subsequent discharge of the infected caseous material. This is inhaled into the lung and gives rise to extensive caseous tubercles which become confluent in a rapidly-spreading pneumonic process. Or reinfection may result from repeated inhalation of large numbers of organisms from the infant's mother.

SECONDARY OR ADULT TUBERCULOSIS OF THE LUNG.—As a result of the primary lesion a varying degree of allergy and immunity are developed. These are to a large extent independent of one another. The degree and type of secondary reaction, to a great extent, depends upon their relative proportions. The secondary reaction differs from the primary by a marked tissue response. Thus, the organism tends to become localized and only rarely are the regional peribronchial lymph nodes involved.

The mechanism by which such secondary tuberculosis develops is still somewhat unsettled. In general, it is accepted that the adult type of tuberculosis represents a secondary or reinfection. This is probably in the great majority of cases exogenous as to source, and results from intimate contact with a person having open, ulcerative tuberculosis. In a small percentage of cases, the infection may well be endogenous in origin, either from the breakdown of a primary, childhood lesion, or from a subclinical, unrecognized, small secondary focus. In any case, the secondary lesion is likely to follow some lowering of resistance as a result of a thousand and one things such as worry, pregnancy, lactation, malnutrition, acute upper respiratory infection or exposure to cold.

Types of Pulmonary Tuberculosis

The lesions of adult pulmonary tuberculosis fall into four major groups both from the clinical and the pathological standpoints: (1) Chronic fibroid phthisis, including quiescent or healed cases; (2) Chronic ulcerative and caseous tuberculosis; (3) Acute pneumonic form (tuberculous bronchopneumonia); and (4) Acute miliary tuberculosis.

Chronic Fibroid Tuberculosis (Fibroid Phthisis). —In a great majority of individuals, coming to autopsy from whatever cause, there is found near the apex of the lung, particularly the right lung, a small, slightly depressed scar, which on section cuts with fibroid resistance and is usually pigmented. It tends to be flattened rather than rounded in shape. The central part may show some caseation or calcification. It is not discrete but sends bands of fibrous tissue into the surrounding lung. The tubercle bacilli may at times be demonstrated by animal inoculation, showing that some of these lesions are quiescent and not completely healed. Such a lesion is probably to be desired, since it appears that resistance to the disease rapidly falls once the body is entirely free of infection. On the other hand, such quiescent lesions undoubtedly may take on renewed activity when the patient's resistance has been greatly lowered, and are responsible for some of the more serious cases of pulmonary tuberculosis.

Histologically, the lesion seems to consist almost exclusively of mature fibrous tissue which has undergone hyalinization and pigmentation. In the deeper layers a small amount of caseation may be seen. Other areas may show calcification. There is no evidence of tubercle formation with the presence of typical "epithelioid" cells or giant cells. A few lymphocytes may be encountered throughout the lesion, but even these are inconspicuous. At the periphery, occasional persistent alveoli, lined with cuboidal epithelium, may be seen within the fibrous tissue. In this chronic type of fibroid tuberculosis, therefore, it is seen that, due to a marked degree of resistance of the host to the presence of the organisms, fibrosis and healing predominate.

Fibrocaseous (Ulcerative) Tuberculosis.—(Fig. 145 and 146) Under this broad term are included the great majority of cases of what we think of clinically as pulmonary tuberculosis. They vary from relatively acute cases with rapid cavitation and spread throughout the lungs within the matter of a comparatively few months, to chronic cases in which fibrosis predominates and which may run a course of twenty, thirty or even forty years, and then succumb to cardiorenal-vascular disease rather than to their tuberculosis. These subdivisions of the tuberculous lesion have been discussed in Chapter XVI.

Roughly speaking, the degree of activity of the tuberculous lesion in respect to its characteristic caseous necrosis, ulceration and cavity formation, depends upon the relative resistance of the host, the size of the dose and the virulence of the infecting organism. Here, as in the case of the true fibroid healed lesion just described, the process begins in the apex of the lung, particularly the right apex, either from activation of a quiescent tubercle, or from a second exogenous infection. The lesion is characterized by slow, progressive caseation and cavity formation accompanied by a variable amount of fibrosis. As the caseous process continues, the lesion extends to involve the bronchi. The central caseous material softens and is evacuated into the bronchus, thus forming the chronic cavity.

Much of this caseous material will be expectorated in the sputum in which the organisms may be demonstrated. A part, however, will be inhaled into adjacent bronchioles, and will result in tiny areas of atelectasis with subsequent formation of tubercles. These tend to coalesce in lobulated, cloverleaf *acinar* lesions. These lesions are at first gray and translucent; later, as caseation advances, yellow and opaque.

The typical cavity is found as an apical lesion, It varies greatly in size from a centimeter or so up to huge lesions involving nearly the entire lobe (Fig. 147, Case 61, Ref. #S-140). The wall is smooth and made up of fibrous tissue which is undergoing caseation. An occasional blood vessel may be seen transversing the cavity as a cord-like structure, probably due to the greater resistance of the elastic tissues to the caseous process. Upon examination, however, it will be seen that the wall of the vessel is thickened and the lumen practically obliterated. More often such bands are simply thickened fibrous septa. The comparative rareness of open hemorrhage in tuberculosis is due to the occlusion of the blood vessels in advance of the caseous process by thrombosis or endarteritis obliterans.

With ulceration, the tuberculous cavity usually becomes contaminated with pyogenic and saprophytic bacteria. This mixed infection results in a more rapid extension of the process. The process may spread to the lower lobe and the other lung, chiefly by way of the bronchi, caseous material being inhaled. The lesions thus formed show abundant exudate and considerable fibrous tissue response. Numerous pleural adhesions are present over the site of the cavity as the result of organization of the associated fibrinous exudate which is usually found. At times the adhesions may be very extensive and involve the entire pleura and result in complete obliteration of the pleural cavity. The peribronchial lymph nodes are usually not involved.

Clinically, such cases may be slowly progressive, or due to treatment, may become stationary, or even regress with much fibrosis. On the other hand, after a chronic course of a number of years, the tempo of the process is likely to be speeded up with a rapid bronchogenic spread, and often accompanied terminally by an hematogenous dissemination of the organisms, with the development of miliary tubercles in the lung, liver, spleen and other viscera.

Histologically, the lesions are characterized by an abundant productive exudate with many "epithelioid" cells, giant cells and lymphocytes. Special staining reveals considerable increase in the reticulum which extends into the areas of caseation. Fibrosis is a prominent feature, and is seen to best advantage in the older lesions. The resistance of the patient is evidenced by the presence of this extensive reaction, by the persistence of the elastic tissues and by the proliferation of the reticulum. Typical miliary tubercles are often formed as the result of the bronchogenic spread of the process.

Acute Pneumonic Form (Tuberculous Lobar or Bronchopneumonia, "Galloping" Consumption).— Clinically, in this type of tuberculosis, the onset may resemble a lobar pneumonia in which, however, the crisis fails to appear. Physical signs of consolidation are apparent over a lobe or even the entire lung. Eventually, the tubercle bacillus is demonstrated in the sputum and the true nature of the process is discovered.

The entire disease may run its course in the matter of a few weeks. In this form of the disease, the resistance of the patient to the organism is very slight. The process spreads throughout the lung with great rapidity. The bronchi become involved, and small cavities may be formed. These may occur anywhere in the lung. Their walls are made up of ragged, necrotic, caseating lung tissue. The process is one of rapid caseation with little or no reaction in the form of exudate or fibrous tissue formation. It spreads by way of the bronchi, and by the lymphatics to other lobes. Terminally, it frequently becomes hematogenous in nature, through ulceration into a pulmonary vein, and the patient may succumb to a complicating tuberculous meningitis.

Histologically, massive caseation of the lung is the dominant feature, but the outlines of the alveoli may still be recognized. Some of the vesicles contain an acute exudate made up of fibrin, mononuclears and occasionally a few polymorphonuclears. Special staining reveals the organisms present in large numbers. In the less extensively involved portions, tubercle formation may be seen but such tubercles consist solely of areas of caseation necrosis around which a few "epithelioid" cells and lymphocytes may be seen.

Weigert stains reveal extensive destruction of the elastic tissue throughout the areas of caseation. There is no proliferation of the reticulum within the lesions as is seen in the usual fibrocaseous form where the resistance is high. The peribronchial lymph nodes usually show caseous lesions.

Acute Miliary Tuberculosis.—In this form of the disease the organisms gain access to the blood stream from some focal primary or secondary lesion. This is likely to be in the apex of the lung or in one of the caseous peribronchial lymph nodes. The lungs, as well as various viscera, spleen, kidney, etc., are studded with tiny miliary tubercles. They are about 1 mm. in diameter, are grayish in color and semi-translucent. In the lung they usually occur in groups and may be palpated as tiny shot-like nodules throughout the lung. Histologic examination of such lesions reveals numerous miliary tubercles with caseation at the center and a few epithelioid cells and lymphocytes at the periphery. Giant cells in some instances may be seen. Death occurs in such cases due either to the overwhelming toxemia or to terminal involvement of the central nervous system in a tuberculous meningitis which is quite commonly associated with this form of tuberculosis.

Syphilis of the Lung

This condition may be congenital or acquired. The *congenital form* is encountered in the "stillborn" and occasionally in infants. The usual lesion is a diffuse process throughout a considerable portion of one or both lungs. There is a diffuse, fibrous proliferation of the stroma, together with an obliteration of the air sacs. Some, however, may persist, and are lined by cuboidal epithelium. When such a lung is expanded, the affected portion remains airless and very pale, since, due to the constriction of the alveolar structure, the blood supply is materially reduced. The term "white hepatization" or *pneumonia alba,* has thus been applied. Special silver staining (Levaditi method) reveal innumerable Treponemata (Fig. 121). It is accompanied by other evidence of syphilis with changes in the spleen, liver, bones, etc. See Chapter XV, Case 58. At times, the lesions may be tertiary in type and consist of miliary gummata.

Acquired Form.—In acquired syphilis of the lung, the most frequent finding is the gumma. It is usually found near the hilus and is commonly solitary. It varies considerably in size, is grayish or grayish-yellow in color, and may show caseation near the center. In old lesions, a dense fibrous tissue with hyalinization is usually present and at times the true nature of the lesion is difficult to determine. A rather unusual type of acquired syphilis occurs in the lung in the form of a diffuse fibrosis, usually beginning about the hilus and extending into the lung. The causative organisms may occasionally be demonstrated. Miliary gummata formation accompanies the condition. A few cases of stenosis of the bronchi, and usually followed by ulceration, have been demonstrated to be of syphilitic etiology. For a detailed discussion of the organism and syphilis in general, refer to Chapter XV.

Actinomycosis

The lesions of actinomycosis in the lung are usually secondary to infection by the fungus about the mouth. However, the organism may be inhaled directly into the lung. The lungs show numerous small areas of liquefaction necrosis, unlike tuberculosis. If the case is of long standing, considerable fibrosis may be present walling off the areas. Within the lesion, the ray-fungus may be seen (Fig. 162 and 164). The lesions are prone to ulcerate into the bronchi or bronchioles. The fungi are seen in the sputum in the form of colonies as tiny, yellowish or grayish masses, about 1 mm. in diameter, and are referred to as *"sulphur granules."* The disease in general, with a discussion of the fungus, has been included under Chapter XVII, Case 63 (Ref. #S-250).

Blastomycosis

Involvement of the lung in infections due either to the American or European variety of blastomyces is common. In some instances the primary lesions are cutaneous. In others the organism is apparently inhaled as spores in dust. The lesions produce a patchy type of consolidation which is soon followed by necrosis and cavitation of the lung, which may be confused with tuberculosis. The necrotic process is usually more acute in nature and liquefactive rather than caseous, however.

Histologically, the lung shows a number of abscess-like lesions scattered throughout the lobe from which a small amount of pus may be pressed out. The surrounding lung seems to be consolidated. His-tologically, the central part of the lesion consists of liquefaction necrosis with numerous polymorphonuclear leukocytes. In the surrounding area the lung is consolidated by fibrinous exudate in which numerous polymorphonuclear leukocytes are present. The budding, yeast-like blastomyces are present in large numbers and are seen as refractile oval bodies. Many show figure "8" formation (Fig. 165 and 166). In the less acute forms of the disease there may be a tendency towards fibrosis and numerous foreign body giant cells containing fungi may be seen. A discussion of the disease in general, together with the morphology of the organism will be found in Chapter XVII, Case 64 (Ref. #S-288).

Other Chronic Infectious Granulomatous Conditions Affecting the Lung

Streptothricosis, Sporothricosis, Aspergillosis, Moniliasis, Coccidiodal granuloma and Glanders have also already been discussed in Chapter XVII in respect to their pulmonary pathology.

PART II

THE PNEUMOCONIOSES

Pneumoconiosis results chiefly from the infiltration of inorganic particulate matter into the lung through the inhalation of various dusts containing the irritant substance. It is a common occupational disease. It is frequently seen in miners, in stone cutters and grinders, and in similar employment. As a rule, pneumoconiosis per se is not a fatal disease. Its importance lies in the ease with which tuberculosis may occur following lung damage from certain forms of dust infiltration. The most important forms are silicosis, asbestosis and anthracosis.

Several other forms of pneumoconiosis have been described; for example, siderosis, a form frequently observed in workers in iron, brass, bronze, tin or copper industries; and chalicosis, occurring among potters, workers in quarries, stone cutters, grinders, etc. Inhalation of organic dust likewise occurs, but the response is mild and the irritant is usually absorbed without serious injury. Such cases are seen among workers in shoddy, in cotton and wool weavers, felt workers and the like.

Silicosis.—Silicosis was originally described as occurring among the gold miners of South Africa. However, it is now recognized that in the above and other similar forms of pneumoconiosis, it is the presence of silicon within the dust that is responsible for the characteristic tissue reaction and the serious injury to the lung.

Grossly, the lungs of silicosis are grayish in color. They vary considerably in size, but usually do not collapse on opening the chest. They are further characterized by the presence of typical, small nodules, which may be palpated throughout the lung. If the lesions have become confluent, that whole portion of the lung may be quite firm. On section, the nodule cuts with fibroid resistance. They not infrequently present a soft, necrotic or caseous center with laminated layers of dense fibrous tissue surrounding. If the lesions are very numerous, there may be evidence of chronic congestion of the lung, and clinically patients may show dyspnea. Silicosis, uncomplicated by tuberculosis, probably never shows extensive necrosis nor cavity formation. The process is usually slow and may require a number of years of repeated exposure to the dust to bring about advanced lesions. On the other hand, well authenticated instances of the disease have been recorded in which the exposure to the silicon was only the matter of a few weeks. The infiltration of the lung parenchyma is of importance because of its apparent effect in lowering resistance to infection by the tubercle bacillus.

Histologically, when the silicon-containing dust is inhaled into the alveoli, the particles penetrate the alveolar wall either directly or through the intermediary action of large mononuclear phagocytes. They are thus conveyed to the lymphoid tissue of the alveolar wall. Within the tissues, the silicon may lead to some irritation mechanically due to its sharp edges. However, it is probable that the major part of the reaction is secondary to irritating substances produced by its solution in the tissue fluids. The first effect seems to be in the form of local necrosis. The area is soon surrounded by mononuclear cells. Fibroblasts proliferate in large numbers about the area and result in the formation of a dense layer of fibrous tissue. This continues to be deposited in concentric layers, walling-off the lesion. The older nodules are made up almost completely of this concentrically arranged fibrous tissue, which may show some necrosis of the central part, and which undergoes extensive hyalinization. These silicotic nodules are characteristic of the process.

Illustrative Case

Case 185. (Ref. #S-297)
Diagnosis.—Lung—silicosis.

Patient was a male of 40 years, who had worked in a Portland cement factory for ten years and was admitted to the hospital with the chief complaint of a chronic cough with considerable sputum.

Present Illness.—The onset of the patient's present illness was totally indefinite. It dated back for a number of years when he had first noted a rather persistent, dry, hacking type of cough which had increased in severity as time went on. In recent months, this had been accompanied by the raising of considerable mucopurulent sputum and on exertion he had noted moderate difficulty in breathing. His appetite had fallen off in the past few months and he believed he had lost perhaps ten pounds in weight. He had had occasional night sweats which had been rather severe, and he believed that he had had some afternoon temperature on occasion. He did not feel acutely ill, but just below par, and was beginning to be worried about his cough as some kindly friend had suggested that it sounded like tuberculosis. Accordingly he entered the hospital for thorough study.

Past Medical History.—The patient had had all the usual childhood diseases. He had never, however, had rheumatic fever so far as he was aware. A review of his systems in general was not particularly enlightening. He had not been unduly subject to upper respiratory infection, and aside from this progressive and persistent cough had not had any symptoms referable to his respiratory tract. He had never been heart conscious. His gastro-intestinal history was of little value in estimating his present illness. His appetite had always been rather variable but up to the present time he had maintained his weight. His genito-urinary history was negative. He denied venereal disease.

Physical Examination.—Patient was a fairly well developed but somewhat underweight middle-aged white male. Head was not remarkable. Eyes, ears, nose and throat were negative. Chest was symmetrical. Expansion was equal but somewhat limited on both sides. On percussion, no actual dullness could be made out, but there did seem to be some impairment of breath sounds and a number of fine crackling râles throughout both lungs on auscultation. Heart was not enlarged. No murmurs were heard. Sounds were of good quality. Abdomen was negative. Extremities were negative except for beginning clubbing of his fingers.

Laboratory Findings.—Red blood cells on admission numbered 4,200,000 cells with 78% hemoglobin. White blood cells, 9,200 with 71% neutrophiles. Urinalysis was negative. Sputum examination was negative for tubercle bacilli on several occasions. Wassermann was negative.

X-ray examination of the patient's chest revealed a mottling throughout both lungs of the type to almost suggest a diffuse miliary or conglomerate type of hematogenous spread tuberculosis. On the other hand, the majority of the lesions seemed to be relatively larger than the usual tubercles and many of them showed calcification. In view of the patient's occupational history, a tentative diagnosis of silicosis was made.

Subsequent Course.—The patient developed a typical diffuse confluent bronchopneumonia within the first forty-eight hours after admission, which apparently had been in its incubation period. He went rapidly downhill and died two weeks after admission.

Autopsy Findings.—The autopsy findings of significance were restricted to the lungs. Both lungs were uniformly studded with hard, shotty nodules varying in size from the head of a large pin to a centimeter in diameter. This was accompanied by marked anthracosis. Lungs were likewise relatively emphysematous and on section suggested a diffuse fibrosis, cutting with markedly increased resistance. There was a diffuse confluent bronchopneumonia involving the left lower lobe, which appeared to be the immediate cause of death. Moderate chronic passive congestion of the viscera was noted.

Microscopic Description of a Section Through the Lung.—(Fig. 425) Histologic examinations of the tissues

Asbestosis.—Asbestosis occurs as a result of inhalation of dust in the processing of asbestos rather than in the mining of the rock. Asbestos is hydrated silica of magnesium with usually small percentages of iron and nickel. Here again we are dealing with a form of silicosis. Following this infiltration, lesions develop rapidly, and death may occur without the complication of tuberculosis. The asbestos appears in the lung as tiny black particles or frequently as elongated, golden-yellow, dumb-bell-like structures with segmented bodies. These structures are probably fragments of asbestos fiber which have been partially digested by the tissue fluids. They are sometimes found in the sputum, and are pathognomonic. Pathologically, the process is usually diffuse. Evidence of pulmonary congestion is marked. There is an associated bronchitis and terminal bronchopneumonia in the fatal cases.

Anthracosis.—Anthracosis results from the inhalation of dusts containing carbon particles. This form of pneumoconiosis is almost universal, particularly in the lungs of city-dwellers, due to the inhalation of carbon particles in the air. In coal miners, an extreme degree of the condition may be encountered. The lungs externally show numerous black or dark gray areas beneath the pleura, which usually are several millimeters in diameter, and in extreme conditions the lungs may be almost solid black. On section, the anthracotic infiltration can be seen studding the lung throughout, particularly concentrated

reveals the characteristic picture of what appears to be uncomplicated silicosis. The general features which are observed consist of a diffuse fibrosis of the entire lung parenchyma with moderate thickening of the alveolar walls in many places. In an attempt to compensate for this change some emphysema of the air vesicles is observed in places. Around the bronchi and bronchioles, there is a characteristic silicotic nodule formation. This is seen as an almost laminated mass of hyalinized connective tissue. Centrally some of these nodules show degenerative changes with actual calcification. For the most part, however, they are seen to consist of simply concentric layer upon layer of collagen in which very few nuclei can be identified. Around this silicotic nodule is a zone of chronic inflammatory cellular infiltration. This consists of a variety of mononuclear cells including lymphocytes, plasma cells and scattered large mononuclear phagocytes. Only rarely is a foreign-body giant cell seen.

in the subpleura, about the bronchi and bronchioles and to a lesser degree, the interstitial tissue throughout the rest of the lung. This forms a network outlining the lymphatics of the lung and pleura grossly (Fig. 37, Case 14, Ref. #S-188, Chapter IV). The peribronchial lymph nodes are usually coal black.

Microscopically, the carbon particles are seen within the lymphoid tissues of the lung. They are contained to a considerable extent within the reticulo-endothelial cells but at times accumulate in large masses apparently lying free within the connective tissue. A moderate degree of such anthracosis is seen in practically all adult lungs without much evidence of other pathologic change. When the condition is extreme, however, there is a considerable increase in fibrous scar tissue in the vicinity of large masses of pigment. Moderate pulmonary congestion may result.

Unlike silicosis, according to recent reports, the incidence of tuberculosis is not much greater among individuals (coal miners) suffering with extreme anthracotic pneumoconiosis than in average adults. In view of the poor hygienic conditions of the average mine, together with a lack of sunshine, this statement would appear to take on added importance. It is explained on the basis that the anthracotic process acts at the outset to prevent the spread of tuberculosis through blocking the lymphatic circulation mechanically until ultimately the condition becomes extreme, and the infection spreads rapidly.

PART III

DISEASES OF THE PLEURA

The pathological processes which affect the pleura are for the most part secondary to some underlying pulmonary or circulatory disturbance, and accordingly have been discussed already to a large extent. However, there are a few conditions encountered in which the clinical picture is dependent chiefly upon the lesion of the pleura primarily. These will be reviewed briefly.

Hydropleura (Hydrothorax).—By this is meant the accumulation of an excessive amount of transudate within the pleural cavity. The process is usually bilateral and is particularly associated with renal and cardiac disease. In the cases associated with renal disease the quantity of fluid is only moderate and both pleural cavities are usually involved to an equal degree. In those cases due to cardiac disease, on the other hand, the process is often unilateral, usually on the right side. If it is bilateral, there is a tendency for the amount to be greater within the right than the left pleural sac. The fluid is usually clear, amber in color, with specific gravity under 1.018 and a protein content of less than four per cent. The few cells obtained by centrifugation are mononuclear in character. These are mainly desquamated endothelial cells. Neutrophiles are usually absent.

Hemopleura (Hemothorax).—Hemorrhage into the pleura may be brought about by traumatic wounds of the chest, such as a fracture of the ribs, stab wounds, or gun-shot wounds, or it may result from rupture of an aortic aneurysm, hemorrhage from malignant tumors, or more rarely blood dyscrasias such as purpura hemorrhagica. Under these circumstances the pleural cavity is more or less completely filled with blood or blood clot. The lesion is usually unilateral. The etiology is easily demonstrated as a rule.

Pneumothorax (Pneumopleura).—By this term is meant the presence of air or gas within the pleura. This results in a degree of collapse of the lung. Etiologically, the great majority of cases result from the perforation of a tuberculous cavity into the pleura. Seventy to ninety per cent of pneumothorax is of this variety according to Boyd. A few cases result from rupture of an abscess or bronchiectatic cavity of the lung which already communicates with the bronchial tree. Occasionally, an emphysematous bleb may rupture. Wounds of the chest, perforation of the esophagus or stomach as a result of malignancy or ulcer, perforation of the diaphragm and pleura in ulcerative carcinomas, and even abscesses of the liver are other less common causes. A pneumothorax may be produced by the growth of organisms of the gas-gangrene group such as Bacillus welchii. This, however, is a very rare occurrence and probably is only associated with traumatic lesions. In the treatment of certain types of pulmonary tuberculosis, an artificial pneumothorax is produced and maintained by the injection of nitrogen to enable the pathological process in the lung to heal.

Pleuritis.—The process may be primary or secondary, acute or chronic, fibrinous, sero-fibrinous or suppurative in type. Most of these have been described in relation to their associated pulmonary pathology, and so will only be reviewed briefly at this time.

FIBRINOUS PLEURITIS (DRY PLEURISY).—This type of pleuritis is usually secondary to pathology within the lung or adjacent organs from which the organism spreads by lymphatics or by direct continuity. Thus, the pleura over an affected lobe in lobar pneumonia will show a fibrinous exudate. Likewise, in bronchopneumonia, infarction and abscess, a fibrinous pleuritis will occur over the affected area. Occasionally, it may accompany a tuberculous lesion of the lung. In a few cases no demonstrable pathology can be shown in the adjacent organs and the process would seem to be primary within the pleura. In some of these the tubercle bacillus may be demonstrated. The condition occasionally occurs during the course of rheumatic fever and may be due to involvement of the pleura by the infecting agent.

Pathology.—The affected pleura is covered by a fibrinous exudate which varies in thickness up to one half inch. If extensive, it may appear shaggy, with adhesions between the visceral and parietal layers. The fluid portion of the exudate is inconspicuous or absent. This exudate, if not rapidly removed, undergoes organization and subsequent fibrous adhesions are produced. In the great majority of cases the removal of exudate takes place by lysis and absorption, but in tuberculosis adhesions usually result and at times go on to obliteration of the pleural sac.

SEROFIBRINOUS (WET PLEURISY).—The serofibrinous variety is characterized by a thin layer of fibrin covering the pleura plus considerable free serous exudate. The fibrinous element is so insignificant in many cases that the condition is frequently simply spoken of as serous. According to Aschoff seventy-five to eighty per cent of such cases are due to the tubercle bacillus. It may occasionally be seen in lobar pneumonia due to the pneumococcus. In streptococcic bronchopneumonia the pleuritis may begin as serofibrinous but very frequently progresses to suppurative empyema. A few cases are associated with rheumatic fever.

Pathology.—Typically the picture is one of a thin fibrinous exudate covering the pleura, and with considerable clear, amber-colored fluid present within the pleural sac. In this instance, the specific gravity is over 1.018 and the protein content greater than four per cent. If the streptococcus or pneumococcus is the etiological cause, polymorphonuclears will be present in the exudate. In the case of the tuberculous variety, the cells of the exudate are mainly lymphocytes.

SUPPURATIVE PLEURITIS (EMPYEMA).—The condition is more common in children than in adults. Pneumococci, streptococci and tubercle bacilli are the most common etiologic agents. The process is usually secondary to lung infection, often as the result of rupture of an abscess into the pleura. In from two to five per cent of lobar pneumonia a suppurative pleuritis due to the penumococcus complicates the picture, the organism apparently extending directly from the pneumonic area. In epidemic influenza, measles, and streptococcal bronchopneumonia with an associated pulmonary abscess in many instances give rise to a suppurative pleuritis. A few cases of empyema are due to wounds of the chest. A few seem to be primary without apparent associated pulmonary disease. In these cases, the organisms must be brought by way of the blood stream. Rarely, the tubercle bacillus is found in empyema.

Pathology.—The surface of the lung is covered by a shaggy fibrinous exudate which may be quite thick and involve the parietal and visceral layers. The lung is partially collapsed due to the presence of varying quantities of pus undergoing liquefaction necrosis. There is a tendency for the empyema to be localized by such fibrinous exudate, as for example, between the lobes, as an interlobar empyema. The pus is usually thick and creamy if the organism is one of the pneumococci. In streptococcic empyema, on the other hand, the pus is rather thin and serous. Amyloid infiltration of the various organs is occasionally seen in empyema. Varying degrees of atelectasis of the lung are produced which may be permanent, as a result of the enormous amount of thickening of the pleura, which follows the organization of the fibrin.

Tumors of the Pleura.—Among the rarer tumors are those of the pleura. They have been discussed in Chapter XXVII dealing with the so-called endotheliomata. It will be recalled that they occur either in a papillary or a solid form, and that their exact histogenesis is still somewhat debatable.

CHAPTER XLV

DISEASES OF THE RESPIRATORY SYSTEM (*Continued*)

LUNG (continued)

TUMORS OF THE LUNG

The problem of cancer of the lung has become of increasing importance during the past two decades as a result of a very striking increase in incidence of the condition. Fried, Simons, and others, in their recent reviews of the subject, have emphasized this curious phenomenon that, whereas cancer of the lung was an extreme rarity scarcely twenty years ago, yet to-day it is rapidly climbing toward the third place among the various forms of systemic malignancy. Historically, however, cancer of the lung has been known for at least over four hundred years, dating back to the time of Agricola. The first adequate description of such a condition was given by Morgagni in 1761, but even as recently as 1912, only three hundred and seventy-four cases had apparently been reported in the medical literature as presented in Adler's monograph. In recent years, however, cancer of the lung has definitely increased until it now represents approximately fifteen per cent of all reported cases as a cause of death.

With this increasing incidence of a condition, naturally speculation turns in the direction designed to attempt to explain it. In Simons' recent review, he records fourteen different etiologic factors, which have been suggested as possibly of some significance. These, he has classified as follows: Heredity, trauma, tuberculosis, influenza, pneumoconiosis, roentgen rays, dust inhalation, inhalation of tar particles, inhalation of motor exhaust fumes, war gases, and various other forms of industrial occupational hazards, the inhalation of tobacco smoke, and the problem of general hygiene, particularly as influenced by vitamin deficiency in the diet. This latter cause has already been mentioned in respect to the changes which could be produced in experimental animals, as shown by Wolbach and Howe on white mice on a deficient Vitamin "A" intake. After an exhaustive

discussion of these various factors, Simons comes to the conclusion that "no single agent is the sole cause of pulmonary cancer. Without exception, all of the fourteen etiologic factors so far suggested have one common quality—the production of chronic pulmonary irritation. Chronic irritation, whether simple or complex, may be (1) chemical, (2) mechanical, (3) bacterial, (4) radio-active or (5) as has not been investigated, but has occurred in several modern industries, thermal." He goes on to state that even heredity requires chronic irritation for the activation of malignancy.

From the clinical standpoint, the problem of diagnosis is often most difficult and uncertain, by the usual routine methods of examination of a patient. In this connection, it is of some interest to note that the incidence of the disease is approximately three times as great in men as in women. The age incidence has been recorded from as young as sixteen months to as old as ninety-one years. The peak incidence of pulmonary cancer, however, is found in the fifth decade, although the sixth decade runs a very close second. It has been incontrovertibly demonstrated that the great majority of tumors of the lung are basically of bronchogenic origin. As such, they tend to arise in the bronchial mucosa, to be slow growing and, therefore, to be late in their manifestations symptomatically. Ultimately, the tumor, in its growth, will tend to occlude the bronchus in which it arises. This, in turn, will be followed by atelectasis of the obstructive acquired type. At this time, x-ray examination of the chest may show such an atelectatic band and may demonstrate some deviation of the trachea or even of the entire mediastinum with the tendency toward their displacement in the direction of the affected side. The tumor, more often than not, is not demonstrable by x-ray due to its rela-

PLATE CII
TUMORS OF THE LUNGS

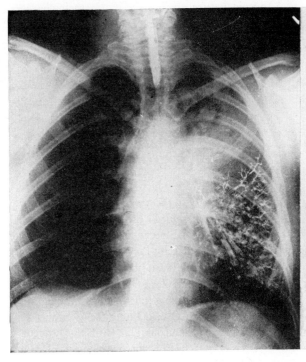

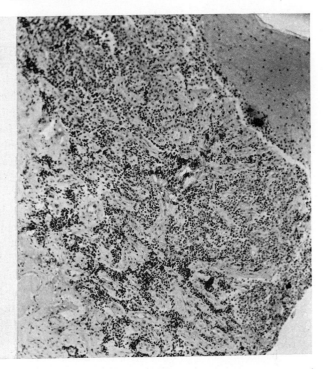

FIG. 432.—ROENTGENOGRAM: CHEST: ADENOMA.—CASE 186.—Lipiodol installation shows almost complete obstruction of left upper bronchus with resultant atelectasis of left upper lobe.

FIG. 433.—LUNGS BENIGN ADENOMA.—CASE 186.—Submucosal neoplasm composed of masses of small hyperchromic epithelial cells showing a tendency toward acinar formation. Structural arrangement and absence of mitoses suggest its benign nature. App. 100 x.

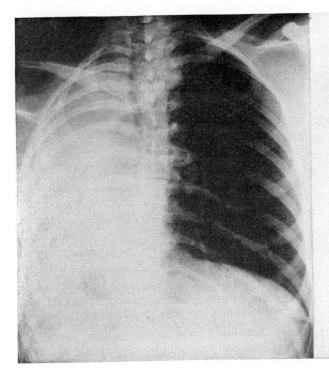

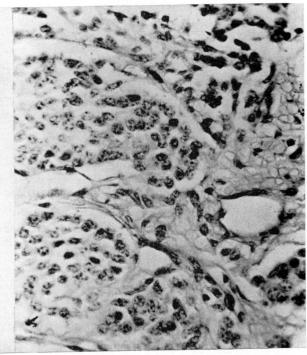

FIG. 434.—ROENTGENOGRAM: CHEST: BRONCHOGENIC CARCINOMA (ADENOCARCINOMA).—CASE 187.—Plate demonstrates complete occlusion of left main bronchus with resultant atelectasis of the lung.

FIG 435.—LUNG: BRONCHOGENIC CARCINOMA (ADENOCARCINOMA TYPE).—CASE 187.—Invasive tumor made up of relatively undifferentiated, atypical, hyperchromatic cells with occasional mitotic figures, and with some suggestion of acinar arrangement. App. 400 x.

tively small size and the fact that the secondary atelectatic changes of the lung overshadow the actual neoplastic lesion. As a result of the atelectasis, not infrequently pneumonia may occur and should serve to warn the alert physician of the possibility of an underlying neoplasm as an etiologic factor in its development. Perhaps even more frequently than pneumonia, a chronic suppurative bronchiectasis is encountered which is very commonly mistaken for tuberculosis. Paralysis of the diaphragm, and aphonia as the result of recurrent laryngeal nerve involvement are other symptoms which point toward this diagnosis.

As a final step in the establishment of the diagnosis of a bronchial or pulmonary neoplasm, bronchoscopy is essential. By the early use of bronchoscopy in the hands of a skilled bronchoscopist, biopsy material from the great majority of such lesions can be obtained for pathological verification of the suspected diagnosis. This is of great clinical importance because certain tumors arising in these tissues are of an entirely benign nature and the treatment should be of an entirely different type than in those instances of frank malignancy. The earlier diagnosis can be established, the more likely success may be had in the surgical treatment of these cases by pneumonectomy. It has been found, through considerable experience, that x-ray treatment is of very uncertain value. On the other hand, the importance of x-ray in the diagnosis of the condition, particularly from the standpoint of whether it is a hilar or central type of tumor, or a peripheral bronchial lesion, is of great consequence. In this x-ray method of diagnosis, the use of artificial pneumothorax may be of considerable value in outlining the size and position of the lesion and of the amount of lung tissue involved. Similarly, the use of lipiodol has been of considerable value in localizing the lesion through the obstructive phenomena and in differentiating malignancy from a simple chronic bronchiectasis.

From the clinical standpoint, the most frequent symptoms found are those of a sharp, stabbing type of pain in the chest, due to early involvement of the pleura. This is often aggravated by percussion. Dyspnea, combined with qualitative pain in the chest and hemoptysis should always incite suspicion in the absence of hypertension or primary valvular heart disease. Repeated small hemoptyses are likewise very suggestive of carcinoma when they occur in the in-

dividual in the cancer age. Cough and expectoration of a mucoid nature are less specific in their characteristics. This is also true of the rather frequent weakness and rapid loss of weight, which not infrequently accompanies the condition. Dry cough, out of all proportions to the physical findings, is definitely suggestive.

Pathology.—In the classification of tumors arising in the lung, we find that there is a considerable variation in the picture. In two recent papers by Jackson and Konzelmann, a series of cases of primary lung tumors was reviewed, which illustrates, in general, the features which we wish to emphasize in this respect. All of these cases were checked by biopsy diagnosis obtained through bronchoscopy. From the pathological standpoint, tumors arising from the bronchi and lung may be divided into five varieties based primarily on their specific histologic features. From the broader standpoint of classification, all tumors of the lung must arise, as Ewing has so aptly stated, from (1) cells lining the bronchi, (2) cells making up the mucous glands of the bronchi, and (3) cells which line the pulmonary alveoli. Thus, it should be theoretically possible to have a simple adenoma which might arise from either type of bronchial epithelial cell, the glandular epithelium or the surface epithelium; or an adenocarcinoma from either of these cells. Inasmuch as there is so little accord among histologists, embryologists and pathologists regarding the nature of the lining cells of the pulmonary alveoli, less certainty can be expressed in respect to the type of tumor which one might be likely to find arising from those cells. From the practical standpoint, it can be said without fear of contradiction that tumors of the alveolar lining cells are extremely rare and might even be open to some question.

Curiously enough, in spite of this theoretical consideration of the possible types of tumor which one might expect to find arising in the bronchi and lungs on the basis of the normal cell make-up of these tissues, the great majority of cases of malignant tumors are of the squamous type, which implies either some metaplasia of these ciliated lining cells, or as Fried has emphasized, a common embryologic ancestry for the epithelium which gives rise on the one hand to the squamous lining of the esophagus, and on the other hand to the ciliated lining cells of the respiratory tree. This is perhaps the simplest way in which to interpret the rather startling pre-

PLATE CIII
MALIGNANT TUMORS OF THE LUNG

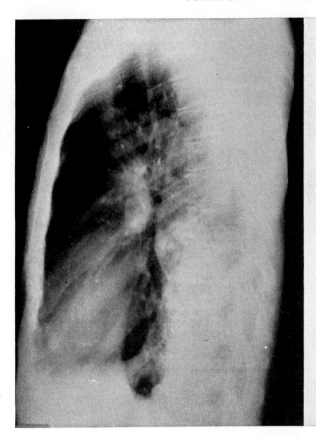

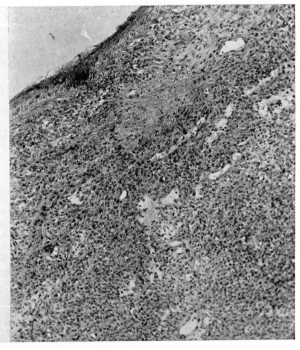

FIG. 436.—ROENTGENOGRAM: CHEST (LATERAL VIEW), BRONCHO-
GENIC CARCINOMA) (SQUAMOUS CELL TYPE).—CASE 188.—Left
lower lobe of lung atelectatic. Dense shadow at apex of atelectatic
lobe suggesting possible neoplasm.

FIG. 437.—LUNG: BRONCHOGENIC CARCINOMA (SQUAMOUS CELL
TYPE).—CASE 188.—Typical squamous cell carcinoma invading lung substance: Composed of pleomorphic, anaplastic
cells showing atypic mitoses but some attempt at differentiation with keratinization and "pearl" formation. App. 100 x.
(Courtesy J. Thoracic Surgery.)

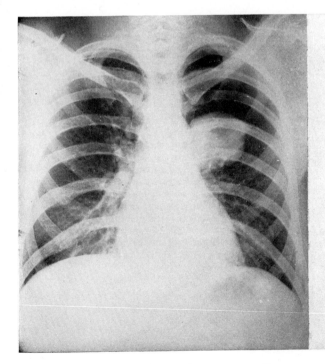

FIG. 438.—ROENTGENOGRAM—CHEST—BRONCHOGENIC CARCINOMA
(UNDIFFERENTIATED CELL TYPE).—CASE 189.—Plate reveals a
mass 2.5 cm. in diameter just above the left lung root, strongly
suggestive of neoplasm.

FIG. 439.—LUNG—BRONCHOGENIC CARCINOMA (UNDIFFEREN-
TIATED CELL TYPE).—CASE 189.—Tumor composed of sheets
of totally undifferentiated cells showing considerable spindling. Many atypic mitoses, areas of necrosis and hemorrhage
all attest to its rapid growth and high malignancy. App. 100 x.

dominance of squamous carcinoma. Practically, we find, as has already been mentioned, at least five distinct varieties of neoplasm.

ADENOMATA.—In a series of nearly seventy cases of bronchial or pulmonary neoplasm, twelve cases were found by Jackson and Konzelmann of this benign type. They are most frequently designated by the term *bronchial adenoma,* or an *adenomatous polyp of the bronchus.* These tumors offer more difficulty, perhaps, to the uninitiated and inexperienced pathologist than almost any other type of neoplasm from the standpoint of diagnosis. They are very commonly considered as malignant tumors and indeed, in the investigation of this problem, the clinical history of certain of these cases was of unquestionable value in the ultimate recognition of the pathological lesion. The tumors, themselves, have little regularity in their microscopic appearance, and show some of the most bizarre histologic features at times, in respect to cytological detail. Their nuclear structure, however, retains a striking degree of normalcy, and the inability of the tumors either to infiltrate or to metastasize is further evidence of their benign nature. From the gross pathological standpoint, and from that of the clinician, particularly the bronchoscopist, it is noteworthy that all of these tumors are endobronchial in origin and tend to protrude into the lumen of the bronchus. The tumor, in general, seems to be a small nodular lesion just beneath a somewhat hyperplastic epithelium, which tends to be of the squamous cell type. The tumor is not infrequently almost encapsulated from the surrounding tissues by a dense zone of hyalinized connective tissue. At times the tumors seem to be arranged in sheets or cords without any specific acinar arrangement and may resemble a basal cell so-called "carcinoma." There is marked variation in the shape and even in the size of the cells at times, but the nuclei remain consistently uniform, usually ovoid, with small nucleoli and only finely scattered granules and rods of chromatin. At times, the acinar arrangement of the tumor may be very striking and in some instances the cells appear to be capable of actual secretion with the formation of mucus. It is striking that mitotic figures are rarely encountered in these tumors. The amount of stroma varies, as is true in other similar benign adenomatous lesions. As was suggested by Kernam, the possibility of these tumors being related to the so-called "carcinoids" of the gastro-intestinal tract has been difficult to rule out on morphologic grounds alone, but those tumors which have been studied by silver impregnation methods fail to show the argentophile nature of the cells.

ILLUSTRATIVE CASE

CASE 186. (Ref. #S-375)
Diagnosis.—Bronchus—benign adenoma.
Patient was a white female of 33 years, admitted to the hospital because of a productive cough of two years' duration.
Present Illness.—The onset of the present illness was insidious. It began approximately two years before the present admission with what the patient thought was a simple acute upper respiratory infection. This was followed by a chronic, dry cough which during the past few months had become much looser in character and associated with the raising of a very considerable amount of sputum. This was occasionally blood streaked. The patient likewise complained of pain in her chest accompanying the more severe coughing attacks. She had had occasional chills and night sweats and ran a regular low-grade temperature every afternoon. She had noted some dyspnea at times, but had had no dysphagia. On the basis of these findings, in spite of the negative sputum, the patient was admitted to a tuberculosis sanatorium where she remained for nine months and gained twenty-two pounds in weight. Repeated sputum examinations during this period were consistently negative. No changes were found in the x-ray studies of the lung, and as a result the patient was finally discharged with the diagnosis of some chronic pulmonary lesion which was probably non-tuberculous. Her cough, however, had persisted and she was referred to this hospital for further study.
Past Medical History.—The patient had had the usual childhood diseases, but nothing of a serious nature until the onset of the present illness. At that time she believed that she had a mild attack of pneumonia with her upper respiratory infection, but this could not be confirmed. The patient was married and had had three children, all prematurely delivered, who died within a few weeks after birth.
Physical Examination.—Patient was a well-developed and well-nourished young white female who appeared to be in excellent health. Head was negative. Eyes reacted normally. Nose and throat were negative. Mouth showed good oral hygiene. She had apparently had a tonsillectomy. A moderate, chronic, granular type of pharyngitis was present. The chest showed a limited expansion of the left upper portion. This was associated with a definitely impaired percussion note over the left upper lobe with diminished breath sounds. Many coarse râles were present. In general, the remainder of the lung sounds were negative. Heart was not enlarged, and showed no murmurs. Abdomen was negative. Extremities: There was slight clubbing of her finger tips, but the extremities otherwise were negative. Temperature, at the time of

admission, was slightly elevated ranging from 97.6 to 100.4°. Pulse and respirations were normal. Blood pressure was 130/80. Bronchoscopic examination revealed an obstructive lesion in the left upper bronchus. This could be readily visualized. It appeared to be submucosal in position with marked inflammatory thickening of the overlying mucosa. A specimen was removed for histologic examination.

Laboratory Findings.—Red blood cells, 4,900,000 with 11.5 gm. of hemoglobin. White blood cells, 13,150 with 51% polynuclears. Urinalysis was negative. Sputum examination was negative for tubercle bacilli and for spirochetes or fungi. There was a scant growth of non-hemolytic staphylococci.

X-ray examination was made with instillation of lipiodol, and almost complete obstruction of the left upper bronchus was found. There was no evidence of bronchiectasis in the remainder of the lung. (Fig. 432)

Subsequent Course.—On the basis of the pathological findings, the tumor mass was removed from the bronchus and found to be relatively limited in distribution. It showed no evidence of invasion of the wall of the bron-

chus, being entirely restricted to the submucosa. The patient made an uneventful recovery from the operation and at the end of a two-year interval had showed no recurrence, appearing relieved of her symptoms.

Pathological Report.—*Gross Description.*—Specimen consisted of a small biopsy fragment from the left upper bronchus. It was reddish-gray in color and rather firm in consistency. It presented no gross features of diagnostic significance.

Microscopic Description of Section Through the Biopsy Tissue.—(Fig. 433) Histologic examination of the material shows a dense fibrous stroma in which some small areas of actual calcification have occurred. In other areas the tissue is relatively cellular. There are masses of cuboidal and columnar cells in a suggestive glandular architectural arrangement. In other places they form solid sheets. The nuclei of these cells are round or oval, and vesicular in character, containing only fine chromatin granules and small nucleoli. On one side of the specimen, a layer of chronic hyperplastic epithelium is seen representing the mucosal surface. Beneath this, there is a rich vascular bed of granulation tissue.

ADENOCARCINOMA.—The adenocarcinomatous type of lesion is seen with much less frequency. It makes up roughly fifteen to twenty per cent of the total number of cases encountered. The lesion is very likely to arise relatively centrally in relation to the larger bronchi. It starts as an endobronchial lesion from the mucous glands of the bronchus and tends to become an annular growth extending beneath the surface mucosa along the bronchus and thus infiltrating the lung to a considerable distance. At other times, it may break through the bronchial wall and invade the lung parenchyma as a solid tumor mass. It likewise may invade the mucosal surface and fill the bronchus not only as a subepithelial growth but as an actual tumor mass within the lumen. Rarely, tumor tissue may be expectorated and a diagnosis made from such fragments.

Histologically, the picture is that of any adenocarcinoma. The tumors vary considerably in their rate of growth, but in general they are of a relatively low grade malignancy, slowly developing and have a striking tendency to remain localized within the lung substance for many months before they extend to involve the regional peribronchial and mediastinal lymph nodes. It is this fact which renders the prob-

lem of surgery in lung cancer a very real method of therapy, which we believe will be employed much more extensively as times goes on and more men become trained in the field of thoracic surgery. The tumors show a variable amount of acinar arrangement, histologically. In places, this is well-defined. In other areas, the cells occur in sheets and cords with very little lumen formation. The nuclei tend to show rather marked hyperchromatism. They vary in size and shape. Their nucleoli, likewise, are irregular in size in relation to the nucleus. Mitotic figures, both typic and atypic are variable in number, but invariably present. The tumors are likely to show considerable necrosis and hemorrhage. The amount of stroma, as in the case of the benign adenomatous type of lesion, varies, but as a rule is less.

From the standpoint of therapy, these cases are extremely discouraging. The tumor cannot be removed by bronchoscopy. It is usually extremely radio-resistant to irradiation therapy and, unfortunately, is likely to be situated relatively near the hilum which renders the problem of lobectomy or pneumonectomy more complicated, and often impossible.

ILLUSTRATIVE CASE

CASE 187. (Ref. #S-377)
Diagnosis.—Lung—bronchogenic adenocarcinoma.
Patient was a white female of 20 years, admitted to the hospital with the chief complaint of weakness of her lower extremities.

Present Illness.—In reviewing the patient's history, in retrospect it appears that the present illness actually began approximately three years before admission. At that time she had a sudden unexplained profuse hemorrhage which was believed to be of a tuberculous nature.

She thought that she had had an intermittent, dry, non-productive cough for a month or two preceding this hemoptysis, but was somewhat uncertain in this regard. Her interval history had been essentially negative except for a rather persistent dry, hacking type of cough. She had been in a sanatorium for a year with the diagnosis of presumptive tuberculosis, but in view of repeated negative sputum examinations for tubercle bacilli, and a general improvement in her condition, she had been discharged. About one month before her present admission, she began to feel a progressive weakness in her ankles and legs. This was not associated with pain. Within two weeks, the condition had progressed to a point where she was unable to walk without help. At intervals, this had been accompanied by a curious, dull, aching pain between her scapulae, especially when sitting in an upright position. The patient became completely bedridden and noticed that there was a definite tingling sensation with subsequent numbness developing in her feet. Two days before admission, the patient again had a severe pulmonary hemorrhage, losing about 500 c.c. of blood. This came on abruptly in conjunction with a mild coughing attack. Since that time she had had ten or twelve other less severe hemoptyses. She became so weak and exsanguinated that she feared she was going to die and called a physician, who referred her immediately to the hospital.

Past Medical History.—The patient had had all the usual childhood diseases, including scarlet fever and diphtheria. She never had had rheumatic fever, however. She had never had any operations other than tonsillectomy in childhood. A review of her systems revealed that she had always been subject to rather severe epistaxis since childhood. At times, this required packing. Her gastro-intestinal history had always been negative. Her genito-urinary history was negative. Her cardio-respiratory system was of significance in relation to the onset of the present illness as characterized by her intermittent attacks of dyspnea and occasional precordial pain in association with a chronic, nonproductive cough of several years' duration. Her menstrual history was essentially normal. Her periods began at the age of thirteen and were somewhat irregular, ranging from twenty-eight to forty day intervals. She had never had any definite menorrhagia, metrorrhagia or dysmenorrhea.

Physical Examination.—Patient was a well-developed, fairly well-nourished young white female who was resting apparently comfortably in bed. Head was grossly negative. Eyes reacted normally. Ears, nose and throat were negative. Chest was symmetrical. Expansion on the right was good, but was very definitely limited on the left. There was a bulging of the intercostal spaces noted on the left side, especially posteriorly. The percussion note over the entire left side, except in the extreme apex, was almost flat, and auscultation revealed marked changes in breath and voice sounds except in the apical region where many râles were heard. The heart seemed to be within normal limits. Abdomen was negative. Extremities: There was almost complete motor paralysis of the lower extremities with considerable disturbances of sensation as well. On the basis of the physical findings and history, a tentative diagnosis of presumptive left-sided pulmonary tuberculosis with extension to the spine as a Potts' disease, was made.

Laboratory Findings.—On admission the red count was 3,400,000 with 63% hemoglobin. White blood cells, 10,600 with 73% neutrophiles. Blood chemistry was normal. Urinalysis was negative. Repeated sputum examination revealed no acid-fast organisms, no fungi, and no spirochetes.

X-ray examination revealed a complete atelectasis of the entire left lung, except for the apex (Fig. 434). There was deviation of the trachea toward the left. There was some scoliosis of the thoracic spine. The body of the third thoracic vertebra was partially destroyed by what suggested a metastatic neoplasm. This had resulted in pathological fracture of the vertebral body producing moderate kyphosis. There was erosion of the fifth and sixth ribs on the left of a pressure type rather than a metastatic infiltrative nature. The x-ray conclusions were stated as showing complete occlusion of the left main bronchus, probably of a neoplastic nature. Nothing was found by x-ray to suggest tuberculosis.

Subsequent Course.—On the basis of the history, physical examination and x-ray findings, a bronchoscopic examination of the patient was made and the left bronchus was found obstructed by irregular soft fungations. Specimens of this tissue were taken for biopsy study and a large amount of secretion was aspirated after making an airway through the bronchus. In addition to the bronchoscopic operative procedure, an exploratory laminectomy was done exposing the first, second, third, fourth, fifth and sixth thoracic laminae. At the level of the third thoracic lamina a telangiectatic, angiomatous mass was found which had apparently resulted from the invasion of the third vertebral body by tumor, and its subsequent compression. It was felt that no further operative intervention was indicated, and with the laminectomy the pressure symptoms might improve. Clinically, the patient did improve. The lung showed moderate expansion subsequent to the removal of the obstructive portion of the tumor. The pressure symptoms were relieved and a moderate return of function in the lower legs followed. The patient was lost sight of at the end of six months so that it is impossible to state how long she lived, but it was obvious from the findings that it was merely a question of time.

Pathological Report.—*Gross Description.*—Specimen from the bronchus consisted of several brownish-red, hemorrhagic, ragged fragments of tissue totaling about 2 c.c. in volume. No gross features of diagnostic significance could be made out.

Microscopic Description of the Bronchial Biopsy.——(Fig. 435) Histologic examination of the tissue shows a mass of rather large epithelial cells arranged in clumps and sheets. Here and there there is a suggestion of lumen formation with the cells architecturally placed around a potential lumen. The nuclei of these cells are peripherally arranged in the mass so that the resemblance to glands is striking, even where no actual lumina are seen. The cytoplasm is slightly acidophilic. The nuclei stain deeply and show hyperchromatic nucleoli. A few mitotic figures are seen. There is only a scant amount of stroma. Considerable necrosis and hemorrhage are also found.

SQUAMOUS CELL TYPE.—The squamous cell type makes up perhaps seventy to seventy-five per cent of the cases of malignant lung tumors. The same tendency toward slow growth is seen, fortunately, in most of the cases. The location of the tumor is, on the other hand, probably a little more favorable than in the adenocarcinomatous group, as they not infrequently will be found to involve secondary and tertiary bronchi rather than the primary or major divisions. The clinical features are similar to those of other forms of pulmonary neoplasm and need not be repeated at this point.

The microscopic diagnosis of this type of tumor is readily made by bronchoscopic biopsy. The tumor arises more often from the surface epithelium, and as such tends to show a thickened mucosal layer. Under the microscope, the great majority of these cases belong, from the standpoint of degree of malignancy, in Grade II, showing as they do rather marked cell differentiation, with epithelial pearl formation, keratinization and many of the features of normal epithelium. The basement membrane is often rather well preserved, and only here and there does any evidence of invasion occur. Mitotic figures are usually present, and there is a variable amount of pleomorphism and anaplasia. There is likely to be a considerable stromal response and to be a marked secondary inflammatory reaction. From the standpoint of irradiation, these tumors are more likely to show some temporary regression than in the group of adenocarcinomata. However, owing to the fact that they are generally so well differentiated, the same problem of resistance to such therapy is found as in similar lesions elsewhere.

ILLUSTRATIVE CASE

CASE 188. (Ref. #S-378)

Diagnosis.—Lung—bronchogenic carcinoma, Grade III. Patient was a white male of 55 years, admitted to the hospital with the chief complaint of a chronic cough of about two years' duration.

Present Illness.—The patient's present illness began as an acute process following the swallowing of a fragment of chicken bone the wrong way. At about the same time, he also broke a tooth and was never able to find the fragment. He was inclined to believe that this likewise was acting like a foreign body. Shortly after this incident, he began to have spasmodic coughing spells and raised considerable mucus. No blood streaking was noted and the sputum had no disagreeable odor to it. For the past three or four months, he noted spasmodic pain in his left side accompanying the coughing attacks, and there had been a somewhat progressive dyspnea which was more marked on exertion. He tended to run a slight afternoon temperature and had had occasional night sweats. He had lost about twenty-five pounds over the preceding four months.

Past Medical History.—The patient's past medical history was apparently irrelevant. He had had the usual childhood diseases, with the addition of malaria and yellow fever. He never had had any serious illness otherwise, and had never had any operative procedure. He was an inveterate smoker and had been more or less subject to what he called a "cigarette cough" for many years. Following the onset of his present illness, the patient was seen by several physicians, and numerous x-rays were taken. These were negative so far as actually demonstrating any foreign body was concerned, but there was a marked atelectasis, which the radiologist felt might well have resulted from such an obstructive lesion by a non-opaque foreign body (Fig. 432). A review of the patient's systems in other respects was negative. He never had any cardio-respiratory difficulties. His gastro-intestinal history was entirely negative. He had had no frequency or nocturia. He denied venereal infection.

Physical Examination.—Patient was a fairly well developed, poorly nourished white male who appeared considerably more than his given age. Head was grossly negative. There was slight internal strabismus of the left eye with an opacity of the lens. The nose and throat were negative. Chest was somewhat asymmetrical. The right side showed normal expansion; the left was definitely impaired with considerable lagging. Breath sounds were diminished over the entire left lower lobe. This was accompanied by impairment of the percussion note and of the vocal fremitus. Occasional râles were heard over the left base. Heart was essentially negative. Abdomen and extremities were negative.

Laboratory Findings.—The red count on admission showed 3,510,000 cells with 72% hemoglobin and 10,500 white blood cells with 66% polynuclears. Urinalysis was negative. Repeated sputum examinations revealed no tubercle bacilli. X-ray examination showed an almost complete atelectasis of the left lower lobe. There was a large, soft tissue mass just above the left main bronchus, which appeared to represent enlarged lymph nodes. There was a somewhat dense shadow measuring about one centimeter in its greatest diameter situated at the apex of the pyramidal shadow of the atelectatic left lower lobe. These findings were somewhat inconclusive in that they might represent a foreign body with secondary inflammatory reaction, or might even suggest the presence of neoplasm. (Fig. 436)

Subsequent Course.—On the basis of these findings, exploratory bronchoscopy was done. The sharply circumscribed mass was not visualized but was moved in the process, suggesting that it was actually a foreign body. Marked thickening of the bronchial mucosa was found and sections were taken for histologic study. The patient was discharged home for x-ray treatment, after the completion of these studies. He died about one year later, according to a report from his family.

Pathological Report.—*Gross Description.*—The gross specimen consisted of four small fragments of grayish-white tissue.

Microscopic Description of Biopsy Specimen.—(Fig. 437) Histologic study of the fragments shows one of them to be covered by a chronic inflammatory, thickened layer of pseudo-stratified epithelium. The submucosa shows marked hyalinization of rather dense connective tissue. In this desmoplastic reaction are found large nests of huge squamous cells. The nuclei of these show varying degrees of anaplasia and of degeneration. The nuclei vary in size and the degree of chromatism. Many of them show extremely large nucleoli. Some slight tendency toward keratinization and whorl formation is noted. Deep epithelial, anastomosing and branching pegs of cells are

seen which terminate in irregular invading masses of tumor cells. Rare intercellular bridges are identified. There are numerous mitotic figures, both typic and atypic. There is obvious erosion of the surface mucosa in places with resultant secondary inflammatory infiltration by leukocytes and mononuclear cells.

UNDIFFERENTIATED CELL CARCINOMA.—Another group of cases is seen which makes up about an equal number, or possibly a somewhat slightly larger group than the adenocarcinomatous variety. This type of tumor might best be considered as an undifferentiated cell carcinoma. There are times when such tumors seem to show a tendency toward alveolar arrangement, and even acinar formation. At other times, there is a very striking suggestion of differentiation toward the squamous type of cell. From the clinical standpoint, it does not seem possible to make these tumors fit in with the concept of Grade IV undifferentiated type squamous cell carcinoma as can be done in the case of the cervix, or other forms of epidermoid carcinoma, as they, too, run a relatively chronic course and fail to show the same degree of invasiveness and metastasis which one would expect to find in such an embryonic-appearing tumor. However, it does remain true that this group of tumors represents the most malignant of these major forms of bronchial neoplasm and that they do tend to invade the lung parenchyma as a

rather more bulky tumor mass than do the adeno, or definitive squamous cell varieties of carcinoma. Peribronchial and hilar lymph node involvement, likewise, is more often encountered in this group than in the others.

From the histologic standpoint, the tumor is made up of almost solid sheets of undifferentiated cells which present no very characteristic cytological details for identification. The nuclei are usually round or only slightly ovoid. They tend to be hyperchromatic and to have a prominent nucleolus. In spite of the high degree of undifferentiation of the cells, there is a curious uniformity in size and appearance of the individual component cells of the tumor. Mitotic figures are relatively numerous and may show marked variation in their histologic features, although the great majority of them appear to be of a normal type. The stromal reaction in these tumors is usually less marked than in the other lesions. There is a rather frequent likelihood of ulceration and the development of secondary infection and inflammatory changes.

ILLUSTRATIVE CASE

CASE 189. (Ref. #S-376)

Diagnosis.—Lung—bronchogenic carcinoma, undifferentiated cell type, Grade IV.

Patient was a white male of 27 years, who was first admitted to the hospital with the chief complaint of a dry cough of several weeks' duration, associated with substernal pain.

Present Illness.—The patient's occupation was that of a spray-painter in a sheet metal plant. His present illness began rather indefinitely several weeks before admission when he first noticed an irritating, dry sort of cough. This, he believed he had had for some weeks but had not paid any attention to it until he began to have substernal pain accompanying it. About three days before admission, he coughed up what he thought was a small fragment of meat, which he believed must have gotten into his bronchial tubes when swallowing, by mistake. This was blood streaked. This raising of material which looked like meat particles occurred again on the day of admission, which was what really brought the patient to the hospital. It had been accompanied by a tired feeling for several weeks, although he did not believe that he had lost any weight. He did not complain of dyspnea nor dysphagia. He commented in respect to his occupation that at the end of his day's work he could usually raise sputum in rather profuse amounts, which

was the color of the lacquer with which he had been working that particular day.

Past Medical History.—The patient had had the usual childhood diseases but did not recall having had rheumatic fever. He had broken his nose on three occasions, but had had no difficulty as a result. He had had psoriasis in a mild form off and on for about fifteen years. He had had no other previous illness of any magnitude.

Physical Examination.—The patient was a fairly well developed and nourished young white male, who appeared to be in fairly good health. His eyes, ears, nose and throat were negative except for marked deviation of the septum in his nose as the result of the previous fractures. His chest was symmetrical and well developed. There was no retraction. The expansion was symmetrical. There was no lagging noted. Percussion was negative. On auscultation a cogwheel type of breathing was heard in the left apical area. The heart was negative. Abdomen was negative. Extremities were normal. Neurologic examination was negative.

Laboratory Findings.—Red blood cells, 4,610,000 with 65% hemoglobin. White blood cells, 11,450 with 64% polynuclears.

X-ray examination: In the left upper lobe of the lung, just above the left lung root, a sharply circumscribed mass about 2.5 cm. in diameter was seen. From its position and appearance, this could be either a hyperplastic lymph node or a neoplasm (Fig. 438).

Subsequent Course.—Repeated bronchoscopy failed to reveal any definite neoplastic process involving any of the major bronchial mucosa. The left upper lobe branch seemed to be congested and somewhat thickened, but no definite tumor could be recognized. The patient again coughed up a fragment of necrotic appearing material, which was submitted to the pathological laboratory for study, and the diagnosis of undifferentiated cell carcinoma was made. With the apparently localized nature of the neoplastic process, it was decided to attempt a simple lobectomy. This was done as a two-stage operation. The left upper lobe of the lung with the tumor was removed and a solid tumor mass about 8 x 10 cm. was identified. This presented certain unusual features in that it appeared almost encapsulated and was much softer than the usual lung tumor.

The patient did extremely well for a period of one and one-half years. This was followed by recurrence of the neoplastic growth in the root of the lung, and extension to the mediastinum with ultimate death of the patient nearly two years after his operation. Autopsy was not obtained.

ALVEOLAR CELL TYPE OF PRIMARY LUNG NEO-PLASM.—The alveolar cell type of primary lung neoplasm is the least common of all forms of respiratory tract tumors. Indeed in our entire series of cases, only one such instance has been encountered. This is perhaps as adequately discussed by reviewing the clinical history as by going into any further

Pathological Report.—*Gross Description.*—Specimen consisted of the left upper lobe of the lung, which was collapsed and measured approximately 12 x 9 x 6 cm. Its surface was covered by a thick, shaggy, fibrinous exudate which showed considerable organization. On splitting the lung, a neoplastic mass occupying about one-half the volume of the lung substance was found. This varied greatly in color, numerous areas of extensive necrosis and hemorrhage being seen. Where the tumor appeared definitely viable, it was of a pale yellowish-gray color. The tumor seemed to communicate directly with one of the relatively larger bronchi. It was indefinitely demarcated from the surrounding lung tissue, but did not show any real encapsulation on sectioning.

Microscopic Description of a Section Through the Tumor.—(Fig. 439) Histologic examination of the tissue reveals a tumor of an extremely undifferentiated cell type. The cells tend to show very marked spindling and in this respect to almost suggest the possibility of a sarcomatous nature. Mitotic figures are numerous and many of the mitoses are somewhat atypical in appearance. There is considerable hyperchromatism and irregularity in the size, shape and staining capacity of both nuclei and cytoplasm. Extensive hemorrhage and necrosis of the tumor tissue is found in many areas.

detail regarding the histologic features of the tumor. It is our impression, from very careful study of this tumor, that it gives added evidence to the thought that the lining cells of the pulmonary alveoli are epithelial in nature rather than either reticulo-endothelial or of a modified connective tissue type as has been suggested (Fig. 430).

ILLUSTRATIVE CASE

CASE 190. (Ref. #S-379)

Diagnosis.—Lung—primary alveolar cell diffuse carcinoma.

Patient was a Negro male of 48 years, admitted to the hospital with the chief complaint of a chronic, non-productive cough of several years' duration.

Present Illness.—The onset of the patient's present illness was very indefinite, but dated back several years. He believed it was initiated by a cold and a possible bronchopneumonia about four years earlier, as he had had an intermittent dry cough since that time. This had become constant during the past year. His immediate problem was related to the fact that he had been losing weight and becoming so extremely weak recently that he had had to give up working.

Past Medical History.—The patient did not remember anything regarding his childhood medical history. Twenty years before his present illness, he had had "walking typhoid." He had been treated for the past ten years as a diabetic. This was obviously of a very low grade, as he did not get into any particular difficulty with dietary indiscretions. A review of his systems revealed that he had been more or less subject to mild upper respiratory infections all his life. He had had no gastro-intestinal disturbances. His genito-urinary history was positive for both gonorrhea and syphilis, but he could not supply any data as to the date of the infections. He had had what

appeared to be a very inadequate amount of treatment for the syphilis.

Physical Examination.—The patient was a middle-aged, adult Negro, well developed, but who showed a marked loss of weight. His mucous membranes and nail beds showed considerable cyanosis and beginning clubbing of his fingers. Head was not remarkable. Pupils were somewhat unequal and reacted sluggishly. Teeth were in poor condition. Throat was moderately injected. Chest was asymmetrical. The right side showed marked limitation of motion. The left side was apparently normal. Lungs: There was flatness over the entire right lung. This was most marked, however, in the upper and middle portions. A few râles were heard at the right base. The left lung sounds were those of a compensatory emphysema. Clinically the lung findings suggested a complete lobar pneumonic type of consolidation. The heart was somewhat enlarged. The apex beat was noted in the sixth interspace. The heart sounds were regular and no murmurs were heard. Abdomen was distended. The liver edge was palpable four fingers' breadth below the costal margin. The genitalia showed an old penile scar. Extremities were negative.

Laboratory Findings.—Red cell count showed 4,100,-000 cells with 72% hemoglobin. White blood cells numbered 12,400 with 73% neutrophiles. Wassermann and Kahn were both positive. Urinalysis showed a three plus sugar, but was otherwise negative. Blood chemistry showed 180 milligrams of sugar. Sputum examination was negative. X-ray examination showed a complete consolidation of the right lung with what was believed to be a bronchial effusion.

Subsequent Course.—Patient was put on a diabetic diet. A right thoracic thoracentesis was done and 350 c.c. of grayish-yellow fluid removed. Subsequent x-ray examination showed the mediastinum shifted to the left. The patient ran a steadily downhill course. He had repeated thoracenteses and died three weeks after admission.

Autopsy Findings.—The body showed marked emaciation. Heart was apparently within normal limits as to size and consistency. No valvular lesions were found. The pleural cavities both contained a transudate. The right visceral pleura was studded with metastatic, grayish tumor nodules. The lungs showed terminal bronchopneumonia and hypostatic congestion of the base. The right lung showed a complete consolidation, which on section suggested the appearance of gray hepatization. The lungs did not collapse on opening the chest. Metastatic tumor tissue was found involving the peribronchial and peritracheal nodes, and in view of the diffuse neoplastic involvement of the pleural and mediastinal nodes, the thought that this consolidation might represent a diffuse neoplastic process could not be avoided. The kidneys showed a benign nephrosclerosis. The liver was not particularly enlarged but had been displaced downward by the neoplastic process of the lung. Microscopically, the gross findings were borne out, a diagnosis of primary diffuse alveolar type carcinoma of the lung being made.

Microscopic Description of a Section Through the Lung.—(Fig. 431a and b) Histologic examination of a section through the lung presents a very unusual picture. The alveolar walls are well maintained. They tend to show moderate fibrosis and dilatation of the capillaries. This is accompanied by some chronic inflammatory mononuclear cellular infiltration. In addition, particularly in the septal areas, lymphatics are noted distended with tumor cells. The most striking feature of the histopathology is seen in a diffuse alveolar type of carcinoma which extends as solid sheets of cells throughout the alveoli. Where the air sacs are seen communicating with one another, this diffuse sheet-like arrangement of the cells is even more striking. The cells themselves are relatively large and polyhedral in form, with large, vesicular nuclei with very prominent nucleoli. The chromatin is scattered as coarse rods and granules. Mitotic figures are innumerable. Most of these appear to be normal in their composition, although occasional atypic figures are encountered. Here and there, some suggestion of lumen formation is seen indicating the possibility that these cells are of actual alveolar lining cell origin with a tendency toward adenocarcinomatous formation. The picture is one of a highly malignant, diffuse, epithelial tumor of the lung, of a somewhat unusual type.

CHAPTER XLVI

DISEASES OF THE GASTRO-INTESTINAL TRACT

CONGENITAL LESIONS

The gastro-intestinal tract develops embryologically from the entoderm and gives rise, through lateral outbuddings, to the digestive glands, the liver and the pancreas. In the course of its development, there is ample opportunity for congenital anomalies to develop through persistence of some of the fetal structures. Among the most important and frequently encountered of these may be cited varying degrees of atresia of the esophagus, of the intestinal tract, particularly of the small intestine, of the bile ducts and imperforate anus. Most of these are incompatible with life unless remedied by surgical treatment almost within the very first few hours after birth. Of the developmental defects which result in the persistence of fetal structures, perhaps the most commonly encountered is the Meckel's diverticulum, due to incomplete closure of the omphalo-mesenteric duct. As a result of failure of the cloaca and allantois to develop normally, we may find the persistence of fistulous tracts between the bladder, the urethra, the vagina and the rectum. These various congenital anomalies are of interest but occur so infrequently that they are not important problems either clinically or pathologically.

MECHANICAL LESIONS

There are several important lesions, the result of mechanical causes, for the most part, which may lead to obstruction, and for that reason become of clinical importance.

Congenital Hypertrophic Pyloric Stenosis.—In a few babies who appear perfectly normal at birth, and who usually have a history of being breast fed for the first five or six weeks of life, there may occasionally develop a symptom complex characterized by persistent vomiting. Physical examination in the more typical instances reveals an olive-like, palpable enlargement of the pyloric end of the stomach. This is the result of hypertrophy of the circular bands of muscle fibers of the pyloric sphincter. Its etiology is unknown and it is at times differentiated clinically with great difficulty from a simple spastic pyloric stenosis in which this anatomical alteration of the musculature is non-existent. In this spastic type the same symptoms of persistent vomiting are present, but they usually may be relieved by modification of the feeding methods and are more frequently seen, incidentally, in bottle-fed babies and at a somewhat later age. In congenital hypertrophic stenosis operative intervention is indicated promptly before dehydration and emaciation make surgery dangerous.

By merely splitting the circular muscle fibers these patients recover almost miraculously.

Intussusception.—By intussusception (Fig. 452) is meant the invagination of a segment of the intestine upon itself. This occurs most frequently at the ileocecal junction with the invagination of the ileum into the cecum. The etiology of this condition is likewise difficult to explain satisfactorily. Differences in muscle tone and peristaltic activity are thought to account for it in some cases. It is more often seen in debilitated individuals and is particularly a condition of infancy and childhood. Its importance lies in the fact that it produces in the great majortiy of instances complete intestinal obstruction with the usual fatal outcome from toxemia if it is not reduced promptly surgically. The mortality from intussusception rises rapidly after the first twelve hours. Its onset is abrupt and accompanied by severe pain. As the lesion progresses it interferes first with the venous circulation. This results in stasis and edema and ultimately in arterial circulatory disturbance with resultant gangrene. This is followed by perforation and secondary peritonitis. In the first few hours, the intussusception can usually be reduced without excision. After the first twelve to twenty-

520

PLATE CIV
DISEASES OF THE GASTRO-INTESTINAL TRACT

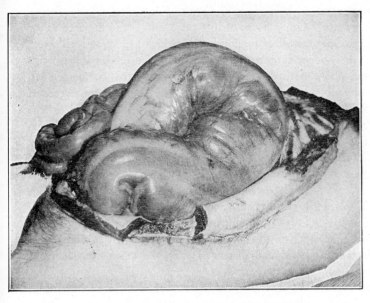

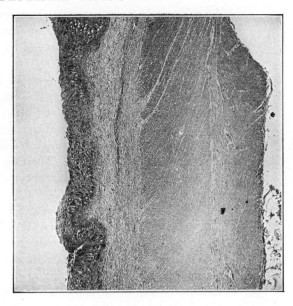

Fig. 440.—Cadaver: Hirschsprung's Disease (Megalocolon).—Case 191.—Enormous enlargement of entire colon both in length and diameter and accompanied by marked thickening of its wall.

Fig. 441.—Colon: Hirschsprung's Disease.—Case 191.—Photomicrograph through thickened wall of bowel essentially produced by hypertrophy of musculature, and by interstitial fibrosis. App. 10 x.

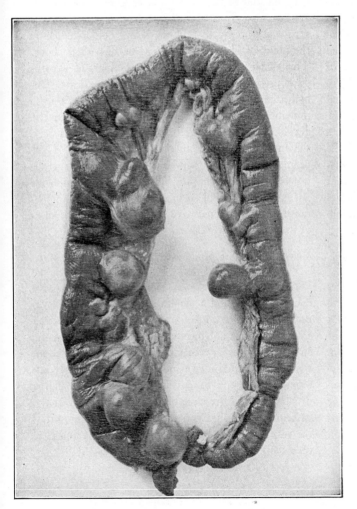

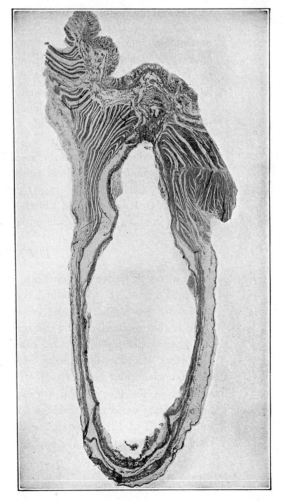

Fig. 442.—Sigmoid: Diverticulosis.—Gross photograph showing a dozen or more outpocketings of the wall of the bowel near the mesenteric attachment.

Fig. 443.—Sigmoid: Acute Diverticulitis.—Case 192.—Section through a diverticulum of the sigmoid near its point of origin in the intestinal wall. Note exudate within lumen. App. 5 x.

four hours, however, resection becomes necessary, but even then death may result from toxemia. Hence the importance of early diagnosis and treatment cannot be overemphasized.

AGONAL INTUSSUSCEPTION.—As an agonal phenomenon it is not uncommon to find single or multiple areas of intussusception along the course of the small intestine. These are of no significance pathologically, except to be differentiated from the true obstructive lesion during life. There is an absence of any circulatory or inflammatory change both grossly and microscopically.

Volvulus.—By volvulus is meant a twisting of a loop of bowel upon its mesentery. This is seen particularly in the sigmoid and in the small intestine. The etiology, again, is uncertain. In some instances developmental defects or anomalies of the various mesenteries may be an important factor, but variation in the muscle tone and hyperactive peristalsis are probably equally significant factors. Its importance lies in the fact that the circulation is cut off by this torsion and secondary necrosis, gangrene, perforation and peritonitis follow, as in intussusception.

Strangulated Hernia.—Another form of intestinal obstruction which may give rise to the same fatal outcome is seen in those cases of hernia, usually of the inguinal variety, in the male, in which a large loop of bowel becomes strangulated in the hernial sac with a shutting off of the blood supply at the ring. This again becomes an acute surgical problem either requiring the reduction of the hernia if the gut is still viable, or its resection if it shows evidence of beginning necrosis and gangrene to prevent toxic absorption and secondary peritonitis. This has been estimated as being the cause of intestinal obstruction in about 70 to 75 per cent of all cases.

Miscellaneous Forms of Intestinal Obstruction.—Other forms of intestinal obstruction are seen as the result of foreign bodies, which have been swallowed, or large gall stones which have eroded into the intestinal tract from an obstructed common duct, bulky tumors, inflammatory lesions of the nature of the so-called "regional ileitis," and strictures, the result of many etiologic agents but particularly seen in women as a result of lymphogranuloma inguinale infection. *Paralytic ileus* is also often included in the group of cases in which the symptoms of intestinal obstruction are present. This is a condition, probably neurogenic in origin, seen not infrequently following major intra-abdominal operations in which peristalsis is obliterated and the bowel becomes paralyzed and distended with the gaseous products of fermentation.

Clinically, the results of intestinal obstruction, whatever its cause, are seen in persistent vomiting which becomes fecal in character and results ultimately in a picture of profound toxemia which is believed due to the absorption of split protein products. In any given case of intestinal obstruction it is a rule at autopsy to find the bowel collapsed below the point of obstruction and to be distended above. This distention may be sufficiently marked to produce pressure upon the diaphrgam and heart. Dehydration as the result of the persistent vomiting is probably one of the most important factors in the development of the toxemia and indeed, it has been shown by many investigators that the lives of experimental animals may be prolonged to a very appreciable extent simply by the administration of adequate fluids. This principle is of practical importance in the post-operative treatment of human cases of intestinal obstruction.

DISTURBANCES OF CIRCULATION

In a consideration of circulatory disturbances which affect the gastro-intestinal tract, we have to deal with two major types of lesion. The first of these is the result of cardiac disease and is part of the general picture of chronic passive congestion. The other lesions represent local disturbances of circulation which may be the result of portal obstruction, as in the case of the esophageal varices or hemorrhoidal varices, or thrombosis or embolism of some branch of the mesenteric arterial circulation resulting in infarction of the bowel.

Chronic Passive Congestion.—In chronic passive congestion, we find a generalized, rather dusky, cyanotic appearance to a uniformly thickened mucosal surface. This is apt to be particularly striking in the stomach and as a result of the slowed circulation, symptoms of qualitative indigestion, particularly anorexia, are prone to develop. Rarely from such a process can the presence of blood be detected in the gastric or intestinal contents. If it does occur, it is the result of some added factor with an oozing type of diapedesis rather than true hemorrhage.

PLATE CV

DISEASES OF GASTRO-INTESTINAL TRACT (*Continued*)

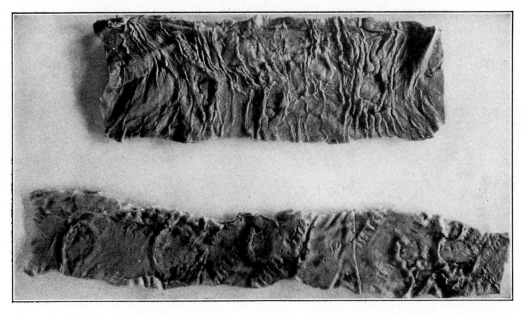

FIG. 444.—ILEUM: TUBERCULOSIS.—CASE 193.—Gross photograph showing typical tuberculous ulcers, whose greatest diameter lies in the transverse axis of the bowel. Edges are undermined; base lined by tuberculous granulation tissue.

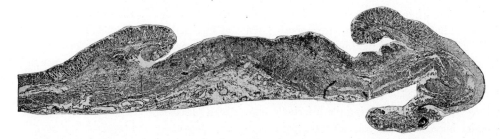

FIG. 445.—ILEUM: TUBERCULOSIS.—CASE 193.—Photomicrograph to better illustrate the diagnostic features of the ulcerative process. Note undermined edges, tuberculous granulations in base and extension to the serosa. App. 10 x.

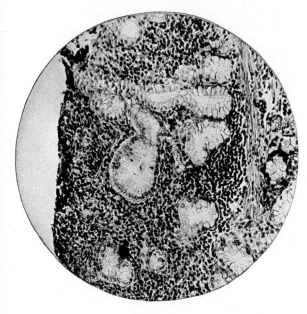

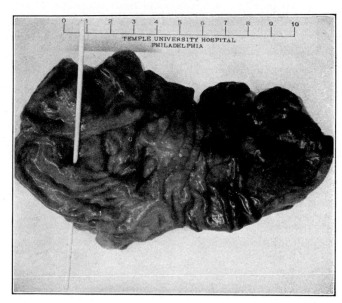

FIG 446.—DUODENUM: PEPTIC ULCER.—CASE 197.—Photomicrograph from the mucosa adjacent to the ulcer shown in Fig. 447. Note marked inflammatory thickening and cellular infiltration. App. 100 x.

FIG. 447.—DUODENUM: PEPTIC ULCERS.—CASE 197.—Two acute ulcers showing typical punched-out appearance, one of them having perforated, shown by a probe passing through the point of rupture.

Esophageal Varices.—In cases of portal obstruction usually associated with a cirrhosis of the liver, although at times caused by local lesions, the esophageal veins become dilated and tortuous. This may even at times be sufficiently marked to be visible in fluoroscopic and x-ray studies of a patient. Not infrequently the actual cause of death in a patient suffering from advanced cirrhosis of the liver is the result of rupture of these esophageal varices and the development of a fatal hemorrhage. It is for this reason that the importance of their recognition becomes apparent.

Hemorrhoids.—A similar mechanism is found in the development of hemorrhoidal varices. These develop particularly as the result of chronic constipation, or other local obstructive mechanisms such as occur during pregnancy through the enlargement of the uterus, or in older men from marked hypertrophy of the prostate. Hemorrhoids pathologically consist of enormously dilated tortuous venous channels which, through their location are subject to considerable trauma and commonly become thrombosed. Indeed, the histologic study of sections of such hemorrhoidal varices often offer one of the best opportunities to study the entire story of thrombosis from the earliest laying down of the intravascular clot to its ultimate organization and canalization. Hemorrhoids occur both as internal and external lesions, the former in association with the superior hemorrhoidal veins; the latter involving the inferior group. Their chief importance is because of the pain associated with their existence when they become inflamed or infected as they not infrequently do, and because of the danger of hemorrhage which, while not usually severe is likely to recur so constantly as to induce a rather marked anemia at times.

Mesenteric Thrombosis and Embolism.—One of the most serious conditions from the standpoint of mortality may result if the circulation to the intestine is interfered with through thrombosis or embolism of branches of the mesenteric vessels, particularly when the lesion involves the superior mesenteric artery because the branches of this vessel are endarteries and have little or no anastomosis with the rest of the circulation. When occlusion of such a vessel occurs clinically it is ushered in with an acute onset, with pain. This is followed by profuse hemorrhage from the bowel. As the process goes on, hemorrhagic necrosis and gangrene ensue, with perforation and peritonitis as terminal events, as in the case of intussusception, volvulus or strangulated hernia.

Hemorrhage.—In the preceding paragraphs, we have enumerated a number of the more striking lesions in which hemorrhage may occur from the gastro-intestinal tract. In addition must be mentioned a number of other lesions which will be discussed subsequently. Ulcerations of a wide variety may be associated with hemorrhage of a severe degree, even at times fatal. This is seen, perhaps best in the chronic peptic ulcerations of the stomach and duodenum, and in the late complication of typhoid fever. Hemorrhage is a significant finding in many of the infectious diseases of the small and large intestine, but does not often occur in severe enough form to be fatal. Thus we find that dysentery, both of the bacillary and amebic forms, chronic ulcerative colitis, parasitic infestations such as that with Balantidium coli, all show the presence of blood either grossly or microscopically in the bowel contents. The various forms of intestinal obstruction which have been discussed are likewise a source of bleeding. Another cause of hemorrhage is seen in the neoplastic diseases of the gastro-intestinal tract. Curiously, in spite of rather extensive ulceration, the hemorrhage at any given time is usually minimal, although constant oozing bleeding from the surface may ultimately result in a marked anemic picture. The presence of gross or microscopic blood from the gastro-intestinal tract, either as hematemesis from the stomach or as hemorrhage from the bowel is a pathological finding which requires some explanation clinically, and some form of treatment designed to control the bleeding.

INFLAMMATORY LESIONS (NONINFECTIOUS)

Among the various inflammatory processes which involve the gastro-intestinal tract are certain localized lesions which are the result of noninfectious agents.

Poisoning.—It is impossible to attempt to cover the wide range of inflammatory processes which result from the swallowing of toxic substances either accidentally or with suicidal intent to say nothing of the ordinary abuse of the digestive tract by most of us in our dietary habits. The changes which result

PLATE CVI

DISEASES OF THE GASTRO-INTESTINAL TRACT
REGIONAL ILEITIS.—CASE 194

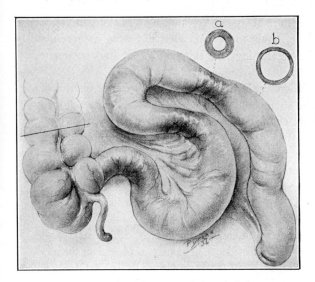

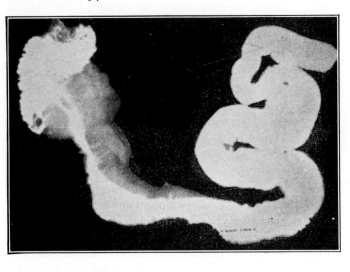

FIG. 448.—ILEUM—Multiple areas of chronic inflammatory thickening of wall of ileum with narrowing of lumen (a) and relative dilatation of uninvolved areas (b).

FIG. 449.—ROENTGENOGRAM—ILEUM—Postoperatively filled with barium to demonstrate the so-called "string sign" and the tendency toward sinus tract formation.

Figures 448 and 449 are reproduced with the permission of the authors, Pemberton, J. deJ., Brown, P. W. and Jackson, R. H., and the Annals of Surgery (1937, 105:855).

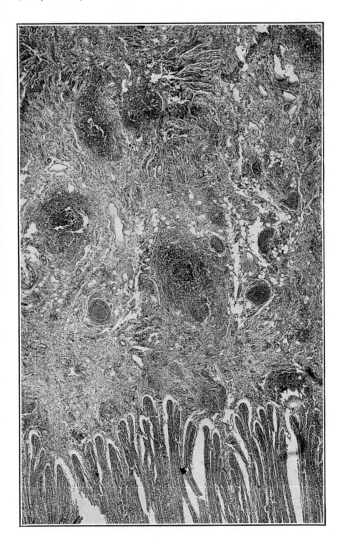

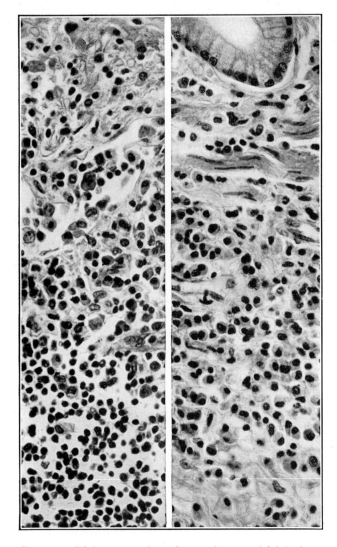

FIG. 450.—ILEUM.—Low power photomicrograph to show the enormous thickening of the submucosa as a result of diffuse chronic monocytic cellular infiltration and fibrosis. Note lymphoid follicular formation. App. 10 x.

FIG. 451.—High power photomicrographs, one (right) from base of mucosa; the other (left) from the deeper tissues. Note inflammatory exudate composed of lymphocytes, large mononuclears and many plasma cells in a proliferating fibrous stroma. App. 200 x.

depend obviously upon the nature of the irritant. Mild substances such as highly seasoned foods, alcohol and the like will produce only mild catarrhal inflammatory changes in the mucosal lining of the esophagus and stomach. On the other hand, strong acids and alkalies or other corrosives such as bichloride of mercury (Case 49; Ref. #S-85; Chapter XIII, part 2) will cause the most profound gangrenous types of inflammation if the patient survives over a long enough period for these changes to take place. If the individual dies within a short time of the swallowing of some such corrosive poison, it will be found that the esophageal and gastric mucosa will appear grayish-white in color. This is the result of the fixation of the cells by these various poisonous substances. Histologically, the cells are perfectly preserved under such circumstances and it is only with the passage of time that the action of proteolytic ferments, the invasion of leukocytes, the occurrence of hemorrhage and edema, and the other evidences of acute inflammation develop. No point is gained by any lengthy discussion of these graded lesions. Suffice it to say that aside from these more severe conditions two varieties of inflammatory change are likely to develop in the stomach, particularly. These are known under the general term "gastritis" and are the result of long-continued irritation and abuse of the gastric mucosa. Two forms are recognized: the "hypertrophic" and the "atrophic" varieties of chronic "gastritis."

Hypertrophic Gastritis.—In hypertrophic gastritis (Fig. 465) we find a tendency for the mucous membrane to undergo marked thickening. This involves the actual mucosal cells in both a hypertrophic and hyperplastic reaction, and also the submucosa, which shows an increase of connective tissue and diffuse chronic inflammatory mononuclear cellular infiltration. At times, this may approach a picture which is so extreme as to be called *polypoid gastritis*. The gradation of such hypertrophic lesions of an inflammatory nature to the true polypoid adenomata and adenoma malignum of the stomach is but a step, and their differential diagnosis at times may be extremely difficult.

Atrophic Gastritis.—In the atrophic form of the lesion, which is seen particularly in chronic alcoholics, in individuals who have been long on a vitamin-deficient diet as, for example, in pellagra in its chronic form, and in pernicious anemia, the reverse

condition is found. The mucosa is markedly thinned. The normal rugae are missing. The organ, as a whole, tends to be somewhat distended as a result of a weakening and thinning of all its component parts.

Microscopically, very few glands can be identified. The submucosa is thinned, fibrosed and is apt to show chronic inflammatory cellular infiltration frequently with a rather prominent number of eosinophiles. The muscle fibers are atrophic and appear separated, and there is some diffuse fibrosis of the wall as well. This atrophic picture may follow the initial hypertrophic type of gastritis as an exhaustion picture. In this latter form, there is almost invariably a complete absence of free hydrochloric acid and experimental evidence in respect to pernicious anemia has emphasized the importance of the anti-anemic factor which is normally present in the gastric mucosa in the development or maintenance of that disease.

Hirschsprung's Disease (*Megalocolon*).—The etiology of Hirschsprung's disease is still debatable. By some authors it is included as a congenital lesion; by others, it is considered among the inflammatory diseases of the gastro-intestinal tract. A considerable literature has sprung up regarding the neurogenic basis of its origin. In a great many instances there is an accompanying megalo-esophagus. Spasm of the sphincter has been thought by many to be the basis of the development of the enormously dilated bowel, but it has been shown both clinically and experimentally that no spasm necessarily exists. More specifically, the neurogenic theory emphasizes the lack of balance between the sympathetic and the parasympathetic nerve supply to the bowel. This results in a non-spastic contracture of the sphincter, which permits the dilatation of the bowel to take place. Invariably, in true megalocolon, however, not only is the bowel dilated, but the wall of the colon shows enormous thickening of all layers (Fig. 440 and 441). This is particularly true of the muscular and submucosal portions where chronic inflammatory productive fibrosis is present to a marked degree. At times this is accompanied by some chronic inflammatory mononuclear cellular infiltration. A point which is stressed by many investigators of this subject is the increase in number of the ganglion cells in the nerve plexuses of the bowel wall. Similar changes have been noted in the esophagus, including both the

PLATE CVII

DISEASES OF THE GASTRO-INTESTINAL TRACT (*Continued*)

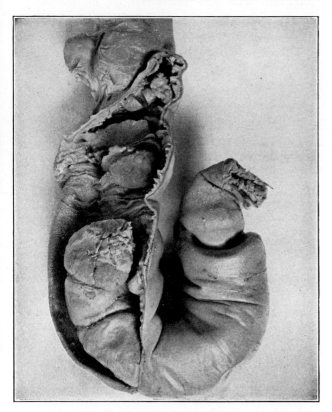

Fig. 452.—Ileum: Intussusception.—Gross photograph to illustrate the telescoping of the bowel into itself, producing complete obstruction.

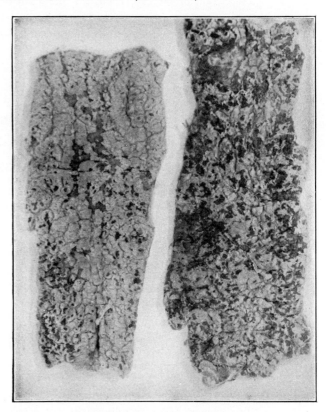

Fig. 453.—Ileum: Acute Bacillary Dysentery (Shiga).—Small intestine showing typical diffuse, hemorrhagic, necrotic, membranous, ulcerative inflammation.

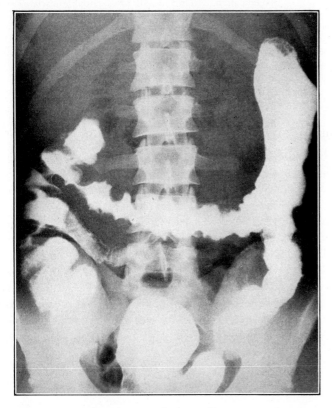

Fig. 454.—Roentgenogram: Chronic Ulcerative Colitis.—Case 195.—Following barium enema the characteristic scalloped appearance resulting from ulceration and hyperplasia of mucosa is revealed.

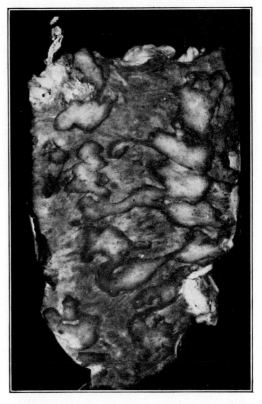

Fig. 455.—Colon: Chronic, Nonspecific, Ulcerative Colitis.—Case 195.—Superficial large serpiginous ulcers with shaggy, overhanging, hyperplastic margins. Intervening mucosa shows marked hyperemia and an excess of glairy, tenacious mucus on its surface.

constriction of the cardia and the dilatation of the esophagus with similar thickening of its wall. Just what part fermentation and the accumulation of fecal material in such dilated coli play in maintaining the vicious circle is unsettled, but it seems self-evident that they must be significant.

ILLUSTRATIVE CASE

CASE 191. (Ref. #S-349)

Diagnosis.—Colon—Hirschsprung's disease (megalocolon).

Patient was a white male of 24 years, admitted to the hospital in a moribund condition.

Present Illness.—The onset of the present illness could not be ascertained with any degree of accuracy. He had been seen in another hospital one year earlier at which time a diagnosis of Hirschsprung's disease was made. At that time he complained of severe constipation and marked enlargement of his abdomen. This was associated with a large, hard mass which occupied most of the abdominal cavity. This condition had been developing over a period of several years.

The patient was transferred to the surgical side of the hospital where, under spinal anesthesia, the lower part of the colon was evacuated manually in the manner of a version. The patient refused more radical surgery and was discharged against advice.

Past History.—The past medical history was likewise very unsatisfactory and incomplete. So far as could be discovered, he had never had any other illness than this condition affecting his gastro-intestinal tract. A point of interest, however, in this respect was that three other members of his family were supposed to be victims of the same condition. Living in a distant city, it was impossible to verify this point, but in view of the more or less commonly held opinion by many gastro-enterologists that the disease is of congenital origin such an observation seems of particular importance.

Physical Examination.—The patient was a fairly well developed but emaciated young white male. His head was not remarkable. Pupils were widely dilated. Nose and throat could not be examined because of his unconscious condition. Chest was symmetrical. Respirations were slow and labored. Heart sounds were imperceptible. Pulse was not elevated. Skin was cold and clammy. Abdomen was enormously distended and tympanitic throughout. No peristalsis was observed. The patient died before any laboratory studies could be made.

Autopsy Findings.—Hirschsprung's disease (Fig. 440) with marked megalocolon involving the entire large bowel from the cecum to the rectum. No corresponding megalo-esophagus was found. As a result of pushing the diaphragm up there was a very striking basal atelectasis. The heart likewise showed compression, being somewhat displaced, as a result, laterally. This was accompanied by diffuse chronic passive congestion of the viscera. There was a terminal meningitis of undetermined etiology involving the lower lumbar and sacral portions of the cord.

Microscopic Description of a Section Through the Wall of the Large Intestine.—(Fig. 441) Histologic study of the sections through the wall of the colon shows a diffuse hypertrophy of the muscular layers. This is accompanied by a very extensive intercellular fibrosis. The large ganglion cells of the nerve plexuses seem unusually prominent in the sections studied. The submucosa is likewise involved in the process. It shows diffuse thickening with considerable fibrosis and chronic mononuclear cellular infiltration. The mucosa itself does not appear particularly involved, although the glands are somewhat distorted as a result of the rather marked submucous inflammation. Many small hypertrophic arborescent glands are noted rather than the typical test-tube type lined by large columnar goblet cells. Most of the hypertrophy appears to involve the muscular wall and the other changes seem incidental to this process.

Diverticulosis.—Another lesion which it is somewhat hard to classify is diverticulosis (Fig. 442). It is quite probable that there is an actual congenital factor in the development of the diverticuli of the gastro-intestinal tract. This defect is apparently in the pattern of the musculature. The contributory factors to the development of these outpocketings of the wall of the gut are associated with intestinal stasis in conjunction with chronic constipation, senile degenerative changes of the wall with loss of muscle tone, and, as has been emphasized by many investigators, a neurogenic factor, as in the case of Hirschsprung's disease. It is of interest to note that diverticuli are found most frequently in the sigmoid where they occur as multiple lesions as a rule. Such diverticuli may vary all the way from slight bulging in the wall of the intestine up to true finger-like projections which, at times, may attain a length of 2 cm. or more. Less frequently, diverticuli are seen in the small intestine, particularly in the duodenum, but even at times in the jejunum or ileum. In these locations they are more likely to be single, but may also occur as multiple lesions. In the large intestine they are usually seen in relation to the fatty epiploic tabs and at first glance may escape recognition on the operating table or even at autopsy. X-ray examination is particularly useful in demonstrating these lesions which fill with the opaque mixture. The importance of diverticulosis lies in the fact that these outpocketings, lined by mucous membrane and having an extremely thin wall of relatively poorly formed musculature and connective tissue are liable to be the seat of an acute inflammatory reaction, which at times may closely simulate ap-

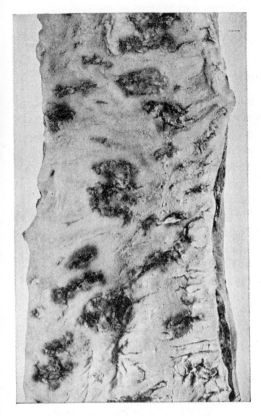

FIG. 456.—COLON: AMEBIC ULCERATIVE COLITIS.—CASE 196.—Gross photograph of colon showing multiple superficial ulcerations with hemorrhagic bases. Intervening mucosa relatively normal.

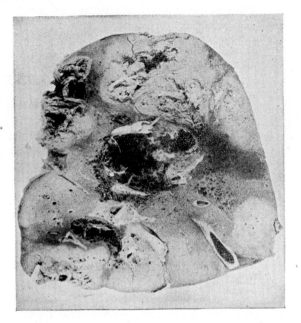

FIG. 457.—LIVER: AMEBIC ABSCESSES.—CASE 196.—Gross photograph of a section of liver with several large chronic "abscess" cavities lined by a ragged, degenerated fibrous capsule.

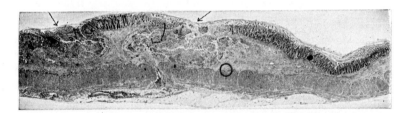

FIG. 458.—COLON: MULTIPLE AMEBIC ULCERS.—CASE 196.—Microtessar photograph to illustrate the typical "bottle-neck" appearance of the ulcer, with the necrotic process extending laterally in the submucosa. App. 10 x.

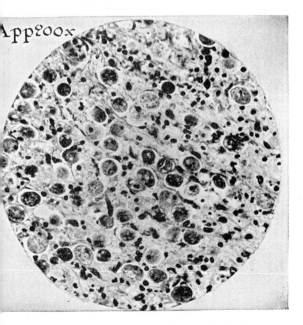

G. 459.—COLON: AMEBIC ULCER.—CASE 196.—High power otomicrograph from circled area in Fig. 459. Note crowd-g of tissue spaces by Endamoeba histolytica (vegetative, tile forms). App. 200 x.

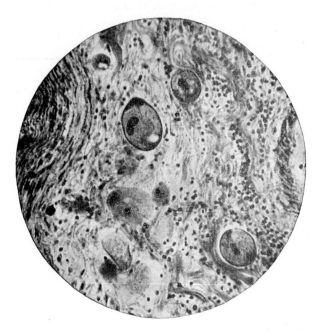

FIG. 460.—COLON—BALANTIDIAL COLITIS.—Photomicrograph of an area of submucosa showing several balantidium coli in their vegetative phase. Note cytosome at anterior end, the characteristic kidney-shaped nucleus and the nature of the inflammatory exudate. App. 100 x.

penditicis. Because of the thinness of the wall of many of these diverticuli, perforation occurs early and secondary peritonitis is particularly prone to follow, especially as a generalized process, because the diverticuli, which are so much more frequently found in the sigmoid area lie free in the peritoneal cavity, although in many instances the infection spreads extensively in the mesentery at first.

INFLAMMATORY LESIONS—INFECTIOUS

The remainder of the inflammatory lesions of the gastro-intestinal tract may be considered as the result of more or less specific infections with the notable exception of the chronic peptic, gastric or duodenal ulcer, which will be discussed separately. For convenience, these lesions must be considered in relation to that portion of the gastro-intestinal tract which is the principal site of the infection. Just as in the case of other infectious diseases, so do we find certain apparent specific tissue localizations for these many bacteria and parasites. From the practical standpoint, there are actually very few lesions which affect the agastro-intestinal tract which are of importance numerically. Appendicitis, diverticulitis, typhoid fever, tuberculosis, bacillary dysentery, amebic dysentery, chronic ulcerative colitis and possibly the recently emphasized so-called "regional ileitis" are deserving of individual consideration. In addition, numerous other types of infections are found in conjunction with the acute gastro-intestinal infections, either occasionally or in epidemic form at times. Among these should be cited briefly the paratyphoid infections, cholera, actinomycosis, Balantidium coli, and other parasitic infestations to say nothing of rare types of infection which usually go unrecognized.

Appendicitis.—Appendicitis has been discussed in our consideration of the general pathological processes in inflammation. It is not a specific infectious disease and may be produced by a wide variety of etiological agents. A considerable proportion of the cases of acute appendicitis are found caused by a variety of Streptococcus. From a large number of cases, only organisms of the Bacillus coli group can be recovered. Parasitic infestations, particularly *Enterobius vermicularis,* are occasional offenders. As contributing factors, we find anomalous positions of the appendix, torsion of its pedicle with interference with the circulation and even very probably actual embolic lesions. The picture varies with the nature of the infecting agents, with the position of the appendix and with the resistance of the individual. It represents the most typical example of acute inflammation with which we have to deal. Therefore, typical examples of this condition in the various degrees of its manifestations have been presented in Case 37 (Ref. #S-7), Chapter XI, Fig. 77 and Case 42 (Ref. #S-6), Chapter XII, Fig. 91, 92, 93 and 94.

Diverticulitis.—Diverticulitis, as has been emphasized, may be defined as an inflammatory reaction involving a diverticulum. Among those should be included cases of Meckel's diverticulitis. It may be caused by any of the bacterial or parasitic organisms which are commonly associated with such lesions in the appendix. Thus, we may have acute forms of the condition, or at times find a more chronic granulomatous type of infection and reaction (Fig. 443).

ILLUSTRATIVE CASE

CASE 192. (Ref. #S-334)
Diagnosis.—Diverticulitis.
Patient was a white woman 35 years of age, who was admitted to the hospital complaining of a history of vague abdominal pains more marked in the left lower quadrant over a period of about ten days. This had been accompanied by some nausea and on two or three occasions the patient had vomited. This had not seemed to bear any direct relationship to the time of taking food. She had had a persistent history of severe constipation which had only been controlled by almost daily use of laxatives. She had had several previous attacks of a similar nature, but not as severe and not previously accompanied by actual vomiting. The present attack was progressive in its nature, with the pain becoming more definitely localized in the left lower quadrant, more severe in character and tending to radiate to the epigastrium.

Past History.—Patient had always been in good health except for the usual childhood diseases. For the past several years had noted that she had had severe constipation with occasional attacks of what she had interpreted as indigestion. Patient was married and had had three normal pregnancies with three living and well children, the oldest being twelve.

Laboratory Findings.—On admission, patient had a temperature of 100.8, a pulse of 96 and respirations of 20. Urinalysis was essentially negative. There were a few leukocytes in the sediment. Blood count: red blood cells, 4,200,000; hemoglobin 83%; white blood cells, 11,200 with 83% polynuclears of which about 10% were non-filament forms.

Physical Examination.—The patient was a well developed, and normally nourished appearing young white adult female, who did not look acutely ill. The head is essentially negative. There is no generalized adenopathy. The heart and lungs on auscultation and percussion seem to be within normal limits. The abdomen is slightly protuberant. On palpation there is some suggestion of generalized lower abdominal tenderness most marked in the left lower quadrant at a point corresponding to McBurney's point on the right. Deep palpation gives a definite muscle spasm which makes examination somewhat difficult. There is an impression of a vague mass in this right lower quadrant. Vaginal and rectal examinations rule out the ovary as the site of the difficulty, as the ovary appears to be normal in size and position. Again, by rectal examination, a vague mass is felt in the left side in the region of the sigmoid. Proctoscopic examination is negative.

A tentative *working diagnosis* of a possible diverticulitis was made and exploration advised.

Operative Record.—A left rectus incision was made and the peritoneal cavity opened. The omentum was found pulled down over the sigmoid to form a rather bulky mass of what appears to be chronic inflammatory tissue. This had a somewhat doughy feeling and there was marked injection of all the vessels in this area with a small amount of fibrin on the serosal surface. A definite diverticulum of the sigmoid was found with acute inflammatory changes which had gone on to almost abscess formation. A number of other diverticuli were found involving practically the entire sigmoid. The sigmoid was resected and the gut anastomosed. The patient made an uneventful recovery and was discharged improved.

Pathological Report.—*Gross Description.*—Specimen consists of a portion of the large bowel apparently sigmoid, measuring 12 cm. in length. In this are found about one dozen small diverticuli, which extend up into the fatty epiploica. One of these is found to be definitely the site of an acute inflammatory process with a very marked peridiverticulous inflammatory infiltration of the tissue. In appearance, this is very similar to the picture seen in acute appendicitis.

Microscopic Description.—(Fig. 443) Microscopic examination presents a tangential section which shows the lumen of the sigmoid and the lumen of the diverticulum. The section does not quite include the ostium of the diverticulum. The wall is thinned and there is evidence of a moderately acute diffuse inflammatory cellular infiltration which extends into the peridiverticular fatty and serosal tissues.

Typhoid Fever.—In like manner, typhoid fever has been discussed and the lesions as they affect the lymphoid structures of the gastro-intestinal tract have been described in detail in the two cases, Case 52 (Ref. #S-124 and S-125), Chapter XIV, Fig. 111 and 114; and Case 53 (Ref. #S-246 and S-247), Chapter XIV, Fig. 113 and 115. It will be recalled that the lesion consists of an inflammatory hyperplasia of the lymphoid elements with resultant superficial ulceration and sloughing of the involved lymph follicles and Peyer's patches, leaving a smooth-based ulcer with sloping sides, which heals without scarring.

Tuberculosis.—Tuberculosis of the intestinal tract is similar histologically to tuberculosis elsewhere so far as its histologic manifestations are concerned. In the chapter relating to the general discussion of tuberculosis, much was made of the fact that tuberculosis might be primary in the intestinal tract, particularly in children as the result of infection from milk. It is likewise true that in somewhere between 90 and 100% of cases of chronic pulmonary tuberculosis with open lesions and having positive sputum, dying of their disease, that ulcerative enteric lesions are found, usually restricted to the lower part of the ileum and cecum. The organism like the typhoid organism tends to invade lymphoid structures, but this is much less striking in the case of tuberculosis. The lesion which is produced is a chronic productive inflammatory reaction with the development of occasional areas of necrosis and the sloughing off of the necrotic tissue. This results in the devolopment of a chronic granulomatous ulcerative bed to the ulcer which tends to spread by way of the lymphatics and thus is frequently encountered as a more or less annular type of ulcer in contradistinction to the ulcers of typhoid fever, which usually parallel the long axis of the small intestine. These ulcers also tend to be undermined with shaggy, hyperplastic, heaped up margins. Furthermore, the lesion is likely to extend through the entire wall of the bowel and to be easily identified from the outside at autopsy due to the presence of definite tubercle formation on the serosal surface. This is the result of lymphatic extension and, indeed, radiating linear thickenings which represent extension of the infection along the lymphatics are commonly found. In the more advanced lesions, actual caseous tuberculosis of the regional lymph nodes draining the affected area may also be found (Fig. 444 and 445).

Less frequently, tuberculosis may occur in the colon in the form of a chronic tuberculous ulcerative colitis. This is often extremely difficult to diagnose clinically as the ulcerative lesions tend to be relatively high in the large bowel toward the cecal end rather than in the sigmoid and rectum where they might be easily inspected by sigmoidoscopy. Also, the search for tubercle bacilli in stool specimens is a discouraging and almost hopeless task unless the infection is overwhelming. X-ray studies are often of more value in respect to diagnosis than the usual laboratory methods.

One form of intestinal tuberculosis is deserving of particular attention. That is the so-called "hyperplastic tuberculosis," which involves the ileocecal valve and cecum usually in young children. Considerable uncertainty has been cast upon the diagnosis of many of these cases by recent studies in relation to regional ileitis, but its existence cannot be denied in others as tubercle bacilli can be demonstrated in many such cases. Characteristically, these patients present vague, indefinite gastro-intestinal symptoms with perhaps some slight discomfort in the right lower quadrant rather than actual pain. Examination reveals a boggy mass in this area. Surgery seems to be the method of choice in respect to treatment, as these cases do not do well under the usual simple symptomatic type of treatment. If such a specimen is removed surgically it shows marked thickening of the entire cecal wall, which prevents its collapse on sectioning. Rarely is any frank ulceration or caseation noted. The picture is one of a chronic hyperplastic granulomatous lesion with at the most some superficial erosion of the mucosa. At times it may even result in obstruction to the ileocecal valve. Simi-

lar hyperplastic changes are seen in the regional lymph nodes in such instances. It is a particularly resistant type of tuberculosis and even operative measures are rarely ultimately successful.

Under the microscope it is difficult to recognize the tuberculous nature of the process as characteristic tubercle formation is only occasionally encountered. The picture is one of diffuse epithelioid cell proliferation accompanied by fibrosis. Only when actual tubercle bacilli can be demonstrated does it seem safe in the light of our more recent knowledge of these enterocolic lesions to assume the diagnosis of tuberculosis.

Aside from the ulcerative lesions of tuberculosis and the hyperplastic type, one other form of infection by this organism is seen which is of some importance. As a complication of tuberculosis low in the rectal area, there may develop a cold abscess in the peri-anal tissues. This tends to slowly break down and ultimately to produce a chronic sinus or fistulous tract communicating with the skin surface. This is lined by a tuberculous granulation tissue. It is extremely resistant to therapy and requires frequently repeated surgical attempts to succeed in repairing the ravages wrought by the infection.

ILLUSTRATIVE CASE

Case 193. (Ref. #S-79 and S-142)
Diagnosis.—Ileum, tuberculous ulcer.

Patient was a colored male of 47 years, admitted to the hospital with a history of chills, night sweats, fever and a productive cough of one month's duration.

Present Illness.—Patient had been in his usual good health until a little more than a month before his admission. At that time he noticed that he was becoming unusually easily fatigued and developing an irritating hacking sort of cough. Following this he had several severe chills and noticed that he felt feverish following these attacks. Almost every night he would wake up with a profuse perspiration. The cough became more and more pronounced and he began to raise a considerable amount of tenacious mucopurulent sputum. He had lost about ten pounds of weight during this month's interval and finally went to see a physician because he felt so weak that he was no longer able to work. The physician made a diagnosis of presumptive tuberculosis and referred him to a hospital.

Past Medical History.—The patient was unable to remember any details of his earlier medical history which appeared relevant to the present illness. He believed that he had had all the usual childhood diseases. He had never been sick enough to be hospitalized, however. A review of his systems gave no undue incidence of upper respiratory infections. His gastro-intestinal history had always been negative until his present illness when he developed a marked anorexia. He gave a history of

having had a chancre 25 years earlier for which he was treated with medicine by mouth, and ointments which he rubbed into his skin.

Physical Examination.—Patient was a well-developed and well-nourished middle-aged male negro who appeared somewhat older than his given age. His head was normal in appearance. His eyes reacted normally to light and distance, pupils were slightly irregular. Nose and throat were negative. There was no marked peripheral adenopathy. His chest was symmetrical. His lungs were clear. His heart was markedly enlarged to the left and downward. The apex impulse was in the sixth interspace in the midaxillary line. There was a typical "water hammer" pulse. His blood pressure was 180/0. His abdomen was negative on palpation, no masses or tenderness could be demonstrated. There was an old healed penile scar. His extremities were negative.

Laboratory Examinations.—Red cell count was 3,-400,000, with 67% hemoglobin. White cells numbered 7,200, with 59% polynuclears. Kahn and Wassermann tests were positive. The sputum was positive for tubercle bacilli. Urine analysis was negative.

X-ray Examination revealed a pulmonary tuberculosis at the left apex with a small cavity. Definite aneurysm of the aorta was likewise visualized. This was in the first portion of the arch.

Subsequent History.—The patient went steadily downhill during the three months that he was in the hospital. He developed a diffuse pneumonic consolidation of the left lung. He was put on intensive antiluetic treatment but to no avail.

Autopsy Findings.—The patient showed a typical luetic aortitis with beginning saccular aneurysm of the aortic arch. (Fig. 126) The lungs: There was a large serpiginous cavity measuring 8 cm. in diameter at the left apex. The walls were lined with a purulent exudate and caseous material. The remainder of the left upper lobe and the left lower lobe contained tubercles of various sizes showing caseation. Both pleural cavities were obliterated by fibrous adhesions. The peritoneal cavity contained about a liter of fluid. The peritoneum was studded with discrete tubercles measuring 1 mm. or less in diameter. The mucosa of the ileum, cecum and ascending colon showed numerous ulcers with undermined edges. The ulcers were oval in shape, with their long axes in the transverse axis of the bowel. On the serous side of the wall of the intestine numerous small tubercles were seen along the lymph vessels producing marked thickening of the serosa.

Regional Ileitis.—Regional ileitis is a term which has been applied in the last few years to a group of lesions which apparently represents a clinical and pathological entity, which was emphasized by Crohn and his associates. The lesion is a non-specific chronic granulomatous one most commonly affecting the terminal ileum (Plate CVI), but which may occur at any point in the intestinal tract from the jejunum to the rectum. Its etiology is unknown, but it is suspected to have a virus as its activating agent coupled with some subacute or chronic secondary bacterial invader. Its relationship to a pre-existing chronic ulcerative colitis or to a group of cases of subacute fibroblastic peri-appendicitis has been emphasized. Its similarity to many cases of unverified so-called "hyperplastic cecal tuberculosis" is also a point of interest.

The lesion grossly is found typically involving the last ten to fifteen centimeters of the ileum and to stop sharply at the ileocecal valve. This limited area of the small intestine may best be described as having the appearance and consistency of a piece of rubber garden hose. In its development it tends to go through several phases. The earliest of these shows

Microscopic Description of a Section from the Ileum Through a Tuberculous Ulcer.—(Fig. 444 and 445) The serosal and subserosal tissues are greatly thickened. They show many tubercles made up of epithelioid cells, lymphocytes, plasma cells, Langhans, giant cells and some early caseation. The muscularis is infiltrated with small round cells, chiefly lymphocytes. The mucosa presents an ulcerated lesion which extends into the submucosa to the muscle layer. The base of the ulcer is made up of tuberculous granulation tissue. The ulcer extends under the mucosa for a considerable distance and in the deeper portion some persistent caseation can be made out, occasional giant cells and a very diffuse epithelial proliferation. Edges of the ulcer are composed of extremely hyperplastic tuberculous granulation tissue which is raised considerably above the level of the remaining mucosa. The epithelium in these areas shows inflammatory hyperplasia but does not suggest malignant degeneration. The picture is typical of a moderately advanced tuberculous ulcer of the intestine.

a rather more acute picture with congestion, ulceration and hemorrhage. As time goes on, the chronic granulomatous thickening develops with persistence of the ulcerative picture and terminally a phase develops in which multiple sinus and fistulous tracts communicating with other loops of bowel or even with the abdominal wall are found. These may be readily demonstrated by x-ray (Fig. 449).

Microscopically, the picture is one of a diffuse, non-specific chronic granulomatous productive fibrosis and mononuclear cellular infiltration of all layers of the intestine. This is accompanied by superficial ulceration of the mucosa. The cellular reaction tends to be of a mononuclear variety with plasma cells, large mononuclears and lymphocytes predominating. Occasional pseudo-tubercles are found with foreign body giant cells. Many of these cells contain foreign bodies of a non-specific nature believed to represent material from the intestinal contents. The muscle layers are equally involved in this process with wide separation of their bundles by productive fibrosis and cellular infiltration. Similarly the serosa shows marked thickening and evidence of the same chronic inflammatory picture (Fig. 450 and 451).

ILLUSTRATIVE CASE

CASE 194. (Ref. #S-292)

Diagnosis.—Regional ileitis.

Patient was a young white woman 26 years of age, who was admitted to the hospital complaining of pain low in the abdomen, radiating to the right thigh and down the right leg on motion.

Present Illness.—This began seven days before admission with pain in right inguinal region on moving her leg. She had vomited twice during the week but had been

able to eat fairly well. Bowels had been moving satisfactorily. She did not think she had had a fever and had no other complaints except "nervousness." This attack was somewhat similar to several which she had had during the past year, which seemed localized for the most part in the right lower quadrant. These had never been severe enough to keep her in bed before. She also recalled a similar acute attack of very severe right lower quadrant pain about two and one-half years ago.

Past Medical History.—Past medical history was essentially unimportant. She had always been of a nervous nature. Following a severe emotional shock four years ago she had had an increase of this complaint, and her health had been definitely impaired. She had lost some forty pounds in weight, dropping from 135 to 94, and complained of feeling run down, easily fatigued, unusually irritable and suffered from insomnia.

Physical Examination.—Patient was a young adult white female, who appeared fairly comfortable in spite of a temperature of 103.5, a heart rate of 168 and respirations of 28. Head examination was essentially negative except for a nervous nystagmus. Chest likewise was negative. Heart sounds were of good quality and the rate was regular. Lungs were clear throughout. Blood pressure was 128/78. Abdomen was normal in contour. No scars or striae were visible. There was a network of superficial veins over the right lower quadrant and upper thigh. Abdomen was generally soft but a sense of resistance was felt in the right lower quadrant. On deep palpation, it seemed as if there was a fixed mass close to Poupart's ligament. There was moderate swelling of the right inguinal region. Regional lymph nodes on the right were enlarged and somewhat tender. Extremities were negative.

Laboratory Findings.—Blood count: red blood cells, 4,460,000, with 83% hemoglobin; white blood cells, 17,000 with 77% polynuclears. Urinalysis was essentially negative. Serology was negative.

A tentative diagnosis of regional ileitis and suppurative lymphadenitis was made and an exploratory operation advised.

Subsequent Course.—A six inch transverse incision entering over McBurney's point was made. A mass of broken down granulation tissue with considerable pus was found walled off just within the peritoneum. This abscess cavity was drained and the patient sent home temporarily to get in condition for more extensive operative procedure at a later date. Three months later the patient was readmitted with a clinical history of very little change in her condition. The sinus which was drained at the time of discharge gradually seemed to be improving but about three weeks before her readmission, she developed a diarrhea of five or six loose motions a day which had continued up to the present time. Physical examination at the time of her second admission was essentially as before with no apparent tenderness in the abdomen in general, but a little in the right lower quadrant. There was a draining sinus from which purulent material could be expressed.

Operative Record.—Patient was operated upon and a more extensive 14 cm. diagonal incision in the right lower quadrant was made and the ileum and cecum exposed. The ileo-cecal mesenteric vessels were ligated and the cecum freed of its attachments. The distal twelve inches of the ileum were hard, brightly injected with walls about five times the average thickness, hose-like in consistency. There was marked enlargement of the mesenteric lymph nodes. An anastomosis of the ileum with the colon was made.

Subsequent Course.—Patient did very well for a considerable period of time, but there was a good deal of trouble with the sutures breaking down and causing local leaking of the bowel and ultimately, after a prolonged and stormy period she developed an acute terminal generalized peritonitis and died two months after operation. The autopsy revealed nothing of additional significance, confirming the clinical picture of terminal peritonitis.

Pathological Report.—Gross Description of Surgical Specimen.—(Fig. 448) Specimen consisted of the cecum and terminal ileum as described operatively. The wall is tremendously thickened with some narrowing of the lumen in the distal 8-10 cm. No ulcerative lesions are made out grossly. About 6 cm. from the ileocecal valve, there is a small opening in the mucosa which burrows beneath the mucosa to enter into a multi-branching sinus tract communicating with the external fistula. On the serosal surface around this area is a focal area of peritoneal irritation. The appendix is included in the specimen and shows a chronic fibrous thickening of the terminal portion.

Microscopic Description of Section Through the Ileum.—(Fig. 450 and 451) There is a chronic inflammatory thickening of the entire wall of the ileum. Some of the mucosa is destroyed but does not represent a real ulcerative picture. The wall of the ileum is interesting in the character of the cellular reaction. As a whole, it is a marked mononuclear picture with many large mononuclear phagocytes as well as lymphocytes and plasma cells. Here and there, several lesions strongly suggestive of tubercle formation are found with typical Langhans' giant cells and a suggestion of radially arranged epithelioid cells. Careful examination of these giant cells shows the presence of foreign material within them, and careful attempts at demonstration of tubercle bacilli by Ziehl-Neelsen technique fail to demonstrate their presence.

In summation, the picture is one of chronic granulomatous lesion of the terminal ileum of unknown etiology, but representing the rather characteristic type of reaction seen in this condition, known as regional ileitis.

Bacillary Dysentery.—The various forms of bacillary dysentery may be considered briefly. The Shiga type of organism is the one which produces the most marked pathological change but, fortunately, is comparatively infrequently encountered as compared to infection by the Flexner, Hiss-Russell and other types. It affects primarily the lower ileum, but in the more extensive cases may extend to involve the cecum and a variable amount of the large intestine as well. It is characterized by the production of an acute gangrenous type of mucositis, usually hemorrhagic in nature, and frequently complicated by the development of a diffuse diphtheritic-appearing membrane. This is composed of fibrin and leukocytes and contains the bacteria in large numbers. The clinical pathological examination of the stool in these cases reveals large amounts of mucus and many pus and red cells. Much of the leukocytic reaction shows extensive degenerative changes. This is in contradistinction to the mononuclear type of reaction of the exudate seen in the amebic form of dysentery. In a disease which presents so much difference in the picture, depending upon the nature of the particular organism, the numbers of the infecting agent and the resistance of the host, no one description can possibly cover the entire field. The ultimate diagnosis must be made by the identification of the particular bacterium (Fig. 453).

Nonspecific Chronic Ulcerative Colitis.—A wide variety of infectious agents likewise may be found in the development of various forms of colitis. These, in general, depend upon the particular character of the organism involved. Beyond this relatively specific group, however, must be considered a variety of colitis in which the infectious agent is still distinctly *sub judice.* This is known as non-specific chronic ulcerative colitis. Bargen has described a gram-positive coccus, usually occurring in the diplococcic form, which he believes to be the etiologic agent. This has not been generally accepted as yet, as it has been impossible to recover this organism from many of the cases which present the characteristic clinical picture. Other investigators are inclined to feel that a virus may be responsible for the initial infection and that other bacteria are the cause of the secondary ulcerative manifestations of the disease.

Another group of workers in this field are inclined to believe that one of the dysentery bacilli is the usual causative agent in the production of this pathological picture. Considerable experimental evidence has been presented by them to support this hypothesis. In small series of cases, as recorded by the adherents of this concept of the etiology of the disease, the dysentery bacillus has been recovered in as high as sixty-five per cent of the cases.

Finally, more recently, the thought that this disease may be the result of an allergic reaction on the part of the individual to a previous sensitization by the causative agent, notably the dysentery bacillus, has been put forward as the most likely explanation for the development of the pathological picture. This might be compared in a rough sort of way to a visceral manifestation of the Schwartzman phenomena, although occurring in a much less dramatic and acute form.

Clinically, it is a condition which occurs at all ages, but is particularly frequently seen in the middle and older age groups. It has a slow, insidious onset with irregularly alternating periods of diarrhea and constipation. Stool examination from such cases shows the presence of variable amounts of blood, pus and mucus. Bacterial investigations have yielded almost every conceivable type of organism at one time or another, but from the numerical standpoint, the gram-positive diplococcus already mentioned has been most frequently obtained. The symptoms persist over weeks and months, often dragging on into years. This results in a debility of the patient, the development of a marked secondary anemia and ultimate death very commonly from intercurrent upper respiratory infection. Not infrequently, secondary liver abscesses and blood stream metastatic abscesses are found.

Pathologically, the area involved may be relatively localized or, in the more severe cases, may include the entire colon. There is superficial ulceration in these areas. The ulcers consist of shaggy, irregularly serpiginous lesions tending to have hyperplastic edges with considerable undermining of the submucosa in the deeper portions. There is usually extensive inflammation of the entire wall as an interstitial cellular infiltration and fibrosis between the muscle bundles and in the subserosa. At times this picture may very closely simulate that of regional ileitis, and differentiation is extremely difficult from the purely pathologic standpoint. Whether such a preexistent colitis may be the antecedent of the regional type of ileitis is one of those unsettled problems, but from the pathological standpoint, their similarity in many respects cannot be entirely overlooked (Fig. 454 and 455).

Microscopically, the changes are those of a nonspecific chronic granulomatous lesion with varying degrees of acute inflammatory change in the actual ulcer and marked mononuclear cellular infiltration accompanied by productive fibrosis of the deeper structures. Focal aggregations of lymphocytes to the extent that actual follicle formation may occur is by no means uncommon. Foreign body giant cell reaction in such lesions is likewise a relatively frequent occurrence.

Treatment of these cases is extremely discouraging. Medical methods usually fail and various surgical procedures have been attempted with variable results. These include actual resection of the bowel, palliative ileostomy or colostomy in an attempt to give the affected portion of the bowel time to heal. Permanent relief is rarely obtained.

ILLUSTRATIVE CASE

CASE 195. (Ref. #S-382)

Diagnosis.—Colon—chronic nonspecific ulcerative colitis.

Patient was a white male of 66 years, admitted to the hospital with the chief complaint of a chronic diarrhea.

Present Illness.—The patient's symptoms were of about three months' duration. He had developed a diarrhea which was accompanied by anywhere from three to eight or nine stools a day. They contained a good deal of mucus and at times appeared blood streaked. During this period he had lost about forty pounds in weight. He had also had malaise, marked anorexia and generalized abdominal soreness. For the week preceding admission he had had a non-productive cough.

Past Medical History.—So far as could be determined, the patient's past medical history was irrelevant. He had had the usual childhood diseases. He had never had any very serious illness requiring hospitalization. He had been in the World War and had had an attack of dysentery while in the service. A review of his systems otherwise was of little help in interpreting his present picture. He had had no more than the usual upper respiratory infections. His gastro-intestinal history, other than an attack of dysentery, was negative. His genito-urinary history was apparently normal. He denied venereal disease.

Physical Examination.—On admission, the patient appeared both badly dehydrated and emaciated. He had a temperature of 101°, pulse of 120 and respirations of 24. Head was negative. Eyes, ears, nose and throat were within normal limits. He had compensated edentia. Chest was symmetrical. There was dullness over the entire left base. Heart was negative. Abdomen was moderately distended and definitely sensitive to palpation. Extremities were negative.

Laboratory Findings.—He showed no leukocytosis, his white cells numbering 7,300, but he presented a moderate secondary anemia with a 3,300,000 red cell count and a 71% hemoglobin content. Urinalysis was negative. Wassermann was negative. Stool examination yielded a mixed bacterial flora, including a Gram-positive diplococcus and a gram-negative nonmotile bacillus, which appeared to belong to the dysentery group.

X-ray examination revealed a rather characteristic, scalloped appearance of the mucosal lining of the colon in relation to the areas of hyperplastic and ulcerated mucosa (Fig. 454).

Subsequent Course.—Patient went rapidly downhill, dying of a diffuse bronchopneumonia one week after admission. During this interval he continued to have a very severe diarrhea of seven or eight mucopurulent-appearing stools a day, occasionally being blood streaked.

Autopsy Findings.—The autopsy findings of significance were limited to a rather atypical chronic ulcerative colitis which involved the descending portion of the colon (Fig. 455), sigmoid and the rectum. This was characterized by a diffuse thickening of the entire wall which extended to involve the mesentery of the sigmoid. The mucosa showed marked serpiginous ulceration, the ulcers tending to be undermined and presenting shaggy overhanging edges. Several of these had a small amount of blood clot in the base of the ulcer. There was a markedly increased amount of mucus which was adherent to the mucosal surface. No evidence of diverticulosis or diverticulitis was found. As the immediate cause of death a diffuse secondary terminal bronchopneumonia, most marked on the left side, was demonstrated.

Microscopic Description of Section Through the Colon.—Histologic examination of the tissue reveals a diffuse hyperplastic overgrowth of the mucosa in those areas adjacent to the ulceration. The ulcers themselves are of a definite chronic type with rather shaggy undermined edges which show chronic granulomatous proliferation of the connective tissue and new capillary blood vessels. There is a diffuse inflammatory cellular infiltration of the submucosa which consists of both mononuclear and polynuclear cells, the former predominating by fat. Among these plasma cells and eosinophiles are prominent. There is no evidence of tuberculosis histologically. No ameba could be found in the deeper portions of the lesion. No evidence of malignancy is present. The picture is one of chronic infection.

Lymphogranuloma Inguinale.—In relation to the inflammatory infectious diseases of the gastro-intestinal tract, it is necessary to include briefly lymphogranuloma inguinale. This infection, which has been shown very conclusively to be due to a specific virus, is usually seen as a primary lesion involving the genitals. It apparently extends by the lymphatics, and due to the anatomical distribution of the lymphatics in the female is not infrequently followed by a localized involvement of the rectum. This, pathologically, is a localized nonspecific chronic granulomatous process causing marked thickening of the wall of the rectum and progressing to an ultimate stricture development. The pathology is nonspecific microscopically likewise and has been confused most frequently with syphilis. The male is much less likely to develop this complication, but some instances of such lesions have been reported.

Syphilis.—The question of whether or not syphilis actually involves the gastro-intestinal tract has been the source of a great deal of argument between clinician and pathologist. In the so-called tabetic crises, which are so characteristic of advanced syphilitic disease, the patient suffers intense cramp-like pains, which have been ascribed to spirochaetal invasion of the stomach, but which apparently can better be explained on the basis of neurogenic involvement. Actually the demonstration of spirochaetes in the gastro-intestinal tract has only been accomplished in a very few rather doubtful instances, although careful search has been made in many thousands of cases of syphilitic infection.

On the other hand, syphilis of the rectum is by no means a rare lesion. This may occur even as a primary infection, but more often represents an extension of the lesion as a secondary process. As in the case of any other similar chronic granulomatous lesion, this results in a marked thickening of the wall in a somewhat asymmetrical but annular fashion. This may proceed to a point of actual stricture.

PARASITIC INFESTATIONS

In line with the infectious lesions must be considered briefly two or three of the more frequently encountered parasitic infestations of the gastro-intestinal tract. These have been considered in the sections devoted to the problem of parasitic diseases in general so need only be referred to at this time. Of the protozoan infestations, only amebiasis and occasional infestation with the Balantidium coli are of importance. From the worm infestation standpoint, a considerable number of the round-worms including hookworm, pinworm, Ascaris and the whipworm are the most frequently seen. Many of these produce very little actual pathological change in the gastric mucosa. Finally, certain of the flukes may be associated with gastro-intestinal disease.

Amebic Dysentery.—(Fig. 456, 457, 458 and 459) As has been brought out in the chapter on parasitic infestations, amebiasis represents one of the most important protozoan diseases. By amebiasis is meant the infestation of the individual by the *Entameba histolytica.* This is not synonymous with amebic dysentery in which we find ulcerative lesions localized almost exclusively to the large bowel caused by the vegetative form of the organism. The parasite gets into the crypts of the glands in the colon and there burrows its way into the submucous tissues. It may become encysted and remain inactive, or it may proceed to multiply and to stir up a local inflammatory response of a rather low grade type. The toxin which is liberated by the amebae is mild and the reaction which follows is largely mononuclear in character with large mononuclear phagocytes predominating. Gradually, however, the inflammatory reaction may cause sufficient tissue destruction to discharge through one or more of the large intestinal glands to the surface, thus producing a definite abscess. Characteristically, the abscess has a relatively narrow opening on the mucous surface, but spreads out in the deeper submucous tissues to form a large, flask-shaped area of necrosis. Secondary infection by the intestinal bacteria follows superficially and a varying amount of leukocytic infiltration takes place with subsequent further proteolytic destruction of the tissue. The lesion, as a whole, remains as a relatively subacute one at its best, and it is here that the organisms can be demonstrated in section. Due to their ameboid activity, they may subsequently migrate into the lymphatics or blood vessels and be carried to the liver where they again set up their local inflammatory reaction.

Typically, the amebae produce the so-called "solitary" abscess of the liver, usually in the right lobe (Fig. 457). This gradually increases in size producing a moderate amount of liver enlargement and tenderness. Due to the mild action of the toxin, it is very slow in its development and often is unaccompanied by sufficient symptomatology to be recognized until well advanced. A connective tissue capsule develops around the abscess wall. The contents of the abscess cavity are of a relatively dry, granular character at first, but later may undergo frank liquefaction necrosis. The amebae tend to become encysted in such lesions and thus may exist for many years. Occasionally, such abscesses may extend directly through the diaphragm and break into the lung. At other times the organism gains access to the blood stream and, with curious tissue selectivity, involves the brain in similar abscess formation. The symptoms here are dependent upon the localization and the rate at which the abscess develops. Less commonly, other visceral lesions develop. Amebic dysentery, fortunately, only develops these complications in a few instances, and the great majority of cases go on as a chronic process with periods of remission and relapse depending upon encystment phases and reactivation of the organism, for periods of many years. Only when the complications ensue is amebic dysentery likely to be a fatal disease, except in overwhelmingly acute infestations, which fortunately are only rarely seen in this country.

ILLUSTRATIVE CASE

CASE 196. (Ref. #S-270, S-271 and S-272).

Diagnosis.—Brain—amebic abscess; colon—amebic ulcer.

Patient was a white Italian male of 50 years, a farmer by occupation, who was admitted to the hospital complaining of profuse bloody expectoration, loss of weight, pain in his chest and marked weakness.

Present Illness.—The patient was perfectly well until six months before admission when he began to develop a dry cough, a feeling of malaise with easy fatigability and weakness. These symptoms increased slowly during the six months' interval and were accompanied by a loss of weight totaling forty pounds. About one month before admission the cough became much looser in character, the patient raising a large amount of blood-streaked sputum. This varied considerably in amount at times totaling over a liter in a twenty-four hour period. During the last few days before admission the bleeding seemed less prominent and the sputum consisted of a large amount of white mucoid and granular-appearing material. Accompanying this cough there had been progressively severe pain throughout the lower right chest and under the sternum. It was noteworthy that the sputum was not foul smelling. The patient had marked anorexia and had developed a tendency toward a mild diarrhea. For several weeks he had noted severe night sweats.

Past History.—The patient had been born in this country of Italian parents and had never been away from a limited district in eastern Pennsylvania. He had worked as a farmer all his life. He did not recall that he had ever had any of the childhood diseases. A review of his systems was essentially negative. He had occasional mild upper respiratory infections, but had never had pneumonia. His gastro-intestinal history was entirely negative. He had always been a heavy eater. Genito-urinary history was negative. He denied venereal disease. He was married and had five children. He had never been operated upon for anything.

Physical Examination—The patient appeared to be a well-developed middle-aged Italian male who showed evidence of marked loss of weight with a wrinkled skin. Head was normal in contour. Conjunctivae: Mucous membranes were pale. Eyes, ears, nose and throat were negative. His chest was symmetrical and showed limited expansion on the right side. Vocal fremitus was progressively diminished until absent over the lower right side of the chest. It was normal on the left. Breath sounds were normal on the left side but were absent over the base of the right lower lobe. Crepitant râles were heard over the right apex. Heart was not enlarged but seemed slightly pushed over to the left side. There were no murmurs. Abdomen: The liver was palpable about 5 cm. below the costal margin. It did not appear to be tender on palpation. The spleen was not felt. There were no masses which could be palpated. Extremities were negative.

Laboratory Findings.—The blood, on admission, showed 3,300,000 red blood cells with 6 gm. (38%) hemoglobin. White blood cells, 16,900 with 82% polynuclears. Urinalysis was negative. Sedimentation rate was increased. Repeated sputum examinations showed no tubercle bacilli.

X-ray examination of the chest showed the presence of a large mass in the right lower lobe, which was associated with considerable atelectasis. This was accompanied by an empyema which made the visualization of the lung field somewhat unsatisfactory. The findings were somewhat suggestive of a neoplasm, but it was recommended that bronchoscopy be done in an attempt to establish the diagnosis.

Subsequent Course.—Repeated bronchoscopies were done and no definite evidence of obstruction to any of the accessory bronchi could be demonstrated. The impression of the Bronchoscopic Service was that the pathology was pleural and parenchymal rather than bronchial. Biopsy material from bronchoscopic examination revealed only a chronic bronchitis.

A rib resection was done and 200 c.c. of pus withdrawn from the pleural cavity. Bacteriologic examination of this was negative. During his stay in the hospital the patient continued to have a mild catarrhal type of diarrhea with three or four bowel motions a day. For this reason, x-ray studies of his gastro-intestinal tract were made. A marked degree of irritability was found in the terminal small bowel and in the colon. Some evidence of ulceration was noted in the region of the sigmoid and transverse colon. Repeated stool examinations were made during this period and no parasites or bacteria were found which seemed responsible for the condition.

In view of the chronic diarrhea, the enlarged liver and the right lower lobe involvement, the question of amebiasis was brought up. Sigmoidoscopic examination of the large bowel was done and several deep ulcerated areas were found from which scrapings were taken. Examination of these scrapings revealed the presence of a few motile amebae of the *Entameba histolytica* variety. Rare encysted forms were found. Three weeks after admission, the patient developed hemiplegia and an exploratory craniotomy was done on the assumption that there was a brain abscess present, as suggested by x-ray. The abscess was exposed and drained. Amebae were recovered from the contents of this abscess. The patient went progressively downhill and died about one month after admission.

Autopsy Findings.—The findings were those of a chronic amebic dysentery with metastatic abscesses of the liver (Fig. 457), lung and brain. The entire colon (Fig. 456) showed multiple ulcers measuring about 0.5 cm. in diameter. The ulcers had a ragged outline and there was undermining of the edges. The lumen of the bowel was filled with blood. The abscess in the right lower lobe of the liver measured about 3 cm. in diameter. It was filled with tenacious green pus. It had eroded through the diaphragm and caused multiple abscess formations in the lower lobe of the right lung. Occupying most of the left parietal lobe of the brain was an abscess measuring about 5 cm. in diameter. It was filled with thick, creamy pus. Motile amebae were recovered from the ulcers in the colon.

Microscopic Description of Section from Wall of Abscess of the Brain.—(Ref. #S-272) Sections microscopically show a central area of necrosis with definite suppuration. Most of the exudate is found to consist of polynuclear leukocytes and large mononuclear cells. The great majority of these cells have undergone degenerative changes with fragmentation of their nuclei and disintegration of their cytoplasm producing true suppuration. Around the edge of the abscess is seen an attempt at reparative gliosis and in the semi-viable area of the abscess wall may be found occasional typical vegetative *Entameba histolytica*. The surrounding brain tissue shows extensive degenerative changes. The microglia has reverted to its phagocytic form as Gitter cells, which will be seen as large ovoid cells with eccentric nuclei and filled with vacuolated or granular material representing cellular detritus and degenerative myelin.

Microscopic Description of a Section Through the Colon.—(Ref. #S-270) (Fig. 458 and 459) The serosa does not show any significant pathological change other than a small amount of subserosal edema. The muscularis is likewise intact. The mucosa shows marked inflammatory hyperplasia with hypertrophy of many of the glandular epithelial cells. Many of these are distended with mucus. There is a small area present where the mucosa is lacking. This represents an ulcer which extends beneath the mucosa almost to the muscular layer. It spreads out beneath the surface epithelium as a flask-shaped lesion with a narrow neck and undermines the mucosa extensively. This undermined mucosal abscess is lined by a mass of semi-necrotic tissue. Considerable fibrin and cellular detritus are present. Toward the surface polynuclears and red cells are seen in increasing numbers. Toward the base of the lesion most of the inflammatory cellular reaction is mononuclear in nature with large mononuclear phagocytes predominating. Deep in the tissues are seen a large number of amebae which at times are difficult to differentiate from the mononuclear phagocytes. As a whole, they are considerably larger. They have a sharp cell membrane and a small round or ovoid eccentrically placed nucleus. Chromatin of the nucleus does not stain well. The amebae are actively phagocytic for the most part, many containing polynuclears and red cells. They are found burrowing deeply into the submucous tissues which surround the ulcerated area. It is instructive to note how comparatively little acute inflammatory reaction is produced by the presence of these parasites even in the enormous numbers in which they occur in this lesion.

Enterobius Vermicularis Infestation.—As has likewise already been mentioned, other parasitic infestations by the various worms may be the cause of some specific clinical syndrome. One of the most frequent parts of the gastro-intestinal trace to be involved by such infestations is the appendix, and the presence of the *Enterobius vermicularis* as an inciting agent in the production of acute infection, particularly in childhood, is quite frequently encountered. Case 79, Chapter XXI, Fig. 212, illustrates this type of lesion.

Balantidum Coli Infestations (Fig. 460).—Occasional infestations of man by the *Balantidium coli* have been reported. A photomicrograph illustrating the nature of the pathological process and the invasion of the submucosa by the parasite is presented (Fig. 460). A more detailed discussion of this infestation may be found in Chapter XX.

CHAPTER XLVII

DISEASES OF THE GASTRO-INTESTINAL TRACT (*Continued*)

PEPTIC ULCER, CARCINOMA

One of the most important problems from the clinical aspect relating to diseases of the gastro-intestinal tract is seen in establishing a differential diagnosis between the so-called chronic peptic ulcer of the pylorus or duodenum and carcinoma particularly of the same region. Entire monographs have been devoted to a consideration of each of these conditions, and unfortunately the question of etiology is still unsettled. The relationship of infection, of chronic irritation, of circulatory disturbances, and of functional alteration in the secretory activity of the gastric and duodenal glands have been emphasized in the past. The influence of neurogenic factors has gained particular prominence in recent years.

Peptic Ulcer

Clinically, ulcer of the stomach may be seen in a wide variety of forms, but the development of the typical chronic peptic ulcer, which may be either gastric or duodenal in location, remains a definite entity apart from these other more acute lesions. In the course of almost any acute infection, it is not uncommon to find follicular ulceration of the mucosa. In poliomyelitis, well over one-third of the cases coming to autopsy show petechial hemorrhages in the submucosa, which in some instances result in superficial sloughing of the mucosa with similar follicular abscess formation. An enormous amount of experimental work has been done in attempting to reproduce the picture of chronic ulcer, but the results in general have been to produce an acute ulceration which heals within a very short period of time, with no evidence of scar formation. MacCallum and others have even removed large segments of the mucosa in the pyloric area with the same result—that repair followed promptly leaving little or no evidence of permanent injury to the lining of the stomach. One of the most widely held views regarding the etiology of this condition was first advanced by Virchow, that the ulceration was the result of embolism of branches of the gastric arteries, usually the right. This idea aided in explaining the localization of these lesions for the most part in the region of the pylorus and along the lesser curvature. Other investigators have carried the theory of embolism one stage further

emphasizing the importance of such emboli being of a bacterial nature, which would result in more extensive tissue changes.

Several neurogenic theories have been advanced; one in which it is suggested that local anemia as the result of stimulation of the autonomic system, not unlike the view expressed regarding the development of Hirschsprung's disease, may be a factor. More recently, Cushing has suggested that gastric ulcer is seen so frequently in association with lesions affecting the basal ganglia and hypothalamus that it seems more than coincidental. This again implies parasympathetic stimulation. This work has been substantiated to some extent by experimental production of ulcer in monkeys by manipulations in the hypothalamic area.

Gregory Cole is perhaps the most persistent proponent of the infected embolus theory. He believes that ulcer results from a local abscess formation in the submucosa as the result of blood-borne bacterial infection. This abscess gradually extends, much as a furuncle would on the skin surface, until it ruptures through the mucosa. He lays great stress upon the fact that in simple peptic ulcer there is usually definite destruction of the muscular layer with retraction of the muscle fibers forming rather sharply sloping sides to the ulcer bed and that the base of the ulcer is composed essentially of granulation tissue. The view generally held in explaining the persistence

PLATE CIX
DISEASES OF GASTRO-INTESTINAL TRACT (*Continued*)
PEPTIC ULCER.—CASE 198

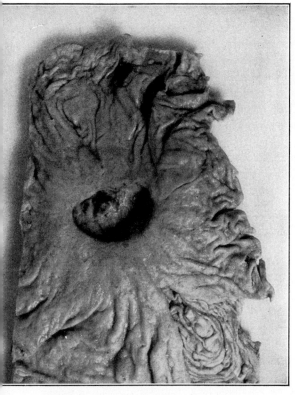

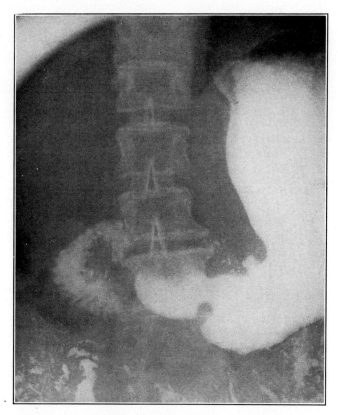

461.—STOMACH: CHRONIC "PEPTIC" ULCER.—Gross photo-
ph of a large 3.0 cm. chronic ulcer of lesser curvature.
margins are thickened due to dense fibrosis. There is con-
rable inflammatory infiltration of the surrounding mucosa.

FIG. 462.—ROENTGENOGRAM: GASTRIC ULCER.—Cf. CASE 198.—Note
characteristic filling defect in mucosal surface of lesser curvature
just above the pyloric ring.

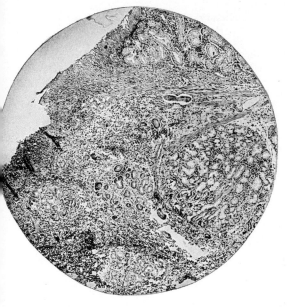

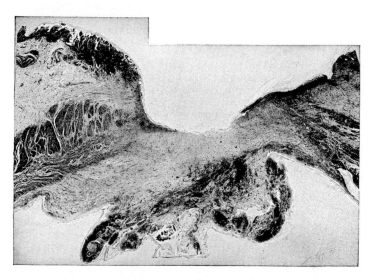

G. 463.—STOMACH: PEPTIC ULCER.—Section from edge of
cer shown in Fig. 464. A few normal glands are present
upper part. Note retraction of musculature and chronic
anulomatous reparative reaction lining the ulcerated area.
pp. 50 x.

FIG. 464.—STOMACH: PEPTIC ULCER.—Microtessar photograph through the
ulcer. Note "punched-out" appearance, the destruction of mucosa and
musculature with retraction of latter, and thickened fibrous base. App.
3 x.

of the lesion is that the autolytic degeneration of the tissues by the digestive juices of the stomach prevents healing and tends to cause the ulcerated area to slowly increase in size. This autolytic digestion of the tissues is at least one factor in the rather common complication, perforation. The development of the lesion might be compared to a river attempting to overflow its banks as the result of flood conditions, with the fibroblasts building up a protective wall around the ulcerated area, much as levees of sand bags are thrown up to prevent the flood from inundating the surrounding area. Upon the degree of this productive fibrosis depends whether or not a given ulcer may go on to perforation. Fortunately, most of these ulcers, being situated on the posterior aspect of the stomach or duodenum, or along the lesser curvature, tend to perforate posteriorly and are backed up by retroperitoneal structures, particularly the pancreas. At other times, however, the ulcers are not so fortunately situated and the perforation may occur into the lesser peritoneal cavity or even into the main abdominal cavity.

Whatever the etiology, there are several clinical features which are extremely suggestive in the establishment of the diagnosis of peptic ulcer. The disease, in general, tends to occur relatively early in life, during the twenties and thirties. It is usually ushered in by a vague, epigastric pain or distress accompanied by marked distention of the stomach and the eructation of large amounts of gas. The pain is apt to be of a gnawing character and to occur two to three hours after the taking of food, and is relieved almost immediately by the taking of food or alkali. Typically, these attacks tend to subside spontaneously after a period of weeks only to recur with greater severity at some later date. Thus, recurrent attacks with periods of remission are in themselves almost diagnostic. Examination of the gastric contents shows an almost invariably increased acidity. The pain becomes more intense and nausea and vomiting are frequent accompaniments of the picture. The pain has been variously explained on the basis of the hyperacidity producing irritation of the more ulcerated mucosal surface, but this explanation to-day is not accepted except as a very mild contributory factor. The pain appears to be due to the hypermotility of the stomach causing pain on the exposed nerve endings in the affected area.

ILLUSTRATIVE CASE

CASE 197. (Ref. #S-273)

Diagnosis.—Duodenum-peptic ulcer.

Patient was a white male, 38 years of age, who entered the hospital with complaint of intermittent attacks of acute abdominal pain of four years' duration.

Present Illness.—The onset of the patient's illness dated back for a period of more than four years. It began with a dull gnawing type of pain in the epigastrium which came on, as a rule, two to three hours after meals. This was associated at times with a moderate amount of nausea, but at the outset, no vomiting. The pain was relieved by the taking of food and by the use of alkalies which his physician recommended. The pain and discomfort was not sufficient to prevent the patient from attending his work but he noted a slow loss in weight over a period of months. By carefully restricting his diet to bland, semisoft foods, this pain disappeared after three to four months. During the past four years he had had several such attacks which lasted longer each time and during which his symptoms became progressively more severe. The last attack he had was about four months before admission and was accompanied by several attacks of vomiting. In at least one such attack he noted that the vomitus was blood streaked. The pain did not come on for four to five hours after taking of food. In this last attack of his, it was much more intense and was accompanied by a great deal of flatulence and gaseous eructation. On one occasion he noted that he had black, tar colored stools for a period of two or three days. He had been put on a modified Sippy regime and had previously done very well under this treatment. Following his last attack, he gained twelve pounds in weight and had felt better than at any time for the preceding four years. The present onset was ushered in by a sudden sharp attack of severe epigastric pain which remained localized but prostrating. He was forced to go to bed and call a physician, who made a tentative diagnosis of ruptured peptic ulcer and sent him to a hospital as an emergency.

Past Medical History.—His previous history was essentially irrelevant. He had had the usual childhood diseases including scarlatina, but had never had a history of rheumatic fever. A review of his systems revealed that he had always been more or less subject to attacks of indigestion and biliousness, even as a child. His genitourinary history was negative. He was married and had two normal healthy children.

Physical Examination.—Patient was a well-developed and well-nourished, young adult white male. His head was negative except that his face showed an extremely worried look. His pupils reacted normally. The nose and throat were negative. His chest was symmetrical. His lungs were clear. His heart was rapid with a rate of 120, but otherwise appeared to be within normal limits. His blood pressure was 105/65. His abdomen was held rigidly and was exquisitely tender under the slightest palpation. It was impossible to examine him more in detail. His extremities were negative.

Laboratory Findings.—Red cell count, 4,600,000 with 83% hemoglobin. White cell count, 28,600 with 84% polynuclears. Urinalysis showed a moderate amount of albumin, otherwise negative.

PLATE CX
DISEASES OF THE GASTRO-INTESTINAL TRACT (*Continued*)
STOMACH

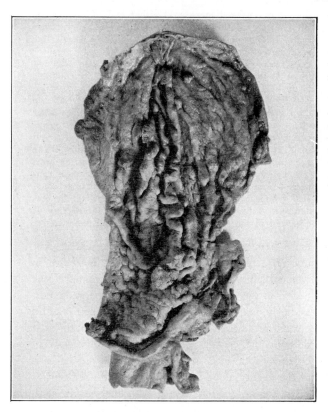

FIG. 465.—CHRONIC HYPERPLASTIC GASTRITIS (GASTRITIS POLY-POSA).—Note thickening of mucosa with exaggeration of the normal rugae, as well as a few localized polypoid overgrowths.

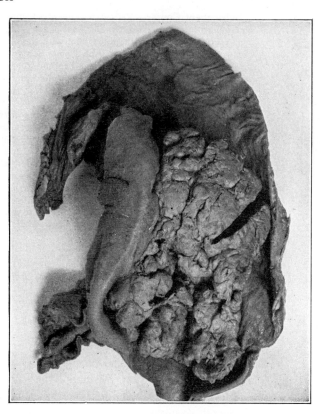

FIG. 466.—PAPILLARY ADENOCARCINOMA.—This large, fungating growth mechanically has caused almost complete obstruction of the lumen. Note its relatively narrow base and comparatively slight invasion of the gastric wall.

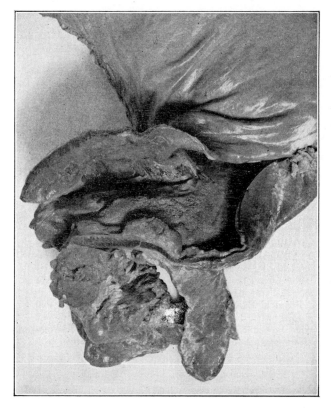

FIG. 467.—ULCERATIVE ADENOCARCINOMA.—Marked, indurated, annular thickening involving the pyloric end of the stomach, with an area of superficial ulceration. Note extensive invasion of wall in contrast to Fig. 466.

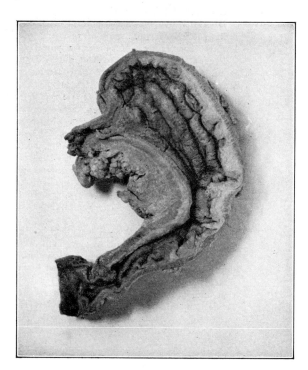

FIG. 468.—DIFFUSE SCIRRHOUS CARCINOMA (LEATHER-BOTTLE STOMACH; LINITIS PLASTICA).—CASE 200.—An almost uniform leathery thickening of the entire gastric wall as a result of diffuse scirrhous carcinomatous infiltration of the submucosa, musculature and serosa. Mucosal surface relatively uninvolved.

Subsequent Course.—Patient was operated upon as an emergency and a perforated duodenal ulcer (Fig. 447) was found. A section of the duodenum with the ulcer and perforated area was removed and a posterior gastro-enterostomy was done. There was a beginning spreading peritonitis which continued to develop in spite of the operative measures and he died five days after operation.

Pathological Report.—Specimen consisted of 7 cm. of the proximal portion of the duodenum. In the first portion there were two ulcers, one measuring 1 cm. in diameter. It was cone-shaped and perforated the duodenal wall. The other was oval, measuring 2 cm. in its long diameter. The edges were smooth, rounded and indurated. The floor was covered with granulation tissue. There was a marked thickening of the floor of the larger ulcer which apparently prevented its perforating.

Microscopic Description of a Section Through the Ulcer.—(Fig. 446) Histological examination of the tissues shows normal mucosa at either end of the section. The mucosa at the edges of the ulcerated area shows some inflammatory hyperplasia. There is a sharp line of demarcation where the mucosa disappears. The ulcer crater shows a slightly shelving edge and extends through the musculature into the serosa. The muscle fibers are seen retracted and invaded by productive inflammatory fibrous tissue. In the ulcerated area all the deep glandular structures, including the typical Brunner glands, are absent. The ulcer crater contains a considerable amount of cellular detritus, fibrin, leukocytes and some red cells. There is a zone of granulation tissue growing from the edges of the lesion and from the base. The ulcer appears to be backed by a thick layer of connective scar tissue which infiltrates the pancreas. Several groups of alveoli are seen which establish the recognition of pancreatic tissue. Some slight fat necrosis is observed in the interstitial structures of the pancreas.

Aside from perforation, the other outstanding complication of peptic ulcer is, as in the case of typhoid fever, erosion of one of the blood vessels at the base of the ulcer with hemorrhage of varying degrees of severity. Hematemesis is one of the emergency problems to be met in the clinical care of such cases, and requires prompt surgical intervention as a rule. Most ulcers bleed to some extent, but more as an oozing hemorrhage from the granulating surface of the lesion. Over a period of time this results in a profound secondary anemia of the hypochromic type.

As has been mentioned, ulcer is particularly commonly seen in the young adult age group. For some curious and unexplained reason, the gastric form is more frequently encountered in males, whereas the duodenal type of ulcer has a higher incidence in women. Likewise, there is apt to be a secondary peak period in the development of ulcer in the male, particularly, which is seen in the fifties and sixties. This creates an added difficulty in diagnosis, falling as it does in the cancer age period. The diagnosis of chronic peptic ulcer should be possible on the basis of the history alone in approximately 80 per cent of cases. In conjunction with gastric analysis, an additional 10 per cent should be confirmed and the remaining cases of doubtful nature, with rare exception, can be definitely proven by x-ray studies. The treatment in the majority of cases is surgical.

ILLUSTRATIVE CASE

CASE 198. (Ref. #S-372)

Diagnosis.—Stomach—chronic peptic ulcer.

Patient was a white male of 55 years, admitted to the hospital complaining of epigastric pain.

Present Illness.—The present illness began about one month before admission and had become progressively worse during this interval. It was characterized by a pain which started in his epigastric region and radiated toward his back, and more or less generally over his lower thorax and upper abdomen. This seemed to have no relationship to the taking of food. This had not been accompanied by any nausea or vomiting and his appetite seemed to be good. The pain had not been severe enough to interfere with sleep. These symptoms seemed to be totally unrelated to his previous medical history which was climaxed approximately one year before his present admission by an appendectomy and cholecystectomy with relief of symptoms.

Past Medical History.—The patient had had an essentially uneventful medical history until about one and one-half years before his present admission. He believed that he had had all the usual childhood diseases. He had never been seriously ill enough to require hospitalization and had not been operated upon except for the appendectomy already mentioned. A review of his systems other than the gastro-intestinal was entirely non-informatory.

In reviewing his gastro-intestinal history, it appeared that about one and one-half years earlier he had noticed vague epigastric pains which used to occur about twenty minutes after meals. These continued almost steadily for a period of an hour or more unless relieved by alkalies. He had never previously noted any qualitative dyspepsia. He had not lost any weight recently and had not noticed any undue amount of constipation. He had had no jaundice. His symptoms were so indefinite that he was admitted to the hospital for study. X-ray examination revealed no apparent defect in the stomach or duodenum. Biliary drainage yielded no significant information, but gave him temporary relief of symptoms for about one month. They then recurred with increased severity and an exploratory operation was done with the removal of a chronically inflamed gallbladder and a routine appendectomy. Following this operation, he had complete relief from symptoms until the onset of his current attack of pain, which brought him to the hospital.

Physical Examination.—Physical examination revealed a fairly well-developed and nourished middle-aged man who showed no particularly significant physical findings. Head was negative. Nose and throat were negative. Eyes

PLATE CXI
DISEASES OF GASTRO-INTESTINAL TRACT (*Continued*)

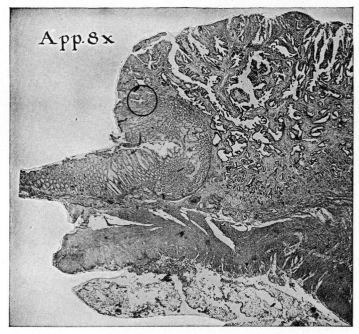

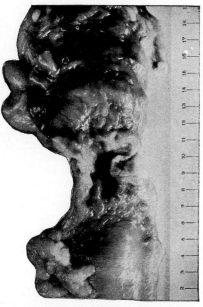

FIG. 469.—SIGMOID—ADENOCARCINOMA (PAPILLARY TYPE).—CASE 199. Microtessar photograph showing the transitional zone with the hyperplastic relatively normal mucosa at left and the somewhat fungating adenocarcinoma at right. (See Figs. 328 and 329.) App. 8 x.

FIG. 470.—COLON—ADENOCARCINOMA (ULCERATIVE TYPE).—(Cf. Fig. 467—Stomach.)—Annular, constricting, obstructive, invasive tumor of colon, showing superficial ulceration.

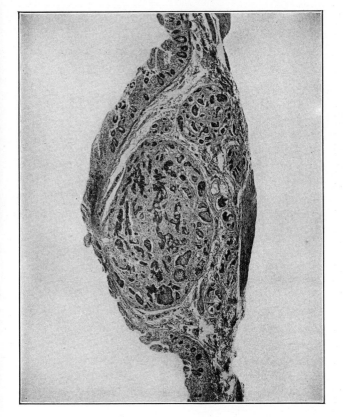

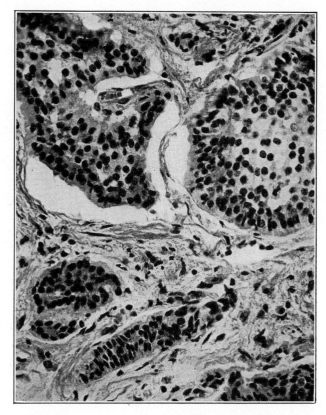

FIGS. 471 and 472.—APPENDIX—"CARCINOID" (CHROMAFFINOMA; ARGENTOPHILE TUMOR).—CASE 201.—Fig. 471, a microtessar photograph showing the relationship of the tumor with its origin in the submucosa (App. 10 x). Fig. 472, a high power photomicrograph showing the characteristic nests of small, round, hyperchromic, argentophilic cells embedded in a generous septate connective tissue stroma (App. 200 x).

reacted normally. Chest was clear throughout. Heart was apparently normal. Abdomen showed the scar of his former operation in the upper right quadrant. His extremities were negative.

Laboratory Findings.—Laboratory findings at this time revealed a red count of 5,000,000 cells with 14 grams of hemoglobin and a white blood count of 10,200 with 76% polynuclears. Urinalysis was negative. Blood chemistry was negative. Wassermann was negative.

X-ray examination at this time revealed a large outpocketing along the lesser curvature of the stomach. The duodenum appeared negative. There was no notable retention of the gastric contents at the end of the four or twenty-four hour period. The conclusions from the x-ray examination were that the patient had developed a penetrating ulcer of the stomach (Fig. 462).

Subsequent History.—On the basis of the recurrent epigastric symptoms and the additional x-ray evidence of primary gastric pathology, an exploratory operation was done and the stomach exposed. A large, punched out, sharply circumscribed ulcer of the lesser curvature was found in the upper third of the stomach. This made any question of the ordinary posterior gastro-enterostomy impractical and instead a subtotal resection of the stomach was done. The patient made an uneventful recovery and at the end of one year was entirely free from any gastro-intestinal symptoms.

Pathological Report.—Gross Description.—The specimen consisted of what appeared to be about two-thirds of a stomach. Along the lesser curvature about 3 cm. from the upper end and 9 cm. from the pylorus, there

was a sharply punched out ulcer measuring 3 cm. in diameter (Fig. 461). Its floor was 1.5 cm. below the mucosal surface. The mucosa ended abruptly at the edge of the ulcer and showed but little induration. The floor of the crater was made up of tough, fibrous tissue covered by a gray, necrotic-appearing, filmy exudate. Over the serosal aspect of the ulcer there was marked fibrous thickening. The mucosa of the stomach as a whole showed a rather striking hypertrophic type of gastritis with a very marked pebbling.

Microscopic Description of a Section Through the Ulcer.—(Fig. 463 and 464) Histologic examination under low power shows the edge of the ulcerated area. The mucosa ends abruptly at the beginning of the ulceration. The ulcer crater shows a dense fibrous tissue base, which is covered by a thin, fibrinous exudate showing many broken down polynuclear cells. There is definite granulation tissue forming at the base and characterized by the production of new capillaries and young fibroblasts. This is accompanied by marked round cell infiltration consisting chiefly of lymphocytes, plasma cells and large mononuclear phagocytes. As in the preceding case of duodenal ulcer, the histologic characteristics which aid the microscopist in differentiating a simple ulcer from a malignant process are seen. The same retraction of the musculature of the gastric wall as seen in the duodenal ulcer is observed, and the entire ulcer bed, both its base and its lateral margins are lined by this dense fibrous granulation tissue. However, in this case, the process appears to be much older in nature and considerable fixation of the retracted muscle fibers is noteworthy.

GASTRIC CARCINOMA

From the clinical standpoint, on the other hand, the story of carcinoma of the stomach is usually quite different from that of the typical chronic peptic ulcer. In general, the cases of carcinoma do not occur until in the older age group. This point is by no means of any great differential diagnostic help, except that in the late ulcer cases there has usually been a previous history of recurrent attacks of a rather characteristic type. In cancer, the course of the disease is usually progressive. Not infrequently, unfortunately, the patient remains symptom-free until the disease is so far advanced as to be inoperable.

The great difficulty in making the diagnosis of carcinoma of the stomach is that a very large proportion of the cases show extensive ulceration. This results in a crater-like lesion by x-ray, which frequently simulates the appearance of ulcer. In some forms of carcinoma, however, the growth extends into the lumen of the organ so that by x-ray there is a very frank filling defect which is readily differentiated from ulcer.

Diagnosis is often established by additional laboratory studies. Typically, gastric analysis reveals a striking diminution or absence of free hydrochloric

acid, in many instances this going on to a complete achylia. Moderate bleeding is much more common in carcinoma than in ulcer, and the stomach contents are usually described as resembling coffee grounds due to the changed hemoglobin. On the other hand, profuse hemorrhage is rarely encountered as a complication and a cause of death.

Pathologically the carcinoma of the stomach with associated ulceration is the one which causes the greatest confusion. It has long been a moot question as to whether or not carcinoma develops upon a pre-existing peptic ulcer. Opinions in the past have varied considerably in this regard. With more careful observation and study of the material it is rather generally believed to-day that not more than 5 per cent of such ulcerated carcinomata arise from a simple peptic ulcer. It is believed that the great majority of the carcinomata start as carcinomata and subsequently undergo ulceration rather than that chronic ulcers undergo malignant transformation. This may be established histologically by the fact that in primary carcinoma the ulcer bed shows definite evidence of neoplasm with tumor cells invading the deeper structures. In those few cases in which a long history of preëxistent ulcer has been known, and which have subsequently developed carcinoma, the neoplastic changes are found involving only the margin of the ulcer. The line of transition from normal mucosa to malignant cells can be followed fairly readily. In such cases, no neoplastic invasion of the ulcer bed can be demonstrated. A microscopic criterion which Cole has suggested is based on the assumption that the tumor causes a desmoplastic reaction of the supportive tissues with resultant fixation of the muscular layer so that muscle cells may be seen extending right to the ulcerated area of the tumor in contra-distinction to the retracted fibers seen in simple ulcer.

These various differential criteria make up one of the most interesting problems in the diagnosis of these two conditions. Chronic peptic ulcer and gastric carcinoma are unquestionably the two most frequently observed lesions of the stomach and cause more difficulty in diagnosis than any others. For this reason we have emphasized the discussion of these lesions rather fully. A consideration of the various forms of neoplasm, as affecting the gastro-intestinal tract as a whole, follows.

TUMORS OF THE GASTRO-INTESTINAL TRACT

STOMACH

In the stomach, we find that there are a considerable number of types of carcinoma, all of which basically have their origin from some portion of the glandular epithelium. The most common site for carcinoma of the stomach is found just above the pyloric ring, most frequently along the lesser curvature.

Ulcerative Adenocarcinoma.—The typical tumor is a sessile annular lesion (Fig. 467) which tends to be ulcerated, not infrequently from the very outset. These tumors as a rule show moderate glandular hyperplasia, frequently with some slight suggestion of papillary proliferation. The line of demarcation from normal mucosa to tumor is readily made out. The tumor is made up of acini of varying form and size with the tumor cells showing little or no restraint and invading the tissues extensively. This invasion may completely ultimately replace the entire musculature in this area and extend to the serosal surface. Metastasis is usually lymphatic in nature and to the liver. Some of these tumors may become very extensive and involve practically the entire stomach wall before any appreciable symptomatology develops.

A comparable lesion is found as the most common form of adenocarcinoma involving the lower bowel, particularly the sigmoid and rectum. An illustrative case of such a tumor from the sigmoid is presented at this point, which compares in all histopathological details to the similar lesion seen in the stomach and shown in Fig. 467.

ILLUSTRATIVE CASE

CASE 199. (Ref. #S-235 and S-383)

Diagnosis.—Sigmoid-adenocarcinoma (Fig. 328 and 329); Sigmoid-adenoma malignum.

Patient was a 70-year-old white female, admitted to the hospital complaining of marked constipation.

Present Illness.—The patient's troubles began approximately a year before admission with alternating attacks of constipation and diarrhea. During the preceding six months there had been no diarrhea and the constipation had become more and more marked until at the time of admission, she noticed that her stools were ribbon-like in appearance. Even with extensive catharsis this same flattened appearance of the stool was noted and it was accompanied by marked difficulty in defecation. The problem was complicated by a marked desire on her part, but inability, to move her bowels. She had also shown a moderate loss of appetite and believed that she had lost some 15 or 20 pounds over a period of a year. She had no pain and had not noted any nausea or vomiting.

Past History.—Her past history was entirely irrelevant. She had the usual childhood diseases. She never had any serious gastrointestinal disturbances. She had never had any operative procedure. She had been married and had had three children. Her catamenia had been normal. The menopause had occurred over 20 years previously.

Physical Examination.—Patient was an emaciated, elderly white woman. The head was negative except for a marked tortuosity of the temporal vessels. The pupils reacted normally. The nose and throat were negative, the mouth edentulous. The neck was negative. The chest was symmetrical; heart and lungs were within normal limits. The abdomen was moderately distended, particularly in the lower portion. Palpation revealed a doubtful mass in the pelvis. Gynecological examination showed a normal senile atrophic uterus and a mass which appeared to involve the rectum. By proctoscopy, a constricting, annular, ulcerated lesion about 15 centimeters above the anal orifice was demonstrated.

Laboratory Examination.—The red cell count was 3,300,000 with 71% hemoglobin. White cells numbered 8,200 with 69% polynuclears. Urine showed a moderate trace of albumin. It was otherwise negative.

Subsequent History.—A diagnosis of carcinoma of the sigmoid was made and a two stage operation for its removal advised. The preliminary colostomy was performed and subsequently the removal of the tumor was accomplished.

Pathological Report.—Specimen consisted of a section of the sigmoid, 25 centimeters in length (Fig. 470). In the central portion there was a raised cauliflower-like growth which encircled the bowel except for one small area. The surface was ulcerated and hemorrhagic with adherent exudate on it. A small button-like lesion was noted in the mucosa about five centimeters above the main tumor mass, and two small pedunculated polypoid tumors were present between these two neoplastic growths.

Microscopic Description of a Section Through the Tumor.—(Ref. #S-235) (Fig. 469) Histologic examination of the tissue shows a normal mucosa at one side of the specimen. The section includes a transitional zone from normal mucosa to the characteristic hyperplastic carcinomatous tissue. The cells present a somewhat papillary proliferation. Individually, they show marked increase in size. The tumor suggests a relatively low grade type of malignancy as there is a striking persist-

ence of the gland arrangement. On the other hand, the cells are quite atypical in places and show a loss of polarity. There is marked hyperchromatism, numerous atypical mitoses and considerable anaplasia. The histology is that of a true adenocarcinoma but it suggests an origin from a tumor of lower grade malignancy, probably from a so-called adenoma malignum. Profuse infiltration of the submucosa and the muscle wall by tumor cells is found, and nests of tumor cells are likewise encountered in the subserosa.

Microscopic Description of a Section of One of the Pedunculated Tumor Masses.—(Ref. #S-383) Histologic examination of the button-like lesion and of the pedunculated tumor mass presents the characteristic picture of the so-called adenoma malignum. There is a moderate hyperplasia of the epithelium with the cells tending to show a papillary arrangement. Except by comparing the tumor cells with the normal, it would be hard to realize the fact that considerable hyperchromatism is actually present. The cells are somewhat increased in size. Many of them show an increased mucous secretion. The glandular arrangement is well preserved. Occasional mitoses are present but they are normal in appearance. The lesion may be classified on the graded basis as showing early malignancy. It would be amenable to surgical excision probably without much likelihood of recurrence, if metastasis had not already occurred but might well progress to frank malignancy if left alone.

Papillary Adenocarcinoma.—A less common type of tumor is the polypoid variety (Fig. 466). This is called by several terms, depending upon the degree of malignancy which it shows grossly and histologically. In the more benign form of the lesion, it is spoken of as a simple polyp or polypoid adenoma. As it begins to show evidence of malignancy it is frequently labeled "adenoma malignum," and in its frankly malignant form, it is spoken of as a "papillary or polypoid adenocarcinoma." Such tumors tend to be large, bulky, fungating, cauliflower-like masses, which in extreme instances may almost fill the entire lumen of the stomach without giving undue symptoms of obstruction, arising as they usually do from the lesser curvature. This permits the passage of food between the surface of the tumor and the greater curvature. As long as actual blocking of the

pyloric ring does not occur, no evidence of obstruction can be demonstrated.

Carcinoma Simplex.—By this term is meant a type of carcinoma which almost invariably arises in the prepyloric area. It may assume a scirrhous form, but more often develops as a lesion more comparable to the medullary or encephaloid carcinoma of the breast. As the tumor grows, it may extend throughout the wall of the stomach. At times, this tumor is spoken of as a "small round cell carcinoma." The tumor frequently arises deep in the submucosa and extends in the submucosa with the surface epithelium remaining intact for a considerable period until subsequent ulceration takes place. This tumor, likewise, tends to metastasize early by way of the regional lymph nodes. It is highly malignant, and has an almost certain fatal outcome.

ILLUSTRATIVE CASE

Diagnosis.—Stomach—Carcinoma simplex, medullary type.

In a case of carcinoma of the stomach occurring in a sixty-eight-year-old white married woman, the findings at autopsy were those of a carcinoma of the stomach of the medullary type, accompanied by regional lymph node metastasis. The immediate cause of death was a terminal pneumonia associated with malignant cachexia and general debility.

Gross Description of Stomach.—The mucosa lost its normal appearance at a point about 5 cm. above the pylorus along the greater curvature of the organ

where the mucosa formed a rough, bosselated ulceration which extended forward into the lumen. The edges appeared indurated and everted, giving the lesion an irregular ovoidal outline. The lesion was approximately 6 cm. in diameter. The underlying muscular and serosal coats were thickened and indurated. The pylorus was not involved. The inferior gastric lymph nodes were enlarged, stony and firm. On cross section, they were mottled, dull gray and smooth.

Microscopic Description of Section Through the Stomach Wall.—Section histologically through the wall of the stomach presents a very unusual picture. There is definite transition noted from the normal glandular mucosa to the neoplastic process. The tumor is characterized as a very diffuse medullary type or solid malignant infiltration of the submucosa which extends through the muscular wall and even invades the subserosa. The cells are apparently derived from the acinar epithelium and in places retain their colloid producing capacity. In places, this almost gives a suggestion of signet-ring cell formation not unlike the type of cell seen

Linitis Plastica (Scirrhous Carcinoma or Leather Bottle Stomach).—The only essential difference between the true linitis plastica type of carcinoma and the tumor just described is one of distribution. The linitis plastica lesion likewise starts in the pyloric area, but extends gradually to involve the entire stomach. It is an extremely slow growing tumor comparable in many respects to the scirrhous carcinoma of the breast. There is a very extensive desmoplastic reaction with marked thickening and contraction of the wall of the stomach to such an extent that its total contents may be less than two ounces

in the so-called Krukenberg tumor. For the most part, however, the cells are round or ovoid with large nuclei, with sharply defined nuclear membranes, prominent nucleoli and hyperchromatic granules within the nucleus. They occur in sheets and masses without much suggestion of lumen formation. They extend as narrow cords or groups of cells between the muscle bundles and are found in similar sheet-like arrangement under the serosal surface of the stomach wall.

(Fig. 468). It is a peculiarly persistent and invasive tumor and is associated with an extremely high mortality from the surgical standpoint. In itself, if left alone, it has a hundred per cent fatal outcome. The difficulty from the surgical standpoint is in knowing how far the neoplastic process has extended, as there is no sharp line of demarcation. An examination of sections from the stomach wall is notoriously difficult to interpret. The desmoplastic reaction is so striking, and the tumor cells so few in number that often in a given section, no tumor cells can be identified. This has led to the belief that some cases are not cancer.

ILLUSTRATIVE CASE

CASE 200. (Ref. #S-268)
Diagnosis.—Stomach-scirrhous carcinoma (linitis plastica).

Patient was a male of 58 years, admitted to the hospital complaining of loss of appetite.

Present Illness.—The onset of the patient's troubles dated back for approximately three to four months when he noticed that his appetite had become progressively poorer. Previously, he had always had an unusually good appetite and had never had any history of any disturbance of digestion. One of the most striking factors in arriving at a diagnosis was found in his statement that if he should eat more than two to three ounces of food at a time, it would produce marked nausea and vomiting. As a result of this inability to handle food, he had shown a marked weight loss of some 30 pounds during the preceding three months. Accompanying his gastric symptoms, he had noted a marked obstipation which he attributed to the fact that he had been unable to take any appreciable amount of food. At no time had he noted any blood either in his vomitus or in his stools and he had never had any pain associated with his difficulties. He had noticed a sense of fullness in the epigastrum following the taking of food, but this had not been accompanied by any undue belching.

Past Medical History.—The past medical history was essentially irrelevant. The patient had a normal childhood with the usual diseases. A review of his systems was negative. He had never had any serious upper respiratory infections. His gastro-intestinal history was negative. His genito-urinary history was essentially normal. He denied venereal disease. He had never had any operations.

Physical Examination.—Patient was a fairly well-developed but somewhat-emaciated elderly male. His head was normal. The eyes were negative. His pupils reacted normally. The nose and throat were negative. His

teeth showed numerous carious stumps. His tongue was coated. His neck was negative. There was no enlargement of any of the peripheral lymph nodes. His chest was symmetrical. His heart and lungs seemed within normal limits. His abdomen was slightly prominent. His liver was not palpable. No masses or tenderness could be made out in the abdomen. Genitalia and extremities were negative.

Laboratory Findings.—His blood count showed a slight secondary anemia. There were 3,700,000 red cells with 71% hemoglobin. His white cell count was 9,400 with 63% polynuclears. Urinalysis was negative. Gastric lavage was attempted but it was impossible to get the tube into the stomach.

X-ray examination showed a very small stomach with a total content of less than 60 c.c. as visualized by barium fluoroscopy. This diminution in size of the stomach seemed to be uniform. The mucosal surface appeared smooth without any well developed rugae, and the walls were markedly thickened from the cardia to the pyloris. Picture suggested a scirrhous carcinoma of the stomach, radiologically.

Subsequent Course.—Patient was advised to have a subtotal gastrectomy as a palliative procedure to improve his nutritional state. At the time of operation, it was deemed necessary to do a complete gastrectomy with an esophago-jejunostomy. This was done and the patient improved clinically for a period of over six months at which time he developed an upper respiratory infection and died of a pneumonia.

Pathological Report.—The surgical specimen consisted of a stomach measuring 13 cm. in length and 6 cm. in width. The serosa was somewhat hemorrhagic. Many discrete, hard nodules, measuring about 0.5 cm. in diameter along both greater and lesser curvatures, were noted. The lesser curvature was infiltrated with firm, nodular tumor tissue. The mucosa appeared hyperplastic, although the normal rugae were lacking. The walls were greatly thickened, measuring 1 cm. on the average. Their cut surface was white, glistening, trabeculated and of cartilaginous density (Fig. 468).

Microscopic Description of the Section through the Wall of the Stomach.—Histological examination of the tissue presents an intact mucosa which shows some slight tendency toward hyperplasia of the superficial portion of the glands. Between the glands and involving the entire submucosa, which is thickened perhaps ten times its normal depth, is found a diffuse, rapidly growing, small cell carcinoma. This is made up of masses of small,

Mucous Carcinoma (Colloid or Gelatinous Carcinoma).—Similar to the mucous tumors of the breast should be mentioned large, bulky, gelatinoid tumors of the stomach. These are characterized by the presence of signet-ring cells similar in appearance to fat cells at first glance. They will be seen, however, on closer examination to be filled with a gelatinous or mucinous material. In other respects, they appear to represent typical adenocarcinomata. They are usually slow-growing, persistent tumors with a high mortality. (Refer to Case 6 (Ref. #S-223), Chapter II, Fig. 20.)

KRUKENBERG TUMOR.—In Chapter XXXV, round or oval hyperchromatic and somewhat anaplastic appearing cells. The nuclei are relatively small and nucleoli relatively large by contrast. There is very little cytoplasm to these cells. Very little suggestion of acinar arrangement can be made out except here and there. The tumor not only spreads along the submucosa, but infiltrates between the muscle bundles, separating many of them widely. In addition, plaques of similar rapidly-growing tumor tissue are seen in the subserosa. Mitotic figures are numerous, but no tumor giant cells are made out. There is a very marked chronic productive fibrosis representing neoplastic desmoplasia.

Case 154 (Ref. #S-162), Fig. 340, the so-called Krukenberg tumor has already been discussed. This we believe to be a variety of mucous carcinoma with the primary tumor arising in the gastro-intestinal tract, most frequently in the stomach. When these tumors occur in women, they are very prone to metastasize to the ovary. It is not generally believed today that these tumors are primary ovarian tumors as they were originally considered by Krukenberg. Histologically, they are likely at times to be confused with the carcinoma simplex type of lesion because of the lack of mucous production of the cells in the more rapidly growing instances.

SMALL INTESTINE

Carcinomata of the small intestine are extremely uncommon. Occasional instances of adenocarcinomata, usually either of a sessile or polypoid type have been described. From the standpoint of frequency, such tumors are more often found in the ileum and duodenum than in the jejunum, but are comparatively uncommon in any of these areas in the digestive tract. Mesothelial tumors also may occur.

APPENDIX

Two tumors are found involving the appendix at times; the adenocarcinoma, which usually arises from a preëxisting mucocele of the appendix; and that curious tumor which is found in the submucosa and is most commonly known as a "carcinoid." The adenocarcinoma needs no further comment. It is an extremely uncommon lesion, but when it occurs follows the course of other adenocarcinomata of the digestive tract. Carcinoid, however, can well be discussed in more detail.

Carcinoid (Chromaffinoma or Argentaffinoma).— This tumor is believed, as the result of Masson's work, to arise from the Kultschitzky cells in the mucosa. These tumors are usually small lesions sharply circumscribed, yellow in color and found incidentally at surgical operation or autopsy in the submucosa of the appendix, usually in the distal portion. Occasionally, these tumors may extend through the wall of the appendix and appear as a dumb-bell or collar-button-shaped lesion—a mass on either side of the musculature connected by a band of tumor tissue. As a rule, the tumor is entirely benign, but some half dozen cases are on record in the literature in which malignant changes have occurred with metastasis. Their relationship or identity with the argentaffin cell neuromata of the appendix is not completely established, but seems highly probable. At all events, the cells of the carcinoid stain intensely with the silver methods as do the cells of the neuromata. It is for this reason that they are called argentaffinomata. Occasionally these tumors may occur elsewhere in the intestinal tract, almost always in the ileum where they behave in similar benign fashion.

ILLUSTRATIVE CASE

CASE 201. (Ref. #S-344)

Diagnosis.—Appendix—carcinoid.

Patient was a white female of 23 years, admitted to the hospital with the chief complaint of dull pain in the right lower quadrant associated with attacks of nausea after eating.

Present Illness.—The onset of the present condition began approximately one month before admission. There had been almost regularly a feeling of nausea following eating and this had been accompanied by practically constant dull pain in the lower right side. At times, a sharper, knife-like pain was felt which began in the epigastric region but radiated to the lower right quadrant. Three days before admission she had a severe attack of nausea and vomiting after her supper. Since that time she had noticed a great deal of gas in her stomach.

Past Medical History.—The patient had the usual childhood diseases, but since that time had enjoyed comparatively good health until the onset of the present illness. A review of her systems was essentially negative. She had no more than the usual number of mild upper respiratory infections. Gastro-intestinal history was negative. Menses began at the age of fourteen and had been regular.

Physical Examination.—The patient was a well developed and nourished young white woman who did not appear acutely ill. Eyes, ears, nose and throat were negative. Chest was symmetrical. There were no abnormalities of the heart or lungs that could be made out. Abdomen: there was superficial hyperaesthesia in the right lower quadrant with some suggestion of tenderness on deep palpation. There was no rebound phenomenon. No palpable masses could be felt. Extremities were negative.

Laboratory Findings.—Red blood cells, 4,370,000 with 90% hemoglobin. White blood cells, 13,300 with 92% polynuclears Urinalysis was negative.

Subsequent History.—The diagnosis of acute appendicitis was made and the appendix removed in routine fashion. The patient made an uneventful recovery and was discharged cured.

Pathological Report.—Gross Description.—Specimen consisted of an appendix which measured 5 x 1.5 cm. The serosa was dull and injected. The end showed a moderate bulbous swelling, somewhat asymmetrical in distribution. On examining the mucosal surface, there was a definite thickened submucosal plaque approximately 0.3 cm. in diameter. This was yellowish-gray in color.

Microscopic Description of a Section Through the Appendix.—(Fig. 471 and 472) Histologic study of the nodule noted in the appendix presents the typical appearance of a so-called "carcinoid." There are small round or polyhedral epithelial appearing cells arranged in cords and nests embedded in a diffuse septate connective tissue stroma. With appropriate silver staining technique, these are found to be argentophil in nature. No mitoses are seen. The neoplastic process is limited sharply to the submucosa, although no definite capsule can be made out. No evidence of malignancy is noted.

LARGE INTESTINE

Next to the stomach, the large intestine is the most common site of the various forms of carcinomata. In general, it may be said that tumors of the polypoid and ulcerative sessile varieties predominate from the numerical standpoint. The diffuse type of tumor, such as the so-called "carcinoma simplex" and "linitis plastica" are not usually encountered. Occasionally, true mucous ("colloid") carcinomata likewise develop, but more often the large, fungating, polypoid type of adenocarcinoma undergoes extensive mucoid degeneration. No further purpose is served by a repetition of the description of these various lesions pathologically, as they correspond both grossly and histologically to the neoplasms already described under the heading of the stomach. (For an illustrative case refer to polyposis, Case 87, Chapter XXIII, Fig. 315.)

Aside from the carcinomata, other varieties of tumors of the gastro-intestinal tract are relatively uncommon. Lymphosarcoma may occur anywhere along the digestive tract from the cardia to the rectum. When such a tumor occurs in the stomach, it develops as a large, fungating mass which can usually be diagnosed by biopsy through direct gastroscopy. Such tumors are extremely radiosensitive and there are a number of instances of permanent cures of more than five and ten years' duration. Curiously, as these lymphosarcomata or reticulo-endothelial sarcomata occur in the small and large intestine, they appear to become increasingly malignant and more difficult to treat either surgically or by irradiation. The mortality is, in a general sort of way, roughly inversely proportional to the distance from the mouth in which they are found.

Myomata and myosarcomata are likewise rare tumors which may arise from the smooth muscle of the wall of the digestive tube. The more malignant lesions are likely to be found around the cardia of the stomach and in the jejunum and ileum. They tend to metastasize to the liver and are a particularly unfavorable group of cases therapeutically.

Miscellaneous odd tumors—fibromata, fibrosarcomata, fibrolipomata, myxomata, chondromata—have all been reported. Their occurrence is so unusual, however, that no further comment need be offered.

CHAPTER XLVIII

DISEASES OF THE LIVER

The liver represents the most important organ of the body in respect to metabolism. As a result it is more subject to injury than any other organ. We have already considered many conditions which affect the liver in the section devoted to general pathology. An organ which has such an extraordinarily generous double blood supply is particularly susceptible to injury through circulating toxins. These many toxic substances act upon the liver cells to produce extensive degenerative lesions. Fatty metamorphosis, granular and hyaline degeneration, disturbances of carbohydrate metabolism as in diabetes with the abnormal deposition of glycogen in the liver nuclei, amyloid infiltration—altogether add up to a significant group of disturbances of liver function. In addition to these general degenerative phenomena there are a number of conditions which affect the liver specifically and which require individual consideration as a result. The pathology of the liver is presented for convenience in the same sequence with which lesions of the other organ systems have been taken up.

CONGENITAL LESIONS

The liver, curiously enough, is more nearly free, perhaps, from malformations which are of functional significance, than any other organ of the body. It is true that there may be a marked variation in the number and arrangement of the liver lobes. It is likewise true that the liver may occur on the left side as part of the general picture of situs inversus. Among all the potential anomalies, there is only one pathological condition which exists of any serious significance.

Congenital Atresia of the Bile Ducts.—The name describes accurately the actual lesion. There is a complete atresia usually of the common duct. This is comparable to the atresias which are found in the esophagus, the small intestine and the rectum in the newborn. Inasmuch as the liver and biliary system develop as an outbudding of the intestinal tract it would seem to imply that some inflammatory processes developed during the course of intra-uterine life and produced an inflammatory reaction which resulted in an obliteration of the duct at or near the point where it enters the duodenum. As a result, after the child is born, bile is secreted, but it cannot get into the duodenum and so backs up into the liver. This produces one of the most striking histologic pictures of bile stasis of the liver imaginable and results in a progressive jaundice, which becomes more and more intense. Terminally the cholemia becomes sufficiently marked to cause central nervous symptoms and ends invariably fatally. From a pathological standpoint, the process is accompanied by a tremendous proliferation of the bile ducts as a compensatory process. With this bile duct proliferation, a corresponding connective tissue stromal response occurs and a picture which might well be compared to the obstructive type of biliary cirrhosis ensues. At times the bile duct proliferation may be so marked as to almost suggest neoplasm. These latter changes are the more striking when the process is not a complete atresia, but a partial blocking of the duct through congenital stricture. Under such circumstances the child may live for a matter of several weeks or even months, which permits the development of these secondary proliferative changes.

ILLUSTRATIVE CASE

CASE 202. (Ref. #S-336)

Diagnosis.—Liver—congenital atresia of bile ducts with obstructive biliary cirrhosis. Erythroblastosis foetalis.

Clinical History.—Patient was a newborn, admitted to the surgical service one week after his delivery because of a progressive jaundice. The pregnancy had been a normal full-term one and the child had been born spontaneously after a relatively short labor. The day following delivery, he showed a rather marked icterus neonatorum. No particular attention was paid to this for

PLATE CXII

DISEASES OF THE LIVER

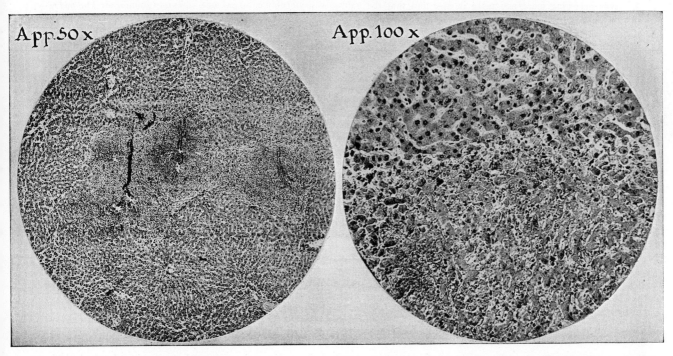

FIG. 473.—ECLAMPSIA—FOCAL NECROSIS.—CASE 3.—Low power photomicrograph to illustrate the distribution of the necrotic lesions, chiefly in the peripheral portion of the liver lobule. App. 50 x.

FIG. 474.—ECLAMPSIA.—CASE 3.—Higher magnification to show the marked necrosis of the liver cells with loss of their nuclei and disintegration of cytoplasm. Note extensive hemorrhage into necrotic areas. App. 100 x. (See also color plate CXIII, Fig. 482.)

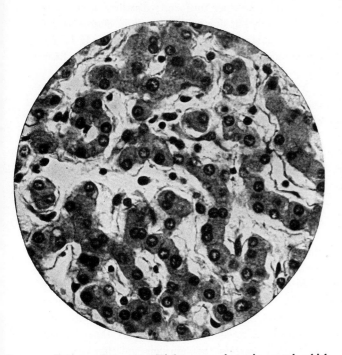

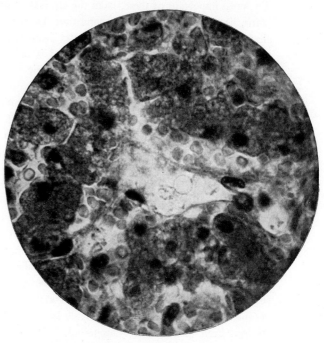

FIG. 475.—EDEMA.—CASE 203.—High power photomicrograph which shows the accumulation of fluid between the liver cells and the sinusoidal endothelium. Liver cells slightly compressed but otherwise normal in appearance. App. 400 x.

FIG. 476.—CHRONIC PASSIVE CONGESTION AND CENTRAL NECROSIS OF LIVER WITH HEMORRHAGE.—Cf. CASE 204.—Liver cells show pyknotic nuclei and marked cytoplasmic degeneration. Red cells have escaped from sinusoids and are seen in spaces between the endothelium and liver cord. App. 400 x. (See also Plate CXIII, Figs. 479 and 480.)

the first few days, but it was noted that the jaundice was becoming more and more intense and that the baby vomited almost regularly after nursing.

Physical Examination.—Examination of the baby showed it to be apparently normal in other respects except that it showed no bile pigment in its stools which, in conjunction with the progressive jaundice, suggested the possibility of an atresia of his bile ducts.

Laboratory Findings.—Blood examination revealed a red cell count of only 2,300,000 cells with a hemoglobin of 43%. There was an apparent white count of 96,000 cells. When this was studied from the standpoint of the blood smear, it was found that the actual white count could be corrected to read approximately 18,000, the remaining 78,000 nucleated cells representing various types of nucleated red cells. Smears showed a marked hypochromic anemia with a tendency toward microcytosis. The most striking feature was the presence of the early red series in the peripheral blood in such large numbers. In view of the clinical picture, it was felt that this represented a typical erythroblastosis fetalis rather than a von Jacksch's anemia.

Subsequent Course.—Operative attempt was made to correct this congenital defect but the operative procedure was too extensive to be tolerated and the baby died less than twenty-four hours postoperatively.

Autopsy Findings.—At autopsy the liver was found considerably enlarged and intensely jaundiced. The operative field was explored and an attempt made to find the atresic duct at its point of entrance into the duodenum. A thickened fibrous cord was demonstrated. The bile ducts above the operative field were dilated and thickened. No other pathological changes than bile pigmentation of the tissues generally were found.

Microscopic Description of a Section of the Liver. —(Fig. 491) Histologic examination of the liver presents a picture which shows a number of striking pathological features. In the first place, there is a very marked bile stasis with dilatation of the small bile ducts and capillaries. Bile pigment is found within the cytoplasm of the liver cells. There is considerable fatty and granular degeneration of the liver parenchyma. The most striking feature of the pathology aside from the bile stasis is an enormous amount of proliferation of the bile ducts as a result of the obstruction. In addition, a secondary fibrosis is observed which creates the picture of a beginning biliary cirrhosis of the pure obstructive type. Finally, countless islands of active erythropoiesis may be identified throughout the liver parenchyma far in excess of the usual picture. These show all stages in the development of the red cell from the relatively undifferentiated megaloblast down to the normoblast.

CIRCULATORY CHANGES

Chronic Passive Congestion.—Among the most striking of the changes which are found in the liver are those relating to the disturbances of circulation. The most important of these, from the clinical standpoint, is represented by the condition known as chronic passive congestion. This results from a disturbed cardiac mechanism ordinarily, and is usually seen as the aftermath of a chronic rheumatic infection of the heart with mitral stenosis. This results in the backing-up of the blood stream, with an initial passive congestion in the lung. This in turn is followed by the same process in the liver and other viscera. The liver, due to its architectural arrangement, is more rapidly susceptible to circulatory changes than is true of any of the other organs. Grossly, the liver in uncomplicated chronic passive congestion is characterized by a marked dilatation of the central vein and of the sinusoids in relation to this vessel (Fig. 477). As a result of the slowing of the circulation, the blood tends to accumulate in these dilated sinusoids and to appear rather darker than is true of ordinary venous blood. Furthermore, because of the increased carbon dioxide in the blood, the nutrition of the cells is impaired. This is followed by rather marked, fatty degenerative changes manifested by a yellow color of the liver parenchyma. The resulting gross picture is extremely striking, the

yellow liver tissue standing out sharply against the dilated sinusoids, giving the so-called "nutmeg" appearance to the cut surface of the organ. Ordinarily this picture is rather uniformly distributed throughout the liver, but due to differences in degree of the circulatory stasis, this is not always true. It is not uncommon to find the peripheral part of the liver less prominently involved.

Microscopically, the picture of chronic passive congestion (Fig. 478) in its uncomplicated form is characterized by enormous distention of the sinusoids which becomes progressively less marked as one proceeds away from the central vein toward the periphery of the lobule. Typically, the liver cells show simple atrophy. The cells are narrowed and compressed; the nuclei condensed and hyperchromatic. The chromatin material seems massed together and it is difficult to find the characteristic nucleolus. Whether this atrophy may be considered as actually of mechanical origin, or whether it had best be thought of in terms of nutritional anoxemia is somewhat of a controversial point. It is our belief that the latter is the more important factor. The picture may be identified microscopically by the fact that the red cells are all *within* the sinusoids and that the sinusoidal endothelium is in close contact to the compressed liver cords. This, in contrast to the picture of central necrosis of the liver complicated by hemorrhage, in which the red cells are found *outside* the sinuses between the sinusoidal endothelium and the liver cells (Fig. 476 and 479).

As a concomitant of chronic passive congestion with circulatory stasis, and often preceding this more marked change, just described, is the picture of *edema* of the liver. A recent review by Klemperer has demonstrated convincingly that the only significant cause of such hepatic edema is found as a result of cardiac pathology, usually associated with the phase of cardiac decomposition. Such edema is characterized by the presence of a fine granular precipitate, microscopically, which is seen lying between the sinusoidal endothelium and the somewhat compressed liver cords. As a result of this edema, the sinusoids themselves may appear relatively bloodless in spite of the fact that there is actually an associated congestive failure of the circulation (Fig. 475).

ILLUSTRATIVE CASE

CASE 203. (Ref. #S-337)
Diagnosis.—Liver—edema.
Patient was a colored female of 61 years, admitted to the hospital with the chief complaint of swelling of the feet and ankles.
Present Illness.—Approximately two years before admission the patient first noticed moderate dyspnea on exertion. This had increased in severity during the interval so that at the time of admission she was practically confined to bed or a chair. For the preceding six months she had had a progressive edema of her lower extremities which was increased on standing. A week before admission she developed a slight productive cough and complained of marked anorexia accompanied by nausea. She became extremely dyspneic, had a sharp attack of pericardial pain, became cyanotic, developed sweating and chilliness and decided she needed medical attention.
Past Medical History.—It was difficult to obtain a satisfactory past medical history. The patient believed she had all the childhood diseases but it was impossible to estimate whether she had actually had rheumatic fever or not. A review of her systems was essentially noninformatory. She had never had any particular upper respiratory difficulty. She had had attacks of qualitative dyspepsia. She had never required any operative procedures. The genito-urinary examination was negative. She had been married and had had one child who died in infancy. This had been followed by two spontaneous miscarriages. She denied venereal disease and had never received any intravenous or intramuscular medication.
Physical Examination.—Patient was an elderly negress who showed marked generalized anasarca. Head was negative. Her chest was emphysematous in type. Breath sounds were heard normally over the left base but were diminished over the right base. The heart was greatly enlarged with the apex 13 cm. from the midsternal line on the left. Blood pressure, 190/60. Heart sounds were irregular and varied in intensity. Only the strong beats apparently reached the wrist as the pulse rate there was 36 as compared to 72 at the apex. The liver was greatly enlarged, a hand's breadth below the costal margin. Abdomen otherwise was negative except for the edema. Extremities showed pitting edema.
Laboratory Findings.—Urinalysis: Albumin, a slight trace on several occasions but otherwise was negative. Blood red count, 3,700,000, white cells, 9,400. Kahn test was negative.
Subsequent Course.—Patient's lungs began to fill up and in spite of all efforts, covering a rather prolonged period, she went steadily downhill and died three weeks after admission.
Autopsy Findings.—There was general anasarca. There was marked edema and congestion of the lungs. The heart weighed 600 gm. and showed both hypertrophy and dilatation, more marked on the left side. The liver was moderately enlarged, intensely congested and firm in consistency. The other organs showed passive congestion.
Microscopic Examination of a Section Through the Liver.—(Fig. 475) Section histologically through the liver presents evidence of several striking circulatory lesions, the most outstanding of which is edema. This edema is characterized by the presence of fluid in the interstitial spaces between the liver cord cells and the sinusoidal endothelium. It is noted as a faint pink-staining granular precipitate. The liver cords showed considerable atrophy largely presumably the result of anoxemia. Owing to the long standing nature of the process, the chronic passive congestive picture is rather striking and some degree of central cirrhosis is found.

Infarction.—Rarely embolic and thrombotic lesions may occur in the liver which result in a picture of infarction. This may be entirely portal in origin, but more usually is seen as a combined lesion affecting both the portal vein and the hepatic artery. Due to the extremely generous double blood supply of the liver, such infarction is extremely rare, and, when it does occur, as has already been commented upon, is seen as a frankly hemorrhagic type. Such lesions are usually found incidentally at autopsy and are rarely recognized clinically, as the liver is capable of such amazing regeneration that it would require much larger areas of involvement to produce any evidence of hepatic insufficiency.

DEGENERATIVE AND INFILTRATIVE DISEASES OF THE LIVER

At this point, it seems logical to refer to the degenerative and infiltrative lesions of the liver. Only brief comment is necessary as these have been considered extensively in the first part of the book in a consideration of the general pathological processes. The liver perhaps is one of the most suitable organs for the study of such changes because of its comparative simplicity of structure anatomically. Among the most obvious are those changes associated with fatty infiltration, fatty degeneration, glycogen storage, pathological glycogen deposition as in diabetes, cloudy swelling, granular degeneration and actual necrosis; and finally, amyloid infiltration in the chronic wasting diseases. These are all illustrated in the first three chapters, to which the reader is referred.

TOXIC LESIONS OF THE LIVER

The most important lesions of the liver are those which occur as the result of the action of circulating toxins upon the liver parenchyma. These toxins cover a wide range of substances, both exogenous and endogenous in origin. They include such toxins as those elaborated by bacteria with the focus of infection elsewhere in the body. They include as well, such chemical poisons as may enter the body by ingestion or inhalation. Among these must be mentioned particularly chloroform, phosphorus, arsenic, usually in the form of one of the arsenicals such as salvarsan, carbon tetrachloride, which is used extensively to-day as a vermifuge, tetrachlorethane, one of the important cellulose solvents used industrially in the manufacture of rayon, and a host of other less important and common poisons. There remain a considerable number of toxic substances, the origin of which is most obscure. Among these may be cited the toxins found during pregnancy, which are associated clinically with the two major toxemias of pregnancy, pernicious vomiting seen in the first half of the gestation, and eclampsia, seen in the latter half. And finally, the condition known as yellow atrophy, either in its acute or subacute form represents a group of cases in which the etiologic toxic agent is unknown.

For convenience, the toxic lesions of the liver may be divided on the basis of the localization of the lesion in respect to the anatomical liver lobule. Thus we find three major anatomical varieties of such necrosis:

1. Central necrosis in which the lesion is found chiefly around the central vein, exemplified by chloroform poisoning.

2. Mid-zonal, or zonal necrosis in which the lesion is found in the middle portion of the anatomical lobule, and usually in relation to some streptococcic infection, and

3. Focal necrosis in which the lesion may be found without respect to the anatomical arrangement of the liver lobule. In this group should be included the many actual focal bacterial lesions, as well as such purely toxic conditions as eclampsia.

Central Necrosis.—As has already been remarked upon, liver cells are particularly susceptible to the action of circulating toxins. Fortunately, however, they are equally capable of regeneration. It has further been shown that a liver can function without evidence of symptomatology so long as approximately one-eighth of its cells remain uninvolved in the degenerative process. The great majority of cases of necrosis of the liver are seen in the form of central necrosis. This is because of the anatomical arrangement of the lobule in respect to its circulation so that circulating toxins are liable to occur in their greatest concentration with chronic passive congestion.

It is believed, on account of the marked anoxemia

PLATE CXIII

Fig. 477.—Liver, Chronic Passive Congestion "Nutmeg Liver." Cf. Case 161.

Fig. 479.—Left, Chronic Passive Congestion; Right, Central Necrosis, Hemorrhage, App. 400 x.

Fig. 481.—Liver, Alcoholic Cirrhosis; Hyaline Degeneration of Liver Cells. Case 208. App. 800 x.

Fig. 478.—Liver, Chronic Passive Congestion. Cf. Case 161. Dilated sinuses, atrophic liver cords. App. 50 x.

Fig. 480.—Liver, Passive Congestion with Central Necrosis and Hemorrhage. Case 204. App. 50 x.

Fig. 482.—Liver, Eclampsia; Focal Hemorrhagic Necrosis. Case 3. (*See also* Fig. 473 and 474.) 50 x.

PLATE CXIII

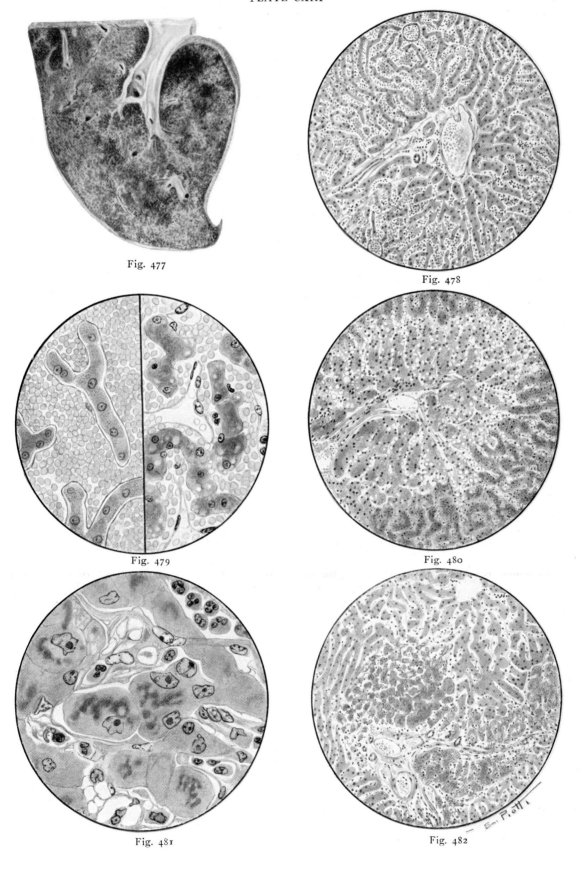

Fig. 477

Fig. 478

Fig. 479

Fig. 480

Fig. 481

Fig. 482

of the tissues which accompany such chronic passive congestion, that the liver cells are particularly susceptible to the action of such toxins, under the circumstances. Accordingly, it is not surprising that necrosis follows, even in conjunction with what might otherwise appear to be minimal toxemia. Indeed, it has been shown that following almost any acute upper-respiratory infection sufficient toxin from the focus of infection in the nose or throat may be absorbed in the blood stream to produce such necrotic changes in the liver to a variable degree.

The most striking example, perhaps, of central necrosis is seen as a result of chloroform poisoning. It is for this reason that chloroform is used much less extensively as an anesthetic than other drugs such as ether, in which this necrotic picture is much less likely to develop. Grossly, the lesion is often difficult to recognize with certainty at the autopsy table except in the more marked instances. It appears as rather opaque, reddish yellow areas, more or less uniformly distributed in relation to the central portion of the liver lobule.

The diagnosis is best established, or confirmed, by microscopic examination of the tissue. The liver cells surrounding the central vein present evidence of varying degrees of fatty and granular degenerative changes to the point of actual necrosis. With the ordinary hematoxylin and eosin stain, these central areas of necrosis stand out prominently as bright pink or red areas in contrast to the purplish red color of the normal liver parenchyma (Fig. 479 and 480). Under higher magnification the nuclei of the cells present karyorrhectic and karyolytic changes. Moderate leukocytic infiltration is seen in an attempt to remove this cellular detritus.

The endothelium of the sinusoids is involved in the process with necrosis as well. This results in actual hemorrhage into the liver substance. This is best observed around the periphery of the lesion. Much of the intense eosin-staining reaction of the necrotic areas is due to the presence of hemorrhage. In the periphery of the lesion, the red cells may be found outside the sinusoidal endothelium, lying characteristically between the liver cells and the sinusoids. This is a distinctive histologic differential diagnostic feature, in contrast to simple, chronic passive congestion.

Around the edges of such necrotic lesions may be found evidence of liver cell regeneration, with occasional mitotic figures and many hypertrophic liver cells. These, it may be assumed, are attempting to take over the function of the destroyed liver parenchyma. As the process goes on, these liver cells continue to regenerate until they completely replace the destroyed tissue, and in most instances restore the normal architectural arrangement of the lobule. Curiously enough, in spite of the extensive necrosis which occurs at times, little or no evidence of fibrous tissue scarring is found, due apparently to the rapidity with which liver cell regeneration occurs.

ILLUSTRATIVE CASE

CASE 204. (Ref. #S-41)
Diagnosis.—Liver—central necrosis with chronic passive congestion.
Patient was a white male of 35 years, admitted to the hospital with the chief complaint of hemoptysis.
Present Illness.—The onset of the patient's current illness was sudden in nature. It was ushered in with a severe attack of cough and dyspnea which was followed by the expectoration of about a tablespoonful of bright red blood. He became dizzy and felt faint as the result of this attack and was sent to the hospital for study. His present illness should be more accurately dated back to the age of fifteen when he developed an acute attack of rheumatic fever which was followed by definite cardiac damage. This had never been severe enough to interfere with his normal activities, but on exertion he had suffered from dyspnea. This had not been improved by a fracture of his nose some ten years previously, which had almost completely obstructed his nose in respect to breathing and had forced him to breathe very largely through his mouth. During the preceding year he had had a number of acute upper respiratory infections and on several occasions had noted blood streaking of his sputum.

Past Medical History.—The patient had the usual childhood diseases, measles, mumps, chicken pox and scarlet fever. As previously commented upon he had had rheumatic fever at the age of fifteen. A review of his systems yielded a few facts of possible significance. He had always been subject to upper respiratory infections. In spite of the fact that he had had rheumatic fever associated with severe tonsillitis, he had not had his tonsils removed. He had apparently not had any recurrence of his rheumatic attacks and the only feature of significance in this respect were related to his occasional attacks of dyspnea on exertion. His gastro-intestinal history was relatively negative although he had never had much of an appetite and was definitely underweight. His genito-urinary history was negative. He denied veneral infection.
Physical Examination.—Patient was a tall, emaciated, white male showing a considerable dyspnea, but no cyanosis. Head externally was not remarkable. There was marked deviation of his nasal septum with complete obstruction on the left. Throat was negative. Teeth were in poor condition. Chest was fairly symmetrical and was somewhat emphysematous in appearance. There was

marked prominence of the intercostal spaces which moved with respiration. There was some slight diminution of expansion on the left side with dullness and bronchial breathing over the left lower lobe. A few scattered râles were heard. Heart was moderately enlarged. Numerous extrasystoles and a loud, blowing systolic murmur were heard over the mitral area. Blood pressure was 132/82. Abdomen: Liver was palpable three fingers' breadth below the costal margin. Extremities were negative.

Laboratory Findings.—Urinalysis was negative. Blood examination showed a red cell count of 3,200,000 with 63% hemoglobin. White blood cells were 19,000 with 92% neutrophiles. Sputum examination was negative for tuberculosis, but showed many type 7 Pneumococci as proved by the Neufeld technique.

Subsequent Course.—The patient developed a typical diffuse pneumonia involving apparently the entire left lower lobe. He went steadily downhill and died four days after admission.

Autopsy Findings.—Autopsy findings revealed a lobar pneumonia of the left lower lobe associated with an acute fibrinous pleuritis. The heart presented a typical healed rheumatic endocarditis with a double mitral lesion showing marked stenosis of the valve. There was a terminal acute fibrinous pericarditis. There was marked hypertrophy of the heart as a whole, but particularly of the right side. The abdominal viscera all showed very marked chronic passive congestion. This was particularly prominent in the liver where the lobules were prominently outlined by the dilated sinusoids. Centrally, they appeared to show actual necrosis, being yellowish in color and rather friable in consistency. There was a coincidental cholesterolosis of the gallbladder.

Microscopic Description of a Section Through the Liver.—(Fig. 479 and 480) Sections histologically show a typical picture of chronic passive congestion. This is evidenced by atrophy of the liver cords around the central vein of the liver lobule. It is accompanied by considerable edema between the sinusoidal endothelium and liver parenchyma in places. Immediately around the central vein the sinusoids appear markedly distended but in the midzonal and peripheral portion of the lobule the edema just noted may best be observed. In a few areas some actual necrotic changes may be seen in the liver cells around the central areas. There is possibly a slight increase of connective tissue in the portal areas as well. There is a moderate amount of hemosiderin, the result of the chronic passive congestion, with stasis and breakdown of the blood pigment which is taken up by the Küpffer cells. Being produced in excess this pigment is also found in the liver cells as part of the functional disturbance as the result of the congestion.

Zonal Necrosis.—More rarely one may find a curious localization of the necrotic process to the mid-zonal or peripheral portion of the lobule, with the central area remaining intact. Opie was among the first to recognize the almost constant relationship of this particular lesion to the action of bacterial toxins, particularly those of streptococci. This is a lesion which is rarely encountered in human cases as the regenerative process has apparently gone on to a point where the recognition of the lesion is at best doubtful, by the time such patients come to autopsy. In the experimental animal, on the other hand, it is extremely easy to reproduce this distribution of the lesion. Various explanations for this phenomenon have been offered. Perhaps the simplest of these is dependent again upon the anatomical relationship of the lobule to the circulatory mechanism.

Focal Necrosis.—In this discussion particular attention will be called to the focal necroses which are produced as a result of various toxemias, the focal bacterial lesions being dismissed with a very brief comment, as they are considered in conjunction with the infectious diseases in which they occur. The most important of the bacterial lesions of this type are seen in typhoid fever (refer back to Case 52, Fig. 114, etc.), and in miliary tuberculosis. Almost any bacterium which gains access to the blood stream may localize in the liver and produce its characteristic cellular response. Thus, it is possible to have focal abscesses as the result of staphylococcus infections. Similarly, actinomycosis may involve the liver in the terminal stage of the disease, wherever its primary focus may have been. Parasitic infestation, such as amebic abscess, likewise represents a type of focal necrosis.

ECLAMPSIA GRAVIDARUM.—Of the outstanding toxic lesions which produce focal necrosis must be mentioned at length the condition known as *eclampsia*. In this disease we find that the entire liver is likely to be somewhat enlarged. Even through the capsule can be seen focal hemorrhagic lesions ranging in size from a millimeter or less up to large areas one or two centimeters in diameter. On cut section of the liver, these focal hemorrhagic necrotic areas will be found irregularly distributed throughout the liver substance (Fig. 482). They bear no relation as far as can be made out to the anatomical architecture of the lobule.

Microscopically, these lesions are seen to consist of two apparently distinct processes (Fig. 473). In the first instance, we have an actual focal necrosis of the liver cells. This presents essentially the same features as necrosis elsewhere. As a part of the picture, but more or less unrelated except secondarily, is the hemorrhagic phase. Due to vascular endothelial injury, the red cells are poured out into the necrotic foci. Both grossly and microscopically, this hemorrhagic picture is by far the more outstanding part

PLATE CXIV

DISEASES OF THE LIVER (*Continued*)

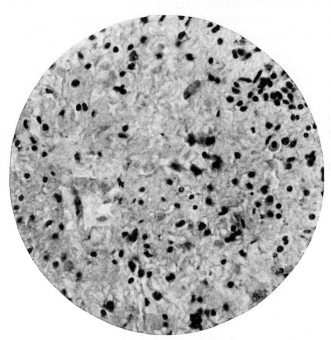

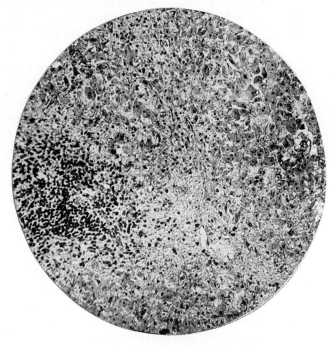

FIG. 483.—LIVER—ACUTE YELLOW ATROPHY.—CASE 205.—High power of Fig. 484. Note extensive necrosis of the liver cells, with loss of nuclei, and cytoplasmic detail, hemorrhage and beginning mononuclear cellular infiltration. App. 200 x.

FIG. 484.—LIVER—ACUTE YELLOW ATROPHY.—CASE 205.—Low power photomicrograph to illustrate the diffuse extent of the toxic necrotic process without regard to anatomical relationships. App. 100 x.

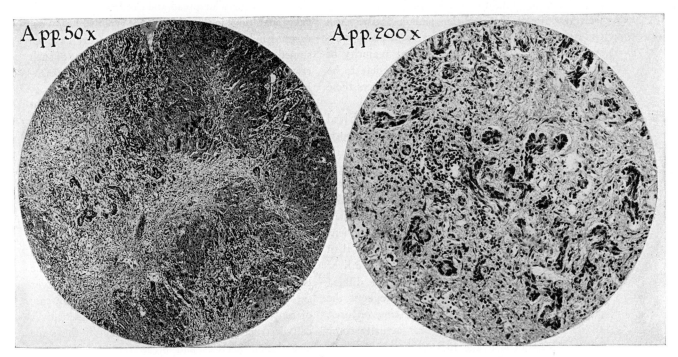

FIG. 485.—LIVER—SUBACUTE YELLOW ATROPHY.—CASE 206.—Low power photomicrograph which emphasizes the replacement fibrosis and abortive attempt at liver regeneration by bile duct epithelial hyperplasia. App. 50 x.

FIG. 486.—LIVER—SUBACUTE YELLOW ATROPHY.—CASE 206.—High power of Fig. 485, which better demonstrates the regenerative efforts of the biliary epithelium, the fibrous scarring and the chronic round cell infiltration.

of the process. The lesions of eclampsia are not strictly anatomically distributed, but it is true that for the most part, they occur in the peripheral portion of the lobule in relation to the portal area. Whether this is because these toxins are carried to the liver by the portal vein, and thus affect the first cells they come in contact with is somewhat problematical. However, it perhaps helps explain the rather characteristic and striking distribution of the lesions (see Fig. 473, 474 and 482).

As a further manifestation of eclampsia, we have already seen the degenerative changes which involve the renal-tubular epithelium (Chapter LV). In addition a variable degree of acute glomerular damage is seen, characterized by cellular proliferation and resultant avascularity of the capillary tuft. By many this is believed to be the more significant renal lesion, with the tubular injury as definitely secondary. At all events, this particular combination of hepatic and renal lesions makes a pathological diagnosis of eclampsia inevitable (Refer back to Case 3, Chapter I; and to Fig. 6, 11 and 548).

ACUTE YELLOW ATROPHY

Acute yellow atrophy is best considered under the general heading of toxic necrosis of the liver (toxic hepatitis), representing as it does a widespread, diffuse lesion, but one which bears no relationship to the anatomical arrangement of the liver. Acute yellow atrophy may be defined as a non-specific type of extreme necrosis of the liver. It is seen most frequently in association with the severe toxemias of pregnancy and for that reason is encountered about ten times as often in women as it is in men. However, being non-specific in its origin, any severe toxemia including certain of the industrial poisons may well give rise to the condition pathologically. Even children at times are not exempt from such widespread liver destruction. In the great majority of cases of acute yellow atrophy it is impossible to be certain what the toxic agent is which produces these changes.

The name applied to this condition was derived from the gross appearance of the liver at autopsy. Typically, the liver is small, often weighing as little as five and six hundred grams. It is of a bright yellow color due to a combination of necrosis, fatty degeneration and bile pigmentation. It is usually flabby in consistency and extremely friable on handling. Actually, by the time the average patient dies, the liver has assumed a rather more red than yellow color due to the fact that much of the liver parenchyma has been destroyed leaving the dilated sinusoids and areas of hemorrhage throughout the persistent liver tissue as the more striking features. In its earlier stages, the liver may actually show some increase in size due to swelling of the cells before the widespread destruction and absorption of the cellular detritus and necrotic tissue has taken place. This has led to confusion in some instances until histologic studies have established the underlying nature of the process.

Clinically, the picture of acute yellow atrophy is characterized by a sudden onset. This is associated with marked nausea and vomiting, which almost invariably goes on to hematemesis. It is accompanied by a rapidly progressing, intense jaundice. The patient goes on to develop a cholemia with delirium, and coma, and often dies within forty-eight hours of the appearance of the first symptoms. A number of cases have been reported in recent years associated with the widespread and careless use of arsenical preparations in the treatment of syphilis. Likewise, cases of industrial poisoning of a like nature have assumed a position of importance in the incidence of such cases. During the World War for example tetrachlorethane poisoning was a not uncommon cause.

Histologically, the liver in these cases shows a practically complete loss of the liver parenchyma. The vascular endothelium and Küpffer cells do not usually become involved. The jaundice is explained on the basis that the Küpffer cells are still producing bile, but the liver cells being unable to utilize it, it is absorbed by the blood stream instead. Likewise, the bile ducts do not become involved in the destructive process and the portal areas stand out microscopically sharply against the mass of necrotic liver tissue. Depending upon the stage at which the liver is seen, one will find varying amounts of liver substance persisting. It might be compared to a case of central necrosis which went on to complete liver cell destruction. The liver cells undergo the same coagulation necrosis and break up into fragments which are gradually absorbed or phagocytized by poly- and mononuclear cells but the distribution of the process is apt to be patchy.

ILLUSTRATIVE CASE

CASE 205. (Ref. #S-39)

Diagnosis.—Liver—acute yellow atrophy.

Chief Complaint.—Patient was a white female, 60 years of age, admitted to the hospital complaining of distress in her lower abdomen.

Present Illness.—The onset was characterized by a feeling of exhaustion and weakness and lassitude which became progressively more severe. A week before admission she began to have pain in the lower abdomen. There was no anorexia nor diarrhea. The patient always had had a tendency to be constipated. A moderate degree of jaundice appeared about one week before admission which had become progressively more intense. This was accompanied by itching of the skin.

Past Medical History.—Her previous history was essentially negative. She had had the usual childhood infections. She had never been operated upon. She had never shown evidence of cardiorenal disease. She had had her menopause at 31. During the past year she had suffered several attacks of rheumatism and for two weeks previous to the onset of her present illness, she had been taking twenty-one grains of cincophen a day.

Physical Examination.—Showed a fairly well nourished elderly white woman with moderate degree of jaundice. She was in a semi-stuporous condition from which she could be roused with difficulty and she was not mentally clear. Heart and lungs were essentially negative. Abdomen was distended but not rigid. Generalized tenderness was noted but especially in the right upper quadrant. The liver was palpable along the edge of the costal cage, but did not seem to be nodular. Spleen was not felt. Extremities were negative.

Laboratory Findings.—The stools were bile stained; urine showed the presence of bile. Blood count showed a moderate secondary anemia and no leukocytosis. Her blood chemistry was negative. There was an indirect, immediate van den Bergh and an icterus index of 90 units.

Subsequent Course.—The jaundice became progressively deeper. The patient became much weaker and stupor developed into true coma in which the patient died three days after admission.

Autopsy Findings.—A fairly well nourished elderly white female with marked jaundice. There were about 2,500 c.c. of bile stained fluid found in the peritoneal cavity. The liver was small and atrophic, weighing 525 grams. On section it was of a mottled golden-brown with patches of dark greenish-red. In the brownish areas there was some nodular elevation of the surface, while in the intermediate greenish areas, the surface of the liver was depressed. No very striking anatomical distribution of this process could be made out. The pericardium and heart were essentially negative except for scattered petechiae in the epicardium. The pleural cavities and lungs were negative except for a terminal congestion and edema of the dependent portions. The kidneys, adrenals and other viscera were essentially negative except for marked albuminous degeneration and congestion.

Microscopic Description of a Section Through the Liver.—(Fig. 483 and 484) Sections microscopically show a picture which varies in different parts of the tissue. There are places where there is very extensive liver cell necrosis and degeneration. There are other areas where there is very marked bile duct proliferation and beginning fibrosis. In the fibrotic areas considerable cellular infiltration, chiefly mononuclear but with a scattering of polymorphonuclears and eosinophiles is seen. The mononuclear reaction is principally lymphocytic, but also some large mononuclears and plasma cells are seen. The outstanding histology is the patchy fibrosis without regard to anatomical distribution in conjunction with the acute degenerative changes of the liver cells. The picture suggests a phase of yellow atrophy in its beginning healing stage obviously following an acute attack of which the etiology is undetermined, but in which cincophen poisoning is strongly suspected.

SUBACUTE YELLOW ATROPHY

In addition to these striking cases of *acute* yellow atrophy which go on to a fatal exodus, usually within forty-eight hours, the condition may exist in a milder, subacute form in which the patient survives. In such cases there is a variable amount of liver cell destruction. The more marked lesions are invariably found in the right lobe. The left lobe may escape appreciable damage. Where the liver cell destruction has occurred, however, practically all anatomical relationships in respect to the liver lobule are lost.

Microscopically, the same basic histologic changes are present varying only in degree and extent. Scattered here and there may be found islands of liver tissue which have survived and regenerated. These take over the function of the destroyed liver paren-

chyma. Such cells are usually hypertrophic in appearance with not infrequently actual evidence of mitoses being present. Bile duct proliferation is striking. There is a very marked relative and absolute increase in connective tissue; relative, because of the loss of liver substance; absolute, because of the actual increase in the amount as the result of the inflammatory reaction. This process leads to a picture spoken of as *toxic sclerosis,* or by some as *toxic cirrhosis.* This is the end picture histologically of a mild, subacute type of yellow atrophy. In this healed stage, the inflammatory cellular infiltration will have disappeared almost entirely. We find a liver which is usually somewhat smaller than normal and irregularly coarsely nodular in appearance as the result of liver cell regeneration as discrete islands. These areas of liver cell regeneration are seen embedded in a dense connective tissue stroma in which bile duct proliferation is most striking. In its essentials, it represents a reparative and replacement fibrosis with some slight secondary inflammatory productive fibrosis. This latter is of minimal extent and significance.

Such a reparative process should not, strictly speaking, be considered as a true *"cirrhosis,"* because by the term, cirrhosis, both the clinician and the pathologist think in terms of a chronic progressive disease. In yellow atrophy, on the other hand, the disease represents a single acute process which might be compared to any acute infectious or toxic process in any other organ, which results in similar healing or scarring as an end picture.

ILLUSTRATIVE CASE

CASE 206. (Ref. #S-338)

Diagnosis.—Liver—subacute yellow atrophy.

Patient was an Italian male of 26 years, admitted to the hospital with the chief complaint of jaundice and abdominal pain.

Present Illness.—Began twelve days before admission with an attack of epigastric pain of short duration and mild character accompanied by the vomiting of some blood-stained material. The following day he noticed jaundice of his eyes and skin. This had become progressively more marked. It was accompanied by sweats and chills and a colic-like type of pain after eating. His stools had become gradually almost clay colored and his urine extremely reddish-brown in color. He had become progressively weaker and thought that his abdomen had increased in size.

Past Medical History.—He had a similar attack approximately a year before which had lasted about six months. There had been no history of digestive disturbance between the two attacks. There was no apparent relationship to his occupation nor was there any suggestion of drug poisoning. He had had a normal childhood with the usual mild infections but had never been previously hospitalized. A review of his systems was essentially negative. He had had a penile ulcer six months before his present illness which was painless and which he had treated himself with salves.

Physical Examination.—Showed a well developed and somewhat under-nourished young adult male. He appeared somewhat distressed but in no acute pain. There was marked general jaundice. His pupils were negative. His cardiovascular findings were normal. His abdomen was distended with slight bulging of his flanks. There was a fluid wave with shifting dullness. The liver edge reached the level of the umbilicus. It had a sharp border and was tender on palpation. The spleen was also palpable but nontender. There was a scar of a penile ulcer present.

Laboratory Findings.—Red cells, 4,490,000 with 68% hemoglobin, white cells, 9,600 with 84% polynuclears, 13% lymphocytes, 2% mononuclears and 1% eosinophiles.

Urinalysis was negative except for a high concentration of bile pigment. Wassermann was positive. Icterus index, 120 with an immediate, very strong, direct van den Bergh and an index of .13 by the indirect method. Blood chemistry showed an albumin/globulin ratio of 0.66.

Subsequent Course.—Patient had a rather prolonged stay in the hospital of some three months' duration, showing considerable variation in his clinical condition, but his jaundice remained persistent and he went gradually downhill and developed a terminal pneumonia of which he died.

Autopsy Findings.—At autopsy the liver was found to be moderately enlarged, intensely jaundiced and extremely firm in consistency. It was irregularly nodular in outline. The more marked changes were found involving the right lobe. On section large areas of scar tissue were seen in which were embedded occasional small islands of liver tissue. There was an associated ascites of about three liters of bile-stained but otherwise clear fluid. All the viscera showed moderate bile pigmentation. The heart showed rather marked toxic degeneration and was acutely dilated. There was a diffuse bilateral basal broncho-pneumonia.

Microscopic Description of a Section through the Liver.—(Fig. 485 and 486) The outstanding feature of pathology histologically is seen to be a marked bile duct proliferation embedded in a mass of inflammatory fibrous tissue. The bile ducts appear in places to be attempting either to unite with islands of liver cells or to be differentiating into liver cells. It is difficult to determine this exact relationship. The liver cells which are present show hyperplasia for the most part with marked granular degeneration of their cytoplasm. The scar tissue is diffusely infiltrated with chronic inflammatory cells, lymphocytes for the most part, although many large mononuclear phagocytes and occasional plasma cells can be identified. There is no evidence of any actual bile duct infection but there is some bile stasis with some of the bile canaliculi distended with bilirubin. The picture as a whole is one of a healing or healed process with some persistence of a chronic inflammatory cellular reaction.

CHAPTER XLIX

DISEASES OF THE LIVER (*Continued*)

THE CIRRHOSES

Cirrhosis of the liver may be defined as a productive fibrosis, usually anatomical in distribution and progressive in nature, which may be produced by a variety of causes, many of them as yet undetermined. The tawny, yellow color, which the name implies, and which was originally used by Laennec to describe the condition, is frequently absent. The classification of the various forms of cirrhosis is obviously unsatisfactory because of our lack of knowledge regarding the numerous etiologic agents and the mechanism involved. On the other hand, the cirrhoses may be conveniently divided into several major types, which are fairly distinctive, both clinically and pathologically. In its simplest concept, the cirrhoses may be divided on an anatomical basis, into *central cirrhosis,* associated primarily with chronic passive congestion of long standing; *biliary cirrhosis* in which the fibrotic process develops in relation to obstruction or infection of the biliary tract; and *portal cirrhosis* in which the cirrhotic process arises initially in the portal areas but becomes a diffuse lesion with little regard for anatomical relationship. By such a classification, however, it is difficult to include some of the varieties which have less obvious anatomical relationships. Among these might well be cited hemochromatosis; syphilitic cirrhosis; tuberculous cirrhosis. and if we wish to include the healed picture of the subacute yellow atrophy, the so-called "toxic"

cirrhosis. Likewise, the condition known as Hanot's hypertrophic biliary cirrhosis becomes a problem from such an arrangement standpoint. It becomes apparent, therefore, that the classification of the cirrhoses is fraught with certain difficulties and dangers. It is perhaps more satisfactory for that reason to present them on the basis of their relative clinical pictures rather than on strictly anatomical grounds. With these thoughts in mind, no suggested nomenclature can be considered as anything more than a working plan until the etiologic basis can be demonstrated and established. The following outline of the cirrhoses is presented for convenience in their discussion:

1. Portal cirrhosis (Laennec's cirrhosis; atrophic cirrhosis; alcoholic cirrhosis; hobnail liver; diffuse nodular cirrhosis and chronic progressive cirrhosis; insular cirrhosis and certain instances of toxic cirrhosis).
2. Biliary cirrhosis (hypertrophic cirrhosis)
   a. Obstructive
   b. Infectious
   c. Hanot's primary hypertrophic biliary cirrhosis
3. Central cirrhosis
4. Pigment cirrhosis (Hemochromatosis)
5. Syphilitic cirrhosis
6. (?) Toxic cirrhosis (subacute yellow atrophy)

Portal Cirrhosis

When the term, cirrhosis, is used clinically, in nine times out of ten the clinician has in mind this particular condition known by the host of synonyms which have been suggested. To our minds, this is true cirrhosis in contradistinction to inflammatory lesions with simple fibrous tissue repair and scarring. Clinically, portal cirrhosis is a chronic progressive disease ending invariably fatally. It goes through at least two distinct phases, the first characterized by enlargement of the liver, with rather vague, indefi-

nite gastro-intestinal symptoms; and the second, a stage in which the liver becomes contracted and nodular, showing no interference with the bile flow, but resulting in portal obstruction and associated ascites. Frequently the development of esophageal and gastric varices may cause death through rupture and hemorrhage. There is usually a concomitant enlargement and fibrosis of the spleen terminally, and in the end stage, jaundice frequently supervenes. The disease is seen much more frequently in males

PLATE CXV

DISEASES OF THE LIVER (*Continued*)

PORTAL CIRRHOSIS (ATROPHIC, LAENNEC, ALCOHOLIC)

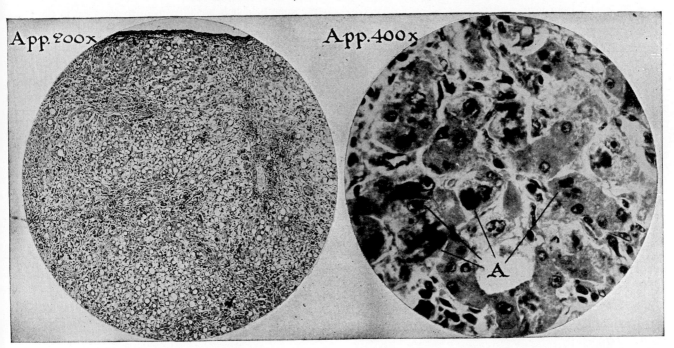

FIG. 487.—CASE 208.—Lower power photomicrograph in which widespread liver damage, with fatty metamorphosis is apparent. Note increased fibrosis with irregular distribution in respect to anatomical lobule.

FIG. 488.—CASE 208.—High power photomicrograph in which the details of the degenerative changes, especially the presence of intracytoplasmic hyaline masses (A) are better illustrated. (See also Fig. 482 in color.) App. 400 x.

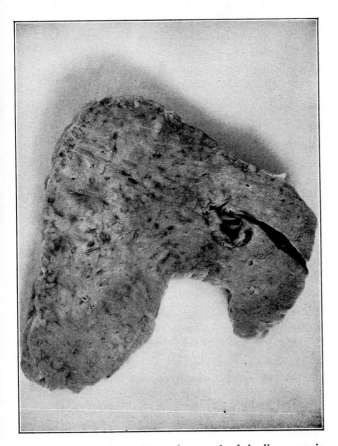

FIG. 489.—Cf. CASE 208.—Gross photograph of the liver seen in cross section, in which the irregular, yellowish islands of parenchymatous cells are outlined by fibrous tissue. Note "hobnail" surface laterally.

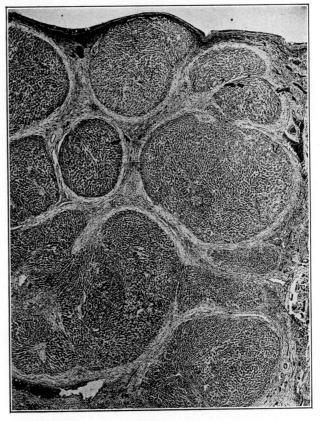

FIG. 490.—Cf. CASE 208.—Microtessar photograph of an advanced case of atrophic, portal cirrhosis, in which an insular arrangement of the liver parenchyma is observed, the result of diffuse fibrosis without regard to anatomical pattern, and the accompanying liver cell regeneration. App. 15 x.

than females. It occurs chiefly in the middle age group from forty to fifty.

At autopsy in these late cases, one usually finds a liver which is smaller than normal, frequently weighing less than 1,000 grams. Its surface is finely or coarsely nodular due to islands of regenerating liver tissue which are elevated above the contracted connective tissue. The liver is apt to be intensely bile stained as a result of the extensive damage to the liver cells. It is usually of a pale, tawny yellow color, and on section it cuts with marked resistance due to the increased connective tissue. The same nodular island arrangement of the cells, separated by bands of connective tissue, may be seen throughout the liver on section (Fig. 489).

Microscopically, the appearance of these cases of portal cirrhosis varies only in degree. The basic histology remains the same. Outstanding is a diffuse fibrosis which, as can be seen in the earlier cases, ordinarily starts with a typical portal distribution but which soon progresses to the point where it cuts the anatomical lobule in every direction and the normal lobular architecture becomes completely lost (Fig. 490). The disease being primarily one of liver cell damage, it is not associated with any noteworthy change in the bile duct apparatus, although occasionally the bile ducts seem to show some evidence of hyperplasia. Usually the prominence of the bile ducts is relative due to the loss of liver substance. The liver cells themselves show a curious degeneration which typically is preceded by marked fatty infiltration and fatty degeneration (Fig. 487). This is followed by the appearance of intensely eosin-staining hyaline droplets or fused masses within the cytoplasm of the liver cells (Fig. 481 and 488). Gradually the liver cells undergo disintegration and are removed by proteolysis and phagocytosis. Within the same field it is not infrequent to see, even in the late stage of the disease attempted regeneration on the part of these damaged liver cells, and mitotic figures are not infrequent. The disease might be likened to a battle in which the liver cell regeneration is attempting in vain to overcome the liver cell destruction as produced both by the basic toxic factor and by compression atrophy of the cells by fibrosis.

The etiology of this condition is completely obscure. Many of the cases being seen in association with chronic alcoholics, the disease acquired the reputation of being alcoholic in origin. It has been impossible by experimental means to reproduce the condition in animals by the use of even enormous amounts of alcohol over long periods of time. The part which alcohol *may* play in human cases is in the production of the initial fatty degenerative changes which ordinarily antedate the actual cirrhosis. The other chief group of agents which has been suspected as of etiologic significance has been the heavy metals. Lead, copper, phosphorus, and more recently arsenic have been incriminated to some extent experimentally. The experimental proof of the part they play is somewhat unsatisfactory because while a variable amount of cirrhosis may be produced in experimental animals by the use of these agents, with their withdrawal the liver regenerates, and the evidence of cirrhosis becomes lost. In human cases, the disease is a definite chronic progressive one, ending fatally. It must of necessity have a toxic etiologic factor, but what this agent is still remains unsettled. The pathological changes are very likely the result of a combination of causes including possibly digestive intestinal toxins, either bacterial or enzymic in nature.

ILLUSTRATIVE CASE

CASE 207. (Ref. #S-138)
Diagnosis.—Liver—portal cirrhosis.
Chief Complaint.—Patient was a white male of 41 years, admitted to the hospital for study.
Present Illness.—The onset of the patient's present illness was rather indefinite. He had had a history of intermittent attacks of arthritis of several years' duration. For a matter of six or more months he had noticed a progressive sense of fullness and heaviness in his upper abdomen. This had been accompanied by weakness and easy fatigability. He had had no very definite gastrointestinal symptoms otherwise. He had not had any nausea or vomiting. His bowel habits had been regular. His stools had been normally pigmented. He had not noticed any jaundice until about a week before admission when he first found his eyes were yellow.

Past Medical History.—The patient's past medical history was largely negative. He had the usual childhood diseases. He had had no more than the usual number of upper respiratory infections. The gastro-intestinal history was negative. He had had lues at the age of 17 and had had an intensive antiluetic course of treatment at that time.

Physical Examination.—Patient was a well developed, somewhat undernourished middle-aged white male. He was moderately dyspneic. He showed a generalized edema of the dependent parts most marked in his lower extremities. He showed a mild jaundice. His head was

PLATE CXVI

DISEASES OF THE LIVER (*Continued*)

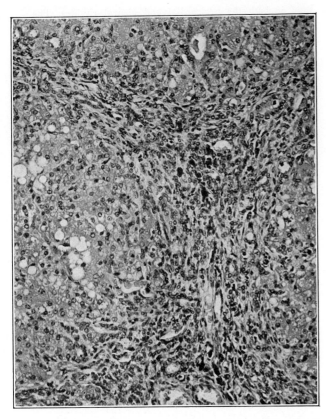

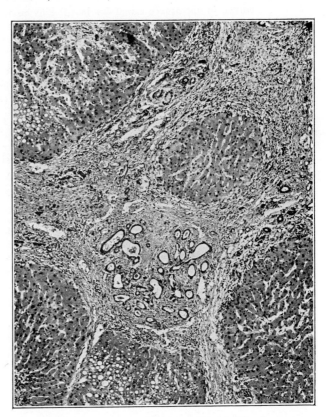

Fig. 491.—LIVER: CONGENITAL ATRESIA OF THE BILE DUCTS, WITH OBSTRUCTIVE BILIARY CIRRHOSIS AND BILE STASIS.—CASE 202.—The striking feature is the extreme bile duct proliferation. (Cf. colored Plate VIII, Fig. 36.) App. 200 x.

Fig. 492.—LIVER: BILIARY CIRRHOSIS, LATE.—Cf. CASE 209.—Marked periductile fibrosis, with some regenerative bile duct hyperplasia and diffuse monocytic cellular infiltration. Note fibrosis is anatomical in distribution extending from one portal area to another. App. 100 x.

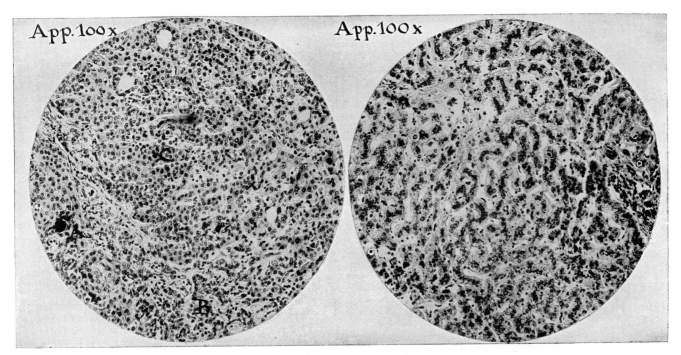

Fig. 493.—LIVER: BILIARY CIRRHOSIS, INFECTIOUS, EARLY.—CASE 209.—Note the beginning fibrosis around the bile ducts (B) and their obstruction, with marked bile stasis (A). Kupffer cells show considerable bile pigmentation. App. 100 x.

Fig. 494.—LIVER: HEMOCHROMATOSIS (PIGMENTARY CIRRHOSIS).— CASE 17.—Outstanding feature of histology is the pigmentation which is seen within the liver and Kupffer cells as well as deposited intra- and extracellularly in the areas of fibrosis. (See also Plate VIII, Figs. 33 and 34.) App. 100 x.

normal in appearance except for jaundice of his sclerae. His nose and throat were negative. His chest was symmetrical. His breathing was somewhat labored and a few râles were heard at both bases. His heart was not enlarged and showed no murmurs. His blood pressure was 140/90. His abdomen was distended. There was a definite fluid wave present. On standing he showed a prominence of his lower abdomen as the result of shifting of the fluid.

Laboratory Findings.—Red cells, 3,600,000, hemoglobin 72%; white cells, 6800 with 62% polynuclears. Urinalysis was negative except for the presence of a considerable amount of bile. Stools were almost clay-colored. Wassermann was negative.

Subsequent Course.—While in the hospital his condition steadily became worse. He had several abdominal paracenteses with the removal of a total of 14,000 c.c. of fluid. This was bile-stained but clear. He developed a double mitral and an aortic murmur which were thought to be the result of stretching of the valves through toxic myocardial changes accompanied by dilatation. His liver was enlarged as determined on examination after paracentesis. He went steadily downhill and died three weeks after admission.

Autopsy Findings.—A somewhat emaciated, middle-aged white male with moderate jaundice. The peritoneal cavity contained a moderate amount of free fluid. The liver was greatly enlarged, weighing 4,500 gm. It was greenish in color. There was a very slight granular appearance to the surface of the liver, which on section suggested a diffuse hyperplasia of the liver parenchyma which was embedded in the connective tissue stroma. There was some polyserositis with a small amount of

fluid in both the pericardial and pleural cavities. The heart showed evidence of chronic mitral, rheumatic endocarditis with numerous bead-like vegetations along the free edge of the posterior cusp. The other organs showed no significant changes. There was a moderate inflammatory reaction about the ampulla of Vater and the duodenum.

Microscopic Description of a Section of the Liver. —(Cf. Fig. 487 and 488) The tissue histology presents a moderate amount of confusion in differential diagnosis combining as it does several of the features of both major types of cirrhosis. There is a basic underlying picture of a typical portal "alcoholic" cirrhosis. This is evidenced by the toxic degeneration of the liver cells associated with marked fatty changes and the presence of hyaline masses within their cytoplasm. There is likewise evidence of liver cell regeneration which ordinarily accompanies this type of picture. The liver lobules are considerably distorted as the result of connective tissue proliferation. In fact there is a beginning arrangement of the regenerated hyperplastic liver tissue as a nodular type of cirrhosis.

To complete the picture there is, however, in addition, an unusually diffuse interstitial fibrosis which, while it has its origin obviously in the portal areas, tends to be associated with marked bile duct proliferation and evidence of biliary obstruction. This would suggest, therefore, the possibility of a combined type of cirrhosis, primarily of the portal type but with a superimposed chronic biliary cirrhosis as the result of secondary infection or possible inflammatory obstruction of the bile ducts. It is this not infrequently encountered complex picture which adds to the diagnostic confusion.

ILLUSTRATIVE CASE

CASE 208. (Ref. #S-228)

Diagnosis.—Liver: Portal cirrhosis—late—with hyaline degeneration.

Chief Complaint.—Patient was a white female, 43 years old, who was admitted to the hospital because of abdominal symptoms.

Present Illness.—The onset of the patient's present illness, she thought, began about nine months earlier with a cold, which persisted for three weeks. It was accompanied by a cough which had continued to the time of admission. About six months before admission, she began having attacks of vomiting. These had increased in frequency and severity. Two weeks before admission, patient felt as if something had "burst" within her, and, after a bowel movement, a large dark blood clot was passed. She developed a progressively increasing jaundice which began one month before admission, and the vomiting had been almost constant following the taking of food or liquids during this period.

Past Medical History.—Patient was a self-confessed chronic alcoholic, drinking about a pint of liquor a day for many years. With this she had had various gastrointestinal upsets, one of which had caused her to seek medical attention previously. She had no good recollection of her childhood in respect to any illness. She had never been operated upon. A review of her systems was essentially negative other than as indicated. She had been married and had had two children who died in childhood. Her husband had deserted her and she had been driven to earn her living as a scrubwoman.

Physical Examination.—Patient was an emaciated, drowsy-appearing, middle-aged woman who was aroused with some difficulty. There was very marked jaundice. Her pupils reacted sluggishly. Her heart and lungs appeared normal. The liver was somewhat enlarged and felt nodular. It was not tender. There was some distention of the abdomen and a definite fluid wave was present. The lower extremities showed moderate edema.

Laboratory Findings.—During her stay in the hospital, she showed a progressive secondary anemia with a gradual elevation of the white cells up to 20,000 with 80% polynuclears. Her urinalysis showed a slight trace of albumin and the presence of bile but was otherwise negative.

Subsequent Course.—She developed a marked ascites which required relief on several occasions by paracentesis. She continued to fail. Terminally she developed what appeared to be pneumonia of the left base and the immediate cause of her death, clinically, seemed to be this terminal bronchopneumonic process.

Autopsy Findings.—At autopsy the body was that of a well-developed emaciated middle-aged white woman. The abdominal cavity contained about 3,000 c.c. of lemon yellow fluid. The liver was unusually firm and somewhat enlarged. It weighed 2,075 grams. There was a fine nodular mottling of the surface on section. The gallbladder appeared essentially normal. The pericardium and pleural cavities both contained a moderate amount of clear, straw-colored fluid. The heart itself appeared normal. Lungs showed terminal edema and in the left lower lobe, there was an abscess 3.5 cm. in diameter. The kidneys showed bile staining and were somewhat edematous but otherwise negative.

Microscopical Description of a Section through the Liver.—(Fig. 481, 488, 490) Histologic examination of the tissue shows a very marked cirrhosis. At first glance it is difficult to identify the tissue as liver because scarcely any normal liver cells can be seen. Those which are demonstrable do not show any very regular lobular arrangement. There is extensive fatty degeneration and infiltration. There is marked toxic necrosis of many of the liver cells. There is a striking accumulation of hyaline droplets and masses within the cytoplasm of the liver cells around the periphery of the most markedly involved areas. The liver nuclei, however, as one looks through the section as a whole, are relatively little involved and except for the actual necrotic areas, the remainder of the liver cells appear viable. Indeed, in places attempts at regeneration may be made out with the presence of mitotic figures. The other outstanding feature of this picture is the development of a marked increase of connective tissue having its origin in the portal areas. This has progressed to the point where the liver lobules are badly cut up and difficult to identify. It represents a very marked example of the so-called "alcoholic" or portal cirrhosis.

BILIARY CIRRHOSIS

Obstructive and Infectious.—Biliary cirrhosis, in contrast to portal cirrhosis, is usually a condition occurring most frequently in children and young adults instead of in the middle age group. It is most frequently *obstructive* in nature, although this may be complicated by infection. Certain cases of congenital atresia of bile ducts seen in the newborn give evidence of this obstructive type of cirrhosis in which the bile is incapable of being excreted and an intense, progressive jaundice ensues (see Case 202; Ref. #S-336; Chapter XLVIII). This is associated with marked proliferation of the bile ducts and a diffuse fibrosis surrounding them, with resultant gradual atrophy of the liver cells from pressure. Just as in portal cirrhosis, liver cell regeneration goes hand in hand with the biliary tract damage.

In general, cases of biliary cirrhosis show an enlarged liver with a smooth surface which only late undergoes any notable nodulation and never develops the coarse hobnail appearance of portal cirrhosis. The somewhat artificial division of biliary cirrhosis into purely obstructive and purely infectious cases is justified by this congenital lesion just described. Milder cases of this type of lesion may be seen following obstruction of the biliary system by cancer of the head of the pancreas or the bile ducts themselves in the older age group. Most of the cases of biliary cirrhosis, however, are associated with infection of the bile ducts. This may be either hematogenous or ascending in nature. In the tropics where gastro-intestinal disease and parasitic infestation of the intestinal tract are common, this condition is very much more frequently seen than in this country. Cases may result from such bizarre conditions as the obstruction of the biliary tract by Ascaris worms (Fig. 209). Another instance of such biliary cirrhosis has been presented in Case 82 (Ref. #S-309)

in Chapter XXI, with *Clonorchis sinensis* infestation. Clinically, in contrast to portal cirrhosis, the outstanding features of biliary cirrhosis are the marked enlargement of the liver, and jaundice, usually of a progressive nature. Only exceptionally, and terminally does the complicating picture of portal obstruction and ascites develop. Likewise, only rarely does enlargement of the spleen accompany the development of biliary cirrhosis.

In contrast to the usually contracted liver of portal cirrhosis, the surface is smooth, the edges rounded, and the color is usually a deep greenish due to the marked retention of bile pigment. On section, a diffuse uniform anatomically distributed connective tissue framework can be recognized which follows closely the markings of the liver lobules.

Microscopically, this relationship is confirmed with persistence of the central veins and a variable amount of connective tissue outlining the liver lobule, arising from the periductile tissues of the portal area. Invariably, inflammatory cellular infiltration is seen in this connective tissue. This may be associated with actual infection of the bile ducts, or may only represent a diffuse chronic mononuclear infiltration. Specific instances of tuberculous cholangitis and resultant infectious biliary cirrhosis are found occasionally, but these represent a rather unusual distribution of the tuberculous infection. In no instance has the characteristic hyaline degeneration of the cytoplasm of the liver cells, so diagnostic when it is found in the portal form, been demonstrated in biliary cirrhosis.

Hanot's Cirrhosis.—This is a condition open to question as to its specificity. It was first described by Hanot as a condition in children in which there was a diffuse generalized fibrosis of the entire liver unlike the usual picture of periductile fibrosis seen in the usual type of biliary cirrhosis. A considerable question as to whether this may not represent a type of congenital syphilitic hepatitis, exists. The differential diagnosis of such a diffuse syphilitic cirrhosis from the so-called Hanot's cirrhosis might easily be dependent upon the finding of the spirochete. It is an interesting curiosity, both from the clinical and pathological standpoints.

ILLUSTRATIVE CASE

CASE 209. (Ref. #S-43)

Diagnosis—Liver—infectious biliary cirrhosis; bile stasis.

Chief Complaint.—Patient was a 23-year-old white woman, admitted to the hospital with a history of a progressive jaundice of one month's duration.

Present Illness.—Her present illness began about two months before admission with a severe gastro-intestinal upset accompanied by nausea, vomiting and followed by diarrhea. However, by going more carefully into the history, it appeared that the patient had had minor gastro-intestinal disturbances for the better part of two years. This was associated especially with the taking of foods high in fat content. She had had several attacks of nausea and vomiting but had not considered them as anything more than mild digestive disturbances from dietary indiscretion. With the onset of the present illness, however, she noticed that it was accompanied by a feeling of marked fullness in her epigastrium and she was under the impression that the size of her abdomen had actually increased. This was determined in relation to her clothing which she had difficulty in wearing. During the few days preceding her admission, she had had a slight temperature and noticed that her pulse was more rapid than usual. This was accompanied by considerable sweating. Her stools had become progressively more and more clay-colored and for the past few days been dry and crumbly in consistency and had been associated with marked constipation.

Past Medical History.—Patient gave no past history of apparent relationship to her present illness. She had an uneventful medical history as a child and a review of her systems was noninformatory. Her menstrual history was entirely negative. Her menses had begun at the age of thirteen and had been regular. She was married but had had no children.

Physical Examination.—Patient was a well-developed, well-nourished young, white female who showed a very intense jaundice. Her head otherwise was negative. Pupils were regular and reacted normally. Nose and throat were negative. Her chest was symmetrical. Her heart and lungs appeared within normal limits. Abdomen was moderately prominent. Her liver was easily palpable a full hand's breadth below the costal margin. No fluid could be demonstrated in the abdominal cavity.

Her spleen could not be felt. Her extremities were negative.

Laboratory Findings.—Blood count: red cells, 3,100,-000, hemoglobin 58%; white cells, 9,800 with 78% polynuclears. The urine was negative except for the presence of bile. The patient showed a direct van den Bergh and a high icteric index. Wassermann was negative.

Subsequent Course.—Patient progressively failed during her stay in the hospital of nearly a month. Jaundice became more and more intense as time went on and was not relieved by any therapy. She gradually lapsed into stupor and coma and died with a typical cholemia.

Autopsy Findings.—The body was that of a well-developed and fairly well-nourished young white woman, showing an intense jaundice. On opening the abdominal cavity there was a small amount of free fluid, bile-tinged in color. The liver was greatly enlarged, about 10 cm. below the costal margin. It weighed 2,850 gm. The capsule was smooth and tense. The liver, on section was seen to be intensely bile stained, having a greenish, discolored appearance. It cut with increased resistance, which suggested a diffuse fibrosis. The remainder of the autopsy findings were essentially negative, or did not bear upon the pathological picture.

Microscopical Description of a Section of the Liver.—(Fig. 493) Histologic examination of the liver shows a marked increase of connective tissue which appears as trabeculae from one portal area to another enclosing the liver tissue of each lobule in a semi-capsule. This increased connective tissue is seen to be periductile in distribution. There is some slight inflammatory cell infiltration noted around the ducts. There is marked evidence of bile stasis with some of the ducts and many of the bile canaliculi being distended with bile pigment. The cause of this obstruction was not noted at autopsy and would appear to be a simple inflammatory reaction of the hepatic duct system. The liver cells show varying degrees of toxic degeneration with cloudy swelling and fatty infiltration. There is none of the hyaline degeneration so characteristic of the alcoholic type of cirrhosis to be found in any of the liver cells. The lesion is definitely anatomical in its distribution and in this case appears to be a combination of infection and obstruction. There is an associated bile duct proliferation of a very marked grade.

CENTRAL CIRRHOSIS (CIRRHOSIS OF CONGESTION)

By this term is meant that curious anatomically uniform fibrotic process which is seen usually in association with long-standing chronic passive congestion. It is characterized by a productive fibrosis arising in the central portion of the liver lobule in relation to the long-standing circulatory changes and particularly following the necrosis of the cells around the central vein. It tends to be of a chronic progressive nature, but should probably best be considered as evidence of a disease of the circulatory system rather than a primary one affecting the liver. It was frequently spoken of by the older school of pathology as cirrhosis of "red atrophy." Essentially it represents a replacement fibrosis.

PIGMENT CIRRHOSIS

Hemochromatosis.—Hemochromatosis is the outstanding example of the so-called pigment cirrhosis. The disease is the result of some disturbance of iron metabolism and is not restricted to the liver. It is characterized as affecting the tissues rather generally, particularly the fibrous tissue of the liver, pancreas, heart and subcutaneous tissues. This results in the curious bronzing of the skin and the clinical picture of so-called "bronzed diabetes," as described in Case 17 (Ref. #S-204 and S-205), Chapter IV, Fig. 33, 34 and 494.

The histologic picture of the liver in hemochromatosis is similar to the picture as seen in typical portal cirrhosis, with the additional factor of the presence of the hematogenous pigment, chiefly hemosiderin and hemofuscin. In the typical case, the pigment is chiefly contained within the large mononuclear phagocytic cells, but due to the large amount is frequently found deposited in the interstitial connective tissue stroma as well. There is further evidence of the disturbed iron metabolism as shown by the presence of large amounts of hemosiderin within the liver cells. The lesion starts as a portal fibrosis and soon develops the characteristic nodular or insular picture seen in advanced portal cirrhosis with the anatomical lobules completely destroyed and replaced by nodes of regenerating liver cells. Unlike simple portal cirrhosis, hyaline degeneration is not observed.

The etiology of this condition is likewise obscure. Again, as in the case of portal cirrhosis, several of the heavy metals have been in part incriminated by experimental methods. The work of Mallory, who was able to reproduce the condition in sheep by the use of small amounts of copper, and more recently in rabbits by chronic phosphorus poisoning, is of interest and possible significance in this respect.

SYPHILITIC CIRRHOSIS

In congenital syphilis, as has been already brought out in the chapter devoted to a discussion of syphilitic disease, Chapter XV, the spirochetes are found in all the viscera. It is an inevitable histological sequence for productive fibrosis to follow. In the liver this results in moderate to marked enlargement of the organ which can be palpated clinically often well below the costal margin. Similar fibrotic enlargement of the spleen may also occur.

At autopsy the liver from such a case presents the picture of a diffuse fibrosis with scattered islands of liver cells which are valiantly attempting to carry on the various hepatic functions. Again, as in the case of subacute yellow atrophy, it does not seem to us that this represents a true cirrhotic process, but rather the productive inflammation and repair picture as seen in any chronic granulomatous type of infection. As such, it should perhaps better be termed "sclerosis" or "fibrosis," and limit the use of the term "cirrhosis" to the more characteristic chronic progressive type of lesion. As a part of the syphilitic picture must also be included those occasional instances of healed gummata. These are localized focal areas of scar tissue formation but are considered by some to fall into the group of cirrhoses, if the use of the word is applied to all productive fibrotic changes of the liver, as many authors seem to feel it should.

TOXIC CIRRHOSIS

The use of the term, "toxic cirrhosis," leads to a great deal of confusion. It applies to two distinct conditions from the clinical standpoint, healed subacute yellow atrophy and portal cirrhosis. That these two conditions may very possibly have a common etiologic factor at times is by no means improbable, but portal cirrhosis is a chronic progressive fatal disease, whereas subacute yellow atrophy, if the patient survives, represents a single incident with healing. The term is merely included in this discussion in the hope of clarifying what seems to us to be an unnecessary confusion.

TUMORS OF THE LIVER

The tumors of the liver have been discussed in the general section of tumors, particularly in Chapter XXXV. The primary tumors of the liver may be divided into two major types; those tumors arising from the liver cells (primary liver cell type); hepatomata, and those arising from the bile duct epithelium, cholangiomata.

Hepatomata.—Of those arising from the liver cells, their general behavior suggests that such tumors may occur both in a benign and a malignant form, although by far the greater number show evidence of malignancy sooner or later. These tumors, as has already been emphasized, may be single or multiple. When they occur as multiple lesions, it is generally held that the condition is one of generalized malignant change in the liver tissue as a whole with multicentric foci of tumor formation rather than the lesions representing metastatic extensions from a primary focus.

Cholangiomata.—The bile duct epithelial type of tumor may occur as a primary lesion within the liver substance from the duct epithelium anywhere. More often, however, the bile duct epithelial type of tumor is found arising in the gallbladder or common duct and extending both by direct invasion and by metastasis along the portal lymphatics to the liver proper. These tumors, likewise, may exist as benign lesions but similarly tend to undergo malignant change relatively early.

Angiomata.—Of the other tumors which are found within the liver, the great majority are metastatic with the exception of the congenital cavernoma. As has already been emphasized, the cavernoma should perhaps better be considered as a developmental anomaly rather than as a true tumor as it ordinarily shows no evidence of increase in size or appearance throughout the life of the individual and is usually found incidentally surgically or at autopsy. Rare instances of primary malignant tumors arising from the vascular endothelium as angiosarcomata have been recorded similar to those occasionally found in the spleen.

Metastatic Tumors.—Metastatic tumors which are commonly found in the liver originate particularly in carcinoma of the stomach, pancreas and lower gastro-intestinal tract, but may have the primary lesion anywhere in the body when blood stream metastases occur. The gastric and pancreatic type of metastases are usually of direct lymphatic extension by contrast to the other blood-borne embolic lesions developing from tumor cells which start new foci of tumor wherever they become implanted.

For illustrative cases refer to Case 151 (Ref. #S-238), Chapter XXXV, page 372, as a case of cholangioma malignum, also Fig. 495; Case 150 (Ref. #S-192 and S-117), Chapter XXXV, page 370, and Fig. 343 as an example of a malignant hepatoma, also Fig. 496.

CHAPTER L

DISEASES OF THE GALLBLADDER

Diseases of the gallbladder make up such a very important group of cases clinically that a rather full discussion of their nature seems warranted. The gallbladder itself is derived embryologically from an outgrowth of the intestinal entoderm as part of the biliary system. Its major function apparently is to act as a storage reservoir for bile during the periods between digestive activity. This is effected through a very delicately balanced mechanism depending upon relative contraction of the sphincter of Oddi and relaxation of the gallbladder itself. This would not in itself be adequate perhaps if it were not for the fact that the mucosa lining the gallbladder is an active physiological agent which is capable of concentrating the bile through absorption of water. Following the ingestion of food the sphincter of Oddi becomes relaxed both through chemical and neurogenic stimulation and bile is expressed from the gallbladder to aid in the digestive processes. That this is a function of the gallbladder is seen by the dilatation of the bile ducts following the removal of the gallbladder surgically, in an attempt to reproduce the storage capacity of the gallbladder itself.

Inflammation of the gallbladder as acute or chronic cholecystitis with or without the production of gall stones represents the most important lesion affecting this organ. Inasmuch as gall stone production is such a prominent factor in the development of the inflammatory lesions of the gallbladder, its consideration will be taken up first.

Cholelithiasis
(Biliary Calculi; Gall Stones)

The underlying etiology of gall stone formation is to a considerable extent theoretical. There are three factors which are thought to be the most important in connection with their formation: (1) Stagnation of bile is emphasized by many investigators as the most important factor; (2) a high concentration of cholesterol in the bile is likewise significant. One of the principal functions of the gallbladder mucosa, as has already been mentioned, is the concentration of the bile. If excess cholesterol is present in this bile, it is obvious that its precipitation may readily occur as the concentration of the bile produces a super-saturated state. (3) Infection is usually stressed as probably the most important single factor. Infection may be caused in the gallbladder by any of the bacteria, but the *Streptococcus,* the *Bacillus coli,* the *Bacillus typhosus* and the *Staphylococcus* are the most frequently encountered organisms. The infection may reach the gallbladder first, by the blood stream; second by the lymphatics and third, by ascending infection of the bile ducts. There are three major types of gall stones found pathologically which correspond in a general way to the three causative factors involved in calculus formation and described above:

Pigment Stones.—These are very small, soft, greenish-black stones which usually occur in large numbers and are made up of concentrated bile pigment (bilirubin). With obstruction of the common duct they may even form within the bile ducts of the liver from stagnation and concentration of the bile.

Cholesterol Stones.—These stones are usually large, oval in shape, pale yellowish-white in color, and on section seem to be composed of radially arranged, stellate cholesterol crystals. They are found about three times as often in diabetics as in other individuals; and also frequently following pregnancy, both of which states are usually associated with a hypercholesterolemia. The incidence is much greater in women than in men.

Mixed Stones.—These are stones composed of a mixture of bilirubin, cholesterol and calcium, laid down usually in concentric, alternated laminae. They may be single, but are more often multiple. When multiple they may show faceted surfaces in appo-

PLATE CXVII

DISEASES OF THE LIVER AND GALL BLADDER

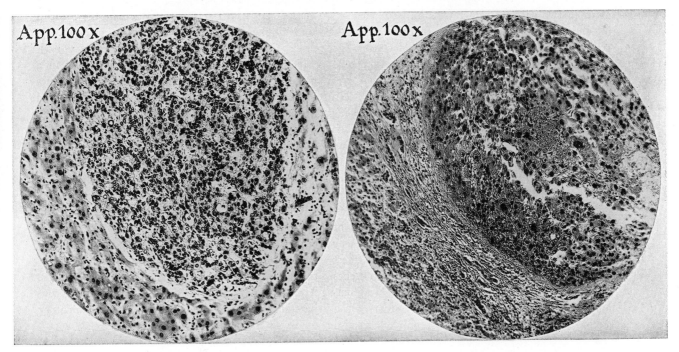

FIG. 495.—LIVER: CHOLANGIOMA MALIGNUM.—CASE 151.—Low power photomicrograph showing an area of the tumor invading the liver parenchyma and composed of cells somewhat resembling bile duct epithelium in morphology and arrangement. Occasional mitotic figures are seen. App. 100 x.

FIG. 496.—LIVER: HEPATOMA MALIGNUM.—CASE 150.—Low power photomicrograph from a nodule of a multicentric primary malignant liver cell tumor. Note large and irregular size of tumor cells; also the associated cirrhosis. App. 100 x.

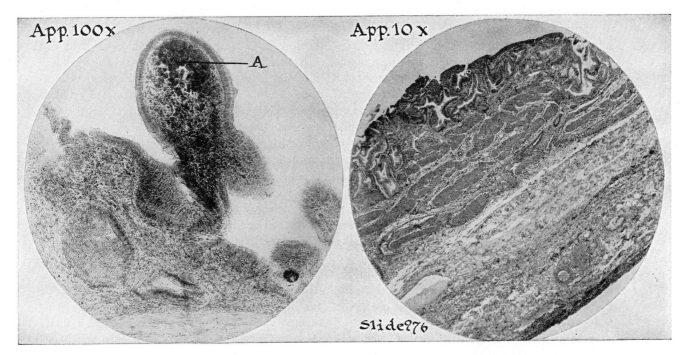

FIG. 497.—GALLBLADDER: CHOLESTEROLOSIS ("STRAWBERRY" GALL-BLADDER).—CASE 211.—Photomicrograph showing one of the papillae of the gallbladder mucosa, the tunica propria of which contains numerous lipoid-laden mononuclear phagocytic cells (Scharlach R stain). App. 100 x.

FIG. 498.—GALLBLADDER: CHRONIC CHOLECYSTITIS.—CASE 210.—Wall of gallbladder markedly thickened due to chronic productive fibrosis, especially of subserosa. Note glandular hyperplasia with beginning erosion and diffuse inflammatory cellular infiltration of hyper-trophied muscular coat. App. 10 x.

sition to one another from pressure, and may also occur in two or three rather uniform sizes, suggesting an inflammatory origin at different times, roughly corresponding to clinical attacks of cholecystitis. On section they are apt to show a central core composed of cellular debris and bacteria, and if the cholesterol is dissolved, a skeleton of coagulated protein is seen to persist, indicative of the exudative nature of the medium in which they developed. Pressure of such stones may produce ulceration and even perforation into the peritoneal cavity or into the duodenum as a choleduodenal fistula.

This very brief presentation gives some indication of the general types which are found in gall stones. The relative importance of the various factors of stagnation, concentration and infection obviously vary extensively in individual cases. It is of interest to note that clinically patients may have gall stones for many, many years without any clinical symptomatology. These are spoken of as silent stones. Such stones are very commonly almost pure cholesterol

in composition. They are apt to occur as a single large stone, which at times may assume the form of the gallbladder itself as a pear-like calculus. At other times, two or three such stones may exist which become faceted, and again together form a cast of the gallbladder cavity. These large stones are particularly commonly seen in the diabetic and because of their size rarely get into the cystic or common duct to produce obstruction with resultant biliary colic, jaundice or infection. Owing to their cholesterol content they may even be difficult to demonstrate roentgenologically and are frequently found only incidentally at autopsy.

On the other hand, small stones which are apt to occur in multiple form may readily get into the biliary tree and produce complete or incomplete obstruction, ulceration of the mucosa, secondary infection, and the picture of acute or chronic cholecystitis. More will be said of this side of the picture in conjunction with the discussion of the inflammatory lesions of the gallbladder.

Cholecystitis

By the term, cholecystitis, is meant an inflammation of the gallbladder. This may be acute or chronic in nature. It may be infectious or non-infectious. The infection may be hematogenous, lymphogenous or contiguous in origin. In a very large percentage of cases of cholecystitis, cholelithiasis exists concomitantly and may play an important part in the development of the clinical picture. The persistence of biliary calculi within the gallbladder cavity tends to complete the inflammatory process, however, as a true chronic inflammation. This is in contrast to the usual type of acute infection such as one sees in appendicitis where the infection is overcome after its initial onslaught and healing by fibrosis and scar formation takes place.

The typical history of the chronic gallbladder patient, who is in a large percentage of the cases a woman in her late forties or fifties, just past the menopausal period, and usually obese, is one of recurrent attacks of vague gastro-intestinal disturbances with some local tenderness over the gallbladder area as a rule. In many instances, the picture simulates that of chronic peptic ulcer or other forms of gastro-intestinal pathology, and particularly, in the absence of jaundice makes the diagnosis the more difficult.

Acute Cholecystitis.—The acute form of cholecystitis, as such, is much less commonly encountered clinically than the recurrent acute exacerbation of chronic gallbladder disease. It is associated in the great majority of instances with impaction of a stone in the neck of the gallbladder or the cystic duct, and is followed by an ulcerative mucositis with secondary infection localizing in the ulcerated area at the outset, but spreading through the wall of the gallbladder rapidly. Grossly such a gallbladder shows a moderate increase in size. The wall is edematous and thickened. The serosa shows acute inflammatory changes, often with actual fibrinous deposition. Under the microscope, dilated capillaries are seen in this area with a typical perivascular leukocytic infiltration such as has been seen already in acute appendicitis and similar acute inflammatory lesions. The fibrinous exudate is of particular significance in this connection because of the tendency for fibrous adhesions to form in the organization of this exudate. The mucosal surface shows ulceration ranging all the way up to actual gangrenous necrosis. The gallbladder may become filled with a purulent exudate made up of pus cells for the most part, which undergo liquefaction necrosis with the development of the so-called *empyema* of the gall bladder. At times this process may become so marked that actual rupture of the gallbladder may occur with the development of secondary peritonitis.

Surgically, opinions vary considerably as to the best method of treatment during this acute stage. The general consensus of opinion to-day is to be relatively conservative as most such acute attacks subside spontaneously within a few days which makes the surgical approach somewhat safer. On the other hand, in the more severe cases, again conservative drainage of the gallbladder rather than its immediate removal is recommended by the majority of surgeons.

Chronic Cholecystitis.—This condition represents the most commonly encountered condition of the gallbladder. The disease may follow an acute attack of cholecystitis. More often the process starts as a mild hematogenous infection of the outer wall which gradually extends to involve the mucosa. The picture is variable, depending on the presence of stones and the development of obstruction to the cystic or common ducts to a very considerable extent. Infection plays an extremely important part in the picture ordinarily, but it is entirely possible for a chronic cholecystitis to develop without infection as a result of simple incomplete obstruction of the cystic duct because of adhesions or stone, which acts in a somewhat valve fashion.

HYDROPS.—If obstruction of the cystic duct is complete, the gallbladder distends with clear fluid secreted by the lining epithelium. The bile pigment is absorbed; and, no more bile entering the gallbladder through the cystic duct, and no fluid escaping, enormous dilatation may result. This is spoken of as *hydrops.*

It brings up the interesting consideration of the functional activity of the bile duct epithelium. We have already seen that the bile duct is capable of absorbing water, producing concentration of bile under normal conditions. When obstruction occurs there appears to develop a safety-valve sort of mechanism whereby the mucosa is activated to absorb the bile pigment from the bile so that it will not be lost to the body, returning it apparently by way of the circulation. Similarly, this process results in a reversal of its activity, in this instance the cells secret-

ing a clear, watery fluid instead of absorbing this material from the bile.

In the ordinary case of chronic cholecystitis, which usually is not associated with complete obstruction of the duct system, the muscle fibers in the gallbladder wall show a striking hypertrophy in a functional attempt to overcome the obstruction and force the bile down the biliary tree into the duodenum where it can take part in the digestive process. Similarly, the connective tissue of the subperitoneal layer increases in thickness again as a protective mechanism, probably to prevent rupture. Not only is this subperitoneal layer involved, but there develops a diffuse interstitial fibrosis of the entire wall, including the muscular layer and the submucosa. Cellular infiltration follows. This varies greatly in its composition depending upon the severity and nature of the inflammatory process. It is usually particularly prominent in the subserosal layer. It consists usually of a mononuclear reaction with histiocytes, occasional plasma cells and lymphocytes. These latter predominate and may even form lymph follicles with germinal centers. The submucosa varies a great deal in its appearance. It is not at all uncommon to find a polypoid hyperplasia of the entire lining mucosa. Under the microscope this appears as a diffuse hyperplastic picture with increase in both numbers and size of the cells. At times, this is so marked as to almost suggest neoplastic adenomatous formation. More often, and particularly in conjunction with stone formation, chronic indolent ulcers are found involving the mucosal surface and the entire mucosal lining becomes eroded with a loss of the mucous membrane and its replacement by what might be termed a chronic granulation tissue.

As has been mentioned earlier, the picture of chronic cholecystitis is apt to be complicated by recurrent acute or subacute exacerbations in which one finds evidence pathologically of the underlying chronic inflammatory process with its productive fibrosis and mononuclear cellular reaction, but complicated by an acute and often ulcerative picture associated with hemorrhage and leukocytic infiltration. No two cases of cholecystitis are identical, but they tend to follow one or another of these patterns which have been indicated.

ILLUSTRATIVE CASE

CASE 210. (Ref. #S-276)

Diagnosis.—Chronic cholecystitis and cholelithiasis.

Chief Complaint.—Patient was a white woman of 34 years, who was admitted to the hospital because of severe colic-like pain in the abdomen.

Present Illness.—Onset dated back approximately one year. This had been accompanied by intermittent attacks of this same colic-like pain which had become progressive in severity during each successive attack. The most recent of these had been about two weeks before admission. By careful restriction of her diet, the pain had moderated but still persisted in the right upper quadrant and tended to radiate to the scapular region. The patient complained of associated flatulence and gaseous eructation.

Past Medical History.—Patient had had an uneventful medical history up to the onset of her present symptoms. She had been through all the childhood diseases including scarlatina. A review of her systems yielded very little additional information. She had had an insignificant upper respiratory tract infectious history. Her gastrointestinal symptoms had largely been those of an occasional attack of qualitative dyspepsia and associated constipation. Genito-urinary history was negative. Catamenic history was likewise normal. She was married and had had three normal pregnancies.

Physical Examination.—Patient was a well-developed, overweight, young, white female. Head was negative. There was a suggestion of an icteric tinge to her sclerae but no definite jaundice of her skin could be noted. Nose and throat were negative. Her chest was symmetrical. Heart was negative; lungs were clear. Abdomen was moderately prominent. There was a definite feeling of tenderness and pain on palpation in the upper right quadrant. Depression of the abdominal wall over this area caused this pain to radiate to the scapula on the right. Extremities were negative.

Laboratory Findings.—The red cell count was 3,800,-000 and hemoglobin, 72%; white cells, 8,300 with 71% polynuclears. Urinalysis was negative. Stools were bile stained. Icterus index was normal, van den Bergh was negative. X-ray examination showed the presence of gall stones.

Subsequent Course.—A diagnosis of cholecystitis was made and the patient was advised to have her gallbladder removed. She made an uneventful recovery and was discharged two weeks postoperatively.

Pathological Report.—Specimen consisted of a gallbladder measuring 4.5 x 2.6 x 0.5 cm. It contained seven faceted cholesterol appearing stones measuring each approximately 0.5 cm. in size. The serosal surface was thickened but smooth. The entire wall appeared thickened on section and the mucosa showed several areas of hemorrhagic ulceration.

Microscopic Description of a Section from the Gallbladder Wall.—(Fig. 498) Histologic examination of the tissue shows evidence of a definite chronic cholecystitis. This is characterized by marked thickening of the entire wall with the more marked inflammatory changes being noted in the adventitial portion of the organ. There is marked fibrosis of the subserosa with considerable cellular infiltration. The musculature shows marked hypertrophy and interstitial fibrosis. The submucosa is thickened and shows likewise considerable fibrosis. The mucosa is hyperplastic and shows marked papillary proliferation. The sections show the mucosa of one of the ulcerated areas to be missing and the ulcerated surface is covered by a fibrinous exudate.

Cholesterolosis
("Strawberry" Gallbladder)

Cholesterolosis of the gallbladder is a form of chronic cholecystitis which is very commonly associated with the picture of hypercholesterolemia and is seen particularly in the younger age group, and especially during or following pregnancy and in diabetes. It acquired its name, "strawberry" gallbladder, from the yellowish cholesterol deposits in each papilla of the mucosa, which simulate grossly the appearance of the seeds of the strawberry as seen against the red pulp of the fruit. It apparently develops as the result of or in association with some lipoid metabolic disturbance. It results in a mild inflammatory thickening of the gallbladder wall. Slight hypertrophy of the muscle bundles is frequently seen. A very mild mononuclear inflammatory reaction is usually present, particularly in the submucosa. The outstanding feature histologically is the presence of hypertrophied villi, which appear in section as pedunculated lesions. The stalk of the villus has a narrow pedicle at its base and expands above this narrowed area as the result of diffuse mononuclear cellular infiltration. Within the cytoplasm of these large mononuclear cells are found droplets of lipoid material. In frozen section this stains typically with the fat soluble dyes such as Scharlach R. In the usual hematoxylin and eosin stained preparation, the lipoid material has become dissolved and only vacuoles remain. With polarized light in unfixed tissue it is found that this lipoid substance is very largely composed of cholesterol. From the pedunculated nature of these lesions it is obvious how the enlarged portion may easily break off and serve as a nidus for the further deposition of cholesterol and the development of typical cholesterol stones. This is one explanation for the existence of this particular type of stone.

The symptoms associated with this condition are, as a rule, vague and indefinite; those usually of a mild chronic gastro-intestinal, qualitative dyspepsia. The treatment by surgery seems warranted, by the resultant loss of symptoms in the great majority of cases.

ILLUSTRATIVE CASE

CASE 211. (Ref. #S-179)

Diagnosis.—Cholesterosis of gallbladder.

Chief Complaint.—Patient was a white female of 45 years, admitted to the hospital because of epigastric pain.

Present Illness.—Her symptoms began with a sudden onset following a rather indiscreet dietary lapse about two weeks before admission. She was seized with severe epigastric pain which radiated to the right scapula and produced a burning sensation in her back. This was severe enough to require morphine for relief. It was accompanied by nausea, but no vomiting. Shortly after the onset of this pain, the patient developed jaundice. This lasted for several days and then disappeared gradually. Since that time, the pain had been constant, but not as acute as in the initial phase. The diagnosis of "cholecystitis" was made by her surgeon who referred her to the hospital for operation.

Past Medical History.—Patient had the usual childhood infections. She had no recollection of ever having had rheumatic fever. A review of her systems revealed very little of diagnostic help in respect to her present illness. She had had the usual mild upper respiratory infections. Her gastro-intestinal history, as a whole, had been fairly negative with occasional mild qualitative dyspeptic attacks and a rather marked constipation. Her menstrual history was negative. It began at the age of twelve and had been regular throughout her life. She was married and had had four normal pregnancies. She never had had any illness severe enough to require hospitalization previously.

Physical Examination.—Patient was a well developed somewhat obese middle-aged white female. Her head was negative. There was no evidence of jaundice. Nose and throat were negative. Chest was symmetrical. Heart and lungs seemed within normal limits. Abdomen was difficult to palpate because of the obesity but the liver did not seem to be enlarged. No definite masses could be made out. There seemed to be some slight tenderness associated with muscle spasm most marked in the right upper quadrant. Gynecological examination was essentially negative. The extremities were normal.

Laboratory Findings.—Blood count, red cells, 4,100,-000, 78% hemoglobin; white cells, 8,700 with 68% polynuclears. Urinalysis was negative except for a trace of bile. Stools were normal. Wassermann was negative. Blood chemistry was normal.

Subsequent Course.—Patient was operated upon with the diagnosis of chronic cholecystitis and the gallbladder removed. She made an uneventful recovery and was discharged ten days postoperatively.

Pathological Report.—Specimen consisted of a gallbladder measuring 6 x 2.5 cm. When opened, the serosa was intensely congested and the wall showed moderate papillary thickening. Each of the villous tips were flecked with yellow. No stones were submitted with the specimen. The picture grossly suggested that of chronic cholesterolosis of the gallbladder.

Microscopic Description of a Section of the Gall-Bladder Wall.—(Fig. 497). Histologic examination of the tissue shows a somewhat thickened gallbladder wall. The thickening appears chiefly in the adventitia where there is some increase of connective tissue accompanied by some mononuclear inflammatory cellular infiltration. The musculature is moderately hypertrophied and there is some interstitial fibrosis. The submucosa likewise is thickened and intensely injected as evidenced by the dilated capillaries. There is a moderate papillary hyperplasia of the lining mucosa. Each papilla is found to contain a variable number of large mononuclear cells, each filled with vacuoles representing lipoid material. Some of this is found free in the tissue spaces as well, where the cells have broken down and liberated their lipoid contents. Frozen section examination of this tissue stained with Scharlach-R confirms the lipoid character of the intracellular material.

A word regarding the newer methods of diagnosis of gallbladder disease is perhaps not out of place at this point. Cholecystography is the term applied to the visualization of the gallbladder by x-ray following the administration of a drug, tetraiodophenolphthalein, which is carried in the bile to the gallbladder. Upon the ability of the normal gallbladder mucosa to concentrate bile depends the success of this method. Under normal circumstances, the gallbladder is well outlined as the result of the concentration of the opaque dye. When gallbladder function is interfered with, then the inability of the mucosa to concentrate the dye results in the failure to outline the organ. The presence of stones is likewise frequently noted, even although they are non-opaque, through the differences in density of the shadow of the dye in the gallbladder as it overlies the stone.

Tumors of the Gallbladder

The tumors of the gallbladder have already been described in conjunction with the tumors arising from the bile duct epithelium as seen in the liver. It is possible to have the formation of polyps within the gallbladder. From the gallbladder mucosa, benign adenomata may occur on occasion. The typical neoplasm of the gallbladder, however, is the true carcinoma, which arising from the high columnar epithelium produces a striking adenocarcinomatous picture. In rare instances, the tumors may undergo squamous metaplasia and appear as highly malignant epidermoid carcinomata.

CHAPTER LI

DISEASES OF THE PANCREAS

Congenital Lesions

The pancreas embryologically develops normally as two entodermal buds—the dorsal portion from the wall of the intestine; the ventral portion from the common bile duct at or near the ampulla. These more or less intimately fuse to form the adult single gland. Anomalies in the usual rotation to the left result in annular glands surrounding the gut. Anomalies in the point of origin give rise to aberrant pancreatic tissue at any point along the entire gastrointestinal tract. The dorsal pancreas makes up the major part of the normal gland including the entire tail and body and the dorsal portion of the head. The ventral pancreas gives rise only to the ventral portion of the head. Each of these retains its own duct, the main dorsal pancreatic duct being called the duct of Wirsung; and the accessory ventral duct being known as the duct of Santorini. These may fuse or open separately into the duodenum. These epithelial outgrowths branch to form the pancreatic

acini and also send out cords of cells which differentiate into the islands of Langerhans. In injuries of the pancreas this same indiscriminate capacity of the duct cells to differentiate either as acinar or island cells is seen, but it is doubtful if there is ever any transition from acinar epithelium to island epithelium or vice versa.

Aside from the congenital anomalies, there are only four major lesions which might be cited as of particular significance in respect to pancreatic pathology. There are no major circulatory lesions of importance. The degenerative and infiltrative changes which occur in the pancreas are seen in association with these more or less major lesions, which will be discussed individually. Two of these are perhaps best included, under our plan of presentation, as inflammatory in nature; the third might be thought of as a toxic or metabolic lesion; and the fourth covering the neoplastic picture as seen in the pancreas.

Acute Hemorrhagic Pancreatitis

This lesion has been described previously in our consideration of the various forms of necrosis in Chapter VII (Case 27, Ref. #S-73 and S-78). The disease is an acute one with a sudden onset characterized by severe abdominal pain. This may or may not be associated with other gastro-intestinal symptoms such as nausea or vomiting. The condition usually is rapidly progressive with the patient passing into shock and coma, and dying within a comparatively short time, rarely more than forty-eight hours after the onset.

The etiology is somewhat obscure. It is believed that a very considerable number of cases is associated with the backing up of the bile into the pancreatic duct as a result of obstruction to the ampulla of Vater. It is possible to reproduce the picture experimentally in animals by this method as Opie has so convincingly shown. On the other hand, there are many cases of acute hemorrhagic pancreatitis in

which this obstruction of the ampulla cannot be demonstrated. These are more difficult of explanation. Rich and Duff have attempted to show that the essential lesion was vascular in nature with necrosis of the vessel wall as the initial lesion. This was followed by tissue necrosis permitting the digestive enzymes to escape by rupture of the acini. In the presence of such tissue changes activation of the enzymes could be accomplished without the intervention of bile. The mechanism is still best explained by the following sequence of events: with the backing up of the bile into the pancreatic duct, the pancreatic proteolase and lipase are activated so that autolysis of the gland and duct cells follows. Depending upon the extent of the necrosis and whether or not erosion of blood vessels takes place, we may or may not find an associated extensive hemorrhage into the pancreatic substance. The pancreatic enzymes tend to spread locally into the retroperitoneal

PLATE CXVIII
DISEASES OF THE PANCREAS

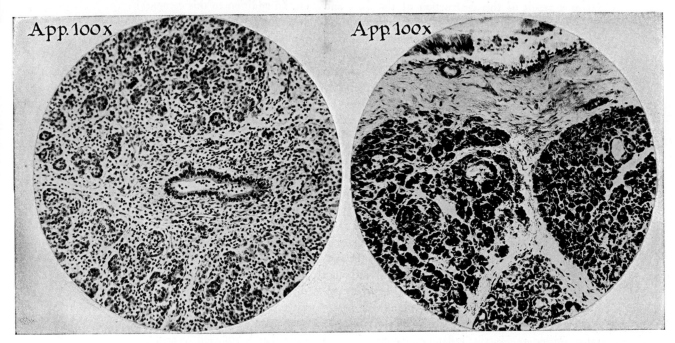

FIG. 499.—PANCREAS: ACUTE INTERSTITIAL PANCREATITIS.—CASE 212.—Greatly distorted histological picture as a result of a diffuse interstitial exudate in which polynuclear cells predominate. App. 100 x.

FIG. 500.—PANCREAS: DIABETES.—CASE 213.—Low photomicrograph to show the extensive interstitial and periductile fibrosis. App. 100 x.

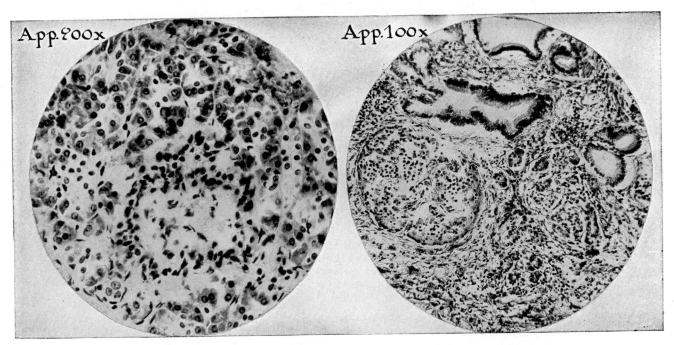

FIG. 501.—PANCREAS: DIABETES.—CASE 213.—High power photomicrograph of one of the islands of Langerhans showing atrophy as the result of extensive hyaline infiltration. App. 200 x.

FIG. 502.—PANCREAS: ADENOCARCINOMA (DUCT TYPE).—Photomicrograph with little recognizable pancreatic tissue persisting (see hyperplastic island of Langerhans at left) due to diffuse infiltration of parenchyma by a carcinoma arising from the duct epithelium. App. 100 x.

fat as a result of this destruction of the duct and acinar epithelial lining. They often may even spread over the peritoneal surface and omentum, producing focal areas of fat necrosis. As the digestive autolytic process extends, inevitably the hemorrhagic picture follows as blood vessels become involved in the proc-

ess. In addition to this comparatively simple process, with autolytic necrosis of the tissues not infrequently the picture may be complicated clinically and pathologically by an added factor of infection. The commonest organisms under such circumstances are the *Streptococcus* and *Bacillus coli.*

Interstitial Pancreatitis

Occasionally we may find evidence of an acute interstitial pancreatitis. This is not unlike the acute lesion seen in the liver as an acute interstitial hepatitis, or in the parotid as an acute interstitial parotitis. It is characterized as a periductile inflammation and usually represents an ascending infection from the excretory end of the duct. When this occurs in the parotid or submaxillary salivary glands, the condition is commonly spoken of as "mumps," although at times, such interstitial parotitis may be of a nonspecific type just as in these other glandular organs under discussion. In the case of the pancreas, the same diffuse periductile inflammatory reaction occurs. This may result from ascending infection along the duct or as in the case of gallbladder disease may have a lymphogenous or hematogenous origin.

Histologically, the ducts are usually filled with mucopurulent exudate. The process tends to spread from around ducts out into the interacinar connective tissue supportive stroma which likewise becomes diffusely infiltrated by inflammatory cells. At the outset, the inflammatory reaction tends to be polynuclear, and focal areas of necrosis are by no means uncommon. As the process heals, the cellular picture becomes mononuclear, characterized by a diffuse, chronic interstitial fibrosis and scar formation. The diagnosis is rarely made definitely clinically as the picture is one of rather indefinite gastro-intestinal symptomatology and difficult to recognize. If the condition is sufficiently acute, it may go on to the development of an acute hemorrhagic pancreatitis, Case 27, Chapter VII. More often, the result is healing of the lesion, which is only found incidentally at autopsy.

ILLUSTRATIVE CASE

CASE 212. (Ref. #S-281)
Diagnosis.—Pancreas—Interstitial pancreatitis.
Chief Complaint.—Patient was a female, nine months old, admitted to the hospital for study.
Present Illness.—One week before admission she developed a sore throat and an upper respiratory infection. This was treated with temporary improvement. The day before admission, her temperature rose sharply and she started vomiting. This became projectile in type and increased in frequency.
Past Medical History.—Patient was a full term normally delivered child who had been breast-fed during the first six months of her life. She had been on a bottle since that time but had had no difficulty until the onset of the present illness.
Physical Examination.—On admission the child was desperately ill and toxic. Her temperature was 105°. Her heart rate was 200. There was marked cyanosis. Respirations were rapid and shallow with a marked expiratory grunt. Examination of the chest revealed a limited expansion with harsh breath sounds throughout, but no impairment of resonance. No râles were heard. The heart was rapid and its sounds were of poor quality. The abdomen was of a peculiar doughy consistency with flatness throughout on percussion but no fluid wave could be demonstrated. The liver was slightly enlarged. Peristalsis was absent. A tentative diagnosis of upper respiratory infection with bronchopneumonia and fulmi-

nating septicemia was made. The question of a secondary peritonitis also was considered.
Laboratory Examination.—Red blood cells, 4,600,000 with 81% hemoglobin. White cells numbered 28,600, with 92% polynuclears. Urinalysis showed a large trace of albumin and occasional red cells. Blood cultures showed the presence of a hemolytic streptococcus.
Subsequent Course.—Patient went rapidly downhill and died twenty-four hours after admission.
Autopsy Findings.—The body was that of a well-developed, well nourished, but dehydrated, female child. The peritoneal cavity was filled with slightly turbid, straw-colored fluid. The liver showed moderate enlargement and toxic cloudy swelling. The spleen presented a picture of toxic splenitis. The pancreas seemed somewhat thickened. The heart was negative. The lungs showed definite evidence of consolidation and were moderately congested and edematous in their dependent portions. The gallbladder showed evidence of acute inflammation with thickening of the wall. There was a somewhat purulent, bile stained material in its lumen.
Microscopic Description of a Section of the Pancreas.—(Fig. 499) Histologic examination of the pancreatic tissue presents a very striking picture of an acute interstitial pancreatitis. This is characterized by a mucopurulent exudate distending the ducts and by a very diffuse periductile and interstitial polynuclear infiltration. The glandular epithelium is undergoing toxic degener-

ative change, many of the cells being swollen and showing beginning evidence of necrosis.

The etiology of this condition is somewhat obscure in relation to the autopsy findings, but suggests, perhaps,

both an ascending infection from the intestinal tract and a hematogenous distribution as part of the picture of septicemia. Whether this may have been secondary to the infection of the gallbladder is likewise a possibility.

Diabetes

From the standpoint of pathology, diabetes is unquestionably the most important disease associated with disturbance of pancreatic function. The cause of diabetes is still obscure, and to-day most of the associated disturbances of metabolism, such as hypercholesteremia, are thought more likely to be the result of the diabetes rather than the causal factor. Endocrine unbalance, a nervous instability of glandular control, some obscure toxemia, possibly of intestinal origin, all have been suggested as hypothetical etiological factors. The symptoms of diabetes are chiefly those of excessive thirst often associated with similar increase of hunger and always accompanied by polyuria. There is a loss of weight which follows rather promptly in the more severe form of the disease, but much later on in the milder diabetic, naturally obese, and in whom the condition does not develop until the late forties or early fifties. From the functional standpoint the symptoms of diabetes are due primarily to an inability of the patient to handle carbohydrates satisfactorily from the metabolic standpoint. As a result marked alteration in relation to the handling of fats and proteins may also ensue. Due to the incomplete combustion of fats, acidosis associated with air hunger, coma and death may occur. From the practical standpoint, the mechanism which is involved in the development of the clinical picture is found as a result of pancreatic inability to manufacture the carbohydrate-splitting enzyme, insulin.

The essential pathology of diabetes is far from satisfactory in its manifestations. One of the most amazing features is that more often than not, one cannot detect any gross or microscopic changes in the diabetic pancreas. Knowing as we do that carbohydrate metabolism is largely controlled by the secretion of the islands of Langerhans, we naturally look first to these structures for evidence of pathology. In the experimentally induced disease, there is marked hydropic degeneration of the Beta cells. On the other hand, no changes have been demonstrated in the Alpha cells other than atrophy late in the disease. These acute degenerative changes have not been seen in human diabetes, but we do not see human diabetes

at the autopsy table at the same stage of the disease process as in the experimental animal.

The most outstanding feature histologically of diabetes is the hyaline degeneration and fibrosis of the islands of Langerhans (Fig. 501), in a small percentage of the cases. Here the question arises as to whether this may not well be the result of the diabetes rather than a manifestation of its cause. It is definitely certain that in tissues removed at autopsy from the majority of cases of diabetes that this feature is usually lacking. On the other hand, it is equally true that if such hyaline degeneration and replacement fibrosis of the island cells does occur in any marked degree, we are surely dealing with a case of diabetes. Such hyaline degeneration is seen in a certain number of individuals past middle age, in association with generalized arteriosclerosis, who do not show necessarily a clinical glycosuria or even any striking degree of hyperglycemia. Such cases must, nevertheless, be considered as latent cases of diabetes.

From the experimental data at hand, we realize that nearly 90 per cent of the true pancreas can be destroyed without the development of any severe diabetic picture and thus it requires comparatively few persistent islet cells to prevent the clinical appearance of the disease. The other changes in the pancreas associated with diabetes are usually those of arteriosclerosis with secondary interstitial fibrosis (Fig. 500). This often results in marked atrophy of the pancreatic tissue, and even of the island epithelium. However, the island cells are capable of regeneration much as the liver cells regenerate. This may be an important factor in maintaining life for the diabetic and may account in part for the gradual ability of the diabetic individual to reduce his dosage of insulin as time goes on. Rare instances of adenomata of the islands of Langerhans have been reported, with clinical hypoglycemia. This has been interpreted as due to an excessive insulin production by the tumor cells.

Vascular Lesions.—Some of the incidental pathology of diabetes has been discussed in relation to some of the other degenerative changes. The two most striking features of diabetic pathology are first of all the disturbances of cholesterin metabolism associated with development of atherosclerosis and generalized arteriosclerosis, particularly of the vessels of the lower extremities. This is followed frequently by diabetic gangrene of the foot. Secondary infection develops very commonly and results in septicemia and death. The diabetic patient to-day usually dies of arteriosclerosis in some form or other, and the problem of the diabetic from the standpoint of life has come to represent the problem of arteriosclerosis. To-day, little excuse exists for a diabetic patient to ever die of diabetic coma; nor with any intelligent study of the individual case should there by any more excuse for his dying of insulin shock. Our real problem to-day is to prevent the premature development of these serious arteriosclerotic lesions and to find some method by which the diabetic's susceptibility to infection may be reduced. Diabetic gangrene

of the lower extremities as a result of arteriosclerosis and endarteritic obliteration of the lumen of the vessels stands first as a cause of death. Cerebral accidents, usually associated with acute hemorrhage following the occlusion of some major cerebral vessel stand second in the group of vascular deaths; and finally, coronary sclerosis with associated myocardial infarction and cardiac decompensation represents the third most common vascular complication.

Incidental Pathology.—The other chief incidental pathological features of diabetes are the result of disturbed carbohydrate metabolism. This is manifested, as has been already brought out in Chapter II, by the withdrawal of glycogen from the normal glycogen deposits; namely, the liver and muscles and its deposition pathologically in the nuclei of the liver cells and in the epithelium of Henle's loop in the kidney. In addition hypercholesterolemia of the spleen may be encountered.

ILLUSTRATIVE CASE

CASE 213. (Ref. #S-177)
Diagnosis.—Pancreas — diabetes — hyalinization of islands of Langerhans.
Chief Complaint.—Patient was a colored male of 74 years, admitted to the hospital complaining of pain in the left foot.
Present Illness.—The patient's symptoms in respect to his admission illness dated back for about one year. Since that time he had noted intermittent attacks of throbbing pain, involving his left foot. This was aggravated upon walking. Two months before admission he noted that his foot had become swollen and several sores broke out on the dorsal surface. These never completely healed in spite of his efforts to cure them by the use of local application of salves. A month before admission the patient showed some evidence of mental deterioration with mild dizzy attacks and some loss of memory for recent events, and a state of mental confusion. The history was somewhat inadequate as it was obtained from a friend who lived in the same boarding house.
Past Medical History.—The past history was entirely unreliable due to the mental confusion of the patient, who was unable to co-operate.
Physical Examination.—Patient was an elderly, colored male in a fair state of nutrition. His head showed no deformity but there was a marked bilateral arcus senilis. The temporal arteries were tortuous and sclerosed. Nose and throat were negative. The chest was emphysematous. The heart was negative. There was an inconstant apical systolic murmur. Blood pressure was 160/110. The lungs were clear. The abdomen was negative. There was a loss of pulsation in the right posterior tibial artery and in the left dorsalis pedis artery. This latter was accompanied by a dry gangrene of the left great toe and two ulcerated areas over the anterior surface of the foot.

Laboratory Findings.—Blood count: red cells, 3,600,-000 with 74% hemoglobin; white cells, 8,200, with 71% polynuclears. Blood chemistry: sugar, 140 mgm. Wassermann was negative. Urinalysis showed a moderate trace of albumin but no sugar. Spinal fluid showed an increase of albumin but was otherwise negative.
Subsequent Course.—Patient progressed rapidly downhill, going into coma, and died one week after admission.
Autopsy Findings.—The body was that of a well developed, well-nourished, elderly Negro. No pathology was noted externally except for the presence of gangrene involving the left foot and extending as a discolored, cyanotic lesion up to about the midleg. There were two superficial areas of ulceration. The heart was slightly hypertrophied. There were no valvular lesions. There were marked arteriosclerotic changes of the coronaries but no definite occlusion. Lungs: Old healed subpleural apical tuberculosis; terminal mucopurulent bronchitis and bronchopneumonia. Kidneys: Chronic nephrosclerosis. Pancreas showed some increase of interstitial stroma and fat. There was obliterative endarteritis of the leg. Microscopically, these vessels showed rather striking atheromatous degenerative changes as well as the usual peripheral Mönckeberg type of arteriosclerosis. This suggested a background of diabetes, although there was no clinical history obtained of its having been present.
Microscopic Description of a Section of the Pancreas.—(Fig. 500 and 501) Section histologically shows diffuse interstitial fibrosis of the pancreas. This is most marked around the ducts (Fig. 500). This is accompanied by considerable catarrhal desquamation of the duct epithelium. The interstitial fibrosis extends into the interacinar tissues as well, tending to separate the acini by bands of connective tissue. Scattered through the section can be seen the islands of Langerhans (Fig. 501). These show varying degrees of hyaline degeneration.

Some of the islands are almost completely obliterated and replaced by hyalinized connective tissue. This process is so extensive as to suggest a typical picture of moder-ately advanced diabetes. In conjunction with the vascular changes of the extremities, the diagnosis seems to be pathologically well substantiated.

Tumors of the Pancreas

Tumors of the pancreas are almost entirely epithelial in nature. Benign lesions of an adenomatous nature may exist as tumors arising from duct, acinar or island epithelium. Only tumors of island epithelium of a benign nature are found from the practical standpoint. These, as has already been mentioned, have been recognized clinically as a result of the associated hypoglycemia, and have even been treated successfully by surgical excision.

Malignant tumors of the pancreas are of the adenocarcinomatous type. They may occur in one of two forms. Statistically, the more common of these two varieties is an adenocarcinoma arising from the acinar epithelium. Theoretically, less often, similar adenocarcinomata arising from the duct epithelium occur. From personal experience, these figures seem to be reversed. The tumors occur most frequently in the sixth decade but many of them are found at a younger age. From the clinical standpoint, the carcinoma of the pancreas represents an entirely hopeless problem. It is an invariably fatal disease. It is not amenable to surgery and both from its location and from its apparent inherent nature is resistant to any form of irradiation therapy. The most common site for its occurrence is seen in the head of the pancreas where, as it grows, it gradually causes pressure upon the ducts with obstruction of the common bile duct and the development of a progressive jaundice. The symptoms at the outset are those of indefinite gastro-intestinal pathology and it is only as the disease advances that a positive diagnosis can be established. It metastasizes by way of the lymphatics to the liver and often extends by direct continuity to the wall of the stomach. Tumors which arise in the tail of the pancreas should be much more amenable to surgery except for the fact that they rarely give rise to symptoms until they are so far advanced that the same problems enter into the picture.

Pathology.—The pathological recognition of the carcinomata of the pancreas depends at times very definitely upon some knowledge of the clinical history as the identification of the cell of origin is frequently impossible. Tumors which arise from the duct epithelium tend to be composed of mucous producing goblet cells which show marked papillary hyperplasia. There is an excessive mucoid secretion and these tumors are often difficult to differentiate from other tumors arising from the gastro-intestinal tract or, in the case of the female, even from the ovary. Where the tumor is of acinar epithelial origin, it is more often easy to identify, although it presents a very much more pleomorphic picture as it becomes more malignant. In these various types of pancreatic carcinomata, we find marked differences in the rate of growth and correspondingly in the histology. Just as in the tumors of the breast and of the stomach, we may find relatively rapidly-growing medullary types of neoplasm or much more slowly growing, sclerosing scirrhous lesions. Statistically, carcinoma of the pancreas is still a comparatively uncommon form of malignancy in this country making up less than two per cent of all malignant tumors.

ILLUSTRATIVE CASE

CASE 214. (Ref. #S-282)

Diagnosis.—Pancreas—adenocarcinoma, duct cell type.

Chief Complaint.—Patient was a white male of 58 years, admitted to the hospital because of headache and dizziness.

Present Illness.—The onset of the patient's admission illness was insidious and difficult to date with any degree of exactitude. He had been subject to mild attacks of vertigo and ringing in his ears over a period of several years. This was believed due to a probable syphilitic infection with vascular involvement. During the year preceding admission he had had fluid accumulate in his abdomen on several occasions. This had been removed several times by tapping but had reaccumulated rapidly. During the week before admission, the patient had developed considerable mental disturbances with confusion, disorientation and a loss of memory, which made it difficult to obtain a more complete history.

Past Medical History.—The past history was unsatisfactory. The patient had apparently been under treatment for syphilis several years previously, but no detailed information regarding this infection could be obtained due to the mental state of the patient.

Physical Examination.—Patient was a fairly well-developed white male about sixty years of age, who showed evidence of recent loss of weight. His head was negative. His pupils were somewhat irregular. Nose and throat were negative. His chest was symmetrical. His abdomen was distended due to the presence of considerable fluid which made palpation of the liver and spleen impossible. There was no jaundice. The heart and lungs seemed normal. No other physical findings of significance were noted.

Laboratory Findings.—Blood showed a mild secondary anemia with a red count of 3,600,000 and 71% hemoglobin; a white count of 11,200 with 79% polynuclears. Urinalysis was negative except for a slight trace of albumin. Wassermann was negative.

Subsequent History.—The patient went rapidly downhill and died five days after admission.

Autopsy Findings.—Body was that of an elderly white male with no external pathology other than distention of the abdomen. Peritoneal cavity contained about 3,000 c.c. of straw-colored fluid in which some stringy white fibrinous material was present. A mass in the region of the tail of the pancreas the size of an orange was felt. The liver was enlarged, weighing 2,100 gm. It was firmly adherent to the inferior surface of the diaphragm on the right by a partially organized fibrous peritonitis. On section several circumscribed nodules appeared in the left lobe. These were roughly spherical in

outline and suggested metastatic tumor tissue. The heart and lungs were negative and the other abdominal viscera showed nothing of significance. A gross diagnosis of carcinoma of the tail of the pancreas with liver metastasis and secondary peritonitis was made.

Microscopic Description of a Section of the Pancreas.—(Fig. 502) Histologic examination of the tissue shows enough normal persistent pancreatic structures to identify the tissue. A few clumps of typical pancreatic acini can be made out, but these are markedly distorted by interstitial fibrosis and mononuclear cellular infiltration. Several pancreatic islands likewise are identified. These appear practically isolated in masses of desmoplastic tumor stroma. The main mass of the tissue is made up of an adenocarcinoma which apparently arises from the pancreatic duct epithelium as many of the acinar structures seen in the tumor are lined by a hyperplastic columnar type of cell. The process is evidently relatively slow in its development because differentiation of these cells is fairly well maintained. Some areas are noted where a loss of polarity, hyperchromatism and anaplasia occur. Mitotic figures are encountered in moderate numbers. There is an extraordinary degree of replacement of the normal pancreatic structures by this tumor tissue.

CHAPTER LII

DISEASES OF THE HEMATOPOIETIC SYSTEM

DISEASES OF THE SPLEEN AND LYMPH NODES

PART I

The Spleen

The spleen arises as a modified lymphoid organ and might well be grouped with the so-called hemolymph nodes. In the developing embryo it plays an active part in general hematopoiesis. By the time of the birth of the infant it has often lost this capacity except in the production of lymphocytes. Ever since the time of Galen it has still remained an organ of mystery. It is not a vital organ as it may be removed surgically, and the individual continues to live out his normal span of years. Its functions have been the subject of an enormous amount of experimental investigation. Perhaps the monograph of Pearce, Krumbhaar and Frazier still better epitomizes our knowledge of the subject than any other publication. The most important function of the spleen seems to relate to its part in the metabolism of hemoglobin through its action upon the red cells as they complete their life span. The spleen has aptly been termed the graveyard of the red cell, for it is here that the red cells undergo disintegration and are acted upon by the reticulo-endothelial cells to break hemoglobin down into the form of bilirubin and its iron constituents. The bilirubin is carried by the splenic vein to the liver where it is resynthesized into bile pigment and in part combined with bile salts as bile; and the iron made available to be re-combined as hemoglobin in new red cells.

The chief activities of the spleen seem to be dependent very largely upon its anatomical structure. An enormous amount of study has been devoted to this in an attempt to evaluate the functional activities of the organ. In recent years, the work of Mac-Neal has done a great deal to clarify this part of the problem. Briefly the circulation of the spleen may be best described as a filter. As the blood enters the spleen from the arterial side it is poured out through anatomical defects in the endothelium of the sinuses into the pulp spaces. From these pulp spaces, venous channels similarly carry the return flow. Thus, barring a few small direct capillary communications from arterial to venous side, which might be considered designed to maintain the nutrition of the organ in the event of clogging of the filter mechanism, all the blood which passes through the spleen must go through this pulp tissue. Aside from this filtration function by which bacteria and other foreign material may be removed from the circulation, and from its functional activity in respect to the destruction of the erythrocytes, most of its other activities are largely hypothetical as the result of indirect evidence through splenectomy.

It has been shown by Barcroft and others that the spleen may act as a reservoir for the storage of blood, which may be restored to the circulation as needed in emergency. Likewise, in the various forms of anemia, it has been shown that the spleen is capable of resuming its fetal activity and take part in the production of red cells and in some instances even myeloid cells. By far the most interesting theoretical function of the spleen is that related to immunity. There has accumulated a considerable amount of evidence to indicate that the spleen is one of the most important structures of the body in the development of antibodies. It has been shown that cases of rheumatic fever in whom splenectomy has been done are more susceptible to recurrent attacks. In cases of secondary anemia associated with splenic enlargement, removal of the spleen again has seemed to reduce the resistance of those individuals for varying periods of time. Gradually, the concept has arisen that it requires a matter of at least six months to a year for the other reticular tissues of the body to take over this immune antibody production, and that such individuals are very prone to intercurrent infec-

PLATE CXIX
DISEASES OF THE SPLEEN

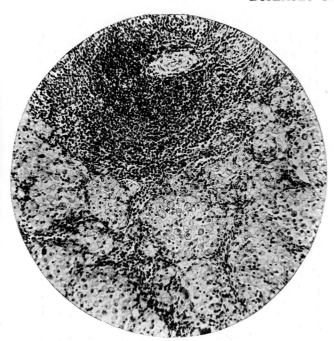

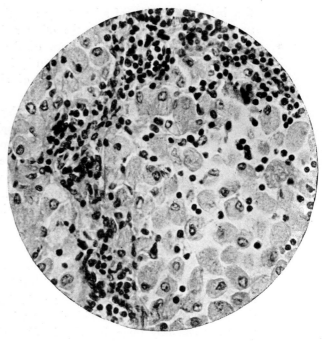

FIG. 503.—SPLEEN: GAUCHER'S DISEASE.—CASE 216.—Low power photomicrograph from an area including a splenic corpuscle. The adjacent splenic sinuses are distended and filled with large, finely vacuolated mononuclear cells. App. 100 x.

FIG. 504.—SPLEEN: GAUCHER'S DISEASE.—CASE 216.—High power detail from Fig. 503 in which the characteristic features of the Gaucher cells can be observed. Note their eccentric, vesicular nuclei, lace like appearance of their cytoplasm, their large size, and the ovoid, polyhedral form. App. 400 x.

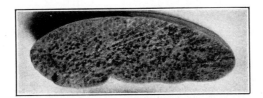

FIG. 505.—SPLEEN: AMYLOIDOSIS.—CASE 13.— "Sago" spleen showing iodine reaction.

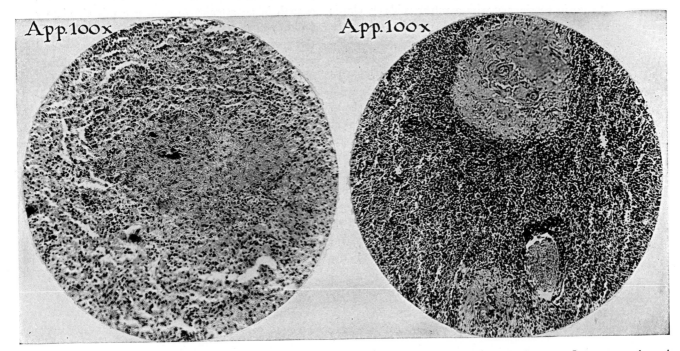

FIG. 506.—SPLEEN: MILIARY TUBERCULOSIS.—CASE 59.—Low power photomicrograph showing an early miliary tubercle with beginning caseation. Note several Langhans' giant cells and marked epithelioid reaction. App. 100 x.

FIG. 507.—SPLEEN: AMYLOIDOSIS.—CASE 13.—Low power photomicrograph to illustrate the amyloid infiltration of a splenic follicle and the wall of a follicular arteriole. App. 100 x.

tion between the time of splenectomy and the assumption of this function by the other reticuloendothelial tissues. Further evidence of the part played by the spleen in infections is seen by its universal involvement in acute infections of almost every sort.

From our practical approach to the pathology of the various organs of the body, the question of splenic enlargement or splenomegaly becomes the paramount issue, and a consideration of some of the more important causes of splenic enlargement involves us in a study of several varieties of disease. These might be grouped under several major headings: First,

those conditions relating to the various degenerative, infiltrative and circulatory disturbances; second, those relating to the various acute infections; third, those concerned with various disturbances of the hematopoietic system in respect to blood formation and blood destruction; fourth, the lipoid storage disturbances; and fifth, the neoplastic group. It is particularly in the disease associated with disturbances of blood formation and blood destruction, and in the disturbances of lipoid metabolism that our major interest lies, as it is in these two groups of clinical diseases that the splenic pathology becomes perhaps the outstanding diagnostic factor.

Degenerative, Infiltrative and Circulatory Disturbances

Degenerative and Infiltrative Disturbances.—The degenerative and infiltrative lesions which affect the spleen are relatively few in number and of little significance. The only one which occurs with any frequency and may cause difficulty in diagnosis is the result of amyloid infiltration in conjunction with the picture of amyloidosis generally.

AMYLOID INFILTRATION.—The problem of amyloid infiltration has been discussed rather fully in one of the early chapters of the section on general pathology and can, therefore, be referred to briefly at this point. Amyloid infiltration of the spleen is seen ordinarily in conjunction with some chronic wasting disease, particularly chronic tuberculous osteomyelitis. It may occur in the course of any chronic disease such as tuberculosis, syphilis, or even long-standing malignancies associated with cachexia. The spleen may be greatly enlarged in this condition. It is firm in consistency with a rather rubbery, elastic feeling. On palpation of its mesial aspect, the notch persists. The spleen cuts with increased resistance and presents a colloid, gelatinous, semi-translucent appearance. The amyloid infiltration may be restricted largely to the follicles in the earlier development of the condition, but later extends to infiltrate the entire splenic structure. The typical appearance of these translucent masses against the deep, congested pulp has been described as the *"sago"* spleen, resembling as it does the grains of sago as seen floating in soup. The various lipoid infiltrations are considered separately in relation to the enlargement of the spleen associated with disturbances of lipoid metabolism. The degenerative lesions are likewise considered very largely in relation to the

changes associated with acute splenitis. For an illustrative case, the reader is referred to Case 13 (Ref. #S-66), Chapter III, page 26, and Fig. 505 and 507.

Circulatory Disturbances.—From the circulatory standpoint, the three lesions which rather consistently show evidence of demonstrable pathology are (a) chronic passive congestion; (b) thrombosis with resultant infarction and (c) rupture of the spleen.

CHRONIC PASSIVE CONGESTION.—In chronic passive congestion, the spleen shows a moderate enlargement, rarely to the degree that it becomes palpable clinically but not infrequently doubling its weight. The capsule tends to be stretched and ultimately is apt to show moderate thickening. The outstanding lesion is a dilatation of the sinusoids due to the circulatory stasis. With this dilatation of the sinuses, there is a stimulation of connective and elastic tissue growth in an attempt to overcome this circulatory failure and to force the blood out of the spleen. As this process continues over periods of months and years, the distention of the sinuses and the diffuse fibrosis results in a marked atrophy of the follicles and lymphoid tissues generally. The end result in such a case may be a small, fibrous, atrophic spleen scarcely half the normal size of the organ. This may best be described from the pathological standpoint as a fibrous splenitis and in a given section it may be difficult to differentiate from the end result in a lesion such as the so-called Banti's disease, or the fibrous splenitis associated with cirrhosis of the liver in the late stage. For an illustrative case of chronic passive congestion, the reader is referred to Case 15 (Ref. #S-68), Chapters IV and V.

PLATE CXX

DISEASES OF THE SPLEEN AND LYMPH NODES

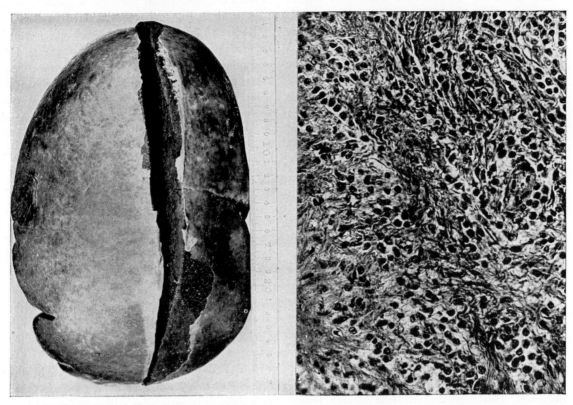

FIG. 508.—SPLEEN: BANTI'S DISEASE.—CASE 215.—Gross photograph of greatly enlarged spleen with thickened, hyalinized capsule. On section, marked atrophy of the lymphoid tissue and diffuse fibrosis of the stroma were prominent.

FIG. 509.—SPLEEN: BANTI'S DISEASE.—CASE 215.—Photomicrograph to illustrate the marked increase of connective tissue and reticulum and the relatively inconspicuous lymphoid structures. App. 200 x.

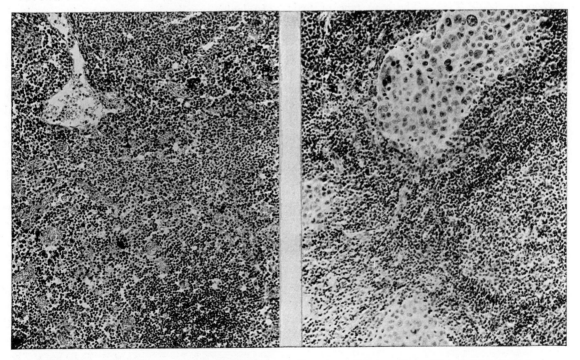

FIG. 510.—LYMPH NODE.—ACUTE SUPPURATIVE LYMPHADENITIS.—Photomicrograph showing diffuse infiltration of lymph node by polynuclear leukocytes. Beginning liquefaction necrosis (center right) may be observed. App. 100 x.

FIG. 511.—LYMPH NODE—METASTATIC CARCINOMA OF BREAST.—Nests of infiltrating tumor tissue composed of large, polyhedral, pleomorphic, anaplastic epithelial cells showing numerous atypical mitotic figures, are seen. Persistent lymph follicle at lower right. App. 100 x.

EMBOLISM OR THROMBOSIS WITH RESULTANT INFARCTION.—Infarction of the spleen has already been described in the chapter devoted to circulatory disturbances in general. It may be produced by a wide variety of causes, but generally speaking, the typical anemic splenic infarct is the result of arterial embolism and is seen especially in such conditions as subacute or acute bacterial endocarditis. Case 2 (Ref. #S-122), Chapter I, page 6, and Fig. 40, illustrates this lesion, as well as Case 162, Chapter XXXVIII, relating to the various forms of endocarditis, including subacute bacterial endocarditis.

RUPTURE OF THE SPLEEN.—The spleen may become ruptured on occasion with resultant fatal intra-abdominal hemorrhage if operative measures are not taken promptly. Such rupture is most frequently of a traumatic nature. Occasionally, however, apparent spontaneous rupture may occur in association with a marked congestion and toxic splenitis. Even here a mild traumatic factor is likely to play a part.

Acute Splenitis
(Acute Toxic Splenitis; Acute Splenic Tumor)

In almost every form of acute infectious disease, and in many parasitic infestations, particularly those of a protozoal nature, the spleen is strikingly involved. This is manifested by a varying degree of enlargement. The capsule becomes tense and stretched. The pulp becomes distended with either red cells or leukocytes or both. Not infrequently the patient may present a feeling of heaviness and even tenderness over the splenic area. If the infection is of such a nature as to cause embolic phenomena, the spleen is commonly the site of such local acute manifestations. This is particularly true in such lesions as subacute and acute ulcerative bacterial endocarditis. The acute toxic splenitis occurs in two forms dependent largely upon the type of organism producing the infection.

Gray or Septic Type.—The gray type of toxic splenitis is seen particularly in conjunction with infections, particularly of the pyogenic variety. One of the best examples is seen in association with a pneumococcic lobar pneumonia, but almost all the coccoid organisms likewise will produce the same picture to a variable degree. The spleen is moderately enlarged, rarely weighing more than double its normal weight. It frequently shows some fibrinous exudate on its surface. In the living patient as seen on the operating table, such a spleen is tense. At autopsy, however, the blood has frequently escaped, leaving the organ somewhat smaller than it was in life and having a soft, mushy consistency. On section, it is a rather uniform, grayish-pink color, and difficulty exists in demonstrating the presence of lymph follicles.

Microscopically this picture is found to be the result of diffuse infiltration of the pulp spaces by leukocytes. In some diseases, such as pertussis, for example, this cellular infiltration is more likely to be made up largely of lymphoid cells. The reaction in a mild infection is so slight as to be overlooked often grossly. Varying degrees of degeneration up to necrosis are found in these cases. The most striking changes, as a rule, are those associated with the germinal centers of the lymph follicles. For an illustrative case refer back to Case 176 (Ref. #S-21) Chapter XLIII.

Red or Typhoid Type.—Typhoid fever illustrates best the so-called red type of acute toxic splenitis. It is difficult to generalize with any degree of assurance, but the bacillary infections, particularly those of the gastro-intestinal tract are more likely to be associated with such red spleens in contra-distinction to the coccoid pyogenic organisms. The red type of splenitis usually shows a greater increase in size, at times approaching three or four times the normal weight. Its capsule likewise is extremely tense. Unlike the gray spleen the red type shows very little difference in size in the living patient and in the dead subject. Mallory and others have emphasized, particularly in respect to typhoid fever, that the endothelial hyperplasia which accompanies such infections tends mechanically to obstruct the outflow of blood from the spleen. This results in the enormous distention of the pulp spaces and of the sinuses by red cells. With such stagnation, the spleen becomes a deep cyanotic red in color and microscopically, evidence of hemolysis with hemosiderin production occurs relatively early. The pathology of the spleen in typhoid fever is presented in Cases 52 and 53, Chapter XIV, to which the reader is referred.

Specific Infections of the Spleen.—In addition to these relatively nonspecific varieties of acute splenitis, occasional instances of specific infections of the spleen may occur. Among these should be mentioned syphilis and tuberculosis.

SYPHILIS.—Syphilis may appear in the spleen either as part of a congenital infection in which instance we see a diffuse fibrosis of the spleen which, except for the demonstration of spirochetes by special staining methods, is essentially indistinguishable from other forms of chronic fibrous splenitis. Occasionally, on the other hand, the tertiary lesion of syphilis in the form of a gumma may be found in the spleen. This is similar in appearance to gummata elsewhere, which have been already described in the section on syphilitic infections. For an illustrative case of gumma of the spleen, the reader is referred to Case 56 (Ref. #S-64), Chapter XV, Figure 123.

TUBERCULOSIS.—Tuberculosis (Fig. 506) rarely involves the spleen except as part of a generalized miliary infection, and just as in the case of tuberculosis elsewhere, under these circumstances we may find lesions of varying size and age representing successive blood stream invasion with metastatic tubercle formation. Other infections such as those produced by mycoses may likewise also occasionally be encountered as part of a blood stream extension of the initial lesion, but by and large, infection of the spleen as a localized condition is comparatively rare. Refer back to miliary tuberculosis, Case 59. (Ref. #S-136) Chapter XVI.

Parasitic Spleens.—In addition to these two major types of acute splenitis are seen those forms associated with parasitic infestations, notably malaria and kala-azar. Due to the persistence of the parasite, the reaction while relatively acute at the outset develops into a subacute and chronic form with the result that such spleens attain a very great increase in size not infrequently. Chronic inflammatory productive fibrosis develops and the spleen becomes extremely firm in consistency and cuts with markedly increased resistance when removed from the body at autopsy. In the case of malaria, the characteristic pigmentation producing a slate-gray color both to the capsule and the cut surface is fairly diagnostic. The demonstration of the parasites makes the diagnosis conclusive. Similarly in kala-azar, the demonstration of the Leishman-Donovan bodies, both intra- and extracellularly establishes the nature of the process.

The spleen in a case of malarial parasitic infestation is discussed in Case 76, Chapter XX. In echinococcic infestations the spleen may be the site of cyst formation, and is spoken of as Zuckerguss hyalitis.

In any case of acute toxic splenitis, it may follow that on account of necrosis of tissue a reparative replacement fibrosis may develop. This is often at the expense of the lymphoid elements and the result may be seen in a moderately or slightly enlarged spleen which shows a diffuse fibrosis on sectioning. Nor infrequently the capsule under such circumstances likewise shows very extensive thickening and due to the inadequacy of the blood supply undergoes marked hyaline change. At times this may approach a picture almost suggesting the frosting on a cake.

Splenomegaly Associated With Disturbances of Hematopoiesis

There are a number of conditions in which we find striking enlargement of the spleen associated with some disturbance of the hematopoietic system. The majority of these are found in relation to various forms of anemia and will be discussed at greater length from that standpoint in the following chapter. Among these should be mentioned pernicious anemia, the hemolytic anemias, von Jaksch's anemia, sickle and oval cell anemia and the various forms of splenic anemia, including the so-called Banti's disease. Of these the only one of particular significance from the differential diagnostic standpoint pathologically in respect to the spleen is represented by Banti's disease. On the other side of the picture in conjunction with increased hematopoiesis should be cited polycythemia vera (Vaquez's disease), although perhaps this should be, strictly speaking, included among the neoplasms as has been emphasized in the chapter relating to tumors of the reticulo-endothelial organs.

Banti's Disease (Splenic Anemia).—The term "splenic anemia" is a generic one, which is applied to a group of conditions in which there is a secondary anemia, usually of the hypochromic type associated with splenic enlargement and for which no specific etiologic agent has as yet been discovered. Among these should be included the condition known as Banti's disease. Whether or not this should be used synonymously with the term splenic anemia is perhaps open to question, and most pathologists refuse to admit the existence of such an entity from the pathological standpoint. Banti, in his original description, defined a series of six cases of splenic enlargement occurring in young adults and accompanied by a moderate anemia. In addition, as the disease progressed, he described the picture of cirrhosis of the liver of the portal type which supervened as part of the end picture of the condition.

ETIOLOGY.—As has been emphasized, the exact etiology of Banti's disease is unknown. It is generally assumed that the development of the splenic picture is the result of some disturbance of circulation associated with an increase in the portal blood pressure. This may be the result of thrombosis of the portal or splenic veins or of pressure from without on these veins. It may be associated with degenerative lesions affecting the blood vessels resulting in dilatation of the portal circulation and relative stasis of its circulation. In the majority of cases, however, no such lesions can be demonstrated. The incidence of atheroma formation, endophlebitis or phlebosclerosis does not appear to be statistically significant. Banti himself was of the impression that the lesion was a toxic one, the result of absorption of a toxin from the gastro-intestinal tract, which he described as fibrogenetic, but confirmation of this theory has not been uniformly successful.

PATHOLOGY.—In typical Banti's disease, the spleen is considerably increased in size, in Banti's original series, rarely beyond 600 grams. In many of the cases which have appeared in the literature since that time, spleens weighing as much as 2,000 gm. or more have been included. This increase in size is largely due to an increase in connective tissue with obliteration of the lymph follicles. In the early phase of the picture, along with an increase of the reticulo-endothelial elements, there is an accompanying diffuse fibrosis which grows in between the reticulo-endothelium and gradually produces obliteration of the normal architecture. This produces what has been described as the siderotic nodule or the so-called "fibro-adenie" of Banti. These nodules, which at times may be seen grossly on the cut surface of the spleen, particularly early in the process, present microscopic evidence of curious focal lesions made up of degenerative elastic tissue fibers on which iron has been deposited in the form of crystals. These do not take any of the usual stains and appear often jointed not unlike the appearance of a piece of bamboo. They have frequently been mistaken for fungi. However, no such organisms have ever been conclusively recovered from any case.

These nodules are, theoretically at least, caused by hemorrhage at the terminal end of an arteriole through the increased portal blood pressure. The hemorrhage is followed by organization and fibrosis. The fibrosis tends to begin around the sinuses and spreads throughout the reticulum until it finally involves the main fibrous trabeculae and the picture becomes one of diffuse fibrous splenitis which, in the absence of the typical siderotic nodule, is indistinguishable from the end result of any such chronic productive fibrotic process.

Either as a result of the increased portal pressure, or the action of some toxin, as Banti originally suggested, the liver becomes secondarily involved in a cirrhosis indistinguishable from any other case of portal origin. This results in the usual picture of cirrhosis accompanied by the development of esophageal and gastric varices with the patient not infrequently dying from a fatal hemorrhage from their rupture. Terminally, many of these cases likewise show a typical ascites but do not develop jaundice as a rule. At this stage it is impossible to differentiate a case of Banti's disease from the usual case of portal cirrhosis and the question as to whether or not they may not represent different manifestations of the same underlying etiological process has often been raised. It is equally true that in the typical case of portal cirrhosis in which the liver enlargement and involvement occurs first, by the time the patient dies there is similar splenic enlargement and fibrosis as in Banti's disease. This remains an attractive speculative hypothesis. One point of difference may be of significance in that the anemia usually develops early in Banti's disease, whereas it is a late sign in portal cirrhosis.

ILLUSTRATIVE CASE

CASE 215. (Ref. #S-290)
Diagnosis.—Spleen—Banti's Disease.
Chief Complaint.—Patient was a female Italian of nine years, admitted to the hospital because of marked weakness and pallor.

Present Illness.—The onset of the patient's present illness was insidious, beginning perhaps a year or more before her present admission. She had had rather vague, indefinite qualitative gastro-intestinal disturbances of digestion and had failed to gain in weight satisfactorily.

Her parents noted that she had been developing a rather sallow, yellow color and had shown increasing lassitude and general weakness.

Past Medical History.—Patient was born normally at full term and weighed 8½ pounds. She was nursed for three months and then put on a bottle. She went along normally, getting on to the family table diet by the time she was a year old. She had had measles, pertussis and varicella during the first three years of her life but had had no serious illness since.

Physical Examination.—Child was fairly well developed but definitely undernourished and had a very sallow color. She seemed extremely apathetic. The head was essentially negative except for the marked anemia. The nose and throat were negative. There was no enlargement of the tonsils. The eyes reacted normally. The sclerae appeared almost blue due to the marked anemia. The chest was symmetrical. The lungs were clear. The heart was not enlarged. There was a soft systolic bruit. The abdomen was prominent. The spleen was enormously enlarged, reaching the symphysis pubis. There was a definite notch felt at the level of the umbilicus. It was extremely firm and had rounded edges. The liver was also moderately enlarged. There was a suggestion of a fluid wave. The extremities were negative.

Laboratory Findings.—The laboratory findings of significance were largely restricted to the blood. The urinalysis was negative except for an increase of bilirubin. The stool likewise showed a relative increase of urobilin. Wassermann was negative. Hematologic findings: The red cells on admission numbered 1,952,000. Hemoglobin was approximately 30%. The white cells numbered 23,000 with 40% polynuclears, 12% large lymphocytes, 30% small lymphocytes, 17% large mononuclears and 1% eosinophiles. The blood smear showed evidence of a very marked hypochromic type of anemia with extreme poikilocytosis, punctate basophilia, achromia and polychromatophilia. There were many cells showing Cabot's ring bodies and Howell-Jolly bodies in addition to a number of megaloblasts and normoblasts. The reticulated red cell count was 5%. The fragility test showed a definite increased fragility, hemolysis beginning at 0.56%.

Subsequent Course.—The patient was followed for a period of two months, being given repeated transfusions to prepare her for a splenectomy. At the time of operation the red cell count was 4,800,000, the white cells, 10,000. The splenectomy resulted in an uneventful postoperative recovery, followed by marked changes in the blood picture. The red cells, after an initial drop, leveled out at about 4,000,000, the white cells increased to approximately 30,000. The fragility dropped in the course of 48 hours so that hemolysis only began at 0.36%. The patient was followed for a period of two years, during which time she continued in the same good health. At that time she moved to another city and was lost sight of.

Pathological Report.—The spleen weighed 1,192 gm. (Fig. 508). It showed marked thickening of the capsule with an almost hyaline degeneration of an old fibrinous exudate. It was a pale grayish-pink in color. It cut with greatly increased resistance. On section no gross evidence of persistent lymphoid structures could be made out. There seemed to be very diffuse generalized fibrosis.

Microscopical Examination of a Section through the Spleen.—(Fig. 509) The spleen microscopically shows evidence of a diffuse fibrosis with resultant replacement to a very large extent of the lymphoid elements. This fibrous tissue proliferation seems generalized but is characterized frequently by curious nests of spindle cells which almost suggest nodular collections of fibroblasts. There is considerable hyaline degeneration of the vessel walls. This is particularly striking with respect to the age of the patient. Nothing else of diagnostic significance can be made out and one is forced to a descriptive diagnosis of chronic fibrosplenitis, which, in relation to the history and hematological findings, seems more consistent with the clinical diagnosis of Banti's disease than anything else.

Polycythemia Vera (*Vaquez's Disease*).—As has already been emphasized, polycythemia vera represents a disease of the red cell series which should perhaps best be considered as representing a leukemic neoplastic overgrowth of these cells. It is accompanied as a rule by marked splenic enlargement. This splenic enlargement is found due to three principal factors. In the first place the spleen has resumed in the majority of instances the function of red cell production so that islands of active hematopoiesis may be recognized with countless nucleated red cells of one variety or another. In the second place, due to the marked increase in the number of red cells and the increased viscosity of the blood, the function of the spleen as a blood reservoir has become emphasized. In the third place, the result of such alteration in the circulatory mechanism with distention of the sinuses and pulp is a productive fibrosis. These three factors, while not absolutely specific for the diagnosis of polycythemia vera make its likelihood extremely probable, particularly if it occurs in an adult in middle life. When such a picture is found in infancy or childhood, the diagnosis of erythroblastic anemia or so-called von Jaksch's anemia must also be considered, although in these latter conditions the anemia is usually a prominent feature.

Diseases Associated with Disturbances of Lipoid Metabolism

In recent years there has been found a considerable number of cases, most of which seem to have a familial background, in which some disturbance in lipoid metabolism appears to be the underlying factor. These are characterized by the curious deposition of lipoid substances in the body tissues, particularly in the reticulo-endothelial organs, although by no means restricted to them. Certain differences in the clinical picture and in the pathology have resulted in the dividing of these conditions into at least six distinct forms, which will be briefly referred to at this point.

Gaucher's Disease.—The etiology is unknown. The clinical picture is obviously associated with some disturbance of lipoid metabolism. The condition occurs principally in children and to a very large extent in children of Semitic origin. It is not infrequently familial, several children in the same family presenting the picture. Symptomatically, the onset is insidious and is frequently first recognized by an increase in the size of the abdomen due primarily to splenic enlargement. It is accompanied by a mild progressive secondary anemia, which is largely the result of replacement of the bone marrow by lipoid-laden reticulo-endothelial cells. It is frequently characterized by the appearance of curious yellowish, wedge-shaped areas of lipoid infiltration of the conjunctiva on both aspects of the eye. Not infrequently, patchy yellowish areas of discoloration of the skin are seen and pains in the bones and joints may occur which are sometimes considered as "growing pains," or in the more severe forms may be mistaken for osteomyelitis. X-ray examination shows rarefaction when this occurs, with a suggestion of fusiform expansion of the lower end of the long bones and flattening of the proximal end. There is no jaundice nor ascites. Liver enlargement may occur late in the disease and is the result of secondary involvement of the Kupffer and reticulo-endothelial cells of that organ. It is a slowly progressive disease which is markedly benefited by splenectomy with apparent cure in some instances. The diagnosis may be established by splenic puncture with the finding of the characteristic Gaucher's cells. In the late stage of the disease, the lymph nodes generally may be involved, and biopsy examination of a peripheral lymph node may likewise be utilized as a diagnostic procedure.

PATHOLOGY.—The spleen is usually enormously enlarged, reaching the greatest relative size seen in any disease with the exception of myeloid leukemia. It cuts readily and is a very pale gray-red in color with yellowish-white patches throughout its substance. It is moderately firm in consistency with a feeling of elasticity. Histologically, the diagnosis is readily established. The lymph follicles tend to be small and replaced by the typical Gaucher's cells. More characteristically the splenic sinuses are found to be enormously distended and lined by large vacuolated cells. Many of these have been cast off into the lumen and fill the sinus. Similar infiltration of the pulp spaces is seen in many areas. A striking alveolar arrangement results from this sinusoidal dilatation. The characteristic Gaucher's cells are enormous in size measuring 20 to 60 micra in diameter. They are extremely pale in their staining reaction. The nucleus is small, round and eccentrically placed. The cytoplasm of the cell is almost completely vacuolated. These vacuoles are filled with a lipoid derivative which has been identified as kerasin (a cerebroside), which requires special staining methods to demonstrate. It will not stain to any appreciable extent with the ordinary lipoid solvent dyes such as Sudan III, Scharlach R or even osmic acid. It is chiefly the presence of these enormous cells which causes the increase in the size of the spleen, although the accompanying fibrosis plays some part. The lesion apparently starts in the spleen, but as the case progresses, subsequent involvement of the liver, lymph nodes, bone marrow and the reticulo-endothelial system in general takes place, as is true of most conditions associated with lipoid metabolic disturbance.

ILLUSTRATIVE CASE

CASE 216. (Ref. #S-69) [Courtesy of Drs. Robert Schless, Herman Epstein, A. Capper, B. Gouley and D. Fishback, Jewish Hospital, Philadelphia]

Diagnosis.—Spleen—Gaucher's Disease.

Chief Complaint.—Patient was a female Jewish child of 10 years, who was admitted to the hospital for splenectomy.

Present Illness.—The child was first seen four years before her present admission when she was admitted to the hospital because of pain and swelling of the *right* thigh just above the knee. This had been of several days duration. A tentative diagnosis of osteomyelitis was made and the right femur was trephined. What resembled "free

pus" was obtained but this was sterile bacteriologically. The wound was drained and healed after a period of about three weeks.

She was readmitted to the hospital one year later because of pain in the *left* thigh of twenty-fours hours duration. At that time she had a temperature of 100.2°, but a white cell count of only 6,000. In view of the previous history, an osteomyelitis of the left femur was suspected and this bone was trephined and drained. Smear and culture from the "pus" were negative. This wound likewise healed satisfactorily and she was discharged at the end of three weeks.

One month later, she was readmitted again because of

perplasia. Among such lesions must be again cited infectious mononucleosis.

Fig. 510 (Ref. #S-74) represents a low power photomicrograph from a section of cervical lymph node in a case of acute hemolytic streptococcic ulcerative tonsillitis. In the midportion of the illustration will be found a wide area of necrosis completely infiltrated by leukocytes undergoing liquefaction necrosis, with the beginning production of an abscess. Around this suppurative area will be seen the hyperplastic lymphoid structures with a portion of the focal infection in the lower right corner.

The neoplastic diseases of the lymph nodes, including leukemia, lymphosarcoma and Hodgkin's disease, represent the most important group of cases diagnostically. They, likewise, have been discussed in the section on those diseases. In addition, metastatic tumors make up another very important group of cases of lymph node enlargement. It is by the evidence of such metastasis that we are able to estimate with some degree of accuracy the prognosis. Typically, when a tumor metastasizes to the lymph node, the metastasis is likely to show much more rapid growth and histologic evidence of a higher grade of malignancy than the original tumor. For that reason, diagnostic biopsies of nodes in suspicious cases are indicated.

Fig. 511 (Ref. #S-369) represents an axillary lymph node from a case of carcinoma of the breast. This was a rapidly-growing neoplasm of the encephaloid variety. The tumor cells may be observed in three areas in the illustration. The rather characteristic pleomorphism, anaplasia, hyperchomatism of many of the nuclei, and atypic mitotic figures may be observed. The germinal center of the lymph follicle is seen in the lower right portion of the picture, and the remainder of the lymphoid structure shows secondary inflammatory hyperplasia.

CHAPTER LIII

DISEASES OF THE HEMATOPOIETIC SYSTEM (*Continued*)

THE BLOOD

HEMATOGENESIS

The most useful concept to hold regarding the blood is that it represents an organ, the cells of which happen to be for the most part relatively mobile units in contra-distinction to the usual fixed tissues. Yet, we must recognize that the bone marrow itself represents the point of origin of the various cell constituents of this circulating tissue under normal circumstances. During embryonic life, we are all familiar with the fact, although it is frequently forgotten, that the spleen, liver and even other tissues play an active part in hematopoiesis. Shortly after birth, this function gradually disappears until the bone marrow alone is capable of maintaining normal blood cell production. In the infant and rapidly growing child, the marrow of all the bones is active in this respect. After adolescence, the demands for new blood cells steadily diminishes until in old age there is almost a complete replacement of the normal hematopoietic active marrow by a fatty fibrous tissue. Such centers of hematopoiesis as are necessary to carry on the normal replacement of cells are largely found in the ends of the long bones. Under pathological conditions as hematopoiesis increases, we find a gradual reversion toward the primitive picture with more and more of the long bone marrow becoming active. Subsequently the vertebral marrow, and in the more marked instances of blood dyscrasias, even a return of hematopoietic function by the spleen and liver takes place. Thus, under normal circumstances, there is a very delicately balanced mechanism, by which the body requirements in respect to hemoglobin and white cells are maintained. When this balance is upset through any cause, then corresponding changes take place within this blood forming tissue.

From the clinical standpoint, these disturbances of blood formation and blood destruction are most readily demonstrated in a relatively crude sort of way by a study of the peripheral blood picture. An increase in the number of leukocytes, known as leukocytosis, is almost "prima facie" evidence of infection. As greater and greater demands are put upon the bone marrow for more and more leukocytes to combat such infections, we find what is spoken of as a *"shift to the left,"* with the appearance of young immature stab forms. In leukemia, as we have seen, with the neoplastic overgrowth of the cells of the granulocytic series, the immature myelocytes, premyelocytes and myeloblasts appear in increasing numbers and the diagnosis of leukemia becomes apparent as these immature cells are found abnormally circulating in the peripheral blood.

On the other side of the picture we may find a reduction in the number of leukocytes. Again, this may signify for us in conjunction with certain other clinical findings that we are dealing perhaps with typhoid fever, with influenza, or with agranulocytic angina for example, and our diagnosis is tentatively substantiated by these peripheral blood findings.

In the same way in the lymphoid series, a sharp rise in lymphocytes bespeaks some pathologic process which may be of an infectious nature such as whooping cough or may suggest the onset of a leukemia. If these lymphocytes are immature and atypic in appearance, the possibility of infectious mononucleosis or of an acute leukemia is raised. Thus, from our examination of the numbers and kinds of circulating white cells in the peripheral blood stream, a considerable range of pathological lesions of a wide diversity of etiology may be indicated.

In similar fashion, a study of the red cell element circulating in the peripheral blood also is of great value in evaluating the nature of the underlying processes which may have induced any variation from the normal. The shape of the cell, the size of the cell as determined by the mean corpuscular volume,[1] the amount of hemoglobin which it contains, as measured by the color index,[2] and by the mean corpuscular hemoglobin concentration,[3] all are factors of extreme importance in demonstrating whether or not some disturbance of erythropoiesis is present. For example, in pernicious anemia, we find that there is marked variation in size (anisocytosis) and shape (poikilocytosis) of the individual cells; but the cells as a whole tend to be larger than normal (macrocytes), and to have a high color index and mean corpuscular hemoglobin concentration as well as a definitely increased mean corpuscular volume although the total count may be greatly reduced.

Another finding of significance is the presence of red cells which show metachromatic staining, indicative of the fact that they have not become completely filled with hemoglobin. Not infrequently accompanying such alteration in morphology of the erythrocytes, we find young forms evidenced by reticulocytes, normoblasts and even megaloblasts under certain conditions. With such abnormal cells in the peripheral blood, we may rest assured that we are dealing with some very fundamental disturbance of bone marrow activity. On the basis of these changes and staining reactions of the peripheral blood cells has been built up a method of classification of the various erythropoietic dyscrasias. This we will try to present in condensed and abbreviated form.

ERYTHROPOIESIS

Erythropoiesis (Fig. 521).—In order to thoroughly understand the changes which occur in respect to the red cells, it is necessary to review briefly the current theories regarding their genesis. This carries us back to a discussion of the origin of blood cells in general. There seems to be little question but what all investigators in this field accept the origin of all the bone marrow cells from the primitive reticuloendothelium. It would seem to serve no particular purpose to go at length into this complex problem other than to say that in general most hematologists to-day believe that the stem cell, or so-called "hemocytoblast," differentiates into three distinct parent cells, the lymphoblast, myeloblast and the monoblast, which in turn each gives rise to its own separate line of white cells. Most currently to-day it is believed that the red cells arise from the actual endothelial lining cells of the bone marrow sinusoids in direct descent from the reticulo-endothelium. This is accomplished by the longitudinal division of the cell, one of the newly-formed cells persisting as vascular endothelium; the other differentiating into a megaloblast. This may be identified by its large vesicular nucleus and its milky, bluish cytoplasm. From this point on, the cell, in the course of its maturation, decreases in size. The chromatin of the nucleus becomes condensed and the cytoplasm more definitely basophilic. This corresponds very closely to the pre- or promyelocyte phase in the development of the white cells. A large number of terms has been applied to this particular stage in the maturation of the red cell. Perhaps the best name to apply to the cell at this stage is the "early macroblast." This is a contraction of the more cumbersome "macroerythroblast." It is likewise spoken of as pre- or proerythroblast, or the pre- or pronormoblast by others.

The next stage of its differentiation is a still further diminution in its size with a rather characteristic arrangement of the chromatin in coarse, spoke-like masses, and a definite basophilic appearance of the cytoplasm. Preferably we feel this cell should be considered as a late maturation form of the megaloblast and simply labeled as a macroblast, but the terms "basophilic normoblast" or "erythroblast" are equally frequently found in the literature. Indeed, it seems to be entirely proper to utilize the term "megaloblast" for all three of these forms, considering them merely as developmental stages from the primitive, undifferentiated cell.

The next stage in the development of the adult

---

[1] The mean corpuscular volume is determined by the following equation:

$$\frac{\text{Hematocrit \% x 10}}{\text{No. of red cells in millions}} = 87 \text{ cubic micra (normal average)}$$

[2] The color index is equal to the following equation:

$$\frac{\% \text{ of hemoglobin}}{\% \text{ of red blood cells}} = 1.0 \text{ (normal average)}$$

[3] The mean corpuscular hemoglobin concentration is determined by the following equation:

$$\frac{\text{Grams of hemoglobin/100 c.c.}}{\text{Hematocrit \%}} \times 100 = 35\% \text{ (normal average)}$$

PLATE CXXI

FIG. 512.—MONOCYTES (ENDOTHELIOCYTES)—DEVELOP-
MENTAL FORMS

Left Column.—Cells 1 and 5.—Primitive monoblasts
(endothelioblasts).
Second Column.—Cells 2 and 6.—Mononuclear endotheliocytes (monocytes).
Third Column.—Cells 3 and 7.—Transitional forms of
monocytes.
Right Column.—Cells 4 and 8.—Segmented forms of
monocytes.

FIG. 513.—ACUTE MONOCYTIC LEUKEMIA (LEUKEMIC
RETICULOSIS)

Cells 1, 2, 3, 4 and 5.—Endotheliocytes (monocytes)
showing transitional and segmented forms.
Cell 6.—Small lymphocyte.
Cell 7.—Large lymphocyte.
Cell 8.—Segmented leukocyte.
Cell 9.—Platelets (thrombocytes).

FIG. 514.—MICROCYTIC, HYPOCHROMIC (SECONDARY)
ANEMIA

Cell 1.—Small lymphocyte.
Cell 2.—Segmented leukocyte.
Cells 3 and 4.—Micro-poikilocytes.
Cell 5.—Microcyte.
Cell 6.—Macrocyte.
Note tendency towards microcytosis on part of red
cells: Some anisocytosis, poikilocytosis and marked
achromia are present.

FIG. 515.—OVAL CELL ANEMIA (OVALOCYTOSIS)

Cells 1, 2 and 3 show marked polychromatophilia.
The red cells generally present a very unusual and
regular ovoid appearance with some slight tendency towards anisocytosis and poikilocytosis.

FIG. 516.—SICKLE CELL ANEMIA (MENISCOCYTOSIS)

Cells 1, 2, 3 and 4 represent normoblasts of rather typical large, intermediate and small forms.
Cell 5.—Sickle cell normoblast, a very rare finding.
Cell 6.—Polychromatophilic macroblast.
Cell 7.—Red cell—polychromatophilia.
As in preceding figure, the striking feature of the
blood film is the tendency towards "sickling" of the
red cells. Variations in size, shape and hemoglobin content are also prominent findings.

[*Courtesy of Dr. Walter J. Crocker, Philadelphia General Hospital—from Atlas of Hematology*
(*in preparation.*)]

PLATE CXXI

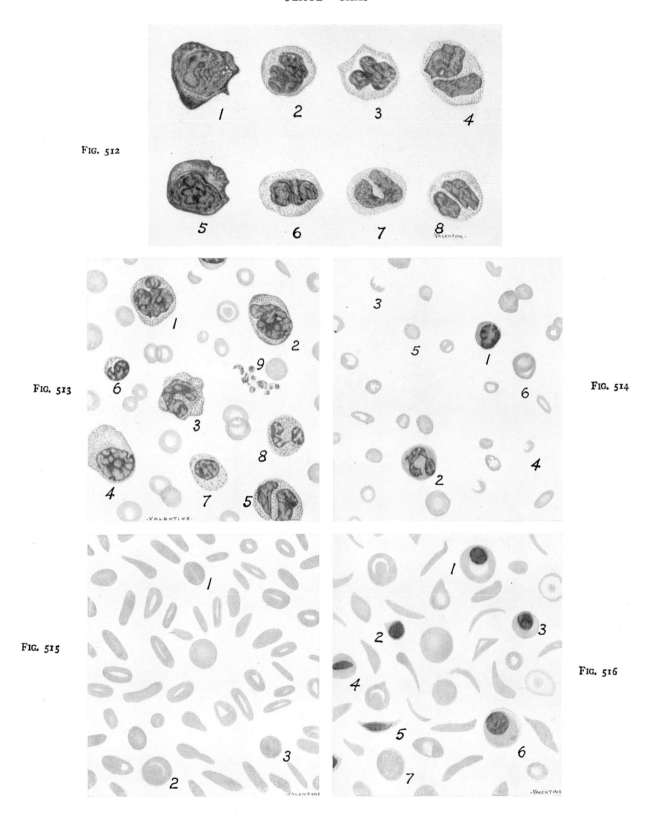

FIG. 512

FIG. 513

FIG. 514

FIG. 515

FIG. 516

red cell is seen as the typical "normoblast." At this stage, the cell has again decreased in size to approximately that of the ultimate red cell which it is forming. It contains a small, densely chromatic nucleus in which little or no arrangement of the chromatin material, as a rule, can be made out. This may be seen in varying sizes, depending to some extent upon whether the ultimate red cell is going to be a macrocyte, a normocyte or a microcyte. At this stage, the cell has accumulated hemoglobin, and for the first time, the cytoplasm appears of a typical orange-pink color in the usual stained preparation.

Gradually, the nucleus disappears from this normoblast either by fragmentation and extrusion of the chromatin material, or by absorption. In this nuclear-free phase, the cell can be demonstrated to contain a basophilic, reticular network when stained with vital dyes such as cresyl blue. This cell is termed the "reticulocyte."

Ultimately, this chromatic material disappears and the adult erythrocyte or normocyte emerges as the final maturation product.

PART I

THE ANEMIAS

We have already concerned ourselves with the neoplastic lesion of the red cell as exemplified by polycythemia vera, and so our further consideration of diseases of the red cell will largely be confined to a discussion of the various types of anemia which are encountered commonly clinically. The classification of the anemias has been a developmental story, and the older terminology of primary, secondary and idiopathic anemia has largely fallen into disuse.

However, in a field in which research is so active, and as our knowledge regarding the etiologic factors in the development of the various blood dyscrasias increases, it must be recognized that any classification is merely one of convenience rather than of an accurate and permanent nature. The following brief classification of the major anemias is followed in discussing the various types seen clinically and pathologically:

I. Anemias due to blood loss, or blood destruction
    A. Anemias due to hemorrhage
    B. Anemias due to hemolysis
        1. Hemolytic jaundice (familial jaundice)
        2. Anemia associated with infectious diseases
        3. Anemia resulting from chemical poisoning
            a. lead poisoning
        4. Sickle cell anemia (sicklemia; meniscocytosis)
            a. Oval cell anemia (ovalemia; ovalocytosis)
        5. Acute hemolytic anemia (Lederer)

II. Anemias due to depressed erythropoiesis
    A. Deficiency anemias
        1. Anemias due to iron deficiency
            a. Nutritional
            b. Defective storage of iron
            c. Defective absorption of iron
    B. Deficiency of the "Anti-anemic Factor"
        1. Pernicious anemia (Addison's anemia)
        2. Anemia associated with extensive gastric carcinoma
        3. Parasitic anemias
        4. Anemias associated with liver injury
        5. Toxic anemias, including the macrocytic anemia of pregnancy, etc.

    III. Miscellaneous "idiopathic" anemias
        A. Aplastic anemia
        B. Erythroblastic anemias of childhood
            1. Erythroblastosis fetalis (icterus gravis neonatorum)
            2. Erythroblastic anemia (Cooley's anemia; Mediterranean anemia)
            3. von Jaksch's anemia
        C. Banti's disease (splenic anemia)
    IV. Myelophthisic anemias

The above classification of the various common types of anemia is based largely upon the suggestions of Castle and Minot, as adapted to the requirements of this rather condensed exposition. Another method of classification is that based wholly upon the size, number and hemoglobin content of the cells. This has proved of considerable practical value, but is open to the criticism that it does not attempt in any way to show the etiologic relationship, which is well established in many forms of anemia. In general, the two methods of classification can be to a large degree correlated in that the great majority of anemias due to hemorrhage or hemolysis tend to be of the hypochromic, microcytic variety. Similarly, the deficiency anemias can be divided into two types: those being the result of iron deficiency likewise being of the hypochromic microcytic variety, while those which are the result of deficiency of either the intrinsic or extrinsic gastric "anti-anemic factor,"

through whatever cause, are similarly of the macrocytic and normochromic or even possibly the hyperchromic type. It is only in the miscellaneous group of anemias which are associated with varying degrees of bone marrow injury and disturbed function that this relationship to normochromic or hypochromic macrocytic or microcytic anemias fails to be apparent.

Finally, in respect to classification, the older terminology of primary, secondary and idiopathic still holds true in certain respects. By *primary anemia* in this older terminology were included pernicious or Addison's anemia, aplastic anemia and any other idiopathic anemia in which no recognized etiology could be established. All other anemias were broadly classified under the heading of *secondary anemia,* which included chiefly those anemias, the result particularly of chronic hemorrhage and of deficient iron intake, absorption or utilization.

Anemias Due to Blood Loss or Blood Destruction

Anemias Due to Hemorrhage.—The anemia which results from hemorrhage may be the result of a sudden loss of a large amount of blood or may occur in relation to some chronic seepage of blood associated with a wide range of lesions, including gastric ulcer, hemorrhoids, endometrial hyperplasia with its associated menorrhagia or metrorrhagia, or in relation to malignancy with its associated blood destruction and cachexia.

In the case of acute hemorrhage, the anemia depends obviously upon the amount of blood lost. The fluid balance is rapidly reëstablished so that estimation of the red cells and hemoglobin content of the blood shows proportional percentage values. This is followed within twenty-four to forty-eight hours by evidence of an actual hypochromic anemia with a stimulation of the entire bone marrow as evidenced by a rapid increase in both the red and white cells. The increase of hemoglobin does not keep pace with

the cell activity so that the count returns to normal well in advance of the corresponding hemoglobin return.

In the chronic type of hemorrhage in which small quantities of blood are lost over a long period of time, the same hypochromic picture is present as a result of actual exhaustion of the bone marrow, which may be actually hypoplastic and appear grossly relatively pale or fatty. There is likely to be marked variation in size and shape of the red cells with considerable poikilocytosis and a definitely diminished mean corpuscular hemoglobin content evidenced by central achromia in the blood film. Typically, there is likely to be a relative increase in size and numbers of the blood platelets. This is a common finding in most of the hypochromic microcytic forms of anemia, apparently as part of the defense mechanism to prevent further hemorrhage and blood loss.

PLATE CXXII
DISEASES OF THE HEMATOPOIETIC SYSTEM
Pernicious Anemia.—Case 219

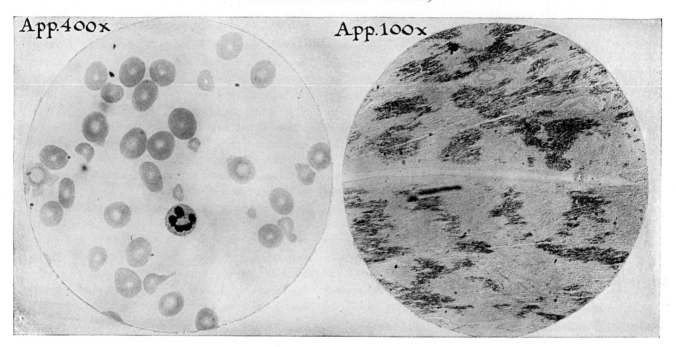

FIG. 517.—BLOOD FILM.—Note marked macrocytosis and poikilo-cytosis; also tendency toward hyperchromic staining of red cells, and the presence of a single multilobulated leukocyte symbolic of the usual leukopenia and shift to the right. (See also Plate CXXIII, Figs. 521, 523 and 524.)

FIG. 518.—HEART: FATTY DEGENERATION (OSMIC ACID TECH-NIQUE).—The fat is revealed as minute black-staining granules within the cytoplasm of the muscle fibers.

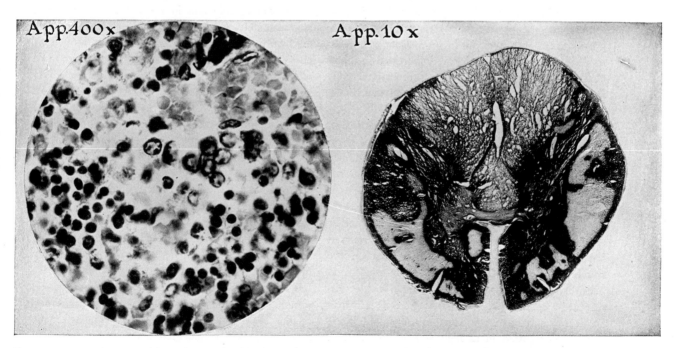

FIG. 519.—BONE MARROW.—Photomicrograph shows an area of active erythropoiesis in which several typical primitive early megaloblasts as well as more maturated forms of the red cells can be identified. App. 400 x.

FIG. 520.—SPINAL CORD: CORD DEGENERATION (WEIGERT MYELIN SHEATH STAIN).—Microtessar photograph which shows the characteristic irregular degeneration of the posterior column and lateral nerve tracts, which stand out as unstained areas as a result of the loss of their myelin. App. 10 x.

Anemias Due to Hemolysis.—HEMOLYTIC JAUNDICE (ACHOLURIC JAUNDICE; HAYEM-WIDAL SYNDROME; MICROSPHEROCYTOSIS; CHRONIC FAMILIAL JAUNDICE).—Hemolytic jaundice is both familial and hereditary in nature. It is characterized by persistent jaundice of variable degree and accompanied by a marked microcytic hypochromic anemia and enlargement of the spleen. The etiology of the disease is unknown, but the necessary elements to perpetuate the condition are successively transmitted according to Mendelian law. An interesting feature of this aspect is that successive generations are liable to show the disease in a more severe form. It was believed for some time that the disease occurred in two distinct forms: one as a hereditary type; the other as an acquired disease. To-day it is believed that the acquired picture occurring in the adult age group merely represents subclinical, latent hereditary cases activated by some acute infectious process.

The basic pathology of the disease consists of a markedly increased destruction of the red cells, chiefly in the spleen as the result of an inherent defect of the red cells themselves. This defect consists of a greatly increased fragility, which is utilized as a diagnostic procedure. Normally, red cells will not show hemolysis in salt solution until the concentration is reduced to approximately 0.45 per cent. In hemolytic jaundice, this hemolysis may begin in concentrations as high as 0.65 per cent. The red cells present a curious alteration in form, being relatively small in diameter but considerably increased in thickness. This is such a prominent feature that the cells are spoken of as "microspherocytes," and the disease is sometimes known as "microspherocytosis."

Clinically, these patients are often more or less able to carry on a normal existence. Many of them see their physician because of the persistent jaundice which shows periods of greater intensity corresponding to periods of greater hemolysis usually associated with some infectious condition or endocrine disturbance. The enlargement of the spleen may be another symptom which annoys them. In females, marked irregularities in respect to the menstrual cycle are common. In the more severe cases, gastro-intestinal disturbances which simulate at times gallbladder disease are seen. Indeed, such gallbladder disease may frequently accompany the condition, and gall stones have been reported in as high as sixty per cent in some series of cases. The anemia is relatively marked with a red count often between one and two million

cells. The white cells are likely to be increased and to show many young forms. The erythrocytes may show a number of nucleated red cells of the normoblast type, but the earlier, more immature cells apparently never are found in the peripheral blood in these cases. Reticulated red cells, however, increase to enormous proportions with counts of twenty, thirty, forty and fifty per cent reticulocytes being by no means uncommon. Additional laboratory findings of some help in establishing a diagnosis are seen in a high icterus index due to the increased bilirubin content of the blood, a positive indirect van den Bergh reaction and an increase of urobilin in both the urine and the stools.

The treatment of the disease is very spectacular. Splenectomy results almost regularly in a clinical cure. Examination of the blood, however, still shows very striking changes. There is no reversion apparently of the red cells to their normal form and microspherocytes persist. They show, almost immediately following the removal of the spleen, a marked improvement in respect to their fragility so that hemolysis may not begin when red cells are placed in varying strengths of a solution of sodium chloride until a percentage of 0.30 is reached. The fragility gradually tends to recur to a limited extent, but rarely approaches the former peak. There is a rapid rise in hemoglobin and in the red cell count until approximately normal numbers are reached. The mechanism is difficult to explain. The immediate effect obviously is the removal of a large amount of reticulo-endothelial tissue and the reduction correspondingly of the amount of hemolysis. As is well known, however, the rest of the reticulo-endothelial system rapidly assumes the functions of the spleen in cases of splenectomy for other conditions, and why relapse does not ultimately result is still a problem for study.

ANEMIAS ASSOCIATED WITH INFECTIOUS DISEASES AND ANEMIA RESULTING FROM CHEMICAL POISONING.—There is a group of similar hypochromic microcytic anemias of the formerly so-called "secondary" type which may follow a wide variety of infectious diseases or chemical poisonings. With few exceptions, no differential features of diagnostic significance can be established from an examination of the blood smear other than to emphasize the features already commented upon.

Lead Poisoning.—A notable exception to this is seen in the anemia associated with lead poisoning, particularly of a prolonged and chronic type. In such an anemia we find the usual diminution in size and numbers of the red cells. There is likewise the usual loss of hemoglobin. The color index may be as low as 0.6. Outstanding among the hematologic findings is the presence of what is spoken of as "basophilic stippling" of the red cells. The origin of this chromatic material is not clear. It certainly does not represent normal chromatin material as nothing comparable to this picture is seen in the normal maturation of the red cells either in the extrusion of the chromatin of the normoblastic nucleus, or in the chromatic material of the reticulocyte. Whether it may not represent an actual lead compound has been suspected. Not infrequently, other variations in the red cells may be seen, notably the presence of Howell-Jolly bodies and Cabot's ring bodies, although these latter are not so common. In addition to the basophilic stippling, there is a considerable degree of polychromatophilia in which the red cells still retain a good deal of their basophilic staining capacity not having yet become completely hemoglobinized.

Clinically, these cases are associated in the acute form with typical abdominal cramps, constipation and peripheral nerve neuritis. In the chronic form, the gastro-intestinal symptoms are often less severe. There characteristically develops a typical *"lead-line"* in the gums at the margin of the teeth.

In recapitulation, a hypochromic, microcytic anemia, associated with basophilic stippling, polychromatophilia, and the presence of a lead-line is diagnostic of lead poisoning.

SICKLE CELL ANEMIA (SICKLEMIA; MENISCO-CYTOSIS).—Sickle cell anemia is again one of the hereditary varieties of hemolytic anemia, which occurs almost entirely in the Negro race. A few instances of its occurrence in the other races have been recorded in which it was difficult to find any trace of possible inherited Negro blood. It is characterized by the presence of peculiar elongated and sickle-shaped red cells as Herrick first observed in 1910. These cells appear to be inherited in the same Mendelian ratio as the microspherocytes are in hemolytic jaundice. In smear preparations from the peripheral blood, the sickling phenomena can be accelerated by preparing hanging drop preparations and reducing the oxygen content of the specimen. It appears to be definitely a disease of red cells rather than of the plasma, as was originally suggested, but which has not been borne out by subsequent studies.

Just as in the case of hemolytic jaundice, the anemic exacerbations seem to be activated by infection. The symptoms are those of anemia with weakness, fatigability and general malaise. The degree depends upon the severity of the process. The lymph nodes tend to be somewhat enlarged as do the liver and spleen, but never to the same degree as seen in hemolytic jaundice. For some unexplained reason, the presence of superficial ulcerations of the skin over the foot and lower leg are very commonly seen in this condition.

The red count is usually somewhere in the vicinity of two million cells or more, although there are cases in which counts as low as one million have been recorded. In the acute stage, there is liable to be evidence of active erythropoiesis of the bone marrow as evidenced by the presence of large numbers of normoblasts and even megaloblasts (see Fig. 516). There is an associated rise in the white blood cells, the platelets and in the reticulocytes. The condition may exist in a relatively latent and almost subclinical form, as has been shown by the recognition of a large number of cases through routine blood examinations of the patients admitted to the hospital for other conditions.

From the pathological standpoint, very little of a specific nature exists. The most characteristic findings are seen in the spleen. Here there is a marked congestion with the pulp spaces and sinusoids packed with the sickled cells. Active hemolysis goes on as evidenced by hemosiderosis. As the acute crisis passes, a diffuse fibrosis of the spleen follows, not infrequently accompanied by the formation of the sidero-fibrotic nodules similar to those seen on occasion in the cases of so-called "Banti's disease." The other visceral changes are those of a severe anemia with particular emphasis to be laid upon the fatty degenerative changes of the heart muscle.

From the standpoint of treatment, splenectomy is not effective in this condition as it is in hemolytic jaundice. Likewise, the use of liver extract and iron is of only relative value. The disease, curiously enough, seems to grow less severe as the patient advances in age; and symptomatic supportive treatment, chiefly by the use of transfusions during the crisis, is about the only method of therapy known at the present time.

PLATE CXXIII

Fig. 521.—Red Cells—Maturation Forms from Bone Marrow

M.—Upper and middle rows, cells 1—10, represent the so-called "megaloblastic" series of red blood cells terminating in macrocytes, as obtained from pernicious anemic bone marrow.

N.—Lower row, cells 11—15, "normoblastic" red cells maturing as normocytes as obtained from normal or the usual secondary anemia type of marrow.

Cells 1, 6 and 11.—Megaloblasts
    (M series Megaloblast A—N series Normoblast A)
Cells 2, 7 and 12.—Early macroblasts
    (M series Megaloblast B—N series Normoblast B)
Cells 3, 8 and 13.—Late macroblasts (erythroblasts)
    (M series Megaloblast C—N series Normoblast C)
Cells 4, 9 and 14.—Normoblasts
    (M series Megaloblast D—N series Normoblast D)
Cells 5, 10 and 15.—Erythrocytes
    (M series Macrocyte—N series Normocyte)

In view of the enormous confusion which exists today in respect to nomenclature of the various stages of the red cell developmental forms, the older, simplified, progressive, schematic presentation has been adopted for convenience, until such time as the newer classification becomes more firmly established, the later terms being given in parentheses.

Fig. 522.—Erythroblastic Anemia (Cooley's)

Cells 1 and 2.—Polychromatophilic macroblasts (early).
Cells 3 and 4.—Polychromatophilic macroblasts (late).
Cell 5.—Normoblast.
Cells 6, 7 and 8.—Polychromatophilic erythrocytes.
Cell 9.—Poikilocyte.

There is a tendency towards macrocytosis and hypochromia of the red cells.

Fig. 523.—Macrocytic, Hyperchromic (Pernicious, Primary) Anemia

Cell 1.—Early macroblast (Megaloblast "B").
Cell 2.—Late macroblast (Megaloblast "C").
Cell 3.—Early macroblast (Megaloblast "B").
Cell 4.—Multilobed segmented leukocyte.
Cell 5.—Red cell—"basophilic stippling."
Cell 6.—Macrocyte.
Cells 7 and 8.—Poikilocytes.
Cell 9.—Polychromatophilic erythrocyte.
Cell 10.—Normocyte.

Note tendency towards macrocytosis and intensity of staining of hemoglobin within red cells. Marked poikilocytosis of the red cells is a feature. Presence of early nucleated red cells, and of multi-lobulated segmented leukocytes is significant.

Fig. 524.—Pernicious (Primary) Macrocytic Anemia

The striking feature is the tremendous increase of reticulocytes (cells 1—10), often up to as high as 15%. Red cells tend to be hyperchromic, and macrocytic. A variable amount of anisocytosis and poikilocytosis is present. Reticulocytes stained vitally with Brilliant Cresyl Blue.

[Courtesy of Dr. Walter J. Crocker, Philadelphia General Hospital—from Atlas of Hematology (in preparation).]

PLATE CXXIII

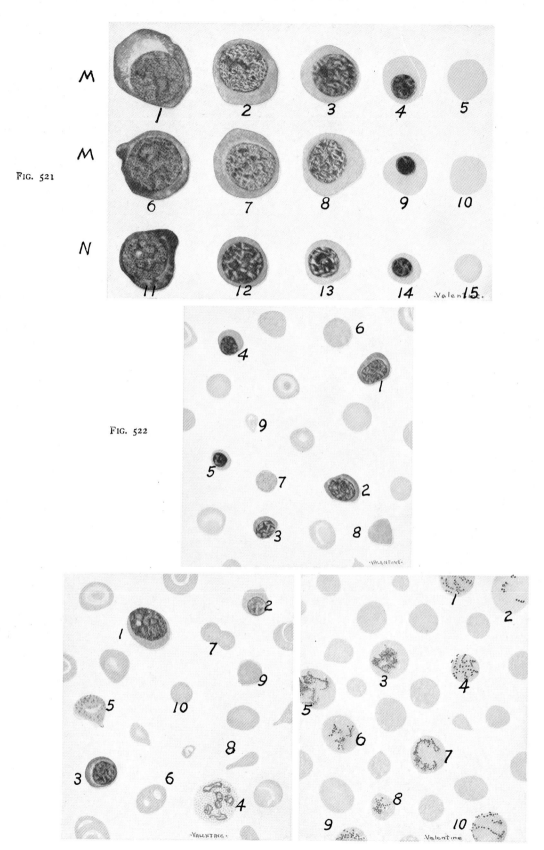

FIG. 521

FIG. 522

FIG. 523

FIG. 524

ILLUSTRATIVE CASE

CASE 217. (Ref. #S-353)

Diagnosis.—Sickle cell anemia; Lymphogranuloma-inguinale (refer back to Chapter XVII.)

Patient was a Negress of 44 years, admitted to the hospital in a state of marked mental confusion following a fainting attack.

Present Illness.—The patient herself was too ill to question and the history which was obtained was provided by her brother. As nearly as he could tell, his sister had been "ailing" for two or three months before the present illness. She had complained of easy fatigability and a feeling of weakness in her legs and arms. She had had definite gastro-intestinal attacks with some nausea and occasional vomiting. She complained of constipation and required frequent laxatives. Three days before admission, she fainted and when she recovered consciousness, she was apparently markedly disoriented and almost maniacal in her speech. She was examined by a physician who thought that she probably had a metastatic cerebral lesion from a neoplasm of the rectum and referred her to the hospital for diagnosis and treatment.

Past Medical History.—Her previous medical history was very unsatisfactory as her brother had only recently moved to this city and did not know much of what had happened to his sister for the preceding ten years. So far as he knew, she was one of seven children, all of whom had all the usual childhood diseases. He did not know of any serious illness which she had ever had which required hospitalization, and believed that he would have been informed if such a thing had occurred.

Physical Examination.—Patient was a fairly well developed, but cachectic-appearing middle-aged, acutely ill Negress. Head showed no deformities. Eyes: Pupils were sluggish; conjunctivae were extremely pale. Tongue was thickened and rather beefy in appearance. Cervical lymph nodes showed moderate enlargement. Chest was symmetrical. Heart and lungs seemed within normal limits on percussion and auscultation. Blood pressure 120/80. Abdomen was essentially negative. Gynecologic examination revealed a white vaginal discharge and marked stenosis of the entire vaginal canal. Rectal examination showed incontinence. There was an irregular hard annular mass palpated in the rectum about a finger's breadth above the anal orifice. This had caused a very marked stenosis. Extremities were negative. Reflexes were normal. Mental examination showed a marked disorientation and confusion.

Laboratory Findings.—Red blood cells, 2,590,000 with 45% hemoglobin (6 grams). White blood cells, 8,150 with 47% polynuclears, 45% lymphocytes, 2% monocytes, 5% eosinophiles and 1% basophiles. Examination of the smear (Fig. 516) showed moderate anisocytosis, poikilocytosis, achromia and an almost universal sickling of the red cells. There were five nucleated red cells found in counting one hundred white blood cells. The fragility was within normal limits, beginning at 0.42% and being complete at 0.34%. Coagulation and bleeding times normal. Platelet count was considerably reduced, the count averaging on several occasions approximately 50,000. The mean corpuscular hemoglobin was 47 micro micrograms and the mean corpuscular volume 95 cubic micra. Urinalysis showed markedly increased albumin with a relatively high specific gravity of 1.022. The sediment contained a few red cells. Wassermann and Kahn tests were negative. Blood chemistry studies were negative.

Subsequent Course.—The patient went rapidly down hill in spite of all that could be done for her. A presumptive diagnosis of rectal stricture and ulcerative proctitis due to lymphogranuloma inguinale, and sickle cell anemia was made. She developed marked nuchal rigidity and a lumbar puncture was done which was essentially negative. This was thought to be the result of a toxic meningismus. The patient died one week after admission.

Autopsy Findings.—There were several areas of softening found in the brain associated with thrombotic lesions of the middle cerebral vessels. The viscera as a whole other than a very marked anemia with corresponding fatty degenerative changes showed very little specific pathology. The heart was somewhat dilated and extremely flabby in consistency with marked fatty change. There was an old chronic enlargement of the inguinal lymph nodes bilaterally, associated with the vaginal stenosis and the rectal stricture. This microscopically showed a typical chronic granulomatous proctitis, presumably in the nature of a lymphopathia venereum.

Oval Cell Anemia (Ovalemia; Ovalocytosis).—This might be considered as a variant of the picture of sickle cell anemia. It is a rare form of similar nature, hereditary in character and of a like hemolytic type. The clinical course is similar to that of the sickle cell variety with occasional exacerbations or crises characterized by a blood picture in which active hematopoiesis is evidenced. The diagnosis is made entirely upon the finding of the characteristic oval-shaped erythrocytes in the peripheral blood (Fig. 515). No recognized therapy exists other than the symptomatic supportive palliative measures used in sickle cell anemia.

ACUTE HEMOLYTIC ANEMIA (LEDERER).—A variety of hemolytic anemia of an acute nature was first described by Lederer in 1925 and bears his name. It is a rare condition seen usually in childhood. It is characterized clinically by a sudden onset with gastro-intestinal symptoms and generalized enlargement of the liver, spleen and lymph nodes. The blood picture is that of a very severe hyperchromic microcytic anemia with marked polychromatophilia and variation in the size and shape of the red cells. Megaloblasts are found in large numbers and there is liable to be a high white count with many immature myeloid cells suggesting a leukemia. It is thought that the cause of this condition is probably of some infectious toxic nature. Recovery is the rule if the condition is recognized, and repeated small transfusions are given the patient to supply the antihemolytic factor. Occasionally cases may go on to an exhaustion of the bone marrow with a terminal leukopenia. The differential diagnosis of this condition lies really in the realm of clinical pathology as there is nothing characteristic about the actual pathological changes found in the blood-forming organs.

Anemias Due to Depressed Erythropoiesis

Deficiency Anemias.—ANEMIAS DUE TO IRON DEFICIENCY.—a. Nutritional; b. Defective Storage of Iron; and c. Deficient Intake of Iron.—In general, the group of anemias which are seen as a result of iron deficiency corresponds to the older terminology of secondary anemia. As has been emphasized in the classification, this deficiency may be the result of a wide variety of etiologic factors, the basis of them all being apparently associated with some nutritional disturbance which results in inability of the individual to absorb iron even although it is taken in excess of the hematopoietic needs as measured by the normal individual; or to a defective mechanism in respect to the metabolism and storage of iron, particularly as relating to liver function; or finally, actually due to a deficient intake of iron in the diet. This group of anemias is seen at all ages, but especially in infants who have been on a prolonged bottle diet, in women during pregnancy as the result of the increased demands of the fetus, and in relation to chronic gastro-intestinal disturbances which may be associated with infections, or simply of a functional nature as the result of achlorhydria.

The clinical picture in all of these cases is relatively comparable. There is a varying degree of pallor of the skin and mucous membranes associated with weakness, easy fatigability, nervous irritability and a variable train of gastro-intestinal symptoms. There is usually no enlargement of the liver, spleen or lymph nodes.

The diagnosis is established on the basis of the history plus an examination of the peripheral blood. The recognition of the general nature of the anemic process as one resulting from depressed marrow function is comparatively simple to establish. There is a variable drop in the total red count, which may range from two to four million cells. This is typically accompanied by a parallel drop in the hemoglobin. There is a considerable variation in size and shape of the cells with microcytes predominating. The presence of polychromatophilia and reticulated red cells can usually be established. The platelets are likely to be moderately increased both in size and numbers. In general, the blood picture may be described as a *hypochromic microcytic type of anemia*. To subdivide these cases on an etiological basis, it becomes necessary to delve fully into the clinical history.

The treatment in all instances consists first of the elimination of the cause of the condition if it can be recognized. In addition, bone marrow stimulation is indicated with the use of iron. The iron requirement of the normal individual is roughly one milligram daily, but this is inadequate in the case of children during the growth period and similarly in women during pregnancy. Iron taken by mouth has to be acted upon by the gastric juices in the duodenum before its absorption is possible. A great diversity of opinion exists regarding the most useful form in which iron should be administered. Simple reduced iron seems to be the least effective. Blaud's ferrous carbonate tablets are among the most popular. More recently the ferrous salts have been shown to be possibly more effective because of their greater absorption, but the ferric salts are often more readily tolerated. In cases with achlorhydria, the supplemental use of hydrochloric acid is definitely indicated and on the chance that there may be some deficiency from the standpoint of the intrinsic gastric factor under such circumstances, the use of liver extract is likewise very generally employed.

Chlorosis.—Among the various forms of such hypochromic microcytic anemia might be mentioned particularly the condition known as chlorosis. This is a condition which usually occurs in adolescent or young women. It used to be a very commonly encountered picture, but in recent years typical cases of true chlorosis are rarely encountered. In view of our more recent knowledge regarding the mechanism and etiology of these various forms of hypochromic anemia, it is believed that chlorosis merely represents one of these varieties of nutritional anemia.

ILLUSTRATIVE CASE

CASE 218. (Ref. #S-355)

Diagnosis.—Idiopathic hypochromic microcytic anemia.
Patient was a white woman of 45 years, admitted to
the hospital with the chief complaint of cough, anorexia
and weakness.

Present Illness.—The patient stated she felt in her
usual good health until approximately one month before
admission when she developed a cold and sore throat accompanied by generalized muscle pain and a feeling of
marked malaise. She developed anorexia and had several
attacks of nausea during one of which she vomited. She
remained in bed for about ten days with the aching pains
of her bones and muscles continuing. She became progressively weaker. About one week before admission she
began to develop a productive cough raising a considerable amount of white mucoid material. This was accompanied by a sharp pain in her right chest which was
increased with inspiration.

Past Medical History.—The patient had all the usual
childhood diseases. She did not recall having had rheumatic fever, however. She was particularly susceptible
to colds and bronchitis and had had several such attacks
almost every year, which had been accompanied by a
cough lasting for five or six weeks. She had likewise had
several attacks of acute tonsillitis but had always refused
operation. Her family history was negative for tuberculosis. The patient's mother had had hay fever. A review
of her systems otherwise was non-informatory.

Physical Examination.—The patient was a fairly well
developed and nourished middle-aged woman who appeared more than her given age. Her lips were slightly
cyanotic. Head was negative. Eyes reacted normally.

Tongue was beefy-red in places and coated in other
areas. Chest was symmetrical. There was no evidence of
consolidation, but there were a few crackling râles at
both bases. Heart was not enlarged. There were no murmurs. There was a hard mass felt in the right breast.
Abdomen was negative. Extremities were negative.

Laboratory Findings.—Red blood count ranged during her stay in the hospital from 3,060,000 to 4,200,000
with her hemoglobin climbing from 9.5 to 11.5 grams.
White blood cells were 8,300 on admission with 72%
polynuclears. This remained relatively constant. Color
index was 0.74. The mean corpuscular hemoglobin was
21 micro micrograms and the mean corpuscular volume
76 cubic micra. There was a moderate amount of anisocytosis with microcytes predominating. There was very
little poikilocytosis. Rare, nucleated red cells were seen in
the blood films (Fig. 514). Blood chemistry studies were
negative. The albumin/globulin ratio was normal. Wassermann was negative. Urinalysis on several occasions
was essentially negative.

X-ray findings showed no evidence of any active pulmonary disease. Two calculi were found in the gallbladder region.

Subsequent Course.—A diagnosis of an idiopathic
hypochromic microcytic anemia resulting probably from
a combination of acute upper respiratory infection coupled
with chronic cholelithiasis was made. The patient was
placed on iron therapy and showed marked improvement
during her stay in the hospital. Therapy was to be continued and the patient was to be kept under observation
in the out-patient clinic until her blood picture had returned to normal.

Deficiency of the "Anti-anemic Factor."—PERNI-
CIOUS ANEMIA (ADDISON'S ANEMIA).—The condition commonly known as pernicious anemia was first
described by Addison nearly a century ago, and is
very generally known throughout the world as Addisonian anemia. The name pernicious anemia or
primary pernicious anemia was given to it in this
country because of the apparently inevitable fatal
outcome of the cases. It was considered as a chronic
progressive disease with periods of remission and relapse, ending sooner or later fatally.

Clinically, the cases showed an achlorhydria,
marked gastro-intestinal disturbances, a very profound anemia with a rather characteristic, ashy-gray,
sallow appearance of the skin, loss of weight and in
some instances marked neurologic symptoms particularly relating to the posterior columns of the spinal
cord.

The term, "pernicious anemia," no longer describes the condition, but it has been so well established in medical literature that its use will probably
continue for many years. To-day, as the result of
the brilliant work of Minot, Murphy, Castle, Whip-

ple, Sturgis and Isaacs, the problem of pernicious
anemia has been solved so far as the clinical side of
the question is concerned. We still have a totally
inadequate conception of the activating mechanism
etiologically which interferes with the normal production of the intrinsic gastric factor. Whether this
is wholly hereditary or whether it may be metabolic
or infectious in nature has not yet been convincingly
demonstrated. Briefly stated, the theory regarding
the mechanism of the development of pernicious anemia to-day is based on the principle that it belongs in
the nutritional deficiency group of anemias.

Hematopoiesis is apparently regulated by an "anti-
anemic factor" manufactured in the stomach and
stored in the liver where it can be withdrawn as
needed to maintain the normal level of red cells. In
the stomach the formation of this "anti-anemic factor" is dependent upon the interaction of an "extrinsic factor" derived from the food and an "intrinsic factor," which is produced by the mucosa of the
stomach. Thus, the picture of pernicious anemia may
result when either the "extrinsic factor" or the "intrinsic factor" is lacking. In general, this deficiency

is seen in respect to the "intrinsic factor." This in turn is definitely related to the almost invariable achylia which is seen in the typical case of pernicious anemia. It is further substantiated by the fact that the disease can be prevented or recovery can be effected by the administration of normal gastric mucosa. More recently, the ingenious experiments of Castle have shown further that remission and recovery can ensue by the administration of normal gastric juice and meat in the diet, which is known to contain the "extrinsic factor." Thus, the picture of pernicious anemia may result from some unrecognized idiopathic etiology or may be seen in association with extensive destructive lesions of the stomach such as are found as the result of carcinoma or the resection of the organ. There appears to be a factor of safety in this respect in that the mucous membrane of the first portion of the duodenum may be able to maintain this "anti-anemic factor" production in the absence of the stomach in such operative cases.

Pernicious anemia is usually a disease of middle life and is seen especially in the temperate zones, chiefly in males, and in the white race almost exclusively. It has been described as representing one of the rather characteristic constitutional diseases and for this reason the possibility of some hereditary distribution of the cases is suggested.

The diagnosis of pernicious anemia is made primarily upon the blood findings, but in conjunction with the clinical history, as it must be remembered that anemias with a similar blood picture may result from other causes. The blood picture typically is that of a macrocytic, normo or hyperchromic anemia. Not only are the red cells generally larger than normal, but they show a markedly increased mean corpuscular volume and hemoglobin content. This is more roughly measured by the color index, which typically is well above the normal figure of 1.0. The red cells tend to be reduced in numbers to unusually low figures, frequently to a million or less. The hemoglobin on the other hand may be relatively high in respect to the number of red cells. Examination of the blood film shows extreme anisocytosis and poikilocytosis with the majority of the cells tending to be frankly macrocytes. Polychromatophilia (Fig. 517, 523 and 524), stippling and the presence of Howell-Jolly bodies and Cabot's ring bodies are often found. There is a striking tendency for the poikilocytes to have a long tail-like process. Typi-

cally, nucleated red cells are present in relatively large numbers. Megaloblasts are seen almost regularly, and indeed many hematologists will not definitely establish a diagnosis of pernicious anemia without their demonstration. They occur, at times, in what is spoken of as "showers" representing crises in the erythropoietic activity. From the white cell side of the picture, very little of help is to be derived. There is a rather striking tendency for a leukopenia to occur and for the granulocytes to show a marked shift to the right, with multilobulated nuclei, often as high as eight or more. On the other hand, these features are often absent, and indeed in the active phase associated with a blast crisis there may even be a leukocytosis and a shift to the left. More notable is a tendency for eosinophilia to occur.

The pathology of pernicious anemia is characterized by several lesions, none of them completely specific, but in combination, extremely important from the standpoint of differential diagnosis. In the first place, there are the changes associated with the actual anemia itself. These include a curious lemon yellow color of the subcutaneous and body fat, the most striking instance of "tigroid" fatty degeneration of the heart muscle (Fig. 518) and pallor of all the tissues. In the second place, there is a rather characteristic atrophic gastritis with small, short glands which seem hypoplastic in appearance. This is frequently accompanied by a moderate submucous chronic mononuclear inflammatory cellular infiltration. In the third place, the very suggestive degeneration of the postero-lateral columns of the spinal cord (Fig. 520) in about a third of the cases, especially in the absence of a positive Wassermann is almost in itself diagnostic. Indeed this may occur before the typical anemia in some instances. It is thought that this neurologic part of the picture may be constitutional and hereditary in nature, just as the achylia seems to be, and that in this respect it may well be a deficiency not in the usual "extrinsic" or "intrinsic" gastric factors, but in one of the vitamins, probably B., in the diet.

Incidental pathologic findings are those of a marked glossitis with atrophy of the papillae and a smooth, shiny mucosal surface, especially on the lateral margins. Moderate enlargement of the spleen often is seen with some hemosiderosis. There is no enlargement of the lymph nodes. The liver may or may not show some enlargement. It is usually of a rather golden brown color due to increased pigmentary infiltration. The Kupffer cells particularly show this pigmentation, but the parenchymatous cells of the liver, especially centrally in the lobule are also often involved in the process.

And finally, microscopically a study of the hematopoietic system reveals a bone marrow which shows active blood regeneration. The bone marrow of the long bones (Fig. 519) is usually of a port red color and of a somewhat gelatinous consistency due to the erythropoiesis. This is in contradistinction to the usually fatty, fibrous yellowish-gray marrow of the same age group. Islands of active erythropoiesis can be recognized and the young red cell forms seen in the sinuses as well as forming part of the regenerative islands.

From the standpoint of treatment, let it suffice to say that while our knowledge concerning this disease is still in the experimental stage, the use of the "anti-anemic factor" in the form of some one of the many varieties of liver extract is probably the most effective method. Supplementing this may likewise be used gastric mucosal extracts. In the milder forms, this anti-anemic factor can possibly be supplied by dietary measures supplementing the routine diet by liver, kidneys and other visceral food, such as calves' brains, sweetbreads and the like. With relapse, more intensive parenteral therapy may be required and in the light of our present knowledge, inasmuch as no knowledge of the etiology of the disease exists, the therapy must be considered in the light of a replacement therapy, and must be maintained for the rest of the patient's life.

ILLUSTRATIVE CASE

CASE 219. (Ref. #S-354)
Diagnosis.—Bone marrow, pernicious anemia.
Patient was a female of 49 years, admitted to the hospital with the chief complaint of unsteadiness of gait and a squirming sensation in the calves of her legs.
Present Illness.—The patient for many years had had vague gastric symptoms with marked anorexia. She had been told that she had anemia and had been taking some sort of "tonic" for years. Six years before admission, she had a severe illness precipitated by a fainting spell. This was followed by apparent paralysis of all four extremities. She was hospitalized at that time and received some form of intramuscular therapy. Following this, the function of her extremities gradually returned over a period of several months. There was a remission of her symptoms of approximately three years' duration. At that time there was a recurrence of the anemia and gastro-intestinal symptomatology. She had a very severe anemia, which was apparently of the pernicious macrocytic type. She received liver therapy at that time and again showed a complete remission of symptoms.

Her present illness was ushered in by a repetition of her original symptoms. There was marked anorexia and the sight of food produced nausea. She had vomited on several occasions and had had marked diarrhea. This was followed by a fever reaching 104°. Her unsteadiness of gait had recurred, and she showed marked weakness of her lower extremities, requiring assistance to walk. She complained of a squirming sensation in the calves of her legs and likewise had noticed that she had developed a very sallow appearance.
Past Medical History.—The patient stated that she had been a strong, healthy child. She had had measles and whooping cough. She never had had any serious illness or operation other than the train of symptoms relating to her present illness. She had been married and had had six children, four of whom were living and well; two of whom had died in infancy. A review of her systems showed little of significance except in relation to her gastro-intestinal tract. She had had intermittent, vague, gastro-intestinal symptoms at intervals over the

six year period. She had no symptoms referable to her genito-urinary system or reproductive organs. Menopause occurred with the onset of her present illness.
Physical Examination.—Patient was a white, middle-aged woman who appeared considerably older than her stated age. She appeared apathetic. She was well-developed, somewhat obese and had a very flabby musculature. Her skin had a yellowish, ashy-gray color but no cyanosis. Hair was gray. Eyes, ears, nose and throat were negative, except for pallor of the mucous membranes. The tongue had a curious pale, pink color with atrophy of the papillae and was extremely smooth, particularly along the lateral margins. Thorax was symmetrical. No cardiac or pulmonary abnormalities were detected. Abdomen was obese and pendulous. No viscera or masses could be felt. The extremities: The patellar reflexes were both absent. There was a positive bilateral Babinski. There was marked muscle weakness of both legs.
Laboratory Findings.—Red blood cells 1,500,000 with 5.3 gm. of hemoglobin. White blood cells, 2,800. The stained film presented the typical picture of macrocytic pernicious anemia. There was extreme anisocytosis, poikilocytosis, moderate basophilic stippling and polychromatophilia (Fig. 523), and a prominent shift to the right of her neutrophile index. Repeated gastric analyses showed a very low total acid curve and a complete achlorhydria. Urinalysis was negative. Wassermann was negative. Spinal fluid was negative.
Subsequent Course.—She was given liver extract parenterally and put on a typical "anti-anemic" diet. Her reticulocytes were followed carefully day by day. On admission, the count was only 1%, but within forty-eight hours, the count had risen to 12%. This dropped again and continued at a level of 1 to 2% for the remainder of her illness. Under intensive therapy, the sensory disturbances of her lower extremities disappeared, but her gait still remained unsteady and she developed a Romberg sign.

Her blood picture improved steadily under therapy, the red cells rising to as high as 3,500,000 and her hemoglobin to 8.5 gm. with the white blood cells likewise increasing to 8,900 with 67% polynuclears. The fragility test was normal. Icterus index gave an indirect van den Bergh of 0.5 mgm. per 100 c.c. Sedimentation time was 29 mm. in 40 minutes. On admission, her mean corpuscular hemoglobin content was 34 micro micrograms and her mean corpuscular volume was 98 cubic micra. Terminally, the patient developed an acute infection with a septicemia.

Autopsy Findings.—The chief pathological findings of significance were those of an extremely hyperplastic red bone marrow, extensive fatty degeneration of the heart, and atrophic gastritis, and postero-lateral sclerosis of the spinal cord—all of diagnostic significance as component parts of the picture of pernicious anemia. The heart presented a typical tigroid mottling comparable to that seen in Fig. 518, which is best brought out by osmic acid staining histologically. This was more striking in respect to the papillary muscles and musculature of the left ventricle. The pathological findings relating to the spinal cord are similar to those seen in tabes dorsalis and will be considered in the chapter on central nervous degenerative lesions. There is nothing characteristic in respect to the atrophic gastritis to warrant an additional description other than the general discussion to be found in Chapter XLVI (Gastro-intestinal Pathology).

Microscopic Description of a Section of Bone Marrow (Sternal Biopsy).—(Fig. 519) Histologic examina-

All Other Forms of Macrocytic Anemia.—
ANEMIA ASSOCIATED WITH EXTENSIVE GASTRIC CARCINOMA; PARASITIC ANEMIAS; ANEMIAS ASSOCIATED WITH LIVER INJURY; TOXIC ANEMIAS.—Other conditions, as has been indicated in the classification of the anemias, may give rise to a comparable macrocytic hyperchromic anemia. These include conditions such as sprue, pellagra, *Diphyllobothrium latum* infestation, advanced carcinoma of the stomach, surgical operations with extensive gastric resections, certain cases seen in the latter half of pregnancy, and the like. These are all essentially diseases which are again dependent upon some break in the production or storage of the "anti-anemic factor." We have seen in typical pernicious anemia that the usual cause is a deficiency in the intrinsic factor. This is likewise true in those cases associated with extensive gastric pathology. In respect to the

tion of bone marrow sections shows it to be extremely rich in cells. All varieties of nucleated red blood cells are encountered. There are some with deeply stained nuclei, the cytoplasm rich in hemoglobin. These are easily recognized as normoblasts. Other cells somewhat larger in size, but still containing hemoglobin are recognized by the pinkish color of their cytoplasm and the heavy, striated arrangement of the nuclear chromatin. These appear to represent late macroblasts.

In addition, under high power, numerous islands of active hematopoiesis may be found in which the early basophilic staining macroblasts and megaloblasts may be identified. Both the characteristic macroblastic, heavily chromatic nucleus and the larger more delicate reticular nucleus of the earlier megaloblast will be found in these cells. Stained by the usual hematoxylin and eosin method, it is impossible to differentiate with any degree of certainty some of these earlier megaloblasts from cells of the myeloid series, but with special staining methods, particularly Custer's modification of the May Grünwald technique, these differences may be more readily observed. The characteristic appearance of these cells by such staining technique may be observed in the colored Fig. 521 and 523.

It is worthy of emphasis that, in the bone marrow removed at autopsy following intensive liver therapy, it was extremely difficult to find megaloblasts as compared to the biopsy during the height of the clinical picture.

various infectious and parasitic varieties of such anemia, the deficiency would seem more particularly to be associated with disturbances in the absorption of the "anti-anemic factor" or in the abence of the "extrinsic gastric factor." In those cases associated with severe liver damage, the storage capacity for the "anti-anemic factor" is destroyed and as a result the control of normal hematopoiesis is interfered with.

From the standpoint of pathology, these various conditions must be considered separately on their etiologic bases, as obtained from the history and other laboratory studies. The blood picture is, in many instances, most confusing in respect to pernicious anemia. Like pernicious anemia, the therapy in this entire group of cases consists of the administration of the "anti-anemic factor" coupled with the removal of the etiologic factor if it is possible.

Miscellaneous "Idiopathic" Anemias

Aplastic Anemia.—Aplastic anemia is a rare form of anemia of which the etiology is unknown. It is characterized by a complete suppression of marrow activity with a resultant rapidly fatal course as a rule, the patient only surviving during the life of the already existent red cells in the peripheral blood. The development of the condition may be relatively insidious over a considerable period of time, but with

a progressive depression of marrow activity until complete suppression supervenes. The cases occur at all ages, but are seen most frequently in young adults.

The diagnosis, in general, is made by examination of the peripheral blood film. It is characterized typically by the presence of a diminished number of red cells, which may toward the end of the disease reach as low a figure as eight hundred thousand. These cells, however, are essentially normal in shape, size and hemoglobin content and the anemia is directly proportional to the drop in the number of cells. There is nothing to suggest a hemolytic process. The white cells are equally affected as the reds, so that the neutrophiles may almost completely disappear from the blood leaving only a small number of lymphocytes, which probably are derived from other sources than the bone marrow.

Pathologically the picture is again one of severe anemia with all the fatty degenerative changes of the viscera which one might expect in association with such anoxemia. Bone marrow is usually, even in children, of a fatty, fibrous nature with only scattered islands of erythropoiesis.

The treatment of this condition is wholly unsatisfactory. By the use of repeated transfusions the patient may be kept alive for a considerable period of time. There is no response to the use of the ordinary anti-anemic agents including liver extract, or iron in any form.

Erythroblastic Anemias of Childhood.—In infancy and childhood, there is a group of anemias characterized particularly by the presence of erythroblastosis. These fall into three subvarieties from the clinical standpoint fairly readily, but are extremely difficult to differentiate in respect to the blood findings alone. All three of these blood pictures are characterized essentially by the presence of large numbers of nucleated red cells and the various intermediate forms in the course of the development of the adult erythrocyte, including reticulocytes and red cells still showing polychromatophilia, stippling, Howell-Jolly bodies and Cabot's ring bodies. The picture is apparently one of generalized active hematopoiesis so that the white cell series is also very likely to be involved, and immature white cells in the nature of juveniles and even myelocytes are seen in large numbers. The white blood cells may arise as high as 75,000 to 100,000. From the blood picture alone, the differentiation from a leukemia in childhood is at times difficult, and as is so frequently true in establishing the diagnosis of any anemia, a complete knowledge of the history and physical findings in respect to the individual patient are quite as necessary as an analysis of the peripheral blood picture.

ERYTHROBLASTOSIS FETALIS (ICTERUS GRAVIS NEONATORUM).—In this condition, the infant may be jaundiced at birth, and invariably goes on to the development of a very severe progressive jaundice. This is accompanied by petechial hemorrhages in the skin, slight enlargement of the liver and spleen, and by a very marked anemia with the characteristic erythroblastosis already described. A great many of these cases go on to fatal exodus within the first few days of life. Others, in whom the picture is not as pronounced, may recover under repeated small transfusions. Not infrequently, this condition seems to be familial in nature and to be associated with a congenital defect in the development of the biliary tract, with a congenital atresia of the common duct. Refer to Case 202 (Ref. #S-336, Chapter XLVIII).

ERYTHROBLASTIC ANEMIA (COOLEY'S ANEMIA; MEDITERRANEAN ANEMIA).—This is a variety of erythroblastic anemia which is seen almost exclusively in children of Mediterranean parents. It is characterized by moderate enlargement of the spleen and lymph nodes and irregularly of the liver. The facies present a curious Mongolian appearance due to rather characteristic bone changes affecting the skull. The disease runs a prolonged chronic course, and in the reported cases ultimately ends fatally as a rule. Splenectomy has been done in a number of instances and seems to be effective in prolonging life, but not in influencing the underlying processes.

The blood findings in this disease are not as striking as in the erythroblastosis fetalis. A hypochromic picture is likely to be present rather than the hyperchromic features of erythroblastosis fetalis. Normoblasts and reticulocytes occur in large numbers. Only rarely are megaloblasts found in the peripheral blood.

The pathology of erythroblastic anemia is particularly striking in involving the long bones and the bones of the skull. This is apparently the result of the hyperplasia of the bone marrow, which occurring as it does in infancy tends to separate the tables of the skull and to interfere with normal growth in the long bones. There are very characteristic radial striations present, which are almost diagnostic in themselves. In the series of cases reported by Wollstein and Coffey, these features have been particularly emphasized. The pathology in other respects is one of diffuse hemosiderosis of the tissues, not unlike that found in hemochromatosis. It has been suggested that the disease may be associated with some disturbance in pigment metabolism on this account.

CASE 220. (Ref. #S-352)

Diagnosis.—Cooley's erythroblastic anemia.

Patient was a 12-year-old Italian boy admitted to the hospital with the chief complaint of anorexia and pain in both legs.

Present Illness.—The onset of the present illness dated back apparently approximately four years at which time he first complained of attacks of intermittent pain in both thigh areas. He seemed to gradually fail from that time on. He developed anorexia, constipation, weakness, easy fatigability and marked lassitude. The parents noted that his color was very sallow. The pains in his legs had become more frequent. They were localized and relatively dull in character, but severe enough to cause him considerable disability.

Past Medical History.—The child had had measles and whooping cough during his infancy, but had never had any of the more severe infectious diseases. He had been in excellent health up to the onset of his present condition. A review of his systems up to that time was entirely negative.

Physical Examination.—The patient was a fairly well-developed and nourished twelve year old Italian male child. He showed marked anemia of all his mucous membranes and conjunctivae. Head showed a slight suggestion of thickening of the parietal and frontal bones with rather marked prominence of the malar eminences. The eyes were negative. Nose and throat other than for the anemia were negative. Chest was symmetrical. Lungs were clear. Heart was not enlarged and showed no murmurs. Abdomen was slightly prominent. Liver was barely palpable, but the spleen was palpable three fingers' breadth below the costal margin. It was freely movable. The descending colon was palpable and seemed somewhat spastic. The external genitalia were negative.

Lower extremities were essentially negative, except that there seemed to be some tenderness over the femora on deep palpation.

Laboratory Findings.—Red blood cells, 3,600,000 with 7.5 gm. of hemoglobin. Color index, 0.8. White blood cells, 5,950 with 53% polynuclears and 39% lymphocytes. Urinalysis, negative. Icterus index, 24. Van den Bergh direct, delayed; indirect, 2 mgms. per 100 c.c. Examination of the blood film (Fig. 522) revealed a rather striking picture of erythroblastosis. Nucleated red cells in varying stages of development were identified. Rare megaloblasts, numerous macroblasts and many normoblasts were found. Reticulocytes were slightly increased, up to 5%.

A sternal puncture was done and histologic examination of this bone marrow confirmed the diagnosis of active erythropoiesis, many immature early red cell forms being found.

X-ray Examination.—Trabeculation of the innominate bone, sacrum and femora was definitely abnormal. It was characteristic of the condition as described occurring in erythroblastic anemia. Similar thickening of the skull bones was observed with thinning of the actual tables and with corresponding increase of the diploë.

Subsequent History.—On the basis of the blood findings, the x-ray findings and the fact that the child was of Latin extraction, the diagnosis of Cooley's erythroblastic anemia was made. He was given three transfusions at intervals of approximately a month and was put on intensive iron and liver therapy. Under this treatment he showed considerable improvement, the red cells jumping to 4,170,000 with 11 gm. of hemoglobin. He was discharged with the advice that he return at frequent intervals for further observation and repeated transfusions as needed.

VON JAKSCH'S ANEMIA.—The nature of von Jaksch's anemia is extremely uncertain. Whether this should be considered as a disease entity or merely representing a very unstable hematopoietic system in association with any of the various forms of anemia as seen in infancy and childhood has been suggested. Many of these cases have been confused with those of true erythroblastic anemia, based solely on the peripheral blood findings and without the confirmation of x-ray studies of the bones. Von Jaksch, himself, originally felt that this was a pseudoleukemia because of the invariable accompanying enlarged liver and spleen and the high white cell count. One thing is certain in respect to von Jaksch's disease, and that is its frequency in relation to severe rickets. Others have suggested the possibility of syphilis as being an important factor in the development of the picture, but antisyphilitic therapy has not shown itself to be of any avail in the treatment of the anemia. There is no recognized therapy for the condition.

Certain of the cases seem to run a self-limited course and recover spontaneously. Others run a progressively fatal course. Splenectomy is not particularly effective, and none of the usual anti-anemic forms of medication seem to affect its course. It is included in this discussion simply from the standpoint of differential diagnosis from the more definite entity of erythroblastic anemia. As time goes on, it is probable that various causes will be found to account for this curious erythoblastic picture associated with anemia and found in infants and young children, which for convenience are still grouped under this rather unsatisfactory term, "von Jaksch's anemia."

Banti's Disease (Splenic Anemia).—The group of so-called splenic anemias, as represented by Banti's disease, characterized by a hypochromic "secondary" type of anemia and by splenic enlargement, have already been discussed in the preceding chapter in relation to the spleen. At this point, it need only be emphasized that they may easily be confused with some of the other forms of hypochromic, microcytic anemias similar to those caused by iron deficiency or to blood loss. For a history of such a patient, the reader is referred to Chapter LII, Case 215.

Myelophthisic Anemias

Under this heading belong a number of pathological conditions represented chiefly by what might best be termed a replacement of bone marrow as the result, particularly of neoplastic infiltration. This results in a crowding out of the normal marrow activity with the corresponding hypoplasia of erythropoiesis. This type of anemia is particularly seen in association with leukemia, with metastatic carcinoma and similar conditions. There is nothing characteristic about the blood picture, it again following in the group of hypochromic microcytic varieties due to a diminished functional capacity of the marrow.

PART II

The Hemorrhagic Diseases

In addition to the various forms of anemia which have been discussed, there are certain diseases which occur that are characterized by hemorrhages. These hemorrhages are likely to occur in the skin, in the joints and in the mucous membranes, especially of the alimentary tract. Certain of these diseases appear to be essential in nature. Of these, hemophilia and essential thrombocytopenic purpura represent the two outstanding examples. In addition to these apparently idiopathic diseases, there are a great many other cases in which similar hemorrhages into the tissues occur. Many of these are believed to be of an allergic nature. Others are suspected to be related to infectious disease, and a small group is possibly accounted for by a vitamin deficiency, notably in vitamin "C," as subclinical scurvy.

In order to understand the mechanism by which these various types of hemorrhagic disease occur, it becomes necessary to establish the outstanding factors which play a part in the development of the picture. It is apparent that all hemorrhagic conditions must be brought about by one of three major factors, either alone or in combination: first, cases which result from an inadequate number of platelets. This is seen in essential thrombocytopenic purpura and in many conditions in which the platelets are decreased as a result of bone marrow disturbance. In the second group are those cases in which some deficiency exists in respect to the various factors which cause normal clotting of the blood. Theoretically, such a picture might exist in a deficiency of calcium, prothrombin, thromboplastin or fibrinogen; or on the other hand, in an excess of the amount of heparin. In hemophilia, some such factor is present as evidenced by the prolongation of the coagulation time. Finally, there are those cases of hemorrhage which occur as the result of increased capillary permeability, which obviously may result from a wide variety of toxic substances. It is in this group particularly that allergy and infection play such important parts.

In those cases of hemorrhage which result from a deficiency in the number of platelets, it is well for us to recall how these curious bodies normally develop. A considerable number of theories have been suggested from time to time in an attempt to explain the source of the platelets or thrombocytes. Wright's brilliant work in recognizing that the megakaryocytes appear to be the normal precursors of the adult thrombocytes is the view which is generally held today by hematologists. The typical primitive megakaryocyte is an enormous cell about forty to fifty micra in diameter. The nucleus is large, with coarsely distributed strands of chromatin. A rather typical bluish cytoplasm and not infrequently many azure granules are present. At times, the nucleus may appear either multilobulated or the cell may actually have several nuclei. The cell has been shown by more recent studies upon bone marrow to be actively ameboid, but rarely passes into the circulation because of its size. The blood platelets, or thrombocytes were believed by Wright to represent the pinched-off pseudopodia as they extended between the endothelial cells lining the sinusoids of the bone marrow. Occasionally in leukemia, or in other severe blood dyscrasias, the megakaryocytes may actually appear in the peripheral blood stream. Other theories regarding the origin of the platelets, which are not as firmly established imply that they are derived from similar pseudopodia of the normoblast or even of the primitive hematocytoblast. For all practical purposes, the acceptance of their megakaryocyte origin seems adequate.

In any disease which crowds the marrow to the exclusion of such megakaryocytic activity and the subsequent maturation of the adult thrombocyte, a resultant thrombocytopenia is bound to follow. Thus, in leukemia or in severe myelophthisic forms of anemia, this condition ensues. In the absence of the platelets, we find that hemorrhage becomes a prominent feature of the clinical picture. This is accompanied by an increased bleeding time, a normal coagulation time, and marked prolongation of the clot retraction.

Hemophilia.—Hemophilia is definitely an hereditary disease which is believed to be restricted to males, but is transmitted by females. Thus, if a normal male and a female carrier marry, one-half the males would be victims of the disease, while one-half of the daughters would carry the stigma and their children might perpetuate the condition. According to Naegli, on the other hand, if a male hemophilic is married to a healthy woman, none of the males from such a union develop the disease, and the condition stops with them. On the other hand, all their daughters are carriers and can thus transmit the disease to one-half of their children. Should a male with the disease marry a female carrier, theoretically, at least, one-half of the daughters might actually be hemophilics.

From the clinical standpoint, the patient afflicted with hemophilia has a very marked tendency for prolonged bleeding following some minor traumatic cut or injury. There is no deficiency in the platelet content of such blood. There is no lack of calcium, nor of any of the other assayable blood constituents which play a part in normal coagulation, including prothrombin and fibrinogen. The process is due, then not to a deficiency in the actual substances, but in the function of some one or more of these various factors. Birch believes that it is an actual hormone deficiency in some one of the oestrogenic agents. The usual explanation for this defect in coagulation has been given by Minot and Lee, who suggest that the platelets of the hemophiliac are unable to release their thromboplastin. This has been shown by a num-

ber of ingenious experiments, by adding the platelets of hemophilic blood to normal blood plasma and obtaining a delayed coagulation time; and at the same time adding normal platelets to hemophilic blood plasma with marked improvement in the coagulation time. More recently, however, it has been shown that the addition of platelet-free *normal* blood plasma will similarly reduce the coagulation time of hemophilic blood. This seems to throw some doubt upon the importance of the platelets as the sole factor in the production of this functional disturbance. At the present moment all we are in a position to say definitely is that the outstanding pathological feature of hemophilia is a delayed coagulation time and that this functional disturbance occurs in the face of adequate amounts of all of the known factors which play a part in normal coagulation and that, therefore, the cause of the condition must be some defect in the mechanism of coagulation through some factor as yet undetermined.

It is seen chiefly in children and young adults. It is associated with a relatively high mortality. Following adolescence, there appears to be a rather definite diminution in the severity of the process, although no actual permanent recovery from the disease is known to have occurred. On the basis of Birch's work in showing that there was a deficiency in the hormone content of the urine in hemophiliac patients, McKhann suggested the use of placental extract as a means of treating these cases. It would be premature to conclude that this is the entire answer to the problem, but there is reason to believe from a preliminary report that a considerable improvement follows such therapy. There is no specific pathology relating to the disease other than the clinical pathological finding of the delayed coagulation period.

The diagnosis is usually established on the basis of family history and repeated attacks of bleeding from the most trivial trauma. Such hemorrhage has been reported as being excited even by overzealous brushing of the teeth, or by the extraction of a tooth; by insignificant cuts of the finger, and the like. Following minor trauma, extensive hemorrhages into the joints are by no means uncommon, the knee being most frequently involved. The anemia which accompanies such repeated hemorrhages is of the usual microcytic hypochromic variety, as might be expected.

The treatment of this condition is, as has already

been intimated, wholly unsatisfactory from the curative standpoint. As in many of the problems of medicine to-day, prophylactic genetics seem to be the most logical attack in advising the members of a hemophilic family.

Essential Thrombocytopenic Purpura (Werlhof's Disease).—This condition was first described by Werlhof two hundred years ago, from the clinical standpoint; but a recognition of its underlying pathology was first demonstrated successfully in 1910 by Duke, who showed that the underlying cause of the clinical picture was a thrombocytopenia. The etiology of the condition is entirely unknown, although many investigators are inclined to the belief that infection is an important factor. Many other contributory conditions which tend to lower general body resistance, such as fatigue, cold, malnutrition and avitaminosis are often suggested. Whether the deficiency of platelets is due to decreased marrow production or to their increased destruction in the spleen, has never been fully established. Splenectomy, however, is extremely effective in increasing the number of circulating platelets very promptly. The figures in a large number of such cases which have been reported vary considerably, but conservatively it can be stated that at least fifty per cent of such patients remain permanently cured. Experience has shown that when splenectomy is attempted, it should be done in an interval between the acute hemorrhagic attacks, and preferably after the patient has been put in condition by multiple small repeated transfusions. The diagnosis of the disease is again made both by the history of repeated petechial hemorrhage and purpuric spots, and by a study of the blood. It has been shown that in this condition, the white cells are usually normal or at times slightly increased in number. The platelets are greatly reduced, usually to less than 100,000 and at times even to twenty to thirty thousand. The coagulation time is normal. The bleeding time is prolonged in contrast to the picture of hemophilia. When blood is drawn into a test tube and allowed to clot, the retraction of the clot likewise is greatly prolonged; and there is a suggestion of increased capillary permeability as shown by the tourniquet test. The difficulty in diagnosis in this condition lies in the distinguishing of true thrombocytopenic purpura from the various other forms which are found in many conditions, including the leukemias, aplastic anemia, certain of the infectious diseases especially meningitis, typhoid fever and

tuberculosis, or many of the allergic food or drug reactions which are accompanied by purpuric hemorrhages. Accompanying any purpura, there is usually a moderate amount of secondary anemia, again of the microcytic, hypochromic type.

Nonthrombopenic (Secondary Purpura).—As has already been intimated in the discussion of hemophilia, and essential thrombocytopenic purpura, there are many diseases in which purpuric manifestations may occur. As such, this purpura represents merely a symptom or sign and should be evaluated with that in mind. There appears to be no particular object in going into these various conditions in detail. Certain terms will be found in the literature applied to rather characteristic varieties of such hemorrhagic diatheses, and will accordingly be mentioned.

HENOCH'S PURPURA.—Henoch's purpura is characterized by the development of acute hemorrhages into the gastro-intestinal tract, with a very striking acute abdominal picture. This shows distention of the abdomen with marked rigidity and tenderness on palpation, not infrequently complicated by volvulus or intussusception. In the absence of skin manifestations of hemorrhage, which unfortunately are not always present, the condition may readily be mistaken for an acute surgical abdomen and an exploratory operation done.

SCHÖNLEIN'S TYPE.—In this form of purpura, the joint manifestations are the more prominent. It is characterized by rather marked tenderness and swelling of the various joints. In any of these various forms of purpura, as they are called, there is likely to be an associated rise in the white blood count and a rise in the temperature, both of which are likely to mislead the clinician into thinking that he is dealing with some acute infectious disease such as rheumatic fever, acute appendicitis or the like. It is for that reason that we have attempted to emphasize the importance of evaluation of the history as well as of the local objective physical findings in these cases.

From the standpoint of therapy in this group, there is nothing that is regularly satisfactory. Probably the most valuable form of treatment is repeated small transfusions in an attempt to stimulate the necessary hematopoietic factors although this is notoriously a failure in many cases. More specifically, a careful search of the history for any possible underlying etiology is of extreme importance. Thus, the presence of an unsuspected, subclinical, latent scurvy may be brought to light. In cases associated with foci of infection, particularly in relation to hemolytic Streptococcus, the elimination of the primary focus is obviously infinitely more important than the local treatment of the hemorrhagic lesions. At times, the study of such cases may require the services of a well-trained allergist in finding the underlying toxic substance, be it food or drug, which may be responsible for the development of the hemorrhagic picture. In the treatment of these cases, a host of therapeutic agents has been employed with variable degrees of success. Most recently, cevitamic acid, snake antivenom and the use of ergot preparations, especially ergotamine tatrate, have been recommended. In general, the mortality associated with these various forms of purpura is relatively low, but many cases run a very prolonged course with repeated periods of remission and relapse. Gradually, as in the case of hemophilia, and essential thrombocytopenic purpura, as the patient grows older the condition tends to become less severe and may ultimately completely disappear. Many of these cases might well be considered as idiopathic in type in that no knowledge regarding their etiology exists. On the other hand, in view of the large number of such cases which occur and in which some specific cause can be demonstrated, it would suggest that the process is fundamentally similar in nature and that it only remains for more thorough investigation to find the actual etiologic factor in every case.

CHAPTER LIV
DISEASES OF THE KIDNEY

The kidney is derived embryologically from two completely separate structures. The kidney proper arises from the metanephros, a derivative of the primitive nephrotome. This gives rise to the glomeruli and the convoluted portions of the renal tubule. The second portion of the kidney is derived from an outpocketing of the cloaca, which normally elongates cephalad to become the ureter. This, in turn, expands and form the pelvis of the kidney, including the major and minor calices and the collecting tubules, which normally fuse with the renal tubule previously described. This embryologic relationship is of particular importance because of the many developmental defects and anomalies which are found.

From the functional standpoint, the kidney is primarily an organ of excretion. It is divided into excretory units or nephrons, each consisting of a glomerulus with its afferent and efferent capillaries; its tubule, which consists of several portions each with its own functional activity, and finally, the collecting excretory tubule. From the functional standpoint, the kidney has an unusually high factor of safety. As is familiar clinically, an entire kidney can be removed with little or no immediate evidence of functional impairment. This is followed by compensatory hypertrophy of the remaining organ until the entire work of the two kidneys is adequately maintained.

Richards and others have shown that the entire kidney does not function uniformly at any given time. It has been demonstrated that only comparatively few of the glomeruli carry on their activity simultaneously. The mechanism of this almost cylic activity of the various parts of the kidney is apparently dependent upon a considerable number of factors among which the neurogenic seems to be the most important. Many questions still remain to be answered regarding the actual mechanism of urine production. It is generally conceded that the glomerulus acts essentially as a simple filter, and that the tubular epithelium, particularly that of the convoluted portions, plays a very important rôle in reabsorption of substances from this initial filtered fluid. It is significant that the arrangement of the glomerulus seems to be so designed as to permit the passage of electrolytes and some colloidal substances, whose molecules are not too large; but to retain the larger molecules, such as albumin. In this way, waste products are eliminated while vital substances for body economy are kept within the blood stream where they may be resynthesized by the liver or other organs.

The tubular epithelium, on the other hand, as has been suggested, plays a very important part in the concentration of these substances. This has been utilized from the clinical standpoint to determine the presence of renal damage. Where such renal pathology involves primarily the renal tubules, an inability on the part of the kidney to concentrate the urine is evidenced by a wide variation in the specific gravity of the excreted urine with constant fluid intake. Thus, it will be seen that while the primary function of the kidney is the simple excretion of waste products, its activities are by no means confined to this. In addition, as Peters has so ably demonstrated, another of the important functions of the kidney has been to maintain a satisfactory tissue water balance. This is of inestimable importance in respect to the whole process of body metabolism and economy, and aids in the control of maintaining blood volume, and by correlary an adequate blood pressure. A third important function of the kidney is dependent upon its capacity for the reabsorption of the excreted electrolytes, particularly the salts, for by this means, coupled with the respiratory exchange, the hydrogen ion concentration of the blood is likewise maintained, and the acid-base equilibrium of the body as a whole is preserved.

With these few introductory comments in respect to embryology and function, we can proceed to a consideration of the various abnormal conditions to which the kidney either as a whole, or in any of its component parts, is particularly subject.

632

PLATE CXXIV
DISEASES OF THE KIDNEY
CONGENITAL LESIONS

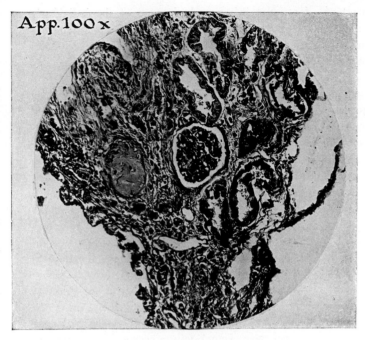

FIG. 525.—KIDNEY: CONGENITAL CYSTIC DISEASE.—CASE 222.—
Photomicrograph of a wedge-shaped vestige of renal tissue between two of the cysts seen in Fig. 526. Note two glomeruli, one
completely hyalinized, and several tubules with epithelial degeneration. App. 100 x.

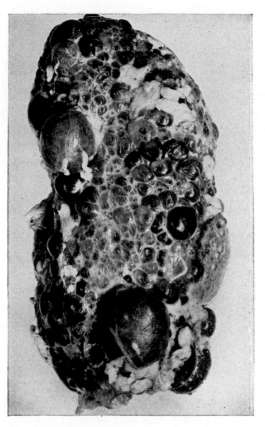

FIG. 526.—KIDNEY: CONGENITAL CYSTIC DISEASE.—
CASE 222.—The kidney is markedly enlarged (1600
gms.) and appears to be composed of numerous
cysts of varying size. On section little resemblance
to renal parenchyma is noted.

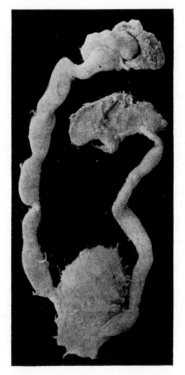

FIG. 527.—KIDNEYS, URETERS, BLAD-
DER AND ADRENALS: HYPOGENESIS.—
CASE 221.—Photograph showing
small underdeveloped kidneys complicated by bilateral hydronephrosis
in a child two years of age.

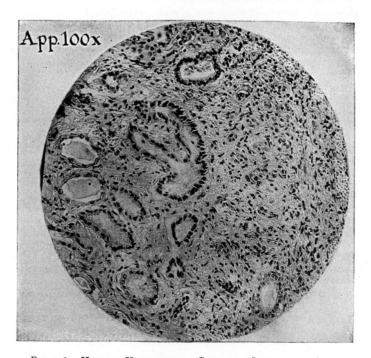

FIG. 528.—KIDNEY: HYPOGENESIS.—CASE 221.—Low power photomicrograph which shows absence of true glomeruli and abortive
attempts through hyperplasia, by the tubular epithelium to take
over glomerular function. App. 100 x.

CONGENITAL ANOMALIES

Due to the complex embryologic development of the kidney, a wide variety of congenital anomalies may exist. Many of these are of little functional significance and are only found incidentally at operation or post-mortem. On the other hand, while the patient may survive uneventfully for long periods of time, nevertheless, such anomalies not infrequently, may result in disturbances of function.

Agenesia.—As a result of failure of the cloacal buds to develop properly, we may have a complete absence of one or the other kidney and ureter; because, with the failure of the ureter to develop, the corresponding metanephron, for some unexplained reason, either atrophies or fails to develop. This complete absence of a kidney is called "agenesia."

Hypogenesia.—Hypogenesia of a kidney is much more common. In this condition, one kidney will be much smaller than the other, depending upon the degree of involvement. This is spoken of as aplasia, or hypoplasia. As a rule, the other kidney shows a corresponding compensatory hypertrophy. This failure of one kidney to develop is somewhat obscure. It is perhaps based upon developmental anomalies of the renal vessels most frequently. Occasionally, such rudimentary renal development may be bilateral in distribution with resultant early death of the infant. Not infrequently because of the individual's inability to excrete phosphates in this condition, they accumulate in the tissues and blood. There follows at times a corresponding lowering of the calcium level, which in turn is apt to be associated with a developmental delay in growth, usually accompanied by rickets. The terms, "renal rickets" or "renal dwarfism," have been applied to this picture implying that the rickets or dwarfism is secondary to the renal disease. These individuals are apt to die early in childhood, or at least by early adult life because of renal failure. The mechanism in these cases is one of incomplete development of the structures of the kidney so that they never become perfect excretory organs. Enough of the parenchyma goes on to complete development and physiological function to carry these individuals for a period through a comparatively normal life. Then either as the result of some sudden toxic or infectious process, or as the demands of later life exceed the power of the kidney to meet them, kidney failure occurs. These cases are constantly associated with sclerosis of vessels and the picture bears much resemblance to the nephrosclerosis of malignant hypertension. It differs from the latter disease in the relatively late appearance of the high blood pressure.

ILLUSTRATIVE CASE

CASE 221. (Ref. #S-335)

Diagnosis.—Kidney—hypogenesis.

Chief Complaint.—Patient was a male white infant of 2 months, who was admitted to the hospital because of increasing cyanosis and dyspnea.

Present Illness.—The onset began approximately two weeks before admission when the mother noticed that the baby was cyanotic following a severe crying spell. This was accompanied by labored breathing. Following this onset, his respirations became rapid and shallow and the cyanosis persisted intermittently since that time. The mother did not think that there had been any fever and there had been no vomiting or diarrhea. The child appeared well otherwise. His appetite was good. He appeared restless and somewhat poorly nourished however, and at times extremely weak and almost prostrated. He had no convulsions.

Past History.—The baby was somewhat premature and only weighed about three pounds at birth. The mother had a normal labor and had been able to nurse the infant successfully.

Physical Examination.—The baby was small but fairly well-nourished; he was extremely dyspneic and somewhat cyanosed generally. He appeared markedly prostrated and was considerably dehydrated. Neurological examination was negative with no abnormal reflexes. His head was normal. Eyes, ears, nose and throat were negative. The chest was symmetrical. Heart was not enlarged but there was a tachycardia with a rate of 140 and a marked sinus arrhythmia. There was a systolic murmur over the base. The lungs were clear and somewhat hyperresonant. There were no râles. Abdomen was prominent and the liver was large. It was palpable just below the costal margin.

Laboratory Examination.—Urinalysis: Acid, cloudy, with a large trace of albumin. Sediment was negative. The blood showed a red cell count of 2,400,000; white cells, 18,000, with a normal differential. Wassermann was negative.

Subsequent Course.—His temperature on admission was subnormal. He was put in a premature jacket but the temperature failed to respond satisfactorily. During the course of the first twenty-four hours he remained in about the same condition. This was followed by the onset of almost continuous convulsions during the next twenty-four hours. During one of these, he suddenly stopped breathing.

Autopsy Findings.—The body showed some subcutaneous edema. The peritoneal cavity contained about 50 c.c. of pale, straw-colored fluid which smelled strongly of ammonia. There was no other evidence of peritonitis. The sigmoid was redundant. The colon was markedly

PLATE CXXV
DISEASES OF THE KIDNEYS

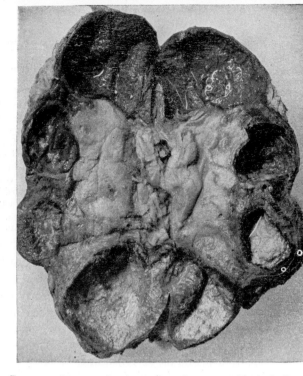

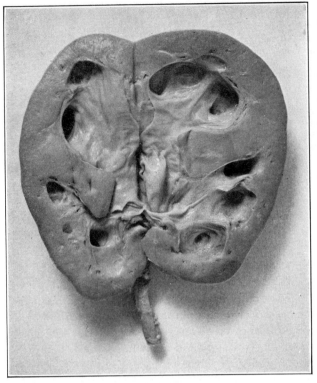

FIG. 530.—KIDNEY: PYONEPHROSIS.—CASE 225.—Marked distention of pelvis with almost complete destruction of renal parenchyma, a mere shell of kidney substance remaining. Note pyogenic granulations lining mucosa.

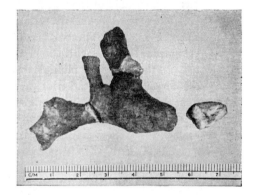

FIG. 529.—KIDNEY: HYDRONEPHROSIS.—Marked dilatation of the pelvis with resultant flattening of calices and atrophy of the parenchyma. Pelvic mucosa is smooth and glistening.

FIG. 531.—RENAL CALCULUS.—CASE 223.—(Courtesy Dr. W. H. Thomas). Large coral-like oxalate calculus forming a cast of the renal pelvis.

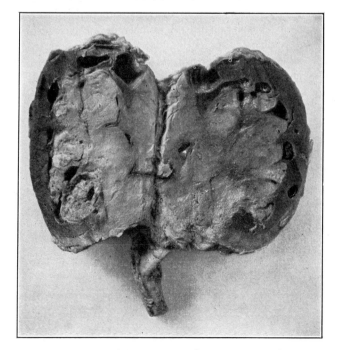

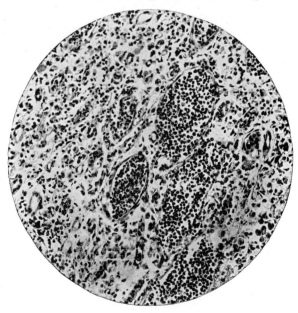

FIG. 532.—KIDNEY—TUBERCULOSIS (RENAL PHTHISIS).—CASE 227.—Chronic caseous tuberculosis involving renal pelvis, parenchyma and ureter. Note evidence of obstruction with hydronephrotic dilatation of nontuberculous portions of pelvis (upper pole).

FIG. 533.—KIDNEY—PYELONEPHRITIS.—CASE 224.—Low power photomicrograph showing several collecting tubules filled with purulent exudate—also diffuse interstitial suppurative infiltration. App. 100 x.

dilated, almost suggesting megalocolon. The ileum contained two small diverticuli, each measuring 2 cm. in length. The ureters were enormously dilated and were first mistaken for loops of bowel. The heart showed a widely patent auricular septum. There was likewise a patent ductus arteriosus. The kidneys were hypoplastic and together weighed only 7 gm. The surface of each kidney was studded with several small thin walled cysts which on section were found to be chiefly cortical in distribution (Fig. 527). The normal architecture of cortex and medulla could be identified but there was considerable distention due to a moderate hydronephrosis in conjunction with the congenital dilation of the ureters, resulting from strictures at the point of insertion into the bladder. The bladder itself showed marked hypertrophy and there was a urethral stricture. The right testis and epididymis appeared as totally separate organs united only by a thin fibrous cord. The left testis was undescended. The case was of particular interest in showing so many multiple, congenital anomalies and particularly in respect to the bilateral hyperplasia of the kidneys.

Microscopic Description of a Section through the Kidney.—(Fig. 528) Section microscopically presents evidence of extremely immature glomeruli in some areas. In other areas there is a curious arrangement of epithelium in the form of dilated or distorted tubules, suggesting hypogenetic glomeruli. The tubules themselves vary considerably in their appearance, some being atrophic, others distended. There is a marked interstitial fibrosis with some slight lymphocytic infiltration.

Horseshoe Kidney.—The so-called "horseshoe kidney" is another comparatively common renal anomaly. The fusion of the kidney substance may occur at either pole but is more frequently seen in the lower pole with the ureters passing anterior to the bridge of renal tissue and frequently showing reduplication with the development of accessory pelves. The opportunity for this fusion seems comparatively simple to explain in the course of the embryologic development, but may in part be due to developmental anomalies of the vascular system.

Miscellaneous Anomalies.—Among the other most common anomalies affecting the kidney are seen developmental defects with double or even triple ureters as the result of multiple outpocketings from the cloaca or a bifurcation of the cloacal outbud at some higher level in its migration cephalad. As a further complication of such reduplication of the ureters, the kidneys may show corresponding double or triple separate pelves, and each may have its own blood supply by independent accessory renal vessels. Not infrequently these vessels overlie one or more of the ureters and produce pressure upon them with resultant hydronephrosis. This, in turn, leads to an unusually high degree of infection in the pelves of such kidneys.

Congenital Cystic Kidney (Polycystic Kidney).—As has been emphasized from our discussion of the embryologic development of the kidney, it is not surprising that occasionally the normal fusion of the individual glomerular tubular unit with its corresponding collecting tubule fails to occur to form the completed renal unit. If this normal process fails, and if the glomerular element goes on to complete functional development, there is no outlet for its product. Thus, fluid tends to accumulate and form a cyst. Occasionally such a single or *solitary cyst* is found, which it is difficult to distinguish from cysts resulting from scar tissue formation with stenosis of one or more of the tubules. Two theories have been advanced to explain the development of the so-called "congenital cystic kidney." The most commonly held view is that the picture develops as a result of the wholesale failure of the metanephric and cloacal derivatives to fuse. The other theory advanced by Kampmeier is that when the ureteral bud meets the renal blastema, it divides, and each such new bud becomes covered by a cap of metanephric tissue which normally would differentiate into a tubule, but pathologically may become detached and persist as cysts. The condition is almost invariably bilateral. It varies a great deal in extent. There may be only a few cysts in the cortices or both kidneys may be composed of almost completely cystic masses, the individual cysts varying in size from a few millimeters to several centimeters. A very high percentage of these lesions are found in the newborn and are sufficiently marked in extent to cause death either from interfering with labor because of the disproportion of the size of the fetal abdomen and the birth canal or because following birth the renal function is inadequate to maintain life. A number of such instances of complete disproportion between the size of the kidneys and the birth canal has been reported with the diameter of the abdomen considerably in excess of that of the head. If the individual survives this initial period because the process is incomplete in its development, then he may well survive until middle life when, as in the case of hypogenesis, either as the result of toxic, infectious or circulatory causes, the demands upon the kidney exceed its capacity, and renal failure occurs.

On section of such a kidney, the individual cysts show marked variation in appearance. Some are filled with clear watery fluid; others with a thick, gelatinoid coagulant; while in still others, hemor-

PLATE CXXVI
DISEASES OF THE KIDNEY

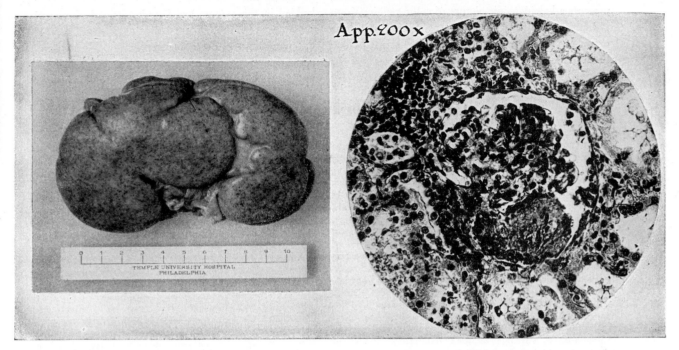

FIG. 534.—KIDNEY: FOCAL EMBOLIC GLOMERULAR NEPHRITIS ("FLEA BITTEN KIDNEY").—Cf. CASE 160.—Kidney in subacute bacterial endocarditis. Capsule removed to better reveal punctate hemorrhages studding the cortex. Note depressed scars of former infarcts.

FIG. 535.—KIDNEY: FOCAL GLOMERULAR NEPHRITIS.—Cf. CASE 160. —Photomicrograph of kidney illustrated in Fig. 534 showing a glomerulus. Within one of the loops of the tuft a hyaline thrombus is seen. App. 200 x.

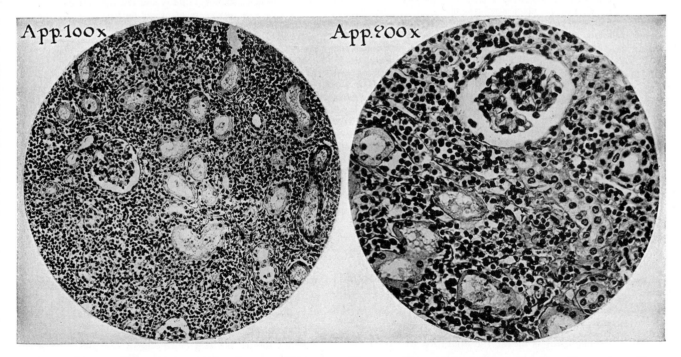

FIG. 536.—KIDNEY—NONSUPPURATIVE INTERSTITIAL NEPHRITIS. —CASE 226.—Lower power photomicrograph to show striking diffuse exudate infiltrating interstitial tissue of the kidney. App. 100 x.

FIG. 537.—KIDNEY—ACUTE NONSUPPURATIVE INTERSTITIAL NEPHRITIS.—CASE 226.—High power photomicrograph to better reveal the characteristic exudate which is seen to be made up almost entirely of mononuclears. App. 200 x.

rhage has occurred which, as the blood disintegrates, presents a kaleidoscopic picture of color ranging from red and purple through the greens and yellows. The organ has been compared to a jewel encrusted stone because of this color distribution. The stroma of the kidney in the typical marked case has an almost lacy or sponge-like appearance separating the cysts. Embedded in this stroma are found scattered glomeruli with their tubules. These show varying degrees of degeneration. In the older-age group, hyperplastic, sclerotic changes affecting the vessels are almost invariably the rule.

ILLUSTRATIVE CASE

CASE 222. (Ref. #S-198)

Diagnosis.—Kidney—congenital polycystic disease.

Chief Complaint.—Patient was a white male of 53 years, admitted to the hospital in coma.

Present Illness.—The present illness really dated back a number of years to several previous attacks similar in kind but less severe which had occurred at intervals. The present attack was ushered in by a sense of vertigo. This was followed by partial loss of consciousness. On recovering consciousness, patient noticed a weakness of his left leg, thickness of speech, drowsiness and considerable difficulty of breathing.

Past Medical History.—Patient had had an uneventful medical history up to the onset of the present history. A review of his systems was surprisingly devoid of information of any importance. He had had the usual quota of upper respiratory infections. His gastro-intestinal history was one of mild qualitative attacks of dyspepsia. He had known for many years that his kidneys were markedly enlarged, but other than occasional disturbances of sensation with a heavy feeling in his abdomen, he had had no direct symptomatic difficulty relating to them. He reported that his urinalysis had always been negative. The only symptom which pointed at all toward his present trouble was the fact that he had developed dyspnea on relatively slight exertion for many years.

Physical Examination.—Patient was a well-developed and well-nourished, middle-aged man lying comatose in bed. He showed a spastic paralysis of the left leg and arm and generalized increased reflexes on the left. His head was negative. His chest was symmetrical. His lungs were clear. His heart was essentially negative. It was not apparently enlarged and showed no murmurs. There was a hypertension of 190/100, however. His abdomen was protuberant. Following an enema, it was possible to palpate two large nodular masses which moved with respiration in both flanks. These were in the position of the kidneys and from their size and general outline suggested bilateral congenital cystic disease of the kidneys. His extremities were negative.

Laboratory Findings.—The red cells numbered 4,500,-000, white cells, 19,500 with 86% polynuclears. Blood chemistry showed a urea nitrogen of 48 mgm. Lumbar puncture yielded uniformly bloody fluid. Urinalysis: specimen was clear, acid, specific gravity 1.018, very slight trace of albumin. Sediment showed an occasional hyaline cast.

Subsequent Course.—Patient went steadily downhill and died forty-eight hours after admission without coming out of coma.

Autopsy Findings.—Heart showed hypertrophy and dilatation. There was a marked toxic myocardosis. The lungs were congested and edematous. There was a suppurative bronchitis. The kidneys: left, weighed 1,250 gm.; right, 1,600 gm. (Fig. 526). Both were tremendously enlarged and the kidney tissue had been largely replaced by cysts ranging from 2 to 30 mm. in diameter and filled with fluid varying from pale amber to a deep chocolate color. The liver showed numerous small cysts on the anterior surface with several large cysts 5-10 mm. in diameter along the portal areas on section. The head was opened and the brain presented a picture of a recent right intracerebral hemorrhage involving the greater part of the thalamus, globus pallidus and the internal capsule. There was some involvement of the nucleus ruber on the right. The hemorrhage had ruptured into the ventricle and had extended into the subarachnoid space through the floor of the third ventricle and the infundibulum.

Microscopic Description of a Section through the Kidney.—(Fig. 525) Histologic examination of the tissue shows some areas of recognizable kidney substance. These contain relatively well-formed glomeruli and tubules. There is considerable distortion of the tubules, however, as the result of pressure by the dilated cysts.

Moderate degenerative changes of the lining tubular epithelium are seen. The cysts are variously lined by cells ranging from flattened, almost pavement-like epithelium to high cuboidal cells resembling epithelial cells. The picture as a whole is one of a multiplicity of cysts of various sizes encroaching upon kidney tissue which is still attempting to maintain normal renal function.

MECHANICAL LESIONS

Hydronephrosis.—In considering the congenital lesions of the kidney, it was noted that occasionally anomalies were found in which obstruction to the ureter existed with resultant hydronephrosis. By hydronephrosis is meant the dilatation of the pelvis of the kidney as the result of obstruction somewhere below that point (Fig. 529). As the kidney continues in excretory function, the fluid accumulates within this dilated pelvis and gradually the dilatation increases with flattening of the calices. This dilatation may proceed until nothing but a membranous sac as big as a child's head remains, and in which little or no kidney substance can be identified even microscopically. Such obstructive lesions may be the result of a number of causes. Among the most important should be mentioned hypertrophy of the prostate with resultant obstruction of the urethra. Under such circumstances the hydronephrosis is likewise accompanied by dilatation of the bladder as well, and the process will be bilateral. On the other hand, the obstruction may be the result of stone or inflammatory stricture of one ureter. In addition, mechnical kinking of the ureter and pressure of aberrant vessels, as has already been emphasized, may produce similar obstruction. Finally, there is a group of conditions resulting from defective action of the autonomic nervous system of the sphincters.

The most marked example of hydronephrosis follows a progressive obstruction, which is not complete at the outset. When the obstruction is sudden, then renal function is shut off more rapidly and the amount of fluid which accumulates is correspondingly reduced. In either instance, however, atrophy and degeneration of the renal tissue takes place with resultant fibrous replacement and scarring of the persistent stroma. Hinman, in his recent monograph, has emphasized the importance of what has been termed *"pyelovenous back-flow"* in this connection. He has demonstrated that the fluid in the hydronephrotic kidney is of a much lower specific gravity than one would expect and is free of all suggestion of odor from protein derivatives. He has shown experimentally in explanation of this phenomenon that absorption of these substances takes place directly into the veins at the base of the pyramids through the minor calices. This probably plays an important part likewise in many other conditions than simple hydronephrosis.

Rupture.—Rupture of the kidney is most frequently seen following severe traumatic injury. It is particularly serious because of the likelihood of secondary infection and the extension of such infection widely in the perinephric soft tissues.

Nephrolithiasis (Renal Calculi).—Just as in the case of gallbladder disease with the production of biliary calculi, so in the case of renal disease do we find the development of renal calculi. Such calculi again depend to some extent upon stagnation of fluid usually in the pelvis of the kidney, of concentration of salts in the urine, and in some instances may be complicated by the added factor of infection. Likewise, as in the case of gall stones, the renal stones may be of three major types: They may be composed principally of uric acid, usually in combination with urates; the commonest form composed mainly of calcium oxalate, known as the oxalate stone; and finally, those made up of a combination of the calcium, ammonium and magnesium phosphates, the phosphate stones. The first two types are usually found in urines of acid reaction, whereas the latter type is associated with alkaline urines. The phosphate type of stone is particularly seen in association with infection and for that reason is more commonly encountered in the bladder than in the kidney first.

In addition to these rather general comments regarding etiology, several added factors have been brought to our attention in recent years, not the least interesting of which is the relationship of parathyroid hyperplasia or actual adenoma. The relationship between parathyroid hyperfunction, the development of renal stones and likewise the possible relationship to renal dwarfism are too frequently encountered to be wholly coincidental. Just what this relationship is still seems somewhat obscure, but depends in part certainly upon disturbances of calcium balance. Vitamin deficiency, particularly of vitamin "A" in the diet has likewise been indicated as of considerable significance. This has been brought out particularly in relation to the geographical distribution of stone formation, it being particularly prevalent in those eastern countries where such dietary deficiency exists. Many other factors, however, need to be considered in this connection. It is rare to find a stone of any one of the three varieties mentioned in pure form when it occurs in the bladder. When it arises in the renal pelvis, as many such calculi do, it is more likely to be fairly pure in type. With the passage of such a stone down the ureter, the patient undergoes one of the most violent forms of pain known to medicine, the so-called renal colic. This may give rise to ulcerative lesions anywhere along the excretory tract including the pelvis of the kidney or the ureter, and to be accompanied by bleeding with the presence of frank blood in the urine. With such ulcerative lesions, secondary infection is prone to follow.

ILLUSTRATIVE CASE

CASE 223. (Ref. #HT-1)

Diagnosis.—Kidney—renal calculi.

Chief Complaint.—Patient was a white female of 32 years, who was admitted to the hospital complaining of severe colic-like pain in the left flank.

Present Illness.—The onset of the patient's illness dated back approximately nine years when she first began to have intermittent attacks of recurrent pain in the left loin region. She was treated at intervals by her local physician during this period with varying degrees of relief. The present attack began acutely with a sharp stabbing pain in the left loin which radiated to the external genitals. The initial attack, nine years earlier, had been followed by the passage of five small stones. The attacks following the first one had never been so severe in character until the present one. The pain had been so severe as to require morphine twenty-four hours preceding admission. This attack had been accompanied by marked hematuria.

Past Medical History.—As a child, the patient had had measles, scarlet fever and diphtheria. The scarlatina was followed by an otitis media which persisted for many years. This had been complicated by mastoiditis and she had had seven operations before this infection cleared up about five years before her present admission. She had also had her appendix and gallbladder removed twelve years previously. She likewise had had a tumor removed from her left breast seven years earlier and had had a hysterectomy with a left oöphorectomy two years before her present illness. She had been married fifteen years and had one normal child who was twelve years old. She had also had three premature children, all of whom died within the first few hours after birth. Her menstrual history began at the age of twelve and had been fairly regular until her hysterectomy.

Physical Examination.—Patient was a young white female who looked considerably older than her given age. Her head showed the bilateral mastoidectomy scars. Nose and throat were negative. There was compensated edentia. Chest was somewhat emphysematous. Expansion was equal. The lungs were clear. The heart was not enlarged and showed no murmurs. The abdomen was obese. There was a long right midrectus operative scar and also a supra pubic scar. No abnormal masses were palpable. There was exquisite tenderness over the left kidney area, especially on deep palpation. The kidney could not be palpated because of the pain and obesity.

Laboratory Findings.—The blood was negative. There was a red cell count of 5,150,000 with 84% hemoglobin, and a white count of 7,850, with 77% polynuclears. Urinalysis showed a blood-tinged turbid fluid with a heavy sediment. It was acid, specific gravity 1.019. There was a large amount of albumin (320 mgm. per 100 c.c.). The sediment showed numerous red cells and pus cells, as well as a great deal of desquamated renal and bladder epithelium and mucous shreds. X-ray examination showed the presence of stones in the upper pole of the left kidney and rather marked dilatation of the left ureter.

Subsequent Course.—On the basis of the clinical history and the X-ray findings, a left loin incision was made and the kidney exposed. The kidney was split, and two large coral-like calculi removed from the upper pole calices (Fig. 531). Patient made an uneventful recovery and was discharged completely relieved of her symptoms.

Pathological Report.—Specimen consisted of two coral-like stones which more or less followed the outline of the pelvis and calices of the upper pole of the left kidney. These were stone-hard in consistency and appeared to be composed of oxalates.

DEGENERATIVE, INFILTRATIVE AND CIRCULATORY LESIONS

The degenerative, infiltrative and circulatory disturbances of the kidney are of very little primary importance. They are usually seen in association with other conditions in which the renal element is only secondary, except in the actual nephritic conditions, which will be discussed separately.

Amyloid Infiltration.—Amyloid infiltration is not infrequently found in the kidney, but rarely except in relation to amyloidosis with infiltration of the spleen, liver and other viscera. Where it occurs, the kidney is usually markedly enlarged and of a grayish-yellow, translucent, waxy appearance on section. It usually cuts with the increased resistance of other amyloid organs. The glomeruli are the first area of the kidney to show such infiltration, as has been already described, but as the condition progresses the entire organ may become involved. Pigmentary in-

filtration of the kidney is seen particularly in those diseases in which marked blood destruction takes place, such as the paroxysmal hemoglobinuria seen in conjunction with malaria. Bile pigmentation likewise occurs as part of the generalized infiltration of the cells in jaundice. (Fig. 18 and 30.)

Chronic Passive Congestion.—Chronic passive congestion as the result of chronic cardiac disease may become a lesion of some clinical significance. On account of the marked stasis of the circulation, the excretion of urine may be very markedly diminished even to the point of almost complete anuria. The urine usually shows an increase in the amount of albumin and many red cells escape passively through the glomerular tuft. At autopsy, in a case dying of cardiac failure associated with generalized chronic passive congestion, the kidney is usually seen to be somewhat increased in size and intensely congested, especially in the medulla. Histologically, a rather diffuse fibrosis is often present, and some thickening of the glomerular tuft as a compensatory reaction. This may proceed to a point of actual fibrous obliteration of the glomerules.

INFECTIONS OF THE KIDNEY

The infectious diseases of the kidney can be very easily and simply classified from the pathological standpoint, but much less readily on a clinical basis.

Infectious Nephritis.—The most important group of infections of the kidney is considered under the general term of "infectious nephritis." This may result from a wide variety of etiologic agents and may well be due in part to tissue allergy as well as to direct infection of the organ. For convenience, these more usual infectious processes in the kidney have been divided into three stages, which merely represent for the most part gradations of the same underlying pathological process. In this discussion, an attempt is made to conform to this clinical concept and explain the terminology on the basis of the demonstrable lesions. The three terms employed in this regard are (a) pyelitis, (b) pyelonephritis and (c) pyonephrosis.

PYELITIS.—By "pyelitis" clinically is meant an acute inflammatory process involving the pelvis of the kidney. This is very frequently unilateral, although it may also be a bilateral lesion. It is particularly seen in infants and young children, and in women during pregnancy. An enormous literature has sprung up in an attempt to explain its etiology. Two major theories still engage the attention of investigators. By far the greater number of pathologists believe that pyelitis is essentially a hematogenous infection, and a number of investigators have shown such inflammatory lesions in the pelvis are always associated with microscopic lesions in the interstitial substance of the kidney. These are frequently so small as to escape recognition grossly and even on routine microscopic study. The other theory as to the development of the lesion is that it is an ascending infection against the flow of urine up the ureter from the bladder. The chief argument in favor of this theory is that the great majority of cases occur in females in whom infection of the bladder by the colon bacillus is comparatively simple from the anatomical standpoint. Furthermore, the great majority of cases of pyelitis are caused by the *Bacillus coli*. A third theory, but one which has largely been discarded, is that direct lymphogenous extension from the intestinal tract by colon bacilli may occur.

In infants this condition may be associated with a high fever, and clinically, in the absence of other explanation for such a temperature, pyelitis should always be borne in mind. From the clinical pathological standpoint, the condition is recognized by the presence of pus in the catheter specimen of urine and at times, the actual catheterization of the ureters may be necessary to establish whether or not the lesion is uni- or bilateral. Therapy in these cases has been largely one of urinary antisepsis by drugs taken by mouth, such as urotropin and hexylresorcinal, and similar compounds, or by the direct irrigation of the renal pelvis. Such infections often are extremely persistent and difficult to eradicate. This is easy to understand if one appreciates that the lesion is really renal and not restricted to the pelvis of the kidney itself.

PYELONEPHRITIS.—By the term pyelonephritis, we commonly mean a diffuse interstitial inflammatory reaction with or without suppuration depending largely upon the nature of the infecting organism, of which the most common are the colon bacillus, the staphylococcus and the streptococcus, with the great majority being due to the colon bacillus. This may give rise to a very extensive inflammatory reaction with diffuse suppuration. Such lesions may be either unilateral or bilateral, but fortunately are more often found involving only a single kidney. As the inflammatory process proceeds, necrosis of renal tissue takes place with abscess formation and liquefaction necrosis. A mechanical factor frequently enters into the picture with the pus being so thick that it blocks the ureter and fills the pelvis causing marked distention. Such a process may go on to the complete destruction of the kidney substance, which is merely represented by a thick capsule or wall of fibrous tissue filled with pus. This is known as pyonephrosis.

PYONEPHROSIS.—Pyonephrosis may arise, as has been just indicated, as a result of the further extension of a diffuse suppurative pyelonephritis, or it may result as the secondary infection of a hydronephrosis. This type of secondary pyonephrosis shows a picture usually complicated by the presence of stone or some obstructive lesion in the ureteral tract which causes stagnation of the urine and secondary infection.

ILLUSTRATIVE CASE

CASE 224. (Ref. #S-329)
Diagnosis.—Kidney-pyelonephritis.

Patient was a white female of 35 years who was admitted to the hospital with the chief complaint of pain in her right side, which radiated down her right leg, and frequency of urination with a scalding sensation.

Present Illness.—The patient had been in comparatively good health until about three weeks before admission. At that time she began to have dysuria and frequency of micturition. She consulted her physician who treated her without apparent improvement in her condition. Her frequency, in fact, increased and was particularly marked at night, requiring her getting up five or six times. The dysuria improved under treatment, but she developed a jumpy sort of pain in her right side, which seemed to radiate down her right leg and across the lower abdomen. This was not constant and not particularly severe. At the onset of her illness, she noticed that her urine had been somewhat reddish in color on several occasions, but this had not been present for the two weeks preceding admission. The patient further complained of a feeling of weakness and easy fatigability and also noted that she had intermittent attacks of vertigo when standing up suddenly. She had had some incontinence on occasion with these symptoms, but it was more the result of urgency than a true incontinence so far as could be determined from her history.

Past Medical History.—She had had the usual childhood diseases, but had never had any serious illness during her entire life. A review of her systems was relatively non-contributory. She had frequent attacks of headache until she had her vision corrected. Her cardiorespiratory system seemed to be entirely negative. In respect to her gastro-intestinal system, she had always been very constipated requiring almost daily laxatives. She had had occasional attacks of qualitative dyspepsia and had noticed that an excess of fatty foods always caused her an upset stomach with considerable belching and flatus. Her genito-urinary history up to the present time had always been normal. She had been married and had had two normal children. Her menstrual history was entirely negative.

Physical Examination.—The patient was a poorly nourished, asthenic white woman who appeared about her given age. Her nose and throat were negative. There was a small nodular growth in the right lobe of the thyroid about the size of a walnut. Her chest was symmetrical. Heart and lungs appeared to be normal.

Abdomen was soft and flat. Liver and spleen were not palpable. There were no definite palpable masses. No pain or tenderness on deep palpation were noted except for a moderate spasm in the right costolumbar angle. Extremities were negative.

Laboratory Findings.—Blood Count: Red blood cells, 3,800,000 with 63% hemoglobin. White blood cells, 8,000 with 66% polynuclears. Urinalysis on several occasions showed a very turbid appearance with a large amount of granular sediment. Specific gravity averaged 1.013. There was a heavy cloud of albumin in the filtered specimen. The sediment showed countless red and white cells, but no casts. Many of these leukocytes and red cells were in the form of clumps, and B. coli were recovered in large numbers from the urine specimens.

X-ray examination revealed a large calculus in the right kidney pelvis. Cystoscopy showed a normal urine coming from the left kidney and a thick, purulent fluid from the right.

Subsequent Course.—On the basis of these findings, a right nephrectomy was urged. This was done and the kidney removed through the usual loin incision. The patient made an uneventful recovery and was discharged greatly improved.

Pathological Report. — Gross Description. — The specimen consisted of a kidney which showed moderate enlargement. It measured 14 x 8 x 7 cm. It weighed 300 gm. The capsule stripped fairly readily except for a few localized areas of adhesion. The pelvis was largely occupied by a coral-like calculus. The kidney substance, on section, showed a diffuse suppurative process with areas of apparent actual necrosis and abscess formation.

Microscopic Description of a Section Through the Kidney.—(Fig. 533) Histologic study of the tissue shows a diffuse interstitial suppurative pyelonephritis. In places, this inflammatory reaction has gone on to actual necrosis and abscess formation. These abscesses tend to conform to the architecture of the kidney, being intertubular in distribution. The glomeruli show varying degrees of secondary inflammatory change. The tubules show extensive degeneration with granular, hyaline, fatty and hydropic degeneration. Many of the lumina are filled with pus cells and these have clumped to form beginning casts. The picture is one of a typical diffuse pyelonephritis, apparently the result of hematogenous infection following interference with renal function through the development of a calculus.

ILLUSTRATIVE CASE

CASE 225. (Ref. #S-341)
Diagnosis.—Kidney—pyonephrosis.

Patient was a white male of 77 years, who was admitted to the hospital complaining of complete anuria of forty-eight hours' duration, accompanied by severe pain in the lower abdomen.

Present Illness.—The patient's present illness dated back about eighteen years to a similar attack of acute retention. At that time, he was treated at another hospital, but refused operation. Since that time he had had difficulty in urinating at intervals and had learned to catheterize himself. He had recently developed a very marked frequency but had been unable to void without

catheterization. He complained of no other symptoms which disturbed him except that with this current attack of retention, he had likewise not been able to move his bowels. He had been unable to introduce the catheter successfully during this period and came to the hospital primarily with the idea of securing help in that respect.

Past Medical History.—The patient was unable to recall anything of significance in respect to his previous medical history. He had never had any serious illness which had required hospitalization except this first attack of urinary retention. A review of his systems was noninformatory. He had had no respiratory, gastro-intestinal or cardiac symptoms.

Physical Examination.—The patient was an elderly male who appeared markedly emaciated and dehydrated. Head showed no deformities. There was very marked arteriosclerosis with tortuous vessels. Pupils were somewhat dilated but reacted normally. Nose and ears were negative. Teeth were carious, with many missing. Chest was definitely emphysematous in appearance, but the expansion was equal on both sides. Breath sounds were barely audible. No râles were heard. Heart was slightly enlarged. There was a systolic murmur heard over the base. Abdomen: Muscles showed decreased tone. There was marked distention of the bladder up to above the level of the umbilicus. Rectal examination showed a markedly enlarged prostate. Extremities were negative. Neurologic examination was negative.

Laboratory Findings.—Blood count on admission showed 3,290,000 red blood cells with 8 gm. of hemoglobin. White blood cells, 11,200 with 83% polynuclears. Blood chemistry showed 165 mgm. of urea and 7.5 mgm. of creatinine. His Wassermann was negative. Urinalysis: Urine specimen was obtained by catheterization and was somewhat bloody in appearance. It was markedly turbid. Specific gravity, 1.011; there was a cloud of albumin present and far too many white and red blood cells to be able to count them. Numerous bacteria were likewise present. A diagnosis of chronic cystitis associated with hypertrophy of the prostate was made.

Subsequent Course.—The patient went rapidly downhill lapsing into typical uremia and died twenty-four hours after admission.

Autopsy Findings.—The autopsy was restricted to an abdominal incision. The liver showed some interstitial fibrosis. The spleen presented a typical picture of senile atrophy. The kidneys were removed with the bladder, ureters and prostate. On section, they both presented the typical picture of a moderate degree of chronic pyonephrosis. They each measured approximately 13 x 5 x 4 cm. The capsule stripped fairly readily except for a few adherent points. The calices were flattened and the pelvis widely dilated and filled with a thick, greenish-yellow pus (Fig. 530). The pelvic mucosa showed replacement by a thick zone of what appeared to be granulation tissue. Similar evidence of chronic infection was noted in the bladder. This was dilated and contained about 1,200 c.c. of hemorrhagic, turbid fluid. The mucosa was markedly trabeculated and hemorrhagic. Numerous areas of erosion of the mucosa were seen. The prostate was greatly enlarged with the typical picture of benign adenomatoid hypertrophy.

Microscopic Description of a Section Through the Kidney.—Histologic study of the kidney shows an almost complete destruction of the renal element in the pelvic portion of the kidney. Distorted, compressed, atrophic tubules are found embedded in a dense mass of fibrous, interstitial tissue. This is diffusely infiltrated by inflammatory cells, both mononuclear and polynuclear. The pelvis is lined by a thick layer of chronic granulomatous tissue. Here and there some of the epithelium is seen to persist and shows marked thickening. The entire pelvic wall is diffusely infiltrated by leukocytes.

FOCAL INFECTIONS.—Aside from this diffuse type of infection which is very largely related to the colon bacillus, we may find on occasion, focal-abscess formation as part of a sytemic septicemia caused by the staphylococcus. This type of lesion is unfortunately usually bilateral. The abscesses are usually restricted to the cortical portion of the kidney where they seem to arise through localization of the bacteria in the terminal arterioles. As is usually true of staphylococcic septicemias, the mortality is extremely high and particularly so with the complication of such pyemic lesions.

Nonsuppurative Interstitial Nephritis.—There is a group of cases which presents a very similar histologic appearance in many respects as the usual findings of pyelonephritis except that the exudate is of a mononuclear variety, and the process rarely proceeds to true suppuration. These lesions are best interpreted as the result of a toxic injury to the vascular endothelium in association with an infection elsewhere. The most classical examples of this type of nonsuppurative diffuse interstitial nephritis are seen in relation to streptococcic infections, notably scarlet fever. The distribution of the lesions tends to be focal, but originates usually around the blood vessels, particularly the venous vessels in the midzone area, as has been emphasized in the chapter on the exanthemata. Occasionally this picture may show some polynuclear infiltration as well. It is the only lesion to which the term interstitial nephritis can be accurately applied as those changes which affect the interstitial tissues in conjunction with the other lesions of the kidney are only incidental, and secondary to the parenchymatous lesion.

ILLUSTRATIVE CASE

CASE 226. (Ref. #S-261 and S-253)

Diagnosis.—Heart—fatty degeneration of myocardium; Kidney—interstitial nephritis.

Chief Complaint.—Patient was a child of 10 years admitted to the hospital unconscious as a result of accident.

Present Illness.—The present illness began acutely with a blow on the head while he was playing football. This resulted in a fracture of the skull over the right orbital region. This was followed by a severe infection of the right ear and mastoid, which required operative intervention and was drained for several months. In addition, the fracture apparently included the right frontal sinus as infection of that area also persisted for the same interval. The child showed a progressive weakness. The picture was one of general toxemia, with a persistent temperature which was intermittent in character, varying with periods of remission and relapse with respect to the sinus infection. He continued to progressively fail and developed a very severe microcytic hypochromic anemia which failed to respond to repeated transfusions.

Past Medical History.—The child had had the usual history of infections in his first five years, including measles, pertussis, varicella and scarlatina. In all other respects he had been an entirely normal boy in his development. He had not shown any complications from his scarlatina infection up to his present illness.

Physical Examination.—At the time of admission, the child showed nothing abnormal on physical examination except for the local fracture. As time went on, however, he showed myocardial failure with marked enlargement of the heart and generalized anasarca. What were interpreted as so-called hemic murmurs were elicited from time to time. Terminally, he developed pulmonary edema and died in convulsions which appeared to be uremic in nature.

Laboratory Findings.—The blood showed a progressive microcytic hypochromic anemia which reached as low as 1,600,000 red cells and was only maintained at higher levels through repeated transfusions. His white cells likewise varied tremendously during the entire period, ranging from 12,000 to 32,000, with an average polynuclear figure of 86%. His hemoglobin reached a low of 32%. Urinalysis likewise showed a progressively more severe nephritic picture with red cells, casts and a considerable amount of albumin.

Autopsy Findings.—At autopsy the most striking picture was found involving the heart and kidneys. The heart was moderately enlarged and acutely dilated. It was extremely pale in color and on section showed one of the most pronounced pictures of tigroid or tabby-cat mottling, indicative of fatty degeneration, imaginable. This was most marked over the papillary muscles of the left ventricle, but involved the entire musculature as seen through the endocardium. In addition, the kidneys were greatly enlarged. Even through the capsule, they showed marked hemorrhagic mottling against a pale yellowish pigmentation indicative of extensive tubular degenerative changes. On section their capsules stripped with considerable difficulty due to innumerable adhesions. Many foci of acute hemorrhagic necrosis were found throughout the cortices. Considerable submucous hemor-rhage was found in the pelves of the kidneys and the ureters were distended with a turbid urine.

Microscopic Description of a Section through the Heart Stained with Osmic Acid.—(Fig. 518) Histologic examination of the heart reveals areas of muscle fibers containing many black globules within their cytoplasm. Intervening groups of cells fail to show this reaction. In sections of tissue stained by hematoxylin and eosin, these fatty changes do not stand out particularly prominently although the areas of degeneration are seen and show fragmentation and marked parenchymatous degeneration. A few cells have a vacuolated appearance, and in these it is easy to make the diagnosis of fatty degeneration. However, osmic acid infiltration of the tissue shows the lesion in a most spectacular way. It will be noted that the involved areas alternate with areas in which only minor degenerative changes are taking place, and it is this alternation of fairly normal and degenerative myocardium which gives rise to the characteristic gross appearance of the so called "thrush breast," tabby-cat, or tigroid mottling of the myocardium.

Microscopic Description of a Section through the Kidney.—(Fig. 536 and 537) Histologic examination of the kidney presents an unusually severe degree of an acute interstitial nonsuppurative type of nephritis. This is most marked in the cortical portion of the kidney although involving the medulla to some extent. It is characterized by the diffuse infiltration of the interstitial tissue by mononuclear cells. These have crowded in in such large numbers as to completely replace the normal tissue. It is extremely difficult to even identify collagen fibers between the inflammatory cells. The result has been an actual interference with the function of both glomeruli and tubules, both of which show rather striking degenerative and atrophic changes. Many of the tubules show very marked granular and fatty degeneration. Some of the glomeruli show marked pericapsular fibrosis and their glomerular tufts tend to be bloodless and nonfunctioning. The blood vessels, likewise, show a compression and the picture is one of generalized ischemia of the kidney except for focal areas where hemorrhage has occurred as the result of the diffuse toxic interstitial process.

Tuberculosis of the Kidney.—RENAL PHTHISIS. —(Fig. 532). The other important infection of the kidney is seen in the form of tuberculosis. Not infrequently from the clinical standpoint, tuberculosis of the kidney may occur as an apparently primary lesion. This obviously is not possible, but a considerable proportion of the cases of renal tuberculosis show no evidence clinically, of any active tuberculosis elsewhere. Careful search at autopsy from such cases, however, will usually reveal a focus of infection elsewhere in the body. The lesion must, of necessity, be hematogenous with the exception of an ascending infection from the bladder. Being hematogenous the lesion is usually from the pathological standpoint almost invariably bilateral. Curiously, however, the tuberculous process usually progresses much more rapidly in one kidney than in the other, which is the justification of the surgical treatment of tuberculosis of the kidney. This statement regarding the bilateral nature of the tuberculous process is not accepted by all clinicians, who believe that many cases of renal tuberculosis are the result of direct extension of tuberculosis of the epididymis along the peri-ureteral lymphatics. This belief is based on the fact that in almost every case of tuberculosis of the kidney, it is possible to demonstrate tuberculosis in the ureter almost regularly, even when the renal lesion is hard to find.

Just as in the case of pyelitis, however, it seems reasonable that the tubercle bacillus is likely, as a hematogenous infection, to localize in the submucosa of the pelvis covering the pyramids and to start up its chronic inflammatory reaction in that location. Clinically, tuberculosis is usually recognized by the presence of unexplained hematuria and increased frequency. The frequency is largely the result of irritation of the trigone of the bladder, which becomes involved early in the tuberculous process. The hematuria is usually the result of ulceration of the pelvic mucosa. Gradually the process extends from a simple ulcerative lesion of the pelvis lined by tuberculous granulation tissue to become a diffuse fibrocaseous mass lesion with complete destruction of the entire kidney. This might well be spoken of under such circumstances as tuberculous pyonephrosis, but much more commonly is known as renal phthisis.

MILIARY TUBERCULOSIS.—As part of the picture of generalized miliary tuberculosis, the kidney likewise may be involved. Such miliary tubercle formation varies considerably depending upon whether one or more showers of tubercle bacilli have taken part in the reaction at variable intervals. Under such circumstances, it is not uncommon to find healed tubercles as well as the more active lesions associated with the terminal clinical picture. Indeed, lesions of several ages may be found in the same section.

ILLUSTRATIVE CASE

CASE 227. (Ref. #S-343)

Diagnosis.—Kidney—renal phthisis.

Chief Complaint.—Patient was a white male of 30 years, admitted to the hospital with the chief complaint of marked frequency of urination.

Present Illness.—The onset began rather definitely about seven weeks before admission when the patient first noticed a marked frequency. Since that time he had complained of having to void almost once an hour even through the night. He had not complained of any particular pain except some slight suggestion of a burning sensation transmitted to the glans penis. He had not noticed that the urine was blood-tinged at any time.

Past Medical History.—Patient had had a rather uneventful medical history as a child. He had never had any of the usual diseases except measles. A review of his systems revealed no more than the usual upper respiratory infection incidence. He had never had any chronic cough, dyspnea, hemoptysis or pneumonia. His cardiovascular history was negative. His gastro-intestinal history had been entirely negative. His appetite had always been good. He had never suffered from indigestion and his bowels had always been regular. Genitourinary history revealed an acute gonorrhea at the age of twenty, which subsided spontaneously in the course of two to three months. Four years before his present symptoms, he had had pain and swelling of both testes. They had been operated upon and removed. He was indefinite in his knowledge regarding the nature of this pathological process but believed that some mention was made of tuberculosis. A review of his skeletal system revealed no evidence of any joint involvement.

Physical Examination.—Patient was a fairly well-developed and well-nourished adult, white male, who did not appear acutely ill. His head was negative. His nose and throat were negative. There was no cervical adenopathy. His chest was symmetrical. His lungs were clear; the expansion was equal. No alteration in voice or breath sounds was heard and no râles were detected. The heart sounds were normal. The abdomen was negative. There was no particular tenderness in the loins. Examination of the genitalia revealed a partial hypospadias with the urethral opening on the under surface of the glands, and an absence of both testes.

Laboratory Findings.—Urinalysis showed a moderately turbid, light yellow specimen with some granular and flocculent material. The reaction was acid; specific gravity, 1.012. There was a moderate trace of albumin.

Examination of the sediment revealed 25 to 30 pus cells and 10 to 15 red cells per high-power field. The pus cells likewise were found in clumps. Examination of the blood revealed a very mild anemia. Red cell count was 4,800,000, hemoglobin 12 gm. (71%), white cells numbered 7,200, 68% polynuclears. Repeated examination of urine specimens microscopically failed to reveal any tubercle bacilli. X-ray showed a large mass of calcific material in the right kidney which involved the lower pole. The left kidney appeared normal in size, shape and position. The picture raised the question of a rather extensive tuberculosis with calcification, or the possibility of some nontuberculous pyonephrotic processes with similar secondary calcific deposition. Subsequent laboratory report: Guinea pig inoculation proved positive for tuberculosis with the urine from the right kidney at the end of a six week period.

Subsequent Course.—On the basis of the positive animal inoculation, a diagnosis of renal tuberculosis was made and the kidney removed by an oblique loin incision. Patient made an uneventful recovery and was discharged from the hospital one month later. It might, incidentally, be remarked that careful x-ray study of the lungs revealed no demonstrable primary focus of tuberculosis.

Pathological Report.—Gross Description.—(Fig. 532)—Specimen consisted of a kidney measuring 11 x 6 x 4 cm. with 3 cm. of the ureter attached to it. On section, at both poles, large fibrocaseous, ulcerative, abscess-like lesions were demonstrated, the largest measuring 5 cm. in diameter. In addition, several small loculated cysts, lined with thick chronic granulation tissue with areas of caseation in the deeper portions could be seen. The central portion of the cortex appeared to have escaped the rather extensive tuberculosis. On cutting, the specimen's marked calcification was noted.

Microscopic Examination of a Section through the Kidney.—Histologic examination of the tissue shows almost complete destruction of the kidney parenchyma. The tissue is taken apparently from the wall of one of the large caseous abscesses and is seen to be composed, for the most part, of typical diffuse tuberculous granulation tissue. In the viable area, characteristic tubercle formation can be made out with many Langhans'-type giant cells and marked epithelioid cell proliferation, diffuse lymphoid infiltration and a moderately extensive productive fibrosis. The cells are arranged in familiar radial fashion around central caseous areas.

Perinephric Abscess.—Strictly speaking, the perinephric abscess is extrarenal, but its origin has been traced in a considerable number of cases, both clinically and experimentally from the renal cortex by way of the capsular lymphatics. Such a lesion may produce a focal abscess, which may attain a very considerable size. This is usually due to a hematogenous staphylococcic infection spreading from some primary focus elsewhere in the body, such as a carbuncle. No explanation has been offered to clarify why in one instance a localized abscess will result, and a generalized septicemia with multiple pyemic lesions throughout the body in another case. Fortunately, however, this localization of the infection with the production of a single abscess occurs with some frequency and is amenable to surgical treatment without even the necessity of removing the kidney as the capsule of the kidney in most instances serves as an effective barrier against the extension of the abscess.

CHAPTER LV

DISEASES OF THE KIDNEY (*Continued*)

NEPHRITIS

A classification of the diseases which are grouped under the general heading of nephritis covers a very wide range of pathological lesions, including changes which, strictly speaking, should not be considered as primarily inflammatory in nature. These renal lesions range all the way from the toxic inflammatory picture associated primarily with diffuse glomerular lesions through the focal glomerular injuries, the essentially degenerative conditions which affect the renal tubular epithelium and the true infectious inflammatory processes, which have been considered in the previous chapter, down to those degenerative changes of the kidney which are the result of circulatory disturbances. Obviously, the term, nephritis, or the older term, Bright's disease, is inadequate to describe such a wide diversity of pathological processes, many of which are degenerative and not inflammatory at all. For this reason, it is suggested that the classification of renal disease, which is based largely upon the now almost classical monograph of Volhard and Fahr should be employed in this connection, and the use of these other terms relegated to the discard. This useful classification, as it is commonly used today, is outlined below with the corresponding terminology which is still found in the older literature.

CLASSIFICATON OF THE SO-CALLED NEPHROPATHIES OR NEPHRITIDES

Current Terminology	*Gross Terminology*	*Older Terminology*
I. Glomerulonephritis		
1. Focal embolic	"Flea-bitten" kidney	
2. Focal, non-embolic or toxic		
3. Diffuse		
a. Acute	Large red kidney	Acute parenchymatous nephritis
b. Subacute	Large white kidney	Chronic parenchymatous nephritis
c. Chronic	Secondary contracted or small, *white*, granular kidney	Chronic interstitial nephritis
II. Nephrosis (tubular nephritis)		
1. Toxic	Large white kidney	Chronic parenchymatous nephritis
2. Lipoid		
III. Nephrosclerosis (vascular nephritis)		
1. Arterial or atherosclerotic (senile arteriosclerotic)		
2. Arteriolar (essential hypertensive)	Primary contracted or small, *red*, granular kidney	Chronic interstitial nephritis
a. Benign (chronic progressive nephritis)		
b. Malignant		

This classification, which is based primarily upon the histopathological changes as they affect the various portions of the kidney anatomically; the glomerulus, tubule, and the blood vessels, represents the most satisfactory concept of the alterations of kidney function. Even this relatively simple anatomical nomenclature, however, fails to satisfactorily fit in with all clinical cases of renal dysfunction. One of

PLATE CXXVII

DISEASES OF THE KIDNEYS

DIFFUSE GLOMERULAR NEPHRITIS

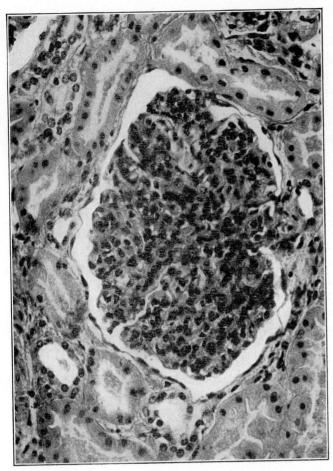

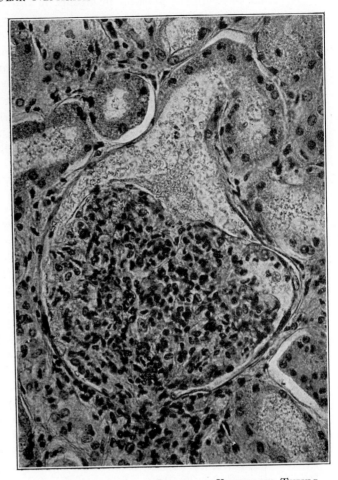

FIG. 538.—GLOMERULUS.—CASE 228.—Showing early changes. The capillaries of the tuft are avascular but the number of cells increased as a result of endothelial and epithelial proliferation. Note early diffuse polynuclear leukocytic exudation. App. 300 x.

FIG. 539.—GLOMERULUS AND PORTION OF URINIFEROUS TUBULE.—CASE 228.—More advanced glomerular lesion with proliferative and degenerative changes. Note albuminous debris and diapedesis of red cells into the capsular space and tubules from increased permeability. App. 300 x.

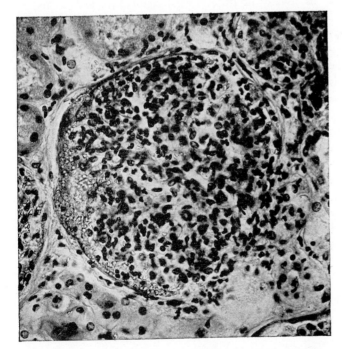

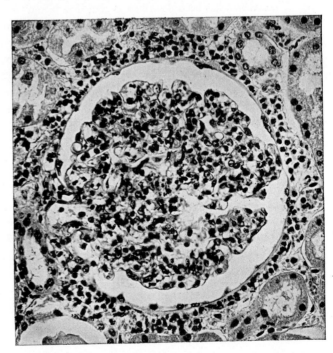

FIG. 540.—GLOMERULUS.—CASE 228.—Photomicrograph showing a glomerulus the site of extensive inflammatory polymorphonuclear exudation. Degenerative changes are conspicuous and hemorrhage has occurred into the capsular space. App. 300 x.

FIG. 541.—GLOMERULUS.—CASE 229.—Photomicrograph showing a striking periglomerular exudate made up of both mononuclear and polynuclear leukocytes. Note also marked exudate within the tuft, the capillaries of which are relatively bloodless. App. 300 x.

the most difficult problems to attempt to correlate on the basis of this purely anatomical arrangement is in respect to edema. In general, edema in renal disease is most striking in relation to the chronic nephrotic lesions which are frequently associated with disturbances in the albumin globulin ratio of the blood proteins. It depends to some extent as well upon salt retention. In the purely nephritic type of edema, the fluid accumulation is characterized particularly by a facial distribution, which is apparently chiefly due to increased capillary permeability. This confusion in respect to the clinical and the pathological interpretation of renal pathology has resulted in the clinician not infrequently accepting a classification of kidney disease on the basis of acute and chronic nephritis, with or without edema, which, if one eliminates the vascular forms of renal involvement, works out fairly satisfactorily in the grouping of the cases as suggested by the anatomical and pathological classification.

GLOMERULONEPHRITIS

Acute Focal Embolic Glomerulonephritis.—Focal glomerulonephritis is frequently the result of a definite embolic process which is seen usually as a complication of subacute or acute bacterial endocarditis. The size of the embolic material determines the extent of the lesion. If the embolus is small enough, we may find only a single loop of the capillary tuft of a glomerulus involved (Fig. 535). Following the blocking of this capillary loop, a thrombosis of the capillary occurs. This produces a small focal infarct, which results in extravasation of blood into the surrounding tissues to a degree that has become visible to the naked eye as a minute, punctate area of hemorrhage (Fig. 534). Due to the distribution of the glomeruli largely to the cortical portion of the kidney, these embolic lesions are seen widely scattered over the surface of the kidney just beneath the capsule. The kidneys as a whole are usually moderately enlarged and of a rather grayish-red color against which these multiple punctate hemorrhagic areas stand out prominently, and give the appearance which has been described as the "flea bitten" kidney.

Under the microscope, these lesions are identified as a mass of rather homogeneous fibrin and coagulated serum and bacteria. There is usually some secondary leukocytic infiltration as the result of the presence of the bacteria, but the cellular reaction is not as marked as might be expected. If the embolus is sufficiently large, we have already seen the more massive infarction which may occur. In the most extreme instances, actual embolism of the main branches of the renal artery may occur with complete renal failure as a result. The diagnosis of the focal embolic variety of glomerular nephritis is often overlooked clinically. It is characterized usually only by the presence of red cells in the urine, with the added appearance of occasional leukocytes and casts during the course of subacute bacterial endocarditis.

At autopsy many of these lesions will be found completely healed with scarred areas sometimes adherent to the capsule where contact with the inflammatory tissue has taken place. The condition in itself is usually of little significance clinically, and is only one of those incidental findings at autopsy in the course of the endocarditis. For illustrative case refer to Case 162 (Ref. #S-267), Chapter XXXVIII.

Acute Nonembolic Focal Glomerulonephritis.—In addition to the frankly embolic variety of focal glomerulonephritis, it is not at all unusual to find instances of a similar focal nature, which apparently arise as the result of the action of toxins from some distant focus of infection upon the vascular endothelium of the glomerular tuft capillaries. Hyaline fibrinous thrombi form in the capillary loops much as in the case of the embolic lesion, but the secondary leukocytic reaction is usually lacking as the lesion is noninfectious. Such a picture is more often recognized at the autopsy table than it is clinically. It is usually of little clinical significance and occurs, probably very frequently, in conjunction with minor acute upper respiratory infections. If careful examination of the urine is made in patients suffering from such infections, it is extremely common to find microscopically a number of red cells which spontaneously disappear without any evidence of renal dysfunction. Such lesions might be spoken of as subclinical glomerulonephritis. That they have existed as true pathological lesions may be shown later at autopsy by the presence of scattered focal glomerular scars.

Diffuse Glomerulonephritis.—By glomerulonephritis is meant a condition in which the primary renal damage occurs in the glomerulus. It may be stated *a priori* that all cases of glomerulonephritis

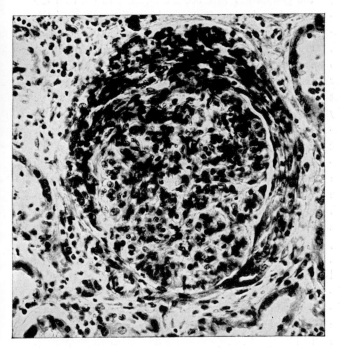

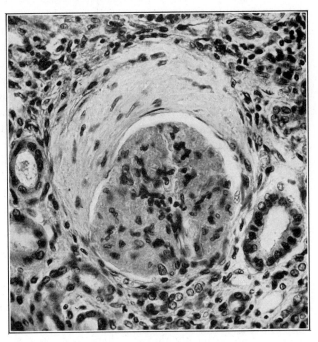

FIG. 542.—GLOMERULUS: SUBACUTE STAGE.—CASE 231.—Photomicrograph revealing the so-called "capsular crescent" the result of eccentric proliferation of the epithelial cells. Proliferative changes may also be seen within the tuft. App. 300 x.

FIG. 543.—GLOMERULUS: SUBACUTE STAGE.—CASE 231.—Photomicrograph showing a later stage of crescent formation. Note fibrosis of the tuft and hyalinization of the capsular proliferation. App. 300 x.

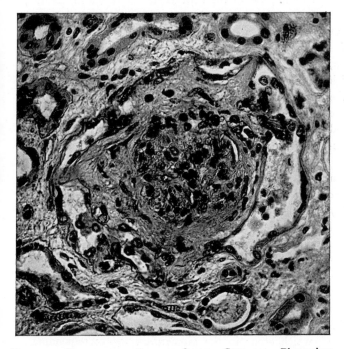

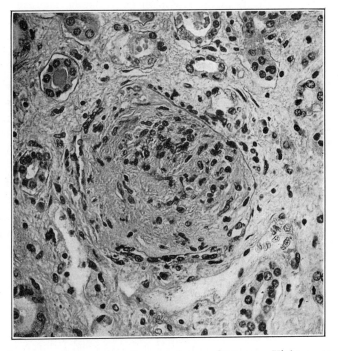

FIG. 544.—GLOMERULUS: CHRONIC STAGE.—CASE 230.—Photomicrograph showing a glomerulus in which the tuft has almost completely been replaced by fibrous tissue. Note adhesions between the parietal and visceral layers of the capsule. App. 300 x.

FIG. 545.—GLOMERULUS: CHRONIC STAGE.—CASE 230.—High power photomicrograph showing almost complete replacement of glomerulus by fibrous tissue. The capsular space is likewise almost completely obliterated. App. 300 x.

represent a lesion the result of infection elsewhere in the body. The infective agent in the great majority of instances is the hemolytic streptococcus. Thus, glomerulonephritis may follow such acute streptococcic infections as scarlatina, erysipelas, acute tonsillitis, streptococcic bronchopneumonia and the like. It is for this reason that the clinician delves into the patient's past medical history to discover whether any of these infections may have existed to account for the patient's condition at the time he is seen by his doctor with symptoms relating chiefly to disturbances of kidney function. From the standpoint of exact terminology, the term nephritis should perhaps be restricted to this group of cases in which the glomerular lesions are the primary ones, but the term is loosely used in relation to any lesion in which renal symptoms predominate and commonly covers the nephroses and the vascular forms of renal disease, to say nothing of the entire group of infectious processes. Glomerulonephritis itself may be divided conveniently into at least three major clinical varieties, as acute, subacute and chronic. From the pathological standpoint, the subacute and chronic merge so frequently that it is hard to draw a sharp line between them, except as seen in the end stage.

ACUTE DIFFUSE GLOMERULONEPHRITIS.—The acute form of glomerulonephritis is seen most typically as the aftermath of scarlatina, approximately two to three weeks following the onset of the disease clinically. As has been shown in the discussion of scarlatina, there is likely to occur also a type of interstitial nephritis, a nonsuppurative, diffuse lesion, which is perivascular in its distribution, and which follows usually from one to two weeks after the onset of the disease. It apparently antedates the more severe glomerular damage and is only encountered pathologically in those acute overwhelming infections, which die during this period.

The more specific glomerular lesions are seen from the clinical standpoint as presenting hematuria either frankly grossly, or more often microscopically. They are accompanied commonly by suborbital edema and not infrequently by a moderate rise in blood pressure up to 160 or 180 millimeters of mercury. As a complication, cerebral symptoms which are usually described as hypertensive encephalopathy supervene. Death in acute glomerulonephritis is quite as often the result of cardiac failure or central nervous involvement as it is due to true renal failure with the characteristic picture of uremia.

Pathologically, in the mildest form of glomerulonephritis, we find that the endothelial cells lining the glomerular tuft become swollen to such an extent that they tend to cut down the caliber of the vessels with a resulting avascularization of the glomerulus. This swelling of the vascular endothelium is indicative of injury to the vessel wall, which renders it more permeable. There follows, logically, the escape of red cells into the capsular spaces. These appear in the urine. This injury likewise extends to involve the reflected epithelial covering cells of the tuft, and considerable cellular debris as a result of necrosis and degeneration of these cells may also be found in the capsular spaces. This granular material may fuse or become adherent to degenerated material in the form of casts, which may also be found in the sediment of the urine. As a result of the increased permeability, albumin may pass readily between the endothelial cells and likewise be found histologically as a fine, pink-staining granular precipitate in the capsular spaces and tubules. It also may be demonstrated in excess in the excreted urine. These changes represent the very earliest which may be identified as representing true glomerulonephritis. With this amount of cell damage, soon there appear inflammatory cells with polynuclears accumulating within the capillaries and migrating into the interstitial spaces of the tuft. Histologically, a markedly increased cellularity is apparent due both to the proliferative hyperplasia of the endothelial and epithelial cells of the glomerular tuft plus the infiltrating exudative inflammatory cells. Hemorrhage becomes more and more prominent. Fibrin precipitates out of the material which passes through the damaged glomerular filter and appears as a layer over the surface of Bowman's capsule, frequently completely obliterating the lumen or orifice of the tubule. In the meshes of this fibrin are seen inflammatory cells and an increase of capsular epithelium, which likewise undergoes inflammatory hyperplasia. These masses of exudate and cellular hyperplasia are spoken of as "epithelial crescents." For some curious and unexplained reason, some instances of glomerulonephritis appear exclusively intracapillary in their reaction while others show a predominance of the capsular lesion. More often, however, the two are found in combination.

As a result of the acute inflammatory changes which occur in the glomerulus, the corresponding tubule undergoes secondary degenerative changes

PLATE CXXIX
DISEASES OF THE KIDNEY
Nephrosis

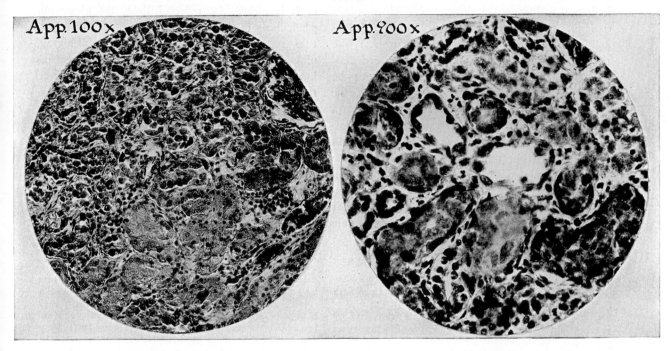

Fig. 546.—Kidney: Acute Toxic Nephrosis (Bichloride Poisoning).—Case 49.—Photomicrograph in which advanced tubular degeneration and necrosis is seen. Note distribution especially to convoluted tubules. App. 100 x.

Fig. 547.—Kidney: Acute Toxic Nephrosis (Bichloride Poisoning).—Case 49.—High power photomicrograph of a field shown in Fig. 546 better illustrating the tubular necrosis. Note lumina filled with desquamated necrotic epithelium in which the nucleus is no longer recognizable. App. 200 x.

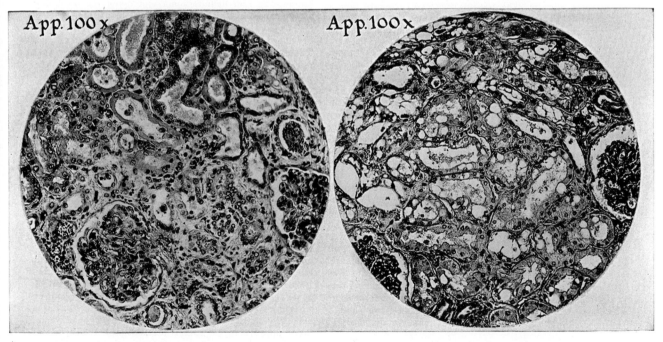

Fig. 548.—Kidney: Acute Nephrosis (Eclampsia).—Case 3.—Advanced fatty, granular and hyaline degeneration of the tubular epithelium. Note cellular debris in lumen which frequently results in obstruction and the ischemic glomeruli. App. 100 x.

Fig. 549.—Kidney: Acute Toxic Nephrosis.—Case 5.—Photomicrograph showing convoluted tubules in its epithelium in which may be seen numerous vacuoles representing hydropic fatty degeneration. App. 100 x.

with swelling of the cytoplasm of the cells, particularly in the convoluted part of the tubule. Fatty, hydropic and granular degenerative changes are striking, and aid in the development of the hyaline and granular casts, which appear in the urine. While the process is described as diffuse, it is, nevertheless, true that the lesion is not uniform throughout the kidney. As has already been emphasized, all the glomeruli do not function simultaneously, and as a result of this protective mechanism, often many glomeruli fortunately escape such extensive damage and persist in sufficient numbers to maintain moderate renal function.

In the acute stage of glomerulonephritis, at autopsy, the kidney may be recognized with a fair degree of accuracy. It is increased in size. Its capsule is tense. It is usually congested and swollen. On section, the capsule almost strips spontaneously as soon as it is nicked. In reflected light, the glomeruli, particularly in the acute exudative phase of the picture, stand out as slightly elevated, reddish-gray, pin-point granules above the surface of the remaining renal parenchyma. This has been compared to the appearance of grains of sand on the cut surface. This picture is the large red kidney of the older terminology. As the acute inflammatory process subsides, the degenerative features in the glomeruli disappear. The tubular degenerative changes, however, become more prominent and the kidney becomes pale in color, but still markedly enlarged. This, the subacute form of glomerulonephritis, gives us the so-called "large white kidney."

ILLUSTRATIVE CASE

CASE 228. (Ref. #S-200)

Diagnosis.—Kidney—glomerulonephritis, acute, diffuse type.

Chief Complaint.—Patient was a white woman of 37 years who was admitted to the hospital with a history of persistent vomiting of one week's duration.

Present Illness.—The onset of the patient's symptoms was believed to be due to an attack of food poisoning although this was never definitely proven. She was under the care of a local physician who was able to give her temporary relief by medication. This only lasted for two or three days and was followed by recurrent vomiting of greater severity. The patient progressed rapidly into a semistuporous condition. On admission she was somewhat disoriented and delirious with a subnormal temperature.

Past Medical History.—Patient was unable to coöperate in providing the data of her past medical history and the information which her husband was able to give was incomplete. As far as he knew, she had never had any previous illness which had been at all serious in nature. There was nothing to suggest a previous history of hypertension. A review of her systems was essentially negative other than the fact that she had occasional attacks of qualitative dyspepsia. Her social history was negative. She had been married fifteen years and had one child, 13 years of age. She had had no other pregnancies.

Physical Examination.—Patient was a semistuporous. acutely ill-appearing woman, with a subnormal temperature of 97.5° on admission. She was somewhat emaciated and dehydrated. She was incontinent and showed marked twitching of the fingers and of the legs. There was marked pallor of the mucous membranes and the nail beds. The eyes reacted sluggishly to light and distance. The chest was essentially negative. The heart rate was about 100. The lungs were clear. Her abdomen was distended and somewhat tense. No definite tenderness or masses could be made out. Her nervous system showed no abnormalities of the reflexes. A tentative diagnosis of uremia was made.

Laboratory Findings.—Red blood cells, 100,000; hemoglobin, 4 gm. White blood cells, 27,000 with 95% polymorphonuclears. Marked secondary anemic picture by smear. Urinalysis: On four occasions this showed a specific gravity ranging from 1.008 to 1.013 with a very heavy cloud of albumin; no sugar; no acetone, and the benzidine test was negative. Sediment: Occasional waxy and hyaline casts with occasional clumps of white blood cells. Blood chemistry: Urea nitrogen 200 mgm.; creatinine 13-15 mgm.; CO_2 capacity 36 volumes per cent; phosphorus 6.1 mgm.; calcium 7.6 mgm.; sugar 150-190 mgm. Urea clearance was approximately one-half of normal. Serology was negative.

Subsequent Course.—Patient proceeded steadily downhill lapsing into definite coma and dying the third day after admission with a typical picture of uremia.

Autopsy Findings.—Body was that of a fairly well-developed, white female, about thirty-five years of age. There was apparently a moderate anemia. Autopsy was restricted to the abdomen. No abnormalities of the viscera generally were found. The kidneys were somewhat enlarged. Their capsules were adherent and when attempts to strip them were made, considerable tearing of the kidney substance occurred. The exposed surface was ragged. The incised surface was pale and faintly striated.

Microscopic Description of a Section Through the Kidney.—(Fig. 538, 539 and 540) Histologic examination of the tissues presents evidence of a relatively acute type of degenerative glomerulonephritis. The glomeruli, as a whole, appear to be relatively bloodless. Many of them show definite hyaline thrombi in the individual capillary loops of the glomerular tuft. These vary in size and accordingly in the amount of capillary tuft tissue which has been destroyed. Some of the glomeruli appear to be very extensively involved. Others seem to have entirely escaped the process. Sections stained for bacteria show no organisms in any of the lesions and the picture, unlike that of acute focal glomerulonephritis appears to be the result of toxic injury to the vascular lining of the glomerular tuft endothelium with resultant thrombosis. Taken as a whole, there appears to be rather marked proliferative overgrowth of the endothelium of the capillaries in the tufts. This has further tended to cut down the blood supply to the secreting units of the kidney. It is difficult to tell whether some of this cellular hyperplasia is endothelial or whether it represents the epithelial covering of the reflected capsule. Very little actual exudation is noted. There is marked congestion and edema of the interstitial

tissue of the kidney as a result of the blocking of the capillary circulation. The tubules show extensive secondary degeneration with fatty, hydropic and hyaline features. Occasional casts are seen within the lumina of the dilated tubules.

ILLUSTRATIVE CASE

CASE 229. (Ref. #S-88)
Diagnosis.—Kidney—periglomerulitis, acute.
Chief Complaint.—Patient was a colored female of 24 years, admitted to the hospital because of loss of weight and weakness over a two months' period.
Present Illness.—The onset of her illness dated back indefinitely to a period about two months before admission when she complained of an annoying cough with a slightly productive sputum. This subsided but she noted that she was losing in weight, became readily tired and felt weak. Two weeks before admission, patient developed a severe cold and sore throat which required bed care for several days. This was accompanied by a high fever. Associated with this she had several attacks of vomiting. She had had a persistent sputum since that time. The last few days she had noted a marked frequency in urination but had had no pain associated with it. Three days before admission, she developed sharp pains in her legs which shot down the calves to her feet. She had a succession of chills and fever with these and had to remain in bed.
Past Medical History.—The past history was apparently irrelevant. As far as the patient could remember, she had never had any serious illness previously. A review of her systems was essentially noninformatory.
Physical Examination.—The patient appeared to be an acutely ill, young Negress. Her head was normal in appearance. Eyes reacted normally to light and distance. Nose showed a slight mucopurulent discharge. Her throat still showed some inflammatory congestion with markedly enlarged tonsils. Cervical glands were slightly enlarged. The chest was symmetrical. The lungs showed some slight dullness at both bases, particularly on the left with harsh breath sounds and occasional coarse râles. Her heart was not enlarged. It was rapid in rate. There were no murmurs. Blood pressure was 130/84. Abdomen seemed to be negative. None of the viscera could be palpated. There was no tenderness. The extremities showed some slight edema of the feet.

Laboratory Findings.—The urine was dark amber, acid, specific gravity, 1.016. There was a heavy trace of albumin but no sugar. Wassermann was negative. Blood count: Red cells numbered 3,800,000; white cells, 29,350; hemoglobin 50%; polymorphonuclears 88%. Blood chemistry findings: urea nitrogen 38 mgms., creatinine 3.8 mgms. Sugar 110 mgms. per 100 c.c.
Subsequent Course.—Patient developed a definite picture of diffuse bronchopneumonia involving the left lower lobe but failed to respond to treatment, which included immune transfusions. She died five days after admission.
Autopsy Findings.—Heart was of normal size. There were two acute vegetations on the auricular surface of the posterior mitral cusp. These vegetations were friable and one small area of ulceration was noted where a vegetation had come away. The valve was thickened generally and suggested a previous rheumatic process. Picture was that of a terminal pneumonia involving the lower left lobe. Kidneys were much larger than normal. The left weighed 220 gm.; the right 260 gm. They were pale yellowish in color. The capsule was thin. On section there was marked edema. The capsule stripped easily leaving a smooth surface. Other findings were negative.
Microscopical Description of a Section of the Kidney.—Histologic examination of the kidney reveals a very striking and somewhat unusual type of acute glomerulonephritis (Fig. 541). This is characterized by very marked periglomerular leukocytic infiltration. In addition, there is definite glomerular involvement with a marked increase of inflammatory cells, both mononuclear and polymorphonuclear, which largely obliterate the lumina of the capillary tuft, leaving relatively bloodless, functionless structures. Here and there, focal, embolic thrombi may be noted as well. There is considerable toxic granular degeneration of the convoluted tubular epithelium. The interstitial tissue shows marked congestion of the blood vessels but the process is too acute for any fibrosis to have developed.

SUBACUTE AND CHRONIC DIFFUSE GLOMERULO-NEPHRITIS.—As was indicated in the general discussion, it is difficult to subdivide accurately the subacute and chronic forms of glomerulonephritis as they represent merely progressive stages in the reparative process. With the subsidence of the acute infection, further damage to the glomeruli likewise ceases, and the reparative process becomes the more prominent feature of the histopathology. From the subcapsular connective tissue stroma and from the connective tissue supportive cells of the glomerular tuft itself, new-formed connective tissue grows in exactly the same way that connective tissue elsewhere proliferates in the repair of any inflammatory

process. As a result of the exudate which fills the capsular spaces in many instances, the epithelial lining is obliterated in places and dense fibrous bands or adhesions form between the tuft and the capsule. The exudative crescent which was commented upon in the acute picture likewise undergoes fibrous tissue organization and appears as a crescentic fibrous tissue scar. The intra-glomerular tuft connective tissue likewise increases in amount with the obliteration of loops of capillaries or, in the more severely damaged glomeruli, the entire glomerular tuft. Abortive attempts to reform the capsular spaces may be seen with the proliferation of the lining epithelial cells just as the serosal cells in acute exudative lesions in the pleura attempt to grow and reform the pleural cavity. In this way, small, isolated, almost cyst-like areas may occur in the glomerulus, which have no relation to any duct. As the process proceeds, the connective tissue increases steadily in amount until the glomerulus may be obliterated and replaced by connective scar tissue. When this occurs, there is a striking tendency for the fibrous tissue to be laid down in parallel concentric layers as it grows out from the capsule, thus producing a picture which has a rather laminated appearance. Such fibrous scarring results in a marked interference with the blood supply and the connective tissue undergoes hyaline degeneration. As an end stage, therefore, the histologic picture of the kidney cortex may be a mass of small, round, connective tissue spherical scars representing the site of previous glomeruli. The amount of renal function which persists depends entirely upon the extent of this process.

Accompanying the obliteration of the glomeruli, from the functional standpoint, is the secondary tubular degeneration and atrophy. Over a period of time the excretory duct system of each destroyed glomerulus gradually disappears entirely. This results in an apparent increase in the connective tissue. This interstitial fibrosis is to a very large extent relative, but there is some actual increase in the amount of such interstitial fibrosis because the inflammatory process is bound to extend to the interstitial tissue as well. Grossly, such a kidney in the end stage of glomerulonephritis is a small, contracted kidney, grayish-white in color and with an adherent capsule. On splitting such a kidney, the cortex is found diminished in thickness; the pelvic fat is increased in amount, and the actual kidney substance may be reduced to one-third or less of the normal amount. The capsule strips with great difficulty leaving a coarsely nodular surface as the result of the contraction of the fibrous scar tissue. This is the secondary contracted, or small white granular kidney of the older terminology.

From the functional standpoint such a kidney shows marked impairment of renal function. There is an attempt by the persistent glomeruli to undergo compensatory hypertrophy to maintain function so far as possible. As a result of the ischemia and the extra load thrown upon the kidney, there is a secondary hypertension. The urinary findings at this stage of the disease are often negligible. The concentrating ability of the kidney decreases so that the specific gravity of the urine rarely exceeds 1.010. There is a urea clearance usually of less than 20 per cent and the nitrogenous products show an increase in the blood.

Glomerulonephritis in itself may be considered very much as any other acute infectious inflammatory process. It consists of a single insult to the renal tissues which, following its removal, is repaired as best it may be by the connective tissue cells. The prognosis and significance of glomerulonephritis lies in the amount of damage which has occurred in the course of this acute process. If the injury is sufficient, death occurs promptly during the acute stage; if the damage is minimal, the patient may live out his normal span of life without any knowledge of renal impairment. Chronic glomerulonephritis really represents an intermediate picture in this respect; where a considerable part of the kidney has been put out of action leaving the remainder without the usual factor of safety which normally exists. Due to this initial inflammatory process the remaining kidney tissue which is under excessive functional strain is more readily damaged by subsequent minor infectious processes elsewhere in the body. Under these circumstances, we can think of chronic glomerulonephritis much as we think of appendicitis or cholecystitis, as representing recurrent acute exacerbations of an inflammatory process with more and more productive fibrosis resulting, until the end stage is represented by the point at which renal function is inadequate to maintain life. This is further complicated, as one approaches midlife by the common vascular changes which further the damage to renal function.

ILLUSTRATIVE CASE

CASE 230. (Ref. #S-89)

Diagnosis.—Kidney, acute, recurrent glomerulonephritis.

Chief Complaint.—Patient was a male Negro of 36 years, who was admitted to the hospital complaining of weakness, feverishness and a severe cough.

Present Illness.—One year ago he was known to have had a hemoptysis following an accident in which he incurred a fractured leg. One month previously, he had had a similar attack. This subsided spontaneously and he continued his work after a few days' rest. He felt fairly well until one week before admission. In the preceding week, he had developed rather acute symptoms associated with a high fever, muscular weakness and a progressive increasingly severe cough. He became dyspneic on the slightest exertion and noted that there was some swelling of his ankles. He had had no urinary symptoms.

Past Medical History.—Patient's recollection of his early childhood was somewhat hazy but he believed he had all the usual childhood infections. He had had several attacks of tonsillitis and on the recommendation of his physician, they were removed three years before the present illness. He recollected that he had had pneumonia as a young man, but was uncertain of the date. He had also had malaria as a boy but had not had any recurrent attacks since he had moved to the north some ten years earlier.

Physical Examination.—Patient was a fairly well-developed and well-nourished, young Negro who appeared acutely ill. He was markedly dyspneic. His head showed no abnormalities. His pupils reacted sluggishly. His nose and throat were negative except for a slight catarrhal infection of his larynx. His chest showed marked impairment of the percussion note over the left apex. This was accompanied by loud bronchial breath sounds. Many râles were heard throughout these dull areas. The heart was not enlarged. No murmurs were heard. Blood pressure was 130/70. Abdomen was distended. No tenderness was present. No viscera could be felt. Extremities showed a moderate edema of the ankles and of the feet.

Laboratory Findings.—Urine: Pale yellow, slightly turbid, acid, specific gravity, 1.018, albumin, two plus. Sediment showed many leukocytes. Blood: Red cells numbered 3,800,000 with 73% hemoglobin; white cells showed marked increase, total 21,600 with 83% polynuclears. Blood chemistry: During the ten days he was in the hospital, the urea nitrogen steadily climbed from 90 to 180 mgm.; his creatinine from 6 to 14.5 mgm. per 100 c.c. The blood pressure likewise rose during this period to 150.

Subsequent Course.—His progress was steadily downhill for the ten days he was in the hospital. Terminally, he went into complete uremic coma associated with clonic Jacksonian convulsions. He died without regaining consciousness.

Autopsy Findings.—Diffuse confluent bronchopneumonia of both lungs with old adhesive obliterative pleuritis on the left. The kidneys were greatly enlarged, each weighing 250 gm. Their capsules stripped readily. Their general appearance was that of the so-called pale white kidney with a cloudy, half-cooked appearance of the cut surface. Other findings were essentially negative, other than generalized toxic degeneration of the parenchymatous organs.

Microscopical Description of a Section of the Kidney.—(Fig. 544 and 545) Histological examination of the tissue shows a very diffuse inflammatory process involving primarily the glomeruli. There are two distinct lesions present; an older one characterized by obliterative fibrosis of many of the glomeruli and associated with areas of scarring in the interstitial tissue. In addition, however, there is a more recent acute reaction involving the glomerular tufts. Glomeruli show hyaline thrombi occluding portions of the capillary loop. Some of these glomeruli thus involved show only acute degenerative changes as evidenced by fading of the nuclei and the bloodless character of the capillaries. Others show marked inflammatory infiltration with polynuclears predominating. The picture suggests an acute diffuse glomerular type of nephritis superimposed on an old preëxisting, healed glomerulitis.

ILLUSTRATIVE CASE

CASE 231. (Ref. #S-199)

Diagnosis.—Kidney—subacute and chronic glomerulonephritis.

Chief Complaint.—Patient was a white female child of 6 years, who was admitted to the hospital with a history of renal disease.

Present Illness.—The onset of the patient's present illness was of about one week's duration. At that time she started having attacks of vomiting and the mother noted that the urine was bloody in appearance. Over the period of a week she had developed progressive drowsiness and had been almost completely anuric with only occasional small amounts of blood tinged concentrated appearing urine. There had been a marked loss of appetite. The present illness dated back possibly to a month earlier at which time the patient had had an otitis media. This was followed by marked frontal headaches believed to be due to acute frontal sinusitis. The original infection appeared to have cleared up until the onset of her present picture.

Past Medical History.—The child had never had any of the usual childhood diseases. Her previous history had been entirely negative except for an attack of pneumonia at the age of two from which she had recovered without any apparent complications or residual symptoms.

Physical Examination.—On admission the child appeared to be in a fair state of nutrition but somewhat anemic. She was semistuporous but could be rather easily aroused, lapsing back to the same state unless her attention was constantly attracted. She had occasional attacks of nausea and vomiting. Her eyes were negative. Her pupils reacted sluggishly to light and accommodation. Her chest was essentially negative with no abnormal heart or breath sounds. Abdomen was relaxed; there was no tenderness. The liver and spleen were not enlarged. Reflexes were negative.

Laboratory Findings.—Repeated urinalysis showed a consistently acid, dark amber urine, which was blood tinged at times. Specific gravity averaged 1.015. There was a heavy trace of albumin on each examination and the test for occult blood was uniformly positive. Sediment showed occasional hyaline and granular casts with clumps of white cells and red cells in varying numbers. Blood chemistry: Urea nitrogen, 160 mgm. rising to 225 mgm. Creatinine 9.2 mgm. rising to 20 mgm. Other findings negative. Serology negative. Cerebrospinal fluid normal.

Subsequent Course.—Patient was in the hospital for a little over two weeks progressing steadily downhill. She developed a marked secondary anemia with a hemoglobin of 10 gm. and a red count of 3,400,000; white blood cells 10,000 to 12,000 with 85% neutrophiles. She became increasingly stuporous and the vomiting became more severe. She was treated with intravenous fluids without improvement and finally lapsed into the typical picture of uremic coma. She died in a typical convulsive seizure associated with marked uremia.

Autopsy Findings.—The autopsy was restricted to an examination of the kidneys. None of the other abdominal organs showed any significant changes. The kidneys were somewhat enlarged, measuring 8 x 5 x 3.5 cm. The capsule stripped readily, leaving a pale, red, smooth surface in which numerous punctate hemorrhages could be seen. The incised surface showed a pale red cortex and beefy red congested pyramids with some edema as evidenced by eversion of the cut edges. The picture grossly suggested an intermediate stage of glomerulonephritis.

Microscopical Description of a Section of the Kidney.—(Fig. 542 and 543) Histologic examination of the tissue shows marked proliferation of the capsular epithe-lium of the glomerulus. There is fibrosis of the glomerular tuft with obliteration of many of the capillary loops. The proliferating epithelium often fills the capsular space as typical epithelial crescents. There are masses of cells that are made up almost entirely of epithelium. These are exaggerated crescents. The glomerulus in some instances consists of only a small fibrous ball with a few capillary channels within it. In other areas the epithelial changes no longer are visible and the glomerulus is represented by a circular mass of connective tissue laid down in concentric rings, the structure looking almost like the cross-section of an onion. These sclerosed glomeruli all show extensive hyalinization. In addition, there are many dilated tubules filled with hyaline casts.

NEPHROSIS (TUBULAR NEPHRITIS)

Nephrosis is a term which has crept into the literature since the turn of the century and has caused a considerable amount of confusion in respect to just what should be included under this name. Essentially, what we try to emphasize in using this term from the pathological standpoint is the fact that the renal damage which has taken place primarily involved the tubules. As has already been emphasized, it is impossible for any one portion of the renal unit to be damaged without secondary involvement of the other two. Thus, secondary glomerular changes and even vascular lesions not infrequently are found in association with such tubule damage. However, there are certain clinical conditions in which this primary tubular renal involvement may be clearly demonstrated and in which the symptomatology is largely the result of such damage. These are best classified under the two subdivisions of (1) toxic nephrosis, and (2) lipoid nephrosis (Epstein's type). Under toxic nephrosis must be considered a wide range of lesions. In the first place must be cited the endogenous toxemias, such as those seen in association with the toxemias of pregnancy, pernicious vomiting and eclampsia, and in conjunction with severe liver pathology such as acute or subacute yellow atrophy; and exogenous toxins which relate chiefly to the heavy metals of which bichloride of mercury poisoning is the most common and most typical. In the second place may be cited the less significant minor tubular degenerative changes seen in association with many infections notably the acute exanthemata, diphtheria and the like. In lipoid nephrosis, we are dealing with a comparatively infrequently met and poorly understood condition, but which presents certain rather characteristic clinical and pathological features.

Toxic Nephrosis.—MERCURIC CHLORIDE POISONING.—Bichloride of mercury poisoning represents the most typical example of the acute primary tubular pathology in the kidney. The drug is usually taken with suicidal intent, but may occasionally be ingested accidentally. As a result of suicidal efforts, the dosage is usually relatively large, and the pathological effects correspondingly great. The drug is taken into the stomach where it is absorbed, moves into the blood stream, and is excreted in a large part by the kidney, but also reabsorbed by the digestive tract so that severe ulcerative gastric and colonic lesions likewise result. In the kidney it apparently passes through the glomerulus without causing undue damage, but in reabsorption from the secreted urine by the convoluted tubular epithelium, it acts upon those cells to produce an acute necrosis.

As one sees these cases clinically, the process has usually gone on for a number of days so that all the evidence of degeneration and inflammation are present. In the experimental animal, it is possible to examine the kidney within a few hours after the action of the drug and there it is seen that the picture presents cell death, but little evidence of inflammation or degeneration. Mercury is a coagulant and, therefore, fixes the tissue cells rather promptly if present in adequate concentration. As time goes on, marked granular changes appear; the cell membrane ruptures; karyolytic and karyorrhectic nuclear degeneration takes place; the cytoplasm of the cells becomes extruded; the cells disintegrate, and the lumen of the tubule becomes completely occluded by this necrotic cellular material. In the milder cases, hyaline casts are formed; in the more severe cases the obstruction is too great for this material to be washed out of the tubules as casts. With these acute degenerative changes, secondary inflammatory cellular infiltration follows. Leukocytic response is fairly marked in an effort to aid in proteolytic degeneration of the necrotic material. As a result of the obstruction to the tubules, the glomeruli become swollen, distended and albumin tends to appear within the capsular space. Gradually the fluid accumulates until the glomerular tuft itself frequently becomes almost collapsed from the fluid content within the glomerular space. Death ensues as a result of renal failure with the development of true uremia and commonly accompanied by convulsions. The nitrogenous elements accumulate in the blood with the nonprotein nitrogen rising at times as high as 300 mgm. In the less severe cases, regeneration of the tubular epithelium occurs and if the patient survives the acute stage, which may last for a period of ten days or more, then recovery is likely to follow as a result of the amazing regenerative capacity of this renal tubular epithelium. Scarred areas may persist in such recovered cases, and where the necrotic tubular material is found, secondary calcification is likely to follow if the material is not excreted through the tubule.

Thus, we find various stages in the course of such mercurial poisoning; the initial stage of acute degeneration of the cells, a secondary stage in which reparative phenomena are engaged in their activity and finally, an end stage which in the more acute form results in death, and in the milder cases in recovery clinically, with pathological calcification of the remaining degenerative material and regeneration of the persistent tubular epithelial cells. The reader is referred to Case 49 (Ref. #S-84), Chapter XIII, Fig. 546 and 547 for the description of the clinical and pathological findings of a typical case.

ECLAMPSIA.—In eclampsia, we have the most striking example of the endogenous toxemias which affect the kidney. This needs be referred to only briefly at this point as the lesions have already been studied in relation to the general discussion of degeneration in Chapter II, and in respect to eclampsia as a clinical entity in Chapter XLVIII. Briefly, the changes are seen as fatty, hydropic and granular cytoplasmic degeneration of the tubular epithelium, which varies, as in the case of mercury poisoning, in degree (Fig. 548). In some instances, these changes may likewise go on to such an extent that the broken down cellular material may occlude the lumina of the tubules and result in renal failure.

More often, the renal pathology is only incidental in the clinical picture.

In addition to the tubular lesions, not infrequently focal glomerular damage may occur which results in fibrous scarring of individual glomeruli. Many pathologists emphasize the glomerular lesion of eclampsia as the more significant describing a proliferative endothelial reaction which results in relative avascularization of the glomeruli and secondary degenerative changes. With this thought in mind, the kidney of eclampsia might well be included in the group of either focal or diffuse glomerular nephritides, but it has always seemed to us that the tubular degenerative changes were the more prominent and significant. Refer to Case 3 (Ref. #S-127).

MISCELLANEOUS FORMS OF TOXIC NEPHROSIS. —As has been intimated in the general discussion, almost any acute infectious process elsewhere in the body may result in mild inflammatory and degenerative changes which affect the tubular epithelium. These are probably rarely of clinical significance. They may be recognized clinically by the finding of hyaline and granular cases, with occasional leukocytes and even red cells in the urinary sediment. Unless they are accompanied by actual glomerular damage, as in the case of the more severe infections, they often pass entirely unrecognized except as an incidental finding at autopsy.

In addition to these more common mild lesions which are represented by the familiar cloudy swelling, occasional instances of death may result from obstruction to the tubules as the result of massive hemorrhagic cast formation with associated uremia. This is seen occasionally following transfusion with an incompatible donor. It is likewise seen in paroxysmal hemoglobinuria. The mechanism is poorly understood in respect to the initial hemorrhage, but the packing of the red cells in the tubules is very striking when it occurs and is comparable to the obstruction seen in the more severe types of nephrosis, such as mercuric chloride poisoning where the tubules become obstructed with the necrotic cellular debris. Refer to Case 5 (Ref. #S-80) and Fig. 549.

Lipoid Nephrosis.—From the clinical standpoint, lipoid nephrosis is characterized by a syndrome in which edema and albuminuria are the two prominent features. Considerable doubt exists among many clinicians as to the actual existence of such a condition. As the term is usually employed, lipoid nephrosis occurs in young individuals and develops insidiously. The blood chemistry tends to show a lower protein level and an increased lipoid content. In the urine, doubly refractile lipoid droplets may be identified by the use of the Nicol prism, and their presence in the face of this clinical picture is considered of diagnostic significance. The disease further is a chronic one running a prolonged course with periods of remission, and the patient may recover spontaneously after months or years. On the other hand, these patients are apparently particularly susceptible to infection and are liable to succumb to upper respiratory disease which under other circumstances, would be considered relatively insignificant.

Pathologically, the condition is likewise on a somewhat insecure anatomical foundation. It is characterized by the presence of extreme lipoid or fatty degeneration of the tubular epithelium. This is not confined necessarily to the convoluted epithelial cells, but may involve the tubule as a whole. Again, the presence of the rather characteristic lipoid substances under the Nicol prism is of some differential diagnostic value histologically. Typically, the glomerular damage is lacking, or is minimal, in contradistinction to cases of glomerulonephritis in which secondary fatty degenerative changes of the tubules exist. Practically, undoubtedly the great majority of cases of so-called "nephrosis" clinically fall into the group of tubular nephroses, secondary to the glomerulonephritis and not, strictly speaking, primary nephrosis.

CHAPTER LVI

DISEASES OF THE KIDNEY (*Continued*)

NEPHROSCLEROSIS (VASCULAR NEPHRITIS)

Cardiovascular Renal Disease

Thus far in our discussion, we have seen that either the glomeruli or the tubules may be the primary focus of renal pathology and that they are frequently seen in combination with each other as part of the picture of true inflammatory disease of the kidney, or nephritis. In this chapter, we turn to a consideration of those changes in the kidney which occur in relation to disturbances in the blood supply. These are ordinarily thought of as degenerative lesions and as such are better described under the newer terminology of *nephrosclerosis* than under the older nomenclature of *vascular nephritis*. The problem of nephrosclerosis carries us unavoidably into a consideration of hypertensive vascular disease in relation to the renal changes. According to vital statistics collected by the various life insurance companies, hypertensive cardiovascular renal disease in some combination is responsible for approximately one-fourth of the mortality in individuals past the age of fifty. For this reason, too much emphasis cannot be placed upon a thorough knowledge of the various factors which play their parts in the production of this eventual hypertension and its concomitant death toll.

From the pathological standpoint, the vascular lesions of the kidney are comparatively simple to classify and identify, but in their relation to hypertension and to cardiovascular disease in general, the problem is not as readily solved. This brings us to a brief review in the consideration of the problem of arteriosclerosis as a whole. In the chapter devoted to diseases of the blood vessels, this has already been discussed in some detail, but it will perhaps serve a useful purpose at this time to review briefly the general concept of this broad term. By the term, arteriosclerosis, are meant two distinct pathological processes. These can be demonstrated both grossly and microscopically. In the first place, the term includes that group of lesions which are characterized,

as Aschoff has so eloquently described, by atherosclerotic changes of the intima. This is the type of vascular pathology ordinarily associated with physiological senile degeneration, but may occur prematurely not uncommonly and may even be found in infancy in a modified form. In this connection, we find a type of renal disease in which the main pathology is found in the larger arterial branches and presents the picture of atherosclerosis.

From the other side of the picture, the general term, arteriosclerosis, includes that condition perhaps better described as hyperplastic arteriolar sclerosis in which the changes are found first in the smaller terminal arterioles and arteries and are characterized by hyperplasia of the subintimal connective and elastic tissues and at times by actual proliferation of the lining intima itself in a rather uniform, symmetrical fashion resulting in narrowing of the lumen even to the point of complete occlusion. This is the term which is applied to the vast group of cases associated with so-called "essential hypertension" and terminating ultimately invariably fatally in renal failure, provided intercurrent infection or some other cause of death does not intervene. This is the condition which we see in a younger age group as compared to the atherosclerotic arterial case, and which has been described by a host of pathological terms. In its usual form in the kidney, it is more familiarly known today as the benign type of arteriolar nephrosclerosis in contradistinction to a malignant form, which is similar in nature but which progresses rapidly, often in a matter of a few weeks, to a fatal outcome.

Arterial (Senile—Atheromatous) Nephrosclerosis.—In old age, as part of the general picture of senile arteriosclerosis, we find not uncommonly that the larger and medium-sized arteries of the kidney become involved in a diffuse atherosclerosis. Indeed, at times this degenerative vascular lesion may be

662

PLATE CXXX
DISEASES OF THE KIDNEY
Cardiovascular Renal Disease: Nephrosclerosis

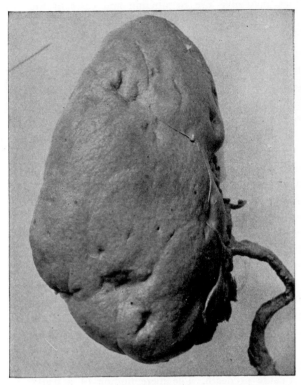

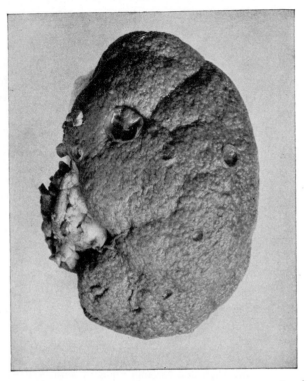

FIG. 550.—KIDNEY: NEPHROSCLEROSIS, ARTERIAL (SENILE) TYPE.—CASE 232.—Gross photograph of kidney showing a number of coarse scars, the remaining surface relatively smooth. Capsular adhesions were present over scarred areas.

FIG. 551.—KIDNEY: NEPHROSCLEROSIS, ARTERIOLAR TYPE (BENIGN ESSENTIAL HYPERTENSION).—CASE 233.—Gross kidney showing the typical finely granular surface with an occasional small retention cyst. Numerous fine adhesions were found between the capsule and the surface.

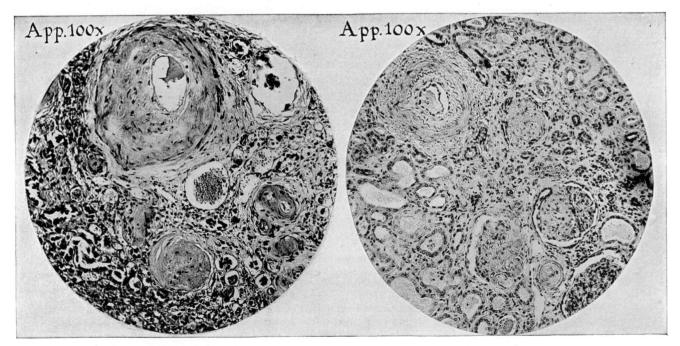

FIG. 552.—KIDNEY: NEPHROSCLEROSIS, ARTERIAL SENILE TYPE.—CASE 232.—Photomicrograph showing a small arteriole with eccentric, fibrous, subintimal thickening of wall, greatly reducing the lumen. Note hyalinized fibrotic glomerulus in foreground, and interstitial connective tissue between tubules. App. 100 x.

FIG. 553.—KIDNEY: NEPHROSCLEROSIS, ARTERIOLAR TYPE (ESSENTIAL BENIGN HYPERTENSION).—CASE 233.—Low power photomicrograph showing a small renal arteriole, the site of concentric hyperplastic sclerosis. Note similar changes with obliteration of arterioles, interstitial fibrosis and glomerular scarring. App. 100 x.

particularly localized to the kidney, just as at other times it seems to be largely restricted to the coronaries, or to the cerebral vessels, or to the peripheral vessels of the extremities, as in diabetes.

This atherosclerotic process is characterized by the infiltration and deposition of lipoid material in the subintima as in the development of atheromata of the aorta or other large vessels. As a result, it is an asymmetrical lesion. If it becomes extensive enough it may gradually occlude the vessel entirely. More often a small channel persists, and not infrequently some calcification takes place. Not infrequently, also, ulceration of these atheromatous plaques in the larger arteries occur. This is followed by thrombosis and the usual reparative organization phenomena. Fragments of these thrombi may break off and embolism of some of the smaller arteries or arterioles may occur. By one or another of these processes, considerable areas of kidney tissue may become deprived of nutrition. As a result of anoxemia, a process comparable to infarction takes place. The lesions are usually multiple and very slow in their development. The end picture in such a case is a scarred and shrunken kidney, because with interference with the blood supply, the kidney parenchyma atrophies and becomes replaced with cicatricial connective tissue. This contracts to form large, wedge-shaped areas of scar formation, between which essentially normal functioning kidney persists. As might be expected in such areas, considerable chronic inflammatory mononuclear cellular infiltration is observed. Lymphocytes, as a rule, predominate even to

the point of follicle formation in extreme instances. From the clinical pathological standpoint, such a kidney may give rise to albumin and casts in the urine. It is associated with but moderate elevation in blood pressure and only in the terminal stages is there evidence of renal failure. The rise in blood pressure in these cases of simple senile atherosclerotic disease is merely the increase in blood pressure which is part of the whole vascular degenerative state accompanied by compensatory activity on the part of the heart and by a wide variety of contributory factors, the result of far-flung senile degenerative changes.

Only rarely does the pressure rise significantly from the standpoint of renal function and only rarely does the individual with this type of kidney pathology die as a result of true renal failure. This is evidenced by the absence of a rise in the nitrogenous substances in blood chemistry studies; by the absence of uremia and by the absence of impairment of renal function as measured by concentration tests. Therefore, from the standpoint of essential renal pathology, the senile arterial nephrosclerotic kidney may be dismissed with but little concern other than that the pathologist learns to recognize its unimportance as a cause of death. The mere finding of a badly scarred and somewhat small kidney with its capsule adherent to these areas of cicatricial tissue is no indication that the kidney was primarily at fault in causing death, and the pathologist will do well to look elsewhere in the body for more significant evidence of disease.

ILLUSTRATIVE CASE

CASE 232. (Ref. #S-87)

Diagnosis.—Kidney—arterial nephrosclerosis (senile atherosclerosis).

Chief Complaint.—Patient was a white male of 72 years, who was admitted to the hospital because of severe pain in his abdomen of a week's duration.

Present Illness.—About a week before admission the patient noticed a progressive localized pain in his epigastric region. This did not radiate in any direction. It was knife-like in character and almost constant. Just before admission, the patient vomited a large amount of blood. He had had almost complete anorexia during the week previous in association with this epigastric pain, and he had been constipated.

Past Medical History.—The patient's history in respect to his present illness yielded the information that five years earlier he had an ulcer of his stomach for which he had been operated upon. He did not know what type of operation had been performed. Aside from this his history pointed more particularly toward pos-

sible genito-urinary disease than to anything else. He had had increased frequency and a marked nocturia which required his voiding five or six times a night. This had existed for several years and had been increasing in degree. It was associated with a sense of urgency and he never felt as if he had completely evacuated his bladder. He had not noticed any definite blood in his urine but had observed that it was very cloudy on occasions.

Physical Examination.—Patient was a well-developed, somewhat undernourished, elderly, white male. His head was negative. His pupils showed a bilateral arcus senilis. There was compensated edentia. His nose and throat were negative. His chest was symmetrical. His heart and lungs were negative. He showed considerable pain and tenderness in the epigastric region. No masses could be felt because of the rigidity with which he held his abdomen. His blood pressure was 110/70. His external genitalia were negative. His extremities showed marked arteriosclerotic changes. His radial arteries and dorsalis

PLATE CXXXI
DISEASES OF THE KIDNEY
Cardiovascular Renal Disease: Benign Nephrosclerosis (Essential Hypertension, Benign).—Case 233

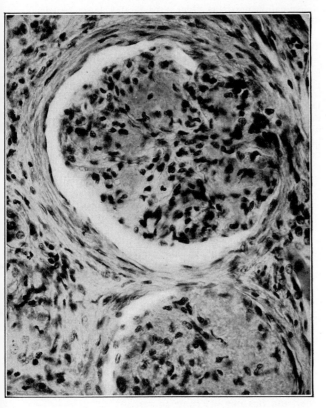

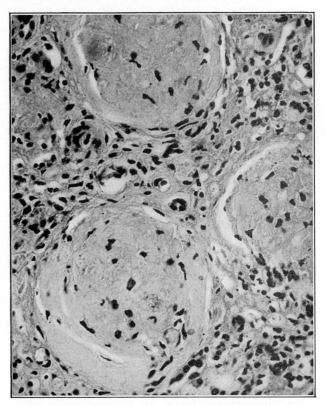

Fig. 554.—Glomeruli.—High power photomicrograph to show the periglomerular subcapsular fibrosis. Note beginning fibrotic changes of tuft. App. 300 x.

Fig. 555.—Glomeruli.—High power photomicrograph of several glomeruli showing complete fibrosis with hyaline changes. Note also interstitial fibrosis and tubular atrophy. App. 300 x.

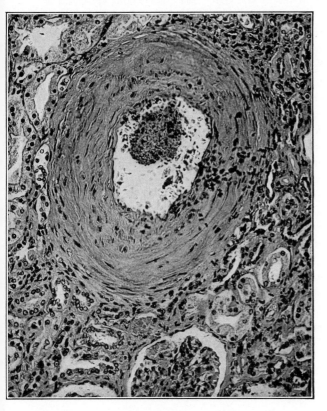

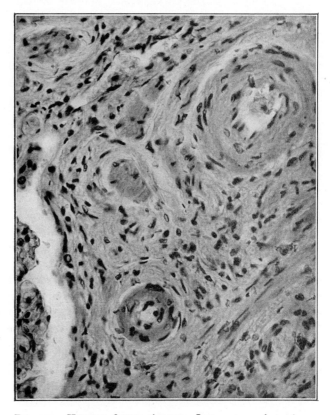

Fig. 556.—Kidney: Arterioles.—The arteriolar lumina are greatly due to muscular hypertrophy and intimal hyperplasia. Note marked interstitial fibrosis. App. 200 x.

Fig. 557.—Kidney: Small Artery.—Low power photomicrograph showing the greatly thickened vessel wall due to hyperplastic sclerosis. Note especially muscular hypertrophy, fibrosis of media and marked subintimal thickening due to fibrous and elastic tissue hyperplasia. App. 200 x.

pedis arteries were almost pipe-stem in character. Rectal examination showed a moderate hypertrophy of his prostate.

Laboratory Findings.—Blood examination: Red cells, 2,400,000, hemoglobin 48%; white cells, 12,600, with 63% polynuclears. Smear showed a slight hypochromic picture but the red cells as a whole were fairly normal. The low count was obviously a result of hemorrhage rather than real anemia. Urinalysis showed a slight trace of albumin, specific gravity 1.010 and a few leukocytes in the sediment. Wassermann was negative.

Subsequent History.—Patient had another severe hemorrhage which apparently came from his stomach, and likewise showed blood in his stool. This blood was fairly bright in color. A diagnosis of bleeding gastric ulcer was made, but before a donor could be obtained, the patient died presumably of exsanguination.

Autopsy Findings.—Autopsy showed a well-developed, emaciated, elderly male with an old midline operative scar. The heart was normal in size. There was marked atherosclerosis of the aorta which increased in degree toward the bifurcation. Coronaries were markedly sclerosed. Kidneys were somewhat small. They weighed but 100 gm. each. Capsules stripped with moderate difficulty due to several depressed sclerotic scars (Fig. 550). The renal artery likewise showed marked atherosclerotic

Arteriolar (Essential Hypertensive) Nephrosclerosis.—Practically it would seem advisable to restrict the use of the term, nephrosclerosis, to this all important condition of arteriolar disease of the kidney. It represents an ever increasing group of cases under the requirements of our modern civilization. The mere fact that from the standpoint of vital statistics the incidence of arteriolar nephrosclerosis occurs in so much greater preponderance in those individuals subject to the greatest degree of mental and nervous strain would point without much question to a psychogenic or neurogenic factor as perhaps the most significant etiologically. It is well recognized that the physician, the judge, the banker, and those individuals who work under particularly high nervous tension die with increasing frequency and at an earlier age of some form of cardiovascular-renal failure than does the phlegmatic, but physically active laborer. The same findings are, in general, true as regards the sex distribution of this condition, the great majority of cases occurring in males, although in recent years a similar increase in incidence has been shown in females engaged in work in which the same type of mental strain exists. These statistical data are a challenge to us, and as a result perhaps no field of endeavor in experimental medicine has been more thoroughly explored in the past two decades. Out of this welter of experimental data, few facts of particularly important practical application have been obtained. It is the old problem of

change. The cause of death was found to be from intra-abdominal hemorrhage from a perforated large gastric ulcer measuring 4 cm. in its greatest diameter.

Microscopic Description of Section Through Kidney.—(Fig. 552) Histologic examination of the kidney tissue presents evidence of a rather marked atherosclerosis involving the larger and medium sized arteries. This is characterized by the development of subintimal atheromatous plaques showing typical lipoidal degeneration. Occasional areas where beginning calcification has occurred can be identified. The lumina of many of the vessels have been considerably decreased in size resulting in a marked ischemia of the renal parenchyma. In places the atherosclerotic process has gone on to complete occlusion of the vessel. In relation to such occlusions, complete atrophy of the nephron supplied by the vessel has taken place. There is a corresponding replacement fibrosis which appears as an interstitial lesion. This has resulted in a wedge-shaped scar which has its base toward the cortex and its apex toward the medulla where the point of obliteration of the vessel has occurred. There is considerable secondary mononuclear cellular infiltration. The rest of the kidney appears almost within normal limits, although here and there some slight arteriolar sclerotic changes are seen in some of the smaller vessels, as might well be expected.

the chicken and the egg, and whether hypertension is the cause of arteriolar disease, or whether arteriolar disease is the cause of hypertension has long intrigued the mind of the experimentalist. The pendulum has swung first one way and then the other and has not yet come to rest.

It is extremely difficult to evaluate the work which has been done over this period of time. The most recent and significant observations appear to be those of Goldblatt and Moritz, who have shown that renal ischemia is apparently the underlying factor in the development of the hypertension and the nephrosclerotic process of the kidney. In the experimental animal such renal ischemia induced mechanically has caused exactly comparable rises in blood pressure and changes in the kidney structure as are found in human cases of essential arteriolar nephrosclerosis. As is true of so many of our experimental studies, the results only answer the question of how, not why, and before the problem can be solved it becomes necessary to go far behind the visible evidence of mechanism to the apparently invisible method of activation of this mechanism. Here the clue seems to lie in the vital statistical data which has been presented. Vasospasm is obviously an important factor in many conditions which affect the circulatory mechanism, but again vasospasm is a mechanistic explanation and does not go back to etiology.

Anatomically, the picture is readily identified by

PLATE CXXXII

DISEASES OF THE KIDNEY

CARDIOVASCULAR RENAL DISEASE: MALIGNANT NEPHROSCLEROSIS; ESSENTIAL
HYPERTENSION, MALIGNANT.—CASE 234

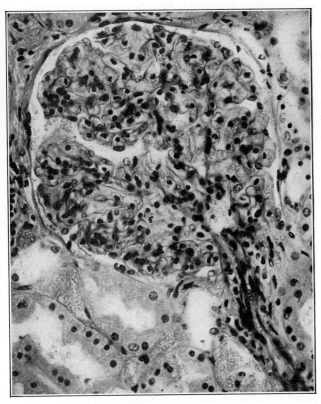

FIG. 558.—GLOMERULUS.—High power photomicrograph with early hyaline necrosis of the afferent arterioles. Glomerular tuft otherwise essentially normal. App. 300 x.

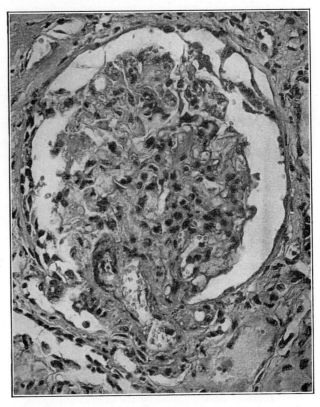

FIG. 559.—GLOMERULUS.—High power photomicrograph of a later stage with definite necrotic arteriolitis, with beginning thrombosis of one of glomerular tuft capillaries and fibrosis of another. App. 300 x.

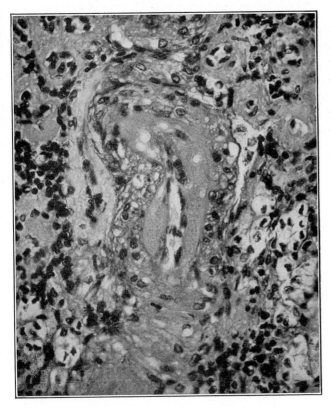

FIG. 560.—ARTERIOLE.—Oblique section in which marked hyaline necrosis of the subintima resulting in almost complete occlusion of the lumen is prominent. Note also proliferative changes of media and adventitia. App. 300 x.

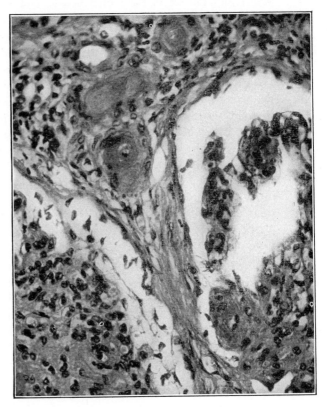

FIG. 561.—GLOMERULI AND AFFERENT ARTERIOLES.—Several small vessels seen in cross section, with their lumina occluded as a result of the necrotizing arteriolitis. Note obliterative changes in glomerular tufts. App. 300 x.

the presence of a diffuse hyperplastic arteriolar sclerosis, which may be a compensatory effort on the part of the blood vessels in an attempt to increase blood pressure in order to promote adequate circulation through the kidney and thus insure adequate elimination. If this is true, then it is just another example of one of those defense mechanisms which works in detrimental fashion upon the well-being of the individual, because as this hyperplastic process goes on the caliber of the arteriolar lumen becomes further and further decreased until ultimately complete occlusion of the smaller vessels results. Whether this is an inflammatory hyperplasia, or whether it is a degenerative process the result of some toxemia with vascular endothelial injury is entirely problematical and hypothetical. We had perhaps best confine ourselves in this discussion to the recognized anatomical factor and pathological features of arteriolar nephrosclerosis than to any further consideration of the innumerable hypotheses associated with the problem. However, it is not out of place to add one or two other comments in this respect.

It is unquestionably true that arteriolar vascular spasm is an integral part of the picture of essential hypertensive vascular disease. This has been unquestionably demonstrated by the ophthalmologists, who are able in the great majority of instances to prognosticate the development of an essential hypertension from their visualization of the spastic changes which they can see in the retinal vessels, and yet, anatomically at autopsy, save in the very extreme instances of essential hypertension with renal failure, rarely can any comparable hyperplastic sclerotic changes of these retinal vessels be demonstrated macroscopically. In similar fashion, studies relating to the peripheral arteriolar circulation have been made in countless cases in the past few years, and in general it may be said that there is little parallelism between the degree of hyperplastic sclerosis which may be found in the peripheral arterioles of the musculature, for example, and in those of the kidney in an established case of essential hypertensive vascular disease. It is true, however, that such hyperplastic changes in peripheral vessels do occur with more frequency in cases of demonstrable nephrosclerosis, as checked by autopsy figures. Furthermore, no correlation between the renal arteriolar changes and those affecting other arterioles or small arteries such as the cerebral vessels, the coronary vessels or the peripheral arterioles of the extremities exists;

and arteriolar disease of the kidney still remains a specific pathological entity in spite of the obvious neurogenic and hypertensive features as they affect the circulation as a whole. In this respect again, the work of Goldblatt is of particular interest in demonstrating the presence of a vasopressor substance, which is apparently derived from the ischemic kidney as shown by experiments consisting of the clamping of a single renal artery with the resultant unilateral ischemia.

From the pathological standpoint, the arteriosclerotic process in this instance is seen as a symmetrical hyperplastic sclerosis of the smaller arterioles of the kidney. This is ordinarily a uniformly diffuse bilateral lesion. The process appears to start in the afferent arteriole of the glomerulus, although even in the milder forms of the condition, involvement of the smaller arterioles before the definite branching of the vessel into its terminal glomerular branch occurs may be demonstrated. Everywhere throughout the kidney, arterioles are thickened and stand out from the cut surface as almost solid cords with but a pinpoint lumen.

In addition to the hyperplastic changes which are apparent in the smaller arterioles and which have resulted from proliferation of the subintimal connective tissue, elastic fibers and intimal endothelium, it will be observed not infrequently that the medium sized arteries also are frequently involved in the pathological process. In these larger vessels, however, the more striking changes are seen in the media where a definite hypertrophy which involves both the musculature and the interstitial connective tissue has taken place. This is comparable in many ways to the diffuse hyperplastic arteriolar changes just described and represents a compensatory effect on the part of these vessels to overcome the resistance occasioned by the diminished caliber of the terminal divisions of the arteriole. Thus, we find that any one of these three pathological changes; intimal proliferation, subintimal connective tissue hyperplasia or hypertrophy of the musculature, may occur separately or in combination as the effective mechanism in the production of the vascular lesions of essential hypertensive nephrosclerosis. Under these circumstances the kidney grossly is very much smaller than normal. On section, the capsule strips fairly readily leaving a uniformly finely granular surface. The cut surface presents a cortex which is definitely narrowed and a pelvis which shows a marked increase of fat. There

PLATE CXXXIII

TUMORS OF THE KIDNEYS

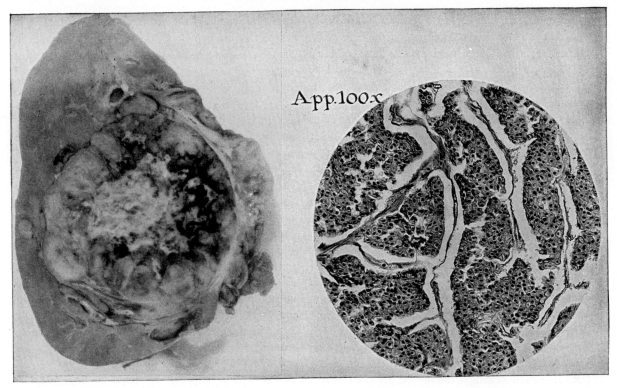

App. 100x

FIG. 562.—KIDNEY: NEPHROMA (HYPERNEPHROMA; RENAL ADENOCARCINOMA).—CASE 236.—Gross photograph which shows the characteristically spheroid, pseudo-encapsulated tumor replacing the parenchyma and invading the pelvis. Note central areas of hemorrhage and necrosis. (See Fig. 565.)

FIG. 563.—ADRENAL GLAND: HYPERNEPHROMA (ADRENAL CORTICAL CELL CARCINOMA).—CASE 271.—Histologically, the tumor is composed of sheets of cells resembling in morphology and arrangement the adrenal cortex. Note delicate stroma (cf. Fig. 342). App. 100 x.

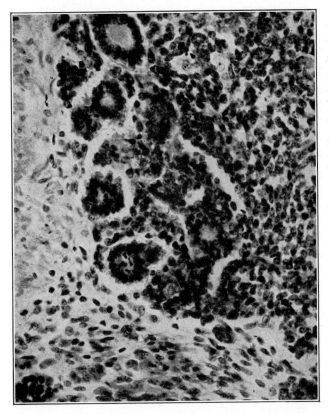

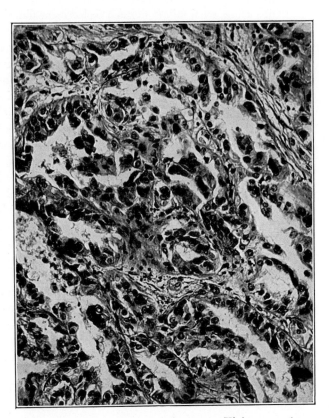

FIG. 564.—KIDNEY: WILMS' EMBRYOMA (MIXED TUMOR).—CASE 237.—High power photomicrograph. Tumor composed of connective tissue and epithelial elements derived from mesoderm. Note abortive tubule formation, occasional mitoses. (cf. Fig. 234.) App. 200 x.

FIG. 565.—KIDNEY: NEPHROMA.—CASE 236.—High power photomicrograph: Cells are large, with relatively clear cytoplasm and hyperchromic nuclei, lining spaces, thus imitating renal tubule formation. App. 200 x.

is a proliferative hyperplastic sclerosis resulting in obliterative endarteritis. The amount of kidney substance may often be reduced to less than one-third of the normal amount and is merely represented by a narrow strip of kidney tissue, which conserves the general architectural arrangement. Such a kidney is likely to show moderate congestion and to be a rather grayish-red in color. For this reason in the older terminology, this type of kidney has long been spoken of as the small red granular kidney or the primary contracted kidney (Fig. 551). This is in contradistinction to the small white kidney encountered in chronic glomerulonephritis.

From the microscopic standpoint, the picture in the usual so-called "benign" form of arteriolar nephrosclerosis is quite characteristic. Obviously, all gradations exist from the early initiation of the lesion up to the terminal picture with the fully developed contracted granular kidney. It cannot be sharply divided into stages as is true of the glomerular type of nephritis, but is best considered perhaps by the term "chronic progressive nephritis." This name has been suggested as comparable to the processes which one sees in the portal type of cirrhosis, or so-called "chronic progressive cirrhosis," in which chronic progressive fibrotic changes gradually result in the loss of liver function in the same way the gradual progressive fibrous tissue changes as the result of ischemia causes renal failure through replacement fibrosis.

In examining the cortex of such a kidney microscopically, it will be noted that the glomeruli show varying degrees of degenerative change ranging from an apparent ischemia down to complete fibrous tissue replacement. Little or no evidence of any acute inflammatory changes is seen. The picture consists of a hyaline degeneration of the wall of the blood vessel with a hyperplastic fibrous tissue proliferation of the subintima and of actual endothelial proliferation. This results in a narrowing of the lumen of the arteriole. The great majority, therefore, of the glomeruli appear relatively bloodless. This is followed by diffuse hyperplastic changes of the lining endothelium of the capillaries and of hyaline degeneration of the tissue between the capillary endothelium and the capsular epithelium. Similar nutritional starvation affects the pericapsular cells and again reparative replacement fibrosis develops with marked thickening of the periglomerular capsular area. In many instances, this actually represents a connective tissue replacement of the lining epithelium of the

capsule. Gradually the connective tissue increases in amount growing in from the sides of the capsule in rather concentric fashion until the entire glomerulus becomes obliterated and replaced by a sphere of hyalinized collagen.

While this process of glomerular obliteration is developing, the tubules undergo corresponding secondary degenerative phenomena. These changes are likewise gradual and progressive in degree. Marked dilatation of many tubules takes place and apparently the tubules even attempt to take over the function of the glomerulus. As Oliver has shown in his dissections of the individual nephrons, these changes which take place are most strikingly encountered in the convoluted portion of the tubule, particularly in the distal part of the convolution. All varieties of degenerative changes may be found affecting these tubules, many of which ultimately undergo complete atrophy and disappearance. There is, as in the case of glomerulonephritis, a tendency toward interstitial fibrous tissue replacement.

From the clinical standpoint, aside from the evidence of hypertension, the renal findings may be recognized by examination of the blood or urine. The urine shows a gradual loss of concentrating power and the presence of albumin. Edema is usually not a significant finding in these cases. There is an absence of anemia until almost terminally in contradistinction to the progressive anemia seen in glomerulonephritis. Retinal spasm and hemorrhages are seen, and typically there is marked concentric hypertrophy of the heart. Terminally there is a progressive increased retention of nitrogen in the blood stream. Not infrequently these cases go on to a typical renal death from uremia, and if seen in that stage for the first time may be difficult to differentiate from the end stage of a chronic glomerulonephritis.

Aside from the renal pathology, it is well for us to recognize that secondary lesions may be found throughout the entire body as a result of the prolonged hypertension and disturbances of circulation. Most striking among these should be mentioned the almost characteristic concentric hypertrophy of the left ventricle of the heart. Indeed, from the clinical standpoint, this picture of left-sided hypertrophy may apparently antedate the renal symptomatology. The changes which follow such hypertrophy as they affect the general circulation have already been discussed in the section relating to hypertrophy and dilatation (Case 164 of Chapter XXXVIII).

CASE 233. (Ref. #S-194)

Diagnosis.—Kidney—nephrosclerosis, benign arteriolar type.

Chief Complaint.—Patient was a colored male of 44 years, admitted to the hospital in semistupor.

Present Illness.—Four days before admission, the patient had a severe chill with a sharp rise in temperature, accompanied by pain in the left chest. He became weak and dyspneic and apparently presented a typical picture of pneumonia. A friend finally insisted on his being seen by a physician, who sent him to the hospital in a critical condition, with a temperature of 103, pulse rate of 140 and respirations of 40. On admission he showed marked mental confusion.

Past Medical History.—It was impossible to secure anything but a very vague story in respect to his previous health. One gained the impression that he had been failing for several months and had shown a marked loss of weight, had had night sweats and a chronic cough with considerable sputum. On several occasions he had noticed the sputum to be somewhat blood-tinged during the past three months. No information of significance with respect to any earlier medical history could be obtained.

Physical Examination.—Patient was an emaciated, dyspneic, weak, cyanotic, critically ill, middle-aged Negro, somewhat irrational and semistuporous. His head was negative. Examination of his chest showed dullness to flatness over the entire left side, accompanied by marked bronchophony and the presence of crepitant, coarse râles. His heart rate was rapid but otherwise negative. Blood pressure was 180/140. Patient died the day of admission and no laboratory findings were obtained.

Autopsy Findings.—A fairly well-developed but emaciated Negro. His heart was negative. Lungs: The left lung showed a diffuse fibrinopurulent pleurisy with beginning empyema formation. Both lobes were involved in a diffuse lobar pneumonia. The right lung showed marked pulmonary edema. The kidneys were moderately enlarged. They were pale in color. Their capsules stripped readily leaving a finely granular surface with several contracted scars. The other viscera were essentially negative. The picture in general suggested, from the clinical history, an old tuberculosis with a terminal tuberculous pneumonia, but autopsy findings showed no evidence of tuberculosis, but a typical left-sided lobar type of pneumonia. The kidney pathology was incidental. (Cf. Fig. 551).

Microscopic Description of a Section Through the Kidney.—(Fig. 554, 555, 556 and 557) Histologic examination of the renal tissue presents the characteristic picture of a typical hyperplastic arteriolar sclerotic process. This appears to be generalized involving not only the arterioles but the medium-sized arteries as well. The vessels show all the changes which have been described in the general discussion of benign nephrosclerosis. There is medial hypertrophy in the arteries in addition to the intimal and subintimal hyperplastic changes which are apparent in the smaller arterioles as well. In some instances, these muscular changes seem to predominate. In other vessels, the intimal proliferation appears more prominent. In all cases where the vessels are studied by the use of elastic tissue staining technique it will be noted that there is marked reduplication of the elastic laminae with considerable fraying of the ends of the elastic fibers as they stretch out into the tissues.

Very characteristically, marked periglomerular fibrosis is seen with a hyalinized thickening of the capsule. This, in places, seems to almost shut off the point where the blood vessels enter. In many places, similar fibrotic changes are seen in association with varying degrees of sclerosis of the glomeruli themselves. Marked sclerosis of the afferent glomerular capillary is almost regularly encountered. In places, the glomeruli are completely replaced by hyalinized spheres of what appears to be dense connective tissue. In a conservative estimate, it would appear that not more than one-third of the glomeruli could be considered as having any functional capacity, the others having undergone such extensive hyaline changes.

Accompanying this diffuse vascular sclerosis is a secondary interstitial fibrosis and scarring of the kidney supportive tissue. Many tubules are found completely atrophied and represented merely by compressed hyperchromatic cells obviously without function. In other places dilatation of the tubules is seen either in an attempt to assume the glomerular function or because of retention of products. Marked desquamation of the lining cells is seen with the development of a few hyaline casts. In other areas, particularly in the convoluted portion of the tubules, typical granular and fatty degeneration are seen. Basically the pathology may be described as of vascular origin in the nature of a diffuse hyperplastic arteriolar sclerosis resulting in the diminution of the renal function, through glomerular obliteration, secondary tubular degeneration and fibrotic scarring of the kidney as a typical picture of a relatively benign example of nephrosclerosis.

MALIGNANT NEPHROSCLEROSIS.—In the malignant form of the disease, the picture differs essentially only in the rapidity of its course and the degree of the changes from the more usual benign form. It has been seen in children as young as eight and is not infrequently the terminal picture in a case of benign hypertensive cardiorenal vascular disease. Its early recognition may be made clinically by observation of the capillary blood vessels in the retina, which typically present marked angiospasm. The renal involvement is only part of the picture, which is basically vascular in nature but results in acute renal failure as the result of a diffuse hyperplastic arteriolarsclerosis. In studying a series of cases, it appears that the earliest lesion occurs in the afferent glomerular capillary. This is characterized by a hyaline necrosis of the wall and as already described, a hyperplastic proliferation of the intima and subintima with gradual complete obliteration of the lumen of the arteriole.

Considerable uncertainty exists as to what should be included under the term of malignant nephrosclerosis. Arbitrarily, if one accepts the fact of hyaline necrosis of the vessel wall as evidence of the malignant nature of the process, then probably all cases of nephrosclerosis which die of *renal* failure will present terminally this picture of a malignant phase to their nephrosclerotic disease. Obviously, therefore, it is a question of interpretation as to definition. It is undoubtedly true that every case of nephrosclerosis would ultimately progress to a fatal outcome from renal failure if he did not die of some other complication such as intercurrent infection, cerebral hemorrhage, coronary disease and the like. From the pathological standpoint, if we accept only microscopic criteria for the basis of differentiation between malignant and benign nephrosclerosis, then, as has been intimated, all cases of nephrosclerosis dying of renal failure must be considered as entering this malignant picture. On the other hand, it would seem preferable from the clinical standpoint to include only those cases which occur in young individuals and run their typically rapid course of only a few weeks or months with an almost steady progression of symptoms, a rapidly rising blood pressure which may reach 350, systolic, and be accompanied by a nitrogen retention which may likewise show values of 20 to 30 mgm. of creatinine, 180 to 200 mgm. of urea and 300 mgm. or more of non-protein nitrogen. This is a question which we must leave for the future. For the present, we must, as in the past, accept our anatomical basis for the classification pathologically of malignant and benign nephrosclerosis.

From the gross standpoint, these cases of malignant nephrosclerosis as they are seen in the younger group in their fulminating form do not have time to develop the same degree of fibrosis with the resultant diminution in size of the kidney, which we see in the more usual benign form of the disease. In this malignant form, the kidney is often normal or even somewhat increased in size. On section, the capsule strips readily and diffuse focal hemorrhagic lesions are commonly found as a result of the necrotic process which affects the vessels. In some respects, they are not unlike the kidneys of focal glomerular nephritis, except the hemorrhagic areas are usually much larger and more diffuse. The renal parenchyma ordinarily is the site of rather marked fatty and granular degenerative changes so that the hemorrhages stand out rather prominently against a yellowish-gray background. When these malignant changes occur as the end stage of the benign process, the added feature of hemorrhage may be present, but due to the marked avascularization of the kidney as a whole, this picture is often absent.

ILLUSTRATIVE CASE

CASE 234. (Ref. #S-126)

Diagnosis.—Kidney—malignant nephrosclerosis.

Chief Complaint.—Patient was a white female of 32 years, admitted to the hospital with the chief complaints of dyspnea, frontal headache, nausea and vomiting.

Present Illness.—The patient had been in her usual good health until a year before the present illness. At that time she noted some puffiness under her eyes and occasional frontal headaches. These symptoms had increased during the year in frequency and severity. For the past two months she had had intermittent attacks of nausea and vomiting, accompanied by marked anorexia and some progressive blurring of vision. She had had no definite urinary symptoms. She estimated that she was three months pregnant at the time of admission.

Past Medical History.—The patient had had measles, whooping cough and scarlet fever as a child. She had been married for eight years and had had two pregnancies; one child dying of pneumonia, the other living and well. She had had no previous serious illness. A review of her systems was entirely negative until the onset of her present illness.

Physical Examination.—Patient showed paroxysmal dyspnea and obvious loss of weight. The peripheral vessels were unusually sclerosed for an individual of her age. The heart showed moderate enlargement. There was accentuation of the second sound and a marked systolic murmur was noted over the base. Blood pressure was 238/152 on admission but dropped before death to 186/128. The pulse rate ranged from 90 to about 110. Fluid balance was very poor with an intake of from 10 to 45 ounces a day and an output of 0 to 12 ounces a day.

Laboratory Findings.—Blood chemistry: Urea nitrogen 100 mgm. on admission, rising to 160 mgm. before death. Creatinine 6.6 mgm. on admission, rising to 11.8 mgm. Urinalysis: specific gravity, 1.013; albumin, 750 mgm. in a single specimen. Sediment showed countless leukocytes and red cells, but no casts. Blood: 7.5 gm. hemoglobin; 3,000,000 red cells; 11,000 white cells with 77% polynuclears. Serology was negative.

Subsequent Course.—Patient went progressively down hill, dying one week after admission.

Autopsy Findings.—There was moderate cardiac hypertrophy, the heart weighing 450 gm. There was moderate thickening of the mitral valve with several atheromatous plaques on its ventricular aspect. The coronary vessels showed rather marked atherosclerosis. The aorta showed progressively increasing atherosclerosis, being most marked at the bifurcation. There was a terminal acute fibrinous pericarditis. The peritoneal cavity contained about 300 c.c. of clear fluid. The lungs were negative. The kidneys were much smaller than normal. Their capsules stripped with some difficulty, leaving a dark red, granular surface. On section the cortex was diminished measuring 3 to 4 mm. in thickness. There was a marked increase in the pelvic fat. The kidney substance was tough and suggested diffuse fibrosis. The arterioles stood out due to thickening. They showed only pin-point lumina. The other organs were essentially negative.

Microscopic Description of a Section Through the Kidney.—(Fig. 558, 559, 560 and 561): Histologic examination of the kidney presents a typical picture of malignant nephrosclerosis. The histology is variable but the predominant lesion is a diffuse hyperplastic sclerosis of the smaller arterioles and the capillaries of the glomeruli. Accompanying this hyperplastic process is seen a very marked hyaline necrosis of the vessel walls accompanied by some cellular infiltration and hemorrhage into the interstitial stroma. As in frequently seen in this condition, there appears to be a secondary glomerular involvement. Some of the glomeruli show a compensatory hypertrophy to make up for the vascular deficiency seen in the many small, sclerosed, obliterated glomeruli, some of which are represented only by concentric fibrous scars. There is marked dilatation of the tubules in many places with the formation of some hyaline casts. Many of these tubules are filled with albuminous debris and desquamative detritus. The tubular epithelium shows very marked secondary degenerative changes. There is marked congestion of the interstitial vessels with some focal areas of hemorrhage. The interstitial tissue is generally characterized by a diffuse increase of connective tissue.

Combined Nephrosclerosis.—There still exists one group of cases which offers a certain amount of confusion both clinically and pathologically. This is the group of cases in which combinations of lesions may occur. It is not at all infrequent to find a marked atherosclerosis present in an individual in his late forties or fifties in conjunction with a well developed hyperplastic arteriolarsclerosis. At times, these two manifestations of arterial disease may be difficult to separate. Similarly, there is no reason why an individual who may have suffered from glomerulonephritis in childhood or as a young adult may not be the victim of benign nephrosclerosis in addition, quite as much as the individual who never had any such previous renal history. Such cases offer particular difficulty in differential diagnosis both from the clinical and from the histopathological standpoints, and when they are found the nephrosclerotic process is usually the more prominent because of the more obvious vascular lesions, so that it is quite possible that many such cases of combined glomerulonephritis and arteriolar nephrosclerosis go down statistically in the latter category. This is probably the more significant feature from the vital statistics point of view.

ILLUSTRATIVE CASE

Case 235. (Ref. #S-86)

Diagnosis.—Kidney—Combined atherosclerotic and arteriolar hyperplastic nephrosclerosis.

Chief Complaint.—Patient was a colored male of 61 years, who was admitted to the hospital because of mental symptoms.

Present Illness.—The onset of the present illness was extremely indefinite. He had shown signs of mental deterioration for approximately a year. More recently he had presented a marked increase of these degenerative phenomena. He would arise in the middle of the night and wander around the house purposelessly. He talked in a disoriented and peculiar manner. He would even attempt to clamber up the walls, and became progressively more and more unmanageable. About one week before admission his ankles began to swell and he complained of pain in his right side. Both of these symptoms had increased in severity during the week.

Past Medical History.—Owing to the patient's mental state, it was impossible to rely upon the history as he gave it. According to the patient, he had never had any serious illness until about six or eight years before admission, when he developed cataracts in both eyes which had been removed, so that he had been practically blind for the preceding four years.

Physical Examination.—Patient was a well-developed, elderly, colored male. Pupils were irregular and opaque. The heart was considerably enlarged and the rhythm was irregular with extra systoles and faint, blowing systolic murmurs over the mitral and aortic areas. Blood pressure was 250/150. The lungs were essentially negative except for a few moist râles at the left base. Abdomen: The liver was moderately enlarged. The spleen was possibly enlarged, although the outline could not be determined. The extremities showed considerable edema of the ankles and legs as far as the knees. There was a very marked peripheral arteriosclerosis with pipe-stem arteries.

Laboratory Findings.—Urinalysis was essentially negative except for the presence of a small amount of albumin and occasional waxy casts. Kahn was negative. Urea 16 mgm.

Subsequent Course.—The patient's mental condition continued to become more and more abnormal and he died one month after admission, apparently of generalized arteriosclerosis with cerebral symptoms predominating.

Autopsy Findings.—At autopsy, the heart showed extensive hypertensive heart disease with left ventricular hypertrophy. There was moderate coronary atherosclerosis. The aorta showed marked atheromatosis. The kidneys showed a marked degree of nephrosclerosis. They were smaller than normal. The capsule was thin and stripped with difficulty. The surface was irregular and granular in appearance with many deep contracted scars. There was generalized chronic passive congestion of the viscera and a terminal bronchopneumonia.

Microscopical Description of a Section Through the Kidney.—(Cf. Fig. 552) Histologic examination of the tissue shows a very complex pathological picture. There is a very striking atherosclerosis of the larger arteries. However, our interest is particularly related to a study of the small sized arteries and arterioles. There is a marked thickening of the wall of these small arteries. This is due particularly to hypertrophy of the muscle and also to hyperplastic thickening of the intima. There is also a marked hyperplasia of the elastic tissue which is brought out by special staining. This is characterized by a series of fragmented and concentrically arranged elastic laminae in the thickened sub-intima. The thickening of the intima leads to a marked diminution in the size of the lumen of the vessel. This hyperplastic sclerosis involves all the small arteries and arterioles. In many of the glomerular afferent arterioles the lumina are completely occluded. Normally, these vessels are barely visible, and their walls are extremely thin. In this condition of hyperplastic sclerosis, these vessels stand out grossly due to the thinning of the entire wall.

As a result of this hyperplastic sclerosis of the arteries, many of the glomeruli have become completely deprived of their blood supply with resultant obliteration. Such glomeruli have been replaced by diffuse fibrous scar tissue which shows extensive hyaline degeneration. In many places this degenerative picture appears as an almost concentric process with a small ball-like hyalinized scar representing the site of the glomerulus. In other areas, the glomeruli have not become so completely involved. Similar hyperplastic scarring of localized loops of the capillary glomerular tuft may be seen and there is also extensive thickening of the capsule as a band of fibrous tissue which shows varying degrees of hyaline change.

TUMORS OF THE KIDNEY

Tumors of the kidney may arise from the various constituent parts of the organ. The embryologic development of the kidney helps us in understanding the curious varieties of neoplasms which are found in this location. They can be divided conveniently into two major types on anatomical grounds; first, those arising from the renal pelvis, and second, those which are found in the cortex.

Pelvic Tumors.—The tumors which arise from the renal pelvis are essentially similar in nature to the tumors which are found in the urinary bladder, both of these structures having the same type of transitional cell epithelium. The tumors range all the way from simple papillomata through various intermediate stages in which alveolar arrangement is noted down to typical epidermoid varieties. The same schematic method of gradation as is applied to other mucous membrane and surface epithelial tumors is applicable to this group.

Cortical Tumors.—MALIGNANT NEPHROMA (HYPERNEPHROMA).—The commonest tumor of the kidney is represented by a neoplasm which is spoken of clinically as a *hypernephroma,* and has been emphasized in the chapter on special varieties of epithelial tumors. The great majority of such "hypernephromata" are actually tumors of renal epithelial origin, and as such should better be termed "nephromata." From the practical standpoint, most of these tumors are malignant in nature and are of the adenocarcinomatous variety. Considerable difference occurs in their morphological appearance. Two major types are found; one, a tumor which presents a very striking papillary adenocarcinomatous appearance and is made up of dark staining granular cells with small, hyperchromatic nuclei, with the cells arranged on rather heavy fibrous stalks; and two, a tumor composed of so-called "clear" cells (Fig. 565). In this latter variety the papillary arrangement is usually absent, although there is a definite attempt on the part of the cells to form acini. These are to be distinguished from the pseudo-acini of the true adrenal cell tumor. These "clear" cells are large, coarsely vacuolated and their cytoplasm is scarcely demonstrable except for the limiting cell membrane. Nuclei are usually large and round, with a well-defined nucleolus and coarse rods and granules of chromatin. The lumina of these acini are frequently filled with a homogenous, pink-staining material. Typically these tumors are extremely vascular and show many areas of necrosis. They lack the well-defined capsule of the adrenal type of hypernephroma and invade the kidney substance much more extensively. Like the true hypernephromata, they commonly invade the renal veins and extend along the vena cava as a thrombus, at times completely occluding the lumen. They likewise metastasize to the lungs and long bones rather characteristically, as do the adrenal cell type tumors.

ILLUSTRATIVE CASE

CASE 236. (Ref. #S-348)

Diagnosis.—Kidney—"clear cell" renal adenocarcinoma.

Patient was a white Italian male of 47 years, admitted to the hospital with the chief complaint of hematuria, weakness and a loss of thirty pounds over a four-month period.

Present Illness.—From the patient's standpoint, the onset of his present illness only dated back about two or three months before admission at which time he first noticed occasional attacks of hematuria. This was very marked when it occurred, with the entire urinary stream appearing bright blood red. At times he would pass a few small clots. The last severe hematuria occurred ten days before admission. Since that time, the urine had seemed clear until the current attack which was almost hemorrhagic in character and brought him to the hospital. This hematuria was not associated with pain at any time, but over the past three or four months, he had noticed that he had been losing weight and developing a marked weakness and easy fatigability on exertion.

Past Medical History.—As a child he recalled that he had had measles, scarlet fever, diphtheria and typhoid fever. Other than these infections in childhood, he did not recall any serious illness except an attack of pleurisy at the age of twenty, which kept him out of work for about three months. This was not apparently diagnosed as tuberculosis and a review of his history at that time gave no other symptoms suggesting it. His gastro-intestinal history always had been normal. Genito-urinary history had been entirely negative up to the onset of his present illness. He denied venereal disease.

Physical Examination.—The patient was a well-developed and well-nourished middle-aged Italian male, who showed some evidence of recent weight loss. The nose and throat were negative. Oral hygiene was poor with many carious teeth. The chest was symmetrical and the lungs clear. Heart was not enlarged and there were no murmurs. The abdomen was prominent, particularly in the upper right quadrant. The whole abdomen was moderately tender to palpation. In the right upper quadrant, a large rounded mass was felt, which was movable on deep palpation and moved with respiration. It appeared somewhat tender. The extremities and external genitalia were negative.

Laboratory Findings.—Red blood cells, 4,800,000 with 60% hemoglobin. White blood cells, 17,400 with 82% polynuclears. Urinalysis was negative. Wassermann was negative.

X-ray examination showed a normal left kidney. There was a large filling defect of the right renal pelvis. This appeared to be due to an intrarenal tumor.

Subsequent Course.—On the basis of the clinical history and x-ray findings, a tentative diagnosis of right renal neoplasm probably renal carcinoma was made, and the right kidney removed by the usual oblique loin incision. A mass the size of a grapefruit was found involving the entire upper pole of the kidney. This was adherent to the ascending colon and had to be separated from this organ. The patient made an uneventful recovery and was discharged greatly improved.

Pathological Report..—*Gross Description.*—Specimen consisted of a kidney with a large tumor mass which together measured 16 x 10 x 6 cm. (Fig. 562). The tumor mass occupied the entire upper pole of the kidney. It appeared partially encapsulated and sharply demarcated from the surrounding kidney structure in the cortex, but showed direct invasion of the pelvis of the kidney. This was accompanied by moderate compression of the calices and renal pelvis in this area. On section, the tumor tissue was of a yellowish-white color with many areas of hemorrhagic necrosis. The picture was typical of so-called "hypernephroma" or renal carcinoma. No apparent invasion of the blood vessels was noted.

Microscopic Description of a Section Through the Kidney Tumor.—(Fig. 565) Histologic examination of the tumor tissue presents a definite glandular structure. In many areas, there is a very well-defined tubule formation. In other areas the tumor is growing more in the form of sheets and trabeculae of tumor cells. The cells are fairly uniform in size with relatively large nuclei containing from one to three nucleoli. The cytoplasm of the cells is distended and swollen and appears finely vacuolated. It represents the so-called "clear cell" type of adenocarcinoma of renal tubular epithelial origin. There is no sharp line of demarcation between the neoplasm and the surrounding renal tissue. The kidney substance itself shows evidence of an old chronic glomerular nephritis with many scarred glomeruli showing adhesions and even obliteration.

CORTICAL ADENOMA.—That tumors may arise from the renal tubular epithelium is well supported by the fact that minute cortical adenomata are not infrequently found in the renal cortex. These are very often multiple. Whether or not these represent embryonic rests is problematical. They remain apparently throughout their life history in this form. There is no particular tendency toward malignant degeneration and in this respect they might be compared to the small fetal (follicular) adenomata of the thyroid. For an illustrative case refer to Case 134 (Ref. #S-10), Chapter XXXII.

EMBRYOMATA (WILMS' TUMOR; RHABDOMYOMATA; ADENOSARCOMATA).—These tumors are found for the most part within the first decade of life. They are usually highly malignant, rapidly growing, large tumors which may attain a size as great as 35 to 40 cm. They are rather solid, whitish tumors which, as they increase in size undergo cystic degeneration. Two major varieties of this group of tumors are encountered; first, the more familiar mixed type of tumor in which both glandular and stromal elements show evidence of malignancy. This was the type of tumor originally described by Wilms, and to which his name has long been attached. The second variety is a type in which striated muscle predominates and is seen in the form of a rhabdomyosarcoma. In Chapter XXVI devoted to a consideration of the group of tumors arising from muscle, such an example was presented in Case 101 (Ref. #S-237). This merely represents a one-sided development of a similar embryonal type of tumor from the undifferentiated renal blastema. Almost any combination of histology may be found, with abortive pseudo-glomerular or tubule formation, with smooth or striated muscle, and with gland-like structures which appear to be secretory. They tend to metastasize early and to extend rapidly throughout the abdomen. They unfortunately have a curious tendency to be bilateral and progress to renal failure relatively promptly. In those instances where the lesion has been unilateral and recognized promptly, several instances of permanent cure have been recorded.

In reviewing the pathological features of the entire group of tumors which arise in the renal substance itself, other than the pelvic tumors, one is gradually forced to the conclusion that all such tumors are basically mesothelial in origin, the kidney representing one of those organs in which the epithelium is derived by differentiation from such mesothelial cells. In reviewing the embryonal tumors, their origin from the renal blastema seems apparent. It has been shown that such cells are capable of differentiation into these bizarre teratoid tumors. It is but a step from this concept to the recognition that the adult malignant nephroma may likewise be derived from the later stage of differentiation of the same renal blastema, as is true of the more complex tumors of the gonads.

ILLUSTRATIVE CASE

CASE 237. (Ref. #S-381)

Diagnosis.—Kidney—embryoma (Wilms' tumor).

Patient was a white female of 63 years, admitted to the hospital with the chief complaint of left lower abdominal pain of four months' duration.

Present Illness.—The onset of the patient's present illness was approximately four months before her admission when she began to have what she thought were abdominal cramps. Gradually this pain localized in the left side and tended to be radiating from the back toward the pelvis. The pains lasted only for a few seconds or so at a time, but occurred six or seven times a day. They did not, apparently, occur at night, or at least they were not sufficiently severe to interfere with her sleep.

Past Medical History.—The patient did not remember with which of the childhood diseases she had been afflicted, but did not recall ever having been seriously ill. About one year before her present admission, she began to have a feeling of weakness and easy fatigability. This was associated with a pain in her left chest. A thoracentesis was done and a clear fluid obtained. This was repeated at intervals of about ten days for five or six times following which she improved in health. A review of her systems was of no particular significance in respect to her present illness. She never had had any cardiorespiratory distress. She had not been subject to upper respiratory infection. Her gastrointestinal history was negative except for a rather chronic constipation. Her genito-urinary history was negative. Menses had begun at the age of thirteen and had been regular throughout her active physiological years. She had had her menopause twelve years earlier. Her family history was negative in respect to tuberculosis and cancer.

Physical Examination.—The patient was a well-developed, well-nourished elderly white female, who appeared to be entirely comfortable, lying in bed. Head showed no abnormalities. Eyes, ears, nose and throat were negative. Chest was symmetrical. Lungs were clear throughout. There was no dullness and no alteration in breath sounds even over the left base where she had had her previous pleural effusion. The heart was not enlarged. The sounds were of good quality. There were no murmurs. The abdomen was moderately distended. There was a large palpable mass about the size of a grapefruit felt in the region of the left kidney area. This was not tender. Extremities were negative. Gynecologic examination showed no significant pathology. There was a laceration of the cervix on the left. Both ovaries could be palpated and seemed normal in size.

Laboratory Findings.—Red blood cells on admission numbered 3,850,000 and there was a hemoglobin of 70%. Leukocytes numbered 7,300 with 64% polynuclears. Urinalysis showed a slight trace of albumin on one occasion and a considerable number of leukocytes on repeated examination.

Subsequent Course.—On the basis of these findings, a cystoscopic examination was done and catheterized specimens from both kidneys were obtained. These were both negative. The bladder showed a moderate cystitis. Pyelography revealed a deformity of the pelvis of the left kidney, suggesting a neoplasm of the body of the kidney. An exploratory operation was done and a large tumor mass found involving the left kidney. This extended as a sheet along the course of the ureter into the pelvis. Because of this extension of the tumor, it was felt that nephrectomy would be of no avail. A biopsy specimen was removed for histologic examination and the establishment of a diagnosis.

The patient was treated by rather intensive irradiation and in a period of less than three weeks the tumor mass had regressed to the point where it could not be palpated through the abdominal wall.

Pathological Report.—*Gross Description.*—Specimen consisted of a wedge-shaped piece of grayish-pink tissue approximately 1 cm. in its greatest diameter. This presented no gross features of diagnostic significance.

Miscroscopic Description of a Section Through the Biopsy Specimen.—(Fig. 564) Histologic examination of the tissue presents the rather characteristic appearance of an embryonal type of renal tumor, the so-called "Wilms', or mixed tumor" of the kidney. Two very distinct types of tissue are recognized in the histologic preparation. In the first place, there are abortive attempts at renal structural formation. These appear as rather isolated small areas in which an attempt at tubule reproduction is apparent. These distorted tubular structures are composed of small cells of a relatively cuboidal form. Nuclei are round or slightly ovoid. They contain rather prominent nucleoli and scattered granules of chromatin. The cytoplasm is rather granular in appearance. The remainder of the tumor tissue is made up of a loose, almost myxomatous-appearing material. The cells tend to be somewhat spindled in form and there is a moderate amount of intercellular matrix, which has the suggestion of fibrillar arrangement. The nuclei here are definitely ovoid or elongated. They tend to be relatively hyperchromic. Occasional mitotic figures are encountered. This combination of connective tissue and epithelial-like structures is extremely suggestive of a primitive embryonal mesothelial tumor arising from the metanephros, and can best be considered in this light.

CHAPTER LVII

DISEASES OF THE MALE GENITALIA

The pathological lesions of importance which relate to the male genitalia are, curiously enough, not very great in number. The congenital lesions which occur are chiefly those relating to the failure of the lower urinary tract to develop normally. Thus, hypospadias, epispadias, ectopia of the bladder, patent urachus and the like are not infrequently encountered. They are of little pathological significance except as they are liable to be involved in secondary inflammatory lesions. From the practical standpoint, the lesions which are of importance pathologically are those relating to inflammatory, hyperplastic and neoplastic lesions of the various organs, particularly the prostate and testes.

BLADDER

The bladder, while more properly belonging to the urinary tract system, because of its pelvic location in relation to the reproductive organs, seems more logically discussed at this point. The really important lesions of the bladder numerically at least, are only two in number, i.e., cystitis and tumors, but there are several other pathological conditions which should be mentioned in connection with this organ.

Congenital Lesions

The bladder, as has been mentioned in the introductory remarks, may take part in a considerable number of pathological conditions relating to the unsuccessful embryologic development of the urogenital tract. The most significant of these is seen in the complete extrophy of the bladder, usually accompanied by incomplete fusion of the abdominal wall with a variable amount of eventration. This is of significance primarily because of the almost inevitable infection of the bladder. It likewise not infrequently may be associated with ureteral defects so that hydronephrosis and renal failure may be incidental complications. It is seen with defective development of the urethral tract and with a wide variety of anomalies relating to the abnormal differentiation of the allantois and lower intestinal tract.

Inflammations

Acute Cystitis.—Acute cystitis may result from infection of an ascending type, especially in the female, or be of a descending variety associated with pyelonephritis. It may likewise complicate the presence of a primary vesicle stone or renal calculi, which have passed down the ureter into the bladder. The most important organism in this connection is the colon bacillus, but many of the other bacteria at one time or another play their part in such acute inflammatory processes. All gradations of acute inflammation may exist ranging from mild catarrhal forms up to extensive gangrenous, necrotic inflammation with actual destruction of the wall of the bladder and diffusion of the infected urine through the soft retroperitoneal and subcutaneous tissues.

Chronic Cystitis.—Chronic cystitis may follow the subsidence of an acute inflammatory attack but may apparently start as a chronic process from the outset. This likewise may be of the chronic catarrhal variety or may show chronic granulomatous features. This is particularly seen in association with the presence of single large stones, which almost fill the lumen of the urinary bladder (Fig. 567).

Cystitis Cystica.—In rare instances of chronic inflammatory involvement of the bladder mucosa, there may appear a marked thickening of the mucosa,

PLATE CXXXIV
DISEASES OF THE BLADDER

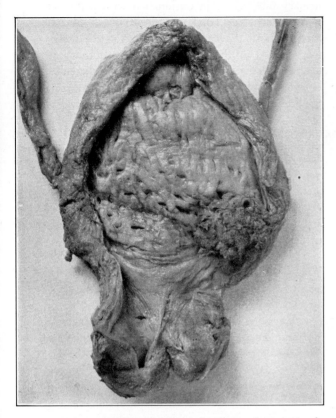

FIG. 566.—BLADDER: BENIGN PAPILLOMA.—Gross photograph of urinary bladder in which a papillomatous tumor may be seen arising in relation to the trigon. Note hypertrophy of bladder wall, beginning pseudodiverticulosis formation.

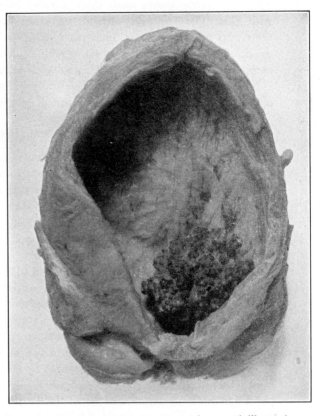

FIG. 567.—BLADDER: CALCULUS.—Gross photograph illustrating a much hypertrophied bladder, containing a large calculus in the neck producing partial urinary obstruction.

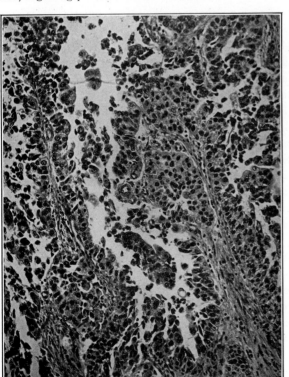

FIG. 568.—BLADDER: MALIGNANT PAPILLOMA.—CASE 134.—Photomicrograph showing two papillae of the tumor covered by atypical, pleomorphic cells, several layers in thickness, with hyperchromic nuclei, and simulating in appearance the normal transitional epithelium. App. 200 x.

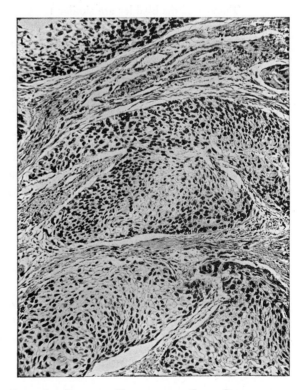

FIG. 569.—BLADDER: TRANSITIONAL CELL CARCINOMA.—CASE 238.—Photomicrograph shows a portion of bladder wall infiltrated by nests of fairly well differentiated transitional epithelial cells. Some hyperchromatism and occasional mitotic figures may be seen. App. 100 x.

which on section shows small cystic cavities filled with fluid. This frequently extends to involve the ureter. Its mechanism is not understood, but it is a condition which has attracted a considerable amount of interest among urologists and pathologists alike.

Tuberculosis.—Tuberculosis of the bladder is usually seen only in the more diffuse forms of genito-urinary tuberculosis in conjunction with a tuberculous ureteritis or renal phthisis in which tubercle bacilli get into the bladder by way of the urine. Here they may set up their typical chronic granulomatous ulcerative lesions. The picture is that of tuberculosis elsewhere and is diagnosed by direct cystoscopy and the finding of the tubercle bacilli in the lesions.

MECHANICAL LESIONS OF THE BLADDER

The wall of the urinary bladder, being made up of interlacing masses of smooth muscle, is capable of an extraordinary degree of distention. This occurs not infrequently as the result of obstructive processes involving the urethral orifice, or as the result of neurogenic influences with paralysis of the musculature. If the process is at all prolonged, there is a tendency for marked hypertrophy of the wall of the bladder to follow. This is characterized by thickening of the bladder trabeculae. Not uncommonly with such distention, a weak point in the musculature of the bladder wall may result in the formation of a diverticulum. This is frequently spoken of as a false or pseudodiverticulum in contradistinction to the occasional true diverticulum, which is congenital in origin and in which the entire wall of the bladder takes part. In the female, as the result of relaxation of the floor of the pelvis in association with repeated pregnancies, the so-called "cystocele" develops, which merely represents the bulging of the organ into the vagina. This may result in marked urinary retention and is one of the important causes of chronic cystitis in the female.

Rupture of the Bladder.—Rupture of the bladder may follow such marked distention, as has been commented upon, or the rupture may be the result of direct trauma upon a moderately distended bladder, or the result of direct perforation as, for example, in traumatic fractures of the pelvis. The chief importance of rupture of the bladder lies in the fact that the extravasated urine is liable to get into the surrounding tissue and set up acute or chronic inflammatory processes leading to the development of fistulous tracts between vagina or rectum.

TUMORS OF THE BLADDER

Tumors of the bladder are similar to those which are found in the pelvis of the kidney. The majority of them occur in three types: first, the benign papillomata; second, the malignant papillomata; third, the transitional cell carcinomata. These three varieties make up at least 95 per cent of all bladder tumors. In addition, certain tumors tend to show an adenomatous arrangement and are spoken of as adenocarcinomata. There are occasional comparatively uncommon tumors encountered of which the colloid carcinoma is one variety. This cannot be differentiated histologically from similar colloid carcinomata of the gastro-intestinal tract. It is generally held that this arises from embryonic rests in the bladder wall during the course of the development of the urinary tract from the cloaca.

Papillomata.—The papilloma arises as a pedunculated tumor from the mucous surface, more often in relation to the trigon than from the fundus (Fig. 566). It may attain a considerable size, almost filling the bladder lumen, but still remaining pedunculated, and involving only a small area of mucosa in its origin.

Microscopically, the tumor consists of delicate papillary stalks of connective tissue and capillaries upon which are arranged typical, transitional epithelial cells, often layer upon layer. They are relatively normal in appearance with well-differentiated nuclei. There persists a well-developed basal membrane. No evidence of invasion of the deeper structures is seen. They do, however, tend to recur and not infrequently may ultimately undergo a malignant transformation into true diffuse infiltrating papillary carcinoma.

Malignant Papillomata.—Carcinoma of the bladder, as has been suggested, may arise from a preexisting papilloma, but may and not infrequently does occur as such from the outset. It is similar in appearance to the benign papilloma except that it is more extensive, usually arises from a larger area of mucosal surface and shows extensive infiltration of the wall of the bladder. It is a large, bulky, hemor-

PLATE CXXXV
DISEASES OF THE PROSTATE

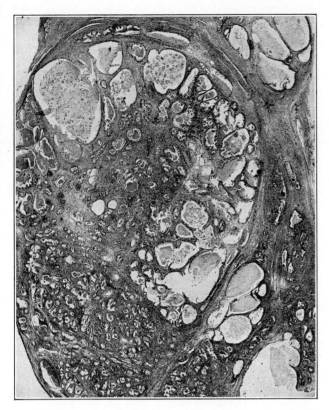

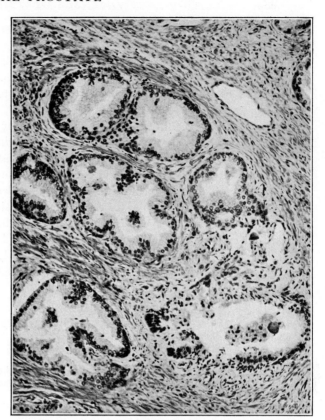

FIG. 570.—PROSTATE: BENIGN HYPERPLASIA (BENIGN HYPERTROPHY).—CASE 239.—Microtessar photograph of a section taken from the enlarged middle lobe showing increase in the glandular and interstitial elements with cystic dilatation of some acini. App. 6 x.

FIG. 571.—PROSTATE: BENIGN HYPERPLASIA.—CASE 239.—High power detail of an area from Fig. 570 to better show the hyperplastic acini lined by several layers of pseudostratified columnar epithelium, which tends to project as papillae into the lumina. App. 100 x.

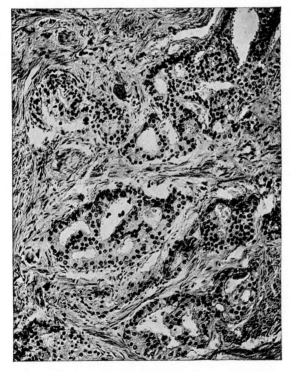

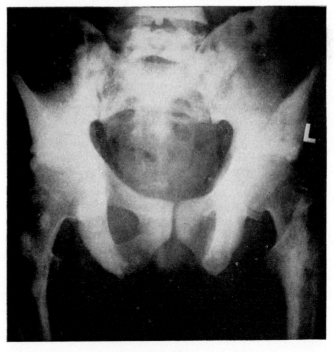

FIG. 572.—PROSTATE: ADENOCARCINOMA.—CASE 240.—Photomicrograph shows a tumor invading the prostate, and composed of aggregations of cells with pseudoacinar formation. Note absence of basement membrane. Cells resemble those of the normal prostate, but lack complete differentiation.

FIG. 573.—ROENTGENOGRAM: PELVIS—METASTATIC CARCINOMA.—CASE 240.—Focal areas of demineralization and rarefaction involving the bones of the pelvis suggest metastatic neoplastic invasion and replacement of bone.

rhagic, necrotic, cauliflower-like growth. On microscopic examination it is found to be made up of anaplastic, pleomorphic, hyperchromic epithelial cells arranged on papillary stalks and showing all gradations of malignancy. The reader is referred to Case 134 in Chapter XXXII, and to Fig. 568.

Transitional Cell Carcinoma.—This variety of tumor represents the type of tumor which one might logically expect as the predominant kind. In most respects, it resembles the squamous-cell type of mucosal epithelial carcinoma, differing from the simpler form in that the cells are of the characteristic transitional type. There is a marked tendency for the tumor cells to grow in massive sheets and to invade the wall of the bladder extensively. Not infrequently the cells are relatively uniform in size with oval nuclei showing a variable amount of hyperchromatism. Mitotic figures likewise vary greatly in number. At times these tumors may become extremely malignant and present all the usual characteristics of anaplasia with the development of atypic mitoses. Efforts at grading this group of tumors have not proven as successful as in the case of the true squamous carcinomata, because tumors which appear relatively innocuous on the microscopic criteria of malignancy are often found to be extremely invasive and of a relatively high degree of clinical malignancy. In general, these tumors do not respond as satisfactorily to irradiation as might be expected from their histologic appearance, but in cases which have gone beyond an operable stage, irradiation is almost invariably of very real palliative value.

ILLUSTRATIVE CASE

CASE 238. (Ref. #S-365)

Diagnosis.—Bladder—transitional cell carcinoma.

Patient was a white male of 42 years, admitted to the hospital because of intermittent hematuria of about one week's duration.

History of Present Illness.—Patient had been in his usual good health up to the onset of the present condition. About one week before admission, he noticed occasionally on voiding, that his urine was blood tinged. This varied in degree and at times appeared to clear up, only to be followed again by a more marked attack. Hematuria was not associated with frequency, burning, urgency, dysuria or pain of any sort. His entire symptomatology consisted of this one feature. It had worried him, however, to the extent that he came to the hospital for study to make sure that there was nothing serious involved.

Past Medical History.—He believed he had had all of the usual childhood diseases. He had had no previous serious illness and no operations. His family history revealed the fact that his mother died of carcinoma of the breast. No other significant facts were obtained. A review of his systems revealed nothing particularly relevant. His cardiovascular system appeared to have been entirely normal. His gastro-intestinal tract showed occasional intermittent periods of constipation, but scarcely more than normal. His genito-urinary history up to the present illness had been entirely negative. He denied venereal infection.

Physical Examination.—Patient was a well-developed, middle-aged white male, who did not appear acutely ill. He showed no evidence of recent weight loss. His head was normal in appearance. Eyes, ears, nose and throat were entirely negative. Lungs were clear throughout. Heart was not enlarged; rate was regular; there were no murmurs. Blood pressure, 130/84. Abdomen was negative. External genitalia were normal. Extremities were negative.

Laboratory Findings.—Red blood cells, 4,800,000 with 85% hemoglobin. White blood cells, 10,200 with 74% polynuclears. Urinalysis: slightly blood tinged, alkaline, specific gravity, 1.020; very slight trace of albumin; no sugar. Centrifuged sediment showed the presence of an occasional white blood cell and a mass of red blood cells, which were so numerous they could not be counted without actual dilution.

Subsequent Course.—On the basis of this painless hematuria, without other symptoms, he was advised to have a cystoscopy for examination of his urinary tract and for possible biopsy diagnosis. The patient was prepared in the usual manner and the cystoscope introduced carefully into the bladder. No abnormalities were noted of the urethra in the passage of the instrument into the bladder. The bladder, itself, for the most part, showed possibly some congestion and edema of the mucous membrane as a whole throughout the organ. In the fundus, there was a large, necrotic neoplasm growing from the mucosal surface. This had a suggestion of a pedunculated base but was integral with the wall of the bladder throughout the greater extent of the lesion.

Pathological Report.—*Gross Description.*—Specimen consisted of a small polypoid mass of reddish-gray tissue removed from the bladder, measuring 1.5 cm. in its greatest diameter.

Microscopic Description of a Section Through the Tumor.—(Fig. 569) Histologic examination of the tumor shows a typical transitional cell type of carcinoma. The cells occur in solid sheets and nests with little or no suggestion of papillary arrangement. On the surface they are seen to be many layers deep. In general, the cells are fairly uniform in size and show moderately complete differentiation into the adult type. The nuclei are round or oval in form with scattered chromatin rods and granules and rather prominent nucleoli. Some disparity in the size of the cells is noted. Occasional mitotic figures are encountered. These all seem to be of the normal variety. At the base of the tumor there is rather striking invasion of the wall of the bladder. The basement membrane is poorly preserved and the tumor has broken through in many places.

PLATE CXXXVI
DISEASES OF THE MALE GENITALIA

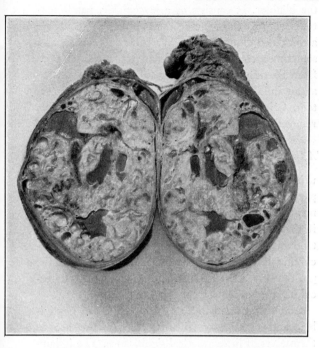

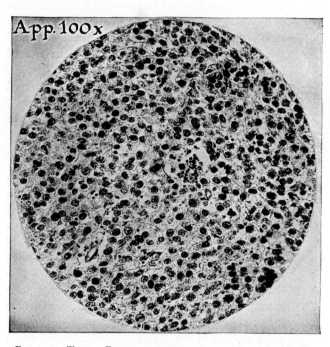

FIG. 574.—TESTIS: TERATOMA (SOLID).—Gross photograph of a unilateral testicular tumor approximately 12 cm. in length, completely replacing the normal testis, and histologically composed of various types of well differentiated tissues.

FIG. 575.—TESTIS: EMBRYONAL CARCINOMA (SEMINOMA).—(Cf. CASE 156 and Fig. 348).—Photomicrograph showing the histological composition of a typical seminoma, with its large, round or polyhedral cells, pale, vesicular nuclei and occasional mitotic figures. App. 100 x.

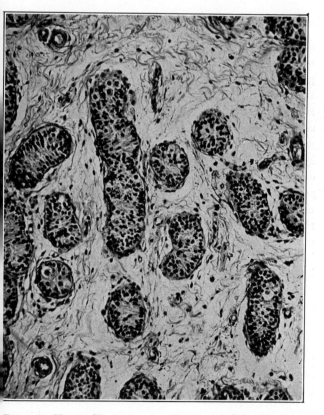

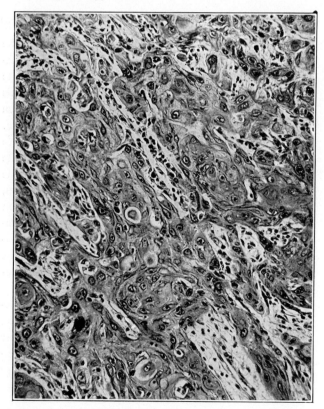

FIG. 576.—TESTIS: HYPERPLASIA IN UNDESCENDED TESTIS (CRYPTORCHISM).—CASE 241.—Photomicrograph illustrates the immature appearance of the reproductive tubules, with their isolation in a stroma of loose, edematous connective tissue. App. 100 x.

FIG. 577.—PENIS: SQUAMOUS CELL (EPIDERMOID) CARCINOMA.—CASE 242.—Low power photomicrograph of a typical squamous cell penile carcinoma which shows some tendency toward adult differentiation. Note large size of cells, atypic nuclei, prominent nucleoli and occasional mitotic figures. App. 100 x.

The other tumors which occur in the bladder are usually the result of direct extension from carcinoma of the prostate or carcinoma of the uterus and as such present a serious complication in the course of those diseases. The bladder is rarely the site of metastatic cancer from other organs.

Urethral Caruncle.—A lesion which might well be considered at this point is the so-called urethral caruncle. This is almost invariably found in the female, within the urethra, just below the neck of the bladder. It consists of a leucoplakic, papillomatous overgrowth of the urethral epithelium, covering a thickened chronic fibrous, vascular submucosa, and sometimes containing glandular structures derived from Skene glands. Whether this should be classed as an inflammatory or neoplastic process is uncertain. Clinically it is a benign process, but requires removal to prevent obstructive symptoms developing.

PROSTATE

The prostate is the male homologue of the uterus, composed chiefly of smooth muscle. It normally develops as three lobes, the two lateral making up the main bulk of the organ with a smaller middle lobe. From the functional standpoint, the prostate contains the ejaculatory mechanism and is provided with a large series of widely arborescent glands which produce the typical prostatic secretion. The prostate gland, although forming an integral part of the lower urinary tract, is a purely sexual organ, and plays no part in the act of urination. Owing to its anatomical situation, however, pathological conditions which in themselves might be regarded as trivial may produce disastrous effects upon the entire urinary system. The prostate enlarges at puberty parallel to the growth of the testes. This enlargement does not occur if the testes fail to develop or if they are removed before puberty. However, castration has no effect upon prostatic hypertrophy occurring later in life. The important diseases of the prostate are acute and chronic inflammation, tuberculosis, benign hypertrophy and cancer.

Congenital anomalies of the prostate are negligible, and circulatory disturbances likewise are in themselves of little practical significance. The inflammatory and infectious diseases of the prostate are almost synonymous with gonorrheal infection and will be discussed on that basis.

INFLAMMATORY AND INFECTIOUS DISEASES

Prostatitis.—The prostate is normally about the size of a large walnut and is of a soft elastic consistency. In the presence of inflammation, the prostate may be acutely swollen and tender. This represents essentially the usual features of acute inflammation elsewhere with all the usual exudative phenomena. Such acute inflammation is almost inevitably due to the gonococcus, which gains entrance to the prostate by direct extension from the infected urethra. The gonococcus, being an acute pus-producing bacterium, is liable to take part in definite abscess formation as well as in the more diffuse inflammatory infiltration of the gland as a whole. The gonococcus becomes relatively readily adapted to existence in the acini of the gland, and due to the anatomical structure of the prostate, is extremely hard to eradicate.

As a result, a high degree of resistance to the organism develops and a chronic inflammatory reaction ensues. This may persist for many months or even years, with the gradual transition of the inflammatory picture from one of an acute exudative nature to a chronic productive fibrosis with extensive fibrous scarring. In many instances, this leads to obliteration of many of the acini and eventually to an atrophic gland. In other cases, compensatory hyperplasia of the acinar epithelium accompanies the inflammatory fibrosis and the gland increases in size. Ultimately, such infections become sterile spontaneously as the resistance against the infection gradually is built up by the patient, and the viability of the organism is diminished. The end result in chronic infectious prostatis is likely to be a dense, tough, fibrosed organ which has lost much of its functional capacity, particularly from the secretory side. While the gonococcus is the prime offender in the great majority of instances, it is not at all uncommon to find secondary infection by other bacteria, including a diplococcus with the morphologic characteristics of the pneumococcus as well as the staphylococcus, the streptococcus and particularly the colon bacillus.

Tuberculosis.—Tuberculosis of the prostate is usually an incidental finding and secondary to tuberculosis of the testis. For some unexplained reason, the prostate itself is almost as resistant to infection by the tubercle bacillus as is its counterpart, the uterus in the female. It is only when the infection is rather extensive and the resistance of the patient distinctly lowered that tuberculosis of the prostate becomes a major problem. More significant in tuberculosis of the genito-urinary tract is the secondary involvement of the seminal vesicle and extension at times to involve the bladder and the ureter, as an ascending infection to the kidney in those cases where this route is followed.

BENIGN HYPERTROPHY OF THE PROSTATE

Benign adenomatoid hypertrophy of the prostate is one of the most commonly encountered pathological lesions in individuals over the age of sixty. In many instances, the condition does not develop symptomatically until past the age of seventy or even eighty. Thus, it is definitely a disease of old age. Its etiology is obscure, but it is probably very closely related to some involutional process which might be considered as corresponding to the menopause in the female. There is considerable experimental evidence which has accumulated in the past few years to establish an endocrine basis for this hypertrophy and it is thought to very probably relate to the balance of the testicular hormone and the production of estrin. In general, it may be compared to the involutional changes seen in the female breast at the time of the menopause in which the same estrogenic factor seems to play such an important role. It has been compared likewise to the changes which take place in the uterus with the development of myomata, but this does not seem to be so definitely comparable, as it is the epithelial hyperplasia which is important rather than the myomatous overgrowth. Attempts have been made to relate this hypertrophy to infection, but it may be said without much fear of contradiction, that any great degree of chronic prostatitis is much more likely to result in atrophy and fibrous scarring of the gland, than in adenomatoid hyperplasia. The hyperplasia is usually symmetrical in its development but occasionally unilateral lobe involvement predominates. Commonly the middle lobe is found undergoing similar hyperplastic changes and results in obstruction to the outflow of urine from the bladder by creating a bar across the urethral orifice. At times this protrudes into the lumen of the bladder as a nodular mass of considerable size.

The effect of such prostatic hypertrophy is chiefly related to this obstructive feature. With such blocking of the urinary passage a residual urine accumulates in the bladder and secondary infection frequently follows with the development of a marked cystitis. If the process becomes advanced, complete obstruction to urinary outflow may occur with resultant anuria and the development of a marked bilateral hydronephrosis. Due to the fact that most such inflammatory processes tend to involve the base of the trigon, considerable irritability of the bladder results with a markedly increased frequency. This is apt to be one of the earliest symptoms of the condition.

The treatment of prostatic hypertrophy is surgical, with the removal of the hyperplastic glandular tissues. This may be done by a variety of techniques either as a perineal operation or by a suprapubic approach and may likewise be performed in a single or a two-stage procedure.

The pathological appearance of such a gland grossly as seen at operation or autopsy is characterized by rather diffuse nodular enlargement of the gland as a whole. Cross section through the prostate reveals these nodules to be discrete adenomatoid areas of hyperplasia more or less indefinitely encapsulated in respect to the gland as a whole. This is particularly true of the very commonly encountered large adenomatoid lesions found in the lateral lobes. Considerable discussion exists in the literature as to whether this should be considered as a true tumor or as a functional involutional lesion. From the gross standpoint, the lesions are strongly suggestive of actual neoplasm, but from a study of their histology and the life history of such cases, one is forced to the conclusion that they are merely functional overgrowths rather than actual neoplasias.

Microscopically, a wide variation in the histology is encountered. The basic lesion is one of diffuse glandular hyperplasia. In many instances the epithelium is thrown up into papillary folds very much as occurs in the normal gland but in exaggerated form. The majority of these hyperplastic glandular structures appears to be isolated from the duct system as a whole and to accordingly undergo varying degrees of cystic dilatation. This results in a loss of the villi and a flattening of the lining cells in the more extreme pictures so that the cysts are seen lined by a flattened layer of epithelial cells with their nuclei tending to be elongated and parallel with the cyst wall. In other areas a much more active hyperplasia of the glandular epithelium can be demonstrated corresponding closely to the hyperplastic picture which one sees in the breast in the active phase of the menstrual cycle. One feature of interest from the histologic standpoint is in the relative frequency with which the characteristic corpora amylacea are found in these glands. Many of the acini are filled with cellular debris, desquamated epithelium and a milky fluid which microscopically appears as a pink coagulant. Hemorrhage occasionally occurs with some hemosiderin production.

The stroma likewise shows very marked variation in the histologic picture. In some places, smooth muscle hyperplasia predominates to the point at times where the lesion is almost wholly one of myomatous overgrowth. There is always a marked desmoplastic reaction and variable amounts of inflammatory cellular infiltration of this stromal connective tissue is found. Such infiltration is largely lymphocytic in nature. Mitotic figures in either the glandular epithelium or in the stroma are practically nonexistent, and there is no evidence of malignant transition in the usual case. Indeed, when carcinoma of the prostate does develop it usually is as a totally independent lesion and follows the simple benign hypertrophic picture in only an insignificant percentage of cases.

ILLUSTRATIVE CASE

CASE 239. (Ref. #S-368)

Diagnosis. — Prostate — benign adenomatoid hypertrophy.

Patient was a white, American male widower of 72 years, brought in to the hospital because of acute anuria accompanied by bleeding from the urethra.

Present Illness.—Two days before admission, the patient began having acute retention of urine. He was seen by a local physician, who catheterized the patient, with complete relief. That night, however, after several attempts, the doctor was unable to introduce the catheter into the bladder and so referred the patient to the hospital as an emergency measure, for treatment, with the thought of probable operative intervention.

Past Medical History.—Patient had no remembrance of any childhood disease. At sixty-one, at the time of the death of his wife, he had a nervous breakdown, which was followed by a bronchopneumonia with persistent pleurisy for some time. He more recently had complained of occasional substernal pain which tended to radiate down the right arm at times. His genito-urinary system was the most pertinent part of his history. He had had four previous attacks of acute retention, the first eleven years ago; the last one being three years before admission. On each of those occasions, he was successfully catheterized with complete relief and a remission of his symptoms. He had complained during this eleven-year period of progressive difficulty in starting and stopping his stream and had had considerable tenesmus at times. There had been marked frequency with a nocturia of two or three times.

Physical Examination.—Patient was a well-developed, elderly-appearing, white male lying in bed in acute distress. Head was essentially negative. Skin was dry and showed moderate atrophy of a senile type. Eyes were negative except for bilateral marked arcus senilis. Nose, ears, and mouth were negative. Teeth were in poor condition—carious, broken and dirty. Throat was negative. Chest was moderately emphysematous. Lungs were clear throughout. Heart was moderately enlarged toward the left. There were no murmurs. Occasional extraventricular systoles were heard. Abdomen was negative. Rectal examination showed marked hypertrophy of the prostate, especially of both lateral lobes.

Laboratory Findings.—Red blood cells, 4,800,000 with 54% hemoglobin. Leukocytes, 21,900 with 87% polynuclears. Catheter specimen: Urine showed moderate albuminuria and the presence of macroscopic blood. In other respects, it was essentially normal. Blood Chemistry: Blood urea, 13 mgm.; creatinine 1.5 mgm.; sugar 100 mgm.

Subsequent Course.—The patient had a two stage prostatectomy, which was carried out in the face of an acute coronary accident with thrombosis and infarction in the interval between the two operative procedures. The patient made a slow, but otherwise uneventful recovery and was discharged greatly improved with the diagnosis of senile, prostatic hypertrophy and coronary disease.

Pathological Specimen.—*Gross Description.*—Specimen consisted of three pieces of tissue, the largest measuring 6 x 4 x 2.5 cm.; the other two being almost equally as large. These apparently represented the two lateral and middle lobes. The tissue on section was grayish-white in color, extremely firm in consistency and somewhat nodular in appearance. There were numerous small cystic areas filled with milky secretion. The largest of these cysts measured 3 millimeters in diameter. The picture was typically that of simple benign hypertrophy.

Microscopic Description of a Section Through the Prostate.—(Fig. 571 and 572) Histologic examination presents the typical adenomatoid hyperplasia of the glandular epithelium and the associated similar increase in the amount of the stromal connective tissue and smooth musculature of benign prostatic hypertrophy. The acini show marked distention in places with some tendency toward flattening of the epithelium. In others, there is marked papillary hyperplasia of the lining cells which are of an unusually high columnar type. A few prostatic calculi are noted. There is considerable epithelial desquamation in places and many of the acini seem filled with granular debris. There is a moderate amount of secondary mononuclear cellular infiltration in the stroma.

CARCINOMA OF THE PROSTATE

Carcinoma of the prostate is almost invariably of the glandular type although rare instances of squamous cancer do occur. Considerable difference of opinion exists as to the relationship of a preceding benign hypertrophy. Some authors quote a figure as high as 15 to 20 per cent of carcinoma cases as developing from a previous adenomatoid hyperplasia. In our own experience this figure seems extremely high. Carcinoma of the prostate is very prone to develop as a middle lobe lesion and to remain as a very small tumor without producing symptoms locally for long periods of time. Indeed, it is a common experience for carcinoma of the prostate to manifest itself first by its metastatic lesions in the osseous system, particularly in the long bones. Spontaneous fracture may be the first indication of the underlying basic pathological process. Such bony metastases are associated with osteolytic changes in the bone and are readily demonstrable by x-ray. Examination of the prostate by rectum is not infrequently negative under such circumstances, although more often a small, firm area in the prostate can be palpated.

Prostatic carcinoma, as has been emphasized, tends to remain localized for considerable periods of time. Due to the anatomical arrangement of the lymphatic circulation it is only in very extensive cases that invasion of the bladder secondarily occurs, and it is much more common for the metastatic lesions of the prostate to involve the seminal vesicles and regional lymph nodes than for it to spread by contiguity. In general, the tumors tend to be relatively scirrhous in type with rather marked desmoplastic stromal development. They can be identified on cross section of the gland by the dense zone of infiltrating fibrous tissue in which small yellowish adenomatoid foci are seen.

Microscopically the picture of prostatic carcinoma, as in the case of benign adenomatous hyperplasia, shows so much variation that it is difficult to adequately descriptively cover the range of histologic pictures. In general there is a tendency toward some slight acinar arrangement of the cells, but equally frequently the tumor cells will be found as nests embedded in a dense connective tissue stroma not unlike the scirrhous carcinoma of the breast without much suggestion of lumen formation. Indeed, the term "carcinoma simplex" might well be applied to a considerable number of such cases. On the other extreme, wildly anaplastic tumors may be found with large cells with hyperchromatic nuclei and atypical mitoses in profusion. No purpose seems to be served by attempting to grade malignancies of the prostate gland as they are uniformly highly malignant so far as the clinical course is concerned. Emphasis has already been placed upon the frequency of bone metastases. Blood borne lesions elsewhere may also be encountered, particularly in the lung. It is often difficult to establish the primary source of the tumor from histologic examination of such a metastatic lesion alone.

Aside from carcinoma of the prostate, other tumors are found with such infrequency as to make their consideration merely a matter of record. Occasional instances of sarcoma of the prostate have been described and almost entirely in age groups well below that of carcinoma. Benign myomata may likewise be found on rare occasions, but these, too, are negligible, numerically.

ILLUSTRATIVE CASE

CASE 240 (Ref. #S-202)

Diagnosis.—Prostate—adenocarcinoma.

Patient was a male Negro of 58 years, admitted to the hospital with the chief complaint of anuria and pain in both legs.

Present Illness.—Four months before admission, the patient first noticed severe shooting pains, which started in the small of his back and radiated down both thighs and legs to his feet. This was accompanied by progressive weakness until he was almost completely paralyzed from the waist down. Three weeks before his admission, he became incontinent and this was accompanied by a definite hematuria. The incontinence alternated with periods of urinary retention which required catheterization. For about two weeks before admission, he had noticed marked dyspnea, even when lying in bed. He had shown complete incontinence of both his bowels and bladder for several days before admission, until the onset of the acute anuria.

Past Medical History.—The patient himself was incapable of giving any coherent story. So far as could be made out, he had never had any serious illness in his childhood. There was a suggestive history of lues in his statement that he had received intravenous medication about twenty years earlier. An attempt to review his systems yielded little additional information.

Physical Examination.—The patient was an extremely ill, well-developed, emaciated, colored male, who was markedly dyspneic and perspiring profusely. Head showed no deformities. Pupils failed to react to light or distance. Nose and throat were negative. Chest showed marked impairment of expansion on the left side. Heart was moderately enlarged with the apex beat felt in the 6th interspace 14 cm. to the left of the midsternal line. There were systolic and diastolic murmurs heard over the apex and a systolic murmur heard over the mitral area. Lungs showed dullness to flatness over the entire left chest posteriorly with increased fremitus and with bronchial breathing over the upper part of the lung. Many râles were heard over the entire right side. Abdomen: The liver was moderately enlarged. The spleen could not be palpated. The bladder was distended up to the umbilicus. Rectal examination showed a dilatation of the anal sphincter. The prostate was moderately enlarged and there were several stony, hard nodules felt in its substance. Extremities showed marked ankle edema, paralysis and loss of sensation bilaterally.

Laboratory Findings.—Red blood cells, 2,600,000 with 58% hemoglobin. White blood cells, 13,500 with 72% polynuclears. Wassermann was strongly positive. Urinalysis: Catheterized specimen showed a moderate amount of albumin and a large number of leukocytes and red cells.

X-ray examination (Fig. 573) showed the presence of extensive metastatic lesions in the bones of the pelvis as evidenced by areas of rarefaction representing neoplastic replacement of the normal structures.

Subsequent History.—It was attempted to prepare the patient for an operation, but his pulmonary condition progressed rapidly. He developed bleeding from his mouth and nose and died forty-eight hours after admission.

Autopsy Findings.—There was a primary carcinoma of the prostate found with metastases to the vertebrae, the spinal cord and the lungs. In addition, a definite luetic aortitis was found.

Microscopic Description of a Section from the Prostate.—(Fig. 572) Histologic examination of the tissue shows a typical adenocarcinomatous picture. The tumor cells occur in nests with some tendency toward acinar formation. There is very extensive mucoid degeneration. The cells are small, hyperchromatic and in many instances actually pyknotic in places. In other areas there is a more diffuse infiltration by the tumor tissue and the cells appear somewhat larger in these parts. There is extensive infiltration of the stroma everywhere. Occasional mitotic figures are seen. In examination of the tissue from the metastases in the lung, the metastatic tumor tissue is seen to be growing much more rapidly with less evidence of alveolar arrangement. There are solid sheets of cells separated only by delicate connective tissue septa and with many mitotic figures. Histologically it is difficult to identify the tissue of origin.

SEMINAL VESICLES

The pathology relating to the seminal vesicles is of very little practical importance. As part of the involutional changes associated with senility, atrophy might be noted. Inflammatory lesions of the seminal vesicles are almost entirely restricted to the various infections, notably the extension of a gonorrheal infection of the prostate and the occurrence of tuberculosis. Tuberculosis occurs with some considerable frequency and is comparable in a rough way to the instance of tuberculosis of the Fallopian tubes producing obstruction and being one of the contributory causes of sterility in the male. Rare tumors arising primarily from the vesicles have been reported, but in general the neoplasms which affect the seminal vesicles are secondary, resulting from extension of tumors of the bladder, prostate or intestinal tract.

TESTIS AND EPIDIDYMIS

CONGENITAL ANOMALIES

Cryptorchism.—The congenital anomalies of the testis consist chiefly of malpositions due primarily to the failure of the testis to complete its normal descent into the scrotal sac. Rare instances of absence of one or both testes are on record. The failure of descent is spoken of as "cryptorchism." It may be unilateral or bilateral. The testis may remain within the peritoneal cavity or its descent may stop in the inguinal canal. This might be considered an almost normal physiological process up to the time of puberty. If the testes at that time do not complete their descent into the scrotum, then they remain in an undeveloped state without spermatogenesis. However, in spite of the failure of the reproductive tubules to develop, the interstitial cells which give rise to the testicular hormone and are intimately associated with the development of the secondary sex characteristics continue their functional activity, and indeed may be present in excessive numbers not infrequently for some poorly understood reason.

ILLUSTRATIVE CASE

CASE 241 (Ref. #S-366)
Diagnosis.—Testis—cryptorchism
Patient was a white, American boy of ten years, admitted to the hospital with a lump in the left inguinal region.

Present Illness.—According to the child's older brother, the lump in the left groin region had been present since birth. The mother, however, had not been aware of the condition until three years ago following an accident when the patient ran into an automobile with his bicycle and injured himself in the genital region. At that time the mother examined the boy and found this mass, which she said had never been tender or caused any pain. She felt that there was a considerable increase in size on a postural basis, it usually being much smaller in the morning and increasing in size toward the end of the day. It never moved from its position. The patient was taken to a doctor, who apparently made a correct diagnosis and attempted treatment with endocrine injections, but without improvement in the condition. As a result the family became dissatisfied and sought another physician, who advised hospitalization.

Past Medical History.—Patient had the usual children's diseases: chickenpox, measles and pertussis. He had an abscess on the left side of his neck in association with suppurative otitis media. Had tonsils removed. These incidents occurred between the fourth and sixth years of his life. Since then he had been entirely healthy with the exception of occasional head colds and the presence of this lump in the inguinal region.

Physical Examination.—Entirely negative except for the local condition. Head was normal. Eyes, ears, nose and throat were negative. Heart and lungs were negative. There were no murmurs or other cardiac abnormalities. The liver edge was slightly enlarged. Abdomen was negative. An examination of the scrotum showed the presence of only one testis on the right side. On the left

Herniae.—As a result at times of congenital failure of the tunica to become obliterated, a direct or indirect inguinal hernia may likewise develop; although the great majority of such herniae occur in later adult life as the result of rupture of the ring through some undue strain. Even such acquired herniae, however, are associated with some congenital weakness in the canal.

There is a group of lesions which affect principally the tunica vaginalis of the testis. These may be congenital in origin, but are apparently more often seen in later life as acquired lesions. They may be the result of trauma or of infection or without determinable etiology. The principal forms of these pathological conditions are briefly reviewed.

Hydrocele.—A hydrocele refers to an accumulation of fluid in the tunica vaginalis or in a dilated portion of the processus vaginalis. It is very commonly found in children and appears to have a congenital origin. It often, however, occurs in later life and is characterized by a rather gradual accumulation of fluid which may reach a total volume of 3,000 c.c. or more. The etiology is not clear. It may follow traumatic injury or may be associated with some disturbance in lymphatic drainage. The fluid is usually clear or slightly opalescent and shows an increase of protein to a degree which suggests that it is of an exudative nature. Treatment of the condition is either repeated drainage with scarification

side, above and to the left of the root of the penis was found a slight, even swelling. On palpation this was of a globular form, which was fixed and did not move on coughing. The mass did not pulsate and was not tender. This was outside the external ring.

Subsequent History.—A presumptive diagnosis of undescended testis was made. In the face of the previous history of unsuccessful endocrine therapy, surgical removal as a prophylaxis against tumor development was advised and carried out with the consent of the mother.

Pathological Specimen.—*Gross Description.*—Surgical specimen consisted of a small, undeveloped testis with its epididymis and a mass of loose, areolar, fatty tissue. The testis measured 2 x 1.2 cm. It was soft and grayish-yellow in color. One could not pick up the tubules with forceps on section as in the normal testis. It showed a definite increase in density due to fibrosis.

Microscopic Description.—(Fig. 576) Section through the testis shows definite atrophy, or perhaps more accurately, a failure of development of the reproductive tubules. The tubules are small and many of them are completely occluded by undifferentiated cells. Here and there, a suggestion of incomplete differentiation but never beyond the stage of primary spermatocyte formation is seen. The intervening stroma shows marked increase of loose areolar connective tissue with an apparent or real increase in the number of characteristic interstitial cells.

of the serosal lining cells in an attempt to obliterate the cavity, or the actual surgical excision of the sac. Microscopic examination of the wall of such a hydrocele sac varies greatly in respect to the amount of inflammatory change present, dependent in turn upon its etiological background.

Hematocele.—By this term is meant hemorrhage into the tunica vaginalis. It is most frequently the result of traumatic injury, but may be associated with some one of the blood dyscrasias or as a complication of a simple hydrocele.

Spermatocele.—Spermatocele in its simplest form, really represents a cystic dilatation of the ducts of the epididymis. This usually follows an old epididymitis with the etiology most commonly gonorrheal. Not infrequently, such a spermatocele may rupture into the tunica vaginalis and produce a spermatic hydrocele.

Varicocele.—The pampiniform plexus of veins in the spermatic cord may at times undergo marked varicose dilatation, and this has been termed a "varicocele." Its etiology is obscure in the great majority of cases. It may be congenital in origin, but usually does not appear until adolescence. It has been suggested that sexual excitement, associated with congestion of the genital organs, may well be of etiologic significance in this adolescent age group. It nearly always involves the left side in later acquired type. This is explained rather unsatisfactorily on the basis of mechanical venous stasis because of the relationship of the angle of entrance of the left spermatic vein to the renal vein. During the war, it was found that approximately 10 per cent of young males showed this lesion to a variable extent. It is readily cured by surgical excision.

Another form of varicocele is an acquired lesion usually the result of pressure upon the intra-abdominal vessels, from a pelvic tumor. Accordingly, any right-sided varicocele occurring particularly in the older age group should arouse suspicions as to the presence of pelvic neoplasm.

INFLAMMATIONS OF THE TESTIS

Acute Orchitis.—The commonest cause of acute inflammation of the testis is as the result of an extension of the gonorrheal process from the prostate and seminal vesicle to the epididymis and testis. The lesion is usually primary in the epididymis but extends both along the tubules by direct continuity and by the lymphatics to the testis as well. This is accompanied usually by suppurative necrosis, which begins in the tubule and extends to the interstitial tissues of the organ. Not infrequently the process will continue to the point where actual abscess formation occurs.

Aside from the gonorrheal type of orchitis, metastatic bacterial infection may occasionally be seen in association with septicemias. Likewise, as a complication of parotitis (mumps), an acute interstitial orchitis develops which very characteristically shows extensive hemorrhage. This apparently is the result of increased capillary permeability and results in extensive cicatricial fibrosis with atrophy of the reproductive tubules resulting in a small percentage of cases in sterility. Traumatic injury of the testis may likewise result in an acute interstitial hemorrhagic type of orchitis with similar scarring. This is more often unilateral in contradistinction to the bilateral involvement in the hematogenous infectious cases.

Tuberculosis.—Tuberculosis of the testis and epididymis is one of the most common localizations of tuberculous infection of the genital tract. This either occurs as a direct hematogenous infection, usually without clinical evidence of tuberculosis elsewhere, or as a secondary direct extension of a tuberculosis of the seminal vesicles. It more frequently begins in the epididymis than in the testis itself, but spreads rapidly by continuity to the testis as well.

Pathologically in the early cases, the lesion seems to start as diffuse, conglomerate tubercules in the interstitial tissue. These tend to fuse to produce large areas of caseous necrosis. The lesion tends further to spread through the tunica vaginalis to cause a generalized tuberculosis of the scrotum which may even extend through the skin as a sinus tract. The lesion, curiously enough, is usually unilateral initially. Almost invariably, however, sooner or later the other testis becomes involved. The condition may run the course of tuberculosis elsewhere with spontaneous healing by fibrosis or calcification in rare instances. There is an unusually high mortality, however, associated in general with this genital type of tuberculosis as it tends to develop into a fatal generalized miliary form of the disease eventually.

Syphilis.—In contradistinction to tuberculosis, which starts in the epididymis, syphilis almost invariably occurs primarily as a testicular lesion when the genital organs are involved. The lesion is of a gummatous nature usually, but may occur, particularly in the younger age group, as a diffuse interstitial fibrosis. As a gumma, it presents the usual features of this type of lesion; namely, avascular caseous necrosis with a peripheral zone of chronic inflammatory cellular infiltration. The cellular reaction consists principally of lymphocytes and plasma cells, and is accompanied by considerable fibrosis. Giant cells are usually lacking.

Occasionally other of the granulomatous infections may involve the testicle, but these are so unusual as to need no particular comment. Among these leprosy is outstanding. It is almost regularly found as part of the general systemic infection in this disease.

TUMORS OF THE TESTIS

The testis may be the site of a rather wide variety of tumors. However, only three varieties are found with any degree of frequency which are of particular importance in respect to this organ. All three of these tumors might well be included under the generic heading of teratoma representing, as they apparently do, merely an origin at varying stages of differentiation of the multipotential undifferentiated cell. These three will be discussed individually.

Embryonal Carcinoma (Seminoma).—This tumor

represents the most commonly found variety of the three above mentioned neoplasms. It may be considered as arising from undifferentiated germinal epithelium. It is a slow-growing tumor which gradually infiltrates and replaces the entire testis. It is potentially malignant and may give rise to distant metastases, but usually relatively late in the course of its natural history. It may best be thought of in terms of the usual malignant type of tumor in which the cells have largely lost their power of differentiation, but have retained their growth capacity. As a result, the tumor is made up of a mass of large round or polyhedral cells with extremely large nuclei and prominent nucleoli. The chromatin is in the form of rods and granules and is rather prominent. Mitotic figures are usually numerous. For the most part they are relatively normal in type but on occasion, atypical mitoses likewise may be found. Rarely are true tumor giant cells encountered. There is a rather striking tendency for these cells to grow in long cords with a suggestion of attempted tubule production. At times, such tumors are seen to arise from cells which have reached perhaps the stage of differentiation of the primary or secondary spermatocytes rather than the more primitive undifferentiated spermatoblast. Under these circumstances, the general morphology is modified, with the cells almost suggesting a tumor which, in the older nomenclature might be described as a "round cell sarcoma." In this variety of tumor, arising as it does from almost completely undifferentiated cells, there is liable to be the production of a considerable amount of prolan in the urine. This may reach as much as 10,000 rat units. Refer back to Case 156 (Ref. #S-263), Chapter XXXVI, Fig. 348, and see Fig. 575.

Teratomata.—(Fig. 574) The teratoid tumors of the testis, which are perhaps as frequently spoken of as embryomata, represent similar tumors in that they arise essentially from the same original type of cell, but usually at a further stage in its differentiation. Thus, we are likely to find in the typical teratoma of the testis tissues which show all three embryonal characteristics with ectodermal, entodermal and mesothelial structures. The tumors tend to be rather more benign in their course than do the embryonal carcinomatous type. Both varieties of tumors are usually unilateral. Such tumors have already been described in the chapter devoted to the mixed and teratoid tumors generally and need no further comment here. In this particular group of tumors, the production of the hormone, prolan, is usually minimal and the more adult in type the tissues appear, the less prolan may be found in the urine. Rarely does this exceed 500 units and it may not be demonstrable in measurable amounts.

Chorio-epithelioma (Choriocarcinoma).—An extremely complex teratoid tumor may occur in the testis in which fetal structures are formed. Such tumors go on to the actual production of abortive chorionic villi and almost invariably undergo malignant transformation. The primary tumor is very apt to be small and often escapes recognition until the marked metastatic lesions in the lung and other viscera make its presence known. In this tumor, as might well be expected, the hormone production reaches its greatest height; in some of the reported instances, as high as 50,000 mouse units of prolan being found in the urine. This tumor has likewise been discussed in the chapter devoted to mixed and teratoid neoplasms, and is accordingly merely reviewed briefly at this point.

PENIS

CONGENITAL LESIONS

There is a considerable degree of variation in the development of this organ, which may well be considered as congenital in nature, but this is usually not of pathological significance. Two or three lesions do occur which are serious problems to the urologist. Of these, *epispadias,* a condition in which the urethra opens directly on the upper surface of the penis and *hypospadias,* in which the urethral opening is on the inferior surface are the most important. These are accompanied by varying degrees of developmental failure of the penile portion of the urethra. They may be seen accompanying extrophy of the bladder as the result of failure of the urogenital cleft to fuse, but may occur independently of this more marked congenital defect. Their relation to developmental defects of the bladder has been discussed.

INFLAMMATORY LESIONS

Phimosis.—As a result of either congenital defect or following acute inflammatory lesions of the penis, the prepuce may not be capable of retraction. This is commonly associated with marked inflammatory features which tend to produce a more or less vicious circle; in the one instance the inflammatory process producing or exaggerating the phimosis; in the other instance, the phimosis itself tending to accumulate secretions which, in turn, produce a secondary inflammatory reaction.

Balanitis.—By balanitis is meant the inflammatory reaction which is seen in conjunction with phimosis. This is usually the result of retained secretions coupled with secondary infection by the colon bacilli or some of the pyogenic cocci, particularly staphylococci. This may go on to the point of actual gangrenous ulceration and is accompanied by marked secondary regional lymph adenitis. Balanitis may likewise be a sequel of an acute urethritis and for that reason is commonly seen in gonorrheal infections. It may be initiated even by intercourse, as a mechanical type of irritation, followed by secondary inflammation and even infection.

Chancroid.—Chancroid is defined as an acute specific infectious lesion caused by the Ducrey bacillus. This is often called the soft chancre in contradistinction to the hard chancre of syphilis. It is usually venereal in origin and is most commonly found among those people with poor habits of personal hygiene. The lesion is characteristically an acute ulcerative process usually rather sharply defined, but not infrequently showing a rather marked undermining. The base of the ulcer is diffusely infiltrated with leukocytes and mononuclear cells. It is apt to be accompanied by a rather marked peri-arteritis. The diagnosis is made by the finding of the bacteria both intra and extracellularly in smears from the ulcerated surface. It is frequently followed by secondary infection from other bacteria and usually results in a rather diffuse scarring. One of the chief complications of this infection is the marked suppurative lymph adenitis which so commonly accompanies the infection and which not infrequently is followed by a chronic draining sinus, which clears up with difficulty.

Syphilis.—The chancre, representing the primary lesion of syphilis has already been discussed in the chapter on syphilis and needs only to be referred to at this time. It is most commonly found on the frenum or glans, although primary lesions of the prepuce or even of the shaft are by no means rare. In the later stages of syphilis, mucous patches may involve the urethra or glans and condylomata may be seen affecting the skin of the shaft and scrotum. Even gummata may occur at times. For an illustrative case, the reader is referred to Case 54 (Ref. #S-296), Chapter XV, Fig. 116, 117, 118 and 119.

TUMORS OF THE PENIS

There are only two tumors of practical importance. One is the benign epithelial papilloma; the other is the squamous carcinoma, which most commonly arises at the mucocutaneous border of the glans. It is usually found in the sixth decade, although it has been reported as early as the age of seventeen.

Benign Papilloma.—The papilloma itself is a comparatively infrequently encountered lesion, which is more often misdiagnosed as some inflammatory verrucous-like lesion. It may, however, attain a considerable size and cause marked discomfort and even difficulty with voiding if the urethra becomes filled with the tumor, as it not uncommonly does. Likewise, malignant degeneration may occur.

Squamous Carcinoma.—More commonly, such hyperplastic mucous membrane lesions are definitely malignant in character. They are likely to show a considerable degree of differentiation of the cells so that on a gradation basis, they most frequently fall into Grade II, if they are seen in the earlier phase of their development. They produce a diffuse, destructive cauliflower-like growth and tend to spread along the urethra as well as to metastasize regionally to the inguinal lymph nodes by lymphatic extension. Fortunately, this metastatic process occurs relatively late in the course of the disease and a very considerable percentage of cure may be expected in such carcinomata of the penis by early amputation.

ILLUSTRATIVE CASE

CASE 242. (Ref. #S-367)

Diagnosis.—Penis—squamous cell carcinoma, Grade III.

A single, white, American male of 35 years, was admitted to the hospital because of a painful ulcer on the penis, associated with painful swelling of the glands in the groin and a loss of weight of fifteen pounds in the past three months.

Present Illness.—Patient was in his usual health until about six months ago when he noticed a somewhat intense swelling of the left inguinal lymph nodes. This persisted for about one week. It was not painful, particularly, except on pressure. About one month later the patient noticed a small "boil" on the left side of the end of the penis. This was painful when it touched his clothing. Several days after he noticed its appearance, this "boil" had broken and discharged what he believed was pus. It had continued to discharge until the present admission. About four months ago he began to have pain in both inguinal regions, but the left side had continued to be the more extreme. A month ago he noticed that this swelling in the inguinal regions was becoming progressively larger and was more distressing in relation to walking.

Past Medical History.—Normal. As a child, he believed he had the usual children's diseases. In addition, he had typhoid at the age of six years. No history of carcinoma, tuberculosis or other familial disease in his immediate family. Denied venereal disease.

A review of his systems was entirely negative in respect to the present history.

Physical Examination.—Head was normal in appearance. Eyes, ears, nose and throat were negative except for marked hypertrophy of the tonsils. Chest: Expansion was equal; lungs were clear. Heart was not enlarged and there were no murmurs. Abdomen: Several large, pigmented moles were seen in the epigastric region. The abdomen was flat and soft. There were no masses except in the inguinal region where the glands were firm and enlarged on the right side to about the size of an olive; on the left to about the size of a lemon. External genitalia: The glans penis was almost completely destroyed, the remaining portion presenting a ragged, grayish, sloughing appearance. The extremities were negative. The patient was advised to have a palliative amputation and a block dissection of the inguinal glands.

Subsequent Course.—On the basis of a tentative diagnosis of squamous cell carcinoma of the glans penis, a midpenile amputation was done with a radical dissection of the inguinal lymph nodes and lymphatics, accompanied by double castration. The patient was discharged improved and at the end of three months had shown no recurrence.

Pathological Report.—*Gross Description.*—Specimen consisted of the anterior half of the penis, both testes and epididymes, and of two masses of adipose tissue in which several enlarged, grayish lymph nodes were found. The end of the glans penis was found as an ulcerative, sloughing, irregular mass of necrotic tumor tissue. The testes appeared essentially negative grossly. The nodes in the adipose tissue were grayish-white in color, firm in consistency and seemed to be made up of tumor tissue which, however, seemed still to be within the capsule, as no invasion of the surrounding structures was noted.

Microscopic Description.—(Fig. 577) The glans penis presents a typical stratified squamous epithelial tumor, which shows moderately well differentiated cells. However, only rare epithelial pearls are present and only occasional intercellular bridges are made out. The cells differ considerably in size and shape. Nucleoli are prominent. Many mitotic figures are seen. The tumor is found infiltrating the corpora cavernosa to some extent. The tumor must be classified on the basis of a Grade III malignancy.

CHAPTER LVIII
DISEASES OF THE FEMALE GENITALIA
UTERUS

A review of the pathological processes which involve the female genitalia covers one of the largest groups of clinical problems which the physician meets. In this presentation only the most outstanding can be discussed. For more detailed consideration of this enormous field, the student is referred to the numerous gynecological treatises. In the present discussion the same general plan of presentation will be followed of congenital, inflammatory and neoplastic lesions, with emphasis laid upon those most commonly encountered and those which are of interest currently in the field of investigation.

CONGENITAL LESIONS

There are a considerable number of congenital lesions which result from imperfect development of the müllerian ducts. The most common of these are seen as a complete reduplication of the vagina and uterus, by the more common bicornuate uterus in its many variations, and finally in the congenital and infantile types of uterus. These are not necessarily of any pathological significance, but often are important in relation to pregnancy, interfering with the normal gestation or delivery of the fetus.

MECHANICAL AND CIRCULATORY DISTURBANCES

Bleeding from the uterus is the most prominent symptom of almost all pathological conditions which affect that organ. Among these must be cited the many variations in position of the organ either as a whole or in respect to the relative position of the fundus and cervix. These are spoken of as anteversion or retroversion in the case of the displacement of the entire organ, or as ante- or retroflexions when the fundus is bent on the cervix. Such malpositions may result in retention of the normal uterine discharge during the menstrual cycle as a purely mechanical phenomenon and be accompanied by severe pain or dysmenorrhea.

A consideration of the various functional disturbances of menstruation in association with endocrine unbalance would, in itself, fill a complete volume. It is well recognized that as the result of estrin formation by the ovary the uterine mucosa is stimulated to the normal sequence of the menstrual cycle. This varies greatly in different individuals. It is characterized in general by a gradual hyperplasia of the endometrial glands with a corresponding overgrowth of the supportive endometrial stromal cells. This is accompanied by marked congestion and ultimately ends in complete desquamation. This is represented by the usual menstrual bleeding. When it exceeds the usual physiological amount, the condition is spoken of as *menorrhagia,* and may be associated with marked endocrine disturbances or even with the development of certain ovarian tumors, such as the granulosa cell type of carcinoma. In contrast to menorrhagia is the condition spoken of as *metrorrhagia,* which represents uterine bleeding not associated with the normal menstrual periods. This obviously may be the result of a wide variety of causes. Among them may be mentioned briefly chronic passive congestion, acute inflammatory lesions and tumors.

INFLAMMATORY LESIONS OF THE UTERUS

Acute Inflammation.—Acute inflammation of the uterus may occur as a limited process involving only the endometrial lining of the organ or may extend as a diffuse involvement of the myometrium, peri-

PLATE CXXXVII
DISEASES OF THE FEMALE GENITALIA
Uterine Lesions

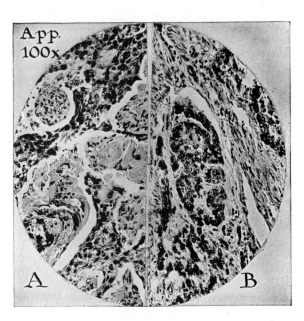

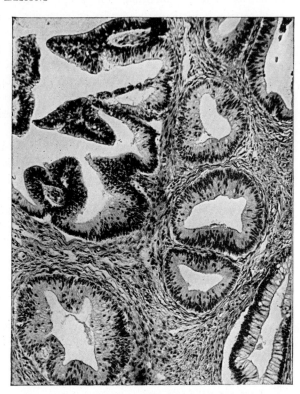

FIG. 578.—CERVIX: SQUAMOUS CELL CARCINOMA.—CASE 246.—Invasion of the myometrium by masses of relatively undifferentiated squamous epithelial cells. Marked hyperchromatism and numerous mitotic figures. "A" represents surface lesion; "B" the deeper portion of the musculature. App. 75 x.

FIG. 579.—FUNDUS: ADENOCARCINOMA.—CASE 245.—Invasion of the body of the uterus by a tumor composed of very large cells derived from the glandular epithelium of the endometrium, which maintain their acinar pattern. App. 100 x.

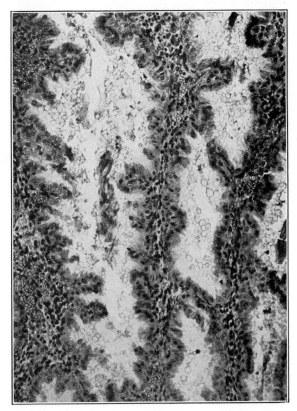

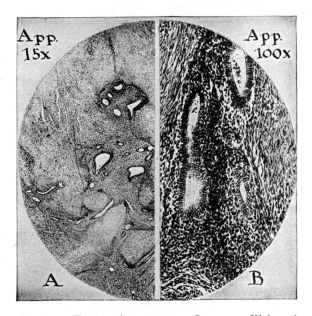

FIG. 580.—ENDOMETRIUM: ENDOMETRIAL HYPERPLASIA.—CASE 243.—Histologic appearance of uterine glands obtained by curettage. Note hyperplasia of lining epithelium with marked papillation, and also increase of stromal elements. App. 100 x.

FIG. 581.—UTERUS: ADENOMYOMA.—CASE 247.—High and low power photomicrograph showing the characteristic interlacing bundles of muscle fibers in which typical endometrial-like glands and stroma can be identified. App. 15 and 100 x.

metrium and parametrium. The simple acute endometritis is particularly seen as an extension of a cervical canal gonorrhea, or it may be associated with retained secundines following delivery of a child, or particularly in relation to incomplete abortions and miscarriages. Such acute inflammatory processes likewise may be seen following various contraceptive procedures, particularly the use of irritating chemical douches.

The uterus itself is obviously much more liable to infection during the puerperium, after the expulsion of the placenta, which leaves open to such infection the vascular sinuses of the endometrial surface. Such a process may go on to complete gangrenous necrotic inflammation and be accompanied by secondary peritonitis and septicemia. The process may extend directly into the fallopian tubes and result in a diffuse bilateral salpingitis. Refer back to acute gangrenous endometritis, Case 51 (Ref. #S-5) Chapter XIII, part 2, Fig. 109.

Chronic Inflammation.—Chronic inflammation may follow the acute inflammatory lesions as in other acute infectious processes. More often, however, it represents a totally independent lesion. From the practical standpoint, the condition known as chronic hyperplastic endometritis or hyperplasia of the endometrium is the most familiar condition which is usually considered in this group of chronic inflammatory processes. However, this lesion should not be thought of as a truly inflammatory one, but is much more likely to be the result of overstimulation of the endometrium by a wide variety of causes, most significant of which would be the endocrine, estrin factor. It is also, a concomitant of chronic passive congestion of the endometrium, which, as has been emphasized, may be the result of malpositions or pelvic inflammation. At times this process may be so marked that actual polypoid overgrowth of endometrium occurs and the differentiation from true neoplasia is extremely uncertain. In the usual pathological specimen, as submitted by the surgeon in the form of uterine curettings, the differentiation of this pathological process from the simple premenstrual hyperplasia is almost impossible.

ILLUSTRATIVE CASE

CASE 243. (Ref. #S-361)
Diagnosis.—Endometrium—chronic hyperplasia.
Patient was a white housewife of 35 years, admitted to the hospital complaining of menorrhagia.
Present Illness.—Patient stated that she had been in her usual health until about eighteen months ago when she had a spontaneous miscarriage. Since that time she had had an almost constant menorrhagia. This had not been accompanied by any undue dysmenorrhea. Between her periods she had noted a foul smelling leukorrhea. This had caused considerable excoriation of the vulva.
Past Medical History.—Her previous history was essentially irrelevant. She had no recollection of any definite childhood diseases. Seven years preceding admission, she had had a gall-stone operation. At the age of fifteen she had her appendix removed. At the time of admission, she had one living child born three years previously. She lost her first child ten years before admission by miscarriage due to a uterine fibroid. At that time she was operated upon and the tumor removed. A review of her systems otherwise revealed nothing pertinent.
Physical Examination.—The patient was a fairly well-nourished and somewhat anemic-appearing young white woman in no apparent pain. Head was essentially negative. Eyes, ears, nose and throat were negative. Mouth showed compensated edentia. Heart and lungs seemed to be within normal limits. Abdomen was somewhat obese with extremely flabby musculature. There was an old right-rectus scar and right lower quadrant appendectomy

scar. No masses or tenderness were noted. Vaginal examination revealed a marked retroversion and a lacerated cervix.
Laboratory Findings.—Red blood cells, 4,000,000 with 78% hemoglobin. White blood cells, 10,100 with 45% polynuclears, 49% lymphocytes and 6% monocytes. Urinalysis negative.
Subsequent Course.—Patient was advised to have a curettage both from a diagnostic and therapeutic standpoint. At the time of curettage, the uterus was found retroverted. The uterine curettings were so extremely profuse as to suggest the possibility either of retained secundines or a polypoid endometritis. The patient made an uneventful recovery and was discharged improved. No recurrence of her symptoms developed.
Pathological Report.—*Gross Description.*—The specimen consisted of about 5 cm. of soft, hemorrhagic, friable uterine curettings.
Microscopic Description of the Uterine Curettings. —(Fig. 580) Histologic study of the endometrial scrapings shows a marked hyperplasia of both the glandular and stromal elements. Many of the glands are dilated and are filled with secretion. The stroma is loose and edematous. There is some slight hemorrhage into the stroma. There is no evidence of decidua nor chorionic villi found. There is nothing noted of a neoplastic nature. The picture is one of simple chronic hyperplasia of the endometrium. This is of such a degree as to almost suggest a polypoid process.

Tuberculosis.—The endometrium is particularly resistant to infection by all bacteria. This includes even the tubercle bacillus. In the more extensive cases of tuberculosis of the fallopian tubes, however, the process may extend from the tube to produce a diffuse involvement of the endometrium. This is likely to occur as multiple subepithelial miliary tubercles, which tend to become conglomerate, and to produce superficial ulceration so that the endometrium becomes replaced by a layer of tuberculous granulation tissue.

The other infectious granulomata including actinomycosis, leprosy and so forth are observed with only great rarity in the fundus of the uterus.

Syphilis.—In syphilis, the cervix may frequently be the site of the primary chancre, just as the cervical glandular tissue is commonly the initial focus of the gonorrheal lesion in the female.

TUMORS OF THE UTERUS

There are four varieties of tumors which occur with great frequency in the uterus and make up approximately 98 per cent of all uterine tumors. These are the polypi of the cervix and endometrium, the leiomyomata, the adenocarcinomata of the fundus and the carcinomata of the cervix, which are usually squamous in type, but may show some glandular arrangement when they arise in the deep cervical glands. In addition, there are occasional other tumors which either arise in the uterus or are related to uterine elements for their origin, and so should be included briefly in the discussion at this time.

Polypi.—One of the most common tumors which is found in the uterus is seen as a polypoid lesion arising most frequently from the endocervix, but not infrequently from the endometrium. These vary a great deal in size and appearance but fundamentally are similar in their histologic make-up. They are very comparable to the adenomatous polypi which are found in the gastro-intestinal tract. They represent a curious, localized inflammatory hyperplasia of the glandular epithelium which protrudes into the lumen of the uterine canal. Owing to the mechanical factors involved, the tendency for these tumors is to grow downward in the canal until they not infrequently protrude from the cervical os as a pear-like mass. Typically in the uncomplicated case, they are covered by epithelium which in many instances extends to show a metaplasia toward the squamous type, particularly on its anterior presenting surface where it is more subject to trauma. However, many such tumors retain the columnar, glandular type of cell throughout their existence. The body of the tumor is made up of connective tissue in which are found acinar structures, some of which appear to communicate with the surface epithelium, and some of which appear to be entirely isolated. The stroma usually shows marked edema and congestion, and a variable amount of chronic inflammatory cellular infiltration. The tumor frequently becomes ulcerated and as a result, secondary inflammatory changes with very marked destruction of the mucosa and secondary leukocytic infiltration occur. Rarely, such tumors may undergo actual malignant transformation and serve as the starting point of a true adenocarcinoma.

ILLUSTRATIVE CASE

CASE 244. (Ref. #S-362)

Diagnosis.—Cervical polyp.

Patient was a white married, American housewife of 45 years, admitted to the hospital because of a profuse leukorrhea.

Present Illness.—For the preceding two months, the patient had complained of a profuse, whitish discharge from the vagina. She had not noticed any foul odor to this, nor had there been any apparent hemorrhage associated with it. She had also complained of a feeling of distention and discomfort in the lower abdomen for the past six or eight months accompanied by low back pain.

Past Medical History.—As she recalled it, measles was the only childhood disease which she had had. She had no other serious illness requiring hospitalization, or operation. She had been married eighteen years and had had two children, seventeen and fourteen years of age. Her husband was living and well. A review of her systems revealed nothing of importance in relation to the present condition. She had had occasional attacks of indigestion with epigastric distress. Cardiac, pulmonary and genito-urinary systems were entirely negative. Menstrual history had always been normal. She had regular periods at twenty-eight day intervals without pain. Her last period was ten days before admission.

Physical Examination.—Patient was a middle-aged, well-nourished, white female, who did not appear ill. Physical examination was essentially negative. Head was normal. Eyes, ears, nose and throat were negative. Upper jaw showed compensated edentia. Chest was negative. Lungs were clear throughout. Heart was not enlarged and there were no murmurs. Abdomen was soft. There was no tenderness or pain. Vaginal examination: There was a mucoid secretion seen coming from the external os. The cervix itself showed a laceration at one side, which was apparently covered by mucosa. A pedunculated mass apparently attached to the wall of the cervical canal was found protruding from the cervix. This was as large as a golf ball. Grossly, it showed some erosion and hemorrhage.

Laboratory Examination.—Blood count was normal. Red blood cells, 4,500,000 with 76% hemoglobin. White blood cells, 6,900 with 42% polynuclears and 49% lymphocytes. Urinalysis was negative.

Subsequent Course.—The cervix was dilated and the polypoid mass excised. A curettage of the uterus was performed. Another smaller polypoid mass was found in the uterine canal.

Pathological Report.—*Gross Description.*—Specimen consisted of two soft, pinkish-gray polypoid-appearing masses, the larger measuring 2 x 1.5 x 1 cm., the smaller 1 x 1 x 0.8 cm. In addition there were about 2 c.c. of small, tough, hemorrhagic endometrial curettings. The polypi both showed some erosion of the surface mucosa with hemorrhage into the substance of the tumor mass as observed on section.

Leiomyomata.—The myomata of the uterus have been discussed in the chapter relating to tumors of muscle cell origin. Briefly, in review, it may be stated that they arise as tumors of the smooth muscle and may occur as subserous, intramural or submucous lesions, depending upon their location. This latter variety tends to become polypoid and to cause marked obstruction of the uterine canal. The tumor is benign in the great majority of instances, only rarely undergoing malignant degeneration (Fig. 594). Occasional instances of so-called "adenomyomata" may be found in which endometrial tissue may be identified incorporated in a tumor in all other respects a simple leiomyoma. In general, it is held that this is the result of some fetal persistence of müllerian or wolffian duct rests. A typical example of the simple myomatous form of uterine tumor is presented in Case 99 (Ref. #S-130), Fig. 229 & 230, Chapter XXVI. See also Fig. 590.

Adenocarcinoma of the Fundus.—The adenocarcinoma is the typical tumor of the uterine fundus, arising from the endometrial glands (Fig. 579). It

Microscopic Description of One of the Polypi.—Histologic study of the tissue shows it to be a typical cervical polyp. The surface is covered for the most part by modified epithelium, which shows a tendency toward squamous development on the surface, with glandular hyperplasia in the deeper portions. In places, there is erosion of the mucosa with hemorrhage into the soft tissues. Scattered throughout the entire mass are found numerous irregular, dilated cystic areas lined by typical tall, columnar glandular epithelium. The surrounding stroma is loose, edematous and shows marked infiltration by lymphocytes and plasma cells. No evidence of malignant, neoplastic change is seen.

varies greatly in extent. As has been emphasized in respect to chronic hyperplasia of the endometrium, at times the differentiation from a polypoid hyperplasia and early neoplasm is extremely difficult. As a matter of practical importance it may be remarked that the fundic carcinoma is usually one of very low grade malignancy characterized ordinarily by merely local invasiveness, and only in the late stages may it extend into the surrounding pelvic tissues and even produce distant metastases.

Microscopically, these tumors are found to be composed of irregular overgrowths of endometrial glandular tissue. This tends to assume a papillary arrangement in many places. There is a variable amount of stroma. The cells show rather well marked adult differentiation for the most part, but are likely to present a considerable number of mitotic figures. There is some loss of basement membrane with local infiltration of the myometrium. The tumor as a rule is accompanied by considerable hemorrhagic and inflammatory cell infiltration of the stroma by both leukocytes and mononuclears.

ILLUSTRATIVE CASE

CASE 245. (Ref. #S-345)

Diagnosis.—Uterus—adenocarcinoma of the fundus.

Patient was a white female of 64 years, admitted to the hospital because of irregular bleeding from the vagina for the past four years.

Present Illness.—The patient had her menopause at the age of forty-nine and ever since that time she would have occasional showing from the vagina which required, on occasions, the wearing of a pad. During the past four years, this has been much more frequent and profuse. Indeed, there had seldom been a day pass in which some bleeding had not been noted. She complained of no other symptoms of any particular significance. She had been under the care of a physician, who had been treating the cervix locally but without any apparent improvement in her condition.

Past Medical History.—The patient had never had any serious illness during her entire life that she could remember, nor had she ever required any operative

treatment. A review of her systems was essentially negative. She had had marked constipation associated with the development of hemorrhoids, but these had subsided under local treatment. Her menstrual history had begun at thirteen, and periods were regular until her menopause. During this period, she had had three normal pregnancies and was delivered of three healthy children.

Physical Examination.—Patient was a well-developed and well-nourished, elderly, white woman who appeared somewhat pale. Head was grossly negative. Eyes, ears, nose and throat were negative. Chest was symmetrical. Lungs were clear. Heart was regular and not enlarged. Abdomen revealed no palpable masses. There was slight tenderness in the lower left quadrant. Extremities were negative. External genitalia negative. The perineum was negative. Cervix was practically absent as a result of the therapeutic procedure. There was a definite sanguineous discharge from the internal os. The fundus seemed slightly enlarged and soft, but this was not very definite in nature. The adnexae were negative.

Laboratory Findings.—Red blood cells, 3,800,000 with 73% hemoglobin. White blood cells, 9,450 with 92% polynuclears. Urinalysis was negative.

Subsequent Course.—On the basis of the long history, it was felt that complete hysterectomy was indicated. This was done and a slightly enlarged uterus with the adnexae was removed. The patient made an uneventful recovery and was discharged, relieved of her symptoms.

Pathological Report.—*Gross Description.*—Specimen consisted of a somewhat enlarged uterus, both tubes and ovaries. The tubes and ovaries were essentially negative showing marked senile atrophy. There were several small cysts of Morgagni present. The uterine fundus measured 8 cm. in diameter when opened. The wall was 2 cm. in thickness. The inner surface was entirely covered by a soft, friable, hemorrhagic cauliflower growth. The cervical canal seemed essentially negative, but the superficial cervix was made up of dense scar tissue.

Microscopic Description of a Section Through the Endometrium.—(Fig. 579) Histologic study of the tissue shows a diffuse, malignant hyperplasia of the endometrial epithelium. The cells are arranged in irregular pseudoacini. They show definite infiltration of the myometrium. The cells vary in size and staining reactions very markedly. Many atypical mitotic figures are observed. In places, the cells are several layers deep. In others, they are flattened out and only composed of a single layer. The picture is one of a typical adenocarcinoma of the fundus of the uterus.

Carcinoma of the Cervix.—In discussing the development of carcinoma of the cervix, we must consider briefly the early inflammatory lesions of the cervix, which seems to predispose to the development of malignancy later. Chronic inflammation of the cervix may well be considered as a contributory factor. Gonorrheal infection, and chronic inflammation as the result of trauma, particularly following the laceration of the cervix at childbirth, are perhaps among the more common causes in the development of such an inflammatory endocervicitis. Superficial erosion of the epithelium not infrequently occurs. Scar tissue is present in considerable volume at times. Glands become shut off from the surface and undergo cystic dilatation when they are spoken of as nabothian cysts. This area of erosion becomes the site of a chronic granulomatous inflammatory tissue production which may gradually become cicatrized or may, on the other hand, go on to the development of a carcinoma. In view of the fact that well over 90 per cent of cases of carcinoma of the cervix occur in women who have had one or more children with the concomitant inflammatory changes of the cervix, little doubt can be cast upon the importance of this chronic inflammatory process in the development of the malignant picture. Recent studies have likewise emphasized the possible importance of endocrine stimulation as the result of pregnancy itself in the production of the pre-cancerous cervical lesion.

The neoplasm grossly usually begins on the lip of the cervix and gradually produces an ulcerated, erosive, shaggy, sloughing mass which extends deep into the musculature of the cervix. In certain varieties, we may find a marked cauliflower-like overgrowth of the tumor tissue, which may even almost fill the vaginal vault. The tumor tends to grow relatively rapidly and to extend by permeation to the parametrium, the bladder, the rectum and around the vagina. The tumor rarely extends to involve the uterine body, and late manifestations may be seen in blood stream invasion with distant metastases.

The tumors vary considerably in their morphology. The great majority of the tumors arise from the squamous epithelium, and as such present the usual picture of squamous or epidermoid carcinoma. It was upon the basis of a study of a large series of such cervical carcinomata that the present method of gradation of the epidermoid carcinomata was suggested. Less often, microscopically, as has already been indicated, the tumors may either arise from the glandular epithelial cells or these cells may become involved in the neoplastic process so that a varying amount of adenocarcinomatous development may be recognized. The tumors as a whole are fairly radiosensitive and particularly so in the more malignant form. As a matter of experience it has been found that the only successful method of treatment of the carcinoma of the cervix uteri is by irradiation in some form. To-day, the method of preference appears to be the use of the x-ray followed by radical surgery in a considerable proportion of the cases when the malignant process has regressed to a point to make surgery profitable. X-ray likewise has been found more satisfactory than radium implantation.

The reader is referred to Case 142 (Ref. #S-322) and Fig. 320 and 324 in Chapter XXXIII for the history of a patient suffering from squamous cell carcinoma of the cervix, Grade IV. Case 246 (Ref. #S-371), presented at this time, represents the same type of carcinoma of the cervix, Grade II.

ILLUSTRATIVE CASE

CASE 246. (Ref. #S-371)

Diagnosis.—Cervix—squamous cell carcinoma, Grade II.

Patient was a white married housewife of 41 years, who was admitted to the hospital because of low back pain and bleeding from the vagina.

Present Illness.—The onset of the present illness dated back approximately between three and four months and began with a feeling of discomfort in the sacro-iliac region accompanied by a bearing-down sensation in the perineum. About one week after this pain started, she noticed intermittent spotting which had no relationship to her periods. She went to a physician, who examined her and made a diagnosis of cancer, and treated her with radium. This resulted in a marked improvement in the pain and a complete cessation of the bleeding for several weeks. About one month before admission, both the pain and bleeding recurred with greater frequency. She was unable to state whether she had lost any weight over this period, but did complain of feeling extremely weak and tired.

Past Medical History.—As a child she had all the usual diseases including scarlet fever and diphtheria. Since that time, however, she had never had any significant illness and had enjoyed unusually good health. She had been married nineteen years and had had seven children, all of whom were living and well. Her menstrual history began at the age of thirteen and was regular at thirty day intervals until the onset of her present illness. A review of her systems otherwise was of no significance in relation to her present illness.

Physical Examination.—Patient was a well-developed, somewhat obese, middle-aged, white woman who appeared to be in no particular distress. Hair was beginning to gray. Eyes were negative. Nose and throat were normal. Teeth were in very poor condition. Chest was symmetrical. Breasts were large and pendulous, but no masses could be felt in them. Lungs were clear. Heart did not appear to be enlarged and showed no murmurs. Abdomen was extremely obese making examination diffi-

cult. Extremities were negative. Gynecologic examination revealed a cervix which showed an excavated, ulcerative surface, which extended toward both fornices. The fundus of the uterus was between two and three times the normal size.

Laboratory Findings.—Blood count on admission showed 4,400,000 red blood cells with 70% hemoglobin and 6,850 white blood cells with 67% polynuclears. Urinalysis was essentially negative.

Subsequent Course.—On the basis of the history and physical findings, a diagnostic dilatation and curettage was recommended with the taking of a biopsy from the cervix. At the time of operation, the uterine cavity was found to be about 13 cm. in length. There was a moderate amount of rather firm endometrial curettings. A wedge-shaped specimen from the cervix was taken for histologic study.

Pathological Report.—*Gross Description.*—Specimen consisted of a small, wedge shaped fragment of tissue, which measured 1.5 cm. in its greatest diameter. It showed an ulcerated surface and it was difficult to make out any line of demarcation between mucosa and underlying musculature.

Microscopic Description of a Section Through the Cervix.—(Fig. 578) Histologic study of the cervical tissue presents a typical picture of a squamous cell type of carcinoma. The surface epithelium has completely disappeared, possibly as the result of the previous radium therapy. However, extending deep into the musculature of the cervix are found long, tongue-like projections and nests of typical squamous cells. There is some attempt on their part toward adult differentiation. A suggestion of basement membrane is seen here and there, but there is definite and frank invasion of the musculature. The cells vary considerably in size and shape and show considerable hyperchromatism of their nuclei. Numerous mitotic figures are encountered. Most of these appear to be fairly normal in type. There is marked secondary chronic inflammatory cellular infiltration of the tissues. Eosinophilic cells are particularly prominent in this instance.

Chorion Carcinoma (Chorio-epithelioma).—This tumor has also been discussed in the section on tumors and so need only be briefly reviewed at this point. It may occur occasionally as a primary tumor in association with pregnancy or as is more often the case, it develops upon the site of a hydatidiform mole. As has already been emphasized, such tumors may be found as a variety of the complex teratomata of the ovary or testis. For a history of hydatidiform mole, refer to Case 157 (Ref. #S-119), Fig. 344 in Chapter XXXVI, and Fig. 586 in this chapter.

Endometriosis.—Neoplasm-like masses of endometrial tissue are found, usually in the form of cystic lesions, not infrequently on the peritoneal surface almost anywhere and particularly on the surface of the ovary. They may likewise be found in the scar

of an abdominal incision following caesarean section. In addition, the appearance of such endometrial tissue in a certain proportion of the myomatous tumors of the uterus has been emphasized. Whether these endometrial-like lesions should be considered as true tumors is highly doubtful. For this reason, the term "endometriosis" has been used rather than the term "endometriomata." So far as the uterine lesions are concerned, it is generally conceded that they probably represent either wolffian body rests, or infoldings of endometrium which have become shut off from the normal endometrial lining of the uterus. In respect to the cystic tumors or implants on the peritoneal surface of the gut, ovary, tube or other abdominal and pelvic viscera, the theory which Sampson advanced that they were the result of an endometrial back-wash during the menstrual cycle

seems the most convincing one. With such endometrial fragments passing into the peritoneal cavity,
they become implanted and continue to grow, repeat-
ing their hyperplasia with each menstrual cycle. Similarly, the implantations in the abdominal wall,
which have followed operative procedures on the
uterus, particularly caesarean section, may also be
explained on the basis of such implantation. For
practical purposes, this seems to offer the most satisfactory explanation of these curious lesions, but that
it has not met with complete accord is seen by the
comment of many other authors. The questions
whether they may not arise as neoplasms from serosal rests, or whether they may not even be ovarian
in origin from ruptured follicular hemorrhagic cysts
are theories currently attracting attention. It does
not seem of sufficient practical importance to go
deeper into this relatively unimportant controversial
discussion.

From the standpoint of the clinician, these lesions
are not considered to be unusual. Indeed, Sampson
has emphasized that they are probably among the
most frequently encountered pelvic lesions of women
below the menopausal age. If they are widely disseminated, they offer a surgical problem in their removal. The removal of the ovaries, or inactivation of
the ovaries by irradiation will result in the great majority of cases in the disappearance of these lesions.

Pathologically, they consist of what appears to be
essentially normal endometrial glands and stroma
(Fig. 581). In many instances there is a tendency
toward actual cyst formation. With each menstrual
cycle the same hyperplastic changes can be followed
in these tissues as in the normal endometrium, with
the result that the cyst increases slowly in size due
to the intracystic discharge of the desquamated blood
cells and endometrium. As a result of this hemorrhage, these cysts tend to be of a chocolate brown
color as the hemoglobin undergoes its usual breakdown and the term "chocolate cyst" is frequently
applied to this lesion. They are not to be confused
with simple follicular cysts with hemorrhage.

ILLUSTRATIVE CASES

CASE 247. (Ref. #S-346 and S-373)
Diagnosis.—Uterus—adenomyoma.
Patient was a white female of 44 years, admitted to
the hospital with the chief complaint of marked dysmenorrhea and metrorrhagia.
Present Illness.—The onset of the patient's present
illness began approximately four months ago with a
rather marked metrorrhagia. She had always complained
of a rather severe dysmenorrhea ever since her periods
first began at the age of seventeen, but this had been
much more marked during the preceding four months. The
flow had been more than twice the normal amount, and
as a result, she had felt weak and unable to do her
housework.
Past History.—As a child the patient had measles,
chickenpox and diphtheria. A review of her systems
medically yielded nothing of significance in relation to
her present illness. She had been married twenty years
ago at the age of twenty-four, but her husband had died
two years later. She had remarried two years before
her present admission. She had had what she believed
was a miscarriage, shortly after this second marriage.
Other than that, she had never been pregnant. Her menstrual history was of significance in that her periods had
not begun until relatively late, at the age of seventeen,
and that they had been at twenty-one day intervals
always associated with marked dysmenorrhea.
Physical Examination.—The patient was a well-developed, well-nourished, middle-aged, white woman who
did not appear acutely ill. Head was negative. Eyes reacted normally. Nose and throat were negative. Chest
was symmetrical. Lungs were clear. Heart was not enlarged. Her breasts were normal in appearance. No
masses could be felt. Abdomen was somewhat prominent.
Liver could not be felt. The uterus was felt about three
fingers' breadth above the symphysis. Extremities were
negative.
Laboratory Findings.—Blood count on admission
showed 4,500,000 red blood cells with 75% hemoglobin
and 7,700 white blood cells with 70% polynuclears. Urinalysis was negative.
Subsequent Course.—On the basis of the history and
the patient's age, it was recommended that she have a
hysterectomy. At the time of operation the uterus was
found to be enlarged to about the size of a large grapefruit. It contained several intramural nodular masses,
apparently fibroids. An ovarian cyst measuring approximately 7 cm. in diameter was likewise found and removed. The patient made an uneventful recovery and
was discharged cured.
Pathological Report.—*Gross Description.*—Specimen
consisted of a uterus and a large ovary containing a cyst.
The uterus measured approximately 15 x 12 x 10 cm. due
to the presence of two large intramural fibroids near the
cornua. These averaged 5.5 cm. in diameter. The ovary
measured approximately 7 x 6 x 5 cm. It contained a
large multiloculated cyst and was filled with a clear,
serous fluid (Fig. 593). On section it was shown to be
frankly multilocular with numerous septal divisions. From
the wall of the major portion of the cyst, typical papillary
proliferations a few millimeters in height could be seen.
They were of a grayish-pink color.
**Microscopic Description of a Section Through One
of the Uterine Tumor Nodules.**—(Fig. 581) Histologic
examination of a wedge of tissue from the uterus shows a
moderately hyperplastic endometrium. The stroma presents
considerable congestion with some actual hemorrhage.
This is accompanied by moderate lymphocytic infiltration. The myometrium appears essentially normal. Section through the myomatous nodule pre-

sents a picture of a typical adenomyoma. This is found to consist of the usual typical whorl-like interlacing bundles of connective tissue fibers and smooth muscle cells. Buried between clumps of such cells are found typical areas of what appear to be endometrial tissue. That this is completely isolated from the actual endometrial surface can easily be established by the encapsulated nature of the tumor tissue. This endometrium shows varying phases of hyperplasia and dilatation of the glands and the stroma, which duplicates that of normal endometrium. It shows considerable chronic inflammatory mononuclear cellular infiltration. This appears to represent a tumor arising from wolffian duct rests in relation to the musculature of the wall of the uterus and is described under a variety of names, the most accurately descriptive of which is adenomyoma or myometrioma.

CASE 248. (Ref. #-293)

Diagnosis.—Abdominal wall—endometrial fistula.

Patient was a single, white woman, aged forty, who was admitted to the hospital because of a draining fistula in the abdominal wall, following an appendectomy.

History of Present Illness.—Patient was well until eight years ago, when she was operated upon for an acute appendix, which had ruptured. She was in the hospital with peritonitis complicating her convalescence for a little over one month. The incision was drained at the time of operation, but subsequently seemed to heal satisfactorily, although causing her some pain. Nearly a year after her operation, she returned to the hospital and was reoperated upon for adhesions. This healed satisfactorily. About two years ago, she noticed a lump in the line of incision following an injury received from running into the corner of a bureau. This was opened with a needle and a bloody fluid was discharged. Since that time, the patient had had a recurrence of this swelling coincidental with her menstrual periods. This had increased in amount until for the last several periods, she had had to wear a pad over the sinus tract. There was no pain at the site of discharge, but before it drained, she had a feeling of tension and discomfort.

Past Medical History.—As a child, she had the measles and chickenpox. Twelve years ago, she had had a thyroidectomy done because of typical hyperthyroid symptoms. She improved after that time and was completely relieved of her symptoms. Nine years ago she had had a tonsillectomy. A review of her systems was of little value in respect to the present history. For the past several months, she had complained of increased "nervousness" and had noted some vague gastrointestinal disturbances, especially associated with fatty foods. Bowels were regular and only required occasional

catharsis. Menstrual history was essentially normal, periods occurring every twenty-seven days, lasting four to five days. Her last period was eleven days ago.

Physical Examination.—Patient was a well-nourished woman in middle age, lying comfortably in bed. Head was negative for the most part. Pupils showed some slight inequality, the right being larger than the left. They both reacted to light and distance, but the right was more sluggish. Neck: no lymphadenopathy. Thyroidectomy scar. Chest: Lungs clear throughout. Cardiovascular: heart negative. Abdominal examination revealed an old appendectomy scar at the lower end of which was a cyst-like enlargement with a pin-point opening from which might be expressed a chocolate colored discharge. What seemed to be a fistulous tract could be palpated beneath the scar. Otherwise the abdomen was negative. The extremities were normal.

Laboratory Examination.—Blood count: On admission, red blood cells, 4,000,000; 83% hemoglobin (13 grams). Color Index 1.0; white blood cells, 8,450 with 73% polynuclears, 19% lymphocytes and 6% monocytes. Urinalysis was negative.

Subsequent Course.—Working diagnosis of endometrial fistula of abdominal wall was made. Operation was recommended and under spinal anesthesia, the fistulous tract was dissected out. It continued as a direct tract through the abdominal wall, down along the external iliac artery to its termination at the right uterine cornu where the stump of the fallopian tube joined it. The fistula and the remnant of the fallopian tube were excised from the uterus by a wedge shaped excision, and the uterine horn closed. At the time of operation, the right ovary was not found and had apparently been removed at the time of previous operation. The left tube and ovary appeared normal. The cecum was freely mobile and showed a puckered scar at the appendectomy site.

Pathological Report.—*Gross Description.*—Specimen consisted of an elongated mass of fibro-fatty inflammatory tissue measuring approximately 4.5 x 4 x 2.5 cm. in length. This included an elliptical piece of skin on one surface with a small sinus opening in the center.

Microscopic Description.—(Fig. 587) Sections show for the most part a mass of chronic inflammatory tissue, which includes some of the muscle fibers of the abdominal wall. Embedded in this mass of dense fibrous scar tissue are seen numerous areas of typical endometrial tissue with characteristic glandular and stromal elements present. These suggest a communicating, potentially cystic cavity as some of the cells seem to be lining empty spaces. The endometrium appears to be in the resting stage as might be expected in relation to the history of the last period being thirteen or fourteen days preceding the operation.

CHAPTER LIX
DISEASES OF THE FEMALE GENITALIA (*Continued*)
PART I
FALLOPIAN TUBE

CONGENITAL LESIONS

The fallopian tubes are likely to show a wide variety of congenital malformations in company with the developmental defects of the uterus. These are of little practical or pathological importance. From the clinical and pathological standpoints, there are only two lesions of major significance, which relate to them: first, salpingitis either as an acute gonorrheal or other pyogenic infection, or in chronic form as tuberculosis; and second, ectopic tubal pregnancy.

Rarely, tumors may arise primarily in the fallopian tube as carcinomata. Myomata may occur arising from the smooth muscle in the wall of the tube. As a complication of tubal pregnancy, chorio-epithelioma may develop. Actually only the inflammatory lesions and ectopic pregnancy are of any significance from the standpoint of numerical incidence.

SALPINGITIS

Gonorrheal Salpingitis.—In gonorrhea, the primary infection is usually found in the cervical canal of the uterus or in the urethra. In the widely branching glands of the cervix this organism finds a most suitable site for its growth and there it produces the characteristic inflammatory changes which have already been described. The endometrium is extremely resistant against all bacterial infection, and the gonococcus passes through the uterine canal not infrequently to become localized in the tubes. The initial infection of the tubes is liable to be in the nature of a very acute process and may clinically be mistaken for appendicitis. However, the process nearly always involves both tubes, although not infrequently in a variable degree. It starts as a mild, acute lesion with edema, hemorrhage, some slight leukocytic infiltration and a marked catarrhal inflammatory hypersecretion on the part of the mucosal lining. This tends to produce blocking of the ostia, and commonly of the isthmus. This results in a cyst-like dilatation of the tube as the inflammatory process continues, and the exudate increases in amount. Due to its anatomical relationship, it becomes twisted on itself until it very closely resembles a distorted sausage. It is accompanied by localized peritonitis of the overlying serosal surface. This in some cases may become generalized, but fortunately more often remains localized. Gradually, the process becomes chronic. It is accompanied by marked fibrous thickening of the walls of the tubes and the gradual inspissation of the purulent exudate. The development of dense fibrous adhesions between the ovary, tube, uterus and the wall of the gastro-intestinal tract follow not infrequently. This condition is clinically spoken of as a pus tube (Fig. 585). Not infrequently a walled-off cavity forms between the tube and ovary in connection with such an infection and because of its anatomical location is best described as a tubo-ovarian abscess. This whole process may extend to involve the ovary as a whole with diffuse infiltration of ovarian stroma and involvement of the graafian follicles. It may undergo necrosis with the development of a huge abscess, which involves the entire ovary and tube as a single lesion. The importance of the acute gonorrheal infection of the tube is that it results in the obliteration of the lumen and with it the opportunity for ovulation to result in the migration of the ovum to the uterine canal. It is, therefore, one of the most important causes of sterility in the female.

Tuberculous Salpingitis.—Tuberculosis of the fallopian tube is the only other infection of importance.

PLATE CXXXVIII
DISEASES OF THE FEMALE GENITALIA

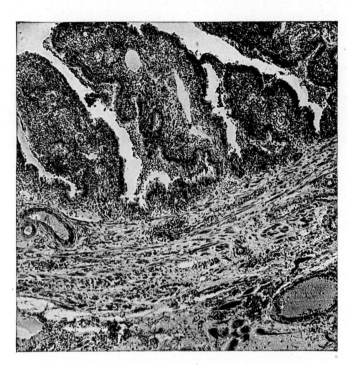

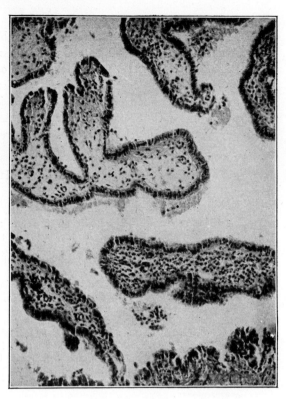

FIG. 582.—FALLOPIAN TUBE: CHRONIC SALPINGITIS (GONORRHEAL).—CASE 250.—Diffuse mono- and polynuclear exudate infiltrating the entire wall and distorted villi, and accompanied by considerable inflammatory fibrosis. A similar exudate is seen within the lumen. App. 100 x.

FIG. 583.—FALLOPIAN TUBE: ACUTE SALPINGITIS.—CASE 249.—Photomicrograph of several edematous villi in which an acute exudate rich in polymorphonuclears and serum is outstanding. App. 100 x.

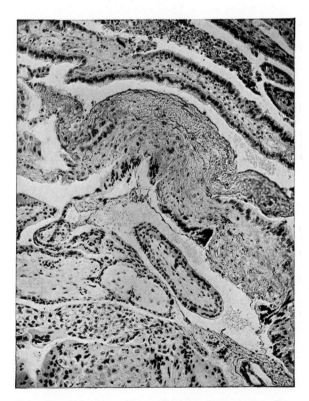

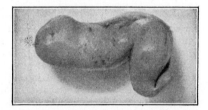

FIG. 585.—FALLOPIAN TUBE: CHRONIC SALPINGITIS, GONORRHEAL (PUS TUBE).—CASE 250.—Sausage shaped, dilated and thickened tube filled with thick, creamy pus.

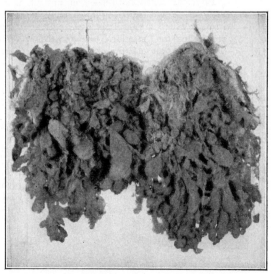

FIG. 584.—FALLOPIAN TUBE: ECTOPIC PREGNANCY.—CASE 251.—Typical chorionic villi and decidual cells in lower part of illustration, intimately associated with adjacent tubal villi in upper part. App. 100 x.

FIG. 586.—HYDATIDIFORM MOLE.—CASE 157 (See Fig. 344).—Cystic villi of varying size occurring in grape-like clusters are seen as the diagnostically characteristic feature of this condition.

It is presumably hematogenous in origin, but may also result from an extension of a tuberculous enteritis. The isthmus and ostia tend to become occluded by characteristic tuberculous granulation tissue and a tuberculous pyosalpinx develops. This consists of a widely distended tube filled with typical thick, caseous material. Secondary infection not infrequently follows with liquefaction necrosis and abscess formation. From the microscopic standpoint, the presence of tubercles renders the diagnosis ordinarily simple. In the earlier stages this may be made by the finding of minute individual lesions in the villi. As the process continues, they become coalescent with the development of a typical chronic picture.

ILLUSTRATIVE CASE

CASE 249. (Ref. #S-363)

Diagnosis.—Fallopian tube—acute salpingitis.

Patient was a white housewife of 43 years, admitted to the hospital complaining of menorrhagia and frequency of micturition of four months' duration, associated with headaches and a generally weak feeling, and with pain in the left lower quadrant.

Present Illness.—Patient had always complained of prolonged and often painful menstrual periods, but for the past four months, this had been almost continuous. She complained particularly of marked frequency, in association with this menorrhagia. Patient had also noted considerable leukorrhea between periods. She had had intermittent attacks of vertigo and headaches. She had secured some relief during the preceding month from a pessary, but her symptoms would return every time it was removed.

Past Medical History.—She was born in Russia. She did not recall any childhood diseases. She was married at twenty-two. She had had five pregnancies, with four normal children and one miscarriage. The patient's first child died, at seven years, of diphtheria, which produced a marked emotional upset in the patient. This was followed by hyperthyroid symptoms, and thyroidectomy was ultimately resorted to the year before admission. A review of her systems showed the following features of possible interest and significance: persistent headaches of a very severe type at frequent intervals; failing vision. Upper respiratory tract: frequent mild colds. Cardiovascular: marked improvement since her thyroidectomy, but still some dyspnea upon exertion. Gastro-intestinal tract: Frequent attacks of dyspepsia, especially with fried foods. Genito-urinary: Some incontinence with anuresis, marked frequency, nocturia and polyuria. She denied venereal infection.

Physical Examination.—The patient was a moderately obese woman lying apparently fairly comfortably in bed. There was still some slight exophthalmus. Pupils were equal and regular. Nose and throat were negative. There was an old thyroidectomy scar. There was no lymphadenopathy. Heart and lungs were normal on percussion and auscultation. Abdomen was obese. There was no tenderness or rigidity. No masses were palpable. Vaginal examination showed a markedly enlarged uterus. Extremities were negative.

Laboratory Findings.—Red blood cells, 4,700,000 with 60% hemoglobin (9.5 grams). Color index, 0.67. White blood cells, 12 to 16,000 with 75 to 82% polynuclears. Urinalysis showed a slight trace of albumin, but was otherwise negative. Wassermann was negative.

Subsequent Course.—The patient was operated upon by a supravaginal incision and a straight vaginal hysterectomy with bilateral salpingectomy was done. The uterine wall was greatly thickened and fibrotic. On section, several small intramural fibroids were noted. The endometrium was hemorrhagic. Two pedunculated polyps were found in the cervical canal. The tubes appeared moderately injected and edematous. The specimen was submitted for pathological examination.

Pathological Report.—*Gross Description.*—The gross features of the uterine pathology, having been described in its essential features in relation to the surgical operation need not be reviewed at this time. The tubes were moderately dilated. They measured 10 cm. in length by somewhat over 1 cm. in diameter. The serosa was very hyperemic. The lumen was filled with a serosanguineous material. There was a large cyst of Morgagni attached to the fimbriated end of one of them.

Microscopic Description of a Section Through One of the Tubes.—(Fig. 583) Histologic examination of the tube shows a typical early, acute, nonspecific salpingitis. The entire wall of the tube shows marked interstitial edema with some slight polynuclear and mononuclear cellular infiltration. The villous folds of the tube are likewise considerably swollen as the result of interstitial edema, and polynuclears are found in moderate number scattered throughout this exudate. There is also considerable exudate present in the lumen consisting of mucoid material, leukocytes and cellular detritus. No fibroblastic reparative activity has yet developed.

ILLUSTRATIVE CASE

CASE 250. (Ref. #S-274)

Diagnosis.—Fallopian tube—chronic salpingitis, gonorrheal.

Patient was a Negress of 23 years, admitted to the hospital with the chief complaint of sharp left lower quadrant abdominal pain.

Present Illness.—The onset of the patient's present illness began ten days before admission while performing her regular household duties. She was menstruating at the time. The pain was so severe that she was unable to continue her work, and this likewise prevented her sleeping. It was more marked on the slightest physical exertion. From that time on the pain was almost constant and had become progressively worse.

Past Medical History.—The patient was unable to give any history which appeared at all relevant in respect to her present illness. She did not recall any of the childhood diseases. She had never been seriously enough sick

PLATE CXXXIX
DISEASES OF THE FEMALE GENITALIA

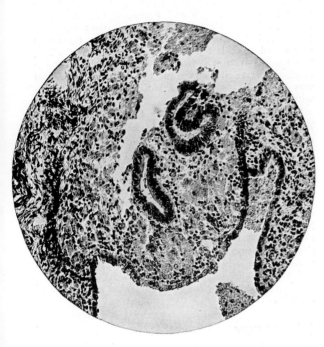

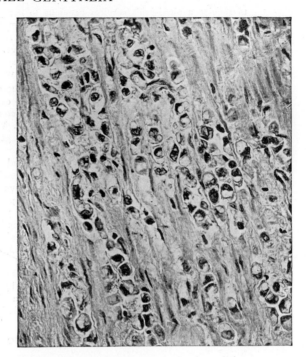

FIG. 587.—ABDOMINAL WALL: ENDOMETRIAL FISTULA (ENDO-METRIOSIS).—CASE 248.—Photomicrograph of an area from a sinus tract lined by typical endometrial glandular and stromal elements, which appear to be in the quiescent, intermenstrual phase. App. 100 x.

FIG. 588.—OVARY: KRUKENBERG CARCINOMA.—(Cf. CASE 154, Fig. 340).—High power photomicrograph. Typical "signet-ring" cells arranged in cord fashion invading ovarian stroma which shows marked distortion. App. 200 x.

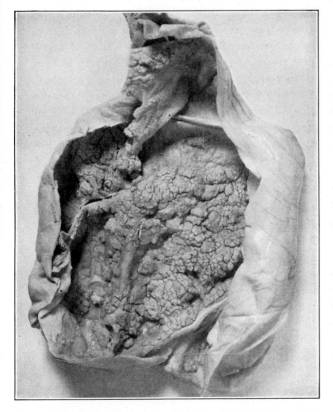

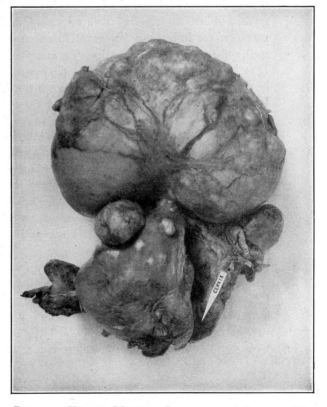

FIG. 589.—OVARY: PAPILLARY SEROUS CYSTADENOMA.—CASE 247.—Gross photograph of a portion of the cyst wall showing typical papillary proliferation of the lining epithelium.

FIG. 590.—UTERUS: MULTIPLE LEIOMYOMATA.—CASE 99 (Fig. 229 and 230).—Gross photograph of uterus with multiple, subserous, intramural and submucous leiomyomata. These have produced marked distortion of the uterine canal with an associated endometrial hyperplasia.

to require a physician's services previous to her present illness. She was married and had had one normal pregnancy. She denied any knowledge of venereal infection.

Physical Examination.—Head was negative. Eyes, ears, nose and throat were negative. Chest was symmetrical. Heart and lungs were normal. Abdomen was held rather rigidly and there was extreme tenderness over the entire lower half. This was most marked over the left lower quadrant. Palpation was unsatisfactory because of tenderness. Extremities were negative. Vaginal examination showed a diffuse vaginal discharge from the cervix.

Laboratory Findings.—Blood findings: Red blood cells, 4,100,000 with 77% hemoglobin. White blood cells, 12,600 with 84% polynuclears. Urinalysis negative except for a slight trace of albumin and occasional pus cells. Wassermann negative. Smears from the vaginal pus contained typical gram-negative diplococci (gonococci).

Subsequent Course.—A diagnosis of salpingitis was made and operation advised. A bilateral salpingectomy and a left oöphorectomy and appendectomy were done.

Pathological Report.—*Gross Description.*—(Fig. 585) The left tube and ovary were bound together by adhesions. There was a tubo-ovarian abscess of a chronic nature filled with inspissated pus and considerable hemor-

rhage. The tubes were both markedly thickened, measuring 12 cm. in length and averaging over 2 cm. in diameter. There were old fibrous adhesions over the peritoneal surface. The fimbriated end of the right tube was closed by old inflammatory adhesions. On the left, this merged with the ovary to form the chronic tubo-ovarian abscess. On section of the right tube, the wall was found greatly thickened with the lumen distended with old inspissated purulent exudate.

Microscopic Description of a Section Through the Right Tube.—(Fig. 582) Histologic examination shows the wall greatly thickened and edematous. On the serosal surface, there is some leukocytic and fibrinous exudate into which hemorrhage has occurred. In the wall of the tube itself there is marked fibrosis, which tends to separate the muscle fibers. There is a diffuse cellular infiltration in which small round cells predominate, although many polynuclear leukocytes are also present. Many of the villi have been completely destroyed. Others are thickened and club shaped. The mucosal lining is missing in some areas and in others shows an inflammatory hyperplasia. The stroma of the villi is edematous and richly infiltrated with leukocytes. Some inspissated purulent exudate is present lying within the lumen of the tube.

Ectopic (Tubal) Pregnancy

The other most common lesion which is seen involving the fallopian tube is that of ectopic pregnancy. Normally, when the ovum is discharged from the ovary, it passes into the fallopian tube where, usually in the vicinity of the isthmus, it meets the sperm and becomes fertilized, then migrates into the uterus where it becomes implanted in the uterine wall and undergoes the normal course of gestation. It so happens at times, however, that the ovum may become impregnated along its course down the fallopian tube and for one reason or another the ovum is unable to continue its migration into the uterine cavity. This may be the result of previous inflammation with narrowing of the isthmus, or through some mechanical torsion of the tube. There are those who would have us believe that there may be an actual hereditary or at least a physiological factor involved as it is not infrequent to encounter a woman who has had one tubal pregnancy to have a second such ectopia. Indeed, there are several cases on record in which such tubal pregnancies have occurred in successive gestations. The ovum becomes implanted into the wall of the tube under such circumstances, instead of in its normal position within the uterine cavity. Instances have been known in which pregnancy went on to full-term successfully, but as a general

thing at the end of a matter of a few weeks, usually somewhere around the fifth to the seventh week, the tube becomes distended to the point where it undergoes rupture. This is followed by profuse intra-abdominal hemorrhage, as a rule, from which the patient may readily die, if the condition is not promptly recognized and emergency surgical measures taken. At other times, hemorrhage may be of a slower, oozing nature, and may not be recognized clinically for some time. Not infrequently, at the time of operation or at autopsy, it is impossible to find the embryonic tissues in the tube as they apparently may have become completely destroyed by the hemorrhagic process. More often, however, atypical decidua and fairly characteristic chorionic villi may be identified. Much less often, actual fetal tissues can be found. The condition is of pathological importance because of its high mortality, unless prompt intervention follows the rupture. The tube, as a rule appears dilated in its middle or distal portion. This may vary considerably in size, at times reaching a diameter of several centimeters. A point of rupture can usually be identified. The remainder of the lumen of the tube is completely filled with blood and in the absence of the fetal tissues, the condition may be confused with a simple hematosalpinx.

PLATE CXL
DISEASES OF THE FEMALE GENITALIA
Ovarian Tumors

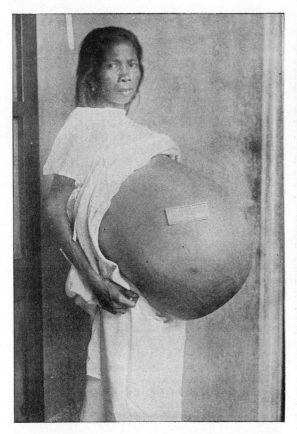

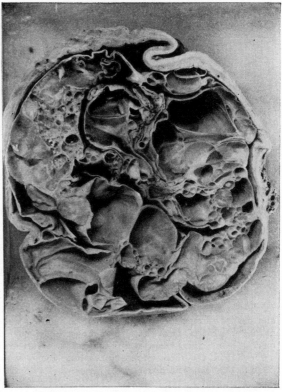

Fig. 591.—Gross photograph of a patient with a huge ovarian cyst similar to that shown in Case 252, Fig. 588. Tumor weighed 84 lbs., was removed surgically with uneventful recovery.

Fig. 592.—Ovary: Pseudomucinous Cystadenoma.—Case 252.—Gross photograph of ovarian tumor in cross section revealing its typical multilocular composition. Some of the cysts may be seen to still contain the characteristic pseudomucinous fluid. (See also Fig. 360.)

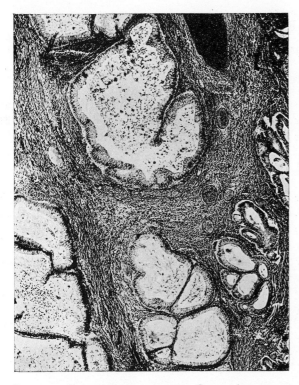

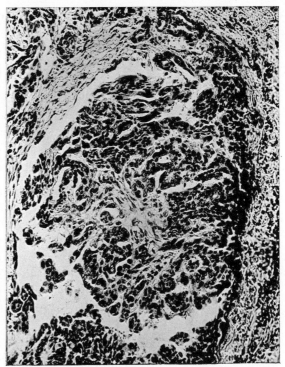

Fig. 593.—Ovary: Pseudomucinous Cystic Adenocarcinoma (Cf. Case 252).—Tumor is composed of cystic, acinar-like structures lined by a columnar epithelium which shows beginning breaking through the basement membrane and invasion of the ovarian stroma. App. 100 x.

Fig. 594.—Ovary: Serous Papillary Cyst Adenocarcinoma.—Case 256.—Photomicrograph showing papillary nature of tumor. Note heaping up of tumor cells, hyperchromatism, occasional mitotic figures and definite invasive nature of the process. App. 100 x.

ILLUSTRATIVE CASE

CASE 251. (Ref. #S-350)

Diagnosis.—Fallopian tube—ruptured ectopic pregnancy.

Patient was a white housewife of 38 years, admitted to the hospital with the chief complaint of sharp pain in the lower abdomen and back of four hours' duration.

Present Illness.—The onset of the patient's present illness was sudden. While she was attending to her housework, she was seized with acute abdominal pain, fainted, and on recovering consciousness crawled to telephone for her physician. In reviewing her history, it appeared that her last normal menstrual period had been eight weeks previously. Her physician made a diagnosis of ruptured ectopic pregnancy and rushed the patient to the hospital for an emergency operation.

Past Medical History.—The patient had the usual childhood diseases. She had always been in good health and had never previously required hospitalization. She had been married for fifteen years and had one previous pregnancy with a normal delivery. Her menstrual history had always been regular. A review of her systems showed that she had had a possible gallbladder attack six years previously, which had subsided spontaneously.

Physical Examination.—The patient was a well-developed, well-nourished white female appearing normal and her stated age. Her eyes, ears, nose and throat were negative except for marked pallor of the conjunctivae and mucous membranes. Chest was symmetrical. Heart was not enlarged and there were no murmurs. Lungs were clear throughout. The abdomen was somewhat distended and tense, and rather tender to palpation. It was tympanitic to percussion, however. It was thought best not to make too thorough an examination for fear of producing further hemorrhage, and the patient was sent immediately to the operating room.

Laboratory Findings.—On admission the red cell count was 2,730,000 with 35% hemoglobin. White blood cells, 12,600 with 80% polynuclears. Urinalysis was essentially negative.

Subsequent Course.—A left ruptured tubal pregnancy was found at operation, and a left salpingectomy was done. The patient made an uneventful recovery following two transfusions to compensate for the extensive intra-abdominal hemorrhage which had occurred. She was discharged cured.

Pathological Report.—*Gross Description.*—Specimen consisted of a fallopian tube, the middle third of which was greatly distended measuring over 2 cm. in diameter while the diameter at the two ends of the tube was only approximately 1 cm. In this distended area there was a perforation 1 cm. in length on the superior surface. The tube was filled with what appeared to be blood clot, and similar blood clot was adherent to the peritoneal surface of the tube. A small, pinkish-gray structure was seen adherent to the mucosal surface of the tube. This grossly suggested placental tissue.

Microscopic Description of a Section Through the Wall of the Tube.—(Fig. 584) Histologic examination of the tissue shows a markedly thickened wall of the tube. This is diffusely infiltrated by both serum and inflammatory cells. Extensive hemorrhage likewise has occurred into the interstitial tissues. The villous processes are thickened and edematous. They also show considerable cellular infiltration. In places, the normal mucosa has disappeared and there is a loose, pseudodecidual reaction which has replaced the underlying stroma. Numerous chorionic villi are found in the blood clot which fills the lumen of the tube. Some villi with their characteristic Langhans' and syncytial cells are found in intimate contact with the tubal lining cells.

PART II

OVARY

CONGENITAL LESIONS

The congenital lesions which affect the ovaries are surprisingly few except inasmuch as they occur in relation to various cystic lesions of the ovary later on in life. Absence of the ovary may occur either as a bilateral or as a unilateral lesion, but so rarely as to scarcely make it worthwhile mentioning.

MECHANICAL AND CIRCULATORY DISTURBANCES

Congestion of the ovary is almost a normal physiological process in relation to the menstrual cycle. Congestion otherwise is usually secondary to some other process, and as such does not affect the ovary as a primary pathological lesion. The only really important lesion of this nature is seen when an ovary becomes twisted on its pedicle with resultant shutting off of the circulation in exactly the same way that a volvulus of the small intestine results in local circulatory failure and secondary gangrene of the area involved. The ovary will undergo similar extensive hemorrhagic necrosis and gangrene. The gangrenous picture is later in its development as it is dependent upon bacterial invasion which does not occur as early as in the case of the intestinal tract where bacteria are normally present in large numbers.

PLATE CXLI

TUMORS OF THE OVARY

App. 100 x

App. 100 x

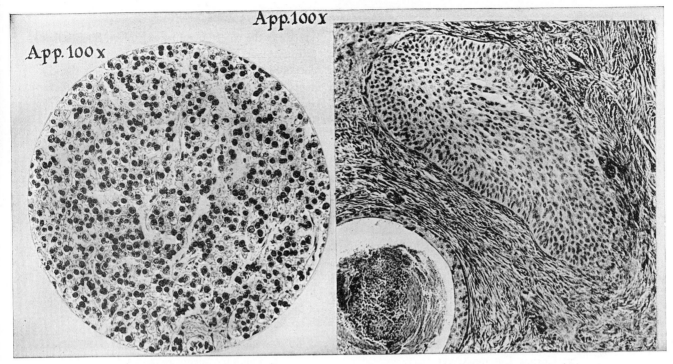

FIG. 595.—DYSGERMINOMA.—(Cf. Case 156, Fig. 348—Seminoma).—Low power photomicrograph showing the characteristic cytology of the undifferentiated gonadal tumor with its large, polyhedral cells with pale cytoplasm and large nuclei, arranged in groups supported by a delicate connective tissue stroma. App. 100 x.

FIG. 596.—BRENNER'S TUMOR (FIBRO-EPITHELIOMA).—CASE 255.—Low power photomicrograph showing a typical nest of relatively undifferentiated epithelial cells and a small epithelial lined cystic area, embedded in dense ovarian stroma. App. 100 x.

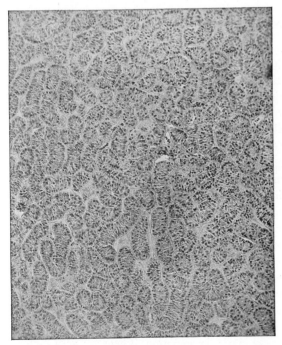

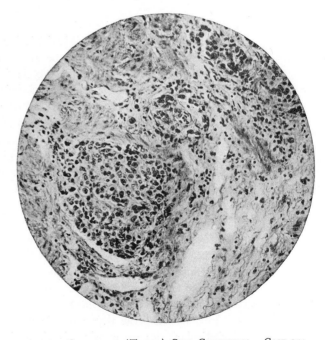

FIG. 597.—ARRHENOBLASTOMA (TESTICULOMA OVARII).—CASE 253.—Tumor composed of uniform tubule-like structures simulating the reproductive tubules of the testis, with a definite basement membrane and a scanty but well-defined fibrous stroma. App. 100 x.

FIG. 598.—GRANULOSA (THECA) CELL CARCINOMA.—CASE 254.—The characteristic arrangement of the typical granulosa cells in masses embedded in a loose, edematous stroma which shows considerable mononuclear cellular infiltration is the outstanding feature of the histology. App. 100 x.

INFLAMMATORY LESIONS OF THE OVARY

Acute Oöphoritis.—The inflammatory lesions of the ovary are likewise relatively unimportant, except in relation to inflammation of the fallopian tube as a secondary process. Acute oöphoritis results from the extension of a gonorrheal salpingitis as a rule, or as part of a puerperal sepsis with a strepto-coccus as the chief offending organism. Such inflammatory processes may be fairly diffuse or may become localized as an abscess, particularly when the contents of a graafian follicle become infected. The relation of such infections to the lesions of the fallopian tube has already been stressed.

CYSTS AND NEOPLASMS OF THE OVARY

The great majority of the pathological processes which involve the ovary are the result of various forms of cystic or neoplastic changes. Some of these are of an entirely benign nature and might almost be considered as exaggerated physiological processes. Others are frankly neoplastic with rather serious prognostic characteristics. The following outline will serve to group these respective lesions conveniently from the standpoint of discussion.

A. Retention Cysts
    1. Follicular Cysts
    2. Corpus Luteum Cysts
B. Cystadenomata
    1. Pseudomucinous cystadenomata
    2. Serous cystadenomata
C. Teratoid Tumors

D. Tumors relating to the secondary sex characteristics
    1. Masculinizing
        a. Arrhenoblastoma (testiculoma ovarii)
    2. Feminizing
        a. Granulosa cell carcinoma (theca cell carcinoma)
    3. Neutral
        a. Brenner tumor
        b. Disgerminoma
E. Carcinoma of the Ovary
    1. Papillary adenocarcinoma
    2. Solid carcinoma
    3. Metastatic carcinoma
        a. Krukenberg tumor
F. Sarcoma

RETENTION CYSTS

Follicular Cysts.—(Fig. 358) The follicular cysts of the ovary apparently arise from the graafian follicles, which following the menstrual cycle fail to completely maturate with the discharge of their ova. Normally, such incompletely matured follicles undergo a simple regressive phase spoken of as atresia. It so happens, however, that some of the follicles fail to go through this atrophic regressive picture and persist as follicular retention cysts. These are lined usually by a thin layer of thecal or stratum granulosum cells, and depending somewhat upon the predominance of one or the other type of cell, they are variously described as *simple follicular cysts, theca luteal cysts* in those cases where the thecal cells show beginning luteinization, or if the involutional changes have gone somewhat further before the cyst develops, they may even be termed *compound lutein cysts.* It is likewise true that a certain number of such follicular cysts apparently arise from follicles which have never undergone any degree of matura-tion. The etiology of such retention cysts is still highly theoretical and we shall content ourselves at this time merely to record their existence and characteristics rather than to delve into any unproductive theoretical considerations. Such follicular cysts are usually multiple and the ovary may be increased in size two or three times the normal. As a result, dragging sensations and discomfort exaggerated at the menstrual period are common symptoms due to the increased weight and congestion of the organ. In many instances symptoms may be relieved by the removal of such cysts or, if the patient is in the menopausal age, by the actual removal of the ovary or ovaries as the case may be. Unfortunately, this process is usually a bilateral one and ultimately is likely to require bilateral oöphorectomy.

Corpus Luteum Cysts.—A similar type of cyst may arise in a fully developed corpus luteum, which undergoes cystic degeneration. These are very commonly complicated by hemorrhage into the cyst, which may accordingly attain a considerable size. Care must be taken at times in differentiating between this intracystic type of hemorrhage as seen in the corpus luteum cyst and the more usual interstitial hemorrhage, which is liable to be found in the simple follicular or thecal type of cyst. Again, the pathological significance of such cysts is relatively slight. Occasionally, rupture of such a cyst may give rise to rather acute pelvic symptoms and require emergency surgical measures. More often, the symptoms are of a chronic, vague nature and tend to subside spontaneously in many instances as organization of this hemorrhagic lesion takes place. They are also not to be confused with endometrial cysts.

CYSTADENOMATA

Two cystic lesions which are particularly frequently encountered fall in this group of cystadenomata, or adenocystomata, as they are variously described. Many of these cysts remain as benign lesions throughout the course of their existence, but on the other hand a considerable proportion of such cystic adenomata undergo malignant transformation after varying intervals of time. The two varieties show a considerable difference in their clinical and pathological features and for that reason will be discussed separately.

Pseudomucinous Cystadenomata.—The pseudomucinous variety of the cystadenomata of the ovary is very prone to be a unilateral lesion. It is the commoner variety and frequently appears as a pedunculated tumor. It is invariably multilocular and may attain an enormous size, extreme instances weighing as much as 70 and 80 pounds. The tumor as a whole is covered by a smooth surface which shows some coarse lobulation, the result of the multiloculated nature of the process. On section, the cystic mass is found to be made up of a large number of cystic cavities varying greatly in size from small lesions a few millimeters in diameter up to large cystic areas several centimeters in diameter. Some of these are intercommunicating; others appear discrete. The contents of the cysts as a whole are composed of a thick, stringy, mucoid material. It is not true mucin, however, in that it does not take the characteristic mucicarmine stain and is not precipitated by weak acids as is true mucin. In some of the isolated cystic areas, it is not uncommon to find cholesterol crystals in large numbers. The color of these cystic areas varies considerably due to the differences in the cyst contents. Many of them show varying degrees of hemorrhagic discoloration with subsequent breakdown of the hemoglobin. Owing to the pedunculated nature of the tumor it is not infrequent to find torsion of the pedicle with resultant acute symptoms from the shutting off of the blood supply. It is in this type of tumor particularly that this problem arises. Likewise, on occasion, certain of these cysts may rupture and their contents become spilled over the peritoneal surface with subsequent implantation of cells and the formation of multiple daughter cysts or the production of masses of this jelly-like fluid which fills the peritoneal cavity and is spoken of as *pseudo-myxoma peritonei.*

Microscopically, the cyst cavities are characteristically lined by a single layer of high columnar nonciliated epithelium. A great many of the cysts may appear to be of the goblet cell variety due to the hypersecretion of the pseudomucinous material within their cytoplasm. The cells are supported on a connective tissue base and the nuclei are basal in position. The nuclei tend to be somewhat flattened with their long axis parallel to the cyst wall. Occasionally some attempt at a minimal amount of papilla formation may be encountered, but papillary proliferation as a whole is not one of the major features of this variety of cyst. The origin of these tumors is obscure. Various hypotheses have been advanced, the two more prominent being first that they represent a variety of teratoid tumor and the second that they are derived from retention cysts of follicular origin.

ILLUSTRATIVE CASE

CASE 252 (Ref. #S-347)
Diagnosis. — Ovary — pseudomucinous cystadenoma. (See also Fig. 360, in Chapter XXXVII, Part 2, devoted to a discussion of Cysts.)
Patient was a white female of 51 years, admitted to the hospital with the chief complaint of inability to void, and a large mass in the lower abdomen.
Present Illness.—The patient stated that she had been in her usual good health until approximately six weeks before admission. At that time she noticed her abdomen

seemed to be increasing in size. About one week before, she began to have difficulty in voiding, and she also noticed that she was becoming increasingly constipated.

Past Medical History.—The patient's past medical history was apparently irrelevant so far as her present illness was concerned. She had had the usual childhood diseases. She had never had any serious illness requiring hospitalization except for a pelvic abscess some twelve years earlier. She believed she had had pneumonia in the influenza epidemic in 1918. A review of her systems was otherwise noninformatory. She had never had any particular upper respiratory pathology other than this attack of influenza. Her gastro-intestinal history was entirely negative. Her cardiovascular history was likewise negative. She had been married in her early twenties and had had three children, who were entirely normal. She had had her menopause about three years before admission.

Physical Examination.—The patient was a well-developed, well-nourished, middle-aged white female. Eyes, ears, nose and throat were negative. Chest was symmetrical. Heart was not enlarged. Lungs were clear and resonant throughout. Abdomen was moderately protuberant and obese. There was a large tumor mass which apparently filled the entire pelvis and lower part of the abdomen up to the level of the umbilicus. This seemed to arise from the left side although it was practically midline in position. Vaginal and rectal examinations yielded no additional information other than to exclude the uterus as the source of the tumor. In order to outline this tumor mass, it was necessary to catheterize the patient as the distended bladder interfered with its palpation.

Laboratory Findings.—Red blood cells, 5,240,000 with 86% hemoglobin. White blood cells, 5,850 with 68%

polynuclears. Urinalysis showed a specimen which was turbid, with a specific gravity of 1.021. It contained a moderate trace of albumin and many red and white cells, but no casts.

Subsequent Course.—A diagnosis of a possible ovarian cyst was made and operation advised. A left oöphorectomy was done. The tumor mass reached nearly 4 cm. above the level of the umbilicus at the time of operation. It was pedunculated and relatively readily removed without rupture.

Pathological Report.—*Gross Description.*—The specimen consisted of a huge cystic ovary. This measured approximately 25 cm. in diameter (Figs. 591 and 592). The serosal surface was fairly smooth, but slightly nodular. The greater portion of the wall measured about 2 mm. in thickness. The inner surface was discolored and partly covered by thick, tenacious, mucoid-like material. There were small cystic areas in the wall projecting into the lumen of the larger cyst for a distance of 3 cm. These were filled with a thick, yellowish, mucinous or cheese-like material. There were some small areas of calcification present. There was also a small, thin-walled cyst of Morgagni submitted measuring 3.5 x 2.5 x 2 cm., and filled with clear fluid.

Microscopic Description of a Section Through the Cyst Wall.—(Fig. 593) Histologic examination of the cyst wall reveals numerous small cystic cavities of varying size, all lined by tall columnar epithelium. Many of the cells are filled with a stringy, mucoid material and the cavities themselves are likewise filled with a similar pseudomucin. Here and there, a few small papillary-like proliferations of the epithelium extend into the lumen of the cyst. No evidence of malignancy is seen in any of the tissue studied.

Serous Cystadenomata.—The serous variety of cystadenomata is very much more commonly bilateral, the lesions being symmetrical. They seldom attain the same degree of enlargement, which is noted in the pseudomucinous variety. They are less uniformly multilocular, many of them apparently consisting of a single cystic cavity. There is a very striking tendency on their part to show a very marked papillary proliferation. At times this may only be noted at one point in the cyst wall and the remainder of the cyst may be a single large cavity filled with a clear serous fluid. At other times, the entire tumor may be composed of these papillary masses of tissue arising uniformly from the entire cyst lining. On section of such a tumor we find it filled with a clear fluid which has a high albumin content. No pseudomucin is found in the typical lesion. As in the case of the pseudomucinous variety, spontaneous rupture of the cyst may occur, or may result from traumatic rupture either from external injury or at the time of operation. In similar fashion a seeding of the cells on the peritoneal surface may take place. Again, this may go on to multiple cyst formation or at times

may result in the persistent functioning of the cells in the production of their fluid so that extensive ascites develops, requiring repeated abdominal paracentesis.

Microscopic examination of these cysts finds them lined by a low columnar or high cuboidal cell, which typically is ciliated. The tumor is usually made up of papillary connective tissue stalks with their capillary blood supply and covered by this same type of epithelial cell, which not infrequently may become heaped up several layers deep in a pseudostratified form. Invasion of the ovarian stroma or cyst wall may result in localized adenomatous formation. A considerable percentage of these cases sooner or later undergo malignant transformation with invasion of the cyst wall and extension of the tumor over the peritoneal cavity. The origin of this particular type of tumor seems to be on a somewhat more secure foundation. It is usually believed to be derived from infolded germinal epithelium. Refer to Case 247 (Ref. #S-373) Fig. 589 in Chapter LVIII for the history of this illustrative case and see the microscopic description following:

Diagnosis.—Ovary—papillary serous cystadenoma.

MICROSCOPIC DESCRIPTION OF A SECTION THROUGH THE WALL OF SUCH AN OVARIAN CYST.—(Fig. 327) Histologic examination of the tissue presents the typical picture of a papillary cystadenoma of the ovary. In places the rather characteristic ovarian stroma can be identified to establish the source of the tissue. Cystic spaces are lined, for the most part, by a single layer of rather high cuboidal or low columnar cells which make up the greater part of the specimen. From one area, a definite papillary arrangement of the cells is found with delicate connective tissue stalks containing nutrient capillary vessels. These papillae are extremely arborescent and are covered by a variable number of layers of similar cells. These, however, show some tendency toward flattening as a result of pressure from the fluid.

TERATOID TUMORS

The teratoid tumors of the ovary have already been discussed in the chapter relating to teratoid tumors in general so they need only be called to attention at this time. These tumors occur in two major varieties, the dermoid cyst [Case 155 (Ref. #S-256), Chapter XXXVI, Figs. 345, 347, 357 and 359] which is almost always a benign tumor and which ordinarily contains derivatives of only two cell prototypes, the ectoderm and mesoderm. It not infrequently is seen as a bilateral lesion and is characterized by being a cystic tumor filled with sebaceous material and hair, and not infrequently showing abortive attempts at tooth formation.

The other major teratoid tumor is the solid variety in which all three embryonal cells are represented by more complex adult structures including glandular organs, brain and gastro-intestinal derivatives. These solid tumors are generally conceded to be of primitive blastomere origin, but it seems highly possible that they may equally likely be derived from one of the undifferentiated totipotential sex cells, as in the case of the testicular teratomata.

TUMORS RELATING TO THE SECONDARY SEX CHARACTERISTICS

These may be divided in respect to their hormonal influence into masculinizing, feminizing and neutral varieties. The great majority of these tumors are, from the clinical standpoint, if not absolutely benign, only rarely of any significant degree of malignancy. When malignancy does exist, it is usually of a very low grade nature and is not accompanied by distant metastases, but merely by local invasion as a rule. They make up a fascinating group of tumors from the clinical standpoint associated as they are with abnormal and precocious secondary sex characteristics in many instances; but they are so comparatively infrequently encountered that any lengthy discussion regarding them does not seem warranted in a volume of this type. A brief review of the three major varieties of these tumors follows.

Masculinizing Tumors

Arrhenoblastoma (*Testiculoma Ovarii*).—This is a rare tumor which is thought to arise from the medulla of the ovary. These tumors are variable in size, one which we have had the opportunity of studying being one of the largest on record. They are composed, in the typical case, of well-differentiated tubules, which it is impossible to differentiate from embryonic testicular reproductive tubules. More often, they show a less well differentiated picture, which at times may simulate an adenosarcoma with hyperplastic changes affecting the stroma as well as the glandular epithelial cells. The tumor occurs chiefly between the ages of twenty-one and thirty-five years. The symptoms are interesting. The earliest sign is usually a persistent amenorrhea with sterility. The breasts atrophy. The uterus and cervix become small and infantile in type. There is an abnormal and excessive development of hair over the body. A beard, necessitating in some cases daily shaving, is usually present. The facial expression is masculine, due to the coarse features and bushy eyebrows. The voice becomes husky and deep. A restoration of the normal female characteristics occurs after removal of the tumor. Normal pregnancy has occurred after operation in a number of the reported cases. Frequently the masculinizing features may be absent. The tumor is of relatively low grade malignancy.

ILLUSTRATIVE CASE

CASE 253. (Ref. #S-360)

Diagnosis.—Ovary—arrhenoblastoma (testicular type).
Patient was a white female of 46 years, admitted to
the hospital with the chief complaint of a mass in the
lower abdomen.

Present Illness.—In reviewing the patient's history, it
appeared that the onset of the present illness dated back
for a matter of at least two years. At that time the
patient noted that she had developed very marked hirsutism, particularly of the face and upper lip, which required shaving nearly daily. She had likewise noted considerable change in her voice, which had assumed an
almost bass quality. There had been rather marked
atrophy of her breasts and a suggestion of redistribution
of the body fat toward the masculine habitus. She had
developed an amenorrhea, which she believed was associated with her menopause and had attributed these
various other visceral changes to the same etiology. These
various objective symptoms had not been manifested by
any particular alteration in emotional or psychic changes.
It was only with the development of the palpable mass in
her abdomen, which had been steadily increasing in size
over the preceding six months that she had become at all
worried.

Past History.—Her past medical history was essentially negative. She did not recall any of the childhood
infections. She had been married at eighteen and had had
one normal child. She had had no particular disturbance
of her menstrual history until the present illness. A review of her other systems was noninformatory in respect
to her present condition.

Physical Examination.—The patient was a well-developed and well-nourished, middle-aged individual who
presented the gross physical features noted in discussing
her symptomatology. A very marked hirsutism involving
her face, chest and with the male distribution over the
abdomen as well as over the extremities was noted. Voice
was deep. Head otherwise showed no deformities. Eyes
were negative. Nose and throat were negative. Chest was
symmetrical. Breasts were almost completely atrophic
and of the male type. Heart and lungs appeared negative.
Abdomen was moderately prominent and somewhat obese.

A large mass about the size of a six months' pregnancy
could be felt in the lower abdomen and pelvis. Extremities other than for the hirsutism were essentially negative.
Vaginal examination showed a somewhat atrophic uterus
with a slight laceration at one side of the cervix. The
pelvic mass apparently had no definite relationship to the
uterus and seemed to be rather more left sided than midline.

Laboratory Findings.—Red blood cells, 4,800,000 with
83% hemoglobin. White blood cells, 8,700 with 63%
polynuclears. Urinalysis was negative. Wassermann was
negative.

Subsequent History.—The patient was advised to
have an exploratory laparotomy; which was done. A
tumor mass approximately the size of a large grapefruit was found arising from the left ovary. The right
ovary appeared atrophic and measured only 1.5 cm. in its
greatest diameter. The uterus was small and atrophic in
appearance. The ovarian tumor was removed easily, being pedunculated, by clamping the pedicle and freeing the
few areas where it was adherent to the peritoneal surface.

Pathological Report.—*Gross Description.*—Specimen
consisted of an irregularly nodular tumor mass approximately 18 cm. in diameter. It was grayish-pink in color
and extremely firm in consistency. On section it was of
a uniform color and denseness. It showed no areas of
cystic degeneration nor hemorrhage. It suggested a diffuse fibroma, but pin-point yellowish areas could be seen
which made one think of the possibility of some epithelial
proliferation.

**Microscopic Description of a Section Through the
Ovary.**—(Fig. 597) Histologic examination of the tissue
shows an almost perfect reproduction of testicular tubules.
Multiple sections taken from all portions of the ovary
show a uniform picture. These tubules are lined by a
relatively undifferentiated type of cell with a typical
large round nucleus with a prominent nucleolus. The cells
vary somewhat in size suggesting that there is some
abortive attempt at maturation. In general, the histology
suggests that of an undescended or pre-adolescent testis,
except that no interstitial cells can be identified. The strana
is relatively fibrous in appearance.

Feminizing Tumors

*Granulosa Cell Carcinoma (Theca Cell Carci-
noma).*—This is again a rare tumor which usually
arises relatively late in life in the postmenopausal period between fifty and seventy years of age. The
origin is disputed. It is believed by many that they
arise from persistent granulosa cell rests, but other
investigators consider that it represents a variety of
teratoid tumor arising from undifferentiated sex
cells. The great majority of these tumors, however, are made up of collections of large cells
resembling the normal granulosa cells of the
graafian follicle. In the typical type of the tumor,
the cells are characteristically arranged in round

or oval masses associated in some cases with cysts.
Occasionally the cellular formation may appear
in solid masses containing areas of hyaline degeneration. Different sections of the same tumor
may show a rather varied histologic picture. The
granulosa cell and Brenner tumors of the ovary are
frequently confused in the literature and even in
textbooks. The cells of this tumor are active in the
production of estrin. When the tumor occurs in a
young child the development of the secondary sex
characteristics is striking, resulting in precocious puberty. There is acceleration of skeletal growth, over-
development of the breasts, growth of hair on the

external genitalia and in the axillæ and the establishment of the menstrual cycle. In the post-menopausal cases, the two most characteristic effects are the reestablishment of periodic uterine bleeding and the production of endometrial hyperplasia. When the tumor occurs during the active reproductive life of the individual, excessive uterine bleeding is quite common, although in many cases the amount of flow is normal, and in others there may be periods of amenorrhea lasting many months. Clinically, the granulosa cell tumors are relatively benign. Only occasionally do they break through the capsule, recurring or metastasizing. Histologically, however, they appear as invasive lesions locally.

ILLUSTRATIVE CASE

CASE 254. (Ref. #S-364)

Diagnosis.—Ovary—granulosa cell carcinoma.

Patient was a white married woman of 42 years, admitted to the hospital because of irregularity in her menstrual cycle, which was causing her considerable worry.

Present History.—The interval between periods was irregular and in general increased to about five or six weeks. The amount of discharge seldom amounted to more than a slight spotting. Coincidental with this irregularity of her menses she had noticed a gradual increase in the size of her abdomen so that the patient believed that she might have been pregnant. A Friedman test was positive. The patient had further noticed a slight increase in the size of her breasts, but there had been no secretion from them. She had experienced no morning nausea. Except for the increase in the size of her abdomen, the patient had been practically symptom-free. She had noted some increase in constipation, to which she had always been subject, but no frequency of micturition.

Past Medical History.—The past medical history was irrelevant. She had had one previous pregnancy, which was associated with slight menstrual bleeding at the theoretical time of each period. This went on to a fullterm pregnancy and she was delivered of a normal child, which only lived, however, for one week, dying of pneumonia. This was twenty years before her present illness, and there had been no interval pregnancies. Ten years earlier she was operated upon for a tumor of the uterus, and apparently a fibroid was removed at that time.

Physical Examination.—Patient was a middle-aged, somewhat obese woman lying comfortably in bed. Eyes, ears, nose and throat were negative. Chest: There were no râles. Lungs were clear and resonant throughout. Heart was normal in size, rate and rhythm. No murmurs were heard. Abdomen: asymmetrical enlargement to the size of about a six or seven months' pregnancy with a bulge to the left, seemingly caused by a hard mass extending to just above the navel. Percussion of this yielded a dull note. No fetal heart sounds nor uterine souffle were heard. No fetal movements nor parts were discerned. Peristalsis was unusually active. Abdomen was tympanitic over other areas. No shifting dullness was noted. Pelvic examination: the cervix showed large, stellate lacerations. No fetal parts were palpated.

Laboratory Findings.—Red blood cells, 4,100,000 with 83% hemoglobin. White blood cells, 5,100 with 58% polynuclears. Urinalysis was essentially negative, except for a slight trace of albumin.

Subsequent History.—A supravaginal hysterectomy, ovariectomy, and the removal of multiple abdominal cystic tumors were performed. The abdomen was found filled with cystic nodular tumors extending from the pelvis, almost to the costal border. Small, miliary nodules on the peritoneum and great omentum were found, as well as larger, cystic masses containing quantities of reddish, brownish, serous fluid and grayish, seminecrotic material. An estimate of 2000 c.c. of such fluid was made. The uterus itself was enlarged to about the size of a five months' gestation and numerous multiple intramural and subserous fibromata were found. The patient made an uneventful recovery and was discharged improved.

Pathological Report.—*Gross Description.*—Specimen consisted of the uterus, both tubes and one ovary. The uterus contained several myomata. The tubes were somewhat thickened and filled with hemorrhagic material. The ovary appeared as a collapsed sac 14 cm. in diameter. It was filled with numerous gray, necrotic masses of tissue, which could be easily scraped off the wall. Many appeared to have been of a papillary nature.

Microscopic Description of a Section Through the Wall of One of the Cysts.—(Fig. 598) Histologic examination of the wall of one of the cystic tumors of the ovary presents a somewhat variable picture. In places there is a thick layer of epithelium, twenty to thirty cells deep lining the cyst. The individual cells for the most part are oval or spherical. The nuclei are enlarged and basket-shaped. The cytoplasm is small in amount and poorly defined. Occasional mitotic figures are seen. Other areas through the ovary show huge collections of cells separated by newly formed connective tissue trabeculae. The tumor is found to have extended into the uterus and to surround the fallopian tube in sections taken from those organs.

Neutral Tumors

Brenner Tumor of the Ovary (Benign Fibroepithelioma).—In 1907, Brenner described a type of ovarian tumor which has since come to bear his name. Macroscopically and microscopically this tumor is now a well-defined entity and has no relation to the granulosa cell tumor. It is believed that they originate from the celomic epithelium near the wolffian body, from which the epithelium of the müllerian duct is derived. The latter may form solid epithelial nodules, or larger formations of indifferent epithelium in abnormal locations, as in the tubes and ligaments. The Brenner tumors may vary in size from a minute nodule, 2 mm. in diameter to a neoplasm as large as an adult's head. The majority, however, are small. The color is white or yellowish-white, distinctly resembling a fibroma. There are two types: a solid and a cystic. The former is composed essentially of epithelial strands in a fibrous groundwork. Small cavities are occasionally seen varying from pinhead to cherry size. The second and less frequent type consists of a solid Brenner tumor in the wall of a pseudomucinous or, rarely, serous cystoma. The tumors are clinically benign, without recurrences, metastasis or fatalities. They produce no clinical symptoms unless the tumor becomes quite large. In fact, most of those reported were incidental findings at operation or autopsy. The tumor is practically always unilateral. Over 75 per cent of the reported cases were found after 40 years of age, and 60 per cent were postmenopausal. The tumor exerts no hormonal effect upon the uterus.

Microscopically, they are composed of a firm, fibrillary connective tissue stroma, with a tendency to hyaline degeneration; occasionally, small calcified areas are found. Embedded in the connective tissue are solid nests and cords of epithelial cells. The cell nests are more or less widely separated. The cells are rather large, irregular, polygonal or oval in shape with a distinct cell membrane. The cytoplasm stains faintly and appears finely granular. The nuclei are oval or slightly irregular. When present the cystic cavitations within the epithelial nests may be quite small or large, single or multiple. The lining cells may be cuboidal in shape, or there may be only a single layer of flattened cells present. The smaller cysts are usually filled with a homogeneous, colloid-like material staining pink with eosin. In the larger cysts the material has more a mucinous character. The tumor as a whole is relatively avascular. It is probably often not even recognized as tumor.

ILLUSTRATIVE CASE

CASE 255 (Ref. #S-278)

Diagnosis.—Ovary—Brenner's tumor.

Chief Complaint.—Patient was a white female of 56 years, admitted to the hospital complaining of pain in her lower back and abdomen.

Present Illness.—The onset of the patient's present illness began approximately five years before admission. with attacks of low back pain and abdominal discomfort. They had been intermittent in character but had grown rather more marked in the past few weeks. This had been accompanied by very persistent constipation but bowel movements tended always to aggravate the pain, so the patient had tended to neglect herself in respect to the treatment of her constipation.

Past Medical History.—The past history was apparently entirely irrelevant. A review of her systems revealed the fact that she did not menstruate until she was sixteen years of age. However, her periods had been regular through her active menstrual life. She had her menopause five years earlier and dated her present illness from that time on. She had not had any bleeding since then.

Physical Examination.—Physical examination showed a well-developed, well-nourished, elderly, white female, who appeared all of her given age. Her head was negative. Her heart and lungs were within normal limits. Abdomen was somewhat obese but a definite mass could be felt in the pelvis, which on vaginal examination was thought to be due to simple "fibroids."

Laboratory Examination.—The laboratory findings were essentially negative. The blood count showed a very

mild anemia with 3,800,000 red cells, 71% hemoglobin; white cells 6,900, with 62% polynuclears. Urinalysis was negative.

Subsequent Course.—On the basis of the symptoms and physical findings, and in view of her age, it was recommended that a panhysterectomy be done. This was done and the patient made an uneventful recovery.

Pathological Report.—Specimen consisted of a uterus which was enlarged about four times the normal size as a result of a dozen or more subserous and intramural fibromata, the largest measuring 3 cms. in diameter. The left ovary appeared normal. The right ovary was moderately increased in size, measuring 4 x 4 x 3 cms. On section, it showed a discrete, grayish-white thickened area at one pole in which a few small cysts could be seen.

Microscopic Description Through the Ovary.—(Fig. 596) There is a dense fibrous connective tissue stroma which somewhat resembles ovarian stroma. Scattered throughout this are numerous large and small, well-outlined nests and cords of epithelial cells. These nests and cords are made up of fairly large polygonal cells, with a light-staining cytoplasm, containing fair-sized, deeply-stained nuclei. Many such cystic areas are seen throughout the section. These are lined by flattened or cuboidal epithelium and contain a pink-staining homogeneous substance. The cysts which are so conspicuous in this case undoubtedly began as small cavitations in these masses of cells and enlarged on finally compress the surrounding cells to a single layer of flat or cuboidal epithelium. There are a few small areas of calcification present in the section.

Disgerminoma.—The disgerminoma is histologically identical with the embryonal carcinoma which occurs in the testis. It is believed to arise from undifferentiated germinal cells which have lost their faculty of sex determination. It is usually found in young girls presenting hypoplasia and underdevelopment of the genitalia. It, like the Brenner tumor, does not exert any hormonal effect upon the genital development. The tumors vary greatly in size. They are characteristically solid, though areas of degeneration and hemorrhage may be seen. In their earlier stages they are well circumscribed, but as they become larger, they tend to become infiltrative, invading the uterus, bladder and other viscera.

The histologic picture is fairly uniform and microscopic diagnosis is much simpler than in the other tumors of the ovary. The cells are rather large, round or polygonal, with clear cytoplasm and large nuclei. A light connective tissue trabeculae surrounds groups of these cells. The tumor may remain quiescent for many years and then metastasize throughout the body.

Refer to Case 156 (Ref. #S-263), Chapter XXXVI, for the histology of this type of tumor as exemplified by an embryonal carcinoma of the testis, and to Fig. 595 in this chapter.

CARCINOMA OF THE OVARY

Papillary Adenocarcinoma.—(Fig. 594) The papillary adenocarcinoma is the most common variety of malignant neoplasm of the ovary. It is derived almost invariably from a preëxisting serous papillary cystadenoma. The same inevitable histologic sequence is seen affecting the histologic detail of the tumor cells as occurs in any other form of malignancy. The cells become hyperplastic, hyperchromatic and pleomorphic in form. They become heaped up on the papillary stalks. The basement membrane is lost and invasion of the stroma and the cyst wall is observed. Extension of the tumor to the surface of the cyst occurs. Local invasion through contact is a common finding. Curiously, however, these tumors, in spite of rather widespread dissemination throughout the pelvis and abdomen only rarely extend beyond this area. If the tumor is unilateral (and it very frequently may be), bilateral oöphorectomy will result in a very considerable proportion showing regression and even disappearance of the metastatic tumor tissue suggesting that there may be some actual hormonal influence necessary for their maintenance. Less frequently, such papillary tumors may arise from the pseudomucinous type of cystadenoma and their history is comparable in all respects to those arising from the serous variety.

ILLUSTRATIVE CASE

CASE 256 (Ref. #S-260)

Diagnosis.—Ovary—papillary cystadenocarcinoma.

Patient was a white female of 43 years, admitted to the hospital with the chief complaint of progressive enlargement of the abdomen, and shortness of breath.

Present Illness.—The patient first noticed that her abdomen was increasing in size about six months before admission. This had not been very marked at first, but in the last two months had grown rather rapidly. There was no pain or other symptoms relating to this condition except for a dyspnea which was more marked on exertion.

Past Medical History.—The patient had had about the average past medical history. As a child she had had scarlet fever, diphtheria and whooping cough. Since that time she had been in fairly good health except for an attack of gallbladder trouble three years previously. She was operated upon at that time and had her gallbladder removed. She had been free of symptoms since then. A review of her various systems otherwise was noninformatory. Her cardiorespiratory system was entirely negative. Her gastro-intestinal history revealed that she had had progressive constipation for the best part of a year. Her genito-urinary history was essentially normal. Her periods had begun at the age of thirteen and had been regular throughout her life. She had been married twenty years, but had never been pregnant.

Physical Examination.—The patient was a well-developed, well-nourished, middle-aged, white female who was lying in bed, apparently in no distress. Head was not remarkable. Eyes, ears, nose and throat were negative. There was compensated edentia of her upper jaw. Chest was symmetrical. Heart and lungs were essentially negative. Abdomen was markedly enlarged to the size of a full-term pregnancy. This enlargement was most marked in the lower part of the abdomen. There was a fluctuant mass, which completely filled the pelvis and extended about three centimeters above the umbilicus. This gave a dull note on percussion. No fetal parts were palpated. No fetal heart sounds could be heard. Gynecologic examination showed no changes in the cervix and no enlargement of the fundus of the uterus. It was felt that the mass represented an ovarian tumor. The extremities were negative.

Laboratory Findings.—The laboratory findings were more or less irrelevant in respect to the present case. Red blood cells, 3,600,000 with 73% hemoglobin. White blood cells, 8,200 with 68% polynuclears. Urinalysis was negative.

Subsequent Course.—The patient had an exploratory incision made and a large, cystic tumor of the left ovary was found. The right ovary could not be identified, and it was thought, very probably, that it had been removed at the time of her previous cholecystectomy for a similar cystic formation.

Pathological Report.—*Gross Description.*—Specimen consisted of a large tumor mass approximately the size of a football. This had a relatively smooth serosal-covered surface which, however, showed several areas of infiltration by tumor tissue. These areas of invasion were of a yellowish-gray color and somewhat irregularly mammillated in appearance on their surface. The tumor on section was found to represent a large, multiloculated, papillary cyst adenomatous type of lesion which even grossly suggested beginning malignant degeneration because of the invasion of the wall. No evidence of extension into the peritoneal cavity or regional tissues could be demonstrated.

Microscopic Description of Section Through the Wall of the Ovary.—(Fig. 594) Histologic examination of the cyst wall presents the typical ovarian stroma at one side, which serves to identify the tissue. This is much more vascular and cellular in appearance than normal ovarian tissue, however. There is a layer of epithelium representing the cyst lining, which is composed of high cuboidal and low columnar cells. This is thrown up into striking papillary folds with marked plication of the lining. These papillae are composed of rather delicate connective tissue stalks containing nutrient capillary vessels. The tumor cells are seen covering these papillae and show marked hyperplasia. The basement membrane in many areas shows a loss of its continuity, and there is definite invasion of the stroma by the tumor cells. The cells tend to be fairly regular in size and to show a rather high degree of differentiation for the most part. Certain of the nuclei show considerable hyperchromatism and occasional mitotic figures may be identified. The picture is entirely representative of the usual early malignant change seen in the simple papillary cystadenoma of the ovary. In view of the fact that the other ovary had already been removed, and that there was no evidence grossly of metastasis at the time of operation, the prognosis should be entirely good.

Solid Carcinoma.—The solid carcinoma of the ovary is usually a slow-growing tumor which in the great majority of cases is unilateral, although bilateral involvement either as a simultaneous neoplastic development or as secondary metastasis not infrequently occurs. The origin of these tumors is somewhat uncertain, but they probably arise from persistent germinal epithelial rests. Like the cystic variety, these tumors tend to extend locally rather than to metastasize distantly as a rule, and are influenced similarly in a small proportion of the cases by surgical removal of both ovaries in spite of the fact that the great majority of the cases occur in the usual cancer age period; namely, from forty-five to sixty years.

Metastatic Carcinomata.—The ovary is particularly prone to metastatic tumor development. Among the most striking of these must be recalled the Krukenberg tumor, which has already been discussed in the section devoted to Oncology. These, it is believed, represent bilateral ovarian metastases from a variety of mucous carcinoma of the gastro-intestinal tract, with the primary lesion most frequently encountered in the stomach. A history of such a lesion is presented in Case 154 (Ref. #S-162), Chapter XXXV, and illustrated by Figs. 340 and 588.

Sarcoma of the Ovary.—Sarcoma of the ovary may occasionally develop on the site of a preëxistent fibroma. They are rare tumors which tend to metastasize by the regional lymph nodes rather than by way of the blood stream, and are of a very low grade malignancy.

The one outstanding feature of practically all ovarian tumors, and particularly as it applies to the malignant varieties is the tendency toward localization to the pelvis or abdominal cavity rather than the diffuse extension to the body as a whole, as is seen in so many other varieties of neoplasm. In the second place, the fact that a certain number of ovarian tumors show definite evidence of functional capacity, especially in relation to their hormonal secretion is another feature of particular interest.

CHAPTER LX

DISEASES OF THE DUCTLESS GLANDS

PART I

THYROID GLAND

The thyroid develops embryologically as a downgrowth in the median ventral line and by two lateral anlages from the so-called fifth pharyngeal pouch. These latter migrate downward to fuse with the median lobe to form the adult thyroid. This is of importance in the consideration of the development of the tumors of the gland.

The function of the thyroid seems to be principally related to the maintenance of normal metabolism. Its interdependence upon the other endocrine glands is not thoroughly understood, but it is definitely affected by alteration in the function of the adrenals and likewise to some extent by the pituitary. The active principle of the thyroid secretion is thyroxin (a tetra-iodine derivative of tyrosine). In addition, iodine is present in an acid-soluble fraction which, when linked with thyroxin and other amino acids is built up into thyroglobulin, which

appears histologically as colloid. There are two main groups of conditions of importance from the pathological standpoint in relation to the thyroid gland: first, those relating to the functional disorders and second, the various types of neoplasm both benign and malignant which occur.

The thyroid may show evidence of a *hypo*-activity or hyperactivity giving rise to two completely different sets of symptoms. The more significant of these is seen in relation to the hyperfunctional activity, in the clinical condition known as hyperthyroidism or Graves' disease, which may or may not be associated with exophthalmos. The hypofunctional cases are represented by the congenital condition known as cretinism, and by myxedema when this occurs in the acquired form in adults. The tumors, on the other hand, only rarely show evidence of functional activity.

Congenital Lesions

There are no significant congenital lesions which affect the thyroid *per se*. There is a considerable opportunity for thyroid rests to become misplaced in the course of the normal migration of the gland to its adult position. These become of significance in later life through position, as substernal thyroid tissue or as possible sources of tumor formation. Similarly, persistence of thyroglossal duct, which normally atrophies, may likewise give rise to aberrant thyroid tissue in the base of the tongue as so-called lingual thyroid, or to the development of a thyroglossal cyst, which is always midline in position. It is reported that occasional instances of absent thyroid have been found in the newborn. This is obviously incompatible with life.

The importance of the thyroid cannot be overemphasized. It might well be described as the governor of most of our body functions as its activity

relates intimately to every phase of metabolic activity. The thyroid has lent itself more readily to experimental investigation than have any of the other ductless glands, and for that reason we feel that we are treading on somewhat safer ground in attempting to evaluate in terms of histologic variation the functional capacity of the organ. In our discussion of diseases of the thyroid gland, we shall make some slight divergence from our usual order of presentation, leaving a consideration of the inflammatory conditions to follow the functional disorders. This is done for two reasons. In the first place, there is considerable relationship between certain of these inflammatory and infectious conditions in respect to functional disturbance; and in the second place, the thyroid gland is notoriously resistant to infection of all sorts and to the usual inflammatory changes, which we see so commonly in other organs, and

PLATE CXLII

DISEASES OF THE THYROID GLAND

Primary Hyperthyroidism

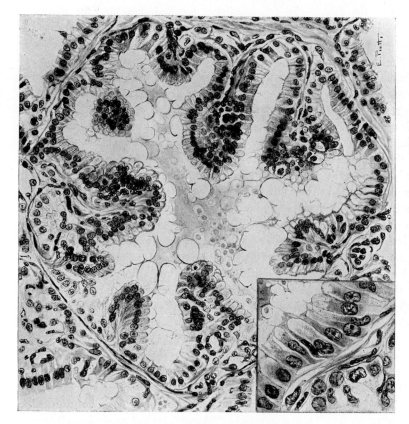

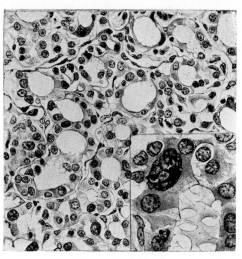

Fig. 599.—Exophthalmic Goitre (Papillary Hyperplasia).—Cf. Case 257.—Drawing of a single greatly enlarged acinus lined by pseudostratified, high columnar epithelium with marked papillation. Note diminished, pale staining, vacuolated colloid in lumen.

Fig. 600.—Primary Hyperthryoidism (Follicular Hyperplasia).—Characteristic increase in number of small acini lined by large, cuboidal, hyperchromic cells, and almost complete absence of colloid.

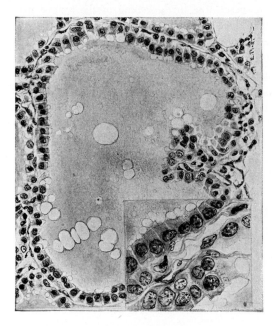

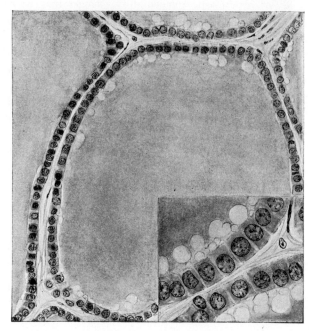

Fig. 601.—Early Involution (Exophthalmic Goitre), Following Iodine Therapy.—Cf. Case 258.—Note decrease in papillation, increase in colloid and reversion of epithelium towards cuboidal type.

Fig. 602.—Complete, Late Involution (Exophthalmic Goitre), Following Iodine Therapy.—Complete return to the normal histologic characteristics of the acinus, evidenced by homogeneous, deep staining colloid and typical low, cuboidal lining epithelial cells.

therefore these lesions are relatively few in number and unimportant clinically.

In general, it may be said that most of the disorders of the ductless glands, from the pathologic standpoint, depend very largely upon the subnormal or excessive functional activity of the particular gland in question. Whether the morphologic changes which are found are causal or the result of such glandular depression or stimulation is somewhat obscure in most instances. However, it is quite possible with experience to interpret the pathologic physiology of the gland clinically in terms of these morphologic changes, with a rather surprisingly high degree of accuracy, and for this reason a consideration of these histopathologic features seems thoroughly warranted.

Cretinism.—As has been already intimated, two clinical varieties of hypothyroidism can be recognized; first, the type which is seen in infancy and childhood as a congenital defect in the functional development of the gland and which is associated with the condition known clinically as *cretinism;* and second, the adult form of deficient thyroid functional activity, known as *myxedema.* In a consideration of cretinism we may find either of two equally characteristic histologic pictures. It may occur in the form of an underdeveloped, hypoplastic gland which appears atrophic. This is much less commonly seen than the other variety. In the more usual type, we have a gland which not infrequently is actually enlarged and in which histologic evidence of hyperplastic compensatory changes may be suggested. Here we are forced to some extent to theorize. It is well known that cretins are prone to be born to parents who suffer from endemic, iodine-deficient, colloid goitre. This has been amply proven experimentally in animals as well.

Under these circumstances, the child may be born with a thyroid, which, during its developmental phase, has been exhausted through the iodine-deficiency of the mother, in its attempt to maintain anything like normal body growth. When such a child is born and his thyroid is thrown on its own resources, the narrow margin which had been provided and maintained through the maternal circulation is lost. As a result, such an exhausted, deficient gland is incapable of producing either an adequate amount of normal thyroid secretion, or produces a defective, deficient type of thyroid product. In either case, we have the development of the clinical picture of cretinism.

In this condition, we find that the body metabolism is lowered, and all body functions retarded, particularly growth of bones and mental development. The interglandular relationship is disturbed and changes which are not wholly thyroid in origin are not uncommonly seen as the result of such disturbed balance of glandular activity. The child's growth is seriously stunted. This occurs particularly in respect to the growth of the long bones as affecting height. There is likewise a tendency for obesity to develop. Marked thickening of the skin, loss of hair, the development of spade-like hands and feet, thickening of the tongue and an impaired circulation, are common accompaniments of such defective secretory activity. Even with the administration of thyroid extract, while considerable improvement may occur clinically, and children who would otherwise have become institutional cases requiring state care may become capable of self-support, yet their development never parallels that of normal growth either physically or mentally. (Fig. 615)

Myxedema.—From the functional standpoint, the acquired form of hypothyroidism is basically the same, but because mental development and physical growth are completed, the alteration in stature and the severe mental changes are not so obvious. There is a marked reduction in basal metabolism, sometimes as much as 50 per cent below normal. The same thickening of the skin; coarseness of the hair; loss of hair; diminution or absence of sweating; and thickness of speech due to thickening of the tongue may be seen. More particularly, we find the patients have a mental torpor; show a marked slowing of the heart and pulse rate (bradycardia), and a resultant clamminess of the extremities through poor circulation. The patients complain of being cold, even in the warmest weather.

Clinically these cases show almost miraculous changes within the course of a few days when their thyroxin requirements are met by the administration of thyroid substance, and a rapid return to normal is to be expected. Usually this replacement therapy has to be maintained throughout the remainder of the individual's life, but because of compensatory hypertrophy and hyperplasia of the glandular tissue, in many cases the amount of medication may be reduced and in some instances even omitted.

PLATE CXLIII
DISEASES OF THE THYROID GLAND

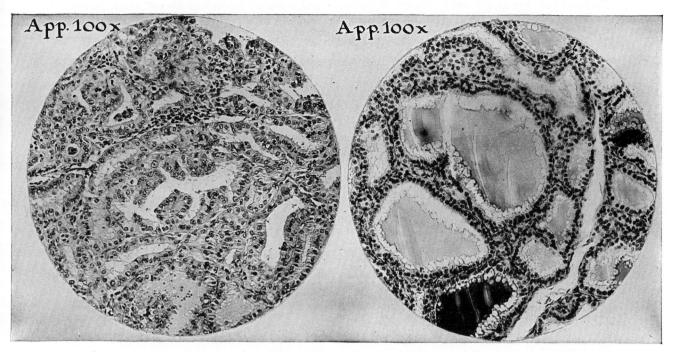

FIG. 603.—THYROID GLAND: EXOPHTHALMIC GOITRE (PAPILLARY HYPERPLASIA).—CASE 257.—Photomicrograph in which the acini show typical increase in size, papillary proliferation of their lining epithelium and a diminution in their colloid content. Note interstitial agregations of lymphocytes. App. 100 x.

FIG. 604.—THYROID GLAND: EXOPHTHALMIC GOITRE (POST-IODINE INVOLUTION).—CASE 258.—Acini present more nearly normal appearance and contain some colloid. However, epithelial cells still show considerable retention of their hyperplastic features. App. 100 x.

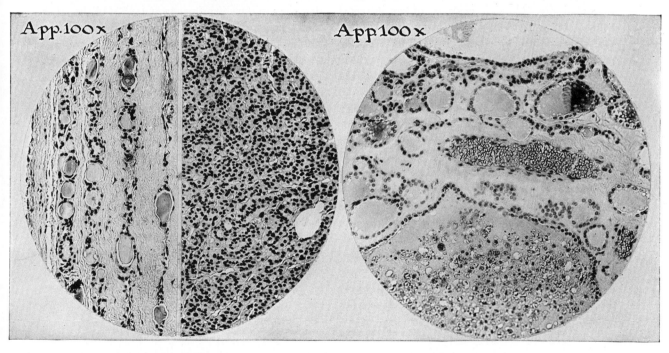

FIG. 605.—THYROID GLAND: FETAL (EMBRYONAL) ADENOMA.—CASE 261.—A tumor composed of cords and trabeculae of undifferentiated thyroid epithelium with a suggestion of lumen formation (right), and surrounded by a pseudocapsule of fibrous tissue with a few atrophic persistent acini (left). App. 100 x.

FIG. 606.—THYROID GLAND: COLLOID ADENOMA.—A localized, encapsulated adenoma composed of acini of varying size and containing relatively normal staining colloid. Note abundant stroma undergoing degeneration. App. 100 x.

Pathologically, the adult cases show this decreased glandular function as the result of some inflammatory or degenerative process which destroys large portions of the thyroid substance. The acini tend to be small. Colloid is reduced in amount and on chemical analysis the total thyroxin and iodine content of such glands is greatly reduced. Such inflammatory conditions usually start outside the gland as for example in association with some severe infection of the larynx and trachea, but occasionally the process may be primarily within the thyroid gland itself.

Microscopically, in hypothyroidism, the picture varies, depending upon the etiology. In the congenital-cretin variety, as has already been emphasized, the gland may actually show enlargement and the individual acini show proliferative attempts at hyperplasia in an effort to compensate for the defective secretion. In the acquired form, the picture is usually one of replacement fibrosis as the result of some destructive inflammatory process. This is accompanied by marked lymphocytic infiltration of the stroma and of atrophy of the acini. Indeed much of this loss of function would appear to be dependent upon the peri-acinar or interacinar fibrosis which prevents the secretion of the thyroid cells from getting into the blood stream normally. As a result of this avascularization, the glandular atrophy follows.

Another variety of hypothyroidism is seen postoperatively in cases of hyperthyroidism in which large amounts of the gland have been removed. This is usually compensated for by hyperplastic changes in the gland over a relatively short period of time and is, therefore, only transitory in nature.

In recent years, total thyroid extirpation has been recommended in cases of coronary disease associated with marked hypertensive features. This results in a lessening of basal metabolism which has been accompanied in a small proportion of the cases by marked clinical improvement. Such complete myxedema, however, requires the reëstablishment of a minimal, basal metabolic rate, which must be supplied ultimately by replacement thyroid therapy. This method of treatment still seems to be in the experimental phase and has not been universally accepted as yet.

HYPERTHYROIDISM

In hyperthyroidism we find the exact reverse picture clinically. There is evidence of an increased metabolic rate which may reach as much as 120 per cent above normal in extreme cases. This is accompanied by evidence of generalized increased body metabolism. There is an increased pulse rate; marked sweating; increased nervousness and irritability. There is a typical fine tremor of the fingers when held in the extended position, and in a considerable proportion of the cases there is a varying degree of exophthalmus. (Fig. 616)

Grossly the gland tends to show varying degrees of increase in size. One may find extreme degrees of primary hyperthyroidism without much increase in size of the gland, but roughly there is a parallelism between the intensity of the symptoms and the increase in the size of the gland.

The etiology of hyperthyroidism is not known. The mechanism of the disease appears to be largely the result of stimulation of the sympathetic nervous system. This is initiated in many instances apparently by some severe emotional or mental shock. The relationship of the adrenals in this connection has been stressed by many investigators. Marine, to whom we owe perhaps more of our knowledge of the thyroid than any one other investigator, believes that the pituitary is primarily at fault. On the other hand, chemotoxic theories ranging all the way from vitamin deficiencies to actual ingested substances are possible factors in the initiation of the condition. In this respect the cyanides have particularly been incriminated, Marine having been able to reproduce the picture of hyperthyroidism even to the point of exophthalmus in many instances in animals by feeding them on a diet largely composed of cabbage, which is particularly rich in cyanides. The relationship of hyperthyroidism to gonadotropic influences likewise cannot be overlooked.

Hyperthyroidism is a disease which affects women in the ratio of six to one as compared to men. It is seen especially at the onset of adolescence and at the menopause. Likewise it may be a complication of pregnancy, and it is a familiar fact that the thyroid increases in size and often in function with almost every menstrual cycle in a very considerable proportion of women.

In our present form of treatment of hyperthyroidism, it has been found that in general, surgery is attended by more uniformly satisfactory successful permanent relief. The use of irradiation in hyper-

PLATE CXLIV
DISEASES OF THE THYROID GLAND

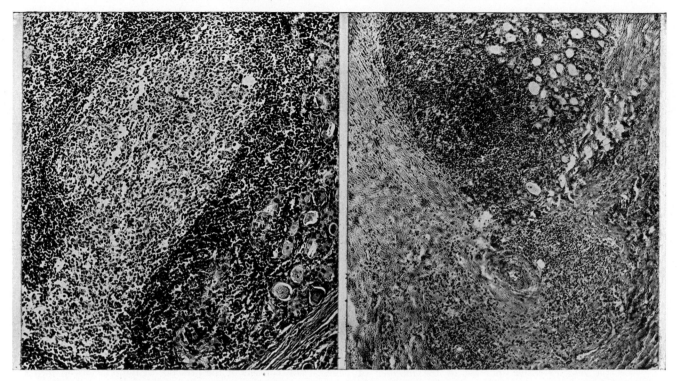

FIG. 607.—STRUMA LYMPHOMATOSA (HASHIMOTO'S DISEASE).—CASE 259.—Almost complete lymphocytic replacement of thyroid tissue and the formation of huge germinal centers are the outstanding features of the histology. App. 100 x.

FIG. 608.—RIEDEL'S STRUMA (CHRONIC LIGNEOUS THYROIDITIS).—CASE 260.—Histologically the pathology is characterized by dense fibrosis with atrophy and disappearance of acini and the presence of large aggregations of lymphocytes and other mononuclear inflammatory cells. App. 100 x.

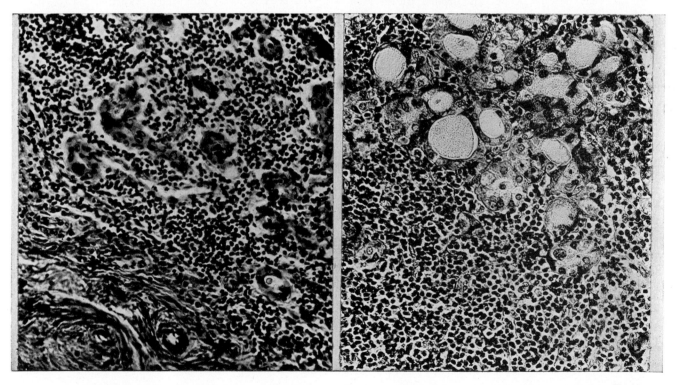

FIG. 609.—CHRONIC THYROIDITIS.—Interstitial, non-suppurative exudation with associated edema has separated and distorted the normal acini. App. 150 x.

FIG. 610.—SMALL ROUND CELL CARCINOMA.—CASE 265.—A small amount of hyperplastic thyroid tissue is seen invaded by a tumor composed of small, hyperchromic, undifferentiated, round cells with many mitotic figures, and little tendency toward acinar formation. App. 150 x.

thyroidism is enthusiastically supported by a few investigators, but except as an adjunct to surgery, or as a substitution for surgery when surgery is contraindicated for some reason, its usefulness seems to be very definitely of secondary importance.

Histologically, two varieties of hyperthyroidism exist: first, the type which is particularly associated with the exophthalmic type of goitre. In this we find the individual acini are considerably increased in *size*. They are lined by an epithelium which has undergone a metaplasia from the usual low cuboidal type to a high columnar type of cell. Not only the transition in cell type is present, but these cells are growing so rapidly that they are thrown into marked papillary folds which often nearly fill the lumen of the acinus (Fig. 599). At the same time, there is noted a marked diminution in the amount of colloid within these acini, which in the more severe cases almost completely disappears. Such colloid as remains shows marked changes in its staining capacity, usually staining very feebly. Likewise, extensive vacuolization of such persistent colloid is noted.

The second type of hyperplasia is represented by a very extensive increase in the *number* of acini rather than in the size of the individual acini. These are relatively small in size. They are lined by a type of epithelium which differs from the normal in that the cells, while still cuboidal are several times the normal dimensions and usually stain relatively intensely with eosin. As in the case of the exophthalmic papillary type of hyperthyroidism, the colloid is reduced in amount and frequently practically absent. This type of follicular hyperplasia is seen often in the more severe cases of primary hyperthyroidism with the highest metabolic rates, but rarely in association with exophthalmus (Fig. 600). At times both features, papillary and follicular hyperplasia, may be seen in the same gland, but they are very apt to remain independent.

Involution.—Both forms of hyperthyroidism, but particularly the papillary exophthalmic type respond temporarily almost miraculously to the administration of iodine. There is a gradual involution of the gland with the epithelium reverting slowly to the cuboidal type and with the deposition of more and more colloid, which gradually becomes normal in its staining reactions. Very striking involution may be seen within a week on the usual iodine therapy of ten to twenty drops of Logol's solution or similar iodine preparations three times a day. This involution is perhaps best explained on the basis that the excess iodine which is administered stimulates the production of colloid, and binds the thyroxin to this newly formed thyroglobulin or colloid. This therapy may not safely be continued indefinitely because a point of saturation will be reached after which no more thyroxin can be bound in this way. There follows once again, a direct outpouring of the thyroxin into the blood stream producing exaggerated symptoms of hyperthyroidism. As a pre-operative procedure to initiate this involution process and thus reduce the metabolic rate and evidence of toxicity, the method is unexcelled. By it, the operative mortality in thyroid surgery has, in general, been reduced from 10 or 15 per cent to less than 1 per cent and today the hyperthyroid patient need not fear thyroid surgery as being more serious than any major abdominal surgical procedure. (Figs. 601 and 602)

In both forms of hyperthyroidism, but especially in the exophthalmic papillary variety, from the histologic standpoint a very striking histologic feature is observed in perhaps fifty to sixty per cent of cases. This consists of the presence of lymphocytes in focal aggregations. Not infrequently actual lymph follicles may be recognized with active germinal centers and broad collars of the small adult type of cell. This has been variously interpreted. Warthin always emphasized its importance on the constitutional basis. He felt that this lymphoid picture was as integral a part of the histology of hyperthyroidism as was the papillary proliferation of the acinar epithelium. In our own experience this has not seemed as significant a finding as fully thirty to forty per cent of cases failed to show this feature histologically. However, it is unquestionably true that such lymphoid hyperplasia does occur with much greater frequency in cases of hyperthyroidism in the thyroid gland than in the thyroid glands of individuals who do not present evidence of this functional disturbance. In this respect, we agree with Warthin that the typical hyperthyroid patient is likely to belong to that group of so-called "lymphoid constitutionality," and in fact we have seen several instances of sudden death among such patients in which the typical picture of status thymicolymphaticus existed simultaneously. We believe, therefore, that this lymphoid tissue is an anatomical feature rather than representative of any chronic inflammatory process as has been suggested.

PLATE CXLV
MALIGNANT TUMORS OF THE THYROID GLAND

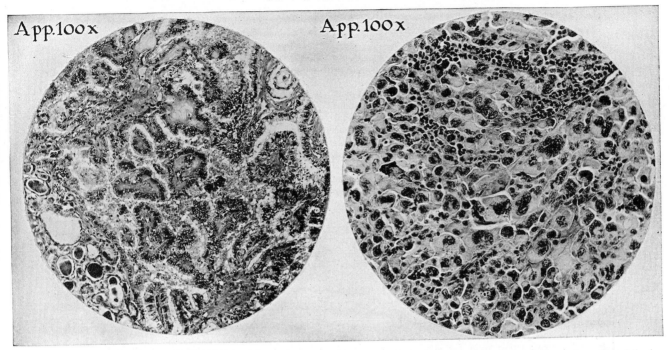

FIG. 611.—PAPILLARY ADENOCARCINOMA.—CASE 262.—Tumor composed of hyperplastic columnar epithelial cells showing marked papillation and evidence of invasion of relatively normal thyroid parenchyma at left.

FIG. 612.—"GIANT CELL" CARCINOMA.—CASE 263.—A rapidly invasive tumor composed for the most part of enormous, pleomorphic epithelial cells, many of the tumor giant cell type, containing intensely hyperchromic nuclei.

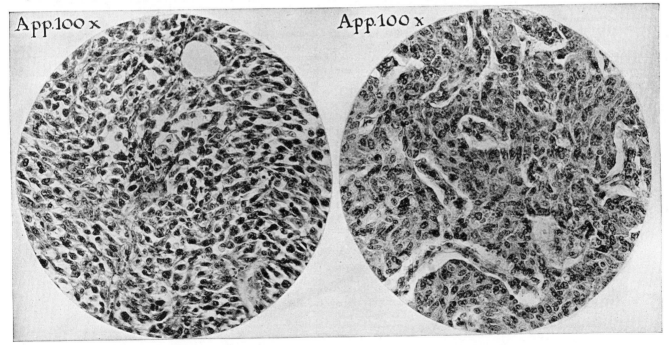

FIG. 613.—"SPINDLE CELL" CARCINOMA.—CASE 264.—Photomicrograph of a field from a less typical portion of the tumor shown in Fig. 614. Note marked "spindling" of cells and the resemblance of the tumor to a sarcoma.

FIG. 614.—"SPINDLE CELL" CARCINOMA.—CASE 264.—Photomicrograph from an area which illustrates the epithelial origin of the tumor, as shown by persistent acinar formation. Certain of the cells are spindle shaped indicative of the transition to the appearance as shown in Fig. 613.

ILLUSTRATIVE CASE

CASE 257 (Ref. #S-236)

Diagnosis.—Thyroid gland—primary hyperthyroidism (exophthalmic goitre).

Patient was a white female of 45 years, admitted to the hospital with the chief complaints of exophthalmos, palpitation of the heart, insomnia and weakness.

Present Illness.—The onset of the present illness was somewhat indefinite but dated back apparently for about two years. During that period she had noted occasional headaches and progressive disturbances of vision. She had not noted any definite protrusion of her eyeballs until about three or four months before admission. About that time she first noticed attacks of palpitation of the heart and suffered from marked insomnia. She used to perspire more freely than normal and became very easily upset emotionally for very minor, trivial causes. Her family complained of an increased nervous irritability. She had a rather distressing, nonproductive, chronic, nervous type of cough. She had no dysphagia or hoarseness. She consulted a physician who sent her to the hospital for study with the diagnosis of probable hyperthyroidism.

Past Medical History.—The patient's past medical history was essentially negative. She had had the usual childhood infections. She had not been unduly subject to upper respiratory infections. Her cardiorespiratory system, up to the present illness, was negative. Gastrointestinal system: Other than for occasional periods of constipation there had been nothing significant until recently when intermittent diarrhea alternated with her constipation. She had been married at the age of eighteen and had had two children, both by cesarean section. Previous to this, she had had two other pregnancies which had ended in spontaneous miscarriage. Her menses began at the age of twelve and had been regular until two years before admission. During this two year period they had been most irregular with the interval between periods increasing. The last period had been six months ago.

Physical Examination.—Patient was a well-developed, well-nourished, middle-aged, white female who did not appear acutely ill. Head was normal in contour. Eyes showed a moderate, bulging exophthalmos with rather dilated pupils. Nose and throat were negative. There was no definite cervical adenopathy. There was moderate fullness of the neck, which on careful palpation seemed to be due to a moderate symmetrical enlargement of the thyroid gland. Chest was symmetrical. Percussion was negative. There were no râles. Heart: Apex beat was forceful and rather diffuse, apparently most marked in the fifth interspace. The rate was increased to 140, but it was regular and there were no murmurs. Blood pressure was 136/80. Abdomen was somewhat obese. A lower abdominal scar indicating her cesarean sections was present. No masses or tenderness could be felt. Extremities: There was a fine fibrillary tremor of the fingers on holding the hands out at full length. Reflexes were generally normal. On talking to the patient, there seemed to be some suggestion of hoarseness of her voice.

Laboratory Findings.—The blood count showed 4,900,000 red blood cells with 78% hemoglobin and a white count of 8,550 cells with 79% neutrophiles. Urinalysis was negative except for a very slight trace of albumin. Her basal metabolic rate was plus 50%.

Subsequent History.—On the basis of the history and elevated basal metabolic rate, the diagnosis of primary hyperthyroidism was made and thyroidectomy advised. The patient was put on pre-operative treatment of 10 drops of Lugol's solution *t.i.d.* for ten days, with the reduction of her basal metabolic rate to plus 28 per cent. Thyroidectomy was done and the patient made an uneventful recovery with the basal metabolic rate dropping to minus 5 per cent a month later.

Pathological Report.—*Gross Description.*—Specimen consisted of two masses of thyroid tissue each measuring approximately 5 x 4 x 2.5. These were beefy red in color. On section there was marked reduction in colloid, the cut surface having lost much of its normal translucent appearance. Considerable increase in the blood supply was noted. There was no evidence of cystic degeneration or calcification. The picture was that of a simple primary diffuse hyperplasia of the gland.

Microscopic Description of a Section Through the Thyroid.—(Fig. 603) Histologic study of the tissue presents the characteristic features of primary hyperthyroidism. There is very marked papillary hyperplasia of the epithelial cells lining the thyroid acini. These have undergone transition for the most part from the usual normal low cuboidal to a high columnar type of cell. They are arranged in what appear to be branching papillae nearly filling the lumina of the dilated glands in many places. This is apparently the result of mechanical plication as a result of the cell overgrowth. There is an almost complete absence of colloid in the great majority of acini. In some, however, it still persists but tends to stain unevenly. For the most part, it is pale, vacuolated and contracted away from the lining epithelium. Here and there individual acini are seen in which as a result of the iodine therapy a moderate degree of involution has occurred. In such areas there is an apparent reversion of the epithelium toward its normal low cuboidal form with the accumulation of colloid in the acinus. This results in marked distention of the acinus so that such glands stand out particularly prominently against the general background of cellular hyperplasia. There is marked dilatation of the blood vessels to a degree which almost suggests a true increased blood supply to the gland. In many areas there are foci of lymphocytes in the stroma. These in places are so numerous as to go on to the development of actual lymph follicle formation. This picture of lymphoid hyperplasia is irregularly distributed throughout the gland. It does not appear to be an inflammatory lesion but rather a constitutional feature of the anatomy.

PLATE CXLVI
DISEASES OF THE DUCTLESS GLANDS

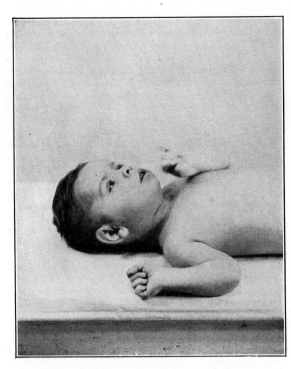

Fig. 615.—Thyroid Gland: Hypothyroidism (Cretin) (Courtesy Dr. G. A. Jervis).—Photograph of patient under thyroid treatment, showing a limited persistence of the typical facies, delayed skeletal growth, and retardation of mental development.

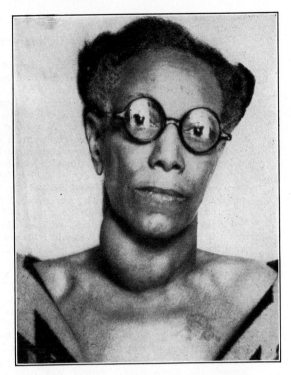

Fig. 616.—Thyroid Gland: Hyperthyroidism.—Cf. Case 257.—Gross photograph of patient showing assymetric enlargement of lobes of thyroid gland, widening of palpebral fissure and moderate exophthalmos.

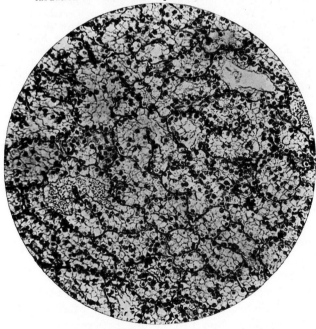

Fig. 617.—Parathyroid Gland: Hyperparathyroidism.—Case 266. (Courtesy Dr. T. B. Mallory).—Note uniform diffuse hyperplasia of gland. The cells present a clear, vacuolated, distended cytoplasm and small peripherally placed hyperchromic nuclei. App. 100 X.

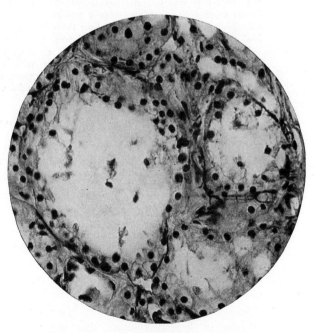

Fig. 618.—Parathyroid Gland: Adenoma.—High power photomicrograph from a case associated with osteitis fibrosa cystica, and showing irregular sized alveoli lined by the several varieties of parathyroid epithelial cells. App. 200 x.

ILLUSTRATIVE CASE

CASE 258 (Ref. #S-279)

Diagnosis.—Thyroid gland—primary hyperthyroidism with moderate involution.

Patient was a white male of 33 years, admitted to the hospital with the chief complaints of increased nervousness, easy fatigability and loss of weight.

Present Illness.—The present illness had been progressive over a two year period. The patient was easily irritated and would get upset over unimportant minor things. He had noticed palpitation of his heart during the last few months on the slightest exertion and complained of constantly perspiring. He had been bothered with a fine tremor of his hands, which interfered at times with his work. He had shown marked increase in appetite, but in spite of this had progressively lost over thirty pounds of weight. For about six months he had had a moderately pronounced exophthalmos. More recently he had noticed that his voice had become somewhat hoarse and he had had some dyspnea and difficulty with swallowing.

Past Medical History.—Past medical history was essentially irrelevant. He had had the usual childhood infections but had never been seriously ill enough to require medical treatment since that time. A review of his systems was negative. He had never previously had any symptoms suggesting hyperthyroidism. He had not been subject to upper respiratory infection. He had never been heart conscious. His gastro-intestinal history was normal. His genito-urinary history was negative. He denied venereal infection.

Physical Examination.—Patient was a well-developed young man who showed a very moist skin and a flushed appearance to his face. Heart was enlarged and the heart rate was considerably increased to about 100. Lungs were negative. There was a massive symmetrical enlargement of the thyroid including the middle pyramidal lobe. Physical findings otherwise were negative.

Laboratory Findings.—Red blood cells, 4,300,000 with 82% hemoglobin. White blood cells, 8,300 with 69% polynuclears. Urinalysis was negative. Wassermann was negative. Basal metabolic rate was plus seventy-four.

Subsequent Course.—He was recommended for thyroidectomy and a subtotal operation was done following a brief preparatory period during which he was given Lugol's solution. He had been taking Lugol's on the outside for about three months with no improvement in symptoms. About nineteen-twentieths of the gland was removed surgically. The patient made an uneventful recovery, being discharged one month postoperatively with marked improvement of his symptoms, including his voice.

Pathological Report.—*Gross Description.*—Specimen consisted of two large pieces of thyroid tissue representing the two lobes, each measuring about 7.5 x 6.5 x 4 cm. The cut surface was of a grayish, beefy-red appearance with some increased vascularity and fibrosis. Colloid could be identified but appeared reduced in amount.

Microscopic Description of a Section Through the Thyroid.—(Fig. 604) Histologically, the thyroid tissue presents evidence of a typical primary type of parenchymatous hyperplasia of the thyroid such as is seen commonly in association with exophthalmic goitre. Here and there acini are seen in which there is some persistence of the rather characteristic papillary hyperplasia described in the previous case. On the whole, however, the cells are of a high cuboidal or rather low columnar type and there is relatively little papillary proliferation. There is a marked increase of the colloid in comparison to the previous case. This colloid shows considerable irregularity in its staining reactions, but again this feature is much less marked in this case. A moderate amount of vacuolization of the colloid is seen. As a whole, however, it almost completely fills the acini without the striking scalloped appearance noted in the preceding case. The interstitial stroma seems reduced and the blood vessels are not at all prominent. Occasional foci of lymphocytic cells are seen, some of which show actual follicular formation. The picture, from the histologic standpoint, is one of marked involutional regression from the primary hyperplastic picture of untreated hyperthyroidism, which in this instance showed features of both papillary and acinar hyperplasia.

COLLOID GOITRE

Before proceeding further with a discussion of thyroid pathology it is perhaps well to define what is meant by the word "goitre." By this term is meant simply enlargement of the thyroid gland. This may or may not be associated with disturbances of function so far as clinical evidence presents. It is unfortunate that this term has crept into the classification of thyroid disease as its connotation usually relates to the hyperplastic syndrome. In the previous two sections we have discovered that both the hypofunctioning gland as well as the hyperplastic type as seen in hyperthyroidism, may show enlargement of the gland and as such be called "goitre." In the same way in the present section, we shall see that the term "goitre" is equally loosely applied to a very large group of cases of thyroid enlargement which are, for the most part, endemic in distribution and result from a deficient iodine intake. In these cases, there is no disturbance of function as evidenced by any clinical alteration in metabolic rate. The enlargement of the gland from the clinical standpoint is to a very considerable extent purely a question of cosmetic appearance and in some instances because of location, especially as substernal thyroids, a question of pressure. More significant than these two factors, however, is the physiological drain upon the gland which has almost no factor of safety. This results, as we have already seen, in a rather high incidence of deficient thyroid offspring among such mothers as compared with those possessing an entirely normal gland.

In colloid goitre, which is the result of a deficient iodine intake, the gland attempts to compensate for this defect by increasing in size, with the deposition of enormous amounts of colloid. Such colloid tends to be defective in some respect, however, and for this reason an even further increase in the volume of this material is necessary to bind the normal required iodine in order to maintain normal metabolism. We can think of the colloid of the thyroid gland roughly in the same way that we can think of the gallbladder as a reservoir, for the storage of thyroxin to meet the body needs, just as the gallbladder stores and concentrates bile to be used in the digestive crises. Thus, in cases of colloid goitre we find two defective factors involved. We find an inadequate iodine intake and a defective colloid production which goes hand in hand with the first of these. As a result, in order to store an adequate amount of thyroxin, the thyroid gland as a whole must increase enormously in size, at times reaching a diameter larger than that of a child's head and becoming almost pedunculated. This at times may be of very serious significance if it produces pressure symptoms. Surgery is not indicated except for the relief of pressure symptoms and for the cosmetic effect. Unlike hyperthyroidism, colloid goitre occurs almost equally between males and females of any given community. A child may even be born with the beginning of such a colloid goitre if the mother is unable to maintain the normal thyroxin globulin balance. It is in this field, particularly that Marine has shown conclusively the part which iodine, or rather the lack of iodine, plays in the development of this pathological picture. In experimental studies upon school children (following his initial work on animals), the reduction in the incidence of colloid goitre in the young age group merely by the iodinization of the water supply of the community was more eloquent and convincing than any amount of written discussion. To-day, endemic colloid goitre in individuals born in the last fifteen or twenty years is only rarely seen in this country.

Pathologically, the typical, simple, colloid goitre is composed of thyroid acini which tend to be many times the normal size. These are lined by a flattened single layer of cuboidal epithelial cells with their rather characteristic hyperchromatic ovoid nuclei and granular dark cytoplasm. The acini are filled with a pale-staining homogeneous, pink-staining colloid which frequently shows some vacuolization along its periphery, but which for the most part fills the acinus much more completely than it does in the normal gland. As a result of this enormous distention of acini, many of the supportive, interacinar blood vessels become compressed and obliterated (cf. Fig. 606). This, in turn, results in anoxemia of the cells and in cystic degeneration, which may be accompanied by hemorrhage. The broken down material in such cystic areas is apt to contain a large amount of cholesterin and secondary calcification is not at all infrequent. As will be explained in the following section relating to multiple colloid adenomatous goitre there is a tendency for irregular nodular hyperplastic involutional changes to occur, which tend to separate clumps of such acini into nodules simulating neoplasm. It is in these nodular areas particularly that such degenerative changes are apt to occur; but for purposes of comparison it is perhaps easier to remember that the uncomplicated picture of simple colloid goitre is evidenced solely by the distention of the acini by a rather poorly stained deficient type of colloid.

Nodular Goitre (Multiple Colloid Adenomatous Goitre)

By the term nodular goitre, which seems to be the preferable term for the condition, is meant a variety of thyroid enlargement which is the result of repeated periods of subclinical functional hyperplasia and involution. It is well recognized that functional hyperplasia in the thyroid is rarely uniform throughout the entire gland, but occurs in patchy, irregular areas. This is not unlike the functional activity of the kidney in which it has been so clearly demonstrated that only a relatively few glomeruli actually take part simultaneously in excretion. Such lesions are seen as borderline cases both in the colloid goitre group and in the hyperthyroid group, developing usually without definite clinical evidence of real symptomatic hyperthyroidism. They occur most frequently in women, and during the childbearing period.

In this connection it should be noted that there is a form of hyperthyroidism which is seen in the period of adolescence. This is usually a self-limited disease and disappears when normal endocrine balance is established, but may at times progress into a typical picture of hyperthyroidism. This group of cases of so-called "adenomatous goitre" may be best considered as a borderline functional group, in which focal areas of hyperplasia and colloid involution have occurred, resulting in isolated nodules which may show extensive colloid formation even to the point of necrosis, cystic degeneration and hemorrhage. These are not true tumors, but represent merely functional aberrations. They are embedded in a pseudocapsule of connective tissue which further heightens their resemblance to tumors and explains much of the confusion which has existed in this respect for many years.

Pathologically, if we examine one of these thyroid glands it is necessary to take multiple sections as the histologic pattern will vary greatly in different portions of the gland. In one of these isolated nodules it is not unlikely that we may find evidence of moderately hyperplastic changes at times even approaching the picture of true exophthalmic papillary hyperplasia, which we associate with hyperthyroidism. In another area where the colloid can be seen with the naked eye, we may find distended vesicles packed with deep-staining colloid and lined by a flattened layer of cuboidal epithelium. Cystic degeneration, hemorrhage, calcification and all the concomitant histopathological changes associated with interference with the blood supply may be demonstrated in one or another such nodules. It is not surprising that in some instances we may have definite toxic symptoms and that in others no evidence of toxicity exists. Varying degrees of lymphoid activity may be encountered as in the usual picture of hyperthyroidism. This is as a rule less marked than in the more severe cases of hyperthyroid disease. This fits in with the theoretical constitutional diathesis which places such borderline lymphoid individuals on the borderline of thyroid dysfunction.

INFECTIONS OF THE THYROID

The thyroid is particularly resistant to the ordinary infectious processes. Even in cases of extensive miliary tuberculosis, it is rare to encounter miliary tubercles within the thyroid substance. Occasional instances of this condition do occur, however, and at times a more massive solitary tuberculoma or diffuse tuberculosis may develop. Only approximately fifty such cases exist in the literature. Even less frequently, the usual pyogenic infections are seen in the thyroid, and such infections as do occur usually result as extensions of acute inflammatory processes of the larynx and trachea. Such cases of acute thyroiditis are easily recognized by the swelling, tenderness and usual picture of inflammation. With their subsidence, not infrequently a myxedema will result (Fig. 609).

INFLAMMATORY DISEASES OF THE THYROID

Hashimoto's Disease (Struma Lymphomatosa).— By Hashimoto's disease is meant a condition in which there is a gradual replacement of the entire thyroid glandular structures by lymphoid tissue. It is particularly impressive in respect to the extraordinary amount of lymphoid infiltration which occurs and for the development of large lymph follicles with enormous germinal centers, many of which are apt to show mitotic figures and evidence of active growth. It is believed by some, notably Graham, that this condition of struma lymphomatosa may lead to the development of a subsequent lymphosarcoma. The etiology of this condition is entirely obscure. It has been suggested that it is part of the lymphoid constitutional picture in an exaggerated form, but no such comparable lesions are ordinarily encountered in the ordinary picture of status lymphaticus. No infectious etiology has ever been described as being consistently present in these cases nor of being capable of inducing the disease in experimental animals (Fig. 607).

Just what follows this initial phase of diffuse lymphoid infiltration and replacement of thyroid gland is somewhat problematical. If, as is true of most such lymphoid reactions it is followed by an inevitable histological sequence of productive fibrosis and scar tissue formation, then it is quite conceivable that this pathological process may represent not a clinical entity in itself, but the initial phase of what at a later time may develop into the condition known as Riedel's struma. The disease is in some instances accompanied by the development of the clinical picture of myxedema, but rarely in a severe or advanced form. This is accounted for by the gradual nature of the process and the fact that the persistent thyroid structures undergo compensatory hyperplasia to the degree necessary to maintain a normal metabolism. In the later stages, however, this balance may be destroyed and clinical myxedema may supervene (Fig. 608).

ILLUSTRATIVE CASE

CASE 259 (Ref. #S-386)

Diagnosis.—Thyroid gland—Struma lymphomatosa (Hashimoto's disease).

Patient was a white female of 49 years, admitted to the hospital because of a palpable mass in her neck.

Present Illness.—The patient first noticed a mass in her neck approximately nine months before admission. This had varied considerably in size. One time it was somewhat tender on palpation. She had not had any symptoms which suggested hyperthyroidism. She had had no increased nervousness, insomnia, sweating or palpitation. There had been no weight loss. She came to the hospital primarily because she was worried that this mass in her neck might be in the nature of a malignant tumor.

Past Medical History.—The patient had had all the usual children's diseases, including diphtheria. She also believed that she had had rheumatic fever at the age of fifteen. A review of her systems otherwise was essentially negative. She had been no more subject to upper respiratory disease than the average individual. She had never been heart conscious. Her gastro-intestinal history was that of the usual story of chronic constipation, but otherwise was negative except for occasional acute gastric upsets. Menstrual history began at the age of twelve and had always been regular. She was apparently going through the menopause at the time of admission, her last period having been six months previously. She had had nine pregnancies, including one miscarriage.

Physical Examination.—Patient was a fairly well-developed and well-nourished middle aged white woman. Head was negative. Eyes reacted normally. There was no exophthalmos. Nose and throat were negative. There was a nodular, hard mass rather fixed in character which involved chiefly the right lobe of the thyroid, but extended to the isthmus. No comparable enlargement of the left side was noted. Chest was symmetrical. Lungs were clear. Heart was somewhat enlarged to the left. There were no murmurs. Blood pressure was 200/110. Abdomen was negative. There was some slight edema of the extremities. Pulse rate was 70, and her basal metabolic rate was plus 9.

Laboratory Findings.—Repeated urinalysis showed occasional slight traces of albumin and sugar. The red blood count on admission revealed 6,000,000 red cells with 92% hemoglobin. There were 9,300 white blood cells with 53% neutrophiles.

Subsequent Course.—On the basis of the history and physical findings it was thought, pre-operatively, that the thyroid lesion was probably in the nature of a neoplasm and excision was advised. At operation, the right lobe was found to be extremely firm in consistency and somewhat irregularly nodular in outline. It appeared adherent to the jugular vein. The entire right lobe and isthmus were removed. The patient made an uneventful postoperative recovery and remained in her usual health for a postoperative observation period of five years.

Pathological Report.—*Gross Description.*—Specimen consisted of a right lobe of thyroid with the isthmus. This showed a diffuse enlargement. It was almost pure white in color and showed no evidence of colloid grossly. It was irregularly nodular on its surface but there was a definitely intact capsule. No evidence of hemorrhage or necrosis was found. Grossly, it was impossible to determine whether or not the picture represented one of neoplasm.

Microscopic Description of a Section Through the Thyroid Gland.—(Fig. 607) The histologic study of the specimen reveals an almost complete replacement of the normal thyroid gland by lymphoid tissue. Here and there evidence of attempted function on the part of the thyroid tissue is seen in the presence of scattered large, hypertrophic-appearing acini. In general, however, the thyroid acini have been replaced by an extraordinarily diffuse infiltration of the gland by lymphocytes. In many places, enormous lymph follicles are present showing active germinal centers, many of them containing mitotic figures. The picture, in general, is that of a diffuse struma lymphomatosa or so-called "Hashimoto's disease." No evidence of malignancy either on the part of the glandular epithelium or on the part of the lymphocytes, all of which appear to be entirely normal, is seen. Whether this represents an inflammatory lesion of unknown etiology, or is the result of some disturbance in thyroid metabolism is impossible to state. In view of the history and the absence of evidence of hyperthyroidism it would seem that this picture is best explained on the basis of an inflammatory reaction of unknown etiology.

Riedel's Struma (Cast-iron Struma; Ligneus Thyroiditis; Chronic Fibrous Thyroiditis).—This is a condition which occurs almost entirely in the older age group, past fifty-five years, and therefore is easily confused with thyroid carcinoma clinically. It is usually unilateral although it may be symmetrical in distribution. It is initiated by a swelling of the thyroid gland, which subsequently becomes replaced by a dense fibrous tissue reaction. This fibrosis is so unusually dense that it is usually described as being of the consistency of iron or wood, from which these various terms have been derived in its nomenclature. It runs a slow, progressive course with the development sometimes of a myxedema. More often, however, the process is so slow in its development that compensatory glandular hyperplasia occurs and no change in the metabolic picture is noted. In some cases it appears to be a chronic progressive condition. In others, it appears self-limited, the process seems to stop and the patient recovers and leads an entirely normal existence. Curiously enough, the patients do better if the involved part of the gland is removed surgically. This would perhaps suggest an infectious etiology in the nature of a virus, although this is by no means established.

Pathologically, the gland is characterized by a dense fibrous scarring replacement to a considerable degree of the normal thyroid acini. There is likewise very extensive lymphoid infiltration and the transitional picture between diffuse lymphoid hyperplasia, Hashimoto's Disease (Struma lymphomatosa) and the fibroid end stage of Riedel's struma suggests that they may be developmental phases of one and the same process, as Ewing believes. The evidence for dividing them into two distinct entities is largely based upon the fact that the Hashimoto picture occurs as a rule in the younger age group and apparently clears up spontaneously in the majority of cases. At all events, the two conditions represent two distinct clinical pictures, both inflammatory in character and suggesting the possibility of some low grade infectious agent as the etiologic initiating agent, not unlikely a virus yet unknown (Fig. 608).

ILLUSTRATIVE CASE

CASE 260 (Ref. #S-387)

Diagnosis.—Thyroid gland—Riedel's struma (cast-iron struma; chronic ligneous thyroiditis; benign granuloma).

Patient was a white female of 49 years, admitted to the hospital because of a swelling of the right side of her neck of about six months' duration.

Present Illness.—The onset of the patient's illness was approximately six months before the present admission at which time she noted moderate swelling of the right side of her neck, which gave her a sense of pressure with certain positions of her head. She was seen by a local physician who believed she probably had hyperthyroidism, and had been treating her with potassium iodide during this interval, but without any noteworthy improvement. She came to the hospital for observation. The diagnosis of hyperthyroidism seemed justified by the fact she showed definite palpitation of her heart on exertion, and had a sense of constriction in her neck accompanied by a nervous type of irritating cough. There had been intermittent hoarseness. She felt that she had been more nervous and irritable than normal, slept poorly and fatigued very easily.

Past Medical History.—The patient's past medical history did not seem particularly significant. She had the usual childhood infections. She had never had any symptoms of hyperthyroidism until her present illness. She had not been subject to upper respiratory infection. She had never previously been heart conscious. Gastrointestinal history was negative. Menses had begun at the age of twelve and had been regular. She had had two children. Her last period had been six months before admission and she believed she was going through the menopause.

Physical Examination.—The patient was a well-developed, somewhat thin type of individual. Head was not remarkable. Pupils were regular and reacted normally. There was no exophthalmos. Nose and throat were negative. There was a marked swelling of the right side of the neck. On palpation this was found to be due to increase in the size of the thyroid on that side. No comparable enlargement was noted on the opposite side, although it did appear somewhat larger than normal. This right sided enlargement was asso-

ciated with considerable fixation of the gland although the skin overlying it was not involved. There was no apparent deviation of the trachea. The chest was symmetrical. The lungs were clear. Heart was not enlarged but the rate was slightly increased to 94. Blood pressure was normal. Abdomen was negative. Extremities were negative.

Laboratory Findings.—The blood count, on admission, showed 3,800,000 red blood cells with 76% hemoglobin. White blood cells, 8,400 with 61% neutrophiles. Urinalysis was negative. Basal metabolic rate was minus ten.

Subsequent Course.—On the basis of the history and physical findings, subtotal thyroidectomy was advised. This was done and the right lobe of the thyroid was removed including a portion of the isthmus. The patient made an uneventful recovery and two years postoperatively was free from symptoms. She showed no evidence of myxedema in spite of a basal metabolic rate, at that time, of minus fifteen, and seemed generally to be in excellent health.

Pathological Report.—*Gross Description.*—The specimen consisted of a considerably enlarged lobe of thyroid measuring approximately 8 x 5 x 5 cm. It was of almost stony hardness. It appeared adherent to the surrounding structures, and it was difficult to identify the true capsule. On section, it was of a grayish-white color. It showed no evidence of necrosis or hemorrhage. From the morbid anatomical standpoint, it was very strongly suggestive of neoplasm, but this was not conclusive and it was felt that the diagnosis would have to be established on a histologic basis.

Microscopic Description of a Section Through the Gland.—(Fig. 608) Histologic study of the tissue presents the typical picture of the so-called Riedel's struma. Under low power it is almost impossible to recognize the tissue as of thyroid origin, as it consists almost entirely of dense connective tissue with areas of lymphocytic infiltration, which here and there shows the presence of actual germinal centers and follicle formation. However, occasional thyroid acini are found embedded in this collagenous tissue, which can be identified by the character of the lining cells and the presence of colloid within them. Much of this acinar epithelium, however, has undergone metaplasia with the formation of large, cuboidal cells with a great increase in the amount of cytoplasm. This stains intensely with eosin. It apparently represents a chronic hypertrophy on the part of the glandular tissue in an attempt to maintain normal thyroid function. The picture, as a whole, suggests one of very advanced chronic inflammation and scar tissue formation.

TUMORS OF THE THYROID

The following abbreviated classification of the tumors which arise in the thyroid is suggested in the hope that it may be of some material assistance in their understanding:

A. Benign tumors
  I. Benign adenomata
    1. Papillary adenomata
    2. Fetal Adenomata
      a. Embryonal (Fig. 605)
      b. Follicular (Fig. 317)
    3. Simple colloid adenomata (Fig. 606)
B. Malignant tumors
  I. Malignant adenomata
    1. Benign metastasizing struma
  II. Adenocarcinomata
    1. Papillary (Fig. 611)
    2. Giant cell type (Fig. 612)
    3. Spindle cell type (Fig. 613 and 614)
    4. Small round cell type (Fig. 610)
  III. Sarcomata
    1. Lymphosarcoma (?)
    2. Fibrosarcoma (?)

Benign Tumors of the Thyroid.—The great majority of the true tumors of the thyroid arise as benign adenomata in one form or another. Among these should be mentioned the papillary type of tumor which has occasioned considerable argument in regard to its origin. We are firmly of the opinion that it is derived from the lateral anlage in its migratory course downward in the neck. This view is held because the tumors which arise in such lateral aberrant thyroid structures invariably tend to show this particular type of papillary hyperplasia. Such tumors are likewise encountered in the lateral lobes of the thyroid gland itself and retain this same distinctive papillary pattern in contradistinction to the usual follicular appearance of those tumors which are derived, we believe, directly from the medial anlage.

Of those tumors derived from the medial anlage, the simplest represents the so-called fetal adenoma. This may occur in several forms depending upon the stage of differentiation of the epithelium at the time the tumor developed. Thus, we find *embryonal* varieties of adenomata in which the tumor is made up of cords and trabeculae of epithelium with little or no tendency toward lumen formation and a complete absence of colloid (Fig. 605). Second, there is the more common *follicular* type of fetal adenoma in which beginning acinus formation is noted as small, discrete acini made up of low, flat cuboidal epithelial cells with the beginning accumulation of colloid in those of the periphery (Fig. 317). Both of these tumors tend to grow centrifugally and to show degenerative changes centrally. Cystic degeneration and secondary cellular infiltration is not at all uncommon. As a third variety of adenoma, we find the simple *colloid* type which, however, is a true adenoma arising from completely differentiated thyroid epithelium. Such tumors are with great difficulty differentiated from the pseudo-adenomata, or localized areas of colloid involution as seen in the nodular goitre.

Malignant Tumors of the Thyroid.—Between ninety-five and ninety-eight per cent of all malignant tumors of the thyroid may be safely said to arise from pre-existing adenomata. For that reason it is still to be considered as good prophylaxis to remove such tumors when they are recognized clinically in their benign stage. Actually, probably not more than five per cent of such benign tumors ever undergo true malignant degeneration, but when malignancy does occur, there is an extremely high mortality rate except in the case of the group of papillary adenocarcinomata.

ILLUSTRATIVE CASE

CASE 261 (Ref. #S-178)
Diagnosis.—Thyroid—embryonal (fetal) adenoma.
Patient was a white female housewife of 45 years, admitted to the hospital with the chief complaint of a lump in her neck which had been increasing in size over a period of two and one-half years.

Present Illness.—The onset of the present illness was quite indefinite, but the patient stated that she first noticed a small lump in the right side of her neck about two and one-half years before admission. This had not been painful at any time. There had been no swelling over the lump nor had it shown any redness. She noticed that it moved every time she swallowed. This had slowly increased in size from a barely palpable nodule to a lump about the size of a walnut during this period of time. Recently she had noticed some slight dysphagia and a little hoarseness of her voice. There had been no dyspnea. She had not noted any increased nervousness. She had not suffered from insomnia. She had not felt any palpitation of the heart and had not been easily tired. She had noticed a loss of about ten pounds in weight during the preceding six months.

Past Medical History.—The patient's childhood medical history was apparently uneventful. She could not recall that she had ever had any of the ordinary childhood infections. She had had no serious illness except for a major abdominal operation for fibroids. A review of her systems was otherwise essentially negative. She had had no undue amount of upper respiratory infection. She had never been heart conscious. She had always been constipated but otherwise had had no gastrointestinal symptoms. Her appetite had always been good. Her genito-urinary history was normal for the most part. Menses had begun at the age of twelve and had been regular. She had had four normal pregnancies. Three years before admission, she had had an operation for fibroids. She had not had any menstrual periods since that time.

Physical Examination.—The patient was a well-developed, middle-aged, white female who did not appear at all ill. She showed no dyspnea or cyanosis but did have some slight dysphagia with solid food. Head was negative. Eyes showed no exophthalmos. Pupils reacted normally to light and accommodation. Nose and throat were negative. She had a compensated partial edentia. There was a swelling of the right side of the neck over the lateral lobe of the thyroid. There was a firm, round mass about the size of a walnut which was not attached to any of the surrounding tissues or to the skin. It moved on swallowing in the perpendicular plane. It was not tender and not definitely fluctuant. Chest was symmetrical. Expansion was equal. Lungs were clear. Heart was

not enlarged. Rate was 84. There were no murmurs. Blood pressure was 140/84. Abdomen: There was an old midline lower abdominal scar. Otherwise, the abdomen was negative. Extremities were normal.

Laboratory Findings.—Red blood cells on admission numbered 4,490,000 with 14 grams of hemoglobin. White blood cells, 6,750 with 61% neutrophiles.

Subsequent Course.—On the basis of these findings, a diagnosis of probable adenoma of the thyroid was made and excision advised. This was done and a small cystic nodular mass was removed from the left lobe of the gland.

Pathological Report.—*Gross Description.*—Specimen consisted of an irregularly spherical mass of tissue measuring 3 cm. in its greatest diameter. One surface of this nodule was smooth and covered by what looked like the capsule of the thyroid. The other surface showed some adherent thyroid tissue where it had been excised. On section there was found a moderate amount of cystic degeneration centrally. The mass had a semblance of a fibrous capsule around its periphery. It was yellowish-white in color in the peripheral portion and showed some hemorrhage into the cystic central area.

Microscopic Description of a Section Through the Tumor.—(Fig. 605) Histologic study of the tumor shows it to be a typical adenoma of the so-called embryonal type. A definite fibrous tissue capsule can be identified in which considerable chronic inflammatory lymphocytic infiltration has occurred. The main bulk of the tumor is made up of closely packed cords and trabeculae of rather large cuboidal epithelial cells separated by delicate strands of connective tissue and small capillary vessels. These cells have relatively large, uniform, round or ovoid nuclei with rather prominent nucleoli and a scattering of coarse chromatin granules. The cytoplasm is relatively pale. Here and there the slightest suggestion of beginning acinar formation is seen. For the most part, the lesion is composed of too young, undifferentiated cells to demonstrate the glandular nature of the tissue.

MALIGNANT ADENOMATA.—Under the term *malignant adenomata* have been described a large number of tumors of the thyroid, which present only one histologic feature suggesting malignancy. This is an invasion of the sinuses or capillaries usually either just beneath the capsule or actually in the capsule itself. In other respects, such tumors maintain the usual morphology of the type of benign adenoma from which they are derived. It has been shown that a small proportion of such tumors may actually metastasize by way of the blood stream as emboli and form new tumor nodules wherever they happen to become implanted. The most common places for such tumor development are seen in the lung and long bones, although the liver and other viscera may at times become involved. The great majority of these tumors, however, which show such vascular invasion never manifest this widespread metastatic picture. It is generally believed that such tumor invasion of the blood vessels behaves more in the nature of a simple thrombus than as a truly malignant tumor and results ordinarily in a re-endothelialization of the lumen of the vessel. Such tumors are malignant only in the sense that distant nodules of tumor tissue may develop from this original site. They do not present the usual evidence of malignancy with local invasion and with the toxic manifestations of cancer generally as exemplified by anemia, cachexia and death.

Benign Metastasizing Struma.—By this paradoxical term is meant a particular variety of the above malignant adenomata in which the metastasizing tumor tissue is derived from a well-differentiated, simple, colloid adenoma as a rule. Thus, when such lesions are demonstrated as metastatic nodules and result as they sometimes may in pathological fractures of the long bones, examination of the tissue reveals an entirely normal-appearing thyroid structure.

If such a lesion had resulted from the blood stream invasion of an embryonal or fetal adenoma, then the same type of relatively undifferentiated thyroid tissue would be found in the metastatic lesion, and the tumor would ordinarily be termed a metastatic malignant adenoma. When the lesion occurs as the result of such a colloid adenoma then it lacks the usual characteristics of true tumor and this somewhat anomalous term of "benign metastasizing struma" has been applied to the metastatic lesion. Occasionally individuals with such lesions show a moderate hyperthyroidism due, presumably, to the fact that these metastatic lesions are composed of essentially normal thyroid tissue, and as a result there may be an actual excess of normal thyroid secretion. Usually, however, this feature of hyperthyroidism is lacking as the normal balance of the metabolic requirements is maintained by the endocrine system as a whole.

ADENOCARCINOMATA.—The adenocarcinomata, as indicated in the suggested classification, are of four major varieties from the histologic standpoint. As has already been indicated, it is believed that well over ninety per cent of such malignant tumors are derived from pre-existing benign adenomata. Rarely, a diffuse adenocarcinoma of the thyroid is found both clinically and pathologically in which this initial adenomatous origin is impossible to detect, just as in occasional instances we may find diffuse tumors of the breast or other glandular organs which are not unicentric in origin.

Papillary Adenocarcinomata.—The papillary type of adenocarcinomata is more likely to occur at an early age in young adults. It is thought that they arise from the lateral anlage of the gland and for some unexplained biological reason possess certain distinctive clinical and pathological characteristics as a result. They are somewhat more radiosensitive than the other varieties of malignant neoplasms. The combination of surgical and irradiation therapy should result in better than an eighty per cent cure. A considerable number of them have been reported as treated surgically alone without subsequent recurrence.

Microscopically (Fig. 611) these tumors are similar in appearance to the benign papillary adenomata, but presenting the usual features of malignant transformation. The cells undergo varying degrees of anaplastic reversion with invasion of the stroma and of the capsule. Mitotic figures are found in moderate numbers. Typically they metastasize directly by the lymphatics as well as by local invasion, and are much less frequently seen invading the blood stream than any other form of thyroid tumor.

ILLUSTRATIVE CASE

CASE 262 (Ref. #S-388)

Diagnosis.—Thyroid—papillary cystadenoma (aberrant thyroid with early malignancy).

Patient was a white female of 20 years, who entered the hospital because of a lump in the right side of the neck.

Present Illness.—The onset of the present illness was only a matter of a few weeks during which she noticed that there was a nodular mass posterior to the lower end of the sternocleidomastoid muscle in the supraclavicular space which had slowly increased in size. These lumps were not tender and gave no subjective symptoms. She could not feel any other similar masses elsewhere.

Past Medical History.—Her past medical history was entirely uneventful. She had had the usual childhood diseases. A review of her systems was negative. Her cardiorespiratory history was uneventful. Gastro-intestinal history was normal. Menstrual history began at the age of sixteen and had been regular since that time. She had had no symptoms of hyperthyroidism.

Physical Examination.—Patient was a well-developed, well nourished young, white female who did not appear in the slightest degree ill. Head was normal in contour. Eyes were negative. The pupils reacted normally to light and distance. Nose and throat were negative. There was a large irregular mass found in the right side of the neck, which appeared to be made up of discrete nodes varying in size from one centimeter to three centimeters. These were relatively firm and elastic in consistency and did not appear fluctuant. They were not tender and did not seem matted together. Chest was symmetrical. Lungs were clear. Heart was negative. Abdomen: No masses or tenderness were felt. Extremities were negative.

Laboratory Findings.—Red blood cells 3,600,000 with 72% hemoglobin. White blood cells 7,600 with 63% polymorphonuclears. Urinalysis was negative.

Subsequent Course.—A pre-operative presumptive diagnosis of tuberculous cervical lymph nodes was made and it was recommended that one of these be removed as a biopsy specimen to confirm the diagnosis. This was done and a diagnosis of a papillary cystadenoma of the thyroid with possible carcinomatous change was made. On the basis of this pathological report, a complete dissection of the lymph nodes of the neck was done. Postoperative irradiation therapy was given, and six years after the operative procedure, no recurrence had taken place.

Pathological Report.—*Gross Description.*—Specimen consisted of an encapsulated tumor mass measuring 2 cm. in diameter. It was irregularly ovoid in outline, purplish red in color and covered with sanguineous fluid. The cut surface consisted of soft, friable, semitranslucent pink tissue which tore easily. It appeared finely papilliferous.

Microscopic Description of a Section Through the Tumor.—(Fig. 611) Histologic study of the tissue shows marked papillary hyperplasia of the epithelium with some tendency to alveolar formation. There is a very fine, loose connective tissue stroma which has taken no active part in the proliferative reaction. In various parts of the specimen, typical thyroid acini which show a tendency toward colloid production are seen. In several places, the hyperplastic epithelium appears to be attempting to break through the capsule. Here and there some calcific deposition may be observed. No mitotic figures are encountered. The cells, for the most part, are of a rather columnar type. The nuclei are uniform in appearance with rare mitotic figures.

Giant Cell Type.—The giant cell type (Fig. 612) of these tumors usually occurs in the late fifties or early sixties and runs a rapidly fatal course, rarely more than six to eight months in duration. These tumors are characterized by the presence of extremely anaplastic appearing tumor tissue in which no suggestion of thyroid architecture as a rule can be recognized. Many large tumor giant cells with multilobulated, hyperchromatic nuclei are found.

There is a striking tendency for perivascular proliferation of the tumor cells with necrosis in those areas removed from the blood supply. They have generally been considered in the past as a form of sarcoma, but in studying a considerable series of these cases it has been shown conclusively that transitional areas showing definite origin from acinas cells may be found, so that their epithelial nature seems indisputable.

ILLUSTRATIVE CASE

CASE 263 (Ref. #S-389)
Diagnosis.—Thyroid gland—giant cell carcinoma.

Patient was a white female, forty-nine years of age, admitted to the hospital with the chief complaint of a mass in her neck which had been rapidly increasing in size during the preceding month.

Present Illness.—The onset of the patient's present illness should perhaps properly date back to a period twenty years previously when she first noticed a lump in her neck. This, however, had remained constant in size during that entire period and had never caused any symptoms until a month before admission when it suddenly started to grow and had increased in size about four times during that interval. It was not particularly painful but was somewhat tender on deep palpation. It had caused considerable discomfort in swallowing and she had noted in the last few days a moderate amount of hoarseness in speaking.

Past Medical History.—The patient's past medical history was essentially negative. She had had the usual childhood infections. She had had no serious illness during her entire life. In reviewing her systems, it appeared she had no more than the usual number of upper respiratory infections. Gastro-intestinal history was characterized by a long-standing chronic constipation. Menstrual history had begun at the age of twelve and had been regular up to the present time. She had been married twenty-six years and had had four normal pregnancies. She had no symptoms referable to her thyroid at any time.

Physical Examination.—The patient was a well-developed, well nourished, middle aged woman who appeared to be resting comfortably in bed. Examination of her head revealed nothing unusual. Eyes were negative and reacted normally. Ears, nose and throat were normal. Teeth were in fair condition. There was a large mass occupying the entire right side of the neck. This was approximately the size of a large grapefruit. It moved with swallowing. Chest was symmetrical. Lungs were clear. Heart was not enlarged and showed no murmurs. Abdomen was somewhat obese. No masses or tenderness were felt. Extremities were negative.

Laboratory Findings.—Red blood cells, 3,800,000 with 78% hemoglobin. White blood cells, 9,400 with 74% neutrophiles. Urinalysis was negative. Wassermann was negative.

Subsequent History.—The patient was advised to have a radical excision of the mass which seemed to involve the thyroid. This she agreed to, and the mass with what remained of the thyroid gland on that side was removed. The patient made an uneventful postoperative recovery, but died three months later of recurrence and extensive generalized metastasis.

Pathological Report.—*Gross Description.*—Specimen consisted of a large, semi-encapsulated tumor mass 12 cm. in its greatest diameter. On section it was found to be filled with soft, crumbling, necrotic tumor tissue. In places, this showed definite invasion of the capsule and of the surrounding relatively normal thyroid tissue.

Microscopic Description of a Section Through the Tumor.—(Fig. 612) Histologic study of the tissue shows it to be made up of a wildly anaplastic, highly malignant, rapidly growing tumor. In many respects this suggests a sarcoma, but on studying carefully multiple sections, the inherent epithelial nature of the cells becomes apparent. There is a very striking tendency for a perithelial arrangement of the cells to be a prominent feature of the slides. The intervening areas show marked necrosis, probably largely the result of avascularization. Enormous multinucleated tumor giant cells are found. Corresponding with these giant cells are found many large, atypic mitotic figures. Mitoses, both typic and atypic, are found in great profusion throughout the tumor. Considerable secondary inflammatory leukocytic infiltration has occurred. Only here and there can some slight attempt at acinar formation be made out.

Spindle Cell Type.—The spindle cell variety (Figs. 613 and 614) of the adenocarcinoma is the most frequently seen of the entire group. It occurs at all ages and particularly in the late forties and early fifties. All gradations of malignancy may be seen from tumors in which the cells show only the earliest pressure changes with a suggestion of conversion to a spindle form up to tumors composed of elongated spindle cells, which resemble closely wildly-growing anaplastic fibrosarcomata. Here, likewise, at times, atypical tumor giant cells may be seen. By the use of differential stains and because of the fact that all gradations from a simple adenomatous type of tumor to this diffuse spindle cell picture have been demonstrated, the epithelial nature of these tumors is likewise established on firm foundations. The mortality in this group varies roughly with the degree of anaplasia. The percentage of recovery correspondingly varies, but the group as a whole may show as high as thirty to forty per cent cure by surgery. Irradiation is of little value, the tumors being highly radioresistant.

ILLUSTRATIVE CASE

CASE 264 (Ref. #S-390)
Diagnosis.—Thyroid gland—spindle cell type of carcinoma from pre-existing fetal adenoma.

Patient was a white female of 57 years, who was admitted to the hospital because of recent rapid enlargement of a mass on the right side of her neck.

Present Illness.—The patient, to her knowledge, had had a lump in her neck for thirty-five years. This had remained the same size until approximately one month before her admission. It had never caused any symptoms either of a mechanical nature or of hyperthyroidism. During the past month the mass had more than doubled in size and had caused some hoarseness and discomfort with swallowing.

Past Medical History.—The patient's past medical history was irrelevant and essentially negative. She had had the usual childhood diseases. She had never had any symptoms pointing toward her thyroid. Her gastrointestinal history had been negative. Menses had begun at the age of twelve and had been regular throughout her active ovarian functional life. She had entered her menopause at the age of fifty-one. She had had three normal children.

Physical Examination.—The patient was a well-developed, somewhat obese, white female about sixty years of age in appearance. Head was negative. She wore glasses. Nose and throat were negative. She had compensated edentia. There was a mass on the right side of her neck in the thyroid region, approximately the size of a small hen's egg. This was not tender, seemed rather firm in consistency, but was not attached to the skin. Its edges were somewhat indefinite. Chest was symmetrical. Lungs were clear. Heart was not enlarged and showed no murmurs. Abdomen was obese. There were no masses or tenderness present. Extremities were negative.

Laboratory Findings.—Red blood cells on admission numbered 4,300,000 with 12.5 grams of hemoglobin. White blood cells, 7,200 with 64% polymorphonuclears. Urinalysis was negative. Wassermann was negative.

Small Round Cell Type.—The fourth variety of these adenocarcinomata is seen as a small round cell type (Fig. 610) of tumor which is very easy to confuse with lymphosarcoma. Typically however, like the giant cell type there is an antecedent history of a preëxisting adenoma with a sudden increase in

Subsequent Course.—A partial thyroidectomy with the removal of the mass was advised and carried out surgically. She made an uneventful postoperative recovery. The tumor recurred within a period of three months, and the patient died at the end of six months with extensive localized infiltration of her neck by the tumor and by x-ray evidence of lung metastasis—this, in spite of postoperative, intensive irradiation therapy.

Pathological Report.—*Gross Description.*—Specimen consisted of the major portion of a lobe of the thyroid measuring 7 x 5 x 4 cm. In the upper pole there was a tumor mass approximately 4 cm. in diameter. This showed some persistence of a capsule, but for the most part this deviation from the normal gland and surrounding structures could not be made out as the tumor had infiltrated the capsule and the surrounding structures. It was of a grayish white color and showed several areas of necrosis and hemorrhage.

Microscopic Description of the Tumor.—(Fig. 614) Histologic study of multiple sections taken from various portions of the tumor nodule shows evidence of a malignant neoplasm which obviously has its origin in a simple follicular fetal type of adenoma. In places, the acinar arrangement of the tumor can be well established. For the most part, however, the tumor shows a marked malignant transformation with the tumor cells having undergone a very striking spindling. In places this was only minimal in degree and a semi-acinar arrangement of the cells can be made out. In other places this is much more extreme approaching the appearance of an actual fibrosarcoma. Differential stains for the demonstration of a possible connective tissue origin for these cells failed to reveal any collagen. Mitoses are found in moderate numbers and principally of a rather normal type. However, here and there, large atypic mitotic figures can be identified and occasional large tumor giant cells are seen. The tumor shows very little stroma, although it has a moderately generous capillary blood supply. (Fig. 613 and 614.)

its rate of growth. There is the same high mortality and rapid course, the average life of the patient rarely exceeding a year after diagnosis is established.

Unfortunately, they are notoriously radioresistant in spite of their histologic appearance. During the past few years, as a result of the uniformly bad surgical results, these more malignant varieties of adenocarcinomata, including the giant cell variety, the more malignant spindle cell type, and particularly this small round cell form, after identification through biopsy, have been subjected to extreme degrees of irradiation with some suggestion that their course may be favorably altered in cer-

tain instances. It is possible that with improvements in irradiation therapy, the mortality may be reduced considerably.

Histologically, these tumors are composed of small round cells which are arranged with a suggestion of acinar formation as they develop. Later in the picture, this acinar arrangement is usually lost and is only faintly suggested here and there in the histologic study of biopsy or autopsy material. Again, by the use of special staining methods, particularly the various trichrome stains, their nonlymphoid nature can be fairly well established although less successfully than in the case of the giant cell or spindle cell tumors.

ILLUSTRATIVE CASE

CASE 265 (Ref. #S-391)

Diagnosis.—Thyroid gland—small round cell carcinoma.

Patient was a white female of 66 years, who was admitted to the hospital because of a mass in her neck of one year's duration which had shown rapid increase in size during the preceding three weeks.

Present Illness.—The patient had first noticed a small lump in her neck on the left side approximately one year before her present admission. This had not been accompanied by any objective symptoms. It seemed to increase somewhat in size during the year's period, but so slowly that she had not paid much attention to its presence. However, approximately three weeks before admission it had suddenly increased in size and had been accompanied by a considerable amount of discomfort. She had noticed an increasing hoarseness and some difficulty with swallowing, but she had not presented any symptoms suggesting hyperthyroidism.

Past Medical History.—Past medical history was essentially negative and irrelevant. She had had the usual childhood diseases. She had never had any history of hyperthyroidism. Gastro-intestinal history had been negative. Menstrual history began at the age of thirteen and had been entirely normal. Menopause occurred at the age of forty-nine. She had had three normal children all living and well.

Physcial Examination.—The patient was a well-developed, elderly appearing woman with iron gray hair. Head was normal in contour. Pupils reacted regularly. Nose and throat were negative. There was an irregular, stony hard mass on the right side of her neck in the region of the thyroid. The thyroid itself could not be well outlined on palpation. Chest was symmetrical. Lungs were clear. Heart was not enlarged. There were no murmurs. Abdomen was negative. No masses or tenderness were felt. Extremities were negative.

Laboratory Findings.—The patient's blood count on admission showed 4,600,000 red blood cells with 83% hemoglobin. White blood cells, 9,600 with 73% polynuclears. Urinalysis was negative.

Subsequent Course.—The patient was advised to have a radical excision of the mass and postoperative radiation therapy. This was carried out, but the tumor recurred within a month of the operation and progressed rapidly with diffuse generalized metastasis. She died four months postoperatively.

Pathological Report.—*Gross Description.*—The specimen consisted of a mass of thyroid tissue including a firm, white, irregular, nodular tumor measuring approximately 5 x 3 cm. in size. The specimen also included a definitely enlarged cervical lymph node 2 cm. in diameter. The origin of the tumor could not be well established grossly as having a definite adenomatous background, as no suggestion of capsule could be found. The tumor tissue merged indefinitely with the normal thyroid tissue which stood out by contrast as a gelatinous, brownish-red color. No evidence of hemorrhage or necrosis could be made out.

Microscopic Description of a Section Through the Tumor.—(Fig. 610) Histologic study of the tumor occasions considerable difficulty in differential diagnosis. At first glance, the tumor very strongly suggests a small cell lymphosarcoma, being composed of masses of small round cells having little or no supportive stroma or demonstrable blood supply. However, on more careful study it is noted that many of these small round cells are arranged in pseudo-acinar fashion with a suggestion of lumen here and there. The cells, furthermore, in places seem to retain a rather suggestive cytoplasm with definite cell membranes unlike the usual picture of a lymphosarcoma. The nuclei are small, round, hyperchromatic, but lack the usual distribution of the chromatin in the peripheral fashion so consistently found in lymphoid cells. Mitoses are very numerous, but show little departure from the normal. The picture is entirely consistent with the diagnosis of a small cell type of thyroid carcinoma, which ordinarily is believed to have its origin from a preëxisting follicular type of adenoma. The fact that the tumor did not respond to irradiation therapy further aids in establishing its diagnosis as carcinomatous rather than lymphosarcomatous.

SARCOMA.—The problem of whether or not sarcoma of the thyroid ever exists is still debatable. Ewing, in his book on neoplastic diseases, notes that no definitely proven case of sarcoma has yet been demonstrated. There are rare cases in the literature, however, which make such a definite statement somewhat hazardous, particularly in the group of small round cell tumors. Certain of these have been reported as following the so-called Struma lymphomatosa or Hashimoto's disease, and have been held by Graham, Warren, and others, to be a variety of lymphosarcoma. This is borne out to some extent at least by the fact that occasional of these small round cell tumors are radiosensitive, which is quite unlike the usual response of the small round cell tumor when it is derived from glandular epithelium. Similarly Zeckwer and others have presented cases as spindle cell sarcoma in which no apparent possible epithelial relationship could be demonstrated. However, the point is still moot and unsettled.

PART II

DISEASES OF THE PARATHYROID GLAND

CONGENITAL ANOMALIES

The problem of congenital anomalies of the parathyroid glands is largely one of numbers. Absence of the glands is incompatible with life but obviously only a minimal amount of parathyroid tissue is necessary to maintain the normal function of these structures. Ordinarily, they are paired organs, four in number placed bilaterally on the posterior surface of the thyroid gland. They are usually not much more than 0.5 cm. in their greatest diameter and merge so with the thyroid tissue that it is almost impossible to identify them. Careful anatomical studies have revealed variations from two to sixteen without evidence of parathyroid dysfunction.

From the physiological standpoint we know that they are intimately related to calcium metabolism. This is manifested by the withdrawal of calcium from the skeletal system as may be demonstrated in the case of diffuse hyperplasia or adenoma formation. With diminished parathyroid activity and corresponding alteration in the available calcium we find that tetany may follow as the result of alteration in the irritability of the neuromuscular juncture. In tetany it is noted that there is a hypocalcemia with a corresponding increased output in the urine with a reversal of the usual phosphorus/calcium ratio. The parathyroid is believed on the basis of indirect evidence largely to be a detoxifier and to prevent tetany, which is induced by some form of nitrogenous protein absorption. The discovery by Collip of a practical method of extracting the parathyroid glands with the production of a substance which is called parathormone has resulted in renewed interest in experimental studies of these glands. With the administration of this parathyroid extract or hormone, the production of marked hypercalcemia by withdrawal of calcium from the bone, and the development of metastatic calcification in the tissues can be established.

Clinically it has been shown that the great majority of cases of osteitis fibrosa cystica are associated with hyperparathyroidism. Indeed, many investigators go a step further and believe that the development of the typical benign giant cell tumor of bone is likewise related to similar hyperplastic activity of these glands. The recent reports of Mallory and his associates have demonstrated the fact that the pathological picture in the parathyroid presents certain rather striking differences in some of these clinical conditions. They differentiate between a simple diffuse primary hyperplasia of the gland and from a secondary type in relationship particularly to renal pathology. In the simple diffuse primary hyperplasia of the gland the cells are converted to the so-called "wasserhelle" or "clear" type. On the other hand, in those cases associated with renal insufficiency due to chronic glomerulonephritis, there is a hyperplasia of the "chief" cells with only comparatively few of the "clear" cells to be found. There is likewise an increase of the oxyphil cells in the secondary type of hyperplasia.

Functional Disturbances

Hypoparathyroidism.—Tetany.—The relationship of tetany to hypoparathyroidism is dependent primarily upon a drop in blood calcium as a result of destruction of the gland by some pathological process. This is seen particularly as a postsurgical complication. As has been discussed in relation to the vitamin deficiency diseases, the parathyroids are not alone the controlling factor in regulation of calcium metabolism. It is likewise dependent to a considerable extent upon Vitamin D so that the tetany of rickets and of osteomalacia is not in any way comparable to the picture of tetany as produced by hypoparathyroidism except as there is often a secondary hyperplasia of these glands as a compensatory mechanism.

Hyperparathyroidism. — In hyperparathyroidism, we have the picture of osteitis fibrosa cystica as the outstanding lesion. This is the result of withdrawal of calcium from the long bones with rarefaction. Marked deformities may result. This is associated with an increased blood calcium up to as high as fifteen to twenty milligrams, with corresponding reduction in the blood phosphorus. The phosphatase, however, is usually increased and this determination, from the clinicopathological standpoint, is one of the most valuable in the recognition of the picture of hyperparathyroidism. Another not infrequent complication of hyperparathyroidism is seen in the development of renal calculus. This is more often associated with adenoma of the gland than with a simple diffuse hyperplasia.

The problem of the relationship of the parathyroid to the kidney is somewhat confusing. It is suggested by Mallory and others that metastatic calcification of the renal tubular epithelium may develop with hyperparathyroidism. This is of sufficient degree at times to cause actual renal insufficiency. In this instance we are dealing with a primary type of hyperplasia; whether of the diffuse type or as the result of tumor formation is immaterial. On the other hand, as has been intimated, the parathyroid may undergo secondary hyperplasia as a result of chronic, long-standing renal disease. This is believed to be activated by the increased phosphorus retention through the renal insufficiency, which in turn stimulates parathyroid hyperfunction to reëstablish the normal balance of calcium and phosphorus. These brief comments emphasize the complexity of the problem but point the way in which experimental work is heading towards its solution.

Illustrative Case

Case 266 (Ref. #S-392) (Courtesy of Dr. Tracy B. Mallory. This case was included in a series reported by Castleman and Mallory in the American Journal of Pathology, 1935, Volume 2, page 1.)

Diagnosis.—Parathyroid gland—hyperplasia.

Patient was a male of 26 years, who entered the hospital because of intermittent attacks of right renal colic over a period of fifteen months.

Past Medical History.—The patient's past medical history was irrelevant.

Physical Examination.—Physical examination was essentially negative.

Laboratory Findings.—Urinalysis: Urine showed many finely granular casts of the hyperparathyroidism type containing calcium phosphate. Blood chemistry: Nonprotein nitrogen was normal. Serum calcium 15.1 mgm. Phosphorus 1.8 mgm.

X-ray revealed the presence of two small stones in the right ureter. Skeletal x-rays were negative.

Subsequent Course.—The ureteral stones were removed. Subsequently a parathyroid tumor just below the right lower pole of the thyroid at the sternoclavicular junction was resected. Directly beneath this lay a second much larger tumor which came from the surface of the prevertebral fascia and the lateroposterior aspect of the trachea and esophagus. This was also excised. The following day the serum calcium was 11.9 mgm. and the phosphorus 2.6 mgm. Two months later, the serum calcium was 10.2 mgm. and the phosphorus 2.3 mgm.

Pathological Report—*Gross Description.*—The first of the above described glands was well circumscribed, encapsulated and smooth. The surface was orange-brown in color and measured 1.5 x 1 x 0.6 cm. The second gland was similarly encapsulated, smooth, ovoid, soft in consistency and weighed approximately 15 grams, measuring 4.5 x 3.5 x 2.5 cm. The surface was reddish-brown. At one pole was a small cyst 0.8 centimeter in diameter filled with clear, colorless fluid. The cut surface was uniformly yellowish or reddish-brown, soft and glistening.

Microscopic Description of Sections from These Glands.—Histologic study of the tissue from the two glands reveals an identical picture. They are made up of large "wasserhelle" cells with no demonstrable "chief" or oxyphil cells present. No normal parathyroid tissue is found. The cells are arranged in true gland formation, in many places producing a characteristic pattern due to the peripherally placed nuclei. The cells are polyhedral in shape, sharply demarcated by a thin, eosinophilic membrane and vary from ten to forty micra in diameter. The nuclei are all approximately the same size averaging about eight micra in diameter. They are round or slightly ovoid, sharply outlined and moderately hyperchromatic, and have an eccentrically placed nucleolus. The cytoplasm is clear except for a little light pink-staining granular material. Many of the granules are composed of glycogen. There is no fat present except for a rare droplet in the stroma. The low power appearance of the sec-tion is so similar to the low power of clear cell renal carcinomata that distinction would be difficult if the source were not known. (Fig. 617)

TUMORS OF THE PARATHYROID

The tumors of the parathyroid are almost invariably of the simple adenomatous variety, although occasional instances of actual adenocarcinoma do occur. The parathyroids, containing as they do both oxyphil and "chief" cells (basophiles), may give rise to tumors in which one or the other variety of cell predominates. As a matter of interest, however, the great majority of these tumors are composed of a mixture of these cells, many of which tend to show marked glycogen distention, which by the usual method of histologic preparation are seen as so-called "wasserhelle" or "clear" cells. The symptoms relating to such adenomatous tumors are those of hyperparathyroidism and have already been discussed (Fig. 618). They are not dissimilar in their varieties to the pituitary tumors.

CHAPTER LXI

DISEASES OF THE DUCTLESS GLANDS (*Continued*)

PART I

PITUITARY

The pituitary gland arises embryologically from two sources. The anterior lobe develops from Rathke's pouch as an outgrowth from the pharynx. Normally, this stalk, just as in the case of the thyroglossal duct atrophies and disappears, but occasionally because of persistence of some of the cells, subsequent cystic or neoplastic development may occur. The posterior lobe is derived directly from the central nervous system arising in relation to the floor of the third ventricle and maintaining normally throughout its existence a few communicating fibers which form a definite pathway to the hypothalamus. In addition to the anterior and posterior lobes, there is an intermediate portion which is known as the pars intermedia. This is usually believed to be derived from the posterior lobe, but it is made up for the most part of basophilic cells which are arranged in a strikingly alveolar and epithelial fashion similar in a considerable degree to the alveolar arrangement of the acidophilic and chromophobe cells of the frankly anterior lobe. Their functional individuality has been emphasized by Cushing.

From the functional standpoint, the pituitary gland is without doubt the most extraordinary structure in the entire human body. Here we have a small, gland-like organ little more than 1 cm. in diameter to which have been attributed no less than ten specific hormonal activities. It is generally conceded that the pituitary regulates growth. It is associated with the development of the reproductive organs and their hormones. To it is likewise attributed a diabetogenic action. Experimental work points strongly to its intimate relationship to thyroid function and to the adrenal glands. It is likewise associated with lactation. Most of these functions have been attributed to the activity of the anterior lobe. The part which the posterior lobe plays has never been thoroughly established other than that from it can be extracted a substance, pituitrin. This is of particular significance in respect to its effect upon smooth muscle particularly as a vasoconstrictor and in its action upon the uterine musculature. Inasmuch as the pars posterior is composed entirely of fine nonmedullated nerve fibers, it has been extremely difficult to understand how these cells could produce a secretion which could be so widespread in its action. In attempting to explain this discrepancy, the usual hypothesis which has been advanced is that the pars intermedia is the secretory portion of the posterior lobe and that its secretions are passed along the pituitary stalk to gain entrance to the circulation.

Ranson has recently shown that the pituitary likewise contains an antidiuretic hormone, which apparently originates in the posterior division of the hypophysis in relation to its innervation by the nerve tract from the hypothalamus. Destruction of this nerve tract produces atrophy of the posterior lobe and the development of diabetes insipidus, and in this way has an important part in the function of body metabolism. Houssay's work over the past five years has definitely established the diabetogenic function of the anterior lobe. This is proven by the fact that animals in whom the hypophyses have been removed are hypersensitive to insulin, and that there is amelioration of pancreatic diabetes by the removal of the anterior lobe of the gland, which is followed by a recurrence of the diabetes by replacement therapy with anterior pituitary extract. It is believed by Houssay that the anterior pituitary controls gluconeogenesis from protein, while Russell, in a very recent review of the problem, suggests that carbohydrate loss is prevented through restraint of oxidation. There is some suggestion that the anterior lobe may likewise promote diuresis so that there is normally a balance between the diuretic

PLATE CXLVII
DISEASES OF THE DUCTLESS GLANDS

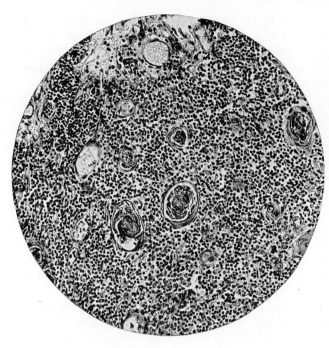

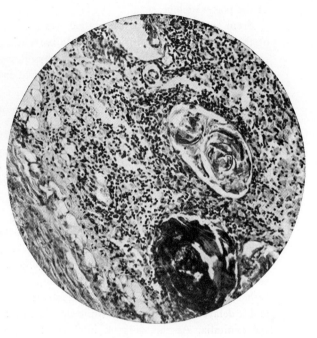

FIG. 619.—THYMUS: HYPERPLASIA—STATUS THYMICOLYMPHATICUS. —CASE 272.—Marked hyperplasia of small round cell element and reticuloendothelial stroma. Hassall's corpuscles relatively small and few in number. App. 100 x.

FIG. 620.—THYMUS: HYPOPLASIA—PERTUSSIS.—See CASE 180.— Relative reduction in small round cell element, prominence of reticuloendothelial stroma, and many large active-appearing Hassall's corpuscles. App. 200 x.

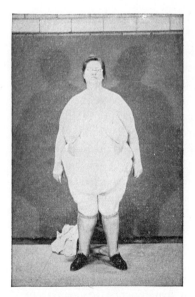

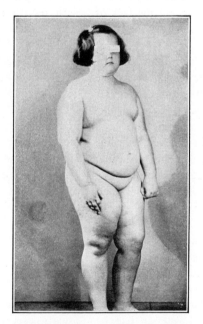

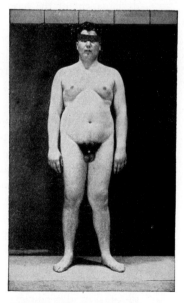

FIG. 621.—Hypophyseal adiposity in an adult female patient. Note distribution of fat chiefly restricted to trunk.

FIG. 622.—Hypopituitarism (Frohlich's syndrome) in a female child. Note extreme adiposity and delayed development of secondary sex characteristics.

FIG. 623.—Hypopituitarism in an adult male. Note feminine distribution of body fat and hair, and infantile genitalia.

action of the anterior lobe and the antidiuretic effect of the posterior lobe.

From the standpoint of the actual histopathology of the gland, there is surprisingly little morphologic change to account for the extraordinary physiological changes which occur in the body. As a matter of fact, very little has been established on anatomical grounds in respect to these functional disturbances. As in the case of the thyroid and the other ductless glands, it seems advisable to consider the pathological features largely on a functional basis, either as hypopituitarism or hyperpituitarism.

HYPOPITUITARISM

Several varieties of change in the body are seen dependent in part upon whether the disturbance of function of the gland occurs before adolescence or in adult life. The most familiar of these is spoken of as *Fröhlich's syndrome* or *dystrophia adiposogenitalis*. This usually results from some injury to the pituitary before puberty and results in marked changes in the appearance of the individual. Typically in the male, it produces the rather familiar picture of extreme obesity during childhood with a rather characteristic feminine distribution of the fat and a delayed or persistent infantile development of the genitalia. As this goes on into adult life, the failure of the secondary sex characteristics to develop is striking. The hair fails to develop and remains as an almost infantile type of soft down. Likewise its distribution persists as of the feminine pattern, with failure of the pubic and axillary hair to appear, absence of hair on the chest and the lack of development of the hair of the face (Fig. 622 and 623).

In the female, corresponding lack of genital development takes place with either the failure of the menstrual cycle to occur at all, or for irregular menses to appear. Particularly striking is the amenorrhea as the individual grows into adult life. The uterus and breasts likewise remain undeveloped. The skin presents a striking picture, likewise remaining almost of an infantile type, being extremely thin and smooth. As the individuals grow older, this soft skin shows a fine wrinkling due to defective development of the corium (Fig. 621). Basal metabolism is usually reduced and there is marked increase of sugar tolerance. Accompanying these physical changes there is apt to be a mental retardation, although this is by no means constant. Indeed, there is a considerable variation in the picture of hypopituitarism depending upon a number of factors. Among these must be emphasized the age at which the lesion appears, to interfere with the pituitary function, and thus modify the nature of the process. In some cases, there seems to be nothing but a depression of the normal function which may be temporary in nature and in these cases, the patient may be markedly benefited by pituitary replacement therapy. In such instances there may be some delay in growth, some retardation or delay in sexual development, or abnormal deposition of fat. In other instances the cause may be a true tumor of the pituitary itself. In these cases it is usually of the chromophobe cell variety. This is more likely to appear in the adult age group or at least not much before the age of puberty. The marked adiposity is apt to be lacking in these cases, but the abnormal distribution of the fat and the sexual immaturity is usually seen. Extra pituitary tumors such as Rathke's pouch, cystic tumors, suprasellar gliomata or tumors of the optic chiasm—all may produce pressure symptoms upon the pituitary with resultant depression of its function or actual atrophy of the gland.

Simmons' Type.—In one rather well recognized variety, the lesion is the result of some embolic process which produces infarction of the anterior lobe of the gland. This results in a curious senile picture spoken of as "progeria." The same lesion may occur in childhood or even in infancy, with the development of this same curious, premature senility, giving an "old-man" appearance to the child.

Lorrain-Erdheim Type.—In certain instances associated with destructive changes of the hypophysis early in life, there may develop a particular type of dwarfism (hypophyseal nanosomia). This has been described as the "Peter Pan" type of child. It is characterized by persistent immaturity, failure of sexual development and likewise failure of skeletal development, the long bones persisting in the almost infantile type without complete osteogenesis. It is usually associated with hypofunction or atrophy of the thyroid and adrenals as well. Curiously enough, however, these children usually show no mental retardation and are often particularly bright. This is

PLATE CXLVIII
DISEASES OF THE PITUITARY GLAND (HYPOPHYSIS)

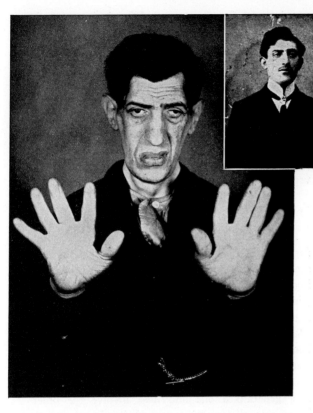

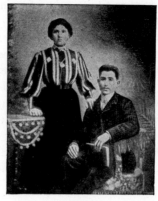
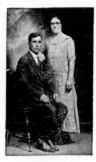

20 years   30 years

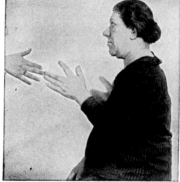
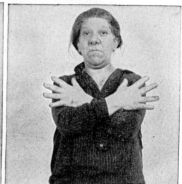

50 years

FIG. 624.—ADENOMA (EOSINOPHILIC): ACROMEGALY.—Cf. CASE 267.—(Case of Drs. A. Ornsteen & B. Gouley, Jewish Hospital.)—Photograph of thirty-year-old male with typical enlargement of facial bones and of the extremities. Insert shows same patient at age of nineteen.

FIG. 625—Progressive series of photographs of a patient at ages twenty, thirty and fifty showing development of typical facial and extremity characteristic of acromegaly. (Case of Dr. Michael Wohl.)

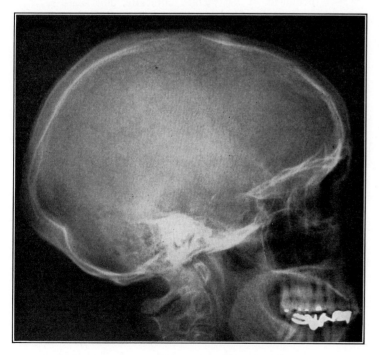

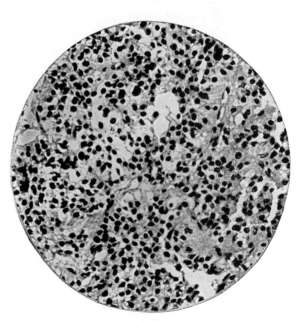

FIG. 626.—ROENTGENOGRAM—SKULL: PITUITARY ADENOMA.—The enlargement of the sella turica with erosion of the clinoid processes characteristic of pituitary neoplasm is well illustrated.

FIG. 627.—PITUITARY ADENOMA (EOSINOPHILIC TYPE) IN ACROMEGALY.—CASE 267.—Photomicrograph shows characteristic pleomorphic eosinophilic staining cells arranged in rather typical pituitary grouping with a delicate stroma. App. 100 x.

frequently spoken of as *pituitary dwarfism* in contradistinction to the Simmons' type of lesion.

Cushing's Syndrome.—In the group of Fröhlich's syndrome, as a subvariety, might well be mentioned the extreme adiposity which is almost entirely restricted to the face and trunk without involvement of the extremities. This is usually found in association with adrenal hyperplasia and indeed this particular picture is said to occur with such adrenal lesions alone. It implies a preadolescent destructive process of the gland. With our present knowledge of pituitary function as a whole, it is extremely difficult to understand this wide variation in picture which results from interference with its activities. There seems to be very little to correlate the variety of injury with the particular clinical picture, with the possible exception of the Simmons' type of hypophyseal senility. We can merely at this time record the observed phenomena and wait until the experimental data has accumulated to be able to evaluate these changes. Clinically such cases are not very frequently encountered.

HYPERPITUITARISM

In the hyperpituitary lesions, we seem to be treading on somewhat more secure foundations. There are only two well recognized varieties of anatomical change associated with such increased activity of the gland, and these are dependent upon whether the overactivity of the gland occurs before puberty or in adult life. Both varieties of change are almost invariably the result of a tumor of the anterior lobe and, rather characteristically, a tumor composed for the most part of the eosinophilic type of cell. Less frequently it may be seen in the preadolescent form, particularly as a diffuse hyperplasia of the gland as a whole rather than as the result of a discrete tumor. The preadolescent picture is spoken of as *gigantism,* while that occurring in the adult is referred to as *acromegaly.*

Gigantism.—In gigantism we are confronted with a marked overgrowth of the entire osseous system, but particularly of the long bones. This is usually followed, as puberty is reached, by a failure of sexual development. The growth phenomena are attributed to the hyperplasia or hyperfunction of the eosinophilic cells of the gland; and the secondary failure of sexual development is believed due to resultant pressure atrophy upon the basophilic cells of the gland, which are generally conceded to be associated with sexual activity. Not infrequently this picture likewise shows disturbances of carbohydrate metabolism which may be followed by the typical picture of diabetes. At operation or at autopsy, it is often noted that the tumor has undergone marked cystic degeneration, which accounts in part for the marked increase in size of the lesion at times, which may be visualized by roentgenologic studies of the sella turcica.

Acromegaly.—(Fig. 624 and 625) In the adult form of hyperpituitarism owing to the fact that the skeleton has become completely ossified, a less striking increase in height occurs. However, the same stimulus to bone production is exerted by the hyperplastic or adenomatous gland and results in this instance in a marked increase in the size of the bones, particularly the long bones. This is especially seen in the prognathous mandible, and in the enormous size of the hands and feet. The process is a generalized one and does involve the other bones as well so that vertebral involvement with the development of kyphosis is often very prominent and enlargement and thickening of the bones of the skull likewise is a not infrequent accompaniment of the picture clinically. For some reason there is usually an associated hyperplasia of all the supportive cells of the body. This is manifested by thickening of the subcutaneous tissues so that the skin becomes thick and coarse, and the lips, nose and ears prominent. The process is slowly progressive over a variable period of years, but sooner or later apparently becomes self-limited with the hyperplastic or adenomatous process causing such marked secondary atrophic changes of the other cell elements of the gland that the picture of hypopituitarism almost invariably follows. These are particularly characterized by the loss of the libido, by the development of adiposity and rather characteristically in a considerable proportion of the cases by mental torpor. Again, as in the case of gigantism, the recognition of the lesion may often be established by x-ray studies of the sella turcica, which usually is greatly increased in size, often with the loss of both the anterior and posterior clinoid processes (Fig. 626).

PLATE CXLIX
DISEASES OF THE ADRENAL GLAND

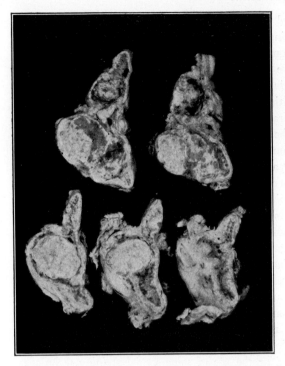

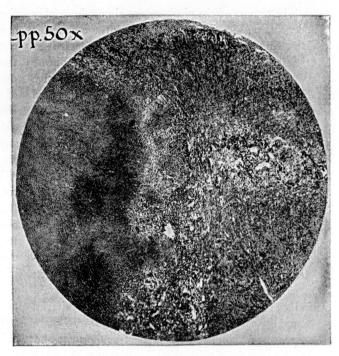

FIG. 628.—ADRENAL GLAND: ADDISON'S DISEASE.—CASE 268.—Gross photograph of cross section of adrenal gland showing the presence of multiple caseous tuberculomata.

FIG. 629.—ADRENAL GLAND: ADDISON'S DISEASE.—CASE 268.—Low power photomicrograph from Fig. 628 to show the characteristic caseous tuberculosis with extensive destruction of the adrenal substance. App. 50 x.

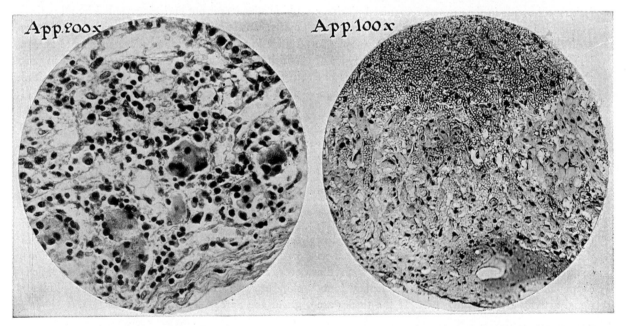

FIG. 630.—ADRENAL GLAND: ACUTE TOXIC DEGENERATION (see text, page 766).—Photomicrograph of adrenal cortex showing extreme destruction of cortical cells and marked secondary inflammatory cellular infiltration. Clinically this was evidenced by fatal adrenal insufficiency. App. 200 x.

FIG. 631.—ADRENAL GLAND—WATERHOUSE-FRIEDERICHSEN SYNDROME.—Photomicrograph showing extensive medullary and cortical hemorrhage and necrosis, associated with overwhelming meningococcemia. App. 100 x.

Tumors of the Pituitary

The tumors of the pituitary are almost invariably adenomatous in type and arise from the anterior lobe. Like many of the other ductless glands, it is at times difficult to differentiate between a diffuse glandular hyperplasia with involutional degenerative changes and a true tumor, but to all intents and purposes they may be considered as true tumors. The great majority of these lesions are entirely benign in nature from the histopathological point of view. The symptoms which they induce are either of a functional nature or as the result of pressure. The pituitary lying as it does in the sella turcica does not have any opportunity to expand or increase in size without coming in contact with the bony walls. Recent studies of pituitary glands taken routinely at autopsy from all types of cases have shown a surprising incidence of discrete lesions which have been described as adenomata. Certain such reports would indicate that as high as fifty per cent of pituitaries generally show such adenomata. These rarely are more than a millimeter in diameter at the most and are not associated with clinical symptoms. Whether they can be considered actually as true tumors or similar to the isolated adenomatoid nodules seen in the involutional thyroid picture is highly problematical. At all events in the cases of recognized pituitary dysfunction, whether of the hyperpituitarism or hypopituitarism type, we are apt to find hyperplastic lesions in which one or another of the cell types of the anterior lobe tend to predominate. This is one of the strongest arguments in favor of their true neoplastic nature.

Chromophobe Type.—By far the great majority of the above mentioned subclinical focal collections of cells as pseudo- or true tumors is represented by this type of cell hyperplasia. The exact function of the chromophobe cell has not as yet been established on sound experimental evidence, and such tumors, when they are found in relation to the various varieties of hypopituitarism which have been discussed in the preceding sections, are generally interpreted as being responsible more through pressure upon the eosinophilic or basophilic cells than from any functional activity on their own part. If the tissues are fixed in Zenker's or Bouin's fluid and stained with ordinary eosin and methylene blue technique, their chromophobe nature can easily be established. Indeed these tumors can usually be recognized even with the ordinary hematoxylin and eosin preparations because of the relatively clear cytoplasm and the rather characteristic arrangement in masses embedded in a rather well defined connective tissue septal type of stroma of the cells. By many it is believed they represent a "resting" stage, and that they may differentiate either as acidophilic or basophilic granular cells as required functionally.

Eosinophilic Type.—The tumor which is found almost invariably in relation to gigantism and acromegaly is seen to be composed for the most part of eosinophilic cells. These occur as almost solid masses of cells with very little interstitial stroma. Scattered through their substance will be found occasional chromophobe and even basophilic cells, but by far the majority of the cells are of this characteristic acidophilic type. These likewise may best be identified by the use of some special staining technique to bring out the inherent acidophilic nature of the cells.

Basophilic Type.—The existence of a true basophilic adenoma is not entirely accepted by all pathologists. Cushing has described a variety of pituitary tumor in which basophilic cells predominate and in which the clinical features already described in part in the preceding sections exist. This is characterized particularly by the localized adiposity of the head and trunk, the development of hirsutism, impotence and amenorrhea. Additional clinical findings of interest in this connection are seen as a rather striking hypertension, the development of erythremia and peculiar degenerative changes in the subcutaneous tissues which result in a rather typical wrinkling of the skin. As has already been emphasized, this picture is not unlike the picture of adrenal virilism and has been reported with almost identical clinical features without any apparent pituitary involvement. However, it does suggest very closely some interrelationship between the basophilic cells of the pituitary gland and adrenal cortical hyperfunction.

PLATE CL
TUMORS OF THE ADRENAL GLAND

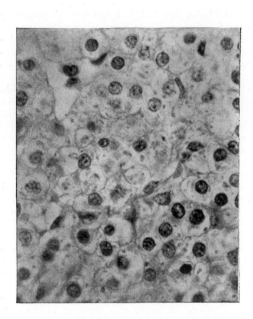

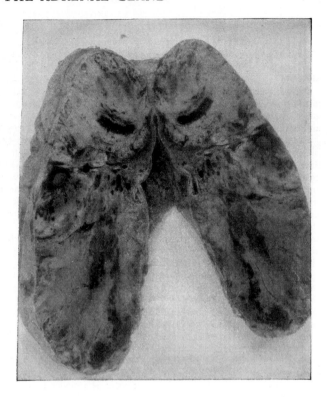

Fig. 632.—Cortical Adrenogenic Adenoma—Adrenal Virilism.—Case 269.—High power photomicrograph showing the histologic structure of the tumor shown grossly in Fig. 633. Note large size of cells, hyperchromatism of nuclei, and typical vacuolated appearance of cytoplasm. App. 300 x.

Fig. 633.—Cortical Adrenogenic Adenoma—Adrenal Virilism.—Case 269.—Gross photograph of large, yellowish adrenal tumor 17 cm. in length which shows numerous areas of hemorrhage and necrosis.

From Trans. of the Am. Ass. of G. U. Surgeons, 1927, 20:179; A. H. Crosbie & L. W. Smith

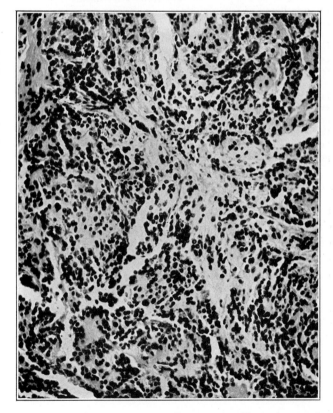

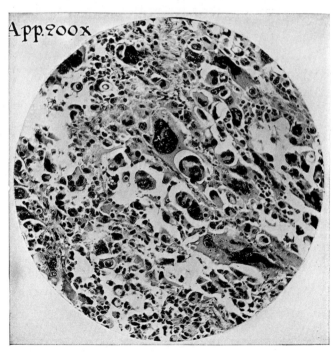

Fig. 634.—Neuroblastoma.—Case 270.—Photomicrograph showing clumps of relatively undifferentiated, small, intensely hyperchromic cells with a fibrillary background, and tending here and there to be arranged in pseudorosette fashion. App. 150 x.

Fig. 635.—Paraganglioma (Chromaffinoma, Pheochromocytoma).—Tumor composed of cells varying greatly in size and shape, staining intensely with chrome salts. In spite of their unusually malignant appearance they tend to remain as small, benign and encapsulated tumors. App. 150 x.

ILLUSTRATIVE CASE

CASE 267 (Ref. #S-221)

Diagnosis.—Pituitary—eosinophilic adenoma (acromegaly).

Patient was a white female housewife of 22 years, admitted to the hospital with the chief complaint of headaches of two years' duration accompanied by amenorrhea and enlargement of the hands, feet and face.

Present Illness.—The onset of the patient's present illness dated back somewhat over two years at which time she began to have attacks of rather generalized headache. These would last for several days at a time and would almost incapacitate her from work. They increased in frequency and severity during the interval since they first appeared up to the time of admission. Shortly after the onset of these headaches she noticed that her menstrual periods had ceased. For several months she interpreted this on the basis of pregnancy and so had not given it any particular consideration. However, when no other signs of pregnancy developed, she could not understand this amenorrhea and sought medical advice. She was treated symptomatically without relief. During the year preceding her present admission, headaches became much more definitely localized over the right fronto-temporal area. They were much more severe in character and would occur perhaps two or three times a month lasting for several days each time. She went to an optician, who gave her glasses for the headache, but this gave her no relief. During the past year she noticed that her fingers and toes, nose and jaw all seemed to be becoming somewhat increased in size. There was also a coarsening of the skin, especially of the face. These changes were not accompanied by any pain. A physician was seen who referred the case to the hospital for complete neurologic study.

Past Medical History.—The patient had always enjoyed unusually excellent health up to the present illness. As a child she had had measles, chickenpox, scarlet fever, mumps and diphtheria. At about the age of nine, she had complained of "growing pains," but these had disappeared after a few weeks. However, she had her tonsils removed at that time. A review of her symptoms was relatively negative. Up to the present illness she had never had headache that she could recall. Her cardiorespiratory system had been entirely negative. Her gastro-intestinal history was uneventful, the patient always having had a good appetite and digestion, and the bowels having always been regular. Menses began at the age of fourteen and had been unusually regular until

the present illness. She had had one normal pregnancy with a child two years old at the time of admission.

Physical Examination.—The patient was a well-developed and well-nourished young white woman who appeared in no immediate discomfort. Head showed no exostoses or sinus tenderness. There was a marked coarseness to her features with a broad nose, a rather grayish, pasty complexion and dry, rather heavy, medium brown colored hair. There was some suggestion of prognathism. Eyes showed thickening of both upper lids, but the reflexes were normal. Nose and throat were negative. Chest was symmetrical. Lungs were clear. Heart was not enlarged and there were no murmurs. Blood pressure was slightly reduced, 90/60. Abdomen was negative. Extremities showed almost spade like hands and large broad feet. Neurologic examination was essentially negative.

Laboratory Findings.—Red blood cells on admission numbered 4,600,000 with 12.5 grams of hemoglobin. White blood cells, 8,500 with 62% neutrophiles. Glucose tolerance test was normal. Urinalysis was negative except for a very slight trace of albumin on several occasions. No Bence-Jones protein was found. Blood Wassermann was negative. Blood chemistry was normal.

X-ray examination: The sella turcica was greatly enlarged, particularly in depth, with thinning of the dorsum sellae and the posterior clinoids. There was some erosion of the anterior clinoids. In view of the symptoms and x-ray findings, the diagnosis of an intrasellar neoplasm, probably a pituitary adenoma, was made.

Subsequent Course.—Removal of a cystic pituitary adenoma was done through a large transfrontal incision by curettage and suction.

Microscopic Description of a Section Through the Tumor.—(Fig. 627) Histologic examination of the tumor shows it to be composed of rather characteristically arranged clumps of cells embedded in a delicate connective tissue stroma. These cells are relatively large and pleomorphic in appearance. Many of them tend to show multilobulated giant cells of the definitely neoplastic type. Sections stained with eosin-methylene blue, after Zenker's fixation, show rather characteristically, the eosin staining granules of the typical acidophilic cells seen in the acromegalic type of adenoma. No mitotic figures, however, can be identified. Considerable hemorrhage and necrosis are present, and the diagnosis is reached only by the characteristic appearance of the individual cells rather than by any anatomical relationship which they possess.

CARCINOMA OF THE PITUITARY

The malignant tumors involving the pituitary gland are extremely rare. According to Cushing they make up less than two per cent of all pituitary lesions. When they do occur they seem to be related more particularly to the chromophobe cells than to either the acidophilic or basophilic varieties. In addition to these extremely rare adenocarcinomatous type of lesions malignant tumors may be found arising in relation to the stalk of the pituitary gland from a rem-

nant of Rathke's pouch. These are apt to be cystic in character because of their origin from the epithelium of the pharynx. They occur in one of two varieties either as an epidermoid type of carcinoma or as a tumor with the general features of the adamantinoma variety of basal cell carcinoma. In either instance they are usually of an extremely low grade malignancy with well-differentiated cells and only rare mitotic figures. There is very little evidence of even a local in-

to the time of his tuberculous infection. Genito-urinary history was entirely negative. He denied venereal disease.

Physical Examination.—The patient was an emaciated, middle-aged, white male who showed rather striking pigmentary changes as noted in his history. This not only involved the skin, but was noted also in the mucous membranes of his mouth. His head was not remarkable. Pupils were regular, equal and reacted normally. Nose and throat were negative. Teeth were in poor condition and showed marked caries. The mucous membranes were pale except for the pigmented spots already commented upon. The chest was symmetrical, but expansion was greatly reduced. The lungs showed dullness over both apices and bronchial breathing over the right upper lobe. The heart was not enlarged. Sounds were of fair quality, but distant. The pulse rate was slow, being only fifty-six. Blood pressure was 90/50. Abdomen was of the scaphoid type. There were no masses or tenderness felt on palpation. External genitalia were negative.

Laboratory Findings.—Red blood cells, on admission, numbered 3,100,000 with 63% hemoglobin. White blood cells numbered 7,600 with 69% polymorphonuclears. Sputum examination was negative on four occasions for tuberculosis, and positive on the fifth attempt. Urinalysis was negative except for occasional faint traces of albumin. Blood chemistry was negative. Wassermann was negative.

Subsequent Course.—The patient continued downhill steadily and died several months after admission.

Autopsy Findings.—Body was that of a fairly well-developed, but extremely emaciated, middle-aged male. The pigmentary changes noted previously had apparently become intensified since their original description. The heart was normal in size but flabby in consistency and pale in color. Lungs: There was an old fibroid phthisis involving the entire upper right lobe and extending to involve a portion of the middle lobe. In addition, there was a secondary involvement of the left apex. The liver, spleen and kidneys appeared normal. The adrenals were markedly enlarged. In the midportion of each there was what almost appeared like a tumor mass. However, on section these were found to represent caseous tuberculomata which had largely replaced both cortex and medulla, and which accounted for the picture of Addison's disease. (Fig. 628)

Microscopic Description of a Section Through Adrenal.—(Fig. 629) The persistent adrenal tissue appears to be fairly normal, although perhaps somewhat atrophic. The regular arrangement of the cortical cells is well preserved, but the medulla is less well defined. At one end of the section will be found a large typical caseous mass which presents the usual picture of tuberculosis with epithelioid proliferation. A few giant cells, moderate fibrosis and considerable mononuclear cellular reaction, chiefly lymphocytic, are noted.

HYPERADRENALISM

Hyperadrenalism is seen chiefly in relation to tumors of the adrenal cortex, but may occur as a simple functional hyperplasia of the gland as a whole. Normally, in the child at birth, the adrenal is found to consist of a relatively hyperplastic-appearing cortex with the thick layer of solid cells spoken of as the fetal cortex. This differs from the subsequent adrenal cortex in that the differentiation into zones has not occurred and the cells are lacking in their subsequent lipoid content. Very shortly after birth, the interval varying considerably in different individuals, this fetal cortex disappears and a gradual replacement by the typical adult type occurs. This curious transition is thought possibly to be due to the withdrawal of the maternal hormone and may be very similar in its mechanism to the termination of pregnancy itself. It is of interest to note that in the anencephalic monster the usual fetal cortex is lacking and the cortical portion of the adrenal is hypoplastic, but of the adult type. It so happens that in some individuals this

cortical replacement goes on at a very much more rapid rate than in others, even to the point of actual multiple pseudo-adenomatous projections of the cortex into or through the capsule of the gland. Many of these are symptomless or at least present only subclinical evidence of hyperfunction. On the other hand, occasional instances are seen in which a diffuse cortical hyperplasia is associated with marked sexual precocity on the part of the child. This sexual precocity is in the nature of a masculinizing action so that in the male the development of the genitals may occur as early as the second year of life in the typically adult form, and even voice changes have likewise been reported. In the female, the picture of pseudo-hermaphrodism is prone to appear. More often, this picture of *adrenal virilism* as it is termed appears in conjunction with a true tumor of the cortex and at a somewhat later age, although chiefly by adolescence. This will be described in greater detail in the following section.

TUMORS OF ADRENAL

Cortex.—ADENOMA.—As has already been indicated, occasional instances of cortical tumors are found in which a picture of adrenal virilism develops. The minor gradations of this picture very possibly

and not infrequently pass unrecognized when the lesion occurs in the male, as evidence has accumulated to show that the cortical hormone is particularly associated with masculinizing secondary sex characteristics. At most, under such circumstances, some exaggeration of the genital organs associated with early puberty is seen. In the female, on the other hand, and particularly when such tumors occur in the post-adolescent period, the features of virilism are much more striking. Under these circumstances one finds a complete transformation of the victim. There is a redistribution of the body fat toward the male type. There is atrophy of the breasts and genitalia. There is a marked hirsutism with hair developing on the face, chest and abdomen with the male pattern. There is often a corresponding change in voice; and more striking perhaps than any of these other features, a prominence of the clitoris, and amenorrhea. This condition is not uncommonly associated with hypertension, and reduction in the blood pressure following the operative removal of such a tumor is likely to follow. An almost dramatic return

to the female habitus follows within a few months after such operative measures. The menses reappear almost immediately and the other physical changes take place more gradually.

The pathology of this condition is usually one of a benign adenoma of the cortex although at times histologic features of malignancy may likewise be apparent. In general, the tumor is well encapsulated, varies considerably in size and may attain a diameter as great as ten centimeters or more. It is composed of typical adrenal cortical cells which may occur in abortive attempts at fascicular, glomerulosa zonal arrangement. The tumor is apt to be extremely vascular and on section shows some cystic degeneration. Like normal adrenal cortex, it contains lipoid material in large amounts and as a result is usually of a yellowish color with areas of hemorrhage emphasizing the pigmented picture.

ILLUSTRATIVE CASE

CASE 269 (Ref. #S-393)
Diagnosis.—Adrenal gland—cortical adrenogenic adenoma.

Patient was a white female of 38 years, admitted to the hospital because of pain in the left side accompanied by chills and fever.

Present Illness.—The onset of her immediate illness was of about one week's duration when she noted a marked frequency of urination associated with scalding. Accompanying this there were intermittent fever and frequent chills. There was a dull pain on the left side of her abdomen. There was no nausea or vomiting and no diarrhoea or unusual constipation.

Past Medical History.—The patient had an uneventful early medical history with the usual childhood diseases. A review of her systems was of great interest and significance in respect to her present condition. She had not been unduly susceptible to upper respiratory infections. She had never been heart conscious. Her gastrointestinal history was essentially negative. Her menstrual history began at the age of thirteen. She had flowed regularly except when pregnant until the age of twenty-nine, when her periods stopped altogether. The patient was married at the age of twenty-two. During the first year of her marriage she had two miscarriages. She apparently had a normal libido, but intercourse was always difficult on account of the size of her clitoris, which had increased over a period of one year or more. At the age of twenty she noted that she began to grow an excess amount of hair on the face, chest and abdomen. This became so extensive that she finally had to resort to shaving at least twice a week. Her voice had definitely changed, becoming much deeper. Breasts had atrophied so that they resembled those of a male. She developed a complete amenorrhea rather suddenly at the age stated, of twenty-nine. Her clitoris had continued to increase in size. As a result of these physical changes, her husband had deserted her, and she had been forced to earn her own living as a saleswoman.

Physical Examination.—The patient, at the time of admission, had a temperature of 103° but did not appear acutely ill. Her head was normal in contour. Voice was deep and of masculine quality. She had a considerable amount of coarse, black hair which had a male distribution over the face, with a well-developed beard and mustache. Her general body build was that of a male. Chest and abdomen were thickly covered with coarse, dark hair. Pelvis and hips resembled those of a man. Skin as a whole was coarse and dry. Chest was symmetrical. Breasts were atrophic and male in type. Lungs were clear. Heart was not enlarged and showed no murmurs. Abdominal palpation revealed a large tumor mass which did not move with respiration. This nearly filled the right side of the abdomen. It was not painful on palpation. Vaginal examination revealed a clitoris four centimeters in length, which closely resembled a penis. The labia were large and edematous. Bimanual examination revealed a normal vagina and uterus in good position. Extremities were negative.

Laboratory Findings.—Blood count on admission showed, 3,800,000 red blood cells with 68% hemoglobin. White blood cells, 14,800 with 86% polymorphonuclears. Urinalysis showed a large amount of pus and the presence of motile bacilli, which proved to be colon bacilli.

X-ray examination showed a normal, left-kidney pyelogram, but on the right side the ureter crossed to the left and the pyelogram showed the pelvis and calices of the right kidney to be below those of the left. The calices were pointed downward and outward. The tentative diagnosis on the basis of these findings was that of a probable pyelonephrosis of the right kidney.

Subsequent Course.—Exploratory operation was done by right oblique lumbar kidney incision. A large fluctuant mass covered with enormously dilated veins was exposed. This was tense. Careful dissection revealed it to have a pedicle of vessels, but to have no connection with the kidney and no suggestion of a ureter. It was assumed that this was a tumor of the adrenal gland on that side. The patient made an uneventful convalescence following its removal and was discharged improved, with her urinary tract infection cleared up.

Three weeks after leaving the hospital she had a normal menstrual period, the first in nine years. One year later she had entirely changed in appearance. The body fat had become redistributed resembling that of a female. Breasts had developed and the hair had disappeared from her face, chest and abdomen. Voice, likewise had risen to its original level. Physical examination at this time revealed no change in the size or appearance of the clitoris, but in other respects she had completely reverted to her normal feminine type.

Pathological Report of the Surgical Specimen.— *Gross Description.*—Specimen consisted of a large, ovoid mass measuring 17 x 12 x 10 centimeters. It was deep purplish red in color and on careful inspection almost suggested an acute splenomegaly. A narrow band represented the pedicle in which the blood supply was found. There was a definite capsule covering the entire mass, which was a rather slaty-blue color. Along the line of attachment of the pedicle, a small, yellowish area was found which suggested possible adrenal cortical chromaffin tissue. On section, the specimen was beefy red in color, extremely hemorrhagic, and showed many areas of cystic degeneration and hemorrhage. The tumor was so vascular that on section it lost approximately one-fourth

of its volume through the outpouring of blood. Numerous yellowish areas were seen around the periphery further suggesting adrenal origin. Centrally the entire tumor seemed to be made up of large, vascular spaces outlined by grayish trabeculae. A presumptive diagnosis of adrenogenic adrenal adenoma was made (Fig. 633).

Microscopic Description of the Tumor.—(Fig. 632) Histologic study of multiple sections taken from various parts of the tumor presents the histology of an adrenal adenoma of cortical cell origin. Many areas of cystic degeneration and hemorrhage are seen in the central portion. The capsule is well defined and shows no infiltration by tumor cells. The cortical portion of the tumor consists of cells which tend to be polyhedral in outline and to show some tendency to reproduce the zonal fasciculata of adrenal cortex. In some places they occur in almost syncytial sheets. The great majority of the cells have a finely vacuolated, foamy appearance which is so characteristic of adrenal cortical cells. The nuclei are fairly uniform in size and have a characteristic scattered arrangement of their chromatin as seen in normal adrenal cells. They have well defined nuclear membranes and nucleoli. Occasional extremely large giant nucleated cells are found with very dense staining nuclei five to six times the normal average size. Rare mitotic figures are seen. The picture as a whole seems to suggest an entirely benign adenoma of adrenal cortical cell origin of the type associated with adrenal virilism.

Medulla.—The tumors of adrenal medulla have already been considered in respect to the tumors of the nervous system arising as they do from the cells of the sympathetic nervous system. There are three varieties of such tumors which depend largely upon the degree of differentiation of the neuroepithelial tissue. These are spoken of as (a) the neuroblastoma or neurocytoma, (b) ganglioneuroma and (c) the paraganglioma (chromaffinoma or pheochromocytoma).

NEUROBLASTOMA.—The neuroblastoma represents a tumor which is almost invariably found as a primary lesion arising in the medulla of the adrenal in infancy or at least under the age of five. This is usually bilateral, or if not bilateral in origin, soon

spreads to the opposite gland. The tumor is likely to grow relatively rapidly and to attain a very considerable size, often filling the abdominal cavity.

Pathologically the tumor is made up of cells which range all the way from immature neuroblasts to fairly well defined adult neurocytes. The neurocyte type of neuroblastic tumor is more likely to be seen in an older age group. Characteristically, the cells are small, deeply-staining, with little cytoplasm and showing a rosette-like arrangement with nerve fibrils pointing toward a potential central area. The presence of such undifferentiated small neuroblasts with the characteristic fibrillary arrangement is entirely specific for this group of tumors, and is similar to the histologic findings of the retinoblastoma.

ILLUSTRATIVE CASE

CASE 270. (Ref. #S-295)
Diagnosis.—Adrenal—neuroblastoma.
Patient was a white male child of 3½ years, admitted to the hospital with the chief complaint of swelling of the eyes and pain in the lower extremities.

Present Illness.—The onset of the present illness dated back for about one month or six weeks. At that time the parents noticed that the child seemed to have had a fever at intervals, usually toward evening. This had been associated with considerable sweating and the development of a marked lethargy. He likewise showed paroxysmal attacks of edema of one or the other eye, which lasted for several days and then subsided. He complained bitterly of sharp shooting pains in the lower

extremities. This had not been associated with any redness, swelling or tenderness of the joints. The most outstanding features from the historical standpoint were the increasing lethargy, fever, and what appeared to be bone pains.

Past Medical History.—The child's past medical history was entirely negative. He was a full-term, normally delivered child, breast fed for the first eight months. He had had no nutritional difficulties and up to the present illness, none of the contagious diseases.

Physical Examination.—The patient was a fairly well-developed, but almost emaciated, young, white male child who showed no cyanosis, jaundice or dyspnea. Head was grossly negative. Ears were normal. Eyes reacted to light and accommodation. There was some mucopurulent discharge from the nares and the turbinates were congested as was the pharynx. There was a slight bilateral cervical adenopathy. The chest was symmetrical. Lungs were clear and resonant throughout. The cardiovascular system appeared normal except for a soft, blowing systolic murmur heard at the apex. This was thought to be hemic in nature. Abdomen was negative. The liver and spleen were not felt. There was no tenderness or rigidity. No masses could be felt in the abdomen. The extremities were normal. Temperature on admission was 103°; pulse 138, and respirations 36.

Laboratory Findings.—The blood count on admission showed 4,690,000 red cells with 10.5 gm. of hemoglobin. The white blood cells numbered, 17,300 with 58% neutrophiles, 33% lymphocytes and 9% monocytes. Urinalysis was negative. The Mantoux test was negative. Sedimentation index was slightly elevated. Because of the marked lethargy, lumbar puncture was done and a clear, colorless spinal fluid under no increased pressure was obtained. Blood chemistry was normal.

Subsequent Course.—Three weeks after admission, an angioneurotic edema of his upper lip developed suddenly in the course of two to three hours. This subsided after a period of three to four days. Shortly after this, a similar swelling occurred in his left eye which took about two weeks to disappear. Five weeks after admission, progressive swelling of the left jaw developed which within forty-eight hours, assumed considerable proportions and was accompanied by a large necrotic area over the mandible on the left side.

X-ray examination taken at this time suggested that the picture was neoplastic rather than inflammatory. Because of its location the thought that it might be some form of adamantinoma was raised. X-ray treatments were given and the tumor subsided almost immediately. However, within two weeks, recurrence had taken place and subsequent x-ray therapy had little or no effect in producing regression in size of the mass.

About two months after admission, a mass was found in the region of the left kidney. This was thought to be probably of adrenal origin and on the basis of the presence of this tumor mass, the interpretation of the jaw lesion was modified to a metastatic tumor, probably a neuroblastoma. The child continued to go downhill rapidly. He developed metastatic lesions which were palpable in the skull. Ultimately he became stuporous and died in one of a series of several generalized convulsive seizures, ten weeks after admission.

In reviewing the x-ray findings it was of interest to note that on admission there was no evidence of pathology in the lung fields, but that two months later the lungs were riddled with metastatic nodules. Similarly, the pelvis, both femora, tibiae and fibulae showed tumor invasion. Involvement of the left radius and of the scapulae and clavicles was found about one week before death, as were lesions in the vault of the skull and lumbar spine.

Autopsy Findings.—At autopsy there was a large tumor mass about the size of an orange, which had completely replaced the left adrenal. This had metastasized widely involving almost the entire skeletal structure of the body as well as the great majority of the viscera. The obvious diagnosis from the gross findings was that of a neuroblastoma of the Hutchinson type. The body was found to show marked emaciation. Several small elevated metastatic nodules could be seen in the scalp. A metastatic process was found involving the greater part of the left mandible. Just below the suprasternal notch was a large, elevated, metastatic lesion which was attached to the underlying sternum. Both lungs showed diffuse metastatic nodules throughout the lung parenchyma and in the subpleural tissues. The liver was composed of multiple masses of pearly white metastatic tumor nodules alternating with compressed areas of liver parenchyma. Some of the tumor nodules showed beginning necrosis and hemorrhage. The primary tumor had invaded the upper pole of the left kidney. No other renal involvement was found. Examination of almost any of the bones of the body revealed the presence of soft, brownish tumor tissue.

Microscopic Description of a Section from the Tumor.—(Fig. 634) Histologic study of a section from the tumor mass presents the rather characteristic picture of a neuroblastoma. The cells are small, round, with little or no cytoplasm as demonstrated by the usual staining technique. There is a tendency for these cells to be arranged in pseudorosette formation with occasional fine fibrillary like structures pointing centrally toward a pseudolumen. In many places the cells are arranged around small capillary blood vessels in similar pseudorosette formation. For the most part, however, they occur in clumps and sheets of cells showing little or no differentiation. There is considerable necrosis and hemorrhage. No adrenal tissue can be identified in any of the sections from the primary tumor itself. A moderate connective tissue stroma is present in some areas, and there is a rather generous blood supply with new capillary formation. The tumor is evidently rapidly growing as seen from the presence of many mitotic figures, some of which are atypic. The great majority of the cells tend to be pyknotic or at least hyperchromatic. The size, shape and arrangement of the cells with the absence of cell membranes and cytoplasm, and the distribution of the metastases identifies the tumor as one of neuroblastic origin.

HYPERNEPHROMA.—The true adrenal cell type of carcinoma or hypernephroma is seen arising in the same way as the simple adenoma from adrenal cortical cells. Unlike adrenal adenoma, it apparently does not usually show any functional activity, but only the usual features of malignancy. The structure varies considerably from massive sheets of relatively well-differentiated, vacuolated, lipoid-filled cells down to extremely anaplastic tumors with cells which may appear as nests or clumps without suggestion of any architectural arrangement and often showing a reversion toward the spindle cell of its ancestry. Tumor giant cells are frequently encountered with large atypical and multilobulated nuclei. Clinically the cases run a course very comparable to those of the renal type of tumor with blood vessel invasion and subsequent bone and lung metastases. Occasionally a simple adenoma with the characteristic clinical features of virilism may undergo such carcinomatous degenerative changes.

ILLUSTRATIVE CASE

CASE 271. (Ref. #S-339)

Diagnosis.—Adrenal gland—primary carcinoma.

Chief Complaint.—Patient was a twenty-five year old white male, admitted to the hospital because of pain and swelling of the right hip region.

Present Illness.—The onset of the present illness was somewhat insidious but, as well as the patient could determine, began about three months before admission. He had seen a physician who thought that the picture was one of some type of arthritis and treated him symptomatically with salicylates, without improvement. The lesion seemed to progressively increase in size and extended beyond the joint area so that the patient was referred to the hospital for x-ray studies.

Past Medical History.—Patient had had an uneventful medical history up to the onset of his present difficulty. He had had the usual childhood infections. He had never had any serious illness. A review of his systems revealed nothing particularly unusual in his history. He had occasional upper respiratory infections but never had any gastro-intestinal disturbances. His genito-urinary history was negative. He had never had any sexual precocity and had had a normal adolescence.

Physical Examination.—Patient was a well-developed, young, white male who showed some evidence of recent loss of weight. His head showed no deformity. His pupils were regular and reacted normally. His nose and throat were negative. His chest was symmetrical. His lungs were clear. His heart was not enlarged. His abdomen was not particularly prominent. There was some rigidity in the right lower quadrant in relation to the pathology in the right hip region. The external genitalia were normal in appearance. The left leg was negative. The right leg showed marked limitation of motion in the hip region and there was a large mass which seemed to involve the hip joint and ilium. It seemed to be integral with the bone.

Laboratory Findings.—The red cell count was 3,600,000 with 77% hemoglobin; white cells, 8,900 with 71% polynuclears. Urinalysis was essentially negative. Wassermann was negative. Blood chemistry studies showed a normal calcium-phosphorus ratio.

X-ray examination revealed an osteolytic process which involved the head and neck of the femur and a considerable part of the right ilium. This had the moth-eaten appearance of metastatic tumor tissue. The possibility of an adrenal tumor was raised but x-ray studies of the kidneys and air injection of the retroperitoneal tissues failed to demonstrate the presence of any definite tumor mass in either of the adrenals or the kidneys.

Subsequent Course.—Patient remained in the hospital for a matter of some six months, showing progressive involvement of more and more of his skeletal system by metastatic tumor. A mass appeared in the scalp about the size of a hen's egg. Another mass appeared to involve the right parietal bone of the skull. Several metastatic lesions were found by x-ray in the lungs, terminally. The patient went steadily downhill and in spite of intensive irradiation therapy, he died.

Autopsy Findings.—At autopsy the body was markedly emaciated with the eyes sunken in their sockets. The scalp showed a scarred, ulcerated area where the metastatic tumor had been removed for pathological study. The right hip region showed marked swelling. There was pigmentation of the overlying skin from the irradiation. Both knees showed similar enlargement and pigmentation. A tumor, approximately 3 cm. in diameter, was found in the right adrenal gland with a small similar appearing yellowish solid mass in the left gland. The lungs were diffusely filled with tumor tissue as discrete circular nodules and as plaques occurring on the pleural surface. There was extensive involvement of the skull, the lower lumbar vertebrae, of both femora and tibiae with invasion of the joint cavities, as well as the large mass involving the right side of the pelvic bones. As incidental pathological features, the presence of several small acute gastric ulcers in the pyloric region was found.

Microscopical Description of a Section from the Primary Adrenal Tumor.—Histologic examination of the tissue shows a rather typical tumor apparently of definite adrenal cortical origin. Here and there, there is a fair reproduction of the general architectural arrangement of the normal gland. The cells for the most part are relatively large with large, pale, round nuclei containing scattered granules of chromatin. The cytoplasm is finely vacuolated, giving a foamy appearance to the cells. There is very little stroma. These consist of delicate strands of connective tissue with capillary vessels. No true acinar formation is noted. Occasional atypical large tumor giant cells are seen. Metastases are fairly numerous. Most of these are typical in appearance but a few are definitely abnormal (cf. Fig. 563).

GANGLIONEUROMA.—This is a very rare type of tumor as its incidence in the adrenal is concerned. It is composed of typical adult ganglion cells often with their characteristic pyramidal form. The tumor more often arises in the sympathetic nervous system elsewhere than in the adrenal itself. A case of this type of tumor has already been presented (Case 130 (Ref. #S-135), Figure 302, Chapter XXXI.

CHROMAFFINOMA (PARAGANGLIOMA; PHEOCHROMOCYTOMA).—This type of tumor likewise is a rare neoplasm which is usually symptomless and is found incidentally, at surgery or at autopsy. It rarely attains a size greater than that of a small hen's egg. It remains encapsulated and is chiefly of interest because in occasional instances of an associated picture of paroxysmal hypertension, these tumors, like the ganglioneuroma, are quite as frequently found in other parts of the chromaffin system as in the adrenal. Grossly they are easily recognized because of their extreme yellow pigmentation and because of their affinity for the chrome salts. As has already been commented upon, they are not infrequently found in association with generalized neurofibromatosis.

Microscopically (Fig. 635) the paraganglioma is characterized by the presence of extraordinary pleomorphism of the cells. The histology is much more alarming than the actual clinical picture. These cells tend to take the chrome salts intensely. They are obviously attempting to reproduce the cell of origin with the most bizarre-resulting morphologic appearance. The cytoplasm in many places shows extensive vacuolization. The nuclear membrane tends to stain rather intensely and to be rather heavy with a considerable amount of rather coarse granular chromatin material within the nucleus. Actual mitotic figures are comparatively rarely found. The diagnosis may perhaps best be made by exclusion, although its appearance is so typical that once such a tumor has been seen, its identification should remain as a comparatively simple problem, as compared to the great majority of malignant tumors.

MISCELLANEOUS LESIONS OF THE ADRENAL

Circulatory Disturbances.—*Hemorrhage* represents one of the most important lesions which occurs in the adrenal gland. It is seen in a wide variety of conditions and may at times be the immediate cause of death. Instances of traumatic hemorrhage of the adrenal at birth in cases of difficult breech delivery in which pressure and traction have been necessary on the fetus are occasionally seen. Allergic phenomena, notably in cases of anaphylaxis, with hemorrhage into the medulla of the adrenal are a very common, if not regular, finding. The so-called *Waterhouse-Friederichsen syndrome* in which massive bilateral adrenal hemorrhage is the outstanding pathological feature is another type of hemorrhagic lesion, which, so far as is known, is always associated with an overwhelming acute meningococcic septicemia (Fig. 631).

In relation to many of the acute infectious diseases, degenerative changes of the adrenal are not at all infrequently encountered. Notable among these are infections elsewhere in the body by hemolytic streptococci, which result in rather striking vascular injury with perivascular cellular infiltration. This occurs chiefly in the medulla and has been particularly commented upon as occurring in scarlatinal infections.

Adrenal hypoplasia is a regular accompaniment of the picture of *status thymicolymphaticus,* as has already been brought out, and it is our belief that the cause of death in this condition is very largely to be attributed to an acute adrenal insufficiency.

Degenerative changes of the adrenal as a result of various other toxemias are likewise of interest. Among these might well be indicted the same toxins which are seen in the production of acute or subacute yellow atrophy and particularly in the toxemias of pregnancy. A case in point relates to a young woman in her early twenties, who developed a picture simulating Addison's disease and who, against the advice of her physician became pregnant. During the first three months of her pregnancy she became progressively worse, but after the third month she showed a continued improvement in her clinical picture. Upon the birth of her baby, within twenty-four hours, she went into complete collapse with adrenal insufficiency and died.

Autopsy showed a small, atrophic adrenal gland which microscopically (Fig. 630) revealed only occasional scattered, degenerated-appearing cortical cells and a fibrotic scarred medulla. It was felt that this patient had survived her gestation period on the adrenal secretion of the fetus. It might be added that the child developed normally during the first year of his life, at which time he was lost sight of.

PART III

DISEASES OF THE THYMUS

The thymus, like the pituitary and adrenal, is composed of cells from two definite sources. In its origin it is largely derived from the epithelium of the third branchial cleft, which migrates down into its adult position beneath the sternum in the anterior mediastinum as a fused midline structure which tends to retain a suggestion of its embryonic two-lobe origin. The second element is very closely related to the lymphoid apparatus. Considerable argument has been spent upon whether or not the small round cell element of the thymus is composed of ordinary lymphocytes or whether these small round cells are of a specific thymic nature. In general, it is believed that they are of lymphoid origin, but that these cells do undergo specific changes which result in their particular functional activities. From the physiological standpoint the function of the thymus gland is very poorly understood. It is not a vital organ, but it plays an important part in the development of the growing animal and seems to have a catalytic effect not only on the physical but the mental development of the child. At approximately the time of adolescence or not later than the age at which skeletal growth is completed the thymus undergoes physiological atrophy, and in individuals past the age of twenty-five, it is difficult to demonstrate thymic tissue as a rule. However, with more careful studies, it has been shown that the thymus is much more likely to persist at least to a limited extent than was formerly believed and it is by no means uncommon to find remnants of thymic structures in a fatty, fibrous type of tissue from the anterior mediastinum in individuals even in their fifties and sixties. This represents one aspect of the lymphoid constitution.

The normal weight and size of the thymus has likewise been a subject of great dispute. Recent work by Hammar has shown that the usual concept is much too low in respect to both weight and size. Her observations would suggest that a thymus of as much as fifteen grams at birth is not unusual or abnormal. It gradually increases in absolute weight until, according to her figures, a weight of thirty-five to forty grams at puberty is not excessive, and then it shows a gradual atrophy until at the age of fifty or thereabouts, it returns to its birth weight. This concept is distinctly at variance with the usual impression regarding the size and persistence of this organ, but the work was very carefully controlled and planned, and only normal individuals dying sudden deaths without evidence of any disease were included in these studies.

From the standpoint of function, we might again be tempted to divide the activities of the thymus into hypo- and hyperfunctional phases, but in a gland in which the function is so obscure, this is not entirely satisfactory. However, the thymus definitely undergoes extensive atrophy in any long-standing chronic condition. Thus we see in infections such as pertussis (refer to Case 180, Chapter XLIII, Part II), which often is prolonged as much as three to four months, and in cases of malnutrition in infants as well as in adults, that the thymus decreases rapidly in size. This is manifested morphologically almost entirely by a disappearance or reduction in the number of the small round cells so that the Hassall corpuscles or epithelial structures become relatively prominent. All gradations of epithelial activity are seen ranging from an apparent atrophy with small, epithelial, pearl-like structures up to enormous focal-like lesions filled with desquamated cellular detritus, the significance of which is not known (Fig. 620).

On the hyperplastic side of the picture, we see again the increase in size is due to an increase in numbers of the small round cells. This is part of the picture of status thymicolymphaticus, which has already been discussed in relation to certain of the infectious diseases, and a case of which is presented below (Fig. 619). As has likewise been indicated, it is part of the so-called lymphoid constitution and is seen almost regularly in cases of hyperthyroidism and in other glandular dyscrasias, which seem to occur more frequently in people presenting this hyperplastic lymphoid picture.

ILLUSTRATIVE CASE

CASE 272. (Ref. #S-201)

Diagnosis.—Thymus—hyperplasia (status thymicolymphaticus).

Clinical History.—Patient was an infant, three days old at the time of death. The delivery was normal and labor was easy, but there was difficulty in getting the child to breathe, and she showed persistent cyanosis. This varied in intensity with periods of relative remission, at which time the color improved considerably. At other times there were attacks of acute cyanosis in which the face became completely livid and marked difficulty in respiration was noted with considerable dyspnea.

X-ray examination of the chest showed a greatly enlarged thymus, both in its anteroposterior and lateral dimensions. X-ray treatment was administered but the child died on the third day before any particular effect could be expected.

Autopsy Findings.—The child was a healthy-appearing, well-developed, and well-nourished, female infant with considerable cyanosis of the head and neck and some postmortem lividity in the dependent portions. The heart was negative, there being no congenital defects and the foramen ovale was essentially closed. The lungs showed a moderate amount of congestion and incomplete expansion. The thymus weighed 37 gm., being approximately between three and four times its normal size. The left adrenal weighed 3 gm., the right weighed 5 gm. There was no apparent coarctation of the aorta. There was moderate hypertrophy of the spleen which weighed 24 gm. and the lymphoid tissue of the mesentery and gastro-intestinal tract showed hyperplasia. To exclude the possibility of cerebral pathology, the brain was examined but no evidence of hemorrhage was found. The cause of death was not well established. A moderate degree of congenital atelectasis coupled with the anatomical findings of so-called status thymicolymphaticus were present as the only demonstrable lesions.

Microscopic Description.—Sections microscopically show a rather marked hyperplasia of the small round cell element of the thymus, and some corresponding hyperplasia of the reticulo-endothelial stroma. The small round cells tend to accumulate in groups forming the so-called "clubs" which are not infrequently seen in these hyperplastic glands. The epithelial element is relatively inconspicuous. Hassall's corpuscles are small and appear fewer in number than normal, although this may be relative due to the marked small round cell hyperplasia (Fig. 619).

TUMORS OF THE THYMUS

There are two varieties of tumors which occur in the thymus from the practical standpoint; first, the so-called *thymoma,* a tumor in which the small round cells play the significant role. This tumor tends to remain localized at the outset and to merely exaggerate the normal architecture of the gland, but gradually undergoes definite malignant transformation with invasion of the mediastinal structures. It produces marked pressure symptoms even resulting in death from asphyxia. As it progresses further, it metastasizes locally to the regional peribronchial and peritracheal lymphnodes and even to distant organs, apparently by way of the blood stream. Histologically, the picture is reminiscent of a lymphosarcoma. The tumor is even more radiosensitive than the or-dinary lymphosarcoma, and a number of permanent recoveries on proved cases have followed such therapeutic procedures. This tumor is usually seen in children or young adults, although it has been reported in the older age groups as well.

The second tumor is a frank *carcinoma* arising from epithelial elements of the gland. It is likely to assume a rather adenomatous appearance. Histologically it does not appear to be highly malignant, but clinically, due to its relatively inaccessible location, it is inoperable; and because of the relatively high degree of cellular differentiation is likewise highly resistant to radiation therapy. Thus, the mortality in this very limited group of thymic carcinomata is uniformly high.

PART IV

DISEASES OF THE PINEAL GLAND

The pineal gland, even more than the thymus, is largely a structure of mystery. Again, as in the case of the thymus, its functional activity is apparently largely restricted to the growth phase. Such experimental evidence as exists suggests that its actions are more or less directly antagonistic to those of the thymus, for its administration results in a retardation in growth physically. On the other hand, if anything, it seems to stimulate the development of the gonads and the onset of adolescence, with the development of sexual precocity. From the clinical standpoint, these effects have been observed occasionally in relation to the development of pineal tumors. In general, however, such tumors, occurring as they do at an early age, develop central nervous symptoms with pressure and death long before any functional disturbances of this organ are encountered. The characteristic tumor of the pineal has been described under the tumors of the central nervous system, Case 126 (Ref. #S-287), Chapter XXX, Fig. 297, page 322, so that it needs only to be mentioned at this time as one of the rare tumors.

CHAPTER LXII

DISEASES OF THE NERVOUS SYSTEM

When it comes to a consideration of those pathological conditions which affect the nervous system, it is obviously impossible to more than briefly outline the lesions found in some of the more important diseases. The various pathological manifestations of disease as it affects the brain, spinal cord and peripheral nerves can best be considered in the same way that other systemic diseases have been taken up; namely, those lesions which are primarily the result of (1), developmental defects; (2) those relating to circulatory disturbances; (3) those caused by various infectious agents, including the several virus diseases which seem to have a specific neurotropic affinity;

(4) the degenerative lesions, which make up one of the most important groups of cases clinically; and finally, (5), the tumors of the nervous system. This latter group has already been discussed in detail in Chapters XXX and XXXI. A thorough understanding of the pathological changes which occur in the nervous system depends on a sound knowledge of the underlying anatomy both from the gross and histologic standpoints. The various cell types which go to make up the central nervous system have been described in relation to the tumors to which they give rise and it will be assumed that the student is familiar with these details.

CONGENITAL ANOMALIES

The great majority of the congenital lesions of the central nervous system might well be considered in teratology, but certain of them are of such relative frequency and importance as specifically representing neurologic problems that it seems well to review the more outstanding of these at this time. Briefly stated, the commoner conditions result from failure of the neural groove to close properly. The lesions which result from such defective fusion of the neural tube are seen ranging all the way from complete *anencephaly* down to the *spina bifida occulta*.

Anencephaly.—In anencephaly, there is a complete failure of the brain to develop. This is likewise accompanied by an absence of development of the cranial bones and often of a defective development of the base of the skull. It is almost invariably associated with a rachischisis of the spinal column of varying degree (for an illustration of this lesion, the reader is referred to Fig. 352 and 353 in Chapter XXXVII). It will be recalled that this condition is likewise associated with an anomalous development of the adrenal glands as of the adult type, although ordinarily being unusually small in size. The relationship of these lesions has not been satisfactorily explained but is well established as being invariably coexistent.

The process may not always be as complete a defect, and recognizable rudimentary cerebellar and brain stem tissue may be found. Under these circumstances there is usually fairly complete development of the base of the skull, and the flat bones may appear in rudimentary form.

Spina Bifida.—The failure of fusion of the spinal column may occur alone as a simple rachischisis. This may involve the entire spinal column, as has been commented upon in relation to anencephaly, or it may occur as a local lesion at any level; more often, however, at either the caudal or cervical ends. When the process is complete, there is likewise an associated failure of the spinal cord to fuse posteriorly, and it may be seen lying in the patent canal as a flat, ribbon-like structure with no attempt at central canal formation. In the incomplete form, which is much more commonly seen at the caudal end of the vertebral column, it is usually associated with the development of a meningocele or meningomyelocele, depending upon whether or not the spinal cord itself is involved in the process. Various interpretations have been placed upon the mechanism involved in this condition. By some authors it has been suggested that the spina bifida is the result of an inflammatory or infectious disease of the central canal, which

PLATE CLI
DISEASES OF THE CENTRAL NERVOUS SYSTEM
CONGENITAL MALFORMATIONS

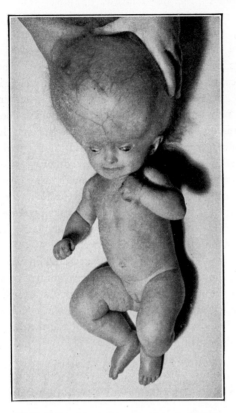 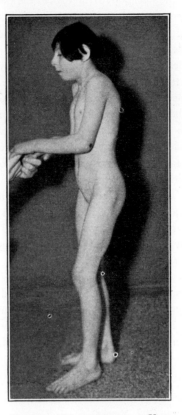

FIG. 636.—CONGENITAL, INTERNAL HYDRO-CEPHALUS.—CASE 274.

FIG. 637.—MICROCEPHALY, 8 YEAR OLD CHILD.—CASE 273.

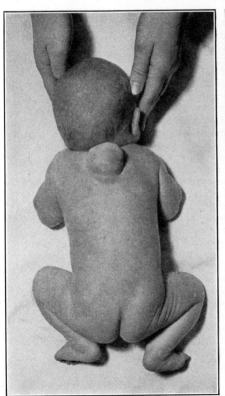 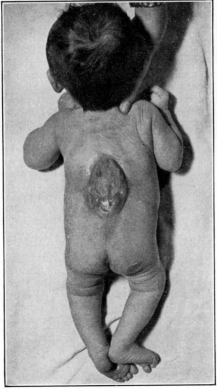 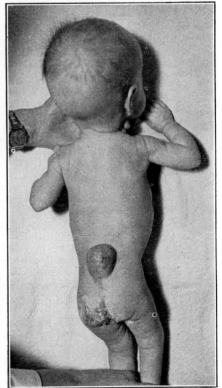

FIG. 638.—SPINA BIFIDA WITH MYELOCELE, THORACICO-LUMBAR.

FIG. 639.—SPINA BIFIDA WITH MYELOCELE, CERVICO-THORACIC.

FIG. 640.—SPINA BIFIDA WITH MYELOCELE, LUMBAR.

results in the pushing out of the cord and meninges against the soft, bony structures in the course of their development, and acting as a barrier to their subsequent fusion. By most observers, however, the bony defect is believed to be primary and the involvement of the spinal cord secondary to the reduced tension over the area where the bony canal has failed to form (Fig. 638, 639 and 640).

In the occult form of spina bifida, the lesion may only be demonstrable by careful physical examination and x-ray studies. It may be suspected, however, by the fact that there is usually an area of pigmentation with hypertrichosis over the site of the skeletal defect. This lesion is often associated with the presence of a pilonidal cyst which, as has been commented upon earlier, commonly becomes infected and breaks through to the surface with the development of a chronic sinus tract, the pilonidal sinus.

Microcephaly.—Other congenital defects of the brain may occur without any apparent defect in the development of the bony structure. The most striking of these is the condition known as microcephaly (Fig. 637). In this condition there is a generalized under-

development of the cerebrum at times approaching the appearance of the lower vertebrates, but usually showing the presence of a well-developed cerebellum. This lesion is likewise ordinarily accompanied by premature closure of the fontanels and cranial bone sutures, which may even be present at birth. Whether the failure of the brain to develop is responsible for this early skull change or whether it is the early fusion of the skull bones which does not permit the brain to develop is a question which has as yet been unanswered. The victim of this pathological lesion is unfortunately usually otherwise normal physiologically and not infrequently may grow into adult life. They often are of a particularly happy, but imbecilic, disposition but usually show varying degrees of motor inability, lying helplessly in bed throughout their entire existence.

Other instances are seen in which this developmental defect is less exaggerated as an underdevelopment of the normal convolutions of the brain. This condition is spoken of as *microgyria* and accounts for a certain proportion of the mentally defective institutional cases.

Illustrative Case

Case 273. (Ref. N-3011)

Diagnosis.—Brain—microcephaly.

Patient was a white, female child of 8 years, admitted to the hospital because of failure to develop properly both mentally and physically.

Medical History.—The patient was a very small, but full term baby, being the seventh child of eight, the others all being normal. The patient was breast fed for one and one-half years and seemed to gain weight normally. She did not develop mentally the way any of the other children had done. She did not start walking until she was over two years of age, and she never had talked. Dentition appeared normal. The patient had a voracious appetite and would eat at any and all times what food was given. She had never had any particular gastrointestinal disturbances, except occasional attacks of mild diarrhea. There was marked enuresis, which had persisted up to the present admission. During the first five years of her life she had measles and whooping cough. She had been immunized against diphtheria and had had no other serious illness. She had always seemed to be strong and healthy physically, but very much smaller than the other children of her age. She seemed to have definite affection for her mother and would laugh and smile at her, imitating the other children, but had never talked.

Physical Examination.—The patient was a slender, wiry, eight-year-old female child with the physical development of a four year old. She had apparently not developed mentally since birth. Head was very much smaller than normal with the following measurements:

Biparietal diameter, 10 cm.; occipitofrontal diameter, 12 cm.; and circumference, 34 cm. There was a depression at the site of the anterior fontanel. There was no asymmetry of the head present. Eyes were normal in appearance and reacted normally, but there was a slight internal strabismus of the left side. Nose and throat were negative. Teeth showed rather marked caries. Examination of the larynx showed no actual anatomical defects, but the child could not speak or cry, and could only make sounds like an animal. Chest was essentially negative, but small, with a circumference of only twenty-one inches. Cardiovascular system seemed negative. Abdomen was negative. Genitalia seemed somewhat underdeveloped for her age. Extremities were negative (Fig. 637).

Neurologic Examination.—Neurologic examination was very unsatisfactory because the patient was constantly moving about. Her gait was uncertain, and she walked with outstretched arms. There was no definite ataxia or spasticity. She stood with a slight kyphosis of the upper thoracic spine. In examining the cranial nerves, vision seemed to be normal. Her olfactory nerve could not be tested, nor could any sense of taste be elicited. The general appearance of the child was that of microcephaly with failure of mental and physical development.

Laboratory Findings.—The laboratory findings were of no significance. The red blood count was normal, showing 5,000,000 cells with 90% hemoglobin. White blood cells, 8,250 with 50% neutrophiles and 40% lymphocytes. Urinalysis was negative. Spinal fluid examination on two occasions was negative.

X-ray Examination: Encephalography was done to see

PLATE CLII
DISEASES OF THE CENTRAL NERVOUS SYSTEM
HEMORRHAGE

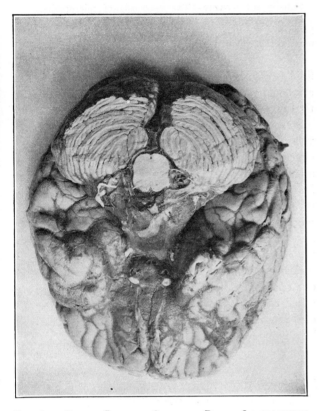

FIG. 641.—BRAIN: INFERIOR SURFACE.—BASAL, SUBARACHNOID HEMORRHAGE.

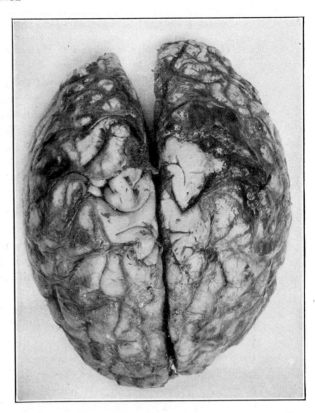

FIG. 642.—BRAIN: SUPERIOR SURFACE.—SUBDURAL AND SUB-ARACHNOID HEMORRHAGE.—Cf. CASE 275.

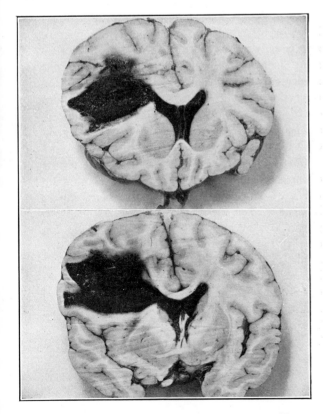

FIG. 643.—BRAIN: CORONAL SECTION.—INTRACEREBRAL HEMOR-RHAGE WITH EXTENSION INTO THE LATERAL VENTRICLES.

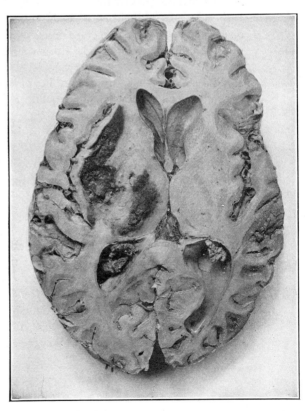

FIG. 644.—BRAIN: HORIZONTAL SECTION.—HEMORRHAGE OF LENTICULOSTRIATE ARTERY WITH EXTENSION INTO LATERAL VENTRICLE.—Cf. CASE 276.

if there was anything of an operable nature, but these studies were negative. The x-ray findings at this time suggested the presence of an accessory ventricle, or a very unusual lobulated enlargement of the third ventricle. The significant finding was an increase in the size of the sella turcica in relation to the other skull

measurements. These measurements were those of a normal adult.

Subsequent Course.—The diagnosis of microcephaly was confirmed. It was felt that nothing could be gained by further hospitalization of the child, and it was recommended that she be sent to an institution for further care.

Porencephaly.—The condition known as "porencephaly" represents again, in its classical form, a congenital developmental failure of the cortical tissue to develop so that there is direct communication between the ventricular and arachnoid systems. The cause of this defect is not known, but at times it may be very marked and the brain consists of only rudimentary lobes. Ordinarily, no such defect is found involving the brain stem or cerebellum. A comparable lesion may occur in the form of a cyst in the cortical portion of the brain, which communicates with the ventricles. This is usually congenital in origin but may follow any severe destructive lesion of an inflammatory or vascular nature.

Hydrocephalus.—By hydrocephalus is meant the accumulation of an excess amount of spinal fluid within the cranial cavity. This may be external to the brain in which instance it is spoken of as "external hydrocephalus," or it may be the result of some obstructive lesion preventing the normal circulation of the spinal fluid from the ventricular system. This variety is known as "internal hydrocephalus" and may result in a gradual compression atrophy of the brain substance until the entire brain may consist of scarcely more than a membrane filled with water-clear fluid. Such lesions may be either congenital or acquired in origin, but may be considered together at this point. The external type of hydrocephalus is comparatively uncommon and is usually congenital in nature and of unknown etiology.

In the internal form of hydrocephalus, it is necessary to review briefly the normal physiology of the cerebrospinal fluid circulation in order to obtain any adequate conception of the mechanism of the process. Normally, it will be recalled, the cerebrospinal fluid is manufactured in the choroid plexus, flows through the third ventricle and the aqueduct of Sylvius to the fourth ventricle where it escapes into the cisterns. It has been traced from the cisternae over the brain stem and past the incisura into the subarachnoid spaces over the cerebrum. Likewise, from the cisternae, it passes freely down around the spinal cord. Various theories regarding its subsequent course have been offered but the most conclusive suggest that the

fluid is absorbed by the large venous sinuses of the arachnoid villi, but may escape to some extent along the course of the nerves.

In order for typical internal hydrocephalus to develop, it becomes apparent that obstruction to this circulatory mechanism must take place. The commonest site for such obstructive phenomena is seen in relation to the aqueduct of Sylvius representing the narrowest point in its course. There may be likewise obstruction in the fourth ventricle. If the obstruction occurs at the mesencephalon in relation to the incisura tentorii, then a type of hydrocephalus spoken of as "communicating" develops, the ventricles still being directly in communication with the spinal canal. Less commonly, a lesion involving one of the foramina of Monro may occur and be followed by a unilateral internal hydrocephalus.

In the congenital internal hydrocephalus, failure of the aqueduct of Sylvius to develop, or intra-uterine inflammatory conditions of the meninges, which result in the occlusion of the foramina of Magendie and Luschka account for a considerable number of the cases. Less commonly, it has been suggested that failure of the development of the arachnoid villi may be of importance. Such lesions may be complete or may be only partial so that the subsequent development of the hydrocephalic picture is gradual. In the milder forms, this condition is not necessarily incompatible with life. Indeed, it has often been pointed out that many of the outstanding men in history, among them Napoleon, have shown minor degrees of such hydrocephalus.

Congenital Hydrocephalus.—The typical picture of the congenital hydrocephalic infant is seen during the first few months of life before the cranial sutures have united and the fontanels closed. At birth, the picture is often scarcely recognizable clinically, but develops rapidly and progressively shortly thereafter. In the more severe instances (Fig. 636), the head becomes enormously enlarged with the cranial bones often completely separated from one another and held together only by a thin, membranous structure. The superficial scalp veins stand out prominently. There is a striking bulging of the forehead over a

PLATE CLIII
DISEASES OF THE CENTRAL NERVOUS SYSTEM

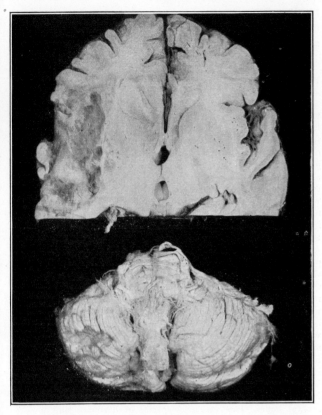

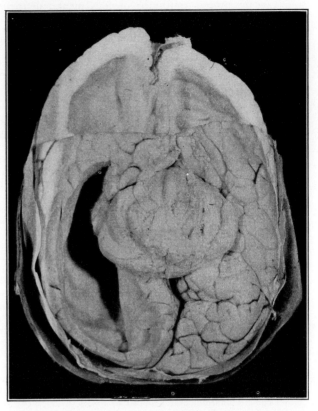

Fig. 645.—Brain.—Section showing an area of gelatinous softening the result of cerebral vascular thrombosis. Cf. Case 277.

Fig. 646.—Brain.—Viewed from the inferior surface, and cut to show marked internal hydrocephalus of the acquired type with compression atrophy of the cortex.

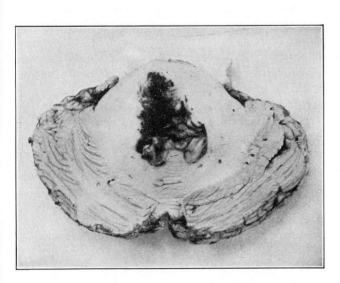

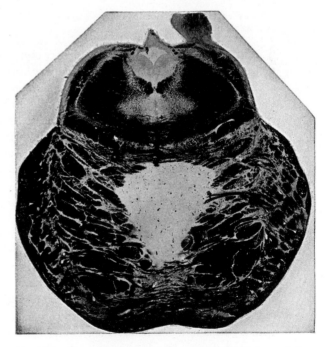

Fig. 647.—Pons.—Gross photograph of typical acute intrapontine hemorrhage with subsequent necrosis.

Fig. 648.—Pons.—Microtessar photograph (Weigert stain) to show area of softening and demyelinization (unstained) as a result of intrapontine hemorrhage.

wizened face. Blindness develops from pressure and as the process continues, obvious mental deficiency follows. Unfortunately, the process is largely restricted to the cerebri, while the structures beneath the tentorium remain essentially uninvolved. As a result, no impairment of function of the basal ganglia or brain stem occurs and the child may live until some fortunate intercurrent infection intervenes.

Illustrative Case

Case 274. (Ref. Ac. No. 2824)
Diagnosis.—Brain—hydrocephalus.

Patient was a female of 11 days, admitted to the hospital because of what appeared to be a paralysis of the face accompanied by closure of the right eye.

Past and Present History.—The child was born after a prolonged sixty-one hour labor and a difficult forceps delivery at home. Shortly afterwards the child was noted to draw the right corner of the mouth down and a swelling was observed behind the left ear. The right eyelid likewise did not open. The child nursed satisfactorily and showed no other gross abnormalities.

Physical Examination.—The head was somewhat enlarged on admission, measuring 40 cm. in diameter. The fontanels were very large but were not bulging. The suture lines were widely separated. The right eyelid was closed and would not open spontaneously. However, the pupils were regular and reacted to accommodation. There was a large hematoma behind the left ear. The chest was symmetrical. The lungs sounded clear throughout. The heart was negative. Abdomen was negative. Extremities were normal. On admission the temperature was 99.2°, pulse 124, respirations 24, and they remained normal throughout the entire period of five months' hospitalization until terminally when the temperature became subnormal and dropped to 91°.

Laboratory Findings.—The red blood count was 3,-200,000 cells with 33% hemoglobin, and the white blood cells were 17,000 with 84% polynuclears. Urinalysis on several occasions was negative.

X-ray examination, on admission, suggested a definite hydrocephalus.

Subsequent Course.—On admission it was felt that the child suffered intracranial birth injury resulting in left facial palsy. Spinal tap was done and the fluid was found to be blood tinged, and with a xanthochromic color on centrifugation. During the child's stay in the hospital the head progressively increased in size. Two months after admission, a corneal ulcer developed in the left eye. A month later, muscular twitchings of a tonic type were noted involving the right arm. The child developed numerous pressure sores over the scalp which became infected. She progressively failed and died five months after admission.

Autopsy Findings.—(Cf. Fig. 636) The body was a picture of nutritional deficiency. The outstanding lesion was a marked hydrocephalus with the circumference of the head measuring 65.5 cm. The midline sutures failed to meet by 8 cm. and over this area, the skin was taut and gave a fluid percussion wave. There was a tremendous bulging of the forehead, and several areas of ulceration were noted involving the scalp, particularly over the mastoid areas. There was a terminal pneumonia found in the right lower lobe with a beginning empyema cavity. On opening the head there was an old extradural hemorrhage found on the left side just above the petron in the region of the junction of the left parietal and frontal bones. This measured 7 cm. in diameter and 2 cm. in thickness and consisted of perhaps fifty to sixty cubic centimeters of clotted and partially organized blood. The entire ventricular system was enormously dilated with the brain cortex appearing as a thin shell of tissue. No apparent involvement of the cerebellum or brain stem was found.

ACQUIRED HYDROCEPHALUS.—A similar obstruction to the cerebrospinal fluid circulation may occur at any time during an individual's existence. Once the skull bones have united, then relatively little change in the size or shape of the head can follow, but the intracerebral pressure increases steadily with a similar atrophy of the brain substance. In the acquired form of the condition, the etiology is more often apparent. In childhood it is particularly seen as the result of an inflammatory involvement of the meninges with adhesions forming over the roof of the fourth ventricle. In adults, a similar inflammatory lesion may be responsible for the picture, but more often perhaps, an intracranial tumor is the immediate cause. Unilateral involvement of one of the lateral ventricles may result from obstruction of the foramen of Monro on one side in conjunction with a glioma or a pinealoma. Tumors arising in the fourth ventricle particularly may similarly obstruct the aqueduct of Sylvius. Large intracerebral tumors may, through pressure, wedge the brain stem at the incisurae, or against the cranium to obliterate the subarachnoid pathways so that absorption of the cerebrospinal fluid is prevented. Adhesions about the arachnoid villi may similarly interfere with absorption (Fig. 646).

From the clinical standpoint, the chief symptoms which point toward such an obstructive lesion are the result of increased intracranial pressure. These are particularly headache, vomiting, mental dullness, choking of the optic disks, a slowing of the pulse rate, not infrequently convulsions and ultimately unconsciousness and coma. These are the more general symptoms relating to intracranial pressure. If the lesion is localized, as in the case of a brain tumor, then in addition to these general symptoms, supplementary localizing symptomatology is likewise present. Thus, typically, in a symmetrical obstructive or communicating hydrocephalus the symptoms are of this general type rather than of a localizing nature.

Hydromyelia.—Just as in the case of the brain in conjunction with a hydrocephalus, so may a similar dilatation of the central canal of the spinal cord occur. This also may be either congenital in nature or acquired later in life as the result of some compression of the cord.

CIRCULATORY DISTURBANCES

Circulatory disturbances of the brain are among the most common pathological lesions which are encountered, especially as some form of hemorrhage. In addition, however, many of the clinical pictures associated with central nervous symptoms are related to alteration in its hydrodynamics. Fay and Chamberlain in several recent studies have demonstrated conclusively the importance of the simple physical relationship of fluid balance functioning as it does within a closed cavity. Even the normal physiological process of sleep is dependent upon variation in the blood supply to the brain. Experimental work has shown that during sleep the brain is in a relatively anemic state and that with increased mental activity, there is a corresponding increase of blood flow to the brain. This variation in the blood volume in the central nervous system must be compensated for by a corresponding loss of cerebrospinal fluid or of tissue compression, which is much less likely to occur. Similarly, if spinal fluid is withdrawn from the spinal canal by lumbar puncture, the intracranial volume is maintained by an instant replacement of the fluid withdrawn by a corresponding increase of blood to the central nervous system. These factors are of inestimable importance in evaluating the clinical picture.

In like manner, Riggs and others have emphasized the importance of an adequate blood supply to the brain to prevent cerebral anoxemia, which appears to be one of the most important factors in the immediate physiological cause of death. It is obviously impossible to go at length into the field of abnormal physiology of the central nervous system other than as it appears in relation to the anatomical lesions which we ordinarily recognize as the manifestations of such abnormal function.

In active hyperemia associated with inflammatory conditions, the problem of maintaining this equilibrium of circulation of blood and cerebrospinal fluid is not infrequently interfered with and results in an edema of the brain. Perhaps even more significant in the development of such cerebral edema are those conditions which are accompanied by passive hyperemia. These may be of a general nature due to underlying cardiac or renal pathology or may be local in character associated with tumor, inflammatory lesions or hemorrhage. In any condition in which this circulatory mechanism is altered, it is common to find an outpouring of serum into the perivascular spaces. This gradually extends between the fibrillary supportive structures to produce edema of the tissues. If this process is generalized, it may result in actual flattening of the convolutions of the brain as they are viewed upon opening the skull at autopsy. If it is local, similar edema and flattening of the convolutions may be seen over an area where a tumor, abscess or cyst is present. In degenerative diseases and toxic lesions such as chronic alcoholism, fluid may accumulate in the subarachnoid spaces in relatively excessive amounts to make up in volume for the atrophy of the cerebral substance which is present.

Edema.—TRAUMATIC EDEMA.—In the condition known as concussion of the brain, one of the outstanding pathological findings is that of cerebral edema. In the more severe cases, this may be associated with multiple petechial hemorrhage or even with more extensive areas of hemorrhage, particularly in the contrecoup position in relation to the site of injury. Fay has shown that the persistence of symptoms following even relatively mild head injuries is dependent upon the persistence of this cerebral edema with resultant increased intracranial pressure. If this be sufficiently marked, the brain may be pushed against the vertex or the tentorium so that obstruction to the cerebrospinal fluid circulation follows. In this way a vicious circle is established and the condition becomes almost chronic in nature. In this connection, Winkleman and Fay's work has conclusively demonstrated that a very considerable degree of actual hydrocephalus can be produced by blocking the arachnoid villi. This may occur as a result of pressure in relation to traumatic injury as suggested. It is very probably an important factor in the development of the picture of edema in association with meningitis, particularly of the tuberculous type, of subarachnoid hemorrhage and in association with syphilitic and other lesions such as chronic alcoholism in which fibrosis of the villi again interferes with normal drainage of the cerebrospinal fluid. Dehydration therapy in these cases by repeated spinal tap and by the use of hypertonic saline solution intravenously, of magnesium sulphate by mouth and even by the simple restriction of fluid intake—all aid in reducing this cerebral edema, with a resultant diminution in the intracranial pressure and subsequent relief of symptoms.

Epilepsy (Idiopathic).—In idiopathic epilepsy, it is likewise highly probable that circulatory disturbances with the accumulation of focalized subarachnoid lakes of fluid are an important factor in the development of the symptomatology. It has been suggested that a similar arachnoiditis with obliteration of the villi in patchy areas may account for the localized accumulation of fluid which is more often seen in the frontal and parietal lobes and is associated with atrophy of the gyri and brain substance, beneath the cerebrospinal fluid pathways. In the *traumatic* type of epilepsy, as a rule, there is actual laceration of the nerve tissue. This is followed by the development of scar tissue composed of both glial and connective tissue cells. This forms a highly vascular scar which produces adhesions between the underlying brain substance and the overlying meninges. As the scar tissue contracts, the ventricle on the side affected may become pulled in the direction of the scar. Penfield has shown that such traumatic lesions are very frequently associated with the jacksonian type of epilepsy which does not appear for several years after the trauma. He has further shown that the surgical excision of such scar tissue, in contradistinction to the tearing of tissues by trauma, and of brain tissue in general is not ordinarily followed by such scar formation.

LEAD ENCEPHALOPATHY.—In cases of lead poisoning, particularly as seen in children, there is very frequently a marked cerebral edema. This is apparently the result of the actual presence of lead within the brain substance, which alters the physiochemical relationships to the extent that fluid accumulates to a surprising degree. The brain itself is markedly enlarged, soft and boggy in consistency. It shows marked flattening of the convolutions due to the edema. On section, not infrequently multiple foci of petechial hemorrhage may be demonstrated.

Histologic examination of the cortex may likewise show rather extensive degenerative changes affecting nerve cells, particularly the large motor cells. This is less frequently encountered in older individuals in whom the picture of lead poisoning from the nervous system standpoint is more often of a peripheral neuritic type. In the more acute, fulminating cases, however, comparable changes may on occasion be seen in this older age group. The diagnosis may be suspected from the appearance of the lead line in the gums and the characteristic hypochromic anemia with basophilic stippling.

Hemorrhage.—Intracranial hemorrhage may occur in a variety of forms and be produced by a wide variety of causes. In general, intracranial hemorrhage is classified on the basis of being either traumatic or spontaneous, and on its extent, as petechial, punctate, or massive. From the anatomical standpoint the type of hemorrhage is classified chiefly upon its location. The hemorrhage may be 1, extradural; 2, subdural; 3, subarachnoid; or 4, intracerebral.

EXTRADURAL HEMORRHAGE.—Extradural hemorrhage is almost invariably arterial in origin and is likewise almost invariably traumatic in origin. It is usually the result of a direct blow on the head. The dura becomes separated from the inner table of the skull by the sudden recoil of the head with the tearing of one or more arteries. The blood pours into this potential space where it forms a clot, which progressively tends to increase in size. At times, such clots may become an inch or more in thickness. It being a rapid process, compression of the brain is marked and increased intracranial pressure causes the development of the almost diagnostic sypmtomatology. There is ordinarily a brief period of unconsciousness as the result of the concussion accompanying the injury. This is followed by a period of mental clarity, which may persist for several hours. This is then followed by the combined general and localizing symptoms of pressure and results, if unchecked by surgical intervention, very commonly in unconsciousness, coma and death.

SUBDURAL HEMORRHAGE.—(Fig. 642) Subdural hemorrhage is by contrast almost invariably venous in type, but also usually traumatic in origin. It follows relatively minor head injury in the great majority of cases. Most frequently it involves the frontal or occipital areas and is produced by a shearing off of one or more of the cerebral veins as they enter the sagittal sinus. The lesion is usually unilateral but may at times be bilateral. The blood works its way through the subdural spaces and forms a massive layer often covering the entire surface of one side of the brain. This varies considerably in thickness at times, from a few millimeters to one or two centimeters.

The clinical history in these cases is often very suggestive. The symptoms are those of intracranial pressure and often do not appear for several weeks after the original trauma except in those cases where the initial hemorrhage is sufficient to produce prominent symptoms of pressure. The hemorrhage in this instance, being venous in type, tends to be arrested spontaneously through clotting. The clot appears as a layer between the pia and the dura in the subdural space. Owing to the curious arrangement of the circulatory mechanism, very little opportunity for the absorption of this clot exists. On the contrary, the clot gradually becomes liquefied centrally and surrounded by a pseudomembrane, which attempts to organize the material. Gradually the entire clot undergoes cystic degeneration, and due to differences in osmotic pressure, fluid tends to accumulate from the spinal fluid into this cyst. This process continues slowly with gradually increasing symptoms of intracranial pressure until such a time as the patient gradually loses consciousness and dies. In this day and age, there is little excuse for a patient to die of subdural hemorrhage as the cases are readily amenable to the surgical removal of the blood clot.

The diagnosis is often established by the finding of xanthochromatic spinal fluid on lumbar puncture due to the fact that a certain amount of the blood pigment is broken down and carried away in the spinal fluid through the action of the tissue phagocytes.

In the newborn, one of the commonest causes of death may be ascribed to extensive subdural hemorrhage as the result of birth injury. In these cases, the hemorrhage usually arises from a tear in the tentorium or the falx, especially in premature infants in whom these structures are still almost embryonic in their composition. Hemorrhagic spinal fluid is very common in this type of lesion as the hemorrhage is often not only restricted to the subdural space, but involves the subarachnoid area as well. Due to the cyanosis which is usually present, the diagnosis of congenital heart disease is not infrequently made in these infants, but the development of Cheyne-Stokes respiration, a slow pulse rate, bulging of the fontanels and convulsive seizures establish the diagnosis. Depending upon the extent of the hemorrhage, the child may die within the course of a few hours or may survive with or without some residue of nervous symptoms. Occasional instances of hemorrhagic disease of the newborn may be confused with this picture of subdural hemorrhage. The importance of clinical pathological studies of the blood cannot be overemphasized as the intramuscular injection of normal whole blood in this hemorrhagic diathesis is followed in the majority of cases by stopping of the bleeding.

ILLUSTRATIVE CASE

CASE 275. (Ref. #S-394)
Diagnosis.—Brain (dura)—subdural hemorrhage with organization.
Patient was a white male of 72 years, admitted to the hospital with the chief complaint of pain in the back of his head.
Present Illness.—The history of the present illness was most unreliable. The patient was more or less irrational at intervals and lapsed into a semicomatose state at times. Apparently, however, the headaches had begun approximately ten days previously with the history of the patient's having fallen and struck his head. At that time he was seen by a physician who considered that the injury was not serious and discharged him without x-ray examination.
Past Medical History.—The past medical history was even more unsatisfactory as it was impossible to secure any coöperation from the patient, and he had no family. All that could be established was that patient had had a prolonged history of alcoholism over many years, and that some fifteen or twenty years ago a physician had given him a number of hypodermic treatments for some condition.
Physical Examination.—The patient was semistuporous and reacted only to painful stimuli. There was marked resistance to the movements of his arms and legs. There was an old scar with slight indentation of the skull over the left parietal region. The pupils were myotic, regular, round, equal and reacted to light. Due to his condition it was impossible to establish their reaction to accommodation. The heart was essentially negative. It was not enlarged. There were no murmurs. Blood pressure was 124/60. Lungs were clear. Abdomen was negative. Extremities showed eversion of the left foot and the suggestion of a Babinski on the right side. Further neurologic observation suggested that there was weakness of the muscles on the left side of his face and a general decrease in activity of the deep tendon reflexes on the left.
Laboratory Findings.—Urinalysis on two occasions was essentially negative. Blood count showed, 4,200,000 red cells with 12 gm. of hemoglobin, and 12,600 white

blood cells with 94% polynuclears. Wassermann was negative. Blood chemistry was negative. Spinal fluid examination showed a moderate increase of globulin, a normal carbohydrate-reducing content, a cell count of twenty-six cells with 6% polymorphonuclears and 94% lymphocytes. Spinal fluid Wassermann complement fixation test was negative.

X-ray examination showed the subdural space on the right side to be increased in size and the subarachnoid space disorganized.

Subsequent Course.—A diagnosis of probable subdural hemorrhage was made and exploratory operation recommended in an attempt to remove the clot. This was done, a large hematoma removed, and a drain inserted. Due to the age of the patient and his general condition, however, this failed to result in permanent improvement. The reduction of pressure locally gave immediate relief, but apparently relieved pressure to the extent where

subsequent intracerebral hemorrhage occurred with the death of the patient.

Autopsy Findings.—At autopsy, nothing of significance was found except in relation to the head. On the right side there was an accumulation of clotted blood adherent to the inner aspect of the dura. This showed considerable organization in its peripheral portions. Sections through the brain substance showed a marked hemorrhage into the internal capsule on the same side (Cf. Fig. 642).

Microscopic Description of a Section Through the Subdural Tissue.—Histologically there is marked hyaline thickening of the dura itself. Beneath this is a mass of blood clot which shows varying degrees of disintegration of the red cells. Centrally, these cells appear almost as shadow cells without any hemoglobin. There is an attempt at organization of this clot as seen by the growth of fibroblasts into the periphery of the clot.

SUBARACHNOID HEMORRHAGE.—(Fig. 641) Subarachnoid hemorrhage, unlike the extra- or subdural types, may be either traumatic or spontaneous. As an accompaniment of many traumatic injuries, subarachnoid involvement is extremely common. Lumbar puncture will reveal a bloody fluid, and while a bloody spinal fluid is not necessarily diagnostic of subarachnoid hemorrhage, as it may occur in any form of hemorrhage which communicates with the cerebrospinal fluid circulation, yet it is the most common lesion in which this picture is found. The spontaneous type is more often seen in children and young adults in association with the rupture of a congenital aneurysm of the circle of Willis, but may also occur in relation to many of the inflammatory conditions affecting the meninges. In those cases associated with rupture of a small miliary aneurysm, the onset of the symptoms is sudden and associated with severe headache and often with other evidence of meningeal irritation which suggests a diagnosis of meningitis. In the less dramatic instances seen in conjunction with various toxic or inflammatory vascular lesions of the meninges, the picture often simulates that of epidemic encephalitis with mental torpor and mild evidence of meningeal irritation. Lumbar puncture in the aneurysmal rupture type of case yields a fluid which appears to be pure blood, as a rule, while in the milder subacute cases, by the time symptoms appear, the fluid may contain only a few red cells but will be definitely xanthochromic in color.

CEREBRAL HEMORRHAGE.—Punctate (Petechial).—By cerebral hemorrhage is ordinarily meant the massive type which is more familiarly known as apoplexy. However, not infrequently in conjunc-

tion with a wide variety of causes, diffuse punctate hemorrhages may be seen throughout the brain substance. In certain cases of acute infectious disease, notably measles and less frequently pertussis, as part of the generalized picture of meningomyelo-encephalitis, injury to the vessel walls may be assumed to take place as they are not infrequently accompanied by rather marked petechial hemorrhage. Similarly, in acute anterior poliomyelitis and in epidemic encephalitis, again both virus infections, similar vascular damage may result in rather extensive extravasation of blood around the smaller vessels filling the Virchow-Robin spaces and even extending into the actual central nervous tissue. Obviously in leukemias, hemophilia and other of the marked blood dyscrasias, similar hemorrhage may occur. In traumatic injuries as the result of minor blows upon the head, such petechial hemorrhage may be found. This is very much more commonly seen in the contrecoup position in relation to the site of injury. In carbon monoxide poisoning, as one of the almost diagnostic features of the disease, bright cherry red punctate hemorrhagic lesions are found. In general, such lesions then may be classed as injuries to the smaller vessels as the result of infection, toxemia or trauma; this, in contradistinction to the more massive types of arterial hemorrhage associated with degenerative diseases of the blood vessels which result in the more striking examples of localized but massive apoplectic hemorrhage.

Massive Hemorrhage (Apoplexy).—By apoplexy is meant a form of cerebral hemorrhage which results from rupture of some one of the intracerebral arteries. The most common site for such hemorrhage is seen in the region of the internal capsule and is usually associated with rupture of the lenticulo-striate artery (Fig. 644). This condition is seen particularly between the ages of forty-five and sixty, and occurs most commonly in males. It is almost invariably associated with hypertension and arteriosclerosis. The hypertension may be of the essential renal type, but more frequently is of the secondary cardiovascular type. A curious paradox in relation to the apoplectic seizure is found in the fact that a very considerable percentage of cases occur while the patient is at rest, sitting quietly in a chair or asleep in bed.

Next in frequency to the lenticulostriate artery to be involved in this picture is some branch of the anterior cerebral artery. Less frequently the hemorrhage is seen in the pons and cerebellum (Fig. 647 and 648). When it occurs in the vicinity of the internal capsule it may be relatively small in extent, but due to its location produces profound symptoms interfering as it does with the major motor neurons above the pyramidal crossing. Thus, there is typically paralysis of the face, arm and leg of the side opposite to that of the lesion. This paralysis is of the spastic type. If the hemorrhage becomes more extensive, it may involve the sensory fibers as well so that there may be hemianesthesia and homonymous hemianopia.

Not infrequently, the hemorrhage may extend rapidly into the lateral ventricle of the side affected (Fig. 643). When this occurs, the patient shows a complete loss of consciousness, a rapid rise in temperature and a loss of the reflexes. Such cases usually die within a comparatively short interval when the hemorrhage occurs in the pons. Again, the symptomatology depends upon the size and location of the hemorrhagic area. Almost regularly, however, a high fever is seen as well as the presence of pinpoint pupils. Paralysis depends upon whether or not the pyramidal tracts are involved. In those much less common instances of cerebellar hemorrhage, the symptoms are those of disturbances of equilibrium with deviation of the eyes to the side of the lesion, nystagmus and a tendency to fall to the affected side. No paralysis is seen.

The outcome of any case of cerebral apoplexy depends upon a number of factors, chief among them being the size and location of the hemorrhage. If the hemorrhage is small in size and does not involve any vital structure nor produce sufficient intracranial pressure to cause death, then recovery may occur. The edema which is invariably associated with the condition may absorb and the patient may improve even to the point of complete return of muscular function. On the other hand, as we have seen, if the hemorrhage extends into the ventricles, death follows promptly.

ILLUSTRATIVE CASE

CASE 276. (Ref. #S-395)

Diagnosis.—Brain—intracerebral hemorrhage, lenticulostriate artery with extension into ventricles.

Patient was a white female of 50 years, who was admitted to the hospital in a semistuporous condition and showing definite hemiplegia.

Present Illness.—The history of the patient's illness was obtained from her daughter. For the year preceding the present admission, she had complained frequently of severe headaches, but other than that her health had apparently been fairly good. The day before admission she was found wandering about the house in a dazed state, limping and unable to use her right arm or leg to any extent. This had progressed in severity until she lapsed into a semistuporous condition. She had not consulted a physician for any of these, feeling that they were merely related to her menopause and that there was nothing which could be done about them.

Past Medical History.—The patient's previous medical history was likewise essentially normal. She was believed to have had the usual childhood infections, but this could not be obtained with any feeling of accuracy. Her daughter, however, was sure that she had never been seriously ill previously. She had been married for twenty-eight years. Her last pregnancy had been four-teen years previously. Her menstrual history, so far as her daughter could tell, had always been normal, regular and without undue dysmenorrhea. She was apparently in her menopause at this time.

Physical Examination.—The patient was a well-developed and well-nourished middle-aged, white woman. Head showed no external deformities. Her vision was apparently fairly good and pupils reacted normally to light and accommodation. There was a definite right facial paralysis. The nose and throat were negative. Heart and lungs appeared normal to auscultation and percussion. Abdomen was lax and obese making satisfactory examination difficult. No masses were felt and no tenderness was elicited. The extremities presented the picture of definite hemiplegia with a relative hyperactivity of the reflexes on the right. The patient's blood pressure was 240/190. Temperature, pulse and respirations were essentially normal.

Laboratory Findings.—Red blood cells, 5,200,000 with 14 gms. of hemoglobin. White blood cells, 17,750 with 94% polymorphonuclears. Wassermann, negative. Urinalysis showed a slight trace of albumin but was otherwise negative. Spinal puncture yielded a clear fluid under no increased pressure. Wassermann and colloidal gold curve were negative. The blood chemistry studies showed a somewhat diminished chloride content but was otherwise normal.

Subsequent Course.—The patient's condition progressed steadily and she died twelve hours after admission with a clinical diagnosis of cerebral hemorrhage.

Autopsy Findings.—The visceral pathology was negligible. Heart showed moderate hypertrophy particularly of the left ventricle with the usual concentric hypertensive picture. Valves were negative. Coronaries were normal. Lungs were essentially negative except for terminal congestion. Abdominal viscera, except for the kidneys were negative. The kidneys presented a relatively early stage of benign nephrosclerosis associated with essential hypertension. The examination of the brain (Fig. 644) revealed a typical large hemorrhagic area in the left internal capsule. This had forced its way into the left lateral ventricle and from there into the third ventricle through the aqueduct of Sylvius into the fourth ventricle. Distention of the left lateral ventricle by blood

Aneurysm.—True intracranial aneurysms are relatively uncommon lesions with the exception of the congenital type. These are found most often in relation to the circle of Willis, but may likewise occasionally be encountered involving the anterior or middle cerebral vessels. It appears to be the result of a defective development of the media with its internal elastic lamina and is usually seen at the point of bifurcation of some one of these vessels. The lesion as a rule is not more than a few millimeters in diameter. Its rupture gives rise to one form of subarachnoid hemorrhage and is likely to be fatal because of its arterial nature. When it arises in the anterior middle cerebral vessels, it not infrequently extends into the brain substance as well. The recognition of the aneurysmal nature of this hemorrhagic process is often difficult to establish even by rather careful dissection. While many of these lesions are true aneurysms, nevertheless the great majority of them are more likely to be false aneurysms which result from oozing hemorrhage into the adventitia as a result of the congenital weakness of the vessel wall.

Less often aneurysms may form as the result of weakening of the vessel wall in association with atherosclerosis or following an infected embolism of an artery. In this latter instance, the condition is spoken of as a mycotic aneurysm in the same way that similar aneurysms are spoken of elsewhere in the body.

Cerebral Thrombosis and Embolism.—In contradistinction to frank hemorrhage of the brain which results from actual rupture of the wall, the more common lesion which is found is related to thrombosis of the cerebral arteries. This is not necessarily associated with hypertension, although a very con-

clot had pushed the thalamus to the right of the midline and the island of Reil laterally to the left. The basilar and vertebral arteries and their branches showed extensive atherosclerosis with asymmetric narrowing of the lumina.

Microscopic Description of a Section Through the Edge of the Hemorrhagic Area.—The histologic findings as a whole are those of a moderate atherosclerotic degeneration of the smaller arteries and arterioles. The point of rupture cannot be found in the histologic sections, but there is very diffuse red cell infiltration of the brain substance. The lesion is so acute that relatively little degenerative change has occurred as yet. However, some demyelinization may be observed, and beginning microglial scavenger cell formation is taking place. Histologically, the changes may be described as the early degenerative changes associated with anoxemia, in this instance as a result of the shutting off of the blood supply through massive hemorrhage.

siderable number of the cases do show secondary hypertensive features, due to the fact that the condition is more prone to occur in the older age group in association with rather marked atherosclerotic changes of the blood vessels. In other instances, a similar picture may be presented in the younger age group in association with cerebral embolism and thrombosis as the result of some condition such as subacute bacterial endocarditis or from sterile material such as may form in the auricular appendage of the heart in association with an auricular fibrillation. The picture which follows any such obstruction to the arterial circulation, whether it be by direct embolism or by the more usual process of thrombosis, will result in a shutting off of the blood supply and what amounts to infarction. In the brain, however, this condition is spoken of as "softening" or *encephalomalacia* due to the inherent nature of the tissue involved. For the purpose of discussion at this point, the typical form of cerebral thrombosis and softening will be discussed. It is obvious that the more acute embolic phenomena will give rise to correspondingly more acute symptoms depending upon the location and whether or not the embolic material is infected. In the latter instance it may well give rise to actual abscess formation.

In simple uncomplicated thrombosis of the cerebral vessels we find typically that, as the blood supply is gradually shut down to an area in the brain, the cells undergo degenerative changes with atrophy and liquefaction necrosis (Fig. 645). The commonest site for such cerebral thrombosis is found affecting the left middle cerebral artery if the lesion is at all massive. Minimal lesions of the same type may be found generally distributed throughout the brain substance and indeed, the process of arteriosclerosis is one of the most important in respect to senile atrophy of the brain. Owing to the vascular pattern in the brain with the comparatively minimal capillary bed, the cerebral vessels in general are thought of as endarteries and thus when they are obstructed, the lesion which occurs is comparable to the anemic infarct seen in the heart, the kidney or the spleen. One of the earliest manifestations of degeneration seen in the brain substance is a demyelinization of the nerve fibers. This is followed by marked changes of the microglial cells which assume their scavenger function. This has already been described in relation to anterior poliomyelitis. These cells are believed to be of reticulo-endothelial origin and possess the same phagocytic capacity as do other cells of this series. They typically lose their glial-like processes and become oval or rounded. They take up the broken down lipoid material and their cytoplasm becomes vacuolated. These are the cells which are variously spoken of as compound granular corpuscles, Gitter-cells and so forth. By many observers it is also believed that in the intermediate form they are identical with the so-called stab cells although some question as to whether this stab cell may not be derived from the oligodendroglia is raised.

In the early stages of this process, the area involved becomes of a soft, grayish-white, creamy appearance. As the process goes on a certain amount of hemorrhage into the area follows. The hemoglobin undergoes breakdown and the necrotic tissue becomes stained with this blood pigment so that it has a distinctly yellow color. Gradually this broken down tissue is absorbed and carried away by the phagocytic cells until an actual cavity is left, filled ultimately with a clear fluid. Around the edges of such areas of softening there is an area of reparative gliosis which tends to form a pseudocapsule. In the end stage this appears as an actual cyst. It is of interest in this connection that typical wallerian degeneration of the nerve fibers below the point of destruction takes place. This can be traced in serial section through the medulla and cord by staining appropriately by the Marchi or Weigert methods.

The chief point of interest from the clinical pathological standpoint lies in the differentiation of thrombosis from true apoplexy or embolism. Roughly speaking, the thrombotic process is more likely to be gradual, but a time comes when the obstruction becomes complete and the clinical picture may very closely simulate that of the more sudden hemorrhagic lesion of apoplexy. Likewise, in many of these cases not only is the initial process gradual, but it is progressive; whereas in apoplexy the onset is sudden and is frequently followed by marked improvement in the symptoms over a period of time. More difficulty may be had in differentiating the acute embolic lesion from that of apoplexy, for in both of these conditions, the onset is sudden and subsequent improvement may follow, provided the picture does not go on promptly to death. Suffice it to say that in respect to the circulatory disturbances of the central nervous system, these two, cerebral thrombosis and cerebral hemorrhage, make up the great bulk of the pathological lesions found at autopsy. They both may have an underlying picture of arteriosclerosis, especially of the atherosclerotic type. In the one instance the process results from the gradual shutting down of the blood supply to a vital area whereas in the other, death is caused by the sudden rupture of the vessel wall coupled with a hypertensive picture and is not infrequently preceded by phenomena suggesting thrombotic changes of the small vessels as an antecedent factor in producing the lesion.

ILLUSTRATIVE CASE

CASE 277. (Ref. #S-396)

Diagnosis.—Brain—Cerebral atherosclerosis and thrombosis with secondary encephalomalacia.

Patient was a white male of 78 years, who was admitted to the hospital because of a hemiplegia.

Present Illness.—The onset of the patient's present condition began ninety-six hours before admission with progressive weakness of his left side and incontinence of his bladder. He had been sickly for a matter of several weeks and had had several fainting attacks with transitory loss of consciousness. He had never been definitely disoriented, however, when conscious. He was referred to the hospital by his physician because he was unable to care for himself in this condition, which had progressed to the point of actual hemiplegia.

Past Medical History.—Past medical history was totally irrelevant. A review of his systems was of no importance in relation to his immediate condition. He had never had any definite cardiac symptoms but had gradually developed a very marked peripheral arteriosclerosis.

Physical Examination.—The patient was a feeble, elderly, white male who on admission was in a semi-stuporous condition. His head was not remarkable. Scalp was bald. Eyes showed marked bilateral arcus senilis. Pupils reacted to light and distance. There was ptosis of the right lid. Ears, nose and throat were negative. Mouth was edentulous. Chest was symmetrical and somewhat emphysematous in appearance. Respirations were rapid and shallow. There was slight impairment of the percussion note over both bases with many coarse, moist râles. Heart was moderately enlarged to the left. Sounds were irregular. There were no murmurs. Blood pressure was 180/94. Abdomen was distended and there was apparently some fluid in the flanks. Extremities were negative in appearance.

Neurologic Examination.—There was a definite weakness of the right arm and leg, but this could not be interpreted as a complete paralysis. Knee jerks were somewhat exaggerated. There was weakness of the entire right side of the face.

Laboratory Findings.—Urinalysis was negative. Blood count showed a normal red count of 4,500,000 cells and a white count of 12,600 with 82% polymorphonuclears. Blood chemistry: Urea 135 mgm.; sugar, 126 mgm.

Subsequent Course.—The patient went steadily downhill and died six days after the onset of his illness.

Autopsy Findings.—The body presented a marked generalized arteriosclerosis with arterial nephrosclerosis.

There was moderate hypertrophy of the heart with considerable parenchymatous degeneration. The most striking lesions found were those involving the central nervous system where multiple areas of cerebral thrombosis with softening were encountered. The cerebral vessels were tortuous and cord-like.

Microscopic Description of a Section Through the Brain.—(Fig. 645) Tissues histologically show evidence of definite atherosclerosis of the cerebral vessels. In places this is accompanied by actual thrombosis, which varies considerably with the age of the process. In some areas, the thrombosis is relatively recent and fresh as seen by typical red thrombus formation composed of fibrin and red cells. In other places the lesions have been present for some time as evidenced by complete organization of the thrombi. Some of the vessels show obliteration of the lumen as a result. Surrounding such thrombosed vessels is a definite encephalomalacia characterized by a loss of myelin of the nerve cells and by the accumulation of "stab" cells and typical well-developed microglial scavenger phagocytes. In places, actual liquefaction necrosis has occurred.

CHAPTER LXIII

DISEASES OF THE NERVOUS SYSTEM (*Continued*)

INFECTIOUS DISEASES OF THE CENTRAL NERVOUS SYSTEM

The infectious diseases of the nervous system may be divided on anatomical grounds into those conditions which are extradural, those which are subdural, and lesions affecting the brain or cord themselves. They may likewise further be divided on the basis of specific etiology into the acute pyogenic infections, chronic granulomata, virus diseases and finally the more uncommon parasitic infestations. Many of these lesions have been discussed in relation to general pathological processes and in respect to a consideration of the specific pathology produced by many of the infective agents. Certain of these, however, stand out so typically as specific clinical pathological problems that it seems well to consider a few of them in detail and to summarize and review briefly the other common conditions.

EXTRADURAL LESIONS

The extradural lesions are characterized by the production of a focal abscess formation, usually as direct extension from an osteomyelitis of the skull, especially complicating compound fractures. They may likewise arise by extension from middle ear, mastoid or other sinus infections and remain entirely localized outside the dura. They are characterized by localized swelling and inflammation of the scalp over the area involved. This was recognized in the English literature nearly two hundred years ago by Sir Percival Pott, and this soft, edematous, inflammatory lesion of the scalp is known as Pott's puffy tumor. Such infections may produce marked pressure symptoms much as similar extradural hemorrhage does.

SUBDURAL LESIONS

The subdural forms of infection usually are seen as the various types of meningitis. By meningitis is meant an infection of the subarachnoid tissue covering the brain. The pia itself acts as a very effective barrier in the great majority of instances in preventing the extension of the meningitic process into the brain substance itself. However, this barrier is not impassable and particularly in tuberculous meningitis, such secondary extension of the pathological process may be found. The meningitides may be divided into two major groups: first, the acute pyogenic varieties which include the cases caused by the *Meningococcus, Pneumococcus, Streptococcus, Hemophilus influenzae* and the occasional other pyogenic bacteria, such as *Bacillus typhosus, Bacillus pertussis, Gonococcus,* and even *Bacillus coli;* and second, the relatively more chronic forms of meningitis produced by the various infectious granulomatous organisms of which the tubercle bacillus is the only common one. In addition, as has been emphasized earlier, rare instances of infection of the meninges by Torula, Monilia and other similar mycotic organisms can occur. In respect to the method by which the organisms may gain access to the meninges, various possible routes have to be conceded, but the hematogenous seems particularly likely. The blood stream seems to be the most important route in certain of these infections, notably tuberculosis and probably meningococcic meningitis. Pneumococcic and streptococcic infections may likewise reach the meninges by the blood stream, but very commonly cause the infection by direct extension from contiguous areas of infection such as occur in middle ear disease, chronic sinusitis, sinus thrombosis and mastoiditis. It is possible that organisms may enter the meninges along the course of the olfactory nerves as is believed by many, particularly in respect to infection by the Meningococcus, as it is known that the organisms are harbored in the nasopharynx of the individual. Again the question of tissue specificity seems to enter into the problem so far as this particular organism is concerned.

PLATE CLIV
DISEASES OF THE CENTRAL NERVOUS SYSTEM

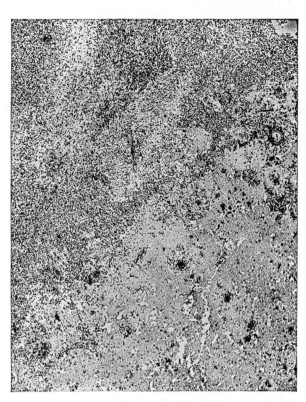

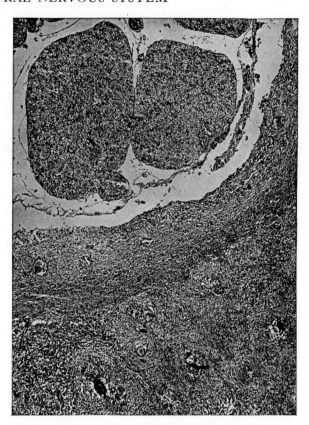

Fig. 649.—Brain: Abscess, Streptococcic.—Case 278.—Photomicrograph showing area of suppuration (upper left) with brain substance (lower right) undergoing degeneration. Note perivascular collars of inflammatory cells. App. 15 x.

Fig. 650.—Nerve Root and Overlying Membranes: Tuberculosis.—Case 279.—Note extensive tuberculosis of membranes with characteristic cellular response and typical giant cell formation. App. 50 x.

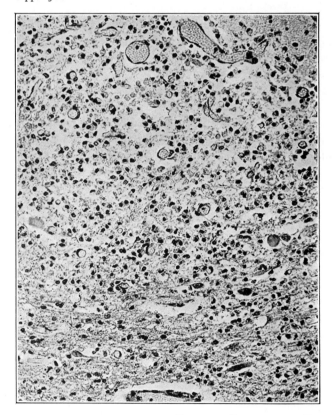

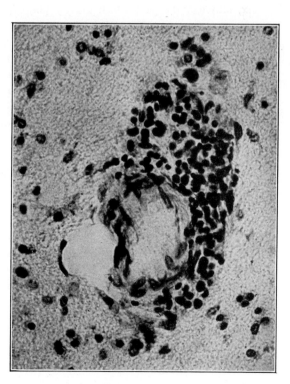

Fig. 651.—Midbrain: Acute Epidemic Encephalitis—Encephalomalacia.—Case 281.—Note congestion; softening, and presence of large numbers of typical microglial (Gitter) scavenger phagocytes. App. 100 x.

Fig. 652.—Brain: Cortex—Acute Epidemic Encephalitis.—Case 281.—High power photomicrograph of a blood vessel with the characteristic perivascular lymphocytic mantling. App. 200 x.

MENINGOCOCCIC MENINGITIS

Acute Pyogenic Forms.—The problem of meningococcic meningitis is not as simple as would appear at first thought. It has been well established that the meningococcus is found in the nasopharyngeal mucosa both in carriers and in human beings infected with the disease. For that reason it has been believed that the meningitis which follows results from the direct extension of the infection through the cribriform plate. However, this does not seem to be well substantiated in view of the findings in some of the acute fulminating cases of meningitic infection in which meningococcemia is the outstanding picture. Indeed, in these severe fulminating cases which are frequently associated, as has been emphasized, with hemorrhagic destruction of the adrenal medullae, as a part of the picture of the so-called "Waterhouse-Friederichsen syndrome," (Fig. 631) the cerebrospinal fluid is very commonly free of organisms; or if organisms are found, they are recovered only from the choroid plexus. For this reason, the suggestion has been advanced that the infection gains entrance to the meninges by way of the choroid plexus and from there, the organisms are carried through the aqueduct of Silvius and the fourth ventricle to migrate into the basal cisterns and from there spread over the surface of the brain. This thought is also somewhat substantiated by the fact that the infection tends to spread from below upward over the vertex, although the part which gravity plays in this respect cannot be disregarded. At the same time it seems difficult to understand why in the great majority of cases the fluid within the ventricular system is sterile while that in the meninges is so heavily infected. It is true that terminally in a certain proportion of cases a severe secondary ependymitis and involvement of the entire ventricular system is found. Many believe this to be a retrograde infection from the subarachnoid spaces.

The diagnosis of meningitis clinically is made as a result of symptoms of increased intracranial pressure with rigidity of the neck, headache, increased motor irritability with exaggerated reflexes and a gradual loss of consciousness. More specifically, the diagnosis is made by the withdrawal of cerebrospinal fluid either from the lumbar region, or in case obstruction around the foramen magnum has occurred, from the cisterna magna. The fluid in these cases is under increased pressure. Its turbidity varies, increasing as the disease progresses. There is an increase of protein and a diminution or absence of the carbohydrate reducing substance. This is believed due largely to the fermentive action of the organism. Typically there is a marked increase in inflammatory cells in the fluid, which are almost entirely of the polymorphonuclear leukocytic type. These vary greatly in number ranging from one or two thousand up to many thousand per cubic millimeter. Characteristically, the smear from such spinal fluid shows the presence of gram-negative diplococci, the great majority of which are intracellular. Curiously these are often only very few in number, although at other times they may be present in enormous quantities. Clinically, the use of antimeningococcic serum introduced into the spinal canal and in the early cases intravenously as well is believed to greatly reduce the mortality and the complications. Recent experimental work has raised the question as to the efficacy of this form of therapy, but it still seems the best means of treatment which we have available. In reported series of cases, as high as ninety per cent to whom serum was administered within the first forty-eight hours of the disease have recovered. A small proportion, treated or untreated probably go on to a fatal exodus.

Pathology.—At autopsy, the pathology, unless the case is of the fulminating meningococcemic type, is largely restricted to the central nervous system. The brain is covered with a purulent exudate which is usually heaviest at the base of the brain and spreads along the normal subarachnoid pathways. Thus, it is found deep between the gyri. This is accompanied by a varying degree of venous congestion so that the meningeal vessels tend to stand out as deeply cyanosed, tortuous channels. (Fig. 99.)

Depending upon the stage of the process, the microscopic picture will vary. (Fig. 100.) In the earlier acute period, a rather marked fibrinous exudate is seen with varying numbers of polynuclears. A little later, the exudate is almost entirely polynuclear in character with the cells showing beginning degenerative changes. Still later, the exudate tends to change toward the mononuclear form with large mononuclear phagocytes appearing first and later, lymphocytes tending to predominate. In this respect the resolution of the meningococcic exudate might well be compared to the process as seen in the lung in pneumococcic pneumonia. In cases in which recovery follows, it is not uncommon to find residual fibrosis and scarring at the base of the brain to an extent which may seriously interfere with cerebrospinal fluid circulation. Actual obstruction of the foramen magnum may occur and incomplete obstruction is comparatively common tending to produce a variable degree of persistent increased intracranial pressure, even to the point of hydrocephalus. Reëstablishment of the cerebrospinal circulation by operative procedures has been almost dramatic in its effectiveness although only a relatively small number of cases respond. For an illustrative history, the reader is referred to Case 45 (Ref. #S-4) in Chapter XIII.

PNEUMOCOCCIC AND STREPTOCOCCIC MENINGITIS

The pneumococcus and streptococcus are the two other most common causes of acute meningitis. These infections very frequently result from direct extension or may occur as a blood stream infection in a similar way as in the case of meningococcic meningitis. The picture is entirely comparable in all respects except in regard to the nature of the inflammatory exudate. In this regard the picture is comparable to that seen in other tissues. In other words, if the infection is caused by the pneumococcus, we are likely to find a very heavy fibrinopurulent exudate which is rather characteristically of a greenish-yellow color. It tends to be more diffuse than the meningococcic picture and to cover the entire surface of the brain as a thick, plastic membrane. The spinal fluid correspondingly shows a much higher leukocyte count, indeed at times the exudate being so thick that it cannot be withdrawn through the diagnostic lumbar puncture needle. On the other hand, in the streptococcic infections, the exudate tends to be more a seropurulent type although the leukocytic reaction may be very marked at times. The use of bacterial antisera in these infections is of little avail and they are usually believed to have an almost hopeless prognosis. However, in recent years, chemotherapy has shown some promise, particularly in respect to the streptococcic group. Sulfanilamide, in the hands of various investigators, particularly Kolmer, seems to be of a very hopeful and promising value.

TUBERCULOUS MENINGITIS

Chronic Granulomatous Forms of Meningitis. —Tuberculous meningitis is usually a terminal event in respect to a generalized miliary tuberculosis. However in a few instances it may appear to be a primary infection. This is particularly true in instances of infantile tuberculous meningitis where no primary lesion elsewhere can be demonstrated. Whether the organism in such cases gains access to the meninges along the course of the nerves or whether it again is a blood stream infection is problematical. Rich believes that in most cases tuberculosis of the meninges is secondary to a tuberculosis of the brain and choroid plexus. He has shown that superficial cortical lesions not more than four or five millimeters in diameter may caseate and rupture into the arachnoid spaces. Just as elsewhere in the body, it is believed that the nature of the reaction is to a large extent allergic. Thus, the mechanism of tuberculous meningitis is still to some extent problematical, but depends primarily upon a hematogenous spread in the great majority of instances.

Pathology.—As in the case of the meningococcic type of meningitis, the lesion is predominantly basilar in its distribution. It is characterized by a curious milky, gelatinoid exudate around the base of the brain, which extends to involve the optic chiasm and olfactory bulbs. It likewise spreads along the subarachnoid pathways, particularly following the course of the middle meningeal vessels where characteristically small miliary bead like tubercles can be seen almost outlining the course of the vessel. The nature of the process varies just as tuberculosis elsewhere. In places it is predominantly a fibrocaseous lesion with severe exudative phenomena. In others the lesion is not unlike the serofibrinous outpouring of fluid which one sees so typically in the pleural cavity. The extent of miliary tubercle formation depends largely upon the acuteness of the process and the degree of reactivity on the part of the individual.

The disease is becoming less common in this country as the incidence of primary infection is reduced. Even so short a time as twenty years ago the bovine type of organism was found to be responsible for a very considerable number of the cases, and Boyd comments that as high as thirty per cent of cases in England are found to be due to the bovine organism. Due to the reduction of bovine infection in this country, this type of infection has almost completely disappeared.

The diagnosis in the case of tuberculous meningitis is made primarily upon the demonstration of tubercle bacilli within the fluid. Clinically, there is the same picture of increased meningeal pressure and irritation. The process, however, is usually slow and progressive, the average case living three to four weeks or more after the onset of symptoms. Repeated lumbar puncture frequently gives great relief during this interval, but gradually unconsciousness ensues. Especially in the marasmic infant, opisthotonos from meningeal irritation is extremely prominent. The spinal fluid is usually almost as clear as water when it is first withdrawn and unless it is compared to a tube of sterile water, it is frequently cast aside as negative. However, it is under increased pressure. Chemical examination of the fluid shows a marked increase in protein content and a tendency for diminution in the carbohydrate reducing substance. More important from the chemical standpoint is the reduction in chlorides which is almost regularly present in this condition. The cell count is of little value. It is usually low, rarely exceeding two hundred cells per cubic millimeter and more often being under one hundred cells. These are usually lymphocytes, although in the more acute fulminating early cases, polymorphonuclears may be present. Upon standing, a characteristic fine network of fibrin forms and examination of this clot is likely to reveal the organism upon which the final diagnosis depends, as the other findings are not sufficiently clear cut to differeniate the condition from lesions such as encephalitis, poliomyelitis, serous meningitis or even presence of some intracranial lesion such as a brain abscess or brain tumor. The reader is referred to Case 59 in Chapter XVI for an illustrative case.

SYPHILITIC MENINGITIS

Syphilitic meningitis, in the absence of central nervous syphilis, is so extremely rare that it need not be considered from the clinical standpoint. At autopsy, the typical case of true syphilitic meningitis is that of a serofibrinous exudate which has a rather characteristic milky appearance. It is usually most marked at the base of the brain and appears to be integral with the brain surface, stripping with difficulty and often resulting in tearing of the cerebral substance. The spinal fluid characteristically shows similar increased pressure and a cell content in which plasma cells and lymphocytes predominate.

The chief point to recall in relation to syphilitic meningitis is that it is merely part of the general picture and is almost invariably associated with vascular syphilis which is seen as a syphilitic arteritis of the meningeal vessels as well as those of the brain substance. Thus, patchy areas of chronic granulomatous scarring are seen in association with the development of miliary gummata quite as often as the above described more acute, diffuse, serous type of meningitis. This serous type of meningitis is perhaps more often seen as part of the picture of congenital syphilis in infancy, whereas the more chronic type of central nervous syphilis is apt to be seen in the middle-aged adult, especially the male, with other evidence of central nervous syphilis.

MISCELLANEOUS CHRONIC FORMS OF MENINGITIS.—In addition to these specific infectious forms of meningitis, there is a variety of inflammation of the meninges which has been shown rather conclusively to be due to a filtrable virus. This is known as *benign lymphocytic meningitis* or lymphatic choriomeningitis. The disease can be reproduced in experimental animals by the injection of a filtrate from the spinal fluid. It is characterized by the production of a markedly increased serous exudate accompanied by a considerable degree of lymphocytic reaction. One such case which we encountered showed a cell count of over one thousand cells, all of which were small lymphocytes. So far as is known, there is no mortality associated with this particular infection. The chief point of interest in the disease clinically is its differentiation from other more serious infections of the central nervous system such as encephalitis. Examination of the spinal fluid may show a slight increase in protein and no alteration in the carbohydrate reducing substance, nor in the chlorides.

Likewise, to be separated from this disease which represents a true infectious process should be mentioned *meningismus,* by which is meant the accumulation of fluid in the cerebrospinal fluid pathways with the development of mild symptoms of meningeal irritation. In a sense, this might be considered as a mild form of external hydrocephalus. It is not uncommonly encountered in acute infectious diseases, such as pneumonia or gastro-intestinal upsets especially in children. It likewise is of little clinical significance except from the standpoint of differential diagnosis.

INFECTIOUS DISEASES OF THE BRAIN AND CORD

Acute Pyogenic Abscess.—The pyogenic infections of the brain are represented by abscess formation which may be either hematogenous in origin or result from direct extension of a local infection such as mastoiditis, middle ear infection, or sinusitis. In the development of such a lesion by direct continuity, there is of necessity likely to be an associated meningitis. This, however, may remain strictly localized and become walled off from the rest of the meninges so that the clinical and pathological picture which we commonly associate with meningitis does not follow. The most common source of infection for a blood-borne metastatic abscess appears to be from some suppurative lesion of the respiratory tract, particularly from a lung abscess. The lesion is likely to be seen as a single abscess cavity and may attain a considerable size. The most common infectious agent is a streptococcus, although staphylococci, and pneumococci are also frequent etiologic agents. A great many of the cases are complicated by a coincidental Bacillus pyocyaneus infection. Rarely do we encounter multiple abscess formation under these circumstances, and even more curious is the fact that no other visceral metastatic pyemic foci can be demonstrated. There is a very striking tendency of such abscesses to become localized and well walled off. They are not very regularly associated with the usual evidence of acute infection as characterized by a rise in temperature or in the white count, although both may be present at times. The lesion tends to become walled off by a thick layer of gliosis and the contents of the abscess cavity may undergo absorption or calcification if the lesion becomes sterilized through phagocytic action on the part of the inflammatory cells. There is liquefaction necrosis. The great majority of such abscesses tend to remain relatively quiescent for long periods of time but to gradually increase in size and produce pressure symptoms. Not infrequently such abscesses have been mistaken clinically for brain tumors. They are usually, except for position at times, amenable to surgical drainage. Ultimately, if left alone the great majority of such abscesses tend to rupture either into the ventricular system or to the surface with the establishment of a severe secondary and terminal meningitis.

ILLUSTRATIVE CASE

CASE 278. (Ref. #S-398)

Diagnosis.—Cerebellum—brain abscess.

Patient was a seven year old white boy admitted to the hospital because of a draining abscess in the right ear associated with mastoid tenderness.

Present Illness.—The onset of the patient's present illness was of forty-eight hours' duration. It began with a severe earache during the course of a varicella infection. The abscess in his ear had apparently ruptured spontaneously with great relief temporarily, but subsequently was followed by swelling and tenderness over the mastoid area.

Past Medical History.—The child had always been subject to upper respiratory infections and had had a previous abscess in the same ear about eight months earlier. He had had whooping cough and measles in addition to his present varicella infection. He had not had scarlet fever so far as his parents were aware.

Physical Examination.—The patient was a well-developed, well-nourished, acutely-ill child lying uncomfortably in bed with his face flushed and groaning with pain. Head showed marked flushing of the skin. There was exquisite tenderness over the right mastoid tip accompanied by considerable edema and reddening. The temperature was 101°. His nose and throat appeared negative. The right ear showed a purulent discharge. The drum of the left ear was bulging and fiery red. Chest was symmetrical. Lungs appeared to be clear. Heart was not enlarged. Sounds were rapid and somewhat distant. Abdomen was negative. Extremities were normal.

Laboratory Findings.—Blood count: red cells, 4,800,-000 with 73% hemoglobin. White cells, 18,600 with 92% neutrophiles. Urinalysis was negative except for a slight trace of albumin.

Subsequent History.—Patient had a radical mastoidectomy done with immediate relief of symptoms, but shortly after, approximately forty-eight hours following operation, there was a sharp rise of his temperature to 104°. This was accompanied by vomiting and the child became irrational. There was considerable rigidity of his neck and a positive Kernig's sign. He developed a definite meningitis with a cloudy spinal fluid under moderately increased pressure. Bacteriologically, hemolytic streptococci were recovered. Repeated spinal drainage, the use of prontylin and of streptococcic antiserum failed to help the child's condition. He went steadily downhill dying two weeks after admission with localizing symptoms, which pointed toward the development of an abscess in the cerebellum.

Autopsy Findings.—At autopsy, multiple small focal abscesses were found throughout the cerebellum and cerebrum, the largest of these being localized in the right cerebellum and measuring approximately 1.5 cm. in diameter. These were fairly well localized by a zone of glial proliferation. They were centrally filled with typical necrotic, broken down leukocytes with the complete picture of liquefaction necrosis.

Microscopic Description of a Section Through the Wall of the Brain Abscess.—(Fig. 649) The gross appearance of the lesion is confirmed by microscopic study. There is a central zone of necrosis with actual suppuration. The polymorphonuclears are present in large numbers, but are for the most part broken down and hard to identify. Scattered bits of chromatin and degenerated cytoplasmic material are seen. With appropriate staining technique for bacteria, the presence of short-chained streptococci can be established. These are most abundant in the edge of the abscess wall. Around the abscess cavity there is a definite zone of glial proliferation which shows extensive leukocytic infiltration. Outside this area, considerable perivascular mantling of the blood vessels is seen, chiefly by lymphocytes, but also including many polymorphonuclears.

CHRONIC FORMS

Tuberculosis.—Tuberculosis of the brain itself, aside from its association with a tuberculous meningitis, is a comparatively uncommon finding. When it occurs it tends to be in the form of a solitary tubercle or tuberculoma. It is usually seen in childhood or in early adolescence rather than in later life and when it occurs, it is most frequently encountered in the cerebellum. Only rarely is such a solitary tubercle found in the brain stem. The lesions are apt to be subcortical in relation to the surface of the cerebellum or cerebrum, and the thought cannot fail to occur to one that they develop by extension into the brain substance from an embolic lesion of the pial vessels. Similar, but much smaller, lesions may be found occasionally involving the substance of the spinal cord. This may push the various nerve tracts aside, but more often tends to invade them with degeneration of the nerve fibers distant to the lesion.

Microscopically the diagnosis is usually comparatively simple. The lesion tends to be almost spherical in outline and to be surrounded by a rather characteristic zone of epithelioid cells with giant cell formation. Centrally caseous necrosis is present although due to the vascular pattern in the brain, this may go on to actual liquefaction. Tubercle bacilli are rarely demonstrated, but animal inoculation with material from the lesion can establish the diagnosis in the great majority of instances. The condition is of grave significance because of its tendency to produce a secondary tuberculous meningitis either spontaneously or as a result of operative interference. The symptoms again are comparable to those of brain abscess or brain tumor, chiefly symptoms of pressure with localizing signs to establish the usual cerebellum involvement. Surgical removal of the tuberculoma may relieve the pressure symptoms in selected cases.

ILLUSTRATIVE CASE

Case 279. (Ref. #S-399)
Diagnosis.—Spinal cord—Compression atrophy; myelomalacia (tuberculous).

Patient was a colored female of 65 years, admitted to the hospital with the chief complaint of pain in the legs.

Present Illness.—The onset of the illness was about six months previously. At that time she began to have dull aching pain in both lower extremities, but especially in the hips and knees. She developed progressive muscular weakness and stated that her legs felt numb; as she described them, "dead." Her physician was inclined to feel that this represented an arthritic problem with focal infection as the etiologic factor. He had her teeth x-rayed and numerous apical abscesses were found. As a result she had all her teeth extracted, but this did not cause any improvement in her clinical picture. About three months before admission, she developed pain in

her chest which was likewise of a dull, aching type rather than a sharp, knife-like, radiating pain. This was almost continuous in character, although varying somewhat in intensity from day to day.

Past Medical History.—The patient had no recollection of her childhood history so far as her infection was concerned. She was married at the age of eighteen and had had six normal, full-term children. She had never had any serious illness apparently, although she said that at times she had been confined to bed at home with the "misery." A review of her systems was essentially negative. She had not been particularly subject to upper respiratory infection. Most of her "misery" was apparently associated with vague gastro-intestinal symptoms, which could not be evaluated. Her genito-urinary history had been negative. Menses had begun, she thought, at the age of eleven; they had been regular. Menopause occurred at the age of forty-six.

Physical Examination.—The patient was a small, senile-appearing Negress lying propped up in bed. She was extremely weak. She did not appear in acute pain. She could move her arms, but not her legs. Head was negative. Eyes, ears, nose and throat were normal. Pupils were equal and reacted to light and accommodation. She was edentulous. Chest was symmetrical and slightly of the senile emphysematous type. Lungs were clear. Heart was moderately enlarged to the left. Sounds were of poor quality. There were no murmurs. Blood pressure 150/84. Abdomen was distended. This distention seemed to be the result of dilatation of the colon. Extremities were negative.

Neurologic Examination.—Memory was extremely poor, but she seemed well oriented. Cranial nerves were normal. Reflexes seemed slightly exaggerated. She was incontinent of urine and feces. There was complete flaccid paralysis of both lower extremities and there was a partial loss of all forms of sensation below the sixth costal interspace.

Laboratory Findings.—Urinalysis was negative except for occasional faint traces of albumin. Blood chemistry showed a definite diabetes with sugar ranging from 170 to 280 mgm. per 100 cubic centimeters of blood. The blood urea was 66 mgm. Red blood cells numbered 3,200,000 with 9 gm. of hemoglobin. White blood cells, 9,400 with 78% neutrophiles. Spinal fluid was negative. Wassermann was negative both in respect to the blood and spinal fluid.

X-ray Examination.—A destructive process which involved the right upper half of the sixth thoracic vertebra was demonstrated with narrowing of the intervertebral space. On lateral view, there was a definite wedge-shaped narrowing of the spinal canal at the level of the sixth vertebra. The lungs by x-ray showed diffuse fibrosis and a number of calcified areas apparently within the hilar lymphnodes. There was no evidence of metastatic tumor in the lungs.

Subsequent Course.—The patient went steadily downhill and died quietly, two weeks after admission.

Autopsy Findings.—At autopsy, a large decubitus was noted over the sacrum. Otherwise, externally, no lesions were demonstrated. Heart was slightly enlarged. The coronaries showed marked sclerosis. On section, evidence of an old infarct in the left ventricular wall with a dense fibrous scar was present. The lungs showed moderate terminal edema. There was no evidence of any active tuberculosis found, but a typical Ghon tubercle five millimeters in diameter, completely calcified, was identified in the lower portion of the left upper lobe. The liver, spleen and other abdominal viscera appeared negative except for moderate parenchymatous degeneration. Examination of the vertebral column showed the fourth, fifth and sixth vertebrae, especially the sixth, were involved in a degenerative lesion accompanied by marked erosion of the vertebral bodies. There was a mass of semisolid, creamy, caseous material in this area which had extended into the spinal canal and enveloped the nerve roots of the cord as they left the foramina. The picture grossly suggested tuberculosis. Examination of the spinal cord showed marked softening and degenerative changes below this point.

Microscopic Description of a Section Through the Spinal Cord.—(Fig. 650) There is a very marked myelomalacia present in the cord as best demonstrated perhaps by sections stained by the Weigert technique. This is most marked in the lower cord where very extensive destruction of both gray and white matter has taken place. The anterior horns cannot be identified as a result of this destructive process, and subsequent gliosis. Secondary degenerative changes, particularly affecting the sensory posterior pathways are present, even in the sections immediately above the compression area. Surrounding the cord there is a typical histologic picture of tuberculosis involving the nerve roots and arachnoid structures.

SYPHILIS OF THE CENTRAL NERVOUS SYSTEM.—Depending upon one's concept of the disease, these central nervous manifestations may be classified either as tertiary or quaternary. It has always seemed to us that they make up a very important group of late lesions which should be considered as a quartanary stage, although we realize that not every untreated case of syphilis will of necessity go on to the development of these central nervous phenomena. It may well be that individual tissue sensitivity may be responsible for this selective manifestation of the disease in a certain group of individuals rather than that the disease must follow a set pattern. It is apparent that syphilis of the central nervous system may be divided into *interstitial forms* of the disease, the so-called "neurosyphilis" or "cerebrospinal syphilis"; and *parenchymatous forms* in which the nerve cells are primarily affected. Levaditi and others have suggested that certain strains of the *Treponema pallidum* have a special affinity for

the central nervous system just as others seem to have a similar affinity for epithelial cells. This theory of the investigative work requires much more experimental evidence than has been brought forward to date, and it seems equally, if not more logical to believe in the constitutional diathesis of the individual in this respect. As a rule, the central nervous manifestations of syphilis do not occur for a number of years after the primary infection, although certain instances have been recorded in which there was a prompt involvement of the brain and cord within the usual time limits expected for the development of the usual tertiary gummatous lesions, and it is for this reason that these various forms of central nervous syphilis are included by many as a tertiary type of the disease. The various forms of central nervous syphilis will be considered separately.

Gumma.—The gumma, like the solitary tubercle, is a lesion which begins usually in the cortex of the brain arising apparently from an infection of the pial vessels. Clinically, also like the tuberculoma, it very frequently gives rise to symptoms simulating brain tumor through increased intracranial pressure, and a number of cases have been established solely through the fact that a positive serologic blood was present.

Pathologically, the gumma of the brain, or more rarely of the cord, is similar in appearance both grossly and microscopically to other gummata. It is a rather firm, dry, grayish-yellow or grayish-white, pseudocaseous area of necrosis. It tends, like the tuberculoma, to be spherical but is likely to be rather larger in size. As an additional differential feature, the lesion is obviously more often seen in adult life.

Microscopically, gliosis and fibrosis are rather characteristic. Lymphocytic and plasma cell infiltration around the lesion is likely to be more prominent than in the tuberculous lesion. There is almost invariably an overlying chronic leptomeningitis.

Interstitial Cerebrospinal Neurosyphilis.—In the diffuse form of syphilis of the central nervous system, we are dealing primarily and essentially with a syphilitic endarteritic process. This presents the usual characterisic subintimal thickening of the smaller blood vessels, not infrequently accompanied by secondary or terminal thrombus formation with the actual occulsion of the lumen of the vessel. Such lesions may be rather widely and uniformly distributed throughout the brain substance, but more often are found as focal lesions which go on to the development of encephalomalacia or softening as in the case of other vascular occulsions. Due, however, to the thickening of the vessel wall, both by the subintimal connective tissue proliferation and the infiltration of the media, as well as the adventitial cellular reaction, hemorrhage into the brain or cord substance is rare in syphilis. Likewise the development of aneurysms is almost negligible in contrast to their development in association with atherosclerotic lesions. In the cord, the focal nature of the process may be manifested by actual segmental distribution of the clinical signs and symptoms. Depending upon the extent of the process, varying amounts of atrophy of the brain or cord substance may follow. As an inevitable accompaniment of the vascular picture is seen an involvement of the meningeal vessels, particularly those of the pia arachnoid. This results in perivascular cellular in-

filtration and resultant fibrosis as the Spirochete tends to stimulate its fibrogenetic activity here as elsewhere. Thus, strictly speaking, the picture of interstitial neurosyphilis should be termed syphilitic meningo-encephalitis.

Diagnostically, the symptoms are so protean in their manifestations that it is worse than useless to attempt to include their discussion in a general pathological outline such as this. In every case in which the diagnosis of the central nervous system pathology is not obvious it is certainly worthwhile to bear in mind the possibility of syphilis—this in spite of the fact that there is a definite decrease in the number of such cases as a result of the intensive campaign against the disease, which has resulted in much earlier diagnosis and more intensive therapy during the past decade. Indeed, it is rare today to encounter gumma of the brain, and many of the cases of central nervous system syphilis which are being seen are in patients who contracted the disease fifteen or twenty years ago and had no knowledge of the significance of their current neurologic symptoms. It must be remembered that syphilis may remain latent for periods as long as twenty years before these late nervous system lesions show up in their true colors. Examination of the spinal fluid in such cases of uncertain diagnosis may be of inestimable value in its establishment. Typically, the spinal fluid will give a positive Wassermann complement fixation reaction and will show an altered colloidal gold curve, which may simulate the paretic picture. The protein content may or may not be increased depending upon the amount of meningeal involvement. The cell count likewise depends on this factor. Where meningitis is a prominent feature the cell count may well rise to several hundred cells, predominantly lymphocytes. On the other hand, chemical and cytological spinal fluid examination may yield essentially normal findings by the serologic reaction and still be of diagnostic significance.

General Paresis, Including the Juvenile Form (General Paralysis of the Insane; Dementia Paralytica; Parenchymatous Cerebral Syphilis).—In this condition, there is a direct invasion of the cerebral cortex by the *Treponema pallidum*. The course which they follow to reach the brain substance is still somewhat debatable. By many, it is believed that they invade the cortex secondarily to a meningeal infection. This is based particularly upon the fact that they are rarely found deep in the brain tissue. Others are equally convinced of their hematogenous spread. It may likewise be of significance that regularly the skull shows thickening rather diffusely over the frontoparietal and temporal areas; that there is marked thickening of the dura and very commonly a diffuse, chronic hemorrhagic pachymeningitis. On opening such a skull the brain invariably shows marked atrophy, especially of the frontoparietal lobes. There is an increase of fluid in the subarachnoid spaces which tends to be somewhat milky in appearance. This is due in part to thickening of the membranes around the sulci. The normal convolutions appear small and the sulci correspondingly widened. The pia is apt to be firmly adherent over the frontoparietal area so that it cannot be separated from the brain without laceration of the cerebral cortex. On cross section the ventricular system is found to be dilated and the ependyma usually granular in appearance. In cross section, it is apparent that the atrophy of the brain is largely due to a diminution in the gray matter rather than the white. The blood vessels stand out prominently and are likely to show a typical syphilitic endarteritic picture similar to that seen in the interstitial form of the disease.

Histologic examination of the brain shows a diffuse cellular infiltration, which is most marked around the basal ganglia in the floor of the fourth ventricle and in the cerebral cortex. This cellular reaction consists of a diffuse, perivascular collar-like infiltration of the tissues by plasma cells and lymphocytes. Other inflammatory cells may be present in variable numbers. Microglial scavenger cells not infrequently will be found in considerable numbers. There is extensive degeneration of the ganglion cells, and various nuclear changes can be seen as well as alteration in the appearance of the Nissl granules. There is a proliferative gliosis, the counterpart of the fibrosis seen in other organs so that the normal architecture of the cortex is completely distorted and the arrangement of the cells appears purposeless. Sections stained by Marchi and Weigert methods show extensive degeneration of the nerve fibers as well. Stab cells representing the intermediate stage in the reversal of the microglia to the typical scavenger or Gitter cell are seen in large numbers in association with the glial proliferation. Not infrequently, as one examines sections of the spinal cord from such cases, secondary degenerative changes of the pyramidal tracts as a result of degeneration of the motor nerve cell of the cortex can be demonstrated.

From the clinical standpoint, general paresis represents one of the most serious complications of syphilis. There is nothing more tragic than to watch the mental deterioration and character change of the individual in whom this lesion is progressing, involving as it does particularly the frontoparietal region. It affects especially judgment and self-control. The patient becomes slovenly in his habits, untidy about his person, coarse in his speech and loses all sense of moral proportion. Not infrequently he gradually acquires delusions of grandeur and ultimately he becomes completely demented. Alteration in speech with tremors of the face and tongue occur. He drools at the mouth and develops a tendency toward epileptiform convulsive attacks in which he may lose consciousness and exhibit a transitory hemiplegia.

Typically, from the diagnostic standpoint, he develops the so-called Argyll Robertson pupillary reflex with inability for the pupil to react to light, although it still responds to accommodation. Lumbar puncture reveals a spinal fluid which is usually clear and may be under a slightly increased pressure. Depending again upon the amount of meningeal involvement, there may or may not be chemical alteration of the protein content and an increase in cells. When cells are present they tend to be of the plasma-cell type. More characteristic is the appearance of the paretic curve by the colloidal gold test and the presence of a positive serologic reaction.

Paresis may occur, not only in the adult in association with acquired syphilis, but may also on occasion be seen in children as part of the picture of hereditary lues. In such instances, it is particularly severe and runs a relatively more rapid course than in those instances occurring in later life.

Tabes Dorsalis (Locomotor Ataxia).—Another of the late neurologic manifestations of syphilis is seen in the degenerative process which affects the posterior columns of the spinal cord and is known as tabes dorsalis. There appears to be a great deal of evidence that the lesion is definitely syphilitic in nature, although spirochetes have rarely been demonstrated except in the perineural spaces. It is generally believed that the primary lesion in tabes dorsalis is a syphilitic meningitis and possibly an endarteritis involving the posterior roots of the spinal cord. These inflammatory changes are so marked it is believed that they interfere with the nutrition of the nerve fibers and result in a subsequent degeneration and gliosis of the posterior columns. In this respect the pathology is unlike that of paresis in which the inflammatory manifestations are the more striking. This theory of secondary degeneration to a chronic inflammatory process of the posterior nerve roots is an attractive hypothesis but one which is subject to considerable criticism. Recently it has been suggested that the focus for this neurolytic toxin may be totally outside the central nervous system and that the toxin reaches the cord by extending along the perineural lymphatics or the axis cylinders of the afferent nerves in the same way in which tetanus toxin acts.

In this instance, we are dealing with what appears to be a simple degenerative process. The disease is one of middle life occurring much more commonly in males. It likewise runs a pitiful course. In this condition the changes are chiefly related first of all to sensory disturbances with a loss particularly of deep sensation. The peculiar manner of locomotion of the tabetic patient is due to this loss of muscle sense, so that the patient is unaware of the position of his feet unless he can watch them. This loss of deep sensation and the vibratory sense results in the characteristic Romberg sign which is of great significance diagnostically. By a positive Romberg test is meant that the patient with his eyes closed and his feet placed together is unable to maintain himself in the erect position. He starts swaying until his balance is completely lost and he falls to the floor unless aided. Such loss of deep sensation is the result of the degeneration of the posterior tracts in which these impulses normally are found. In addition to this incoördination with the typical ataxic gait there are associated sensory disturbances. Among these should be mentioned the shooting pains in his legs, of which the patient complains. In the same way, the reflex arc of the Achilles and knee jerks are broken and these normal reflexes are typically absent. As in the case of paresis, there is an Argyll Robertson pupil through extension of the lesion to the floor of the aqueduct of Silvius. As the condition progresses, the optic nerve may become involved in the same type of inflammatory neuritis as noted in the posterior nerve roots so that ultimately blindness may follow.

Among the more outstanding symptoms of tabes are the acute abdominal attacks of pain spoken of as the "tabetic crises." This has been explained in various ways. In general, it is believed to be a sympathetic nervous system manifestation very possibly the result of vascular distention. In the more advanced cases, it not infrequently follows that the development of a trophic type of arthrosis occurs with degenerative phenomena of the bones and joint surfaces resulting in a flail joint. The knee is perhaps the most commonly involved. This is thought to be due primarily to the fact that there is an analgesia present so that the patient is not aware of any undue strain upon the joint surface. It has been shown experimentally that by cutting pain fibers, or in other conditions in which similar loss of pain sensation has occurred, similar trophic changes may occur in a joint. These need not necessarily be syphilitic in nature, but from the clinical standpoint, the Charcot joint is more often of this associated syphilitic origin. The cerebrospinal fluid examination in tabes again is usually of very little value except in respect to its serology and its colloidal gold curve which is of the luetic type. In the earlier, more acute stages of the process it is not uncommon to find an increased cell count which may rise to several hundred and which may include many polymorphonuclears.

From the pathological standpoint, sections taken at various levels of the spinal cord and stained by Marchi or Weigert technique will present a regular sequence of events. There is usually a varying degree of inflammatory thickening of the pia over the posterior aspect of the spinal column. The columns themselves appear somewhat concave rather than convex due to the degenerative loss of tissue. Similarly the posterior nerve roots are atrophic as compared with the normal anterior roots. In the early stage of the disease it can be demonstrated that there is a marked demyelinization as seen by the fat droplets, which stain intensely with Scharlach R, or by Marchi's method. Soon the axones themselves become involved in the degenerative process and gradually disappear. There follows a replacement proliferation of the glial cells, notably the astrocytes. The process varies in extent, the more marked lesions usually being found involving the lumbar part of the cord.

If only these lower segments are involved, then sections through the cervical spinal cord will show only degeneration of the mesial column of Goll, whereas if the upper extremities and trunk as well are involved in the pathological picture, then both sensory columns, including that of Burdach will also show similar demyelinization and varying degrees of gliosis (Fig. 659).

ILLUSTRATIVE CASE

CASE 280. (Ref. #S-283)

Diagnosis.—Spinal cord—tabes dorsalis.

Patient was a white male of 43 years, admitted to the hospital with the chief complaint of periodic attacks of vomiting accompanied by severe cramps in his stomach.

Present Illness.—The onset of the patient's present symptoms dated back eighteen years when he first began to have occasional attacks of stomach cramps associated with vomiting spells. These came on about one hour after eating and lasted fifteen to twenty minutes. They persisted for a period of about three years and increased in severity. During this time the patient's weight decreased by over seventy-five pounds. He was treated as a case of gastric ulcer at that time.

For a brief period the symptoms seemed to improve, but they recurred with greater frequency. At that time he went to a hospital where he was studied more thoroughly and a diagnosis of syphilis was made. The gastric symptoms were felt to be tabetic in nature. He was given three courses of neoarsphenamine and bismuth treatment and likewise underwent hyperpyretic treatment by induced malaria. Again, with each series of treatments, his symptoms improved, but they always recurred after varying intervals and usually with greater severity. His last course of treatment was about four years ago and his attacks of vomiting and gastric pain had recently recurred once more. The attacks seemed to be precipitated by any form of anxiety or excitement, but did not seem to bear any direct relationship to the taking of food. Nothing would relieve the pain except morphine.

Past Medical History.—The patient had the usual childhood diseases. He had not had scarlet fever, typhoid or diphtheria. He had had influenza during the 1918 epidemic. He had never been particularly subject to upper respiratory disease. His cardiovascular system seemed to be normal. His gastro-intestinal history had been reviewed in relation to his present history. His urinary history was negative. He admitted syphilitic infection at the age of sixteen with the development of secondary lesions shortly after the appearance of his chancre. At that time the symptoms were of a mild nature and disappeared spontaneously. He did not receive any adequate treatment during the early stages of his infection, a local physician having treated him wholly by what probably was mercurial inunction.

Physical Examination.—Patient was a fairly well-developed and nourished, middle-aged white male. Head showed no abnormalities. Pupils were regular and equal, somewhat dilated and did not react to light, but did to accommodation (Argyll Robertson pupils). Nose and throat were negative. Chest was symmetrical. Lungs were clear. Heart was not enlarged and there were no murmurs.

Abdomen was essentially negative. There were no areas of tenderness or rigidity on palpation. There was a small penile scar. The extremities were negative.

Neurologic Examination.—The neurologic examination showed a positive Romberg and a somewhat ataxic gait. Sensation was markedly disturbed over both lower extremities. The knee jerks were absent.

Laboratory Findings.—Blood count revealed, 4,400,000 red cells with 11 gm. of hemoglobin, and 5,250 white blood cells with 67% neutrophiles. Urinalysis was negative. Blood Wassermann and Kahn were negative, presumably as a result of his intensive therapy. Chemistry was normal. Cerebrospinal fluid was clear and colorless and showed ten cells, all lymphocytes. Globulin was not increased. Sugar was negative. Wassermann was doubtful. Colloidal gold gave a typical tabetic curve. Gastric analysis showed moderate hyperacidity.

X-ray studies of the gastro-intestinal tract showed no evidence of ulcer, carcinoma or any obstructive lesion anywhere along its course.

Subsequent Course.—The patient was followed over a period of about one year and showed a persistence of gastric crises in spite of intensive therapy which was directed not only from the antisyphilitic standpoint, but with the addition of high caloric and high vitamin diet, and liver therapy. He was taken acutely ill with a typical lobar pneumonia and was readmitted to the hospital where he died on the seventh day of his illness.

Autopsy Findings.—The immediate cause of death was a very extensive right lower lobe lobar pneumonia in the stage of gray hepatization. This was caused by type-3 pneumococcus. Heart showed moderate myocardial degeneration. There was no evidence of any syphilitic involvement of the aorta or cardiovascular system in general. The abdominal viscera were negative. The stomach showed a moderate hypertrophic type of gastritis. The outstanding pathology in respect to his syphilitic history was seen in microscopic studies of the spinal cord. Grossly the cord appeared somewhat diminished in size. This diminution in size involved the posterior columns so that the surface was almost concave instead of convex.

Microscopic Description of a Section Taken from the Spinal Cord.—(Fig. 659) Sections taken from various levels of the cord show typical tabetic distribution of the pathology, which was restricted to the posterior columns of Goll and Burdach. Here, practically complete demyelinization of the nerve fibers has occurred, which has been followed by a replacement gliosis. By the Weigert staining method, this is readily demonstrated as pale-staining areas where, due to the lack of myelin, the tissues do not stain.

VIRUS DISEASES

As has been brought out in an earlier chapter in discussing virus disease in general, there are a considerable number of such infections which seem to be primarily neurotropic in character. Among these must be included anterior poliomyelitis, encephalitis of the epidemic type, rabies, herpes of both the simple and zoster types, post-vaccinal encephalitis and possibly the encephalomyelitis which is seen in relation to some of the acute infectious diseases, particularly measles and pertussis. The essential pathology of most of these has been considered in relation to the changes which occur in poliomyelitis in Chapter XVIII, and accordingly will only be reviewed briefly at this point for the sake of convenience.

Rabies.—Rabies has already been discussed in Chapter XVIII (Virus Diseases), and so need only be referred to at this point. It will be recalled that it is a specific virus infection, which seems to travel by way of the axis cylinders from the point of inoculation. The virus is ordinarily present in the salivary glands of the infected animal, either dog or cat, and thus is more often transmitted by the bite of such an animal than in any other way. The incubation period is extremely variable, ranging all the way from three weeks to over a year, with eight to ten weeks being about the average period.

The pathology is characterized by the presence of the so-called Negri bodies in the nerve cells of the brain and cord, but are commonly found particularly in the greatest numbers in the ganglion cells of the hippocampus major and in the Purkinje cells of the cerebellum. An illustrative history has been presented in Chapter XVIII, Case 69 (Ref. #S-159).

Herpes.—Similarly, herpes has likewise been discussed. The ordinary cold sore or fever blister (herpes simplex) represents the most familiar type of such herpetic virus infection. Shingles (herpes zoster) presents a similar etiology. The work of Goodpasture over the past ten years or more has emphasized the specificity of these neurotropic viruses. It will be recalled that they remain latent in the tissues until activated by some febrile disturbance. The point of greatest interest in respect to the herpes viruses is their possible relationship to encephalitis. It will be recalled that spontaneous encephalitis of rabbits may be reproduced experimentally by the injection of herpes virus. The similarity of the virus "B" of the St. Louis encephalitic type of infection is likewise believed by many to be closely related to this group of herpetic viruses. There is urgent need in the investigative field of ex-

perimental medicine to clarify the complex situation which exists in respect to this entire group of clinical and pathological conditions.

Acute Encephalomyelitis.—In conjunction with a number of the acute infectious diseases, but particularly in association with measles, less regularly in pertussis and influenza, and at times in association with some of the less typical upper respiratory infections, there is seen an associated acute encephalitic picture characterized by mental confusion and a wide range of neurologic symptoms. In a very small number of cases, this proceeds to a fatal outcome. In the great majority of instances, recovery is the rule and no residual symptoms or pathology are found later in life. In the fatal cases, the picture is usually one of acute congestion, often associated with diffuse petechial hemorrhage. In addition, nerve cell degeneration may be found with similar changes to those already described in poliomyelitis or encephalitis; namely, disintegration of the Nissl granules and degenerative changes of the nucleus with its ultimate disappearance, swelling of the cytoplasm of the cell and a loss of its normal protoplasmic process. A third feature of such encephalomyelitic pictures is seen in a definite demyelinization of the nerve cell structures. This can best be demonstrated by special staining methods such as Sudan III or the use of the Marchi technique. In the severe cases, this is followed by microglial proliferation of the scavenger cells. Whether these represent true virus infections or whether they represent the effect of toxins which have elaborated at the site of infection and carried to the central nervous system is problematical. The experimental induction of such lesions has not to date been notably successful. The relationship of such lesions to some of the more strictly degenerative diseases of the central nervous system is likewise problematical. In general, however, it seems fair to state that these acute encephalomyelitic lesions are apparently inflammatory in character rather than degenerative, and that if the patient survives the initial acute process, repair and clinical recovery follow almost invariably.

Anterior Poliomyelitis.—Anterior poliomyelitis may be defined as an acute specific infectious disease caused by a filtrable virus, which has a predilection for the motor ganglion cells of the spinal cord and brain stem. It will be recalled that the chief portal of entry seems to be the nasopharynx by way of the olfactory nerve endings, through the cribriform plate and along the axones to the central nervous system. Except in unusually severe infections, the cerebrum shows but little evidence of involvement either clinically or pathologically. It will likewise be recalled that there is considerable evidence available to suggest that the disease is a diffuse systemic infection with a very marked reticulo-endothelial response as well, definite hyperplastic and degenerative changes being found in the germinal centers of the lymph follicles of the gastro-intestinal tract, the regional mesenteric lymph nodes, the spleen and not infrequently also the tonsils, and an almost regular accompaniment of thymic hyperplasia. The neurologic manifestations are those of motor nerve cell destruction with neuronophagia by the scavenger microglial cells, which results in loss of motor function of the peripheral muscles. This is usually most marked in the lumbar region of the cord. The pathology is further characterized by marked edema and congestion of the cord and by a rather characteristic perivascular mantling by lymphocytes, which frequently fill the Virchow-Robin spaces. The disease is transmissible to monkeys most readily by direct intracerebral inoculation, but also by intranasal instillation of the virus. For illustrative histories, refer to Case 67 (Ref. #S-157) in Chapter XVIII, representing an acute stage; and to Case 68, (Ref. #S-158), the history of a late stage (270 days) of the disease.

Epidemic Encephalitis.—Epidemic encephalitis, like anterior poliomyelitis, is generally believed to be due to a filtrable virus. The disease is seen in various forms during different epidemics, and there is considerable uncertainty as to whether the infection is due to a single virus as modified by conditions from time to time, or whether there are a number of related strains of virus which give rise to somewhat similar clinical and pathological pictures. Since the first major pandemic of the disease, which occurred in the lethargic form in 1917, several major, more localized epidemics have been seen. The outbreak which followed the initial lethargic pandemic tended to be of the myoclonic or hyperkinetic type with extraordinary mental activity and motor irritability resulting in myoclonic convulsions. However, a very large proportion of these cases ulti-

mately went on to a lethargic state, and the late manifestations of the disease as seen anywhere from a few months to two or three years after the acute attack were similar in nature. Most spectacular among these late sequellae is the condition known as *postencephalitic paralysis agitans* in which the rather characteristic parkinsonian mask-like expression and mental torpor are the outstanding symptoms. As might well be expected, because of the widespread involvement of the brain in the inflammatory process an almost endless variety of clinical pictures and neurologic manifestations may be encountered. These range from mild sensory disturbances with pain to actual palsies and are likewise accompanied at times by marked character change, suggesting extensive frontoparietal involvement.

More recently in the St. Louis epidemic of 1933, a virus was obtained which shows certain features which distinguish it from the earlier and more severe forms. In this particular outbreak there was a negligible mortality. The picture was more of the hyperkinetic myoclonic form with convulsions, but with an absence of actual paralysis. A point of special significance and interest in this particular outbreak is seen in the fact that a virus could be recovered which would reproduce the picture when inoculated into experimental animals by either the intracerebral or intranasal routes. In the earlier epidemics, the inoculation of filtrates from emulsified brain and spinal fluid yielded very irregular results. Likewise, unlike the previous epidemics, inoculation with serum from the St. Louis virus protected animals against subsequent infection. As a result of these rather striking differences, both in respect to the clinical picture and low mortality, and of the behavior of the virus, the condition has become known as encephalitis "B." In many respects, this outbreak was similar to one which occurred some ten years previously in Japan, but again there appears to be some inherent difference in the two viruses as animals could not be protected by convalescent serum of one type against the other strain.

Pathology.—The pathology of epidemic encephalitis has already been described to some extent. Briefly, it may be said that the lesions are essentially indistinguishable from those of anterior poliomyelitis, except as to distribution. In poliomyelitis, the pathology is largely restricted to the cord and brain stem whereas in encephalitis, the lesions are chiefly found in the midbrain and cerebrum. Only in the more severe cases do they involve the cerebellum. The same edema and congestion of the central nervous tissue is found as in poliomyelitis. Similar perivascular mantling by lymphocytes is encountered. Not infreqently, petechial hemorrhage takes place, especially into the Virchow-Robin spaces. Comparable nerve cell degeneration to that found in poliomyelitis may be recognized, but is much less striking. Likewise, as in poliomyelitis, it is not at all uncommon to find rather marked changes affecting the reticulo-endothelial system and evidence of toxic injury to the vascular endothelium as manifested by petechial hemorrhages, especially of the serosal membranes of the pleura, pericardium, peritoneum, and even the joint cavities.

From the standpoint of diagnosis, the picture is often extremely confusing. As has already been commented upon, the mental and neurologic manifestations are too variable to be of much help except by exclusion from other more readily established diagnoses. A point of some value is the fact that the disease is a febrile one at the outset, ordinarily with a moderate elevation of the temperature to perhaps 100 or 101 degrees. Examination of the spinal fluid is essentially negative as in the case of poliomyelitis, except for a slight increase in the number of cells of the lymphocytic series. These rarely exceed forty or fifty per cubic millimeter, whereas in poliomyelitis they may reach as high as one hundred to two hundred. Very little change is found in the chemical examination of the fluid. There is no fibrin clot formed in encephalitis whereas in poliomyelitis it very frequently may be found. The colloidal gold curve in encephalitis is often normal, but may present a luetic curve. This is of little value as a similar reaction is not infrequently seen in poliomyelitis as well.

The inherent neurotropic nature of the infection in both poliomyelitis and epidemic encephalitis accompanied by essentially comparable pathological changes except in respect to the distribution of the lesions has raised the question in many investigators' minds as to whether or not the two diseases may not be protean manifestations of the same underlying infection. The whole problem of this group of virus infections is in a state of tremendous confusion at the present time. It has been shown by a number of investigators that, with the exception of encephalitis "B," the antiviricidal titre of serum from convalescent cases is of very little significance in respect to protecting the experimental animal or human being from infection. In other words, while both of these conditions may cause the development of a relatively high titre of humoral antibodies, this is not any indication of the amount of tissue immunity which that particular individual possesses. If the prophylactic or therapeutic use of serum in these diseases is to be of actual value, the dosage employed must be very much greater than that in current usage. We believe that it requires no less than 200 c.c. to be of even theoretical value.

ILLUSTRATIVE CASE

CASE 281. (Ref. #S-401)
Diagnosis.—Brain—acute epidemic encephalitis.
Patient was a Filipina of 20 years, who was admitted to the hospital because of the development of progressive stupor accompanied by mild clonic choreiform muscular contractions of the extremities.
Present Illness.—The onset of the illness began approximately ten days before admission. At that time the patient showed evidence of mental excitability, began talking almost incessantly and showed marked emotional instability. Within forty-eight hours, these mental symptoms subsided and those of apathy supervened. However, accompanying this second phase of the picture there developed curious muscular twitchings of the fingers, arms, and of the head on the neck. These progressed to almost convulsive myoclonic contractions and were complicated by curious choreiform, athetoid movements of the extremities. The apathy increased until a state of semistupor supervened at which time the patient was taken to the hospital.

Past Medical History.—The patient's previous medical history was uneventful. She had never had any serious illness requiring hospitalization previously. She had not had a history of antecedent influenza. A review of her systems was essentially negative. She was not subject to upper respiratory disease. She had not been heart conscious. Her gastro-intestinal history was characterized by several attacks of diarrhea which had subsided spontaneously. Her menstrual history was negative. Menses began at the age of ten and had been regular from that time.
Physical Examination.—Patient was a well-developed, well-nourished, young Filipina. Examination was somewhat complicated by intermittent myoclonic seizures. Head was not remarkable. Pupils reacted to light. Nose and throat appeared negative. Chest was symmetrical. Lungs were clear. Heart was not enlarged. Abdomen was negative. Extremities were negative.
Neurologic examination showed hyperactive reflexes generally and a condition of semistupor existed from

which the patient could only be aroused temporarily by strong stimuli.

Laboratory Findings.—Urinalysis was negative. The blood count on admission showed 4,190,000 red blood cells with 78% hemoglobin. White blood cells, 10,000 with 87% neutrophiles. Spinal fluid was under slightly increased pressure. It was clear on inspection and showed a slight increase of protein, and no change in its carbohydrate reducing capacity. The cell count was twenty, all lymphocytes.

Subsequent Course.—The patient went on rapidly downhill dying five days after admission.

Autopsy Findings.—The body was negative externally. The heart showed marked congestion. There were no valvular lesions. Lungs showed terminal hypostatic congestion at the bases. The liver showed marked toxic degeneration of the parenchyma. Spleen presented the picture of moderate toxic splenitis. Kidneys showed marked congestion and toxic nephrosis. The brain weighed 1162 gm. There was moderate edema and congestion of the meninges and of the brain substance itself. Sections through the brain showed marked congestion of the smaller vessels even to the point of actual petechial hemorrhage. Focal areas of degeneration could be seen in the corpus striatum, medullae, pons and in the region of the dentate nucleus of the cerebellum. The spinal cord showed similar edema, congestion, and a few focal areas of degeneration accompanied by petechial hemorrhage. The anatomical diagnosis of acute encephalomyelitis was made.

Microscopic Description of a Section Through the Brain.—(Fig. 651 and 652) Histologic study of multiple sections shows a very marked edema, particularly around the blood vessels. The vessels are intensely congested and in many places, actual petechial hemorrhage is seen. Particularly in the midbrain there is very extensive perivascular mantling of the blood vessels by small round cells most of which appear to be lymphocytes. In the cervical cord there is a very striking diffuse infiltration of the gray matter especially of the posterior horns by small round cells. These appear to be chiefly microglial scavenger cells. In the midbrain particularly, but also involving the cortex, and to a less extent the cervical cord, actual nerve cell degeneration can be observed. This is comparable to that seen in poliomyelitis, but less extensive. The degeneration is of the chromatolytic type accompanied by swelling of the cytoplasm and nucleus. Neuronophagia is occasionally observed. Histologically, except in respect to the positional distribution of the lesions in the central nervous system, it is impossible to definitely distinguish them from those of other specific neurotropic virus infections, notably poliomyelitis.

PARASITIC INFESTATIONS

Of the parasitic infestations of the central nervous system, only two need be mentioned. These have already been discussed in Chapters XX and XXI in relation to the general pathological picture which the particular parasite produces. These two are first, *Endameba histolytica* and second, *Taenia echinococcus*.

Endameba Histolytica.—In *Endameba histolytica* infestation of the gastro-intestinal tract, it has already been noted that the commonest complication of this disease is the development of amebic abscesses. Most frequently, such abscess formation is found in the liver as the result of direct extention of the ameba either by the portal circulation or lymphatics to the liver tissue. Less commonly, but representing the next most frequent site of such solitary abscess formation is the hematogenous-borne brain abscess. This has already been described in Case 196 (Ref. #S-272), Chapter XLVI, in which it will be recalled that there is a liquefaction necrosis centrally surrounded by a zone of chronic glial proliferation and fibrosis and that the organisms may be found either in their active or encysted forms within the abscess cavity.

Taenia Echinococcus.—In *Taenia echinococcus* infestation, similarly, blood-borne parasites may localize in the brain as in other organs and produce their characteristic cyst formation. In both such parasitic lesions, the picture is usually one of intracranial pressure and is to be distinguished chiefly from brain tumors, because of the localizing symptoms which usually exist without evidence of infection such as one might expect to find with the ordinary type of pyogenic abscess formation.

CHAPTER LXIV

DISEASES OF THE NERVOUS SYSTEM (*Continued*)

DEGENERATIVE LESIONS OF THE CENTRAL NERVOUS SYSTEM

There are a considerable number of degenerative lesions which affect the central nervous system, which are entirely obscure in their particular etiology. Many of these are associated with specific spinal cord nerve tract degenerations and follow a rather uniform anatomical pattern. Others are much less regular in the distribution of the lesions. Among the most important of these various conditions from the clinical standpoint must be mentioned multiple sclerosis, amyotrophic lateral sclerosis in its upper, lower or combined neuron forms, encephalitis periaxialis diffusa (Schilder's disease), subacute combined degeneration of the spinal cord, especially as seen in relation to pernicious anemia, Friedrich's ataxia, Landry's ascending paralysis, progressive lenticular degeneration (Wilson's disease; hepatolenticular degeneration)

and syringomyelia. In addition, there are paralysis agitans; the two forms of chorea, Huntington's and Sydenham's; Little's spastic paralysis; birth palsy; Pick's convolutional atrophy; and the whole group of muscular dystrophies or myopathies in which considerable evidence is gradually accumulating to suggest that the basic disturbance is neurogenic, possibly as a result of endocrine disturbances. Likewise, to be complete, any discussion should include the various forms of lesions affecting the peripheral nerves; and finally, simple atrophic degenerative changes as they affect the brain and the remainder of the nervous system should not be overlooked. A very brief review of the outstanding pathology in the more important of these degenerative conditions of the central nervous system follows.

SENILE ATROPHY

In a great many conditions affecting the central nervous system, one may find both gross and microscopic evidence of extensive degeneration of the gray and white matter, especially the latter. Among the most important of such conditions should be mentioned first of all the simple senile atrophy which results from a diminished blood supply to the entire brain in conjunction with a generalized arteriosclerosis. This results in a gradual gross atrophy of the entire brain substance so that at autopsy such a brain appears relatively small and shrunken by contrast to the normal adult brain. The convolutions are atrophied and separated by wide sulci. There is a variable amount of increased interstitial connective tissue in the subarachnoid spaces. The surface of the brain as viewed through the membranes has a cloudy, milky appearance due to this thickening of the subarachnoid membranes through which the cerebrospinal fluid can be seen as if through a film. The picture is very comparable to that which is seen in chronic alcoholism

and not unlike that seen in certain cases of paresis. (Fig. 654.)

Under the microscope, such brains show extensive degenerative lesions, particularly of the supportive cells. Many of the actual nerve cells likewise are involved in these regressive changes and alteration in the size and distribution of the Nissl granules, swelling of the cytoplasm of the cells with a loss of their protoplasmic processes and alteration in the appearance of the nucleus going on to pyknosis or karyolysis may be seen. In the supportive interstitial tissue of the brain and cord themselves, a picture is found which is extremely characteristic of such degenerative phenomena. The lesion consists of the presence of varying numbers of globoid bodies varying somewhat in size and tending to stain intensely with methylene blue in routine eosin-methylene blue preparations. These lesions are spoken of as "corpora amylacea," as "colloid degeneration," or as "hyaline degeneration." They are somewhat larger than the size of the

PLATE CLV
DISEASES OF THE CENTRAL NERVOUS SYSTEM

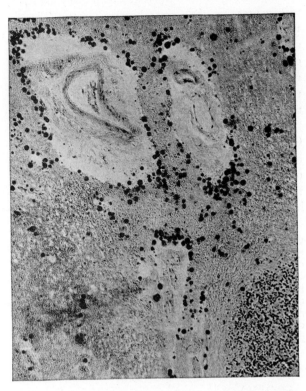

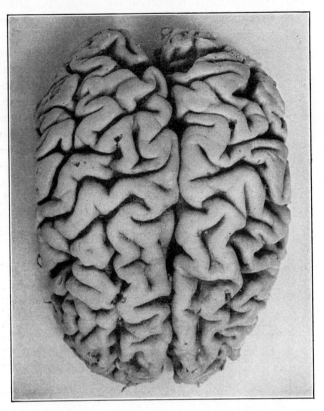

FIG. 653.—BRAIN: CORTEX—SENILE ATROPHY.—Cf. CASE 277.—Note the presence of typical hyaline ("colloid") bodies, believed to represent degenerated oligodendroglial cells for the most part. App. 50 x.

FIG. 654.—BRAIN: SUPERIOR SURFACE—SENILE ATROPHY.—Cf. CASE 277.—Gross photograph from which the pia arachnoid has been removed to better show the marked convolutional atrophy.

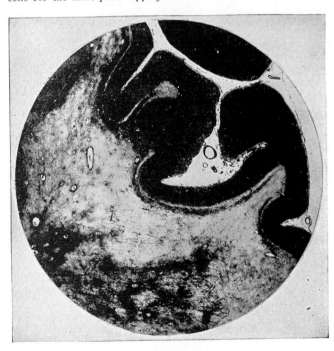

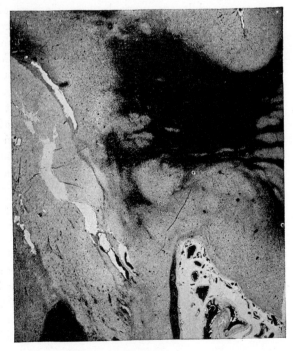

FIG. 655.—BRAIN: CORTEX—SCHILDER'S DISEASE (ENCEPHALITIS PERIAXIALIS DIFFUSA), WEIGERT STAIN.—CASE 284.—Microtessar photograph to show the characteristic subcortical demyelinization. App. 5 x.

FIG. 656.—BRAIN: LENTICULAR NUCLEUS—WILSON'S DISEASE (PROGRESSIVE LENTICULAR DEGENERATION), WEIGERT STAIN.—CASE 285.—The typical demyelinization and replacement gliosis may be noted. App. 3 x.

oligodendroglial nucleus on the average, but recent work suggests that these bluish-black staining bodies represent actual hyaline degeneration of the oligodendroglial cells. These bodies have been the source of a great deal of confusion in the past as it was felt that they represented infiltration of some pathological material, the nature of which was not known. However, with these latter studies the picture seems to be comparable to the same hyaline degeneration with the production of "colloid granules," which we have seen in the more marked examples of hyaline degeneration of the renal tubular epithelial cells. These hyaline bodies, as it has already been suggested, are seen not only in senility, but in association with chronic toxic degenerative lesions notably in chronic alcoholism and not infrequently in association with the degenerative lesions associated with many inflammatory processes of the central nervous system. Thus, they may be encountered in various forms of neurosyphilis, epilepsy, encephalitis and a host of other conditions. All that may be said regarding the significance of this picture is that it is definite indication of some rather severe degenerative lesion of the central nervous system.

For an illustrative case, the reader is referred to Case 277 (Ref. #S-396), page 782, of cerebral atherosclerosis and thrombosis with secondary encephalomalacia, which also demonstrates the condition of senile atrophy of the brain. Fig. 653 shows the histopathology, a description of which follows.

Diagnosis.—Brain—senile atrophy (colloid degeneration).

Microscopic Description of Sections from the Cortex.—(Fig. 653) Sections from the cortex show a very striking example of the so-called "colloid degeneration." This is perhaps most commonly encountered in such senile degenerative lesions as cerebral thrombosis. The outstanding histologic feature is seen in the presence of almost innumerable numbers of varying sized dark, bluish-black, globoid bodies. These, by careful search, can be identified as being derived from degenerating glial cells, apparently almost entirely from the oligodendroglia, and certain of them still show the persistence of the nuclear structure which swells up and becomes this curious homogeneous substance. It apparently represents a curious form of hyaline degeneration associated particularly with the avascularization of the supportive framework of the central nervous system.

MULTIPLE SCLEROSIS (DISSEMINATED SCLEROSIS; INSULAR SCLEROSIS)

Multiple sclerosis is a chronic disease of the central nervous system, which occurs chiefly in the young adult age group between the ages of fifteen and thirty-five. It runs a prolonged course, often characterized by periods of remission and relapse clinically. The etiology is not known. Certain investigators believe it to be a specific infectious disease probably due to a filtrable virus. This theory is based on indirect evidence, dependent in part upon the similarity in certain respects to some of the acute forms of encephalomyelitis in association with other infectious diseases; and secondarily because of a curious geographical distribution, being relatively common in Europe and North America, but rarely encountered in South America or the Orient. This thought is possibly furthered by the fact that many cases apparently date their onset from some acute infectious episode. On the other hand, Putnam is convinced of the vascular nature of the disease and that the lesions are the result of focal thrombotic occlusion of the small blood vessels. This might also be explained on an infectious basis or even on toxic injury to the vascular endothelium comparable to that which we have described in scarlatina and similar streptococcic infections. However, there is no conclusive evidence that the disease is definitely infectious. Syphilis seems to be ruled out, although for many years it was thought to be an important factor.

From the clinical standpoint, the chief symptoms are weakness, spasticity and ataxy of the legs accompanied by alteration in speech, nystagmus, tremors, and not infrequently optic atrophy. These tremors are likely to be of the intention type and are often one of the most distressing features of the disease to the patient. The speech defects are particularly described as of the scanning or staccato type. Often, emotional instability is an outstanding symptom with the patient laughing or crying on wholly inadequate stimulation, but withal a rather striking euphoria tends to persist throughout the progressive course of the disease.

Pathology.—The pathology of the disease is perhaps best seen under the low power in sections stained by the Weigert method to bring out the patchy nature of the scarring which is found. The distribution of the lesions is often spoken of as "shotgun," no one

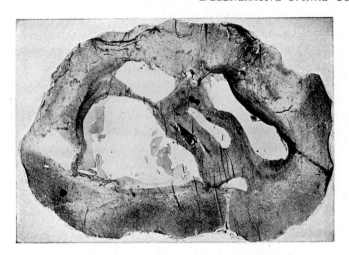

FIG. 657.—SYRINGOMYELIA.—CASE 286.—H & E Stain.—Note cystic degenerative changes. App. 5 x.

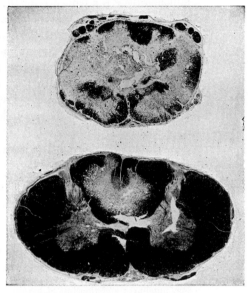

FIG. 658.—TRAUMATIC INJURY WITH CORD COMPRESSION.—Weigert Stain.—Note resultant degeneration. App. 5 x.

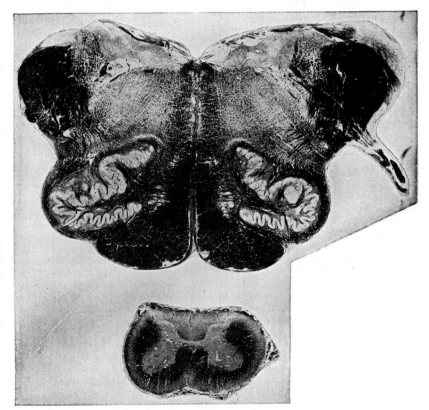

FIG. 659.—TABES DORSALIS.—CASE 280.—Weigert Stain.—Note posterior column degeneration. App. 5 x.

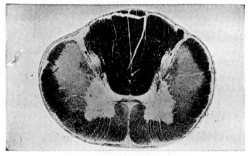

FIG. 660.—AMYOTROPHIC LATERAL SCLEROSIS—CASE 283.—Weigert Stain.—Note demyelinization of lateral columns. App. 5 x.

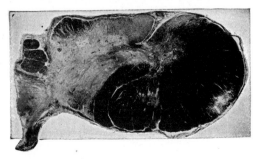

FIG. 661.—SCAR: STAB WOUND.—Weigert Stain.—Note unilateral healed lesion. App. 5 x.

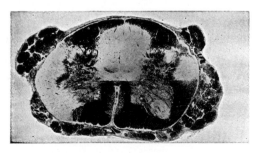

FIG. 662.—MULTIPLE SCLEROSIS.—CASE 282.—Weigert Stain.—Note patchy, irregularly distributed areas of demyelinization. App. 5 x.

tract necessarily being involved throughout its length, although there is a tendency for the pyramidal tracts to be affected more often than other areas. The lesions in the brain are as a rule more extensive than those in the cord. They appear as discrete, sharply outlined areas which fail to take the myelin stain due to the loss of myelin in these areas. Histologically, these lesions are found to represent multiple neuroglial scars around the small blood vessels, many of which appear thrombosed. The actual axis cylinders are often preserved, but because of the loss of their myelin insulation resulting short circuits in the transmissibility of impulses are likely to occur. In the early and more acute stages of the disease, marked cellular infiltration may be observed around the blood vessels as in other forms of inflammatory disease of the central nervous system. The great majority of these cells, however, seem to be microglial scavenger cells which are actively engaged in removing the degenerated myelin. Thus, we see that the picture of multiple sclerosis is a confusing one with certain features suggesting a possible infectious etiology, but with the main lesions of a degenerative nature and usually accompanied by circulatory disturbances particularly by thrombosis of the small vessels.

ILLUSTRATIVE CASE

CASE 282. (Ref. #S-285)

Diagnosis.—Spinal cord—multiple sclerosis.

Patient was a white male of 37 years, admitted to the hospital with the chief complaints of difficulty in walking, numbness and tingling of his fingers and pain of his right hip at certain positions.

Present Illness.—The onset of the patient's illness was approximately eight years before his present admission. It started with a numbness and tingling in the feet which progressed to involve the legs. By the end of a year these same alterations in sensation had extended to reach the scrotum and perineum. He was treated by a physiotherapist with some form of electrical therapy, which had rather definitely beneficial results for a while, but subsequently failed to give him any relief. About two years before the present admission, he attempted to secure relief by chiropractic methods, without success. At about this time, he began to notice for the first time a tingling in his fingers. He felt that he had lost a good deal of strength from his left hand. He was studied thoroughly about six months previously, even to the point of encephalography, but without any improvement subjectively, his symptoms still persisting.

Past Medical History.—His past medical history was of no significance. He had had the usual children's infections, but had never been seriously ill other than this neurologic condition. A review of his systems was entirely negative. His gastro-intestinal history was normal. His genito-urinary history yielded no information. He denied venereal infection in any form.

Physical Examination.—The patient was a well-developed, somewhat undernourished, adult, white male. Head showed no external deformities. Eyes were negative and reacted normally. Nose and throat were normal. Chest was symmetrical. Lungs were clear. Heart was not enlarged and showed no murmurs. Abdomen was negative. No viscera or masses were felt. No tenderness was elicited. Extremities appeared normal.

Neurologic examination showed no evidence of cranial nerve palsies. Mentally, he was extremely euphoric. The deep tendon reflexes in the upper extremities were somewhat exaggerated and the upper extremiteis showed moderately good motor power. He was slightly ataxic in the finger to nose test. Abdominal reflexes were absent. The lower extremities showed marked ataxia and the patient walked with a wide base, but showed no actual palsy. Reflexes were hyperactive. Position and vibratory sense were markedly diminished in the lower extremities, but pain sensation was acute everywhere.

Laboratory Findings.—Urinalysis on several occasions was negative. Blood examination showed a red cell count of 5,420,000 cells with 83% hemoglobin, and a white blood count of 7,000 cells with 64% polymorphonuclears. Blood Wassermann was negative. Spinal fluid was under slightly increased pressure, but was otherwise normal. There was a cell count of three lymphocytes. Spinal fluid Wassermann was negative and the colloidal gold curve was as follows: 3 3 4 3 3 2 1 0 0.

Subsequent Course.—The patient ultimately died of a lobar pneumonia and autopsy was performed in an undertaking parlor.

Autopsy Findings.—Autopsy findings were essentially negative except for his right lower lobe pneumonia with generalized toxic changes affecting most of the parenchymatous organs. Brain and cord showed moderate edema and congestion grossly, but nothing that was of diagnostic significance until histologic sections were studied with the use of Weigert staining technique.

Microscopic Description of Section Through the Spinal Cord.—(Fig. 662) Sections histologically present evidence of a diffuse sclerosis of the brain and cord. This follows no very strict anatomical distribution, but tends to involve the cord irregularly. In some places, the lateral pyramidal tracts are involved. In other areas the sensory columns are degenerated and replaced by a diffuse gliosis. The brain similarly shows scattered focal areas, chiefly subcortical in distribution. Microscopically, these areas are seen frequently in association with obliterated blood vessels. Some of these suggest a previous thrombotic process which has undergone complete organization. In other areas, some canalization of the vessel is seen. Most of the lesions are so advanced that no evidence of any acute demyelinization is found, but in places there are still some microglial scavenger cells visible. Because of the scattered, irregular, patchy distribution of the lesions, their apparent relationship in some instances, at least, to vascular occlusion, the demyelinization which is the outstanding histologic feature, and the reparative replacement gliosis, the diagnosis of multiple sclerosis is readily established.

AMYOTROPHIC LATERAL SCLEROSIS

In contradistinction to multiple sclerosis, this disease is one which generally appears in middle life. It is characterized at the outset by wasting of the small muscles of the hands. This gradually extends to involve the muscles of the extremities.

From the standpoint of etiology, nothing definite is known. Certain cases have been seen in association with central nervous syphilis and for that reason, lues has been considered as a probable factor in its development. However, the majority of cases show no clinical evidence of syphilis and the disease appears to be a frankly degenerative one without recognized cause. It is, like disseminated sclerosis, progressive in nature and runs a very much more rapid and uniformly progressively fatal course, the patient dying ordinarily within three years of its onset.

Pathology.—The pathology of the disease appears to be a combined upper and lower neuron lesion by the time the patient dies with bulbar paralysis as the immediate cause of death. The lesion is one of the anterior horn cells. The earliest manifestations of the disease occur in the form of amyotrophia. As the disease progresses, we find involvement of the descending tracts of the anterolateral columns particularly in the pyramidal portion. This is associated with the corresponding degeneration of the Betz cells in the motor cortex. With this upper neuron degeneration, spasticity and exaggerated reflexes appear, and as has already been commented upon, ultimately there is regularly a bulbar paralysis. Glial and fibrous tissue proliferation as scar tissue formation may be seen, by the time the patient comes to autopsy.

From the clinical standpoint, this neurologic picture may occur in several forms. It may be seen as a simple lower motor neuron lesion with the development of anterior horn cell degeneration alone and be characterized clinically simply by muscle weakness through loss of individual lower motor neurons. On the other hand, the disease may be seen in its upper neuron pattern as a primary progressive bulbar paralysis. More commonly, however, the disease is seen in its combined progressive manifestations beginning as a muscular atrophy and ultimately developing the combined lower and upper motor neuron pattern with progressive bulbar paralysis. No explanation has been offered for this curious selectivity in the distribution of the lesions. From its histopathology, the entire picture appears to be one of a simple unexplained degenerative nature, but this curious focal distribution still bears the hallmark of other specific neurotropic infections, especially of the virus group, and it will not be surprising in the future to discover that such an infectious agent may be responsible for the disease.

ILLUSTRATIVE CASE

CASE 283. (Ref. #S-403)
Diagnosis.—Spinal cord—amyotrophic lateral sclerosis.
Patient was an unmarried white female of 38 years, who was admitted to the hospital for neurologic studies.
Present Illness.—Six months before admission the patient had an attack of laryngitis from which she did not seem to entirely recover. A month before admission, she completely lost her voice temporarily. Since that time she had had recurrent attacks of aphonia which would last anywhere from a few minutes to a few hours. At about the same time, she developed a severe headache, which persisted for ten days or more, but which had subsided at the time of admission. Her immediate difficulty was a sensation of "fullness" in her throat so that she gagged and coughed almost constantly. Recently she had noticed that her hands and feet would get numb at times and be accompanied by a feeling of chilliness. If she moved suddenly, she would have a definite feeling of vertigo, and she also noted a certain difficulty in walking up or down steps. She had had several attacks of dyspnea during the preceding few weeks accompanied by hiccough. She also had had a good deal of difficulty in picking things up or holding them in her hands, and would drop a glass, or a fork, or a pencil for no apparent reason. Her appetite had been poor. Her mother reported that she seemed emotionally very easily upset and would have fits of laughing and crying at times for no reason, and be unable to stop. In summary, the patient had a wide variety of relatively unrelated neurologic and mental changes which were transitory in nature, but had tended to increase over a period of several months.

Past Medical History.—Patient had the usual diseases of childhood. She was very ill as a child with pertussis at the age of three and was rather sickly until she was eight or nine years old. She had had influenza in the 1918 epidemic. She had always been subject to sore throats and tonsillitis, and had finally had her tonsils removed, eight years before admission. This gave her some relief, but she still had recurrent attacks of bronchitis almost every year. A review of her systems otherwise was noninformatory. Her gastro-intestinal system was negative except for the tendency to chronic constipation. Genito-urinary system was negative. Menses began at the age of twelve and had always been regular and unaccompanied by pain.

Physical Examination.—The patient was a well-developed, fairly well-nourished, middle-aged white female. She acted as if she had something pressing on her trachea swallowing frequently while talking. Head was normal in contour. The skin was of a fine texture, but there was deep pigmentation around the eyes and a suboral pigmentation of a lesser degree. Eyes showed slight exophthalmos and reacted slowly to light and accommodation. There was a slight horizontal nystagmus on looking to the right. Ears, nose and throat were essentially negative except for the fact that the tongue protruded slightly to the left and showed a fine tremor. She gagged very readily making examination of her throat difficult. Thyroid was moderately enlarged and quite firm. Chest was symmetrical with equal expansion on the two sides. The breasts were somewhat underdeveloped. Heart and lungs were negative. Abdomen showed moderate tenderness about the umbilicus and on the right side of the lower abdomen. The liver seemed slightly enlarged. The hands and feet appeared small in proportion to the size of the limbs.

Neurologic Examination.—Neurologic examination showed exaggeration of the biceps, triceps, radial and ulnar reflexes. There was a positive Hoffman sign. The right palpebral fissure was slightly larger than the left. The right pupil was slightly larger than the left. There was a definite left facial peripheral type of weakness, but no actual palsy. There was objective impairment of hearing on the left. There was no cerebellar asynergia or dysmetria. The deep tendon reflexes of the lower extremities were markedly increased. There was bilateral clonus.

Laboratory Findings.—Red blood cells, 4,110,000 with 12 gm. of hemoglobin. White blood cells, 7,100 with 60% neutrophiles. Urinalysis was negative. Cerebrospinal fluid was essentially negative. Colloidal gold curve

was normal. Wassermann was negative. There was only one cell seen, a neutrophile. There was no increase in globulin or albumin and the carbohydrate reducing substance was normal.

X-ray examinations were noninformatory.

Subsequent Course.—On the basis of the clinical history and the neurologic findings, a tentative diagnosis of amyotrophic lateral sclerosis was made. The patient went on in the usual progressive fashion and died about eighteen months later.

Autopsy Findings.—At autopsy the body was found in a state of marked emaciation. Marked atrophy of the small muscles of the hands was particularly prominent with scarcely any suggestion of thenar or hypothenar prominences. Similar atrophic changes were noted affecting the peripheral musculature of the extremities. The heart and lungs showed very little pathology other than a terminal congestion and edema. The abdominal viscera were negative. The chief pathological interest centered in an examination of the central nervous system. The more striking changes were those found involving the spinal cord, but on careful examination of the brain there likewise appeared to be definite degenerative changes with atrophy and loss of a considerable number of the large motor nerve cells of the cortex with sclerosis.

Microscopic Description of a Section from the Spinal Cord.—(Fig. 660) The cord lesions were best demonstrated by subsequent staining of the tissues by the usual Weigert method, but routine hematoxylin and eosin stained preparations show definite loss of the anterior and lateral horn motor nerve cells. There is marked sclerosis of the cross and direct pyramidal tracts.

ENCEPHALITIS PERIAXIALIS DIFFUSA (SCHILDER'S DISEASE)

This condition is one which has only been recognized in this country for approximately the past quarter of a century. It is usually a disease of childhood, or at the latest of early adult age. In many respects it bears points of similarity to multiple sclerosis except that the demyelinization process which is found in the disease is definitely restricted to the cerebral hemispheres and does not involve the brain stem or spinal cord.

The etiology of this condition is also unknown. In many respects it suggests an infectious disease, but so far as the actual pathology is concerned, the lesions are those of degeneration rather than inflammation. The typical case shows an acute onset with a relatively rapid progression varying from a few weeks up to possibly three years. It is thought that mild cases may occur which do not necessarily prove fatal and which may account for some of the curious spastic lesions seen in later life and dating from childhood. Typically, the degenerative process begins in the occipital lobes symmetrically and extends gradually forward until the entire white matter of

the brain has undergone demyelinization. As a result, the patient presents progressive symptoms of spastic paralysis, mental deterioration and loss of vision, hearing and sense of position. This is frequently accompanied by convulsive seizures.

Pathology.—On opening the skull of such a case at autopsy, the brain is apt to appear somewhat atrophied, although if the course of the disease has been sufficiently rapid, this diminution in size of the brain may not have had time to develop. In either case, on section of the brain substance, the entire white matter will be seen as a curious soft, grayish-white, gelatinous, translucent-appearing tissue. This may be somewhat patchy in distribution, but in general appears to be rather uniform except that the more marked lesions are likely to be found in the occipital areas. The lesions likewise are bilaterally symmetrical. Histologically, the picture again varies depending upon the stage of the process. In the earlier, more acute phase of the picture, the beginning degenerative changes can be seen affecting the myelin. This may be identified by the usual Marchi staining technique. Accompanying this breaking down of the myelin sheath will be found very extensive secondary microglial phagocytic scavenger cell activity. As the lesion further progresses, secondary axonal degenera- tion likewise follows. In the milder cases who survive a long enough period of time for the reparative phe- nomena to become apparent, there is a secondary progressive gliosis of a fibrillary nature.

ILLUSTRATIVE CASE

CASE 284. (Ref. #S-404)

Diagnosis.—Brain—Schilder's disease (encephalitis periaxialis diffusa).

Patient was a white male child of 10 years, admitted to the hospital because of progressive neurologic symptoms.

Present Illness.—The onset of the patient's present illness was approximately three years before admission. It appeared to have been initiated by a fall down some stone steps, but in retrospect, the neurologic picture probably antedated and was responsible for the fall rather than the fall being responsible for the develop- ment of the neurologic picture. He appeared definitely weak and apathetic after this accident and it was noted that his speech acquired a nasal twang. This was ac- companied by a rather marked rhinorrhea. Shortly there- after he began to drool almost constantly and to have curious athetoid motions of his arms. About three months later he began to act abnormally in school and by the end of a year after the fall he showed a definite spastic- ity of his right leg. Three months later he lost all power of speech and became definitely bedridden. The condi- tion continued to progress with increasing stiffness and rigidity of his extremities. By the end of the second year after the onset he had had several attacks of decerebrate rigidity. These kept becoming more frequent and more severe.

Past Medical History.—As a child, before the age of five, he had had the usual measles and whooping cough. He had never had any other of the contagious diseases. At the age of four he had had a retropharyngeal abscess which had drained for several weeks. At the age of five he had a head injury with a mild concussion for a few hours. There was no actual fracture, but he was kept in hospital for several weeks. His mother stated that one other child had died of spinal meningitis at the age of six.

Physical Examination.—The patient was a fairly well-developed but emaciated white, male child, who ap- peared about ten years of age. Physical examination was somewhat difficult to make because of the condition of the patient. He tended to hold himself in a position of marked opisthotonos accompanied by decerebrate rigidity. These attacks would come on in waves preceded by a hoarse, crescendo moan. The upper extremities were fully extended at the side and externally rotated. Hands were flexed on his wrists and fingers were clenched. Legs alternated between attacks of extreme flexion and hypertension. So far as could be determined, the cranial nerves were negative except that they showed bilateral optic atrophy. Pupils were moderately dilated and re- acted to light. Eyes were turned upward and outward during the attacks. Nose and throat were essentially negative. Chest was symmetrical. Lungs were clear. Heart was not enlarged. The rate was rapid but there were no murmurs heard. Abdomen was negative. Ex- ternal genitalia were normal.

Laboratory Findings.—The blood count on admission showed 5,240,000 red cells with 14 gm. of hemoglobin.

The white blood cells numbered 6,900 with 35% neutro- philes, 48% lymphocytes and 14% monocytes. Urinalysis was negative. Blood chemistry showed a normal calcium/ phosphorus ratio. Wassermann was negative. Spinal fluid examination showed a cell count of five lymphocytes and a normal chemistry. Wassermann was negative. Colloidal gold curve gave a slightly midzone reaction of 0 0 0 1 2 3 2 2 1 0.

X-ray Examination.—The patient had several roent- genologic studies including a ventriculogram. There was an obliterative subarachnoid fibrosis suggested over the right hemisphere. A communicating hydrocephalus with extensive atrophy of the brain was also demonstrated.

Subsequent Course.—In spite of almost every con- ceivable effort to improve the child's condition, he went steadily downhill and died six months after admission.

Autopsy Findings.—The body was that of a fairly well-developed but emaciated white male child. Head showed no gross deformities. Pupils were regular and equal in size. The heart and lungs were negative except for terminal edema and congestion. The abdominal viscera showed toxic degenerative changes. The ex- tremities were wasted, but otherwise negative. A large sacral decubitus was noted. The brain was markedly shrunken in size and there was a corresponding increase of fluid overlying it. The brain was fixed before sec- tioning to preserve its relationships to the ventricular system. After fixation on gross section it was found that there was almost a complete gelatinoid appearing de- generation of the white matter which was responsible for the reduction in size of the brain. This had ap- parently begun in the occipital lobes as a symmetrical lesion, as the atrophy was most marked in these areas. Toward the frontal lobes, the gelatinoid appearance of the degenerative process was more in evidence, whereas in the occiput replacement gliosis was marked.

Microscopic Description of a Section from the Brain.—(Fig. 655) Sections of the cerebellum, taken at various levels, and stained by Weigert's method, show a complete demyelinization and corresponding gliosis of almost all of the white matter. With the routine hema- toxylin and eosin stains, various stages in the develop- ment of this degenerative process can be recognized. In sections from the occipital lobe, the picture is almost one of complete replacement gliosis. In the frontal areas, axones can still be identified, but extensive demyeliniza- tion of the nerve fibers is apparent. Marked microglial scavenger cell invasion of the tissue is seen, particularly in the frontal areas. The etiology suggests that the proc- ess starts as a demyelinization as the result of some un- known etiologic factor. This ultimately has gone on to actual axone degeneration. The degenerative material has been removed largely by the action of the scavenger cells, which incidentally include apparently many of the ordinary large mononuclear phagocytic cells as well as those of microglial origin; and finally, the end stage has become one of replacement gliosis, which readily ex- plains the marked clinical picture.

SUBACUTE COMBINED DEGENERATION OF THE CORD

This condition is one which occurs for the most part in the middle-age group and particularly in males. It is almost invariably accompanied by a hyperchromic macrocytic anemia of the so-called "pernicious" type. From the clinical standpoint, the disease starts as a mild spastic or ataxic paraplegia, but ultimately goes on if untreated to the development of a generalized, diffuse, flaccid paralysis. The etiology of the disease is still obscure. Formerly it was believed to be one of the complications of pernicious anemia, but not infrequently the neurologic symptoms may actually precede the development of the anemic picture. In the light of more recent investigative work in the field of the anemias, the suggestion has been raised that possibly the cord degenerative lesions which are seen in this condition are the result of the same deficient factor which produces the anemia. To further complicate the picture, the condition has been found associated with certain instances of hypochromic microcytic anemia and likewise to accompany in rare instances neurosyphilis. The differentiation of this condition from a combined tabes and lateral sclerosis is under such circumstances extremely difficult. The more generally held view to-day regarding this symptom complex and pathological cord lesion is that it probably relates to or is the result of some type of deficiency disease.

Pathology.—The pathological picture in this condition is best visualized by the same myelin staining technique and atrophy of the posterolateral columns including the pyramidal tracts is the outstanding feature. Under the microscope, this is found to be a demyelinization just as the other degenerative lesions have been. One does not usually have an opportunity to study these lesions in the acute stage and by the time the patient comes to postmortem, little evidence of cellular activity is found. There is a mild degree of replacement gliosis, but this is usually not as marked as in the other degenerative lesions studied thus far. (Fig. 520.)

FRIEDRICH'S ATAXIA (HEREDITARY ATAXY)

In this disease, there is a strong familial tendency although it is rarely transmitted directly from one generation to the next. The disease is furthermore one of childhood, usually appearing by the age of puberty and often at a much earlier date. The etiology of the condition is, like that of most of these degenerative lesions of the central nervous system, entirely obscure. Not infrequently some acute infection seems to initiate the degenerative process, but it cannot be said with any assurance that infection is of any real significance in this respect. The picture, being one of a rather extensive, progressive, diffuse degeneration and sclerosis of the posterior, lateral and direct cerebellar tracts of the cord and of the pyramidal tracts at times, the symptoms are those of muscular weakness, with a profound ataxia due to the cerebellar involvement. One of the most significant diagnostic findings is the development of foot deformities which may first be observed as a rather clumsy motion of the arms or legs. As the pyramidal tract degeneration proceeds, the balance of the muscle pull on the toes is lost so that the arch of the foot becomes exaggerated and the toes have the characteristic "hammer toe" appearance. There is usually a slow, lateral nystagmus with a slurring speech. Unlike tabes, there is no Argyll Robertson pupil and no evidence of any of the sensory disturbances such as shooting neuralgic pains and gastric crises. From the standpoint of pathology, the lesions are identical with those already described except in respect to their distribution. They are almost invariably symmetrical and as already commented upon involve particularly the cerebellar and pyramidal tracts. In the later stages of the disease, reparative gliosis may be observed. This disease is one of the group to which the title of "abiotrophy" was originally applied by Gowers to indicate the premature atrophy of certain structures. This appears as a rather pronounced familial trait, not unlike many other neurologic conditions.

LANDRY'S ASCENDING PARALYSIS

By Landry's paralysis is meant a rapidly progressive motor neuron paralysis which begins in the feet and rapidly extends up the trunk and arms to involve the bulb and results fatally. At times the paralysis appears in descending fashion instead of the usual ascending manner. Clinically, it is more often seen in the third decade. The clinical picture is characterized by progressive muscular weakness with paralysis of the intercostals, diaphragm and finally of the respiratory center.

The pathology is usually relatively minimal. It is characterized by motor nerve cell degeneration which, because of the rapidity of the process, often is hard to demonstrate. Likewise, because of the short time interval involved, none of the usual inflammatory features of perivascular cellular infiltration, demyelinization and microglial proliferation are seen. The condition is believed by many to be a virus infection and may well be simply an abortive form of anterior poliomyelitis or a fulminating variety of amyotrophic lateral sclerosis, although its experimental induction has not yet been accomplished.

PROGRESSIVE LENTICULAR DEGENERATION (WILSON'S DISEASE; HEPATOLENTICULAR DEGENERATION)

This disease of the central nervous system likewise tends to be familial. It is a comparatively uncommon condition which occurs chiefly in young individuals. It was first described by Wilson in 1912 and since that time has borne his name. From the clinical standpoint, the principal symptoms are those of tremors of the parkinsonian type, muscular rigidity, and pain and difficulty in swallowing. More striking, perhaps, are the disturbances of emotional balance which are often extremely marked. The disease runs a relatively rapid and progressively fatal course. It is of interest particularly because of an almost invariable association with a chronic type of cirrhosis of the liver, more or less of the usual portal type, although never proceeding to the extent of producing symptoms. Wilson regarded the cirrhosis as the primary pathological process and felt that this was responsible for the lenticular degenerative lesions which are found at autopsy.

Pathologically, there is bilateral degeneration of the lenticular nucleus involving the entire putamen, but not involving the thalamus. In the more marked cases, actual degenerative changes of the pyramidal tracts may follow.

ILLUSTRATIVE CASE

CASE 285. (Ref. #S-405)

Diagnosis.—Lenticular nucleus—chronic progressive lenticular degeneration (Wilson's disease).

Patient was a girl of 18 years, admitted to the hospital with the chief complaints of tremors of the head and upper extremities, and disturbance of speech.

Present Illness.—The onset had been gradual and dated back for a period of about one and one-half years when the patient first noticed that her head would shake involuntarily. Shortly after this, she began to develop a marked intention tremor of her upper extremities. This increased in severity until at the time of admission she was unable to feed herself. Her speech defect began approximately one year before admission and had been progressive. She had complained of stiffness of her legs, but there was no actual paralysis. The patient's mother reported a definite change in the patient's personality, the patient becoming moody, introspective, quarrelsome, readily excitable and even violent at times. Recently the patient noticed that her breathing had become somewhat irregular and jerky.

Past Medical History.—The previous medical history was of interest in that she had had a severe "catarrhal" type of jaundice at the age of nine from which she apparently made a complete recovery. She had had the usual childhood diseases before that. She had not had rheumatic fever. Menses began at the age of fifteen and a half, and had always been irregular with a very scanty flow. Her family history was pertinent in that a brother had died following an illness characterized by the parkinsonian picture with intention tremors and an associated jaundice and euphoria. At autopsy a hypertrophic cirrhosis of his liver and a fibrous splenitis were found. One sister had died of pulmonary tuberculosis and another of Banti's disease. Her father and mother were living and well. A review of her systems otherwise was negative.

Physical Examination.—Patient was a fairly well developed and nourished young girl with marked secondary sex characteristics. The skin showed a peculiar pigmentation which was diffuse over the entire body and accompanied by many freckles of the addisonian type. Head was not remarkable. Eyes, ears, nose and throat were negative. Chest was symmetrical. There was a supernumerary nipple on the left. Heart and lungs were negative. Blood pressure was 98/70. Abdomen was negative. The liver was thought to be reduced in size as determined by palpation and percussion. No enlargement of the spleen was noted. Extremities, other than for neurologic symptoms, were negative.

Neurologic Examination.—Speech was jerky, scanning and tremendously slow and labored with little control over the volume of the voice. There was a coarse, rhythmic intention tremor of the hands and arms. There were also coarse flexion and extension movements of the left leg when muscles were on the stretch. A coarse, oscillatory tremor of the lower jaw appeared on speaking. Incoördination was seen with marked clumsiness in attempting any fine movements with her hands. There was no definite rigidity of any of the muscles. The deep reflexes were diminished. There was nystagmus on turning the eyes upward. At the sclerocorneal junction almost surrounding the cornea was a well-marked ring of brownish pigmentation.

Laboratory Findings.—Red blood cells, 4,740,000 with 75% hemoglobin. White blood cells, 5,750 with a normal differential count. Kolmer, Kahn and Kline tests were negative. Blood chemistry was normal. Basal metabolic rate was minus eleven. Liver function test showed increased dextrose tolerance, but a normal galactose tolerance and a normal bromsulphalein test.

Subsequent Course.—The patient went progressively downhill and died approximately three years after the onset of her symptoms.

Autopsy Findings.—At autopsy, the outstanding findings were a terminal edema and congestion of the lungs with a possible beginning bronchopneumonia. The liver presented the typical picture of cirrhosis of a somewhat indefinite type but simulating that of the more usual form of portal Laennec's nodular type. The spleen was moderately enlarged and likewise showed a diffuse

fibrous splenitis with a relative atrophy of the lymphoid elements. The remainder of the viscera were normal in their gross appearance. The brain was moderately edematous and congested. Sections, after hardening, showed rather marked focal areas of encephalomalacia in the region of the lenticular nucleus.

Microscopic Description of a Section Through the Lenticular Area.—(Fig. 656) Sections stained by the usual Weigert method show definite areas of demyelinization and replacement gliosis. With other staining methods, there can be identified definite degenerative changes of the nerve cells, not only in the lenticular nucleus, but to a less extensive degree involving the large Betz cells of the cerebral cortex. It is characterized chiefly by chromatolysis and disappearance of the Nissl granules. Considerable edema and congestion are present. In some areas, actual petechial hemorrhage has occurred with the deposition of pigment, which is largely contained within phagocytic cells.

This association of liver and lenticular disease unquestionably must have some underlying simple etiologic basis, but to date, no satisfactory explanation for

this curious combination of lesions, a chronic type of cirrhosis and degenerative changes in the lenticular nuclei, has been advanced.

PARALYSIS AGITANS (PARKINSON'S DISEASE; SHAKING PALSY)

This neurologic syndrome occurs almost entirely in late middle life and affects males about twice as frequently as it does females. The disease has been recognized for well over a century. The clinical picture is characterized by the gradual onset of weakness, tremors, and rigidity of the body which is held in a position of flexion.

As is true of most of this group of degenerative diseases of the central nervous system, no definite etiology can be attributed to its development. Head injuries, emotional shocks and even profound worry are believed to be contributory factors. As has already been mentioned, a condition closely simulating that of paralysis agitans may be seen in the postencephalitic complication in the younger age group. Such cases frequently follow the progressive clinical course of the more classical instances of the disease going on to a fatal conclusion over a variable period ranging from a year or two up to as long as ten or fifteen years. Because of the similarity in the clinical picture as a result of encephalitis the thought that the disease is essentially one of infection is difficult to

overlook. Other suggestions in respect to etiology have laid stress on the possibility of some toxic lesion similar to that which may be the cause of Wilson's progressive lenticular degeneration such as nephritis or liver disease playing a contributory part. As the disease progresses, the patient gradually becomes as rigid as a statue and ultimately speech and swallowing become impossible.

Pathology.—In view of the extraordinarily marked clinical features of the disease, the extent of the pathology seems relatively slight. The essential lesion is one of degeneration of the large motor nerve cells of the corpus striatum, particularly of the globus pallidus. No definite involvement of the pyramidal tracts occurs so that in spite of the marked muscular rigidity, there is no true paralysis. Other changes which have been described in relation to this condition have been those of increased interstitial fibrosis and edema of the periaxial tissues. Not infrequently there is an associated vascular sclerosis and the presence of "colloid" droplets and degenerated oligodendroglial cells may be found.

CHOREA

Two forms of chorea are well recognized from the clinical standpoint; (a) the usual Sydenham type

associated with rheumatic fever, and (b) the adult type known as Huntington's chorea.

Sydenham's Chorea (St. Vitus's Dance).—This nervous disease is a condition chiefly of children between the ages of five and fifteen and occurs very much more frequently in girls than in boys. It is characterized clinically by the presence of involuntary choreiform purposeless movements of the extremities with a varying degree of muscular weakness and incoördination. Not infrequently some mental symptoms are observed. The disease is believed to be one of the manifestations of rheumatic fever, although it is not necessarily preceded by any joint symptoms. It has been reported following acute streptococcic sore throat, which again may represent the onset of the rheumatic attack. The etiology of chorea is obviously the same uncertain etiologic agent which produces rheumatic fever. Ordinarily, the disease runs its course spontaneously in periods varying from a few weeks to a month. Occasionally it becomes progressive in character and is followed by a fatal outcome. The pathology is relatively insignificant. It is obviously an inflammatory lesion when any changes can be demonstrated. There is usually hyperemia and some edema. Not infrequently a perivascular mononuclear cellular mantling of the vessels is found not only in the brain substance, but in the pia as well. Occasionally, thrombosis of the small vessels is observed and degenerative changes of the nerve cells in the cerebral cortex and basal ganglia as well as the neostriatum are seen.

Huntington's Chorea.—This variety is apparently an hereditary disease and can often be traced through several generations. It rarely appears until late middle life. From the clinical standpoint the symptoms are those of choreiform movements and ataxia associated with mental degeneration, which goes on to actual insanity.

The pathology is not well established, but degenerative changes with atrophy of the cells of the neostriatum have been found. In this instance the globus pallidus does not seem to be involved. Likewise, cortical nerve cell atrophy has also been reported, which is supposed to account for the mental deterioration.

LITTLE'S PARALYSIS (CONGENITAL SPASTIC DIPLEGIA)

In Little's disease there is a weakness of a moderate degree which typically is confined to the legs. Clinically it is characterized by a typical "scissors" cross-legged gait in walking. There is usually muscular weakness and marked rigidity of the extremities and hyperactive knee jerks. Commonly, there is an associated involuntary type of athetoid movement of the upper extremities, which at times may be confused with the less severe choreiform motion. Mental impairment is common and may be so marked as to be classified on the basis of congenital idiocy. Articulation in the more severe cases is likewise interfered with and not infrequently, epileptiform convulsions are seen in association with the diffuse spastic picture.

Generally, the term, "Little's disease," is restricted to the minor manifestations of this condition in which the etiology appears to be an arrested development of the motor areas during intrauterine life. On the other hand, a variety of spastic paralysis may occur which is more commonly spoken of as "obstetrical paralysis." In this condition, the lesion is the result of actual evulsion of the brachial plexus, particularly the fifth cervical root as the result of a difficult labor. All gradations of this condition of obstetrical paralysis are seen, ranging from simple internal rotation and extension up to flaccid paralysis of the entire extremity. The lesion may be either unilateral or bilateral in rare instances.

Pathologically, the picture is one of traumatic injury to the nerve plexus with resultant reparative fibrosis and scarring.

SYRINGOMYELIA

Syringomyelia is a disorder of the central nervous system which is usually seen in early life and is believed by many to be congenital in origin as the result of failure of normal development of the spinal cord. This maldevelopment of the spinal cord may well be the result of intrauterine inflammation or vascular disease, or it may be the result of scar formation with subsequent liquefaction necrosis and cystic degeneration. In typical syringomyelia, the cystic degeneration of the cord, which is found, bears no relationship to the central canal. The cavities vary greatly in size, shape and position, but are usually found in the gray matter, often extending well out into the anterior horns. The walls of the cavities are lined by a thick layer of glial cells. This cavitation may extend the entire length of the cord, even up into the brain stem. Not infrequently, the lining of the cavities may be composed of ependymal-like cells which tend to differentiate from the more primitive glioblasts. The lesions are more commonly found in the cervical and upper thoracic parts of the cord and are likewise more frequently encountered posterior to the central canal, thus producing interference with the pain fibers in the gray commissure. From the clinical standpoint dissociated anesthesia with loss of pain and temperature sensation, but with the preservation of the tactile sense is almost pathognomonic of the disease. As has been explained, this is due to the interruption of the pain and temperature fibers which normally cross in the brain commissure. Other symptoms which are usually found in these cases are spasticity of the lower extremities and muscular atrophy, particularly of the upper extremities. Not infrequently vasomotor and trophic nerve changes are present. These latter are not readily explained by the nature or distribution of the pathological lesion. Among them may be cited the Charcot joint, which again, as has already been emphasized, may occur in any joint where there is loss of sensation, and as such is not a specific lesion for any particular condition. The muscular paralysis may well be the result of pressure upon the anterior horns with resultant atrophy of the motor neurons, although this is often hard to demonstrate.

Clinically, the cases run a rather tragic, prolonged course occasionally dying of the disease itself, but more often dying of some secondary infection.

ILLUSTRATIVE CASE

CASE 286. (Ref. #S-284)

Diagnosis.—Spinal cord—syringomyelia.

Patient was a white female of 17 years, admitted to the hospital with the chief complaint of a severe burn of her hand, which had developed without any sensation of pain.

Present Illness.—About eighteen months before admission, the patient noticed that she began to have some weakness in her hands and would have difficulty in picking up objects. She often dropped things and had very little control over the muscles of her fingers. About the same time she noticed that she seemed to lose any feeling of pain in her fingers and on several occasions burned herself to some extent. Her hands always seemed to feel cold. All of these symptoms and signs seemed to become progressively worse over the period of a year and a half, up to the present admission. It was accompanied by an actual atrophy of the muscles of her hands with loss of the thenar and hypothenar eminences. The joints seemed somewhat thickened and rather irregular in shape.

Past Medical History.—The patient's past history was essentially negative. She had had the usual infections of childhood. She had no knowledge of having had scarlet fever or rheumatic fever. A review of her systems was relatively noninformatory. She was not unusually subject to upper respiratory disease. She had never been cardiac conscious. Her gastro-intestinal history was normal. Menstrual history began at the age of twelve and periods had been regular until the three months preceding admission when the interval between periods had been prolonged.

Physical Examination.—Patient was a fairly well-developed and well-nourished young white girl who did not appear acutely ill. Head was not remarkable. Eyes reacted normally to light and accommodation. There was no cervical adenopathy. Chest was symmetrical. Lungs were clear. Heart sounds were normal and no murmurs were heard. Abdomen was negative on palpation. Extremities were of interest particularly in relation to their neurologic changes. There was marked atrophy of the interosseous and other small muscles of the hands.

Neurologic Examination.—There was marked atrophy of the small muscles of both hands, but more prominently on the right. This resulted in weakness in spreading and opposing the fingers. Biceps were absent. Triceps were markedly impaired. On the other hand, ankle and knee jerks were hyperactive. There was no Babinski reflex. Abdominal reflexes were missing. Vibratory sense, joint and touch were normal. There was impairment to pin prick over the hands and wrists reaching a little higher on the right. Heat and cold were definitely impaired up to the shoulder on the left and over the chest on the right side.

Laboratory Findings.—Urinalysis was negative. Blood count was within normal limits. Wassermann was negative. Spinal fluid showed a normal pressure. The fluid was clear. There was no increase of cells. Wassermann and colloidal gold curve were negative. X-ray examinations were negative.

Subsequent Course.—The patient's condition slowly progressed over a period of nearly three years, with more marked dissociation of sensations of heat and cold extending to the lower segments of the cord. There were found progressive muscular atrophy and the development of considerable ataxia suggesting extension of the degenerative process to the sensory columns as well as to the gray matter of the cord. She ultimately became bedridden and developed a terminal hypostatic pneumonia. This had been complicated by the development of a number of decubiti over the bony prominences.

Autopsy Findings.—At autopsy, the chief findings grossly were those of marked muscular atrophy with a generalized appearance of inanition. The heart seemed normal. The lungs showed rather extensive hypostatic congestion and beginning pneumonia of both bases. Abdominal viscera were essentially negative. The brain showed moderate congestion. The most striking lesions, however, were found in the spinal cord where after fixation numerous cavitations were noted, chiefly in the gray matter and extending in tube-like fashion almost the entire length of the cord up into the bulb region. Some of these were more in the nature of smaller cysts. Some of them communicated with one another, while others tended to run up and down the cord as a single lesion. Both gray and white matter were found extensively involved.

Microscopic Description of a Section Through the Spinal Cord.—(Fig. 657) Microscopic examination of the tissue showed degeneration of both anterior and lateral horn cells, and marked gliosis around the cavities and cystic areas. These were filled with a clear, gelatinous-appearing substance apparently representing coagulum from the fluid within the cysts.

Traumatic Injuries of the Cord.—There are a considerable number of cases which show very extensive degenerative changes in the cord as the result of severe traumatic injury. Such injuries may occur as the result of stab wounds in which case the degeneration may be relatively localized and unilateral (Fig. 661). Identical changes occur as in some of the more familiar clinical pictures, with complete loss of the neuron below the point of injury and wallerian degeneration above. This is manifested by the same loss of myelin and replacement gliosis as seen in tabes, multiple sclerosis and similar conditions. In the second group, complete compression myelitis occurs which involves the entire cord. This is a common occurrence in traumatic injuries, particularly associated with fracture of the vertebral bodies. Similar changes may be seen in relation to the compression myelitis which follows the kyphosis of tuberculosis of the spine or other acute destructive bone lesions, including neoplastic infiltration of the vertebrae. An example of such compression myelitis with diffuse myelomalacia is seen in Fig. 658. Here, the major nerve tracts below the point of compression have been completely destroyed. With the Weigert staining method, this is evidenced by a failure of the tissue to stain due to the absence of the myelin. Above the point of compression, a variable amount of secondary degeneration may be observed to have taken place. These changes are best seen in the upper figure in the illustration.

CHAPTER LXV

DISEASES OF THE OSSEOUS SYSTEM

Our knowledge concerning the pathological processes which affect bone is still rudimentary, largely because of our relatively limited information regarding its normal physiology. It is too obvious to more than mention, that the chief function of the bony skeleton is supportive, but in addition to this mechanical background, the bones, as such, serve as a reservoir for calcium in helping maintain the normal metabolism of salts in the body. The regulation of the calcium/phosphorus and other mineral ratios appears to be a highly complex mechanism regulated in part by the vitamins, notably D and C, and by certain of the ductless glands, especially the parathyroids. Nor can the kidneys be disregarded in this respect, as has been brought out in the discussion of hyperparathyroidism and so-called "renal" rickets in a previous chapter.

From the standpoint of the actual pathological conditions which we specifically encounter clinically or at the autopsy table as involving bone, five major groups of lesions can be readily differentiated: (1) the congenital, such as spina bifida and other teratological defects, as well as certain of the osteodystrophies; (2) the traumatic, notably fractures; (3) the infectious, including acute and chronic osteomyelitis, osteitis, and periostitis whether suppurative or granulomatous in nature; (4) the constitutional, metabolic disturbances or osteodystrophies, which make up perhaps the most interesting of all the bone lesions, and cover a wide range from rickets and osteomalacia to osteitis deformans (Paget's disease) and osteitis fibrosa (von Recklinghausen's disease); and finally, (5) the neoplastic diseases, which have been taken up in some detail in Chapter XXV.

CONGENITAL LESIONS

Among those lesions of bone which should be thought of as strictly congenital in nature must be included a very considerable number of conditions of defective skeletal development which have already been discussed in Chapter XXXVII in relation to teratology. Anencephaly, microcephaly, hare lip, cleft palate, the various rachischises, particularly spina bifida, club foot, congenital dislocation of the hip, extra ribs, accessory digits, localized gigantism and many other pathological processes are among the more important and more frequently encountered. With the exception of anencephaly, these disturbances of development all are consistent with life, and accordingly become problems of diagnosis and therapy.

Certain other lesions of a congenital nature may not be so apparent at birth, and perhaps should not necessarily be considered as representing primary bone pathology. Chief of these must be mentioned congenital syphilis in which the skeletal defects are secondary to disturbed bone growth. In this group, likewise, must be mentioned the congenital form of hydrocephalus. Again, defective growth of bone is seen in certain of the so-called "osteodystrophies," notably the dwarfism associated with the clinical condition known as *achondroplasia*. For convenience, this will be considered later in the chapter in relation to the other constitutional diseases which produce bone changes, many of which, such as rickets, cretinism and osteitis fibrosa, are obviously secondary to disturbances of function of the endocrine glands, or to nutritional deficiencies.

ILLUSTRATIVE CASE

CASE 287. (Ref. #R.R.—38055).
Diagnosis.—Bones—achondroplasia.
Patient was a white, female child of 7 years, admitted to the hospital with the chief complaints of weakness and pain in her legs.

Clinical History.—The patient's condition should be considered as a congenital developmental problem, so that the immediate onset of her symptoms are only incidental. She was born at full term and by a normal delivery. She was breast fed for fourteen months and then

PLATE CLVII
DISEASES OF THE OSSEOUS SYSTEM

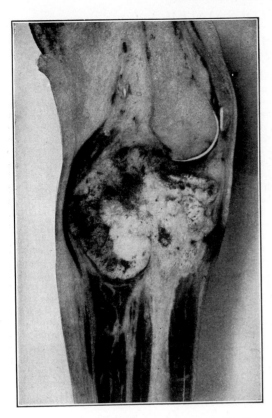

FIG. 663.—TIBIA: OSTEOGENIC SARCOMA.—Cf. CASE 95.—Gross photograph showing a malignant tumor arising from epiphyseal end of the diaphysis and invading the surrounding soft tissues, including the joint.

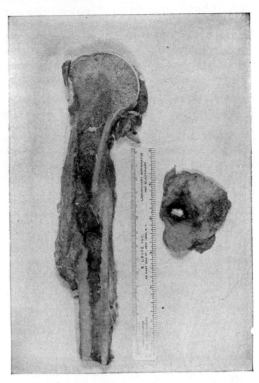

FIG. 664.—HUMERUS: METASTATIC CARCINOMA.—Gross photograph showing the site of a metastatic tumor which has destroyed the cortex with resultant pathological fracture. Note attempt at healing with callus formation.

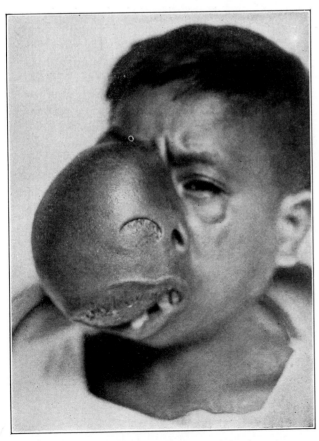

FIG. 665.—JAW: DENTIGEROUS CYST.—CASE 295.—Gross photograph which illustrates the extent of deformity which may result from neglect of an otherwise entirely benign process.

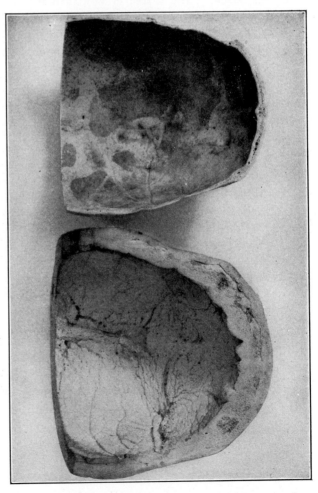

FIG. 666.—SKULL: PAGET'S DISEASE (OSTEITIS DEFORMANS).—CASE 291.—Gross photograph of calvarium showing the extreme thickening and marked porosity, characteristic of Paget's disease (lower) as compared with a normal skull (upper).

put on a mixed diet. She began to walk and talk at the normal average age. Her local physician made the diagnosis of marked rickets at the age of eighteen months, but due to the family's economic condition, the child did not receive vitamin therapy and the rachitic picture seemed to progress.

Since the age of two, the child had failed to grow in stature as she should, and this was attributed to the dietary deficiency as part of the rachitic picture. More recently, she has developed the symptoms for which she was admitted, namely marked general muscular weakness and the occurrence of pain in the legs, particularly around the knee joints.

Physical Examination.—Physical examination showed a typical achondroplastic picture with characteristic shortening of the hands, feet, forearms and thighs, a less marked shortening of the upper arms and lower legs. Marked knocked-knees were present. There was a very prominent lordosis which made the buttocks appear unduly disproportionate in size. The child's arms reached slightly below the crest of the ilium.

In other respects the child's physical examination was essentially negative. The body was in a state of fair nutrition. The child seemed mentally alert. Head was of the brachycephalic type, with a rather short base to the skull. Ears were normal. Eyes reacted normally to light and accommodation. Nose and throat were negative. Tonsils were moderately enlarged and cryptic.

Chest was symmetrical. Lungs were clear. Heart was not enlarged. There were no murmurs present. Abdomen was negative.

Laboratory Findings.—Red blood cells, 4,900,000 with 11 gm. of hemoglobin. White blood cells, 8,450 with 25% polymorphonuclears, 73% lymphocytes and 2% monocytes. Urinalysis was negative. Blood chemistry studies yielded 12.5 mgm. of calcium and 5.04 mgm. of serum phosphorus. Wassermann was negative. Basal metabolic rate was minus two per cent.

X-ray Studies.—The findings by x-ray were characteristic of achondroplasia. The tubular long bones are all much shorter than normal and show marked widening of their epiphyses. The appearance of the epiphyseal lines was adequately explained on the basis of achondroplasia rather than rickets. The skull appeared normal. There was no defect of the sella.

Subsequent Course.—The child was put on a mixed glandular therapy and at the end of eighteen months, some increase in stature was found, but this appeared to be the result of growth of the vertebral column rather than of the long bones. The child's measurements taken at this period were approximately the same as those on the initial admission. The value of hormone therapy did not seem to be very well established, but from the experimental standpoint it was recommended that, in the absence of any other known means of treatment, it be continued.

TRAUMATIC BONE LESIONS

The major lesion of traumatic origin relating to the osseous system is seen in association with *fracture*. Less severe injury may result in a simple periostitis. In either case the essential pathology is comparable. The problem of bone repair was touched upon briefly in relation to reparative phenomena as a whole in Chapter XI. Accordingly it will be reviewed at this time in rather cursory fashion. Bone repair is observed most readily perhaps in a fracture of one of the long bones. Hemorrhage promptly takes place at the site of fracture and blood clot fills the intervening gap between the fractured ends of the bone. Repair of the fracture is accomplished by a progressive replacement of this hemorhagic exudate by the proliferation of fibroblasts and new capillaries in much the same fashion as any granulating surface wound. Simultaneously, the osteoblasts, which form a solid layer beneath the periosteum and are found similarly lining the endosteum and the haversian canals to a considerable extent, proliferate to form either osteoid tissue or true bone. If osteoid tissue is first formed, this undergoes secondary calcification and ossification in much the same way that normal membranous bone develops. The end result is the replacement of the blood clot by an excess amount of relatively soft,

new-formed bone. This is spoken of as a callus and is visualized as a more or less symmetrical, fusiform lesion, both by x-ray and by palpation.

The subsequent steps in the development of the final end picture are accomplished by absorption of the excess new bone callus. This absorption is accomplished by two mechanisms, which usually occur together, but may be seen singly. The more important of these processes is that of simple bone absorption through increased vascularity of the tissue. New blood vessels form in the developing haversian canals and through distention cause actual pressure upon the bony tissue. Presumably, some endocrine stimulation exists which causes the withdrawal of calcium from these areas. In the other method of absorption, the osteoblasts are the prominent factor. These, as it will be recalled, are large multinucleated cells of reticulo-endothelial origin and comparable to the large mononuclear phagocytes as seen in the development of foreign body giant cells. Their function is the actual absorption of bone, which is accomplished in a manner which suggests the gnawing away of the excess bone in much the same way that a mouse gnaws away at food. Gradually new lines of stress are established and in an uncomplicated fracture in which no serious displacement of the ends

PLATE CLVIII
DISEASES OF THE OSSEOUS SYSTEM
OSTEOMYELITIS

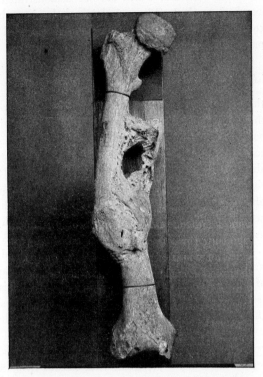

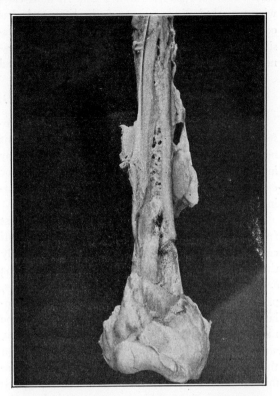

FIG. 667.—FEMUR: OSTEOMYELITIS, SECONDARY.—
Femur, the site of chronic osteomyelitis, the result
of a compound fracture with subsequent pyogenic
infection. Note marked involucrum.

FIG. 668.—HUMERUS: OSTEOMYELITIS, ACUTE.—Cf.
CASE 288.—Gross photograph showing an extensive
osteomyelitis involving the greater part of the shaft.

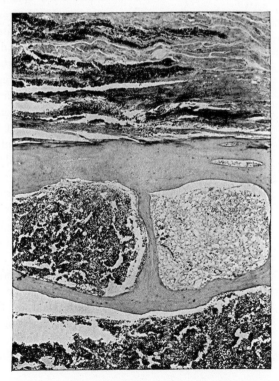

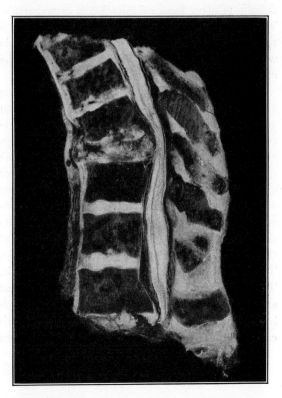

FIG. 669.—BONE: ACUTE OSTEOMYELITIS.—CASE 288.—
Microtessar photograph showing periosteum and adjacent cortical bone which is undergoing caries. Note
exudate infiltrating the periosteum and composed almost entirely of polymorphonuclear leukocytes. App.
15 x.

FIG. 670.—VERTEBRA: POTT'S DISEASE; TUBERCULOUS
OSTEOMYELITIS.—CASE 289.—Gross photograph showing kyphosis as a result of caseous tuberculosis of
the second and third lumbar vertebrae. Note compression of adjacent cord.

of the fracture has occurred, ultimately little or no trace of such a fracture can be found. In those cases where marked displacement of the bone ends has occurred, the process of repair is similar, but excessive bone persists to fill the gap so that some permanent deformity remains and can be demonstrated clinically both by physical examination and by x-ray. These are the obvious changes which occur in the repair of bone and which may be demonstrated by histologic methods. The underlying mechanism which controls this extraordinary functional purposeful repair process, however, is still obscure.

INFECTIOUS DISEASES OF BONE

Osteomyelitis.—By osteomyelitis is meant an infection of the medulla of the bone with subsequent necrosis of the cortex, and usually accompanied by involvement of the periosteum. It may be *acute* or *chronic,* dependent upon the nature of the infecting organism and the resistance of the host.

ACUTE OSTEOMYELITIS.—The acute form is most frequently seen in children and in the majority of cases is due to one of the staphylococci, ordinarily, the *Staphylococcus aureus,* but occasionally the *Staphylococcus albus.* In a small number of cases, particularly in infants, a streptococcus may be isolated. The organism usually gains access to the medulla of the bone by way of the blood stream, although in certain instances direct infection through trauma, especially with compound comminuted fractures, may occur. This latter type is seen as a rule in an older age group. A furuncle, suppurative middle ear disease, and the like may be the apparent primary site. In other cases no such definite primary focus of infection is demonstrable. The condition is, therefore, usually spoken of as a primary infection. Rare instances are recorded in which the *Bacillus coli* or *Bacillus typhosus* are the offenders.

Clinically, the child suddenly develops the picture of septicemia with chills, fever, a rapid heart action and often actual prostration. This is usually accompanied by a marked leukocytosis. There is exquisite pain locally in the affected bone. The most common sites for such acute osteomyelitis, in order of frequency, are tibia, femur and humerus. Less often, the ulna, fibula or metatarsal bones are involved. A history of trauma is usually given. Its significance, however, is questionable, but may at times help explain the localization of the process. The initial lesion ordinarily begins in the metaphysis. This is explained on the basis of the rather curious arrangement of the blood vessels in this area, which because of their sharp angulation tend to mechanically aid in the localization of bacterial emboli. From this metaphyseal focus, the process tends to spread through the medulla and extend through the cortical bone by way of the haversian system, eventually reaching the subperiosteum. There, a subperiosteal abscess forms with elevation of the periosteum. It is this stretching of the periosteum and the pressure of the exudate within the cavity of the bone which accounts for the unusually severe pain which is usually present.

Due to the actual pressure of the exudate and to toxic damage to the vascular endothelium because of the bacterial nature of the process, there is a tendency toward the development of rather extensive thrombosis of the vessels. In this way the blood supply to the involved area is interfered with. This results in actual bone necrosis. This necrotic bone separates from the persistent vital osseous tissue and is spoken of as a *sequestrum.* Sooner or later, the periosteum is likely to perforate and the suppurative process, after extending through the soft tissues ruptures through the skin surface. Such openings are known as *cloacae.* The sequestrum may be spontaneously discharged and repair proceed uninterrupted. If the sequestrum is too large to be discharged spontaneously, it may gradually be absorbed and repair again take place without further complication. On the other hand, such sequestra may persist as foreign bodies, tending to act as a chronic irritant in maintaining the infection. If removal of the sequestrum fails to take place, the infection may extend throughout the medulla of the bone producing extensive liquefaction necrosis of the marrow and of the bone itself and resulting in further sequestrum formation. In such cases, operative interference with the removal of as many of the sequestrated bone fragments as possible and the establishment of adequate drainage is indicated.

The reparative phase of the process is comparable in many respects to the simple repair of bone as seen in a fracture. There is proliferation of the osteoblasts, chiefly of the periosteum, but likewise of the endosteum and of those cells lining the haversian canals. A marked thickening of the bone occurs as the result of this new bone formation. It is found chiefly at the site of the previous periosteal involvement. This new bone formation is comparable in many respects to the development of the callus in simple bone repair, but in conjunction with the infectious process, this new bone is spoken of as the *involucrum.*

Brodie's Abscess.—A less acute, localized type of osteomyelitis is occasionally encountered. This is known as a "Brodie's abscess" and presents a very distinctive x-ray appearance. In these cases the infection remains localized to the medulla of the bone, usually at one end of the shaft. It does not extend to invade the cortex or periosteum. It tends to become walled off and chronic in nature. The treatment is local drainage surgically.

Osteomyelitis may also occur secondary to compound fracture or other injuries leading to infection of the bone from without. Sometimes, the extraction of an infected tooth with injury of the jaw bone leads to the development of such a lesion. This variety is usually spoken of as secondary osteomyelitis in contradistinction to the primary variety just described. It is a frank suppurative process with considerable destruction of bone, both cortical and medullary. Not infrequently it is complicated by invasion of the blood stream by the causative organism and results in a fatal septicemia. It is most commonly seen in adults. (Fig. 667.)

CHRONIC OSTEOMYELITIS.—By the term chronic osteomyelitis is ordinarily meant a chronic pyogenic infection of bone. This may follow an acute osteomyelitis through a gradually acquired resistance of the patient against the particular organism, but inadequate to completely overcome the infection. It may result from improper treatment of a case, such as occurs when sequestra are not removed and thus keep the infection alive. Occasionally, the condition might be termed "chronic" almost from the outset in the case of an infectious agent of low virulence. Perhaps properly tuberculosis and the other granulomatous infections of bone should be included under this heading of chronic osteomyelitis, but it is customary to consider them separately, as they present such characteristic clinical and pathological features. Brodie's abscess should also be included among the chronic forms of the condition.

In the chronic suppurative instances of osteomyelitis cited above, there is a striking tendency for the process to become relatively localized and walled off. It may continue to discharge fragments of sequestra and exudate through a sinus tract for many years. Similarly, involucrum formation continues at the same slow rate to produce the most extraordinary distortion of the normal architecture, yet always with a purposeful functional regard. Thus, new lines of stress develop; and dense ebonization occurs, to give added structural strength to the bone which persists. Commonly, saprophytic putrefactive organisms complicate the picture so that the discharge may be extremely unpleasant at times.

Eventually, *amyloidosis* may result from the long continued chronic suppurative process. As will be recalled in discussing amyloid infiltration of the viscera, particular emphasis was placed upon chronic infectious and wasting diseases, especially those affecting bone as being the most significant etiologic factor clinically in the production of this pathological condition.

ILLUSTRATIVE CASE

CASE 288. (Ref. #S-289)
Diagnosis.—Bone—necrosis; acute osteomyelitis.
Patient was a white female of 7 years, admitted to the hospital because of marked painful swelling of the right leg.
Present Illness.—Five months before admission, there was a history of trauma, a hundred pound cake of ice having fallen on her right foot. She did not complain of any serious pain at the time other than momentarily, and was able to walk without any limp immediately after the accident. She had no disability for the following three days, but then began to complain of soreness of the leg and inability to move it. The lower leg was very painful to touch and began to swell, but no bruise over the involved area could be seen. She was sent to a hospital

where the diagnosis of acute osteomyelitis was made. She was operated upon, and an incision into the tibia was made.

The child remained in the hospital for several weeks and the wound gradually closed over. She seemed to be relatively free of any local symptomatology relating to the leg for the following three months. However, during this period the mother noted that the child was listless, pale, and had no appetite. She fatigued unduly readily and was extremely restless in her sleep. A week before her present admission, she developed marked swelling of the right lower leg, which was exquisitely tender on touch and caused complete restriction of motion because of pain. The mother stated that the child's temperature seemed elevated and that she was acutely sick.

Past Medical History.—Her past medical history was essentially irrelevant. The child was normally delivered and was breast fed for the first year. She had had measles and whooping cough. She had not had rheumatic fever. She had not been subject to sore throats, but was told by her school physician that her tonsils were in poor condition and should be removed. Otherwise, she had developed normally.

Physical Examination.—The child was fairly well-developed but somewhat undernourished and appeared definitely pallid. She was resting comfortably in bed as long as her leg was held immobile. Head was symmetrically developed with slight frontal bossing. Eyes reacted normally to light and accommodation. Nose was negative. Mouth and throat showed a rather pale mucous membrane, the teeth in poor condition and moderate hypertrophy and inflammatory hyperplasia of her tonsils. Chest was symmetrical. Lungs were clear. Heart was not enlarged. The rate was rapid but regular. There were no murmurs. Abdomen was negative. No masses were palpable. The genitalia were negative. Upper extremities: The arms were negative except for bilateral antecubital scars from previous transfusions. Lower extremities: The left leg was negative. The right leg was swollen to twice its normal size. Anteriorly there was a reddened, edematous area extending from the lower border of the tibia to the tubercle. On the inner aspect was a long ulcerated lesion which extended down to the bone and from which escaped a thin, serosanguineous exudate.

Laboratory Findings.—Red blood cells numbered 4,-000,000 with 66% hemoglobin. White blood cells numbered 9,950 with 49% neutrophiles, 46% eosinophiles, 2% monocytes and 3% eosinophiles. Urinalysis was negative on several occasions. Wasserman was negative. Bacteriologic culture of the wound revealed the presence of a *Staphylococcus albus*.

X-ray Examination.—A large sequestrum of the right tibia was demonstrated. This involved practically the entire diaphysis. It was surrounded by massive involucrum formation.

Subsequent Course.—A radical excision of the sequestrum of the tibia was done separating it from the two epiphyseal ends. The leg was put in a cast to maintain position while the involucrum developed. The wound was treated by ultraviolet therapy to clean up the infection and subsequent skin grafts were used to fill in the surface epithelial defect. The patient made an uneventful recovery.

Pathological Report.—*Gross Description.*—(Cf. Fig. 668) Specimen consisted of a tibial sequestrum measuring fifteen centimeters in length. The osseous structure was ragged, thickened and grayish in color. The marrow portion of the bone was filled with soft, grayish, pultaceous, foul-smelling material, which could be readily scooped out.

Microscopic Description of a Section from the Bone.—(Fig. 669) Histologic examination of multiple sections taken from the involved bone shows definite evidence of infection. The potential marrow cavity is largely replaced by an acute polynuclear cellular exudate which shows what might well be interpreted as actual necrosis and abscess formation. The bone likewise has undergone necrosis. No normal bone cells can be seen. The haversian canals are replaced by fibrous tissue or necrotic material. No osteoblasts can be identified in the necrotic areas.

Non-suppurative Forms of Osteitis, Osteomyelitis and Osteochondritis.— SCLEROSING OSTEITIS. — There exists a group of cases, which in recent years has occasioned considerable interest in respect to etiology and treatment. These cases have been recognized for many years under a variety of names. Perhaps the most apt term to apply is that of "sclerosing osteitis." The lesion is characterized by thickening and ebonization of the cortical bone in a local area, usually in one of the long bones of the lower extremity, or occasionally involving the bones of the feet, particularly the os calcis. The cortex is markedly thickened and appears by x-ray to possess an unusual density. Not infrequently, slight irregularity of the periosteal surface with bone spicules can be observed. Frequently there is a concomitant osteoporosis of the medullary portion of the bone. The lesion, at times, radiologically simulates that of actual osteogenic tumor.

Etiologically, there is a very definite impression held rather generally that the lesion is in the nature of a localized chronic or subacute type of osteitis, possibly an actual osteomyelitis. The clinical picture is one of intense and exquisite pain of a progressive nature. There is frequently an antecedent picture of local trauma, but this is by no means always established.

Treatment consists in the reëstablishment of circulation to the area involved by multiple perforation of the thickened bone cortex to allow new vessel development. This, in turn, results in gradual absorption of the excess bone and recovery of the patient clinically.

Pathologically, tissue removed from such lesions presents the picture of excessive dense bone formation with a disappearance of the haversian system and obliteration of the blood vessels which normally supply the cortex through the haversian canals.

OSTEOCHONDRITIS DEFORMANS JUVENILIS (LEGG-PERTHES'-CALVE'S DISEASE, COXA PLANA). —Another form of non-suppurative bone pathology which probably belongs in this group of lesions is the curious process which is seen affecting the head of the femur in children between the ages of five and ten. Clinically, pain is usually very slight, and limp is the most outstanding symptom. Not infrequently the condition is confused with tuberculosis. By x-ray, there is an extraordinary flattening of the head of the femur with shortening of the neck. Pathologically, the lesion consists of a slow caries of the epiphysis with marked osteolysis and subsequent new bone formation. Sequestra may form in the more marked instances. No actual pus is present and the lesions are usually sterile bacteriologically.

Similar lesions have been described in other bones. The condition known as Osgood-Schlatter disease differs only in its location, in this instance involving the tubercle of the tibia. The term "Kohler's disease" is applied to the condition when it involves the tarsal scaphoid bone, and Kienboch's name is usually given to those instances in which the os lunatum is involved. The lesion seems in every instance to start in relation to the center of ossification. No explanation can be offered for this localization other than the relatively greater vascular supply in these rapidly growing areas.

OSTEOCHONDRITIS DISSECANS.—Another variety of non-suppurative caries of bone and cartilage is seen in the condition known as *osteochondritis dissecans*. Spontaneous detachment of segments of the articular cartilage and overlying bone takes place, this tissue being liberated as a loose foreign body into the joint cavity. An explanation which has been offered in respect to etiology is dependent upon the curious arrangement of the nutrient vessels, which because of their angulation are prone to thrombosis and occlusion. With such interference with the nutrition of the tissue in a fashion comparable to that of infarction elsewhere, the area supplied by the vessel undergoes degeneration and separates from the surrounding healthy structures. This is aided by the mechanical motion of the joint.

Tuberculosis of Bone.—Tuberculosis of the osseous system should properly be considered as a chronic granulomatous form of osteomyelitis. Due, however, to its extremely characteristic clinical and pathological features, it is customary to consider tuberculosis of the bone as a separate entity. Curiously enough, the great majority of cases of bone tuberculosis are from the clinical standpoint, primarily infections with no clinical evidence of tuberculosis elsewhere in the body. By careful x-ray examination of such patients, not infrequently a minimal lesion, usually of the hilus lymph nodes may be recognized or suspected, but little suggestion of activity in such lesions is ordinarily demonstrable. At autopsy, even in patients who present the picture of bone tuberculosis it is often impossible to demonstrate successfully any apparent focus of infection from which the bone lesion developed. Yet, it appears obvious that tuberculous infection of the bone can occur only by the hematogenous route, which, a priori, implies the existence of a primary lesion elsewhere in the body.

It is of significance that the great majority of cases of bone tuberculosis are found in children, which implies a relative lack of resistance against the infection. In this country, the great majority of cases of bone tuberculosis are caused by the human type of the bacillus. Only rare instances of bovine infections are encountered. On the other hand, in certain parts of Europe and the British Isles, such bovine tuberculosis is comparatively common. For some curious and unexplained reason, when such bovine infection does occur, it very frequently involves the diaphysis of the long bones whereas in the human type of infection the lesion usually starts in the metaphysis or actual epiphysis and extends rapidly to involve the joint surface. From the clinical standpoint, the bone involvement is often much less significant than the tuberculous arthritis which follows the initial bone infection. As in most infectious diseases, there seems to be a certain predilection of the organism for particular sites of localization. Thus tuberculosis of the spine (Pott's disease) (Fig. 670) and tuberculosis of the hip, knee or ankle joints are by far the most common sites. Less often, tuberculosis may involve the small bones of the hands or feet, or other of the long bones.

The pathology of bone tuberculosis is one of caries of the cancellous portion and the development of an abundant productive tuberculous type of exudate. Caseation is not a particularly prominent feature of the process. Giant cells, however, are likely to be frequently encountered in histologic preparations. As is true of tuberculosis elsewhere, the nature of the process varies dependent upon the resistance or allergic reaction of the individual to the infection. Thus, in some instances, caries proceeds much more rapidly than in others and caseation becomes more marked than does the productive inflammatory reaction. It is in such cases where the process is relatively more rapid that extension of the tuberculosis from the actual bone into the soft tissues with the development of the so-called "cold abscess" occurs.

When joint involvement in tuberculosis takes place, there is usually rather marked swelling of the joint and peri-articular tissues. This is often spoken of as *white swelling* due to the absence of the usual reddening of the tissues seen in acute inflammation. Often there is little or no pain present. The muscles at the outset tend to be spastic in an effort to restrict motion. Through disuse, they are likely sooner or later to undergo marked atrophy. In young children it is not at all uncommon to have rather sharp, severe attacks of pain, usually at night as a result of the relaxation of the muscles which tend to immobilize the disease joint surfaces, the pain being produced by sudden spastic contraction of the muscles, and forceful engagement of the diseased parts. This is often associated with a curious animal-like cry of pain, the so-called "night cry," which is almost diagnostic clinically.

Pathologically, when the joint is first involved, the process is manifested by miliary tubercles in the synovial membrane together with exudate into the joint, producing the swelling so frequently seen in the early stages. As the process spreads, tuberculous granulation tissue covers the synovial membrane and spreads to the adjacent articular surfaces. The synovial membrane may become redundant and show polypoid fringes consisting of fat, or edematous fibrous tissue. Within the synovial fluid, tiny white bodies, the so-called "rice bodies," are frequently seen. These consist of fibrin or tabs from the synovial fringes. The joint capsule may be invaded by the tuberculous process. These tissues tend to undergo caseation and the joint cavity becomes filled with such caseous exudate.

POTT'S DISEASE (TUBERCULOSIS OF THE SPINE). —In tuberculosis of the spine, the tuberculous process usually starts in the actual vertebral body. Typical caries with tuberculous granulation tissue production is found. By x-ray, the tuberculous process is largely a destructive osteolytic one with relatively little bone proliferation, although reparative efforts on the part of the bone are often manifested with new bone formation. This is in contrast to the lesions caused by the Treponema pallidum in syphilis, where the productive bone reaction exceeds the osteolytic destructive process. As the tuberculous lesion extends, it tends to involve the intervertebral discs and frequently invasion of the subarachnoid spaces occurs

with the development of a subsequent tuberculous meningitis. The weight of the patient's body produces compression of the diseased bodies of the vertebrae, giving rise to a characteristic angular deformity of the spine known as *kyphosis*. The lumbar and thoracic vertebrae are the most frequently involved. Occasionally, the cervical vertebrae likewise become the site of the primary lesion.

As a result of the kyphosis, plus the presence of excessive tuberculous granulation tissue, compression of the spinal cord may occur. This may lead to complete spastic paralysis and extensive degeneration of the cord below the site of injury. Refer to Case 279 (Ref. #S-399) in Chapter LXIII.

In other instances, the tuberculous infection may be confined to the cancellous portion of the vertebrae, and as in the case of pulmonary tuberculosis, undergoes spontaneous sterilization with eventual healing and calcification. The deformity of the vertebral bodies with the resulting kyphosis, however, is permanent unless orthopedic treatment has been instituted early enough to prevent the development of such changes. Fusion, which is known as *ankylosis* of the infected vertebrae is the aim of such therapeutic measures.

At other times, the tuberculous process extends anteriorly or laterally into the soft tissues, and particularly behind the iliopsoas muscle with the development of the so-called "cold abscess." If the lesion involves the lumbar vertebrae, the abscess may extend along the sheath of the iliopsoas muscle and point on the inner side of the thigh. If the lesion occurs in the thoracic area, the "cold abscess" usually "points" along the lateral border of a rib. In the case of cervical spine tuberculosis, such a "cold abscess" points in the lateral aspect of the neck. With the rupture of any such "cold abscess" to the surface, the development of a chronic tuberculous sinus tract follows, and a persistent discharge of thick, creamy, yellowish or grayish-yellow pus-like material continues to take place. Histologic examination of such material shows it to be made up of necrotic debris, usually without any actual cells present which can be identified. In the great majority of instances, such exudate is also sterile, even as established by guinea pig inoculation.

ILLUSTRATIVE CASE

CASE 289. (Ref. #RR.-42648)

Diagnosis. — Vertebrae — Pott's disease (tuberculous osteomyelitis).

Patient was a white female child of 6 years, admitted to the hospital because of a painful kyphosis of her back.

Present Illness.—The apparent onset of the patient's present illness was first noted two months before admission, but the child had complained on a number of occasions of a sore back for at least a year. These pains occurred principally on the right side and always at night. With the more acute manifestations, two months before admission, the child complained of pain on pressure over the small of her back. Shortly thereafter the mother noticed that there was a protrusion of the bones of the spine in that area. During this period the child lost weight steadily and her appetite was definitely impaired. The difficulty with her back was not sufficient to interfere seriously with her physical activities, however.

Past Medical History.—The patient was a full-term, normally delivered child who was breast fed for the first ten months of her life. She had had no gastrointestinal upsets of any significant degree. She had had scarlet fever two years previously, and measles six months before admission. The immediate family history was negative in respect to tuberculosis except that the mother's sister had developed tuberculosis, and had visited the child's family on one occasion for several days, over two years before the onset of the child's illness.

Physical Examination.—The patient was a fairly well-developed, but very much undernourished, female child who appeared her given age. Her head was normal in contour. Skin was rather fair and of fine texture. Lips were rather bright cherry red in color. Pupils were dilated but reacted fairly well to light and accommodation. There was a moderate protrusion of the second and third lumbar vertebrae. Chest was symmetrical and of the narrow, long type. Lungs were clear throughout. No dullness was observed. Heart was negative. Abdomen was scaphoid. No masses or tenderness were felt. Extremities were negative. A presumptive diagnosis of tuberculosis (Pott's disease) was made and the child referred to the orthopedic service for treatment.

Laboratory Findings.—Red blood cells numbered 4,-500,000 with 67.5% hemoglobin and 12,300 white blood cells with 69% polymorphonuclears. Sedimentation rate was increased. Urinalysis was negative. Mantoux test was strongly positive in both the human and bovine forms in the dilution of 1:1,000 at the end of 48 hours.

X-ray Examination.—There was a typical tuberculous osteomyelitis of the second and third lumbar vertebrae present. This had produced complete destruction of the cartilaginous discs between the bodies of these vertebrae and had resulted in apparent fusion of the two segments. A definite psoas abscess could be visualized on the left due to marked calcification. The primary focus of the infection could be demonstrated in the right upper lobe of the lung where several partially calcified nodules could be seen.

Subsequent History.—In spite of the orthopedic treatment, the pulmonary lesion lighted up and a diffuse widespread tuberculous bronchopneumonia developed of which the child died.

Autopsy Findings.—At autopsy there was a diffuse tuberculosis bronchopneumonia with evidence of a primary, partially calcified tubercle in the right apex. Generalized miliary tuberculosis of the viscera likewise present as well as a terminal tuberculous meningitis. The most outstanding lesion was an extensive tuberculosis of the lumbar spine with extension of the tuberculous process as a psoas abscess on the right side and moderate compression of the lumbar cord (Fig. 670).

TUBERCULOSIS OF THE LONG BONES.—When tuberculosis involves one of the long bones, it almost invariably begins at the epiphyseal end of the bone. The lesion is similar to that described in the previous section in respect to tuberculosis of the spine in that caries of the cancellous portion of the bone occurs. It differs from tuberculosis of the spine in that almost invariable extension of the process to the joint cavity takes place with the development of a chronic tuberculous granulation tissue to replace the normal synovial membrane. The joint surfaces become destroyed with roughening of the articular cartilaginous surfaces. Early in the process, the joint is frequently swollen due to the accumulation of effusion within the synovial cavity. Pain is a variable symptom and in the majority of cases is likely to be relatively slight although at other times it may be almost incapacitating in severity. The muscles tend to be spastic and tense in an effort to restrict motion in the affected joint. As in the case of tuberculosis of the spine, spontaneous fixation of the joint by ankylosis may occur through calcification. In the milder cases this may be prevented by early orthopedic care with the separation of the joint surfaces through traction. The use of the joint may be preserved to some extent with a variable amount of limitation of motion. In the more severe cases in which extensive destruction of the joint surfaces has occurred, ankylosis will be the preferred solution and likewise may better be accomplished through the use of orthopedic apparatus to secure early fixation of the joint in the position of greatest usefulness.

Syphilis of the Bone.—Syphilitic infection of the osseous system may be seen both in a congenital form and in acquired syphilis. In either instance, the changes which occur in the bone may well be considered as a manifestation of syphilitic osteitis or periostitis, singly or in combination. Syphilis in general has been discussed in some detail in Chapter XV, and the reader is referred to Plate XXXI accompanying that discussion for illustrations of the more characteristic bone lesions.

CONGENITAL SYPHILIS.—In congenital syphilis in infants, the long bones are most frequently involved and the lesion is primarily one of epiphysitis. If a bone such as the femur, tibia or humerus is examined by longitudinal splitting, the epiphyseal line will be seen to be irregular, thick, opaque, much wider than normal and usually of a yellowish-gray or white color. X-ray examination similarly shows marked changes in the epiphyseal separation of the epiphysis from the shaft of the bone in the more marked cases.

Histologic examination of such a lesion shows marked disturbance of bone formation at the epiphyseal junction. In the milder case, the irregular zone noted grossly along the line of ossification appears to be the result of destruction of the cartilage and bone cells by a diffuse, pseudo-gummatous, syphilitic inflammatory reaction. Thus, the osteocartilaginous junction, instead of forming a narrow, regular line, is made up of prolonged projections of cartilage showing irregular calcification. This results in the broadening and alteration in appearance which is seen grossly. In the more advanced cases the cellular reaction is even more abundant. Actual caries is seen with extensive plasma cell infiltration of the surrounding tissues and a productive fibrosis. The caseous necrosis which is present in this zone gives rise to the yellowish color of the tissues noted in the gross specimen. If, as a result of intensive antisyphilitic therapy the child lives, the exudate and necrotic debris may gradually be absorbed and replaced by a diffuse fibrosis. Regenerative efforts on the part of the bone and cartilage occur so that healing takes place. Even under such conditions, however, considerable disturbance in the growth of the long bones persists, resulting in various deformities.

ACQUIRED SYPHILIS.—In the acquired form of syphilitic infection of bone, either an actual gumma develops, or more commonly, a syphilitic infection of the periosteum of the long bones is encountered. Clinically, this is likely to be characterized by painful localized swelling, most often found on the anterior surface of the tibia, but at times involving the other long bones, especially the femur, humerus and ulna.

From the pathological standpoint, there is a chronic granulomatous lesion which lies immediately beneath the periosteum and extends to involve both the cortical bone through the haversian system, and the periosteum and surrounding soft tissues by direct extension. A variable degree of rarefaction of the bone occurs through an interference with the blood supply, both as a result of pressure of the exudate upon the vessels and by actual syphilitic involvement of the vessels themselves.

The lesion may become localized as a typical gumma with erosion of the surrounding tissues. This may even extend to involve the skin with the development of a deep, ragged ulcer, the base of which is made up of necrotic bone. On the other hand, the syphilitic lesion may go on to complete healing with the formation of dense bone and accompanied by marked thickening of the periosteum. In this respect, the proliferative reaction of the bone cells may be compared to the usual fibrogenetic stimulation of the spirochete in soft tissues. The essential difference depends solely upon the fact that the osteoblasts, as connective tissue derivatives, are stimulated to the production of their end product, bone.

In general, such instances of syphilitic osteitis or osteoperiostitis are very diffuse lesions which tend to involve the major portion of the shafts of the long bones. As has been already commented upon, in the earlier stage of the picture, considerable osteoporosis occurs as a result of the diffuse granulomatous reaction with relative avascularization of the tissues. Later, as the healing process goes on, new bone formation occurs with marked thickening of the cortex, which encroaches on the medullary canal as well as involving the periosteal surface. The development of this syphilitic involucrum by the periosteum is apt to be very irregular so that the surface of the bone is markedly roughened. Such tibial irregularities as seen at autopsy are more often luetic in nature than the result of any other cause, although it must be conceded that traumatic injury of the periosteum or other forms of periosteal infection may give rise to such irregular roughened surfaces.

This syphilitic involvement of the bone is by no means restricted to the long bones of the body but may also occur in the flat bones of the skull and not uncommonly in the bones of the nasal septum and the hard palate. In the skull, the process may be quite comparable to that seen in the tibia with the development of a similar thickened, irregular periosteal surface. In the nasal septum and hard palate, the lesion is much more likely to be in the nature of a localized gumma. This not infrequently goes on to actual perforation of the bone and results in the development of the typical saddle-back nose. Such a lesion is again one of the rather more frequently encountered bone manifestations of syphilis in its congenital form. Likewise, in congenital syphilis, involvement of the long bones may occur particularly again involving, as in acquired syphilis, the tibia. This results in such instances through the remarkable degree of productive osteitis which occurs in the condition, in an apparent anterior bowing of the bone as a result of the extensive thickening. This is described in the older texts as the typical "sabre shin" of syphilis.

THE OSTEODYSTROPHIES

Rickets.—Rickets is one of the deficiency diseases of infants caused by a lack of vitamin "D." This results in a defective ossification of bone, particularly involving the epiphyseal ends of the long bones at the line of growth. From the clinical pathological standpoint, there is a definite impairment of calcium and phosphorus metabolism with the normal ratio of these salts being seriously altered. The blood calcium is invariably reduced, but even more significant is the usual drop in the phosphorus, both of which elements are necessary for the development of normal ossification. As was discussed in the chapter on deficiency diseases, the source of vitamin "D," the controlling factor in the regulation of calcium metabolism in this respect has been emphasized and the part which ultraviolet light plays in activating the production of Ergosterol from the cholesterol of the body has likewise been shown.

From the standpoint of the bone pathology it may be said in general that there is a striking tendency for a lowered calcium content of the bones as a whole to occur. With such softening of the bones, many deformities are likely to follow, the most prominent of which are seen in (1) the familiar bowing of the legs, (2) deformities of the chest as a result of pulling of the softened ribs at the point of insertion of the diaphragm with the development of the so-called "chicken" or "pigeon" breast and the flaring of the lower part of the costal cage, (3) the presence of nodular thickenings at the costochondral junctions as the so-called "rachitic rosary," (4) widening of the long bones of the epiphyses with prominence of the ankles and wrists, and (5) actual curvatures of the spine.

The bone lesions, from the histologic standpoint, may be divided into two groups, the first representing those which are the result of the softening of the bones due to their diminished calcium content; and the second, those lesions which result from excessive osteoid tissue formation at the various centers of ossification, particularly at the epiphyseal ends of the long bones. In the first group, the various deformities which have been described should be included, although it is a mechanical factor of weight or tension which produces the actual clinical manifestations of this defective bone development. In the second group, the lesions are best studied in the epiphyseal ends of the long bones, including the costochondral junction.

If the epiphysis of such a long bone be studied carefully, it will be seen that instead of the sharply defined narrow line of ossification which should be present that the rachitic bone presents a wide, irregular band at that point. Frequently this is apparent not only in the long axis of the bone, but may be observed in the transverse axis as a result of excessive osteoid tissue production around the periphery of the epiphyseal line. Thus, there is marked widening of the joint surface as well as thickening of the epiphyseal line. If the child is of weight-bearing age, such flaring of the bone may become even further exaggerated from pressure. Grossly, the lesion presents a grayish, translucent appearance with occasional whitish opacities scattered throughout. These are gritty and represent areas of calcium deposit. The thickening of the epiphyseal line may reach as much as 1.5 cm. or more. This thickening is due primarily probably to the failure of calcium to be deposited in the newformed osteoid tissue rather than because of the excessive production of cartilage, although this point is not entirely settled.

Histologic examination reveals the epiphyseal cartilage to be invaded by numerous small blood vessels and to show considerable absorption as a result. The adjacent cartilage extends in long, tongue-like projections toward the medullary canal where it is undergoing slow conversion into osteoid tissue. This osteoid tissue shows markedly irregular calcification and true bone formation with subsequent ossification extremely poorly carried out. The irregular appearance of the epiphyseal line is due to this excessive osteoid tissue. Frequently whole islands of cartilage may be seen which are completely surrounded by such osteoid tissue. As the area of mature cancellous bone is approached the osteoid tissue assumes the normal trabecular appearance of bone, but still remains uncalcified.

Rickets is a self-limited disease which is rarely seen in its active stage beyond the second year of life. Thus, when healing eventually occurs, as it invariably does in these cases, the osteoid tissue becomes calcified and the bones assume a normal density, but the various deformities are likely to be permanent. The epiphyseal line tends to straighten out and lose its irregularity and ultimately may present a fairly normal line of ossification. Even the fusiform nodulation of the costochondral junction, the so-called "rachitic rosary," may gradually undergo absorption to a considerable extent. As the child grows, the bowing of the tibiae may become to a considerable degree reduced through the production of new bone and the development of new lines of stress. More serious, however, are the deformities of the pelvis, which not infrequently result from such rachitic conditions. These may lead to serious dystocia at the time of childbirth in the female.

Osteomalacia.—Osteomalacia is believed by many investigators to represent the adult counterpart of rickets. It is difficult to explain on the basis of vitamin deficiency in all instances, and it very possibly may have a endocrine factor, presumably parathyroid in nature as a concomitant etiologic agent. The condition is seen principally in females, and usually those who have given birth to a large number of children in relatively rapid succession. The process pathologically is one of generalized osseous decalcification with resultant softening of the bones. It is possible that such factors as the excessive draining of calcium from the bones through the course of repeated pregnancies in supplying the fetal requirements, inadequate nutrition on the part of the woman as is suggested by the fact that the majority of such cases occur in the lower income groups and accordingly, even actually the lack of vitamins in the diet should all be considered as significant in the development of such cases. In several instances of osteomalacia, the most extraordinary degree of deformities may be seen. The lower extremities may be almost of a rubberlike consistency and show extensive bowing. The pelvis may undergo similar extensive deformities. The vertebral bodies may become compressed with

alteration in the normal curvature, resulting in kyphosis, scoliosis and the like.

Histologically, the pathology is very comparable to that of rickets. There is a gradual resorption of the calcium of the bone and the normal bone trabeculae are replaced by osteoid tissue with only scattered areas of calcification. Often a diffuse fibrosis is present which may lead at times to some difficulty in differential diagnosis histologically from conditions such as osteitis fibrosa or osteitis deformans.

Osteogenesis Imperfecta (Fragilitas Ossium; Osteopsathyrosis).—This is one of those osteodystrophies which might well be included among the congenital lesions of bone as the condition usually is found either at birth or shortly after. Indeed, it may exist as an actual intrauterine condition, and the child may be born with bones which show multiple fractures in various stages of healing. Commonly, under such circumstances, the child is likely to be premature and at times stillborn. In some instances, multiple fractures occur at the time of delivery, even to the degree that death may follow from such injuries.

Nothing is known regarding the etiology of this curious condition in which the bones of the body generally are so brittle that they are predisposed to fracture through the most trivial trauma. Only one fact seems to be definitely established—that there is a tendency for the disease to be familial and to be transmitted to the offspring. The lesions are by no means restricted to the long bones of the body, but also involve the flat bones of the skull. These cranial bones are frequently thin and membranous in appearance with only small islands of calcification. The patients are likely to have a very striking appearance of their sclerae with a curious blue color, which is almost pathognomonic of the disease. Fortunately, the condition appears to be usually self-limited and gradually diminishes in degree as the patient increases in age. By adolescence, this tendency to what one might almost think of as spontaneous fracture has largely disappeared and rarely does it exist beyond the age of twenty-five. Unfortunately, however, about this time, in a considerable proportion of the cases, true otosclerosis with resultant deafness is likely to follow.

Pathologically, there is little that one can find microscopically to identify the condition. The diagnosis is perhaps more readily made by x-ray where the bones, particularly the long bones of the body show marked osteoporosis generally with extremely thin cortices and delicate, cancellous bone in the medullary portions. Bone regeneration and repair with the production of callus formation occurs rapidly and often with excessive callus production. X-ray

of such infants may show as many as twenty or thirty such fractures in various stages of healing.

Microscopically, the delicate bony trabeculae with a rather generous vascular supply in the haversian system are the only features which might lead one to suspect the underlying process.

ILLUSTRATIVE CASE

CASE 290. (Ref. #R.R.-31,809)

Diagnosis.—Hypopituitarism (Simmond's disease) combined with osteogenesis imperfecta.

Patient was a white female of 38 years, admitted to the hospital with the chief complaint of asthmatic attacks of nineteen years' duration.

Present Illness.—The patient's present illness represented an exacerbation of her asthma, being so marked in intensity that she was worried that she was not going to be able to get her breath at all. These attacks of asthma had increased in frequency and severity over a period of nearly twenty years. They had been accompanied by a moderate amount of expectoration. During this interval there had been a gradual but notable loss of weight, and this had been accompanied by a poor appetite and more recently by general weakness. The attacks had not been influenced by seasonal changes.

Past Medical History.—The patient was a full-term, normally delivered infant, the last of eight children, the mother being fifty years of age. She was breast fed for the first year of her life and had never had any nutritional disturbances until the onset of her asthma. She had had the usual childhood infections, she believed. A review of her systems proved to be of considerable significance and interest in respect to her present condition. She had not been unduly susceptible to upper respiratory infection, but because of her history of asthma and the possibility of focal infection playing a part in its origin, she had had her tonsils removed about fifteen years previously. Similarly, seven years before admission, she had had her teeth extracted with no improvement in her symptoms. As a child of twelve, she recalled that she had had some trouble with her hip joint and was hospitalized for several months. During the past eight years she had had a series of fractures involving her ribs, her right fourth toe, her left thigh and her left forearm, and recently her left femur. These had occurred at intervals without any significant causative trauma. She had had no symptoms relating to her urinary tract. Her menstrual history was of significance in that her menses did not begin until the age of eighteen and had always been scant, although regular for several years. She had had complete amenorrhea for the past nine years.

The patient's history in relation to her weight was likewise of significance. She had not grown in height since she was twelve years of age, measuring only fifty inches. At the age of twelve, she weighed approximately ninety pounds, which she maintained until some three or

four years before her present admission. During this latter interval she had steadily lost weight until at the time of admission she weighed only forty-seven pounds.

Physical Examination.—The patient was a small, emaciated, white female who appeared much older than her given age. Her skin was of a fine, delicate texture with transparent veins. The skin temperature over her entire body seemed markedly reduced. There was no disparity in the relationship of the extremities to the trunk. Head was of normal contour and had a good growth of fine textured hair. There was an absence of axillary hair and almost no pubic hair. Her eyes reacted normally to light and distance. Nose and throat were negative. She had compensated edentia. Thyroid was not palpable. The chest was symmetrical and showed equal expansion. The lungs were hyperresonant except for a slight suggestion of dullness in both bases. Moist râles were present at both bases likewise, and there were scattered sibilant and sonorous rhonchi throughout both lungs. Heart was not enlarged. Sounds were of fair quality. The rate was somewhat increased. There were no murmurs. Abdomen was flat. No masses or tenderness were felt. The genitalia appeared somewhat underdeveloped. The breasts were likewise small and atrophic. No masses or tenderness could be elicited.

Laboratory Findings.—Red blood cells, 4,480,000 with 11.5 gm. of hemoglobin. White blood cells, 9,350 with 77% neutrophiles, 14% lymphocytes, 2% eosinophiles and 4% monocytes. Urinalysis was negative on several occasions. Wassermann was negative. Blood chemistry, on admission, showed a calcium of 8.8 to 9.5 mgm. and a phosphorus of 1.7 to 3.3 mgm. Blood cholesterol was 128 mgm. Basal metabolic rate was plus-two per cent.

X-ray examination of the chest showed old chronic pleural thickening at both bases with obliteration of the costophrenic angles. There was a suggestion of bronchiectasis, but this could not be established without lipiodol instillation. X-ray examination of the skull showed no abnormality of the sella turcica. The long bones were unusually small and somewhat demineralized, but there was no evidence of cystic disease. The left femur showed evidence of an old neck fracture. Likewise an old healed fracture of the left tibia was observed.

Subsequent Course.—The patient was put on pituitary extract and showed moderate improvement over a period of eighteen months, with a gain in weight but no increase in height. The asthma, during this period, showed marked improvement under this form of therapy.

Osteitis Fibrosa (von Recklinghausen's Disease).—Osteitis fibrosa is a form of bone disease which may be either general or local in distribution. It is frequently associated with cystic degeneration of the

bone and in the general form at least is usually found in conjunction with definite evidence of hyperparathyroidism either as a diffuse primary hyperplasia of the gland or as a solitary adenoma. In the local form, which is usually found in children and young adults not much past the adolescent age, no such endocrine relationship can be definitely established. It is this local form which is often seen as the precursor of subsequent benign giant cell tumor formation in bone. The inherent similarity of the process in the diffuse and local forms leads one to the inevitable suspicion that a related fundamental etiologic agent must be at work, and it may well prove to be true that endocrine unbalance will ultimately be successfully demonstrated in the focal type.

GENERALIZED OSTEITIS FIBROSA.—Clinically, osteitis fibrosa is a disease of adults, chiefly between the ages of thirty-five and fifty-five, and occurring at least twice as frequently in the female as in the male. The first symptoms are usually those of pain in the bones, especially in the lumbar region, pelvis and legs. The condition is frequently accompanied by excessive thirst and polyuria, which lead to the suspicion of a beginning diabetes insipidus. At times, fracture of one of the long bones without adequate trauma may be the first incident to point toward the existence of the disease.

From the clinical pathological standpoint, a study of the blood chemistry shows a marked increase in the blood calcium which may range from twelve or fifteen milligrams up to as high as sixty milligrams per hundred cubic centimeters. The serum phosphorus, on the other hand, tends to be reduced to one or two milligrams. Simultaneously, there is a marked increase in the plasma phosphatase, which is credited with being an active bone producing enzyme. Urinalysis reveals a markedly increased calcium output, and because of the not infrequent renal calculus formation, hematuria may be a feature.

Pathologically, the disease is characterized by multiple areas of rarefaction of the bone with actual cyst formation at times. Not only is the decalcification of the bone restricted to local areas, but it becomes rather widespread with a definite softening. This results in marked deformity from the usual pressure factors. Bowing of the legs may become extreme. Shortening of the trunk through vertebral involvement is likewise often present. Longitudinal section of such a long bone reveals a medullary canal which is markedly increased in size relatively in respect to the cortex. Actual cystic degeneration may be present at times, these cystic areas being filled with a gelatinous or serous material. The bones, as

a whole are porous, and the cortices tend to be thinned. The haversian canals are enlarged and replaced by masses of fibrous tissue. This fibrous tissue is usually poorly vascularized and undergoes degeneration, which probably accounts for the cyst formation. Histologically, one may find evidence of irregular attempts at osteogenesis with numerous osteoblasts and the production of a soft, poorly calcified osteoid tissue. In other areas, actual osteoclasis is seen with many typical large multinucleated osteoclasts. The lesions are likely to be most marked in the upper end of the tibia, femur and shaft of the humerus. As a result of the osteoporosis, fracture is a common accompaniment of the condition clinically and is characterized by an excessive callus formation of a rather poorly formed osteoid tissue. As part of the picture, secondary extensive calcification of the blood vessels occurs. These may even be visible by x-ray. This arteriosclerotic process is most marked as a rule involving the vessels of the lungs and kidneys.

From the standpoint of etiology, the relationship of the parathyroids has been indicated. This has already been discussed in a preceding chapter relating to the various glandular dystrophies.

LOCAL OSTEITIS FIBROSA.—In children, before bone growth has become completed, focal areas of osteolysis usually at one or the other end of one or more of the long bones are seen. In a rather high percentage of such instances, the bone shows definite cystic degeneration which may be visualized by x-ray as multiloculated lesions central in position and tending to produce a rather uniformly fusiform dilatation of the bone with extreme thinning of the cortex. Here, as in the more diffuse form, spontaneous fracture is often the first evidence of the disease clinically. Many such cases go on to actual benign giant cell tumor formation.

From the clinical pathological standpoint, no alteration in serum calcium, phosphorus or phosphatase is found, and no demonstrable changes in the parathyroids ordinarily occur. This condition has been discussed already in Chapter XXV relating to tumors of bone.

Osteitis Deformans (Paget's Disease).—By Paget's disease is meant a condition which affects the skeletal system rather characteristically during the latter half of life. It is particularly prone to affect the skull and the long bones, although Schmorl found that actually the sacrum and vertebral column were more often involved than any of the other bones. Clinically, one of the earliest features of the disease is the increase in size of the head, which is frequently followed by an actual decrease in stature. As the disease progresses, more marked deformities occur with posterior angulation of the spine, flattening of the head of the femora and tibiae, and progressive enlargement of the skull with the bones of the face usually escaping except in that rare form known as *"leontiasis ossea."* In this latter condition which is generally believed to represent an unusual manifestation of the same general process, the bones of the face particularly are thickened, producing the characteristic lion-like facies. While in the more common variety the disease tends to be progressive, not infrequently, sooner or later, subsequent calcification of the bones occurs in the deformed position. The victim of this form of osteodystrophy presents an ape-like picture. The disease rarely goes on to a fatal outcome, except in those instances where osteogenic sarcoma develops, as it occasionally does.

Pathologically, the picture appears to be one of marked thickening and simultaneous softening of the various bones of the body. In the more marked instances, this softening is so extreme that the bones can actually be cut with a heavy knife. In spite of this extreme apparent decalcification of the skeleton, it is rare to find any appreciable alteration in the blood calcium or phosphorus. On the other hand, there is an extremely high blood phosphatase, which is usually even greater than that found in osteitis fibrosa. In the present state of our knowledge, it is impossible to definitely assign any parathyroid relationship to the condition, although one is sorely tempted to hypothecate such an underlying etiology in spite of the absence of demonstrable parathyroid hyperplasia or neoplasia. With our present limited knowledge regarding the mechanism controlling calcium metabolism in the absence of apparent hyperparathyroid activity or vitamin deficiency, speculation as to any possible cause for such a profound osteolysis becomes a very difficult problem.

Microscopically, the process appears to be one in which there is extensive absorption of normal bone, chiefly by osteoclastic activity although probably aided in part by absorption from increased vascularity. This is simultaneously accompanied by the deposition of enormous amounts of rather poorly formed new bone trabeculae. This new bone formation is found both subperiosteally and likewise within the medulla. This gives rise to the marked thickening of the bone. The line between the packed cortical bone and the loose cancellous bone of the medullary canal is completely lost, as is true also in respect to the membranous bones of the skull. This new formed bone is poorly calcified and extremely soft, which leads to the deformities mentioned in the preceding paragraph. The two processes going on hand in hand give rise to a curious mosaic pattern which in itself is diagnostic of the condition, both from the radiologic and from the histologic standpoints. Between these new-formed bony trabeculae, an enormous amount of rather loose connective tissue is laid down so that it may at times be difficult in a given section to differentiate this type of fibrous tissue proliferation from that seen in osteitis fibrosa. However, the myxomatous degeneration and cystic formation rarely occurs in osteitis deformans, and when it does, the cystic areas are almost microscopic in size.

ILLUSTRATIVE CASE

Case 291. (Ref. #S-410)
Diagnosis.—Bones—Paget's disease.
Patient was a fifty-four year old white male laborer admitted to the hospital as an accident case.
Present Illness.—The patient was engaged at his usual work of transporting heavy bales of waste paper on a hand truck. He caught his foot and fell backward down an elevator shaft about fifteen feet, landing on his back. He was knocked unconscious temporarily and was unable to get up by himself when he came to, and was sent immediately to the hospital.
Past Medical History.—His past medical history was entirely irrelevant. He had had the usual childhood diseases, including scarlet fever, which had left him stone-deaf from the age of six. A review of his systems was of considerable interest. He had not been unduly susceptible to upper respiratory infection. His cardiac history was negative. He had had very little gastro-intestinal disturbance. His genito-urinary history was negative. During the past year or more, however, he had noticed that he seemed to be losing stature and that his head was slowly increasing in size so that he had had to get a larger hat on two occasions. He had had no pain at any time relating to his head.
Physical Examination.—The patient was a well-developed and nourished middle-aged white male who was lying semistuporous in bed complaining at intervals of pain in his back. Head was somewhat disproportionate in size with a rather prominent forehead in respect to the size of his facies. His eyes reacted normally to light. There was no evidence of hemorrhage from his eyes, ears, nose or throat. He was totally deaf. Chest was

symmetrical. There was no evidence of rib fracture. Lungs were clear throughout. Heart was not enlarged and the sounds were of good quality. Abdomen: There was a moderate amount of distention. No tenderness or rigidity was present. The back showed a tender area over the lumbar spine. Pain was present also with pressure over the iliac crests. Extremities showed some bowing of his legs.

Laboratory Findings.—Red blood count showed 5,600,000 cells with 12 gm. of hemoglobin (71%). This was evidence of hemoconcentration as part of the picture of shock. White blood cells were elevated to 26,000 with 95% polynuclears. Urinalysis showed a slight trace of albumin, but was otherwise negative. Blood chemistry studies were subsequently made and showed no divergence from the normal. Wassermann was negative.

X-ray Examination.—X-ray examination of the pelvic region showed multiple fractures of the pelvis on the right side through the ischiopubic ramus and at the iliopectineal line. On the left side, there were three fractures of the innominate bone; one through the fovea centralis at the acetabulum. In relation to this latter fracture, there was a marked valgus deformity.

Osteopetrosis (Marble Bone; Congenital Osteosclerosis; Alber's-Schönberg Disease; Chalky Bones).—At the other end of the picture from osteogenesis imperfecta, which is characterized by osteoporosis, is found the comparatively rare condition in which increased density of the bones of the skeleton is encountered. This disease, of which less than one hundred cases have appeared in the literature as reviewed currently by Lamb and Jackson, is one largely of a familial and hereditary nature. It would seem, from what data is available, that this represents recessive genetic mendelian characteristics. The number of cases is about equal in males and females so that there is not a definite sex hereditary factor. Klemperer has suggested that the disease is an inherited one with a perversion of normal development of the undifferentiated mesenchyme, which results in an excessive growth of osteogenic tissue.

Pathologically, the bone changes may be summarized briefly as showing slight retardation of growth with expansion and clubbing of the ends of the long bones, and increased density arising in the diaphysis. A striking feature is the presence of alter-

In addition, there were compression fractures of the bodies of the first and fifth lumbar vertebrae giving a cuneiform appearance to the vertebral bodies. The pelvic bones showed a marked thickening and rarefaction with a curious mosaic pattern. On the strength of these preliminary studies a diagnosis of Paget's disease was made and supplementary x-ray examination of the skull and long bones was done, which confirmed the diagnosis.

Subsequent Course.—The patient developed a terminal hypostatic pneumonia and died ten days after admission.

Autopsy Findings.—At autopsy, the clinical diagnoses of Paget's disease and terminal hypostatic bronchopneumonia were confirmed. The most striking skeletal changes were those of the skull (Fig. 666), which showed marked thickening with a curious moth-eaten demineralization, as may be observed in the illustration.

Microscopic Description of Bone Section.—Histologic examination of the tissue shows it to be made up of trabeculae of poorly ossified bone, but showing considerable osteoblastic proliferation. There is diffuse fibrosis of the intervening areas with a rather inadequate vascular supply.

nating bands of increased and decreased density paralleling the epiphyseal lines and through which not infrequently spontaneous fracture occurs. In the head, the skull lesions are much more extensive and of greater importance than those of the base of the brain. Not infrequently the condition is accompanied by a hydrocephaly, and pressure upon the pituitary gland and optic chiasm are features worthy of comment. In addition to the immediate bone changes is the apparent involvement of the reticulo-endothelial system through obliteration of the marrow spaces and haversian canals by the increased bone production. There is usually an accompanying microcytic type of anemia which, it has been suggested, is a part of the disease affecting the undifferentiated mesenchyme rather than a reciprocal myelophthisic reaction.

From the clinical pathological standpoint, the blood chemistry studies have not been uniform in respect to the calcium content. There is a rather pronounced tendency, however, toward somewhat elevated levels with corresponding low phosphorus figures, not unlike the findings in hyperparathyroidism.

TUMORS OF BONE

For a discussion of the neoplasms of the osseous system the reader is referred to Chapter XXV in the section on Oncology where the more common tumors of bone are considered.

CHAPTER LXVI

DISEASES OF THE JOINTS

Perhaps even more important than the bones from the standpoint of function are those lesions which affect the joints, as serious disability is seen so frequently in conjunction with changes affecting the cartilaginous surfaces and serosal lining of the joints. It is obvious that because of position, these structures are particularly subject to trauma and injury of one sort or another. This is furthered to a significant degree by the fact that the blood supply to the joints is relatively poor. This may be of very definite importance in respect to the chronicity of many of the lesions which we find involving the organs of movement. The more important diseases of the joints may be placed in one of two groups: (1) those in which the process is apparently inflammatory in nature in which the condition is ordinarily termed "arthritis"; and (2) that group in which the degenerative changes are the more prominent pathologic feature, which are usually spoken of as "arthrosis." The inflammatory group is made up of a rather wide number of lesions ranging from traumatic injuries of the joint through the various infectious lesions, both suppura-

tive and nonsuppurative, up to chronic forms of joint inflammation including the chronic granulomatous diseases, such as tuberculosis. At times, such lesions may be minimal, apparently only involving the actual synovial membrane. At other times the process is more extensive and includes the articular cartilaginous tissues as well. These lesions, however, are relatively well defined and have an established etiologic background.

On the other hand, we have the so-called degenerative group of osteo-arthritis or osteo-arthrosis in which these lines of demarcation, of etiology and of pathology are by no means so well established, and in many instances seem to definitely overlap. They include conditions which are frequently spoken of as arthritis deformans, osteo-arthritis, osteo-arthrosis, Charcot joints and the like. It is in this group that so much confusion exists and in which so much further research is indicated in an effort to not only aid the patient materially, but to find some more fundamental factor by which these crippling lesions may be prevented.

ARTHRITIS

Acute Traumatic Arthritis.—Injury to the joint itself, or to its associated tendons, muscle or bones from trauma frequently results in acute inflammatory changes. As a rule, the process is chiefly restricted to the synovial membrane. From the clinical standpoint, the joint is swollen, painful, often reddened; and as a corollary, function is invariably impaired. The swelling is principally due to the accumulation of fluid within the joint cavity as a result of stimulation of the synovial membrane to pour out its normal secretion in excess to act as a buffer and prevent further injury. This may be classed with some of the major protective mechanisms of the body. To a lesser degree, the swelling is due to an actual edema of the synovial membranes themselves.

The fluid, as obtained from such a joint, is usually serous in nature, although in some instances it may appear serosanguineous. The cell count of the fluid

ordinarily establishes the non-infectious nature of the process, as the total cell count, according to Collins, usually averages about four hundred cells per cubic millimeter, of which only twenty per cent are polymorphonuclears. This compares to normal synovial fluid which contains anywhere from ten to two hundred white cells per cubic millimeter, of which ninety to ninety-five per cent are ordinarily large mononuclears. If the fluid is not examined immediately, just as in the case of spinal fluid there is rapid autolysis of the cells so that fluids which have been reported from autopsy cases usually show much lower figures.

Acute Infectious Arthritis.—Acute infectious arthritis may occur in both suppurative and nonsuppurative forms dependent upon the etiologic factor. Thus, if the lesion is caused by one of the pyogenic bacteria, we will find a definite suppurative process. On the other hand, if the infection is

PLATE CLIX
DISEASES OF THE JOINTS

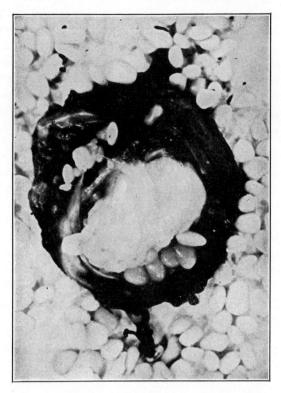

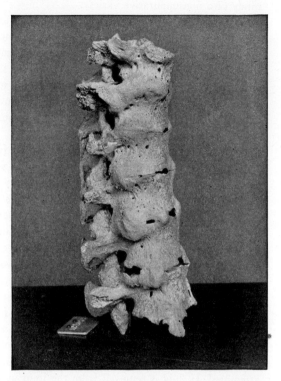

Fig. 671.—Knee Joint: Synovial Fringe—Rheumatoid Arthritis.—Cf. Case 293.—Gross photograph showing numerous pedunculated tabs made up of edematous fibrous and fatty tissue. Some of these have become detached within the joint cavity as so-called "joint mice."

Fig. 672.—Vertebra: Spondylitis Deformans.—Cf. Case 294.—Gross photograph showing the ankylosis of the vertebra due to ossification of the spinal ligaments and intervertebral discs producing the so-called "poker spine."

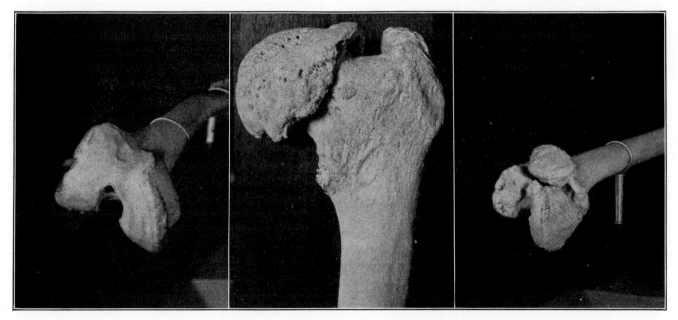

Fig. 673.—Femur: Rheumatoid Arthritis. —Cf. Case 293.—Gross photograph in which the uneven and eroded articular surface is seen resulting from inflammatory changes and subsequent fibrous ankylosis of the joint.

Fig. 674.—Femur: Rheumatoid Arthritis.— Cf. Case 293.—Gross photograph showing the head of the femur with the inflammatory changes which resulted in roughening of the articular surface. Note involvement along the intertrochanteric line.

Fig. 675.—Femur: Degenerative Osteo-Arthritis.—Cf. Case 294.—The articular surface is considerably increased as the result of proliferative changes within the joint membranes and subsequent irregular ossification or calcification.

associated with rheumatic fever, the lesion is definitely of a nonsuppurative variety.

ACUTE SUPPURATIVE ARTHRITIS.—Suppurative arthritis ordinarily results from infection by one of the pyogenic bacteria, particularly streptococci, staphylococci or pneumococci. The *Gonococcus* likewise may produce such a suppurative arthritis with frank pus within the joint cavity, but more often the exudate in this infection is curiously of a serofibrinous type at the outset.

These organisms may be brought to the joint from without as in the case of traumatic injuries with perforating wounds. A suppurative process may extend from adjacent structures such as occurs occasionally in association with osteomyelitis. However, in the greater number of cases the organism is brought to the joint by way of the blood stream in the course of a septicemia, particularly in association with subacute bacterial endocarditis, puerperal sepsis, broncho- or lobar pneumonias, otitis media, meningococcemia, and more rarely in typhoid fever and acute bacillary dysentery. Clinically, in such cases, the infected joint becomes markedly swollen, reddened and painful, particularly when motion is attempted. If fluid is removed from the joint at successive intervals during the development of the inflammatory process, it will be observed that it is serous in appearance early in the course of the disease, but rapidly becomes purulent in nature.

Pathologically, the process begins as an inflammation of the synovial membrane which becomes swollen and infiltrated by many cells, the great majority of which are polymorphonuclear leukocytes. The inflammation extends to the articular cartilages, which not infrequently become softened and eroded. The lining cells of the synovial membrane become desquamated. The actual bone itself may become exposed through destruction of the cartilage and a suppurative osteitis result. Rupture of the capsule may occur in some instances with diffusion of the infection into the soft tissues around the joint and even result in extension to the skin surface with the development of a sinus tract. In some cases the infection may clear up spontaneously by sterilization of the infected joint cavity through cellular activity. Under such circumstances, healing will take place and result in varying degrees of disability dependent upon the amount of destruction of the joint. If only slight erosion of the cartilaginous surface and syn-

ovial membrane has occurred, then fibrous adhesions may be the extent of the permanent injury. Such adhesions will produce some limitation of motion spoken of as *false ankylosis*. On the other hand, if the cartilages have been eroded and the bone itself involved, the healing process will result in the development of true bony ankylosis through osteoblastic activity and the laying down of dense osseous trabeculae.

Gonorrheal Arthritis.—Gonorrheal arthritis usually occurs in the early weeks of the infection following acute urethritis or cervicitis. The earliest manifestations are often seen in several joints simultaneously, but as the disease advances, it seems to localize to a single joint. The joints affected in their order of frequency are the knee, wrist, elbow, shoulder, hip and ankle. Clinically, gonorrheal arthritis is accompanied by fever, moderate leukocytosis, swelling and reddening, and extreme tenderness both on the slightest motion and upon palpation.

Pathologically, the swelling of the joint is due both to an increase in the amount of fluid within the joint cavity and to actual swelling of the synovial membrane. The exudate in this instance is serofibrinous in nature at the outset, but like other forms of suppurative arthritis, it rapidly becomes purulent. The polymorphonuclear exudate almost invariably extends to infiltrate the periarticular structures, and fluid removed from the joint cavity by aspiration usually contains the organism in pure culture. The lesion is very apt to be extensive in nature with marked erosion of the cartilaginous surface of the two opposing bones of the joint. In healing, as a result, true ankylosis very frequently takes place. At best, extensive fibrous adhesions occur with marked limitation of motion.

RHEUMATIC (NON-SUPPURATIVE) ARTHRITIS.— One of the most significant clinical features of acute rheumatic fever is the polyarticular arthritis which is seen during the course of the disease. This is particularly true in those cases which occur for the first time in late childhood or early adult life. In young children the joints frequently escape, and tonsillitis, chorea and early endocardial involvement are more likely to occur.

The arthritic process in rheumatic fever is in the nature of an acute, non-suppurative lesion, which is largely restricted to the synovial membrane. Clinically, the disease is apt to be polyarticular with several joints being attacked successively, the inflammatory process apparently migrating from one area to another, one joint subsiding from its acute manifestations while the process is developing in the new location. The joints most frequently affected in their order of frequency are the knee, ankle, shoulder, wrist, elbow, hip, hand and foot. The affected joint becomes considerably swollen due to effusion into the joint, as well as to the presence of inflammatory edema within the synovial membrane and periarticular structures. It is extremely painful upon motion. It is feverish on palpation and shows some reddening. If the joint is tapped, the fluid will usually appear to be slightly turbid. The cell count is moderately increased. According to McEwen, it ranges from eight hundred to forty-seven thousand per cubic millimeter, varying considerably depending upon the stage and severity of the process. Polymorphonuclear leukocytes predominate early while later there is a gradual transition to large phagocytic mononuclear cells. Keefer, Myers and Holmes, in studying the fluid from a series of cases, report that the higher the count, the greater the relative number of polymorphonuclears. According to these latter observers, the fluid from such joint cavities was invariably sterile.

Pathologically, the process is usually confined to the periarticular and subsynovial tissues, in which typical Aschoff bodies are often found. There is an accompanying inflammatory edema and a moderate mononuclear cellular infiltration. As a rule, the inflammatory process subsides without any involvement of the articular cartilage itself. Thus, in healing, ankylosis is not a usual complication. Some impairment of function with stiffness of the joint occurs at times as a result of thickening of the periarticular structures by fibrosis. This is especially true in those cases in which rheumatic nodules can be demonstrated, which may be taken as an indication of a rather more severe reaction.

Chronic Infectious Arthritis.—Just as in the case of other infectious processes elsewhere in the body, so may the joint cavities become involved in a true chronic infectious reaction, which is usually associated with one of the granulomatous infectious agents, of which tuberculosis is the only really important member.

TUBERCULOUS ARTHRITIS.—Tuberculous arthritis as a clinical condition, apart from tuberculosis of bone, is a very rare lesion. It is said that instances of simon-pure joint infection do exist in adults. Under such circumstances the infection is obviously hematogenous in origin and represents an infection of the synovial membrane with extension of the inflammatory process to the joint cavity. The great majority of cases of tuberculous arthritis, however, are the result of tuberculous epiphysitis with extension of the tuberculous process from the bone through erosion of the overlying articular cartilage into the joint cavity. Even in those cases in which the infection appears to be limited to the joint at the outset, many observers are inclined to believe that the initial infection was actually a minimal and unrecognized epiphyseal infection. This is a difficult problem to prove conclusively one way or the other as in such instances it is not at all uncommon for the lesion to have extended through the articular cartilage to involve the underlying bone, and how anyone can say with assurance which was the primary focus of infection appears highly debatable.

The problem of tuberculosis of bone and its extension to the joint cavities was discussed in the preceding chapter and so will not be reviewed at this time.

SYPHILITIC ARTHRITIS.—Just as in tuberculosis, involvement of the joints may occur in syphilis, both in the congenital and acquired forms of the disease. The pathological picture is one of a nonsuppurative, chronic synovitis in which the joint cavity becomes somewhat distended with serous fluid. Not infrequently the condition is polyarticular. The process is not uncommonly confused with early tuberculosis, but as in the bone involvement, the productive inflammatory changes are more marked in contradistinction to tuberculosis.

Gout (Gouty Arthritis).—Gout is a disease, the etiology of which is entirely obscure. It is seen most commonly in plethoric males in the older age groups. It is found particularly among the heavy meat-eaters and for that reason has generally been held to have a metabolic basis. This, however, is extremely difficult to establish. It seems to be dependent to a large extent upon some constitutional diathesis, and there appears likewise to be an hereditary factor involved although spontaneous cases of gout are seen in which this hereditary background is apparently lacking. Clinically, the disease is characterized by marked painful swelling of one or more joints, most commonly the metatarsal phalangeal joint of the great toe. The condition shows periods of remission and relapse with acute exacerbations during which the patient suffers extreme pain upon the slightest pressure upon, or motion of, the affected joint.

Pathologically, the lesion is seen to consist of the precipitation of sodium biurate crystals within the articular cartilage, the joint capsule, the surrounding ligaments and the synovial membrane. This is accompanied by a serous synovitis with the accumulation of a clear fluid within the joint. The result of this increased pressure and the biurate precipitation, which apparently interferes to some extent with the blood supply of the joint, is often accompanied or followed by varying degrees of necrosis of the articular cartilaginous structures. The lesion is ordinarily restricted to the cartilage, the actual bony epiphysis escaping entirely. Examination of fluid aspirated from the joint after the process is well developed reveals the presence of similar biurate crystals within the fluid.

As the disease progresses, the accumulation of these crystals leads to the formation of nodular bodies or *tophi*. These are composed of sodium biurate crystals around which a varying degree of necrosis of the tissues has occurred which in turn is accompanied by a secondary inflammatory reaction. Occasionally, calcification of such lesions occurs with the deposition of calcium carbonate and phosphate in the tophi. This is probably the result of the secondary degenerative necrotic tissue changes. For some totally unexplained reason, similar gouty tophi are also commonly found in the eyelids, the lobes of the ear, and not infrequently in the tissues of the nose. No conception of the underlying mechanism involved in this curious process exists, although it has been shown in some cases that the deposition of these salts is more prone to occur during a period in which the blood uric acid content is high.

ILLUSTRATIVE CASE

CASE 292. (Ref. #S-411)
Diagnosis.—Tophus—gout.

Patient was a white male 45 years of age admitted to the hospital because of severe pain in his right foot.

Present Illness.—The present illness dated back to a period about three years previously when the patient had his first attack of acute joint pain in his right foot. This involved the metatarsal phalangeal joint and was characterized by swelling, redness and exquisite tenderness. No other joints seemed to be involved at the time. The patient was treated by his physician as a case of acute arthritis and the inflammatory process subsided. Since his initial attack, he had had four other similar acute episodes, each becoming progressively more severe in character. During the past several months the patient had noted lumps which were forming in the subcutaneous tissues of the lobes of his ears and at the angle of his nose. These were not painful. His present attack of arthritis was much more severe than any of the previous ones and he came to the hospital to have a thorough study made in the hope of relieving the situation permanently.

Past Medical History.—His past history was not particularly enlightening in respect to his present condition. The patient had had a normal childhood with the usual contagious diseases. He had never had any serious illness that he could recall. He was rather subject to mild upper respiratory infections. His cardiovascular system had never given him any symptoms. He had always had a very hearty appetite and had been particularly fond of rare meat. His genito-urinary history was negative. He denied venereal disease.

Physical Examination.—The patient was a well-developed, somewhat florid middle-aged white male. Head was normal in contour. Scalp showed marked thinning of his hair which was gray. Eyes reacted normally to light and distance. Ears had several rather characteristic tophi present in both lobes. Similar tophi were noted around the nose at the angle of the alae. Mouth and throat were negative. Chest was symmetrical. Lungs were clear throughout. Heart was not enlarged. There were no murmurs heard. Abdomen was negative. External genitalia were negative. Extremities: Upper extremities were negative. The left lower extremity was normal. There was an acute swelling of the right foot over the metatarsal phalangeal area. This was reddened and felt definitely hot on palpation. It was exquisitely tender.

Laboratory Findings.—Red blood count on admission showed 4,300,000 cells with 87% hemoglobin. White blood cells numbered 12,600 with 78% polynuclears. Routine urinalysis was negative. Wassermann was negative. There was a negative complement fixation test for gonorrhea. Blood chemistry gave the following figures: sugar 128 mgm., urea nitrogen 16 mgm., nonprotein nitrogen 38 mgm. and uric acid 5.6 mgm.

X-ray examination of the foot showed a moderate demineralization of the bony structures in the vicinity of the lesion. There was marked swelling of the soft parts. A few flecks of calcium could be seen within the joint cavity suggesting some pathological calcification.

Subsequent Course.—On the basis of the history, the characteristic localization of the arthritic process, the presence of tophi in the subcutaneous tissues of the face and a high uric acid in the blood, the diagnosis of gout was made. The patient was treated locally for the acute flare-up of his joint symptoms and was put on a restricted diet on his discharge.

Biopsy material was obtained for confirmation of the diagnosis and fluid likewise was removed from the joint cavity by aspiration. This was found to contain sodium biurate crystals.

Pathological Report.—*Gross Description of Biopsy Specimen.*—Specimen consisted of a small mass of material removed from the subcutaneous tissues. This was soft in consistency and was chalk-like in appearance. Smears from this material showed the presence of typical sodium biurate crystals.

Microscopic Description of the Tissue.—(Fig. 679) Histologic study of the tissue surrounding the periphery of the tophus presents a chronic inflammatory picture. Considerable increased connective tissue and a marked mononuclear cellular infiltration consisting principally of lymphocytes and large mononuclear phagocytes are present. Many foreign body giant cells are seen, some of which appear to contain crystalline material.

ARTHROSIS
(Chronic Arthritis; Arthritis Deformans; Osteo-arthritis; Osteo-arthrosis)

Arthritis deformans is a generic term applied to a variety of lesions affecting the joints, which are chronic in nature and lead to marked deformity and disability of the involved part. Great difficulty has been encountered in the classification of this group of diseases since the pathology varies considerably. The subject has been further confused by the failure of the investigators in this field to adopt a uniform classification. However, it would appear that the various types described fall into two major groups, as suggested by Baker, Nicholls, Richardson and others: (1) *Rheumatoid arthritis,* a condition in which the process resembles a chronic infection, the end result of which may be a fibrous or bony ankylosis and in which the process is essentially an inflammatory one involving the synovial membrane and associated cartilaginous structures; and (2) *Osteoarthritis,* a type which seems to be purely degenerative in nature without evidence of inflammation and which terminates in marked deformity of the joint without ankylosis. Impairment of motion, however, may be brought about by the production of bony excrescences about the joint. A brief description of the more important features of each follows.

Rheumatoid Arthritis (Proliferative Arthritis Deformans; Chronic Progressive Polyarthritis).—This disease is characterized by inflammatory changes in the synovial membrane and periarticular tissues together with the presence of varying amounts of fluid within the joint cavity. The disease may be ushered in with fever and pain in the joints, although in many instances the onset may be gradual and insidious. As a rule the process is polyarticular, the joints of the hands and feet being usually affected in association with the process in one or more of the larger joints, such as the knee and shoulder. The hip joint is rarely affected. Women are more commonly afflicted than men. In a series of five hundred cases reported by Garrod, about eighty per cent were found to occur in women. The age incidence appears to lie chiefly between the third and fifth decades. Only twenty-five per cent of Garrod's series were below twenty years of age.

Subcutaneous Nodule.—The presence of one or more subcutaneous nodules adjacent to the affected joint occurs in a small number of cases. These are usually described as enlarged lymph nodes. These nodules were found in seven per cent of the series of cases reported by Collins. Figures as high as twenty-nine and one-half per cent have been recorded by Clawson and Weatherby.

These nodular lesions vary considerably in size ranging from one-half to three centimeters in diameter. They are hard, painless and freely movable in the subcutaneous tissues. They occur principally over bony eminences. Collins suggests that their occurrence in such locations may indicate a traumatic or pressure factor in their development. Probably the most common location is along the subcutaneous border of the ulna two centimeters from the olecranon. The nodules may persist for many years.

Negative results have been obtained on aerobic and anaerobic culture of these nodes by Collins, Dawson, Olmsted and Boots. On the other hand, Clawson and Weatherby claim to have isolated a Streptococcus in twelve out of seventeen cases. In many respects, these nodules resemble those found in rheumatic fever.

Pathology.—The subcutaneous nodule of rheumatoid arthritis is made up of several foci of circumscribed aggregations of cells and fibrous tissue which may fuse to form one conglomerate lesion. In this respect it resembles the subcutaneous nodule of rheumatic fever, which consists of Aschoff bodies. Histologically the individual lesion of rheumatoid arthritis is characterized by a central area of necrotic fibrous tissue around which is a corona of closely packed mononuclear cells. These consist principally of fibroblasts and a few large cells containing prominent, pale-staining nuclei with a delicate reticulum of chromatin together with a few lymphocytes, some of them of the "owl eye" type. Palisading of the cells of the corona is common so that the fibrillae of the fibroblasts intermingle as they approach the central area of necrosis. Dawson and Klinge have now shown the presence of a silver-staining reticulum present around the edge of the necrotic material, the strands of which are continuous with the protoplasmic fibrillae of these marginal connective tissue cells. The outermost portion of the nodule is made up of more mature fibrous tissue. As the rheumatoid lesion develops, this adult type of connective tissue becomes more and more predominant until eventually the entire lesion appears to consist of mature connective tissue with considerable collagen. The central portion of the node shows no evidence of vascularization, the vessels being confined to the outermost portion of the lesion. These arterioles frequently show obliterative endarteritis, particularly in old lesions.

ETIOLOGY.—Although this nodule closely resembles that of true rheumatic fever, according to Collins, the primary picture is one of proliferation of fibroblasts with secondary necrosis of these newly formed cells, whereas it will be remembered that in the case of the Aschoff body the pathology is primarily that of hyaline necrosis of mature collagen derived from the organ affected and followed by secondary cellular infiltration to form the Aschoff body. The similarity of the lesions, however, is noteworthy and the possibility of identical etiology of the two diseases cannot be ignored. The etiology of rheumatic arthritis is still unknown.

Various predisposing factors show great variation in reported cases. In view of the associated clinical findings, together with the pathological picture, the process would seem to be one of chronic infection. Many attempts have been made to culture a specific organism from the synovial fluid. The results have mostly been negative. Some investigators, however, have reported positive findings. Cecil, Nicholls and Stainsby claim to have obtained a typical strain of Streptococcus from the joint fluid of rheumatoid arthritis. Blair and Hallman demonstrated a variety of organisms from the synovial fluid in cases of arthritis, but attached no particular etiological significance to them. Forkner, Shands and Poston reported Streptococcus viridans in eleven out of sixty-three fluids. In spite of the generally negative and otherwise conflicting evidence respecting the Streptococcus as the offender in rheumatoid arthritis, there is still a tendency to regard this organism as the most probable etiological factor, the process possibly being brought about as a result of the presence of only a very small number of organisms, or through the absorption of bacterial toxin from some focus of infection such as the teeth, tonsils, gallbladder and the like. The possibility of rheumatic fever and rheumatoid arthritis having a common etiology and representing merely a variation in the allergic expression of the tissues to the action of a similar agent is a theory which bears further investigation, particularly in view of the similarity of the histopathology of the subcutaneous nodules.

The affected joints are swollen, and on palpation are soft and doughy in consistency. X-ray examination reveals no evidence of osseous nodules about the joint and the bones in general seem somewhat rarefied. The process apparently begins within the synovial membrane within the cartilage. As a result of inflammation, the lining synovia becomes covered by a layer of vascularized granulation tissue. This gradually spreads over the articular surfaces thus forming a covering or *pannus*. In addition to the fibroblastic proliferation, an exudate composed chiefly of lymphocytes and plasma cells may be seen within the synovial membrane. This is further complicated by marked edema. These changes extend to involve the periarticular structures and joint capsule.

The synovial fluid is increased and the total cell count is elevated with a predominance of polymorphonuclear leukocytes which may reach as high a figure as eighty per cent. If the process subsides at this stage, fibrous adhesions will be formed between the two granulating surfaces giving rise to fibrous ankylosis which somewhat limits the joint function to some extent. Fibrous thickening of the capsule and periarticular structures further tends to limit motion in the joint.

In other cases, the cartilage becomes softened and necrotic with resultant exposure of the epiphysis. The degree of erosion in different parts of the cartilage varies. In many cases the articular cartilage may be completely separated from the epiphysis as a result of a layer of vascularized connective tissue which forms within the marrow of the bone and proceeds to grow between the bone and cartilage. Thus, it will be seen that the erosive action and damage to the cartilage takes place from both the joint and bone sides. As the result of healing of such severe lesions, again the ankylosis may be only fibrous in nature, or may result in actual bony union.

ILLUSTRATIVE CASE

CASE 293 (Ref. #R.R.38,291).

Diagnosis. —Rheumatoid arthritis.

Patient was a white female of 60 years who was admitted to the hospital because of joint pain of about one year's duration.

Present Illness.—The onset of the patient's present illness dated back approximately one year at which time she first noticed pain in the left foot. She thought this was due to faulty shoes and bought herself a pair of the so-called orthopedic type. This did not relieve the condition, and indeed it extended to involve the left ankle, which showed a moderate amount of swelling, tenderness and limitation of motion. Within a comparatively few weeks she noticed involvement of both ankles, knees, shoulders, hands, wrists and even her neck. The symptoms were migratory in nature and showed definite periods of exacerbation and relative remission. She consulted a physician, who recommended the use of vaccines. She received such injections over a period of six months, but did not feel that they helped her materially. On a high intake of salicylates she showed the more marked improvement subjectively. During practically the entire year she had had to remain at home almost bedridden, except for the brief periods of remission. During the preceding two months she had been receiving physiotherapy and massage. This had seemed to give her more relief than any other form of treatment, but by no means was entirely successful in overcoming her pain and disability. Her immediate hospitalization was the result of increased symptoms pointing toward her neck, in which she had extremely limited motion for the preceding four or five weeks.

Past Medical History.—Her past medical history was apparently not particularly significant in relation to her present arthritic picture. She remembered that she had had measles as a child but did not think she had had any other acute infection. She was sure she had never had rheumatic fever. She had had her tonsils removed, however, at the age of thirty because of repeated sore throats. She had likewise had a hysterectomy at the age of thirty-two for profuse menorrhagia and metrorrhagia. There was no family history of any rheumatoid condition so far as she was aware. A review of her systems was essentially non-informatory. Her gastro-intestinal history showed a poor appetite, moderate constipation, and she believed she had lost several pounds during the preceding year. Her genito-urinary history was negative.

Still's Disease (Rheumatoid Arthritis; Arthritis Deformans of Children).—A rapid fulminating variety of rheumatoid arthritis occurs not infrequently in children and occasionally in adults. In addition to the articular manifestations, there is marked enlargement of the spleen and lymph nodes. The onset is sudden, usually ushered in by chills and fever. The joint symptoms are characterized by stiffness of one or more joints which gradually become swollen. The process begins in the synovial membrane and spreads to the ligaments, joint capsule and other periarticular structures. The synovial membrane becomes thick-

Physical Examination.—The patient was a fairly well-developed and nourished, elderly appearing white female. She held her head and neck in a markedly rigid position with her head drawn somewhat forward and down on her chest. Eyes reacted normally to light and accomodation. Ears were negative. Nose and throat were apparently normal. Examination of her neck showed no enlargement of her thyroid. There was apparent rigidity of her neck, but when this was tested definitely against measured resistance, there was no actual limitation of motion. Chest was symmetrical. Lungs were clear. Heart was not enlarged. There were no murmurs. Blood pressure was 160/76. The peripheral vessels showed very little sclerosis. Abdomen was moderately protuberant. There was an old midline scar below the umbilicus. No masses or tenderness were elicited. Extremities: There was a fusiform swelling of the joints of the fingers and toes. There was swelling of both wrists and ankles with considerable tenderness over the left ankle. There was marked limitation of motion of the joints of the hands, wrists, feet, ankles, knees and shoulders. This was accompanied by considerable secondary muscular atrophy through disuse (Cf. Fig. 677).

Laboratory Findings.—The blood count on admission showed 3,680,000 red cells with 10 grams (63%) hemoglobin and the white blood cells numbered 6,800 with 60% polynuclears, 29% lymphocytes, 9% monocytes and 2% eosinophiles. Urinalysis was essentially negative except for occasional very slight traces of albumin. Blood chemistry showed a blood sugar of 120 milligrams and a urea Nitrogen of 9 milligrams. The blood sedimentation rate showed a slight increase above normal. Bacteriologic studies showed no significant numbers of streptococci from the nose and throat.

X-ray examination showed an early picture of progressive atrophic rheumatoid arthritis. Films of all the joints showed relatively little change other than a demineralization. There was some deformity of the metacarpal phalangeal joints of both hands. Some hypertrophic bony fringes were seen in the case of the cervical spine, wrists and ankles (Cf. Figs. 673 and 674).

Subsequent Course.—The patient was continued on an intensive program of salicylates, physiotherapy and nonspecific vaccine therapy with no significant improvement except for transitory periods of remission of her symptoms. The pain and disability referable to the cervical spine has persisted and appears to be progressive.

ened, roughened and covered by a layer of granulation tissue. This is frequently redundant and forms villus-like processes which extend into the joint cavity. The reaction may involve the articular surface of the cartilage as well, but extensive erosion is usually not present. Upon healing, fibrous adhesions and thickening of the joint capsule and periarticular structures may lead to considerable dysfunction. Bony ankylosis is exceptionally rare. Not uncommonly, these villus-like processes may become pinched off and act as foreign bodies within the joint cavity. These are sometimes spoken of as "joint mice."

Degenerative Osteo-arthritis (Osteo-arthrosis; Degenerative Arthritis Deformans).—In this form of chronic arthritis, the onset of the disease is usually insidious. There is a lack of the acute manifestations so commonly seen in the rheumatoid type. Fever and leukocytosis are not present, nor is there any other evidence of infection.

The disease is one rarely seen until late middle life and is particularly encountered in the older age group. It is much more commonly seen in males than females. In the majority of cases, the process is polyarticular, although a mono-articular form involving the hip joint is not infrequently encountered. Gradual deformity of the joint occurs with the production of bony nodules (Heberden's nodes), which are almost regularly found. The process does not result in ankylosis, although the function may be impaired due to these bony excrescences which are typically formed about the joint. These are best seen in the joints of the fingers and toes, the nodules producing the familiar "gnarled knuckles" so often seen in elderly individuals.

The pathological picture is one of a degenerative nature which apparently first involves the articular cartilage rather than the synovial membrane. As a result of this degenerative change, the major portion of the articular cartilage becomes eroded and extension of the degenerative process to the actual bone may follow. There is no tendency toward the formation of granulation tissue as in the rheumatoid variety of arthritis. Therefore, fibrous or bony ankylosis does not usually occur. There is, however, proliferation of the cartilage along the edge of the joint with subsequent ossification, which tends to enlarge the articular surface and gives rise to the bony excrescences which are so characteristic a feature of osteo-arthritis.

When the joint is opened in the early stages of the disease, the cartilage is seen to be roughened and resembles plush or velvet. This degenerative cartilage is so soft that it is apparently worn away by pressure. This erosion is unequal, being more marked and occurring earlier centrally than around the periphery. This is explained on the basis of a more abundant blood supply to the peripheral area. In time the central portion of the cartilage becomes entirely eroded and the underlying bone acts as the joint surface, the two opposing bony surfaces coming in contact with one another. The degenerative erosion continues to affect this new bony articular surface, which likewise tends to wear away unequally. Thus, in ball and socket joints such as the hip joint, one side of the head of the femur is commonly much more markedly involved than the other. As a result, dislocation is a common complication of the disease.

There is little tendency toward repair of the bone. The worn surface may appear rather coarsely trabeculated. In other instances, the uneven wear of the bone may lead to the formation of parallel grooves, the harder portions of the bone becoming ebonated and acquiring a high polish. The cartilage which persists around the edges of the joint tends to proliferate. It is due to the ossification of this proliferated cartilage that the bony nodules previously described are created.

The synovial membrane tends to become redundant and shows fringes of edematous tabs of fatty, fibrous tissue. Some of these develop cartilage. Occasionally, calcification of these tabs may occur. One or more of these may become detached as a loose foreign body within the joint cavity. These, as in rheumatoid arthritic cases, are spoken of as "joint mice."

The joint fluid differs strikingly from the rheumatoid variety in that the cell count is very much lower and the percentage of polymorphonuclears rarely exceeds ten to fifteen per cent.

Etiologically, the process appears to be caused by nutritional changes as a result of a deficient blood supply to the joint. This is evidenced by extensive atherosclerosis of the vessels.

ILLUSTRATIVE CASE

CASE 294 (Ref. #R.R.31,022)
Diagnosis. — Degenerative Osteo-arthritis (Osteoarthrosis; degenerative arthritis deformans).

Patient was a white male of 66 years, admitted to the hospital because of severe pain in the region of his right loin of three weeks' duration.

Present Illness.—The onset of the patient's present illness dated back approximately twelve years at which time he had his first attack of arthritis involving his knees, hips and lower back region. These attacks of joint involvement became increasingly frequent as time went on and were associated in many instances with marked disability and limitation of motion. The immediate cause of the patient's hospitalization was the fact that he had developed severe pain in the right loin, which had been increasing in severity during the three weeks preceding admission. This radiated down his side toward the symphysis. The pain had been constantly present but had been aggravated by motion, particularly stooping.

Past Medical History.—In general, the patient disclaimed any previous illness of significance. He remembered no childhood diseases. He believed he had typhoid fever as a young man, but he had always considered himself unusually healthy until the onset of his arthritic condition. In attempting to review his systems, no additional data of significance was obtained. He definitely denied venereal disease. He had never had any operations or accidents. During the past few years he has had to wear glasses for reading and had developed a certain amount of bilateral deafness. He had had all his teeth extracted in an attempt to relieve his arthritis and had two artificial dentures. During the last few years he had had moderate nocturia, but no other renal symptoms.

Physical Examination.—Patient was a moderately obese, elderly, white male who appeared more than his given age. He was lying on his side in bed complaining of pain. Head was essentially negative. His hair was gray and thin. Pupils reacted normally. Mouth was edentulous. Nose and throat were negative. Ears were negative. Chest was somewhat emphysematous in appearance and on percussion and auscultation was generally hyperresonant. Heart was slightly enlarged to the left. Sounds were normal. There were no murmurs. Blood pressure was 154/90. Abdomen was obese. No organs were palpable. There was bilateral costovertebral tenderness. Extremities: The peripheral vessels showed marked arteriosclerosis. There was considerable prominence of the ends of the femora and tibiae. There was some apparent limitation of motion of both the knees and the hips.

Laboratory Findings.—On admission, the patient had a red blood count of 4,380,000 cells with 14 grams of hemoglobin. White blood cells 6,200 with 57% neutrophiles, 32% lmyphocytes, 10% monocytes and 1% basophiles. Urinalysis was negative. Wassermann was negative.

X-ray examination: There was a marked fringe formation about the bodies of the lumbar spine due to trophostatic osteoarthrosis. Similar changes were seen involving the femora and tibiae with broadening of the articular surfaces (Fig. 675).

Subsequent Course.—It was felt that nothing definite could be done to improve this patient's condition other than the usual prescribed forms of physiotherapy. He was not a suitable case for hospitalization in a general acute service and was accordingly discharged to a convalescent home where he might receive continued care, together with suitable physiotherapy.

Spondylitis Deformans.—The deforming type of polyarthritis involving the joints of the spine is a kind of osteo-arthritis in which the spine may become rigid due to the ossification around the joint. The condition may be seen in association with a similar degenerative process affecting the other joints of the body, or it may occur independently. Two varieties have been described: (1) Von Bechterew's type; and (2) the Strumpell-Marie type. In the former, the process is confined to the joints of the spine and is associated with symptoms of extreme pain from pressure on the nerve roots. In the Strumpell-Marie variety the spondylitis deformans is usually accompanied by joint involvement usually of the hip and shoulders, and in this disease the nerve root symptoms are not prominent.

The process in both types, like that described in the joints affecting the long bones, is characterized by degenerative and hyperplastic changes. Ossification of the spinal ligaments, and in extreme instances actual bony ankylosis of the vertebrae occur. The earliest changes appear to be in the form of ossification of the anterior spinal ligaments, with less marked ossification of the entire vertebral tissues. In extreme cases, the intervertebral disks undergo degeneration comparable to the articular erosion seen at the ends of the long bones. This is eventually followed by ankylosis of the vertebral bodies so that the spine becomes absolutely rigid and is often spoken of as the "poker spine." The ossification of these structures tends to produce an anterior curvature of the spine, thus throwing the head forward upon the chest. The costovertebral joints may also be involved with fixation of the ribs and resultant abdominal breathing.

Etiologically, the disease appears to be both degenerative and inflammatory in nature, unlike the lesions which are seen in the typical osteo-arthrosis of the long bone joints. It is particularly prone to occur in males in the sixth and seventh decades, especially in those who have done heavy manual labor. Thus, trauma may play a part in the etiology, although this is difficult to prove. Certain of the proliferative changes which are found simulate the inflammatory reactions seen in rheumatoid arthritis and thus point toward a possible infectious origin. Apparently, normally, a certain degree of calcification and ossification of the anterior spinous ligaments is manifest in many individuals with the advance of years. Many of these cases present no symptoms, but on x-ray examination such calcification or ossification may become apparent. Such individuals show no evidence of osteo-arthritis of any of the other joints of the body.

THE CHONDRODYSTROPHIES

Chrondrodysplasia Fetalis.—Of the two recognized forms of disturbance of cartilaginous development, the fetal or hereditary chrondysplasia is the less common. It represents a complex disturbance of bone formation which is usually apparent at the time of birth. It is more frequently seen in males than females. It is characterized by irregular failure of the bones to grow normally through some retardation factor and by the complicating presence of multiple enchondromatous nodular cartilaginous overgrowths. These areas, which usually are seen in relation to the periosteum, frequently subsequently become ossified and tend to produce marked bony deformities. The condition appears to be self-limited and usually stops at a time when bone growth is completed, leaving a wide variety of deformities.

Achondroplasia.—Both the congenital chondrodysplasia and achondroplasia might well be included in the discussion of the congenital anomalies of the skeletal system representing as they do lesions which are usually present at birth or are progressive with skeletal growth. The condition appears to be congenital, likewise hereditary in nature, and to have a definite familial background. The great majority of the so-called "dwarfs" seen in the usual circus sideshow are individuals afflicted with this disease. In this instance the defect in skeletal development consists of a curious failure of the cartilage of the long bones to grow. As a result the individual grows up with a normal sized head and trunk and with short, stunted arms and legs. Similar defects in the bones of the hands and feet are seen with resultant short, broad hands and feet. As a rule, another deformity which is noted is a saddle type of nose due to failure of the base of the skull to develop normally.

Pathologically, the diagnosis of the chondrodystrophies, particularly this type of achondroplasia, might well be suspected on microscopic examination of the cartilaginous line of the epiphysis. The cells here present a wild disorder with marked variation in their size and shape and a tendency toward macrocytosis. No mitoses, however, are in evidence. Little or no suggestion of osteogenesis is found either as adult bone or as osteoid tissue. The microscopic picture is almost one of neoplasia as compared to normal orderly cartilaginous growth.

The other various forms of dwarfism have been discussed in some detail in the chapter on ductless glands, notably those forms associated with pituitary dysfunction. Whether or not some such endocrine basis for the chondrodystrophies may be established is still problematical.

Hypertrophic Pulmonary Arthropathy (Marie-Bamberger Disease).—This condition is manifested by symmetrical enlargement of the bones of the extremities, particularly the distal phalanges of the fingers and toes. Clubbing of the fingers or Hippocratic fingers may be considered a manifestation of this disease. Such clubbing of the fingers and toes may occur alone or in conjunction with a similar process in the other long bones. From the clinical standpoint, there is a marked bulbous swelling of the digits accompanied by curvature of the nails, both in the lateral and in the antero-posterior planes.

Pathologically, this enlargement is usually due to thickening of the soft tissues, particularly of the connective tissue of the corium. This presents an almost myxedematous picture. As the process goes on, actual bone involvement with thickening of the phalanges occurs as the result of proliferation of the periosteum and subsequent new bone formation.

Etiologically, the syndrome is usually associated with chronic pulmonary disease either alone or accompanied by cardiac pathology. It may accordingly be encountered in long standing chronic pyogenic infections of the lung, such as abscess, bronchiectasis or empyema. Less often, it is seen in association with chronic fibroid phthisis. In instances of congenital heart disease where the pulmonary valve particularly is involved, similar changes may occur. The pathology is apparently dependent very largely upon anoxemia of the tissues, although it may well be supplemented by chronic absorption of various bacterial toxins. In a case recently reported by Konzelmann, a very striking thickening of the peripheral arterioles was observed, suggesting a possible vascular factor in the mechanism of development of this condition.

CHAPTER LXVII

DISEASES OF THE MUSCLES

The pathological processes which relate to the skeletal musculature are among the most difficult to classify because so little is known regarding the etiology of the majority of such lesions. It is impractical to attempt to group these disturbances of muscle in the usual way based on congenital inflammatory and neoplastic criteria, except in a very broad manner. Actually there are very few lesions which primarily affect the muscles and the great majority of such disturbances are secondary. In this text, accordingly, the various lesions will be discussed more particularly from the standpoint of functional disturbance. The most important type of disturbance which occurs is seen in relation to the various forms of atrophy, the great majority of which are recognized clinically as distinct entities. In general, it will be said that atrophy is characterized by a diminution in size of the individual muscle fibers with corresponding decrease in their functional capacity. The muscle cells tend to become narrower with apparent condensation of their striations. If the process be extreme, eventually the major portion of the muscle fiber will disappear leaving only the sarcolemma with persistent groups of muscle nuclei arranged in cord-like fashion along the almost collapsed sheath. Ultimately, even these structures disappear and the muscle becomes replaced by connective scar tissue. Grossly, as one sees such muscles at operation, or in the autopsy room, they present a variable picture. In the early stages of such atrophy, they appear soft and flabby and tend to be darker than normal in color. Gradually, as the muscle fibers become replaced by connective tissue, they assume a grayish color.

The causes of muscular atrophy are many and varied. In those cases in which a definite etiology has been established, the lesion is spoken of as *secondary atrophy*. This group of cases is particularly associated with disturbances of the central nervous system, such as anterior poliomyelitis and amyotrophic lateral sclerosis. If, on the other hand, the atrophy results from some unestablished etiologic factor, but appears as a primary pathological process in muscle, then the atrophy is spoken of as *primary*.

SECONDARY MUSCULAR ATROPHIES

Simple Atrophy from Disuse.—Muscular atrophy may result from disuse alone. If a muscle or muscle group is inactivated for any reason, and is accordingly unable to function, there follows progressive wasting. Such atrophy may be accentuated by pressure in the case of fracture of a bone, where the extremity is immobilized therapeutically to permit healing of the bone. The corresponding muscle groups show a variable amount of atrophy which is dependent upon both disuse and pressure. The amount of atrophy which follows is to a very large extent dependent upon the time factor and is not necessarily permanent when function is resumed.

Such disuse atrophy is in part nutritional in character because where a muscle is immobilized and inactive, the circulation is likely to be stagnant and actual degenerative changes may not infrequently be demonstrated in such muscles.

Atrophy of the muscles surrounding a joint which has undergone ankylosis or which is the seat of some inflammatory process is a frequent finding. The atrophy in such a case is due not only to the factor of disuse, but again probably in part to degenerative changes resulting from the action of toxins either directly upon the muscle or indirectly through its nerve supply.

Senile Atrophy.—As part of the generalized picture of senility, atrophy of the muscles is frequently seen in the aged. This is evidenced both by a decrease in size of the muscle and by a diminished functional capacity. Such atrophy is comparable to the senile or brown atrophy of the viscera, which has already been described and is due very largely to a decrease in nutrition as a result of impaired circulation, together with a decrease in the functional demands.

PLATE CLX
DISEASES OF JOINTS AND MUSCLES

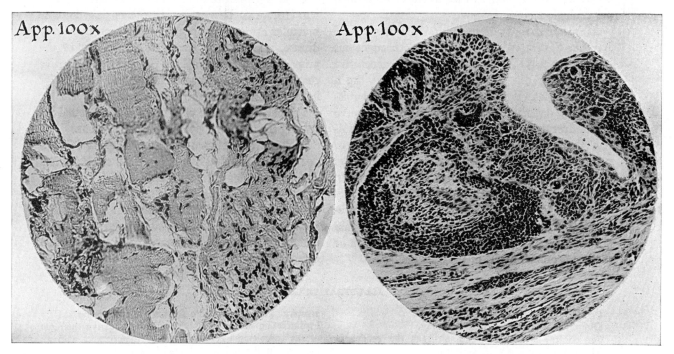

FIG. 676.—MUSCLE: ATROPHY, POLIOMYELITIS.—See CASE 68.— Low power photomicrograph from deltoid muscle showing degeneration and atrophy of muscles with subsequent fibrous replacement. App. 100 x.

FIG. 677.—KNEE JOINT: CHRONIC RHEUMATOID SYNOVITIS.—Cf. CASE 293.—Inflammatory changes consisting of edema, mononuclear cellular infiltration, together with proliferative fibrosis beneath the synovia and extending into the deeper layers, characterize the histologic picture. App. 100 x.

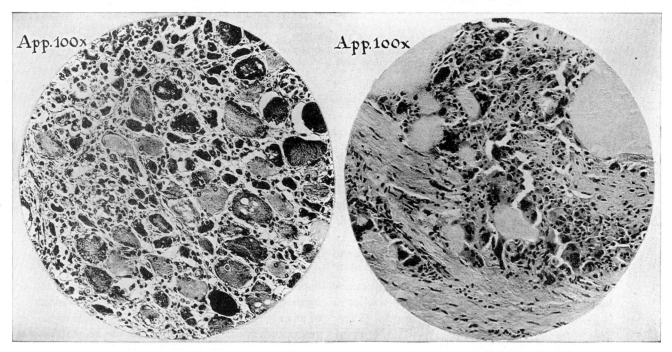

FIG. 678.—MUSCLE: ACUTE MYOSITIS, NON-SUPPURATIVE.—Observe marked interstitial edema and chronic mononuclear cellular infiltration, also the atrophy, necrosis and degenerative changes of the muscle fibers. App. 100 x.

FIG. 679.—TOPHUS: GOUT.—CASE 292.—Photomicrograph showing marked chronic inflammatory reaction characterized by extensive fibrosis, mononuclear cellular infiltration, and giant cell formation, many of which contain crystalline material (sodium biurate). App. 100 x.

Thus, we have a relative disuse as one of the principal etiologic factors.

Muscular Atrophy Secondary to Pathology of the Nervous System.—As has already been brought out in Chapter LXIV, in discussing the degenerative lesions of the central nervous system, there are a number of pathological processes which are characterized by degeneration or destruction of the nerve cells. Muscular atrophy is particularly prone to follow those conditions in which the lower motor neuron is involved. Thus, the most striking changes are seen in such conditions as *anterior poliomyelitis, Landry's paralysis* and the various stages of *amyotrophic lateral sclerosis,* including the simpler progressive muscular atrophic form and the late progressive bulbar paralysis with the degeneration of the motor cranial nuclei of the medulla.

FAMILIAL SPINAL MUSCULAR ATROPHY (WERDNIG-HOFFMAN DISEASE).—In this curious form of muscular atrophy we are dealing with an hereditary disease, which rather closely resembles one of the primary muscular dystrophies. However, degenerative changes have been demonstrated both in the anterior horn cells and in the peripheral nerves to account for the secondary atrophic changes which are found involving the muscles supplied by these neurons.

PROGRESSIVE NEUROMUSCULAR ATROPHY (CHARCOT-MARIE-TOOTH DISEASE).—This condition is a similar muscular atrophy which is also hereditary in nature and begins early in childhood. It differs from the familial spinal type in that it is usually localized and results in the development of acquired clubfoot. Here again, a primary cord lesion has been demonstrated.

ILLUSTRATIVE CASE

CASE 68 (Ref. #S-413)

Diagnosis.—Striated muscle—atrophy.

For clinical history and case abstract, the reader is referred to Chapter XVIII, Case 68.

Microscopic Description of a Section Through the Deltoid Muscle.—(Fig. 676) Histologic study of the musculature from this late case of anterior poliomyelitis reveals a very striking degeneration and atrophy of the individual muscle fibers. Here and there in sections from the deltoid, one may observe muscle fibers which appear essentially normal or even hypertrophic as a compensatory effort on their part to take over the function of the atrophic cells. The great majority of the muscle fibers, however, show varying degrees of degeneration and atrophy. The degenerative features are characterized by hyalinization of the cytoplasm and by abortive attempts of the sarcolemma cells to undergo hyperplasia with an increase in the number of nuclei at times. The process in this particular instance has gone on so long that most of the acute degenerative changes, fatty and hydropic, have largely disappeared. Many of the muscle fibers cannot be identified other than by their sarcolemma sheaths. All gradations of size representing the various stages of atrophy of the cells may be observed among the other fibers. There is a replacement interstitial fibrosis which is likewise rather striking. There is very little evidence of any inflammatory change although a few mononuclear cells may be found in the stroma.

PRIMARY MUSCULAR ATROPHIES

(Primary Myopathies and Muscular Dystrophies)

As was stated in the introductory comment regarding atrophy in general, there is a group of cases in which the muscular weakness and atrophy seems to be the result of a primary atrophy of the muscle itself and without evidence of any etiologic basis other than the fact that these diseases are prone to occur in childhood and seem to have an hereditary or familial predisposition. A brief discussion regarding the more common and better clinically established varieties of these various conditions follows.

Pseudohypertrophic Muscular Dystrophy (Pseudohypertrophic Muscle Paralysis).—This form of muscular dystrophy is definitely hereditary in nature and restricted apparently to male children, although it is, like hemophilia, transmitted through the female members of the family to their male offspring. From the clinical standpoint, the usual story is that the calf muscles show progressive and disproportionate enlargement. However, this is not associated with increase of functional power and indeed is sooner or later followed by definitely decreased function. The process is not restricted to the gastrocnemius and soleus muscles, but also commonly involves the extensors of the thigh. Accompanying this apparent hypertrophy, there is a definite atrophy or wasting of other muscles, very commonly the opposing muscle groups such as the flexors of the knee and thigh. The muscles of the upper extremity are also not infrequently involved with pseudohypertrophy of some and corresponding atrophy of others, notably the muscles of the shoulder girdle. As the disease progresses, the pseudohypertrophied muscles likewise tend to become smaller in size so that in the end stage of the process, the patient shows marked atrophic changes in various muscle groups. At times, the disease may develop without the initial pseudohypertrophic stage, and the atrophic picture predominates throughout its course. Two clinical variations of the condition are commonly recognized (a) *the Landouzy-Dejerine type* in which the primary changes are seen in the muscles of the face with subsequent involvement of those in relation to the scapula and humerus. This is usually referred to as the *facioscapulohumeral type*. Clinically, because of the involvement of the shoulder girdle muscles, there is marked prominence of the scapulae and wasting of the arm muscles. This variety more commonly begins in childhood but occasionally does not occur until adult life; and (b) *the Layden-Moebius and Simmerlin type* in which form of the disease the process almost invariably begins with the muscles of the lower extremity, especially the extensor groups. It is the more common variety and is frequently spoken of as the *thigh muscle type*.

Pathologically, in pseudohypertrophic muscular dystrophy, if biopsy examination of the muscle tissue be made histologically at varying intervals during the course of the disease, a rather characteristic sequence of events can be demonstrated. Early in the disease it will be found that the muscle fibers are essentially normal in their histologic appearance. The increase in size of the muscle as a whole is apparently due to extensive fatty infiltration between the muscle bundles. As the disease progresses the muscle fibers become narrowed and atrophic in appearance, but do not show any appreciable loss of striation until late. Various retrogressive changes may occur with fatty and hyaline degeneration of the cytoplasm of the cells. Accompanying this degenerative and atrophic picture there is a considerable increase in the fibrous stroma between the muscle bundles. In the end stage when gross atrophy of the muscle is apparent, the muscle fibers may be replaced very largely by fibrous tissue and those fibers which persist are likely to show marked atrophy, fatty degeneration and loss of their striae.

Congenital Myotonia (Thomsen's Disease).— This, like most of the other muscular dystrophies, is an hereditary condition which particularly affects male children. Clinically the disease is first evidenced by stiffness of various of the muscles of one or more of the extremities at the time that voluntary muscular movement is attempted. Rather characteristically, the child, when he attempts to walk, moves slowly with obvious deliberation. This is apparently the result of a delayed contractility and is followed by a similar prolonged period of relaxation. After several contractions of the muscle, the normal function is seemingly restored, but the process recurs after even a brief period of rest. The affected muscles appear larger than normal, but their functional capacity, however, is certainly no greater than average and as a rule is rather diminished.

Histologically, studies of the muscle from such cases show an initial hypertrophy in the size of the fibers, particularly as seen in the transverse axis. In addition, rather marked fatty and hyaline degenerative changes are usually present. Not infrequently there is an increase of muscle cell nuclei as compared to the normal. The condition is not infrequently accompanied by somewhat delayed mental development as well.

The disease is extremely uncommon in the United States, and the majority of cases have been reported from northern Europe. Such geographical distribution of any disease always makes the problem of etiology more difficult. Thus far, nothing specific has been suggested as a positive causative factor other than hereditary developmental defects.

Atrophic Myotonia.—This form of myopathy corresponds rather closely to the congenital myotonia of childhood, differing chiefly in the fact that it usually first appears in the adult group between twenty and thirty years of age. Like the other forms of muscular pathology, the condition is seen much more frequently in males than females.

Clinically, the process is characterized by a similar delay in muscular contraction and relaxation as observed in the congenital form. Typically, it is further characterized by a slow, progressive atrophy of the involved muscles. The process most frequently affects the muscles of the face, neck and muscles of the shoulder girdle, although it may also involve the muscles of the forearm and even of the leg, as reported by Duncan, Margulis and Yung.

Histologically, the muscle fibers show marked atrophy accompanied by considerable degeneration of the cytoplasm of the cells and a diffuse interstitial fibrosis. The atrophic changes usually dominate the histologic picture.

Congenital Amyotonia (Oppenheim's Disease).—
In this condition, which is congenital in nature and
usually present at birth, the pathological picture is
characterized by a curious muscle weakness in which
actual atrophic changes are not particularly prominent. The muscles of the extremity are the most
frequently affected. Only rarely do the muscles of
the face become involved.

The etiology is obscure as in the other forms of
muscular dystrophy. Forbes, Wolf and others have
described central nervous cord changes, particularly
a reduction in the number of motor neurons of the
anterior horn. In these cases, the muscle cells appear generally small and embryonic in type. The
muscle cells vary considerably in size and in many
instances show imperfect development of their striations. In the majority of reported cases, no demonstrable lesions of the spinal cord or peripheral nerves
have been found, so that whether this condition
should be thought of as a secondary atrophy in respect to developmental defects of the nerve cells of
the anterior horn, or whether it should be considered
as a primary myopathy is problematical. In some of
the reported cases, marked variation in the size of
the muscle cells has been found, some of them being apparently actually hypertrophic and showing
an increase in the number of nuclei. Not infrequently there is an increase of connective tissue between the muscle fibers, and a variable amount of
fat infiltration in the supportive stroma is likewise
found on occasion.

Myasthenia Gravis.—This is again one of those
mysterious conditions which are frequently claimed
by the neurologists as being of nervous origin.
Pathologically the lesion would seem to be primarily
one affecting the musculature. Unlike most of the
other myopathies, both males and females are affected, the condition being most commonly seen in
middle age in males, but before the age of twenty-
five in females.

Clinically, the picture is characterized by an extraordinary degree of muscle fatigability upon the
slightest effort. This requires a very considerable
rest period to bring about recovery to the point
where contraction can again occur. Muscular
atrophy, from the gross and clinical standpoints, may
or may not exist to a recognizable degree. The disturbance is more particularly one of function than
necessarily of anatomical change, although very commonly as a result of the disturbed function, atrophy
follows.

From the microscopic standpoint, the muscles may
show very little pathologically. In certain cases there
are seen collections of lymphocytes, which occur
within the muscle bundles. This is spoken of as *lym-
phorrhagia*. With this cellular reaction there is
usually present a demonstrable atrophy of the muscle
fibers and not infrequently rather striking pigmentation.

From the etiologic standpoint again, little positive
information exists. In some cases a persistent or
hyperplastic thymus has been demonstrated, and in
several of the reported cases an actual thymic tumor
was present. McCrae has suggested that the disturbance might be one affecting the myoneural junction
with the liberation of acetylcholine, thus interfering
with the activity of the nerve impulse. According to
Gibson, Martin and Buell, there is at times a definite
reduction in the blood sugar level and a diminution in the glucose tolerance suggesting the possibility of some endocrine factor associated with the
condition etiologically.

HYPERTROPHY

True hypertrophy, that is, an increase in the size
and functional power of a muscle or muscle group,
is the most common response to repeated increased
demand for work. It probably should be considered
a perfectly normal and physiological process, the degree depending upon and limited by an adequate
blood supply. The muscles of the trained athlete are
examples of such true hypertrophy. In a previous
chapter the hypertrophy resulting from increased
work placed upon the heart has been described. In
either case, the muscle fibers are enlarged in size
and possibly, in number.

Among the examples of hypertrophy, it used to
be customary to place such conditions as pseudo-
muscular hypertrophy, and congenital myotonia
(Thomsen's disease) because it was assumed that
there was an actual hypertrophy of the muscle
fibers because of the increase in size of the muscle as
a whole. However, with the possible exception of
certain cases of Thomsen's disease, no pathological
hypertrophy of muscle actually occurs. Thus the
various muscular dystrophies have been discussed
under a previous section in this chapter, relating to
atrophy.

RETROGRESSIVE PROCESSES

The various forms of degeneration, which have been discussed in the first three chapters of the book, including fatty, hydropic, granular and hyaline changes may occur in voluntary striated muscle just as they do in myocardium and in the various viscera. The changes are similar in nature and are seen particularly in association with general toxemias and septicemias, or in connection with inflammation of the muscle or adjacent structures.

Histologically, the muscles first lose their transverse striations and tend to be granular and swollen, the process being accentuated in patchy areas throughout the muscle. If the process is severe, tiny fat globules may appear within the muscle cell. In some instances the degenerative change produces a hyaline or vitreous appearance, in which the muscle fibers histologically become refractile and take the eosin stain intensely.

Zenker's Degeneration (*Hyaline Necrosis*).—In certain severe toxemias and bacteremias, particularly in severe typhoid fever, and sometimes in influenza and lobar pneumonia, the voluntary muscles undergo a hyaline degeneration and necrosis frequently accompanied by hemorrhage. It is most commonly found in the recti muscles of the abdomen. This process has already been described in Chapter III on retrograde processes. Such a muscle appears pale, semitranslucent and somewhat resembles fish flesh. Hemorrhagic areas stand out in marked contrast. Histologically, the normal striations are lost, and patchy areas of hyaline necrosis are seen in which the muscle fiber is swollen with interruption or fragmentation of the cytoplasmic elements (Fig. 24). The sarcolemma, in these cases, is usually intact, and if the patient recovers, regeneration may take place without marked scarring.

For an illustrative history, the reader is referred to Case 12 (Ref. #S-213) in Chapter III.

CIRCULATORY CHANGES

So far as circulatory changes are concerned in relation to the muscles, the most important lesions are seen in relation to thrombosis and embolism. However, hyperemia may occur in association with increased activity of a muscle and likewise in the early stages of inflammation. Chronic congestion of a muscle is seen accompanying thrombotic lesions of the veins, as part of the picture of generalized venous congestion such as occurs in thrombophlebitis involving the vessels of an extremity.

Thrombosis, Infarction, Necrosis and Gangrene. —As a result of thrombosis, infarction of muscle tissue may occur with resultant necrosis or gangrene provided the collateral circulation is not adequate. As part of the picture associated with the various forms of gangrene of the extremities, the muscles supplied by the involved vessels likewise undergo necrosis together with the adjacent subcutaneous and deeper structures. If the obstruction is not complete and if the collateral circulation is maintained to a partial degree, there may result a variable amount of atrophy. Such atrophy, as has already been commented upon, is grouped with the secondary forms of atrophy. If the arterial supply is cut off by embolism or thrombosis, actual *coagulation necrosis* of muscle may occur. *Liquefaction necrosis,* although rarely beginning in muscle is seen at times in association with the extension of some suppurative process from adjacent tissue. Similarly, *caseation necrosis* as a result of tuberculous involvement of muscle tissue is uncommon as a primary process, but follows at times from extension of the tuberculous lesion in adjacent tissues, particularly in relation to tuberculosis of bone. The characteristic psoas abscess is the most familiar example of this type of lesion.

Congenital Wryneck (*Torticollis*).—By congenital torticollis is meant a process which usually results from the shortening of the sternocleidomastoid muscle pulling the head to one side. At times, the trapezius may also be involved. The contracture is often not noticeable until the child is three or four years old, at which time the neck tends to grow in length and thus makes the shortening of these muscles more apparent.

In such cases, frequently a history may be obtained of a swelling on one side of the neck, which takes place shortly after birth. This is rather firm on palpation and often somewhat sausage shaped. This swelling persists for a variable time, but usually disappears before the end of the first year. Examination of the muscles and tissues of the neck at this time presents evidence of hemorrhage into the muscle associated with considerable laceration. In the later stages, histologic examination shows the muscle tissue to be replaced to a very great extent by fibrous tissue.

From the standpoint of etiology, several theories have been advanced to explain the development of the lesion, among which the following seem most pertinent:

(1). Excessive traction on the neck muscles during childbirth is believed to result in laceration of the sternocleidomastoid muscle, which subsequently undergoes cicatrization;

(2). Intra-uterine trauma as the result of malposition of the fetus in utero through interference with the arterial blood supply of the muscle has been suggested as a possible cause; and

(3). Prolonged labor with excessive venous dilatation and resultant thrombosis is believed by Middleton to lead to the degeneration of the muscle with subsequent atrophy and fibrosis.

In summary, it is generally believed that either direct trauma or degenerative changes associated with interference with the blood supply of the muscle through malposition or prolonged labor are the important factors in the production of this disabling lesion.

Volkmann's Contracture.—This condition is one in which the venous circulation of the muscle is interfered with as the result of the prolonged use of a tourniquet or pressure of an improperly applied splint. Again, venous thrombosis is the apparent significant factor in the development of the lesion. The muscles at the outset appear firm, swollen and tender. As time goes on they undergo secondary atrophy and fibrosis with resultant contracture of the cicatrix. This lesion is ordinarily found in relation to the upper extremity. Etiologically the process is very similar to that seen in congenital torticollis. Occasionally compound fractures with hemorrhage into the antecubital fossa may exert sufficient pressure upon the tissues to compress the veins and lead to interference with the return venous circulation of the part.

MYOSITIS

Primary inflammatory changes of the muscle are relatively rare. However, acute suppurative or non-suppurative instances of myositis do occasionally occur. The great majority of these result from the extension of an inflammatory process in adjacent tissues.

Acute Suppurative Myositis.—As part of the picture of a generalized septicemia, particularly in infections by the staphylococcus, focal metastatic abscesses may occur in the muscle. Occasionally in severe cases of typhoid fever, in addition to the more usual Zenker's hyaline necrosis, actual infection of the muscle with abscess formation may also be found. In general, however, the acute suppurative forms of myositis are the result of extension of some suppurative process of the subcutaneous tissues or adjacent structures. The usual features of such inflammation may be demonstrated under these circumstances. The muscle fibers show marked fatty, granular and hyaline changes and may eventually undergo liquefaction necrosis.

GAS GANGRENE.—As a rather special type of myositis should be mentioned the gangrene which occurs as a result of infection of the muscle by one or another of the anaerobic gas-producing bacteria, the most frequently encountered of which is the Welch bacillus. This has already been discussed in the section devoted to necrosis and gangrene, from the standpoint of general pathology, but is reviewed briefly at this point because of the frequency with which the muscles are involved in such infections. The process is usually associated with deep wounds in which considerable destruction of tissue has taken place and which have been contaminated with soil or street dirt containing the spores of one of the anaerobic gas-producing bacilli. As a result of the breaking down of carbohydrates within the tissue, gas is formed by the saccharolytic members of the group to produce the tissue crepitus, which is so characteristic clinically. Other anaerobic saprophytes which possess a proteolytic enzyme bring about the lysis of the tissue. Thus, the destructive process spreads rapidly. Grossly the muscles are at first pale and soft and have a typical putrefactive odor. The necrotic tissue later becomes dark reddish brown in color with the breakdown of the myoglobin. Small gas bubbles are encountered on sectioning such muscles.

Microscopic examination reveals extensive necrosis with autolysis of the muscle fibers, the presence of typical large gram-positive bacilli and vacuoles representing the gas bubbles noted grossly. A variable amount of inflammatory cellular infiltration is seen with polymorphonuclear leukocytes predominating.

Acute Nonsuppurative Myositis (Acute Poliomyositis).—There exists a curious form of non-suppurative inflammation of the muscles, the origin of which is undetermined. The process usually involves a considerable number of the skeletal muscles. Clinically, the disease is ushered in by a rise in temperature and painful localized enlargement of the muscles. In the more severe cases, death may follow with involvement of the respiratory group of muscles.

Histologically, a marked inflammatory edema is observed in the interstitial tissues between the muscle fibers. This is accompanied by a round cell exudate in which lymphocytes predominate. The muscle fibers themselves show varying degrees of degenera-tion with patchy areas of fatty, granular and hydropic changes.

DERMATOMYOSITIS.—By dermatomyositis is implied a pathological process which is very similar to that of the simple nonsuppurative poliomyositis, but is accompanied by degenerative and inflammatory changes in the subcutaneous tissue and an associated dermatitis. The condition is not confined to any age group.

Clinically it, like poliomyositis, is ushered in by an acute febrile attack with painful swelling of the muscles which subsequently become firm and inelastic. The process tends to improve spontaneously after an interval of a week or more, but repeated recurrence is the rule. Ultimately a variable degree of muscular atrophy follows. The most common skin lesion seen in association with this picture is a rather marked erythema, but occasionally urticaria is likewise present. Rarely, other skin lesions have been described.

MYOSITIS OSSIFICANS

Unfortunately the term myositis ossificans is used to apply to two totally different conditions which bear no relationship to one another other than the fact that ossification of muscle occurs. In the one instance the disease is a localized lesion dependent upon trauma. In the other, it is a progressive generalized process which ultimately ends fatally.

Local Myositis Ossificans.—The most familiar form of this local type of ossification in muscle is seen in the abductor muscles of the thigh where it is known as "riders' bone." This is believed due to repeated trauma to this muscle with degenerative changes and subsequent fibrosis and ossification. Similar lesions are found in the shoulder muscles, particularly of soldiers, again presumably the result of traumatic injury to the muscle as the result of carrying a heavy rifle. The ossification in these cases is apparently a metaplastic process, the connective tissue undergoing a change with ultimate formation of bone.

General Progressive Myositis Ossificans.—This form of myositis ossificans is one which begins usually in early life and progresses steadily until practically complete ossification of the entire skeletal musculature takes palce. Death usually results with involvement of the respiratory group of muscles. The disease is extremely rare and the etiology is entirely unknown.

Clinically, the onset is accompanied by a rise in temperature and by swelling and tenderness of the involved muscles. As the acute process subsides, small local areas remain in the muscle which become firm in consistency and subsequently undergo actual ossification.

Histologic examination of the muscles reveals the fact that true bone is being deposited in the fibrous tissue sheaths and septa of the muscles. This ossifying process continues until the muscle becomes completely immobilized. The disease usually begins in the erector spinae group of muscles.

PARASITIC MYOSITIS

Infestation of the skeletal musculature by the Trichinella spiralis and the Cysticercus cellulosae may occur at times. These infestations have already been discussed in Chapter XX and will only be referred to briefly at this point.

In trichiniasis, during the febrile stage, an acute nonsuppurative myositis develops. Coincidental with the invasion of the fibrous tissue of the musculature by the larvae, the muscle becomes swollen, painful and tender. On histologic examination of biopsy material, a considerable inflammatory edema of the interstitial connective tissue is seen together with the presence of an exudate made up chiefly of round cells, eosinophiles and occasional polymorphonuclears. These tend to surround the parasite and are scattered rather diffusely throughout the affected muscle. The muscle fiber undergoes marked degeneration and loses its transverse striations. Later there is an attempt at regeneration on the part of the muscle fiber with an increase in the number of nuclei. Ultimately the larvae become encysted, surrounded by a fibrous capsule, and undergo calcification.

In the case of *Cysticercus cellulosae,* the inflammatory reaction to the encysted embryo is similar to that seen in trichiniasis, but is usually more local and less extensive.

TUMORS

Primary tumors of the striated muscle are among the rarest of neoplasms. They are spoken of as "rhabdomyomata" and are more frequently seen in the heart muscle than in the actual skeletal striated muscle. They are almost invariably malignant in nature when they do occur.

Tumors arising from the supportive stroma and blood supply of the muscle as fibromata, myxomata, lipomata, or hemangiomata are occasionally encountered. Metastatic invasion of the skeletal muscle is rarely seen except in the case of malignant melanomata. Extension of a carcinoma or sarcoma, particularly osteogenic sarcomata, to the adjacent musculature is, however, a common occurrence and may at times cause some confusion in correct interpretation.

CHAPTER LXVIII

DISEASES OF THE TEETH AND RELATED STRUCTURES

The pathology relating to diseases of the teeth obviously cannot be discussed in this brief chapter in any completeness or detail. However, in the light of recent investigation, various conditions affecting the teeth should be considered because of their bearing upon general systemic disease. Among the most significant of such lesions as playing a part in the etiology of certain diseases such as rheumatic fever, subacute bacterial endocarditis, occasional instances of peripheral neuritis and the like, are the several infections of the teeth and peridontal structures which serve as foci in the development or maintenance of such clinical pictures. Thus, the ever debatable problem of focal infection injects itself into any such discussion. Caries, with secondary infection of the tooth pulp, periapical abscesses, chronic infectious odontitis and similar conditions become significant as possible reservoirs for bacteria. From such a focus the organism may either gain access directly to the blood stream or discharge its toxin into the circulation to bring about allergic sensitization of tissues at a distance from the site of the actual infection.

The practitioner of medicine should likewise be interested in the pathology of the teeth because of the diagnostic significance which may be attached to certain specific changes which may occur under given conditions. In congenital syphilis, for example, the "Hutchinson's teeth" are so characteristic that the diagnosis of syphilis can almost positively be made from their appearance. The lesion from the pathological standpoint represents a developmental defect which affects the incisors and first molars leading to the classical notching of the incisors and to the formation of the small crowned molar in which the cusps of the crown are almost fused. In certain of the deficiency diseases, also, characteristic changes are frequently manifested in connection with the teeth and gums. In *rickets*, dentition is commonly delayed and the teeth are apt to be extremely soft with very deficient enamel development. Thus, they are liable to extensive caries. Likewise defects in the formation of the jaw and palate are frequently encountered in rickets as a result of the process as it affects bone development. In *scurvy* hemorrhage into the gums around the teeth with the development of a typical cyanotic, spongy appearance and bleeding are characteristic. In diseases such as *lead poisoning,* the deposit of the oxide of the metal within the tissues produces the almost diagnostic bluish discolored area along the gingival margins known as the "lead line," which is again emblematic of the condition. In cases of *phosphorus* and *radium poisoning,* the loosening of the teeth together with the associated degenerative changes of the gum and bone are likewise almost pathognomonic. Most of these lesions have already been discussed in relation to the various disease conditions in which they occur and so in this chapter have only been outlined as briefly as possible.

DENTAL CARIES

One of the most important and common pathological processes which involve the teeth is known as *dental caries*. This is not to be confused with the type of caries which occurs in bone so characteristically in osteomyelitis. In the teeth, caries is a process not of inflammation but of demineralization with subsequent secondary infection. In bone, on the other hand, it will be recalled that the process is primarily infectious and that the removal of lime salts with resultant softening of the bone is secondary.

The etiology of dental caries is a problem which would seem to be dependent upon a considerable number of factors, the relative importance of which is variously stressed by different authors. Among the more important theories in this regard should be mentioned the following:

Defective Enamel.—In the development of the individual, for some poorly understood reason, there may be a congenital defect in the development of the enamel organ of the tooth, which results in the occurrence of microscopic crevices or actual defects in its formation. This seems to occur during the formative period of tooth development. At times, it appears to be the result of certain intercurrent childhood diseases such as severe scarlet fever, measles and the like;

Bacterial Infection.—A great many bacteria have been incriminated at one time or another in respect to the development of dental caries. Apparently the most important among these are the saccharolytic organisms of which the *Bacillus acidophilus* is the most important. Next in significance appear to be certain of the Streptococci, on the basis of the frequency with which they are recovered from such lesions. The *Bacillus acidophilus* breaks down carbohydrate rapidly by fermentation with the resultant acid formation. The bacillus is prone to develop in plaques of mucinous material and food particles which adhere to the teeth. The significance of the acid production is seen in the fact that demineralization of enamel can take place in such an acid medium and where crevices or defects in the enamel exist, extension of the process to the deeper structures of the tooth is readily brought about;

Diet.—The effect of diet has been stressed by many observers from a variety of angles. Vitamin deficiency, notably deficiency of "A," "B" and "C" are important factors. Such vitamin-deficient diets seem to increase the frequency with which caries develops in the teeth. Other dietary factors likewise seem to be of definite importance in this respect. Thus diets high in carbohydrates are much more likely to be followed by dental caries than those which are well balanced and have a minimum of carbohydrate in relation to the protein and salt content. In this connection it is interesting to note that the teeth of the Eskimos were particularly free from caries until the advent of modern civilization. With such a change in diet, caries is frequently seen. Similarly the Negroes of Africa in their native state rarely show any evidence of caries, whereas the Negroes in this country show no such exemption from the disease; and

The Reaction of Saliva.—The relation of the chemical reaction of salivary secretion to dental caries has long been a subject of debate. In spite of attempts to correlate the importance of any altera-

tion from the normal, very little evidence has been brought forth to prove that a shift to the acid side is of very great significance. However, it may be said that any reaction in the chemical composition of the saliva which favors the growth of acid-forming bacteria tends to encourage and increase the incidence of dental caries.

PATHOLOGY OF CARIES.—Caries of the teeth usually is initiated by the growth of acid-forming organisms such as *Bacillus acidophilus* within crevices or defects of the tooth enamel. These organisms are apt to accumulate in such areas because of the presence of food particles which furnish pabulum, and from which the acid is produced by fermentation. It has been demonstrated that it is possible for enamel to go into solution in such concentration of acid as may be produced by these organisms. The destruction of the enamel takes place slowly with demineralization and softening. This forms a cone-shaped area of caries, the base of the cone being at the surface of the tooth, the apex towards the dentine. Gradually this process extends to involve the dentine. Here the destructive action goes on more rapidly. The carious degeneration tends to follow the line of juncture between the enamel and the dentine, extending more slowly as it progresses towards the tooth pulp. In the vital tooth, a reaction around the edge of the area of caries is produced in which the tubules of the dentine are occluded by material which closely resembles this structure itself. This, to some degree, delays the rapidity of the extension of the process. In the devitalized tooth, this protective reaction is not seen, and the caries spreads rapidly to the deeper structures. In the well developed lesion, various bacteria including saprophytes are commonly found.

Once the carious process has involved the dentine, the spread is rapid and almost invariably the pulp will become secondarily infected, as a result of which degeneration and inflammatory changes take place with extension not infrequently to the root and periapical tissues. The pain produced is the result of inflammatory edema and swelling with subsequent pressure upon the nerve endings, or from actual involvement of the nerve filaments in the inflammatory process. The former being probably a more common cause than the latter.

PERIAPICAL INFECTION

This may exist in the form of an acute localized suppurative process brought about as a result of extension of an infectious process from the pulp to the periapical tissue, thus producing a *peridontitis*. Such abscesses may progress with necrosis of the adjacent tissues and the accumulation of varying amounts of pus. They may even point on the gingival surface either on the labial or lingual side of the tooth and rupture spontaneously, with the discharge of the purulent exudate. Not infrequently this results in the development of a chronic fistulous tract which remains until the pyogenic membrane which forms is removed with the abstraction of the tooth.

Depending upon the nature of the infecting organism and the individual's resistance, many such an apical abscess remains localized, more or less encapsulated, and thus acts as a focus of infection for long periods of time. It is from such lesions that bacteria or their toxins gain entrance into the blood stream and produce the extensive distant systemic manifestations of disease, which are so familiar in association with such focal infections. Not infrequently, periapical abscesses in devitalized teeth may be essentially silent and unsuspected by the patient but still constitute an important source of focal infection. Thus, the importance of the periodic examination of the teeth by x-ray cannot be overemphasized. While it is quite true that unquestionably many such periapical abcesses around devitalized

teeth may never cause any definite trouble, yet from a prophylactic standpoint, the advisability of the removal of such teeth and the drainage of such abscess cavities cannot be disputed.

At times, such peridontal and periapical inflammatory processes may develop as the result of bacteria brought to the alveolar structures by the blood stream. In very severe suppurative processes about the tooth, there may be an extension to the adjacent bone with the development of an acute osteomyelitis. In the upper jaw, a periapical abscess may eventually perforate the antrum with secondary suppurative sinusitis. In some instances, the periapical inflammatory process is of low grade virulence and tends to be chronic from the onset. This results in the development of a chronic inflammatory reaction of a granulomatous nature. There is considerable associated inflammatory edema and cellular infiltration of a mixed type with large phagocytic mononuclears, plasma cells, lymphocytes and a few polymorphonuclears. Such lesions are usually referred to as *dental granulomata* or *chronic productive peridontitis*. Due to increased vascularization and pressure, there may be considerable absorption of the alveolar process. Cultures of such dental granulomata usually yield nonhemolytic streptococci, although other organisms have been reported. At times cystic degeneration may take place within such a chronic inflammatory mass with the formation of a pseudocyst.

PYORRHEA ALVEOLARIS

As has been indicated above, infections involving primarily the periapical region are usually initiated as a result of an infectious pulpitis or bacterial embolism. However, infection may occur as a result of a primary involvement of the gingival margins about the neck of the tooth, which gradually extends toward the root and eventually leads to a considerable absorption of the alveolar process together with marked loosening of the teeth. This inflammatory process is known as *pyorrhea alveolaris* or *peridontoclasia*. It begins with injury of the gingival margin of the tooth leading to separation of the peridontal membrane from the dentine at the neck with subsequent infection and suppuration. There is proliferation and extension of the oral epithelium into this area of separation. As the disease progresses the

suppurative process extends deeper giving rise to considerable absorption of the alveolar process as well as adjacent bone, so that eventually the teeth become loose and fall out.

Grossly, the gums are swollen, dark reddish in color, somewhat painful and bleed easily. A small amount of purulent exudate containing many organisms can be found in the pockets produced by the separation of the bone from the associated tooth. The organisms found in this lesion are quite varied. The *fusiform bacillus* and *spirillum of Vincent* are almost always found, together with non-hemolytic streptococci. Occasionally, the *Endameba gingivalis* may be present. However, the exact role of these organisms is still a matter of much debate. Fusiform bacilli and spirilli of Vincent are found in many mouths unassociated with pyorrhea. Likewise, *Endamoeba gingivalis* is apparently non-pathogenic. Thus, it would seem that the etiology of pyorrhea alveolaris is probably one in which the process is initiated by some local irritation or injury. This leads to a primary separation of the gum from the enamel and cementum at the neck of the tooth, thus forming a primary pocket which through secondary infection by bacteria initiates the process which is progressive. The extension of the gingival epithelium to line the separated area makes the separation permanent even when the secondary infection clears up spontaneously, or by treatment.

Although the lesion may extend to involve a number of the teeth and may even involve the root of the tooth, the individual with pyorrhea alveolaris is as a rule healthy, and the infection is probably not of great importance as a focal infection. This possibly may be explained by the presence of a pyogenic membrane which successfully prevents the extension of the bacteria into the adjacent tissues and blood stream.

TUMORS OF THE JAW

The other group of lesions which is of particular importance in relation to dental pathology is made up of the various cysts and neoplasms which arise in relation to the teeth and jaw bones. Considerable confusion exists concerning their classification. In general, it seems simpler to think of the entire group as arising from epithelial rests in the course of the development of the teeth. These epithelial structures were spoken of as peridontal epithelial rests by Malassez fifty years ago, and no better explanation concerning their source has been propounded since that time. The great majority of such tumors, therefore, are epithelial in nature and tend to show varying degrees of cyst formation.

Geschichter, in his review of the various tumors of bone, classifies the strictly dental lesions as (1) radicular cysts, (2) follicular or dentigerous cysts, (3) adamantinomata and (4) odontomata. In addition, the other most common tumor of this region is seen as the *epulis,* a giant cell tumor, which is benign in character, and similar histologically to those found in the long bones. Considerable argument exists as to whether they arise from the peridontal structures or whether they are derived from the bone itself.

In addition to these more strictly regional tumors, not infrequently neoplasms arising from the epithelium of the buccal cavity and from the connective tissue derivatives of the jaws are found. These include fibromata, which show a tendency toward ossification very commonly, true osteomata, osteogenic sarcomata, endotheliomyelomata (Ewing's tumor), basal and squamous cell carcinomata. These latter groups of epithelial and connective tissue cell tumors are essentially similar in their behavior in these locations as elsewhere in the body. They have already been thoroughly discussed in the respective chapters in the section devoted to Oncology, and so are merely reviewed at this time for the sake of completeness.

Of more concern to us at this point are those tumors which are strictly dental in origin. The four major types as outlined by Geschichter seem to merit individual consideration, and a word concerning the epulides likewise is pertinent.

Radicular Cysts.—The radicular cyst is believed to be derived from the root of a devitalized tooth, usually following definite chronic inflammation such as is seen in association with periapical abscesses and the like. The majority of these lesions occur curiously enough in relatively young adults, although they are seen at all ages. They usually affect the molar rather than the incisor teeth. Malassez believed that these cysts develop from proliferation of the deeper peridontal epithelial rests which include, in his opinion, the atrophic von Brunn's sheath, which represents the continuation of the undifferentiated enameloblast over the root of the tooth. The lesion grows slowly and gradually expands the jaw bone, with demineralization. In the more marked instances, there is a thin, parchment-paper-like wall to the cyst. The cyst is usually monolocular and does not contain any suggestion of tooth structure, which distinguishes this type of lesion from the less common, but true dentigerous cyst. A rather large proportion of such tumors ultimately undergo malignant change, although at their outset they are usually entirely benign.

Dentigerous (Follicular) Cysts.—The dentigerous cyst is thought to arise from the enamel organ in the course of the development of the tooth before its eruption. These lesions are likewise slow in their growth. They are almost invariably seen in children or young adults. They vary considerably in size and in position. The majority of them are monolocular, but at times they may appear multilocular, usually as the result of fusion of several such cysts involving more than one tooth. Likewise the great majority of these tumors may be recognized and differentiated from the radicular type because of the presence of one or more imperfectly developed teeth in the wall of the cyst. The cyst wall is usually lined by a transitional columnar type of epithelium representing the undifferentiated enameloblast (ameloblast).

ILLUSTRATIVE CASE

CASE 295 (Ref. #S-412)

Diagnosis.—Dentigerous cyst.

Patient was a twelve-year-old Filipino, who was admitted to the hospital because of progressive swelling of his upper jaw of two years' duration.

Present Illness.—The onset of the patient's illness dated back approximately two years at which time it was first noted that his right upper jaw seemed to be slowly increasing in size. This was not particularly painful and did not seriously interfere with the child's appetite or ability to eat. He suffered no other symptoms than those relating to this disfiguring enlargement of his jaw. By the time of admission to the hospital, it had reached a size where it definitely interfered with breathing and occasioned him a great deal of difficulty in eating anything but soft solid and liquid foods.

Past Medical History.—The patient's past history was essentially irrelevant. He had had a normal childhood and his parents did not recall whether or not he had had any of the usual contagious diseases. Nobody had noted anything unusual about his teeth until his present condition became apparent.

Physical Examination.—The patient was a fairly well-developed, somewhat undernourished, but otherwise healthy appearing young Filipino. Head: The most outstanding feature of his physical examination was seen in relation to an enormous swelling of his right upper jaw, which had completely distorted the entire right side of his face. It had extended to involve the nares so that they appeared as buttonholes against the rounded surface of this tumor-like mass (Fig. 665). The eye on the right side, likewise was practically closed. It had stretched the mouth and upper lip so that they were badly distorted.

The remainder of the physical examination was essentially negative. It was impossible to get a good view of his throat because he could not open his mouth sufficiently to be able to visualize the fossae. There was no lymphadenopathy. The chest was symmetrical. Lungs were clear. Heart was negative. Abdomen was somewhat scaphoid. Genitalia were immature. Extremities were negative.

Laboratory Findings.—There was a mild secondary type of hypochromic anemia. The red blood cells numbered 3,200,000 with 68% hemoglobin. White blood cells 8,400 with 67% neutrophiles. Urinalysis was negative.

Subsequent Course.—A diagnosis of dentigerous cyst or a cystic adamantinoma of the jaw was made and excision advised. At the time of operation, an orange-sized cyst with a thin, parchment-paper-like capsule as its wall was found. The fluid was removed and the cyst wall curetted out. Three poorly formed molar teeth were found in the wall of the cyst. The fluid contents was of a serous nature. Six months postoperatively, no recurrence of the mass had taken place and secondary plastic surgery was done in an attempt to improve the cosmetic result, following which the patient was lost sight of and no information is available as to the final outcome.

Pathological Report.—Specimen consisted of nearly a handful of fragments of tissue, most of which had a crackling, eggshell consistency. Three partially formed molar teeth could be identified in the material. Other fragments seemed to form the cyst wall.

Histologic examination of these fragments showed the cyst wall to be made up of rather undifferentiated osteoid tissue and lined by a layer of high columnar transitional epithelium.

Adamantinomata.—The adamantinoma or ameloblastoma, as it has more recently been termed, is the malignant counterpart of the dentigerous cyst. Historically, the recognition of this type of tumor dates back to the report by Broca in 1868. Like most of the other tumors of dental epithelial rest origin, they occur most frequently in late childhood and young adult life. They are much more frequently encountered in the lower jaw than in the upper; according to Geschichter, in the ratio of approximately six to one, and like the dentigerous cysts, are more prone to involve the molar regions. The rate of growth is usually extremely slow, several instances being reported in which the duration exceeded thirty and forty years.

It has been suggested that nutritional disturbances, notably rickets, with its vitamin deficiency, may be an important factor in the development of the tumor. In experimental rickets, it has been shown that the layer of enamel forming cells presents much the same irregularities which are seen in the epiphyseal ends of the long bones. This results in isolation of groups of such epithelial cells as might well go on to neoplastic development. This relationship to rickets is particularly emphasized by the relative frequency with which these tumors are found in the Negro, in whom rickets is notoriously common, as compared with the white race. On the other hand, it is just as easy to explain the development of an adamantinoma by Malassez's peridontal cell rest theory.

The tumors, as has been emphasized in Chapter XXXV, may occur either in solid or cystic form, with all intermediate pictures. Robinson, in a recent paper, emphasizes the fact that the development of the tooth bud is from an area of thickening of the oral epithelium along the alveolar ridge. From this area, the primitive dental lamina is formed, which in turn differentiates into typical ameloblasts and the stellate reticular cells of the pulp. As the enamel organ forms, it has been shown that dentine must be laid down by the mesodermal odontoblasts before actual enamel production occurs. It is at this point that the dissimilarity between the normal developmental picture and the neoplastic transition takes place. The normal enamel organ proceeds to lay down enamel while in the tumor the enamel organ degenerates to a nonfunctional cystic mass.

These tumors, as has been intimated, are of a very low grade malignancy growing extremely slowly and again, through expansion, causing marked destruction of the bone. Radical surgical excision of the mass should result in a very high percentage of cure, in Geschichter's series reaching eighty per cent.

As a curiosity, it should be mentioned that aberrant adamantinomata have been recorded in the ovary, tibia and hypophyseal duct region. In the ovary, such tumors should be thought of as teratoid. In the tibia, it has been suggested that the overlying surface epithelium invaginates the bone in much the same way that the epithelium over the alveolar process of the jaw invaginates to form the enamel organ. Thus abortive attempts at tooth formation as adamantinomata occur in such locations. Some five or six such cases have been reported in the literature, the most recent one by Bishop. In the hypophyseal area, these tumors are believed to be derived from the cleft between the pituitary lobes.

Odontomata.—The odontoma is believed by some to be a solid adamantinoma; by others, merely an exaggeration of the simple follicular dentigerous type of cyst. These tumors are characterized by the formation of masses of abortive teeth, which vary greatly in appearance and consistency. In many instances the individual type of tooth may be recognized. In others, this similarity to the normal structure is less apparent. In many of the tumors, the enamel is lacking. These are spoken of as soft odontomata. The tumors almost invariably occur in the lower jaw and usually in the younger age group. They outnumber all other tumors of the tooth-forming organs in the ratio of two to one and are usually found arising at the site of an unerupted tooth.

Microscopically, the tumor appears to be composed of a matrix of rather loose areolar connective tissue in which dentine, enamel and cement-like structures may be recognized. In general, the odontoma may be considered as a benign tumor although in the more undifferentiated soft variety, there is a striking tendency for the lesion to recur and to infiltrate locally.

The Epulides.—The term *epulis* has come to be employed commonly for almost any tumor arising from the gums. As such, it is of value in differentiating the regional location of the tumor, but in respect to differentiating the numerous varieties of such neoplasms, it is of very little clinical or pathological significance. In general, the use of the term is especially applied to that group of giant cell tumors which occur, often upon the site of some chronic inflammatory granulomatous lesion of the gum, but also may be derived, as are similar benign giant cell tumors elsewhere, from the bone. Thus, they may occur as tumors of the mandible or maxilla, arising centrally in the medullary canal or more commonly from the periosteum.

Histologically, they present the same characteristic features that have already been described in the section devoted to tumors of the bone in Chapter XXV.

INDEX

INDEX OF ILLUSTRATIVE CASES

(1)